Modern Nutrition
in
Health and Disease

Modern Nutrition

in

Health and Disease

Dietotherapy

Fifth Edition

Edited by

ROBERT S. GOODHART, M.D., D.M.S.

*Director, Office of Medical Education
and Executive Secretary,
Committee on Medical Education
New York Academy of Medicine,
New York, New York*

MAURICE E. SHILS, M.D., Sc.D.

*Attending Physician,
Memorial Hospital for Cancer and Allied Diseases;
Associate Professor of Medicine,
Cornell University Medical College,
New York, New York*

Lea & Febiger · Philadelphia

FIRST EDITION, 1955

SECOND EDITION, 1960

THIRD EDITION, 1964
Reprinted February, 1966

FOURTH EDITION, 1968
Reprinted March, 1970
Reprinted July, 1971

FIFTH EDITION, 1973
Reprinted September, 1974
Reprinted April, 1975

Published in Great Britain by Henry Kimpton Publishers, London

Library of Congress Catalog Card Number: 77-175460

PRINTED IN THE UNITED STATES OF AMERICA

ISBN 0-8121-0384-X

Preface

This edition, the 5th, of *Modern Nutrition in Health and Disease* is the first to be published without the editorial advice and help of Michael G. Wohl, M.D., F.A.C.P., whose *Dietotherapy*, first published in 1945, evolved into this book. Dr. Wohl died June 20, 1970, at the age of 81, after a distinguished career as a medical educator and practitioner. At the time of his retirement, shortly before his death, he was Chief of The Nutrition Clinic, Philadelphia General Hospital; Clinical Professor of Medicine Emeritus, Temple University Medical Center; Consultant in Medicine, Albert Einstein Medical Center, and Chairman, Committee on Nutrition and Metabolism, Philadelphia County Medical Society. We enjoyed his friendship and miss both his help and his company.

We also note with regret the recent deaths of two eminent contributors, Doctors David Y. Hsia and Carl Moore.

As was true of the previous editions, this volume has been designed to serve both as a textbook on nutrition and as a ready reference book for students and practitioners in the fields of nutrition, medicine and public health. It has been restructured to group the various topics in nutrition into major areas which take the reader from basic nutritional science, through problems in safety and adequacy of food supply, interrelations of nutrients and metabolism, diagnosis and manifestations of nutritional deficiencies, nutrition problems during stress, to considerations of nutrition in the prevention and treatment of various disease states. Diet standards, diets, formulas, recipes, and food composition tables are now to be found in the Appendix. We believe that this arrangement will prove to be a great convenience to the user while increasing the readability of the text.

All chapters but one have been revised, most of them quite extensively. Updating has been assisted by the introduction of 32 new contributors with this edition. The section on Abnormalities in Serum Protein Metabolism-Amino Acid Effects, and the chapters on Nutrition and Cell Growth, Clinical Manifestations of Certain Vitamin Deficiencies, and Prolonged Parenteral Nutrition ("Hyperalimentation") are a few of the important additions and modifications in the 5th edition.

The importance of nutrition to clinical medicine is basic. We hope and believe that the breadth and depth of these contributions will reinforce this belief with concrete evidence and assist in spreading this understanding.

This edition is made possible by their expenditure of time and effort and by the expertise of the contributors; our indebtedness to them is great. We also wish to acknowledge our obligation to the staff of Lea & Febiger for their indispensable help.

New York, New York   ROBERT S. GOODHART
New York, New York   MAURICE E. SHILS

Contributors

LILLA AFTERGOOD, Ph.D., Research Biochemist, Environmental and Nutritional Sciences, School of Public Health, University of California, Los Angeles, California.

ANTHONY A. ALBANESE, Ph.D., Director, Nutrition and Metabolic Research Division, The Winifred Masterson Burke Relief Foundation, White Plains, New York.

ROSLYN B. ALFIN-SLATER, Ph.D., Professor and Division Head, Environmental and Nutritional Sciences, School of Public Health, University of California, Los Angeles, California.

GUILLERMO ARROYAVE, Ph.D., Chief, Division of Physiological Chemistry, Institute of Nutrition of Central America and Panama (INCAP), Guatemala City, Guatemala, C.A.

A. E. AXELROD, Ph.D., Professor of Biochemistry, School of Medicine, University of Pittsburgh, Pittsburgh, Pennsylvania.

COLONEL EUGENE M. BAKER, Ph.D., Assistant Chief, Chemistry Division, U.S. Army Medical Research and Nutrition Laboratory, Fitzsimons General Hospital, Denver, Colorado.

HERMAN BAKER, Ph.D., Professor of Medicine and Preventive Medicine, Director, Vitamin Laboratories, College of Medicine and Dentistry, New Jersey Medical School, East Orange, New Jersey.

THEODORE B. BAYLES, M.D., Associate Clinical Professor of Medicine, Harvard Medical School; Senior Associate, Peter Bent Brigham Hospital; Visiting Physician, Robert B. Brigham Hospital, Boston, Massachusetts.

ABBY STOLPER BLOCH, M.S., R.D., Head Dietitian, Metabolic Research Kitchen, Memorial-Sloan Kettering Cancer Center, New York, New York.

JO ANNE BRASEL, M.D., Associate Professor of Pediatrics and Chief, Division of Growth and Development, Institute of Human Nutrition, Columbia University, College of Physicians and Surgeons, New York, New York.

SELWYN A. BROITMAN, Ph.D., Associate Professor of Microbiology, Boston University School of Medicine; Associate in Medicine, Harvard Medical School; Associate in Medicine, Thorndike Memorial Laboratory; and Research Associate, Mallory Institute of Pathology, Boston City Hospital, Boston, Massachusetts.

JOHN E. CANHAM, M.D., Commander and Director, U.S. Army Medical Research and Nutrition Laboratory, Fitzsimons General Hospital, Denver, Colorado.

RALPH R. CAVALIERI, M.D., Chief, Nuclear Medicine Service, Veterans Administration Hospital, San Francisco, California.

C. L. COMAR, Ph.D., Head, Department of Physical Biology, New York State Veterinary College, Cornell University, Ithaca, New York.

CHARLES S. DAVIDSON, M.D., Professor of Medicine, Harvard University, Associate Director, Harvard Medical Unit, Boston City Hospital, Boston, Massachusetts.

H. F. DeLUCA, Ph.D., Professor and Chairman, Department of Biochemistry, University of Wisconsin, Madison, Wisconsin.

PHANI DHAR, M.D., Research Fellow, Gastrointestinal Research Laboratory, Mallory Institute of Pathology Foundation; Clinical Fellow, Harvard Medical Service; Clinical Associate, Klondyke Memorial Laboratory; Instructor in Medicine, Harvard Medical School, Boston City Hospital, Boston, Massachusetts.

ALBERT B. EISENSTEIN, M.D., Chief of Medicine, Gouverneur Hospital, Beth Israel Medical Center; Professor of Clinical Medicine Mt. Sinai School of Medicine, New York, New York.

NANCY ERNST, Chief Nutritionist, Lipid Metabolism Branch, National Heart and Lung Institute, Bethesda, Maryland.

HARRY D. FEIN, M.D., F.A.C.P., Associate Professor of Clinical Medicine, New York University School of Medicine; Attending and Chief of Gastroenterology, Lenox Hill Hospital; Associate Visiting Physician, University Hospital; Associate Visiting Physician, Bellevue Hospital; Consultant in Medicine, Manhattan State Hospital, New York, New York.

V. J. FONTANA, M.D., Professor of Clinical Pediatrics, New York University College of Medicine; Associate Attending, New York University Medical Center, University Hospital; Director of Pediatrics and Pediatric Allergy, St. Vincent's Hospital and Medical Center of New York, New York, New York.

OSCAR FRANK, Ph.D., Associate Professor of Medicine, Co-Director, Vitamin Laboratories, College of Medicine and Dentistry, New Jersey Medical School, East Orange, New Jersey.

GERALD J. FRIEDMAN, M.D., F.A.C.P., Associate Clinical Professor, New York University College of Medicine; Chief of Metabolism & Endocrinology, Attending Physician in Medicine, Beth Israel Medical Center; Attending Physician in Medicine, Bellevue Hospital; Attending Physician in Medicine, University Hospital, New York, New York.

ROBERT S. GOODHART, M.D., D.M.S., Director, Office of Medical Education and Executive Secretary, Committee on Medical Education New York Academy of Medicine, New York, New York.

FRANCISCO GRANDE, M.D., Professor of Physiological Hygiene, School of Public Health, Laboratory of Physiological Hygiene, University of Minnesota, Minneapolis, Minnesota.

HERMAN GROSSMAN, M.D., Director of Pediatric Radiology, Professor of Radiology and Professor of Pediatrics, Duke University Medical Center, Durham, North Carolina.

D. M. HEGSTED, Ph.D., Professor of Nutrition, Harvard School of Public Health, Boston, Massachusetts.

VICTOR HERBERT, M.D., Clinical Professor of Pathology, Columbia University College of Physicians and Surgeons; Medical Investigator, Veterans Administration, V.A. Hospital, Bronx, New York, New York.

ROBERT W. HILLMAN, B.S., M.D., M.P.H., Professor of Environmental Medicine and Community Health, State University of New York, Downstate Medical Center, College of Medicine, Brooklyn, New York.

ROBERT E. HODGES, M.D., Professor, Department of Internal Medicine, Chief, Nutrition Section, University of California at Davis, Davis, California.

L. EMMETT HOLT, JR., M.D., Professor of Pediatrics, New York University School of Medicine, New York, New York.

M. K. HORWITT, Ph.D., Professor of Biochemistry, St. Louis University School of Medicine, St. Louis, Missouri.

DAVID YI-YUNG HSIA, M.D., Late Professor of Pediatrics, Northwestern University Medical School, Chicago, Illinois.

ROBERT M. KARK, M.D., Professor of Medicine, Rush Medical College, Chicago, Illinois.

ANCEL KEYS, Ph.D., Professor Emeritus, School of Public Health, Laboratory of Physiological Hygiene, University of Minnesota, Minneapolis, Minnesota.

W. A. KREHL, M.D., Ph.D., Professor and Chairman, Department of Community Health and Preventive Medicine, Jefferson Medical College, Philadelphia, Pennsylvania.

RACHMIEL LEVINE, M.D., Executive Medical Director, City of Hope Medical Center, Duarte, California.

ROBERT I. LEVY, M.D., Chief, Lipid Metabolism Branch; Head, Section on Lipoproteins; Chief, Clinical Services Molecular Disease Branch, National Heart and Lung Institute, Bethesda, Maryland.

TING-KAI LI, M.D., Professor of Medicine and Biochemistry, Indiana University School of Medicine, Indianapolis, Indiana.

NAN S. T. LUI, Ph.D., Senior Research Associate, Lamont-Doherty Geological Observatory, Palisades, New York.

JEAN MAYER, Ph.D., D.Sc., Professor of Nutrition, Department of Nutrition Harvard School of Public Health, Harvard University, Boston, Massachusetts.

MORTON A. MEYERS, M.D., Department of Radiology, New York Hospital, Cornell Medical Center; Associate Professor of Radiology, Cornell University Medical College, New York, New York.

O. MICKELSEN, Ph.D., Professor of Nutrition, Michigan State University, East Lansing, Michigan.

MARTHA H. MILES, Formerly Head Dietitian, Metabolic Research Kitchen, Memorial-Sloan Kettering Cancer Center, New York, New York.

CARL V. MOORE, M.D., Late Busch Professor of Medicine and Head of the Department of Medicine, Washington University School of Medicine; Late Physician in Chief, Barnes Hospital, St. Louis, Missouri.

ROBERT A. NEAL, Ph.D., Associate Professor, Division of Nutrition, Department of Biochemistry, Vanderbilt University School of Medicine, Nashville, Tennessee.

ROBERT E. OLSON, M.D., Ph.D., Professor and Chairman, Department of Biochemistry, St. Louis University School of Medicine, St. Louis, Missouri.

J. L. OMDAHL, Ph.D., Assistant Professor, Department of Biochemistry, University of New Mexico, Albuquerque, New Mexico.

MURRAY ORATZ, Ph.D., Assistant Chief, Nuclear Medicine and Radioisotope Service, Veterans Administration Hospital; Adjunct Associate Professor of Biochemistry New York University College of Dentistry, New York, New York

LOUISE A. ORTO, M.S., Assistant Director, Nutrition and Metabolic Research Division, The Winifred Masterson Burke Relief Foundation, White Plains, New York.

BERNARD L. OSER, Ph.D., Chairman Food and Drug Research Laboratories, Inc., Maspeth, New York.

JOSEPH H. OYAMA, M.D., Assistant Professor of Medicine, Rush Medical College, Chicago, Illinois.

WILLIAM N. PEARSON, Ph.D., Late Professor of Biochemistry, Vanderbilt University School of Medicine, Nashville, Tennessee.

H. T. RANDALL, M.D., Professor of Medical Science (Surgery), and Section Leader, Section on Surgery, Division of Biological and Medical Sciences, Brown University; Surgeon in Chief, Department of Surgery, Rhode Island Hospital, Providence, Rhode Island.

MARCUS A. ROTHSCHILD, M.D., Chief, Nuclear Medicine and Radioisotope Service, Veterans Administration Hospital; Associate Professor of Medicine, New York University School of Medicine, New York, New York.

OSWALD A. ROELS, Ph.D., Professor, The City College of the City University of New York, New York, New York.

HAROLD H. SANDSTEAD, M.D., F.A.C.P., Director U.S. Department of Agriculture, Agricultural Research Service Human Nutrition Laboratory; Research Professor in Biochemistry and Medicine, University of North Dakota, School of Medicine, Grand Forks, North Dakota.

HOWERDE E. SAUBERLICH, Ph.D., Chief, Chemistry Division, U.S. Army Medical Research and Nutritional Laboratory, Fitzsimons General Hospital, Denver, Colorado.

SIDNEY S. SCHREIBER, M.D., Attending Internist, Nuclear Medicine, Veterans Administration Hospital; Associate Professor of Clinical Medicine, New York University School of Medicine, New York, New York.

JAMES H. SHAW, Ph.D., Professor of Nutrition; Director of Training Center for Clinical Scholars in Oral Biology, Harvard School of Dental Medicine, Boston, Massachusetts.

MAURICE E. SHILS, M.D., Sc.D., Attending Physician, Memorial Hospital for Cancer and Allied Diseases; Associate Professor of Medicine, Cornell University Medical College, New York, New York.

SANT P. SINGH, M,D., Associate Endocrinologist, Brooklyn-Cumberland Medical Center; Assistant Professor of Medicine, Downstate Medical Center —SUNY, Brooklyn, New York.

SELMA E. SNYDERMAN, M.D., Professor of Pediatrics, New York University School of Medicine, New York, New York.

JOHN J. STERN, M.D., Attending Ophthalmologist, St. Lukes Memorial Hospital Center and Utica State Hospital, Utica, New York.

MARGARET B. STRAUSS, M.D., Formerly Director, Allergen Laboratories, Dome Laboratories Division, Miles Laboratories, Inc., West Haven, Connecticut.

EDWARD A. SWEENEY, D.M.D., Associate Professor of Pediatric Dentistry, Acting Chairman Department of Pediatric Dentistry, Harvard School of Dental Medicine; Senior Associate in Pediatrics, Children's Hospital Medical Center, Boston, Massachusetts.

J. C. THOMPSON, JR., Associate Professor, Environmental Radiation Biology, Cornell University, Ithaca, New York.

BERT L. VALLEE, M.D., Paul C. Cabot Professor of Biological Chemistry, Harvard Medical School, Boston, Massachusetts.

FERNANDO E. VITERI, M.D., D.Sc., Chief Biomedical Division, Institute of Nutrition of Central America and Panama (INCAP), Guatemala City, Guatemala, C.A.

DONALD M. WATKIN, M.D., M.P.H., Chairman, Technical Committee on Nutrition, Chairman, Panel on Nutrition of the Post-Conference Board, White House Conference on Aging, Washington, D.C.; Physician, West Roxbury Veterans Administration Hospital, Boston, Massachusetts.

ROBIN C. WATSON, M.D., Chairman, Radiology Department, Memorial Hospital for Cancer and Allied Diseases; Associate Professor of Radiology, Cornell University Medical College, New York, New York.

PAUL WING-KON WONG, M.D., M.Sc., Professor of Pediatrics The Chicago Medical School; Director, The Infant's Aid Perinatal Research Laboratories, Mount Sinai Hospital, Chicago, Illinois.

MYRON WINICK, M.D., Professor of Pediatrics, R. R. Williams Professor of Nutrition and Director, Institute of Human Nutrition, Columbia University College of Physicians and Surgeons, New York, New York.

M. G. YANG, Ph.D., Assistant Professor, Foods and Nutrition Department, Michigan State University, East Lansing, Michigan.

NORMAN ZAMCHECK, M.D., Chief, Gastrointestinal Research Laboratory, Mallory Institute of Pathology Foundation, Boston City Hospital; Associate Clinical Professor of Medicine, Harvard Medical School; Visiting Physician, Harvard Medical Service, Boston City Hospital; Research Associate in Pathology, Boston University School of Medicine, Boston, Massachusetts.

Contents

PART I. THE FOUNDATIONS OF NUTRITION

Part II. SAFETY AND ADEQUACY OF THE FOOD SUPPLY

Part III. INTERRELATIONS OF NUTRIENTS AND METABOLISM

Appendix

PART I

The Foundations of Nutrition

Chapter

1

Body Weight, Body Composition and Calorie Status

ANCEL KEYS

AND

FRANCISCO GRANDE

The body is, in the most literal sense, the product of its nutrition. Though the transformations are profound, nutrition begins with the foodstuffs and proceeds to the material end result, the living body and its functions. The most elementary, but certainly not the least important, aspect of nutrition is the gross mass of tissue it produces and maintains. The most obvious, and in many populations perhaps the most common, nutritional defects are those caused by gross calorie imbalance.

Calorie undernutrition is the most common form of malnutrition in underdeveloped countries but, even in the midst of plenty, starvation caused by disease is common because many illnesses interfere with the appetite or the assimilation of food. In the simplest of societies obesity may be rare, either because of chronic food shortages or because physical exercise is an effective preventive, but as society becomes more specialized, more prosperous and more sedentary, an excessive accumulation of body fat tends to be the rule unless it is consciously combated.

Except for changes in hydration, gain of body weight over a period of time is an expression of positive calorie balance, that is, an excess of calorie intake over expenditure and, conversely, weight loss is an expression of calorie deficit. But it must be borne in mind that, as discussed later, there is no simple relationship between calorie balance and the rate of weight gain or loss at a given

time. Finally, it is possible to maintain constant weight and still be in positive calorie balance; this can happen when muscle is replaced by fat and when body water is lost in the presence of positive calorie balance.

Until recently, besides the impressionistic methods of gross inspection and digital feel, gross body weight, sometimes supplemented with a few measurements of external dimensions, had to suffice for studies on living man. Fortunately, new methods are now at hand for analysis of the body mass into metabolically distinct components.[78,120] These, together with the more widespread application of statistical methods and concepts, provide increasingly useful and precise norms for guidance in calorie nutrition.

BODY WEIGHT

The gross body weight *per se* has some direct metabolic significance. To the extent that it represents the size of the cell mass of the body it determines the Basal Metabolic Rate. The metabolic cost of physical activity is determined by the body weight since most of the energy cost of physical activity is expended in simply moving the body around. With a fixed amount of activity—number, extent, speed and force of movements—energy expenditure tends to be directly proportional to gross body weight.[50,74]

Actually, grossly overweight persons tend to be relatively inactive; the movements they make are expensive in calories but they make

1

fewer movements than persons of average weight. Many recent studies show that overweight persons are not characterized so much by large food consumption as by physical inactivity.[71,88,91] However, when a heavyweight has to move quickly there is an excessive demand for energy and this may mean a strain on one or more vulnerable organs or functions.

Insurance companies report an excessive death rate of overweights from a variety of causes, including accidents. A heavy body is an impediment in avoiding many accidents simply because it is harder to move or to change the direction of movement of a heavy body. Further, the damaging force in a fall is increased with increasing body weight.

Nevertheless, the major importance of the body weight is its association with body fatness. The amount of fat in the body may be considered as an expression of the calorie balance status. It is a common error to regard overweight and obesity as identical. Obesity means excessive fatness and it is essential to adhere to this definition.[69,78] Athletes are often overweight but underfat.[11] It is safe to conclude that a middle-aged man who is 30 or more pounds heavier than the average man of the same height is obese, that is, overfat. But, at lesser degrees of overweight, the relationship between obesity and overweight is not close, particularly at younger ages.[24,25,26]

Many sedentary persons are excessively fat but not overweight, while the opposite condition, overweight without being fat, is common among people doing heavy physical work. The two conditions are, in fact, metabolic opposites, the one tending to result from the lack of activity, the other from excessive activity. Attention to this discrimination discloses differences in characteristics pertinent to circulation and health.[129]

Besides distinguishing between fat and muscle in the gross body weight, variations in the water content of the body must be considered. In ascites 5 to 10 kg of fluid in the abdominal cavity may be encountered and much larger totals of edema fluid are not rare. One of Simonart's[119] starved patients lost 20 kg in a week while his nutriture was improving. Extreme edema is readily detected but more moderate variations in hydration are not easily recognizable. Clinical recognition of the presence of edema requires an accumulation of the order of 5 to 10 per cent of the total body weight as excess water.[78,80] The variable contribution of water to the total body weight of clinically healthy persons is reflected in the weight fluctuations seen on reducing diets under controlled conditions.[97]

Another contributor to confusion about the meaning of the total body weight is the variable weight of the body skeleton. The mineral mass in the adult skeleton averages something like 6 per cent of the normal body weight of the adult but, in different persons, it may be as low as 4 per cent or as high as 9 per cent.[78]

Perhaps a more important contribution of the skeleton to the body weight is through its form. Overweight and underweight are commonly computed on the basis of weight for height. But a broad and short skeleton automatically means a large body weight per unit of height and, so far, no system has been devised to allow for this in a practical manner. The body "frame" types discussed below are theoretical concepts devoid of real utility in the absence of agreed methods of measurement and classification.

The "Constancy" of Body Weight. The literature on body weight contains only limited information about daily weight changes. Rapid fluctuations of body weight do, however, occur with no apparent relation to changes in calorie intake, energy expenditure or health status. These short-term fluctuations are difficult to understand but they should be taken into account in metabolic experiments, especially when they involve limited periods of time. In a group of 44 men living under highly controlled conditions, Durnin[38] observed day-to-day changes of body weight up to 1 kg. Similar observations have been reported by Edholm.[40] Elkinton and Danowski[44] measured body weight of a man on 53 out of 56 days and found a standard deviation of ± 0.86 pound, equivalent to ± 0.51 per cent of his weight. Taggart[127] studied the body weight of a nonpregnant woman for a period of 80 days. The body weight during the period changed from 61.5 to 63.9 kg with daily fluctuations up to

0.8 kg. These changes were not related to the menstrual cycle.

Most of the short-time fluctuations of body weight can be explained by changes in the water content of the body. These fluctuations, however, do not detract from the fact that over periods of a week or more food intake and energy intake are closely balanced and the body weight remains relatively constant.[40]

Considerable changes in body weight can be produced by retention of water associated with deposition of glycogen in muscle and liver. Olsson and Saltin[100] have reported a mean weight gain of 2.4 kg in 19 young men after 4 days of feeding a carbohydrate-rich diet. Total body water, measured by dilution of tritiated water, rose in the 4 days by an average of 2.2 liters. Muscle glycogen had been previously depleted by intense arm and leg activity while consuming a diet of fat and protein for 3 days just before the carbohydrate diet. From determinations of muscle glycogen it was estimated that the glycogen content of the body increased by some 500 gm, which means that 3 to 4 gm of water are bound with each gram of glycogen deposited. The meal eating pattern has a marked effect on body weight in the rat, but Swindell et al.[126] found changes of body weight in young women unrelated to the frequency of meals.

Body Weight Standards. Until lately almost all statistical evaluations of calorie status, obesity, emaciation, and gross nutritional health have been based simply on the gross body weight as related to height. Comparison of a person's actual weight, M, with his "standard (tabular) weight," S, is the most widely used criterion of leanness-fatness. The degree of over- or underweight may be expressed as the percentage deviation of the actual from the standard weight, $\Delta\% = (M - S)/S$, or as "relative body weight," $R = 100\ M/S$. It should be stressed again that body weight is not a very reliable criterion in the diagnosis of obesity. Thus in a recent study of 1761 healthy U. S. Army veterans Seltzer et al.[114] found that only a minority of the extreme relative body weight categories (120, 125 or more) were frankly obese by skinfold measurements. In the United States the standard of reference has long been the tables of average weight for height and age originally published by the Association of Life Insurance Medical Directors and the Actuarial Society of America in 1912 under the title, "Medico-Actuarial Mortality Investigation" (New York). They are summarized in Tables 1–1 and 1–2.

Elsewhere[75,77] we have discussed the limitations of these tables which merely give the average values for men and women of specified ages who obtained life insurance policies at standard premium rates from 1888 to about 1905, mostly in urban centers on the eastern seaboard. The heights and weights were recorded as for "ordinary clothing";

Table 1-1.   Graded Average Weight in Pounds of Men of Different Statures at Various Ages*

Height, Inches	Age, Years							
	20	25	30	35	40	45	50	55
60	117	122	126	128	131	133	134	135
62	122	126	130	132	135	137	138	139
64	128	133	136	138	141	143	144	145
66	136	141	144	146	149	151	152	153
68	144	149	152	155	158	160	161	163
70	152	157	161	165	168	170	171	173
72	161	167	172	176	180	182	183	184
74	171	179	184	189	193	195	197	198
76	181	189	196	201	206	209	211	212

* Davenport, C. B.: Body Build and Its Inheritance. Publication 329, Carnegie Institute of Washington, 1923.

Table 1-2.   Graded Average Weight in Pounds of Women of Different Statures at Various Ages*

Height, Inches	Age, Years							
	20	25	30	35	40	45	50	55
56	106	109	112	115	119	122	125	125
58	110	113	116	119	123	126	129	129
60	114	117	120	123	127	130	133	133
62	119	121	124	127	132	135	138	138
64	125	128	131	134	138	141	144	144
66	132	135	138	142	146	149	152	153
68	140	143	146	150	154	157	161	163
70	147	151	154	157	161	164	169	171
72	156	158	161	163	167	171	176	177

* Davenport, C. B.: Body Build and Its Inheritance. Publication 329, Carnegie Institute of Washington, 1923.

what this means today is questionable. However, for men at least, similar values may apply approximately to the undressed state, that is, in socks and shorts, because the heel height (about 1 inch) roughly counteracts the clothing weight customary half a century ago. For women the application is more difficult because of the variability of heel height and the great reduction in female clothing weight over the intervening years.

More recently, tables have come into use which list body weights for the same height under three headings: "light" or "small frame," "medium frame," and "heavy" or "large frame." The medium frame values correspond to the averages in the older tables and the "light" and "heavy frame" weight values are simply some 5 to 8 per cent smaller or larger, respectively. Unfortunately, there is no accepted system for deciding who has a "light frame," and no actual evaluations of frame size were made in developing the tables. Apparently the observed frequency distributions of the weight values used for the original tables of 1912 (where frame was not considered) were merely divided into thirds. The lighter third of men of a given height and age was arbitrarily defined as having a "light frame" and the mean weight of this group was then considered to be the average body weight of men of "light frame" of the given height and age. In other words, these tables have no basis in measurement and are useless and misleading except to indicate that a single "average" body weight for given height and age is inadequate and that differences in skeletal type may explain some of the variability observed in clinically healthy persons of the same height, age and sex.

Still more recently, the Metropolitan Life Insurance Company has popularized the idea enunciated by Fisher and Fisk[49] that the observed body weights for the average of the population are not necessarily those most conducive to health. In the United States and many other countries it is usual for body weight to increase long after body length growth is finished. But it is possible to argue that the usual gain of weight beyond age 25 or 30 is undesirable, or at least may be unnecessary. Accordingly, tables of "desirable body weight" (at first labeled "ideal") have been provided.[91] Tables 1–3 and 1–4 specify "frame-size," with no more precise definition than indicated above, and they indicate a "desirable" range (of 7 to 18 pounds for different frames and heights) within each height and frame class. But age is not specified, since the theory is that no weight change with advancing age is desirable. The values are, in fact, merely a rearrangement of the 1912 tables but limited to persons of 25 to 30 years of age.

The actual averages and standard deviations for clinically healthy persons of specified age, sex and height in the United States at present are largely unknown, and the further

Table 1-3. Weight in Pounds According to Frame (in Indoor Clothing)*

Height with Shoes 1-inch Heels		Small	Medium	Large
Feet	Inches	Frame	Frame	Frame
		Desirable Weights for Men Aged 25 and Over		
5	2	112–120	118–129	126–141
5	3	115–123	121–133	129–144
5	4	118–126	124–136	132–148
5	5	121–129	127–139	135–152
5	6	124–133	130–143	138–156
5	7	128–137	134–147	142–161
5	8	132–141	138–152	147–166
5	9	136–145	142–156	151–170
5	10	140–150	146–160	155–174
5	11	144–154	150–165	159–179
6	0	148–158	154–170	164–184
6	1	152–162	158–175	168–189
6	2	156–167	162–180	173–194
6	3	160–171	167–185	178–199
6	4	164–175	172–190	182–204

* For nude weight, deduct 5 to 7 lbs. (male) or 2 to 4 lbs. (female).
Prepared by Metropolitan Life Insurance Company. Derived primarily from data of the Build and Blood Pressure Study, 1959, Society of Actuaries.

Table 1-4. Weight in Pounds According to Frame (in Indoor Clothing)*

Height with Shoes 2-inch Heels		Small	Medium	Large
Feet	Inches	Frame	Frame	Frame
		Desirable Weights for Women Aged 25 and Over		
4	10	92– 98	96–107	104–119
4	11	94–101	98–110	106–122
5	0	96–104	101–113	109–125
5	1	99–107	104–116	112–128
5	2	102–110	107–119	115–131
5	3	105–113	110–122	118–134
5	4	108–116	113–126	121–138
5	5	111–119	116–130	125–142
5	6	114–123	120–135	129–146
5	7	118–127	124–139	133–150
5	8	122–131	128–143	137–154
5	9	126–135	132–147	141–158
5	10	130–140	136–151	145–163
5	11	134–144	140–155	149–168
6	0	138–148	144–159	153–173

* For nude weight, deduct 5 to 7 lbs. (male) or 2 to 4 lbs. (female).
Prepared by Metropolitan Life Insurance Company. Derived primarily from data of the Build and Blood Pressure Study, 1959, Society of Actuaries.

specification of "optimal" or "ideal" weight is still more uncertain. For estimating present averages, without regard to what may be "desirable" values, a few data have been obtained from Selective Service records[43] and studies of the Quartermaster Corps.[98,107]

The average white registrant for Selective Service just before World War II was 26 years old, and was, unclothed, 68.5 inches tall and weighed 152.2 pounds. From the old 1912 tables a *clothed* weight of 152.0 pounds would be predicted for the average 26-year-old man whose height *in shoes* is 68.5 inches. Unfortunately, the Selective Service data are not analyzed for other ages and heights, and the data for men after several years in the Army differ from those of men when first called up for service. An analysis in 1946 and 1949 of data on men leaving the Army after several years indicated that, in both white and Negro men, the body weights are higher than would be expected from the 1912 tables.[98] The white separatees averaged 104.4 per cent and the Negro separatees averaged 105.0 per cent of the values listed in the Medico-Actuarial tables of 1912.

For women the actual averages for the population are still more uncertain. No samples generally representative of the population have ever been studied. A sample of about 8,500 women in the Women's Army Corps and in the Army Nurse Corps averaged 26.9 years old, 63.9 inches tall and 130.9 pounds in body weight; the 1912 tabular weight figure would be 128.5.

A national survey in Canada, covering some 22,000 persons in a carefully selected stratified sample of the entire country, provides more acceptable modern data which may be applicable to the United States as well as to Canada.[106] The average weights for specified heights found in the Canadian survey are given in abbreviated form in Table 1-5. These weights are for persons in "ordinary" indoor clothing, without shoes.

What, then, may be concluded about standard, desirable and "ideal" weights? In the first place, it is obvious that the available data are inadequate to describe the actual weights of "average" members of the population or to specify what weights would be most conducive to health. If anything, the young men of today may be heavier, at the same height, than 50 years ago and this may possibly be true of young women as well. The average body weights of older

Table 1-5. Average Weights (pounds) for Height and Age of Canadians in "Ordinary Indoor Clothing, without Shoes." Abbreviated and Adapted from Table 2 of Pett and Ogilvie (1956)

MEN

Height in inches	Age in Years				
	25	35	45	55	65 and over
60	128	139	136	137	130
62	135	146	144	145	140
64	142	152	152	152	149
66	150	160	161	160	158
68	156	167	169	168	167
70	163	174	177	176	177
72	170	182	186	184	186
74	185	189	194	191	195

WOMEN

Height in inches	25	35	45	55	65 and over
58	113	124	131	137	128
60	118	128	135	142	136
62	123	132	139	146	144
64	128	135	143	151	152
66	133	139	147	156	161
68	138	143	151	160	169
70	143	146	154	165	177

persons are much more uncertain, though there is no doubt that weight, in the United States, tends to change with age in something like the same manner as at the turn of the century.

Weights and Heights During Growth. The present discussion is primarily concerned with adults and space does not permit detailed consideration of the situation during growth, that is in infants and children. Far more data are available on children than on adults. Height-weight data for the United States have been summarized recently[67] and Garn and Shamir[60] have reviewed anthropometric methods, including fat estimation, in the study of growth. The extensive data on height and weight at different ages in the United States have been analyzed by Falkner[46] and are given here in Tables 1–6 and 1–7.

Table 1-6. Heights and Weights of Boys Aged 4 to 18 Years. Values of the 5th, 50th (Median) and 95th Centiles. Data from Falkner[46]

Ages (yrs)	Height (inches)			Weight (pounds)		
	5th	50th	95th	5th	50th	95th
4	38.3	40.8	43.3	30.0	36.1	42.2
5	40.3	43.4	46.4	33.0	40.3	47.6
6	42.8	45.9	49.0	36.0	44.7	53.4
7	44.8	48.1	51.4	40.3	50.9	61.5
8	46.9	50.5	54.1	44.4	57.4	70.1
9	48.8	52.8	56.8	48.0	64.4	80.4
10	50.6	54.9	59.2	51.4	71.4	91.4
11	51.9	56.4	60.9	53.3	78.9	102.5
12	53.5	58.6	63.7	60.0	86.0	113.5
13	55.2	61.3	67.4	65.3	98.6	131.9
14	57.5	64.1	70.7	75.5	118.8	148.1
15	61.0	66.9	72.8	88.0	124.3	160.6
16	63.8	68.9	74.0	97.8	133.8	169.8
17	65.2	69.8	74.4	106.5	139.8	174.0
18	65.9	70.2	74.5	110.3	144.8	179.3

Table 1-7. Heights and Weights of Girls Aged 4 to 18 Years. Values of the 5th, 50th (Median) and 95th Centiles. Data from Falkner[46]

Ages (yrs)	Height (inches)			Weight (pounds)		
	5th	50th	95th	5th	50th	95th
4	38.1	40.7	43.3	28.8	36.1	43.4
5	40.6	43.4	46.2	32.2	40.9	49.6
6	42.8	45.9	49.0	35.5	45.7	55.9
7	44.5	47.8	51.1	38.3	51.0	63.7
8	46.4	50.0	53.6	42.0	57.2	72.4
9	48.2	52.2	56.2	45.1	63.6	82.1
10	49.9	54.5	59.1	48.2	71.0	95.0
11	51.9	57.0	62.1	55.4	82.0	108.6
12	54.1	59.5	64.9	63.9	94.4	124.9
13	57.1	62.2	66.8	72.8	105.5	138.2
14	58.5	63.1	67.7	83.0	113.0	144.0
15	59.5	63.8	68.1	89.5	120.0	150.5
16	59.8	64.1	68.4	95.1	123.0	150.1
17	60.1	64.2	68.3	97.9	125.8	153.7
18	60.1	64.4	68.7	96.0	126.2	156.4

At given age during the growing years, both sexes in the United States have been getting taller and heavier during at least the last 50 years.[13],[66]

Body Weights in Other Countries. Compared with the United States information on average and desirable body weights in many, but not all, other countries is as deficient, or worse. Older data, often of doubtful statistical merit, are summarized by Krogman.[82] Useful data are available for Great Britain and Japan. There is no doubt that, at the same height and age, Britons tend to be lighter than Americans and the age-increment in weight is smaller.[73] In Japan, not only is the relative weight smaller but the age-increment in weight is much smaller than in Americans.[137]

A continuous rise in body weight with age, such as is the situation in the United States, is not inevitable. Among relatively primitive people on islands in the China Sea there is no increase of average body weight after 25.[30],[57] It is interesting that most of the usual age-increment in body weight common among adults in the Western World rapidly disappears in populations on short rations who are not actually starving.[78] A relatively moderate reduction in the food supplies available for the entire population tends to produce the greatest loss of body weight in the older, fatter individuals and the health records of World War II suggest that this may be beneficial.

In recent years we have been able to measure heights and weights of substantially all men aged 40 to 59 in selected areas in Italy, Yugoslavia, Finland, Greece, and the Netherlands and have compared these with the findings on statistical samples of United States railroad employees. In terms of the Medico-Actuarial standards (Table 1–1), the medians for relative body weight of different categories of United States railroad employees ranged from 101 to 106 per cent; the corresponding figures for men in the foreign samples were below 100 per cent in all samples except one group in Italy. It is notable, too, that in all of the foreign samples the relative body weight decreased with age from 40 to 44 to 55 to 59 years. In other words, these European men tended to gain less weight

with age than did the Americans. The inference is that American men tend to excessive fat accumulation with advancing age.

Somatotypes. Human bodies differ in type or shape and recognition of gross differences in the body type is not possible solely from measurements of relative weight or of fatness. The idea that particular body types are dominant among patients with certain diseases is of long standing, but there is lack of agreement on the definition of body type and the distinction between body type and relative obesity is not very clear.

Sheldon[115] proposed a scheme of "somatotypes" which is supposed to represent the basic body characteristic, relatively independent of body fatness, and this has been rather widely used. However, it is clear that these types are not, in fact, independent of the state of nutrition.[77],[83] Studies on experimental starvation in man have shown that, when starved, the endomorph is so changed that he will be easily classified as an ectomorph. "Endomorphy" and "ectomorphy" appear to be primarily impure expressions of the obesity-emaciation continuum, while the meaning of "mesomorphy" is uncertain. The fact that Sheldon's somatotypes are related to body fatness and to skeletal shape does not confer any special value to somatotyping; better estimates of these items are available by other and less esoteric means.

Optimal Characteristics. All the foregoing discussion leads to the conclusion that the specification of "optimal" or "ideal" weights is hazardous business. For body weight and relative obesity, at least, the only point on which there will be full agreement is that major departures from the population average should be avoided. There is no doubt that there is an excess mortality penalty in later life associated with marked overweight at the time of application for life insurance.

Insurance experience indeed shows increasing mortality rates with increasing degrees of overweight, but there are serious questions about the samples compared and the interpretations. The fact that insurance companies charge extra premiums to overweight persons probably results in biased samples. Moreover, overweight and obesity, though correlated, especially at the extremes, are far from being identical. Obesity, that is body fatness, has not been measured in the insurance studies and an excess of weight for given height may reflect bone, muscle or body shape as well as, or instead of, actual obesity.

Physicians and the general public alike are under the pressure of constant propaganda about the health dangers of obesity in general and in regard to the development of cardiovascular disease in particular. However, to suggest that the major national health obstacle in the United States is obesity because perhaps a tenth of the population may be 10 per cent or more above the average body weight is more than can be sustained from present evidence. Is there actually any serious health hazard necessarily associated with 10 per cent overweight? At what ages? And can we disregard the question of obesity versus overweight? Much more research is needed before scientifically acceptable answers to these questions will be at hand. One thing seems certain. The elimination of gross overweight among Americans cannot, by itself, be expected to bring our adult mortality to a level to compare favorably with that of such countries as the Netherlands and the Scandinavian[75] countries. A more penetrating analysis of obesity, rather than mere body weight, might reveal more scope for improvement.

BODY COMPOSITION

The development of methods for estimation of the gross composition of the human body *in vivo* has provided an important tool for metabolic analysis and the evaluation of nutritional status. The application of these methods makes possible estimation of the main gross components of the human body and, in particular, the measurement of its fat content. Validation of these indirect methods depends on data obtained by the direct analysis of human bodies: this is the final reference on which indirect computations must be based. The discussion of indirect methods of body composition analysis must start, therefore, with a consideration of the existing data from direct analyses of human bodies.

Direct Analysis of Human Bodies. Technical and legal complications of direct analysis of the main components of whole human bodies are such that few results have been reported in the century since attempts began in this direction. The early work was summarized in the first and subsequent editions of Vierordt's Tabellen[134] but the technical methods then available severely limit the utility of the older data.

In Table 1–8 are summarized the most reliable modern data on the gross composition of three adult male bodies. Two of these can

Table 1-8.[22] Body Composition from Direct Chemical Analysis of 3 Male Cadavers Examined by Mitchell et al.,[93] Widdowson et al.,[135] and Forbes et al.[55]

Reference	Age (years)	Height (cm)	Total weight (kg)	Per cent*				Water % of fat-free weight
				Water	Fat	Protein	Ash	
Mitchell et al. 1945	35	183.0	70.6	68.2	12.5	14.5	4.8	77.9
Widdowson et al. 1951	25	179.0	71.8	62.0	15.0	16.6	6.4	72.9
Forbes et al. 1953	46	168.5	53.8	56.0	19.6	18.8	5.6	69.6
Mean	35.3	176.8	65.4	62.6	15.3	16.4	5.7	73.9

* Computed as per cent of the body weight accounted for by water, protein and ash, comprising 99.7 per cent of the total body weight.

be considered representative of normal bodies, but the body of the 46-year-old man is not free of suspicion of abnormality.

There is a good deal of variability in the total fat content of these selected bodies. Equally significant is the variation in the ratio of ash to protein and in the water content of the fat-free mass. Clearly, the concept of a constant composition of the fat-free portion of the body finds no support from the only direct data we have for man. The data from animals are far more numerous but they also show considerable variation among individuals.

The Compartments of the Body. Metabolically, the most elementary analysis of the body mass begins with the differentiation between the part of the body that is relatively active in energy metabolism and the relatively non-active part. In the latter category are the body fat, the extracellular fluid, the mineral portion of the bony skeleton and a negligible part of the horny epidermis, the nails and the hair.[77,120] The body fat tends to be the most variable compartment, though the extracellular fluid mass may increase considerably in cases of edema.

If, from the total mass of the body, the non-active masses of fat, extracellular fluid and bone mineral are subtracted, the remainder may be termed the "active tissue mass"[110] or "cell residue." This mass, primarily cells of course, may represent anything from perhaps 30 to 65 per cent of the total body weight, but it accounts for substantially all the energy consumption. The highest values for cell mass, as a percentage of body weight, will be found in lean very muscular men in a state of dehydration; the lowest values will occur in sedentary women who are both fat and edematous. The foregoing subdivision of the mass of the body into the four "compartments"—fat, extracellular water, cell residue and bone mineral—is not only metabolically reasonable, it also corresponds to some degree, as we shall see, with the availability of practical methods of measurement *in vivo*. The distribution of the four main chemical components of the body among the four main "compartments" is described in Table 1–9.

It will be observed that this system pays little attention to the traditional classifications of the body into kinds of parts—bony skeleton, cartilaginous skeleton, voluntary muscle, and so on, or into systems—skeletal system, muscular system, nervous system and

Table 1-9.[22]   A System of Symbols Used in Describing the Body Compartments and the Main Chemical Components of the Body

	Chemical components			
Body compartments	Water A	Fat F	Protein P	Minerals M
Fat (F)	—	F	—	—
Extracellular water (A_E)	A_E	—	—	—
Cell residue (C)	A_C	—	P	M_C*
Bone (osseous mineral) (M_o)	—	—	—	M_o
Total body weight	$W = A + F + P + M = F + A_E + C + M_o$			
Total body water	$A = A_E + A_C$			
Total body mineral	$M = M_o + M_c$			
Cell residue	$C = A_c + P + M_c + W - (F + A_E + M_o)$			
Total non-fat solids	$S = P + M$			
Cell residue solids	$(M_s) = P + M_c$			

* Note: M_c refers to the mineral content of the "cell residue" and represents by definition all mineral that is not osseous ($M_c = M - M_o$) *i.e.* the mineral in the "cells" and in the extracellular fluid.

so on. Partly this is because the first focus is on gross metabolism; equally important, however, is the fact that currently no practical methods are available or even conceivable to provide reliable measurements of the living human body in these other terms. Furthermore, when the center of interest is nutrition, and especially changes in nutritional state, some questions about organs and organ systems are only of subordinate interest. For example, the mass of the brain and nervous tissue is relatively insensitive to nutritional effects, at least after growth is finished. Mental and nervous functions may be greatly affected, but this is not at all closely related to the mass of the brain and nerves; the mass itself is remarkably constant in the face of starvation or of gross overnutrition of the body as a whole.[78] How much the adult skeletal mass responds to changes in nutrition is unknown, but in any event the change is relatively small and slow. On the other hand the masses of some organs and organ systems seem to respond alike to gross nutritional changes. In starvation, the percentage reductions in the masses of the heart, voluntary muscles, kidneys, testes and many other organs are similar.[78]

In the partition system just described it will be observed that there are no places, as such, for blood, skeleton or adipose tissue. The estimation of total blood volume (and hence its mass) is not difficult and a combination of the dye method (T-1824 dilution) or labeled erythrocyte injection, with a hematocrit, for example, provides estimates of both circulating blood plasma and cells. These measurements are useful and provide additional detail but they are not essential in the first stage of metabolic analysis. The total mass of the blood is not a large part of the total body mass and it accounts for only an infinitesimal part of the total energy metabolism of the body. The plasma (or rather the plasma water) which normally comprises more than half of the blood volume and makes up about 4 per cent of the body weight, is included in the calculation of extracellular water. The cellular components of the blood account for only about a thirtieth of the total body weight; they are included in the "cell residue" compartment,

which also includes the plasma proteins and the plasma minerals in our system of partition.

The skeleton is a large mass and in the living (i.e. fresh, wet) state may average a sixth of the total body mass. In 64 young white men who averaged 70.7 kg of living weight, the dry defatted skeletal weight was 4,259 gm or 6 per cent of the gross body weight.[7] The bone minerals account for only a fraction of the total skeletal mass, and the water, protein and fat components are included in the estimates of the total body content of these substances, or in the corresponding compartments (extracellular water, cell residue and fat). From the data of the analyses of the three cadavers listed in Table 1-8 we have estimated the mass of bone mineral (after transformation of ash into bone mineral, see 22) as 4.8 per cent of the total body weight.

Fat is defined in this chapter as pure fat obtained after ether extraction of the whole body. Adipose tissue is not, as it is sometimes supposed, pure fat. From Bozenraad's old studies[17] it often is concluded that human adipose tissue is 80 to 85 per cent pure fat. Actually he merely reported that when drying samples of adipose tissue in an oven they lost an average of 15 to 20 per cent of their weight. Bozenraad was well aware of the fact that adipose tissue contains connective tissue, blood vessels and cell walls and he did not suggest that this dried adipose tissue was simply fat. He found the water content of adipose tissue in emaciated persons to be considerably greater than in well-nourished persons. In 7 emaciated bodies water averaged 31 per cent of the abdominal "fat," 33 per cent of the heart "fat," and 25 per cent of the kidney "fat." The corresponding averages for 14 well-nourished subjects were 12, 18 and 14 per cent respectively.

Densitometric Determination of Body Fat. Principles: The relative proportions of the components of a system consisting of an additive mixture of two substances of different density can be calculated if we know the density of each of the components and that of the mixture. Let W_1 and W_2 be the masses of the components, d_1 and d_2 their densities, and D the density of the mixture. D will be

$$(1) \quad D = \frac{W_1 + W_2}{\left(\dfrac{W_1}{d_1}\right) + \left(\dfrac{W_2}{d_2}\right)}$$

If we make $W_1 + W_2 = 1$ and represent the component W_1 as a fraction (w_1) of the total mass we can write

$$(2) \quad D = \frac{1}{(w_1/d_1) + (1-w_1/d_2)}$$

solving for w_1

$$(3) \quad w_1 = \frac{1}{D} \cdot \frac{d_1 d_2}{(d_2-d_1)} - \frac{d_1}{(d_2-d_1)}$$

$$(4) \quad w_1 = \frac{\left(\dfrac{d_2}{D} - 1\right)}{\left(\dfrac{d_2}{d_1} - 1\right)}$$

The application of this equation to the estimation of fat in the living human body requires, then, the measurement of its density, the definition of the two components W_1 and W_2 and assigning values for their densities d_1, d_2.

An early application of densitometry was made by Kohlrausch[81] who used it to demonstrate changes in the body composition of dogs resulting from alterations in nutritional state and in physical exercise. General interest in this method developed later as a result of the pioneer work of Behnke and his colleagues in weighing men under water.[9,10] The development of theory and applications is presented by Keys and Brozek[77] and by Siri.[120] We have published a revision of the constants and assumptions involved in the application of the densitometric method to the determination of body fat in man.[22] The density of the human body is obtained from estimates of the total mass and volume of the body. The measurement of the volume of the living body can be made with considerable accuracy by either of two methods. The Archimedean principle of weighing the body under water provides a sensitive measure of body volume, but it requires that an estimate be made of the air in the lungs and respiratory passages at the time of weighing.[77] Measurement of this residual air is not particularly difficult with the nitrogen washout method. In the alternative method, first used by Kohlrausch,[81] the body volume is estimated from the application of the gas laws of Boyle and Gay-Lussac to the body in an air chamber of known capacity. The considerable technical difficulties of the latter method seem to be largely overcome by the use of a foreign gas, such as helium, of which a known amount is injected into the gas chamber; the free space is then estimated from a gas analysis on the dilution principle.[120]

Lean Body Mass Versus Fat-free Body. Behnke[9] proposed partition of the body into two parts, (1) fat and (2) "lean body mass." The latter was conceived of as the body with the least amount of fat compatible with health and was considered to include the "essential fat," amounting to 10 per cent of its weight. This definition was later revised so that the "lean body mass" was held to include 2 per cent of its weight as fat. Since it is impossible to decide how much fat is really essential and since no methods are available to separate body fat into essential and nonessential parts, more recent investigations have either re-defined the "lean body mass" as the body devoid of all fat[87] or, better, have abandoned the term and deal with the fat-free body and the body fat, the latter being the sum of ether-extractable substances in the body.

Pace and Rathbun[101] considered the body to be made up of a non-fat portion and pure fat and assumed the densities of these two parts to be constant. They then provided a numerical solution for equation number 4 which has been fairly widely used. However, it is now known that their value for fat density is incorrect for living men and that the value for density of the fat-free body is neither a constant nor is it precisely known for any given situation.[77,120] Moreover, such an equation cannot be accurate because when the body becomes fatter it does not do so merely by adding fat to the preexisting mass. Numerous observations in controlled experiments have shown that, in men making large changes of body weight induced by dietary alterations, the density of the tissue gained or lost is never that of pure fat; in other words the density of the non-fat part of the body changes with nutritional status.[76]

The Density of Human Fat. Human body fat, as extracted by ether from adipose tissue removed at surgery from the living body, has a density of 0.9000 gm per ml at 37° C.[48] Variations in fat density are small between the sexes and among individuals and locations in the body. This low variability, as well as the low absolute value of the density, provides the basis for estimating the proportion of fat in the body from the density of the living person.[9,77,120] It should be noted, however, that the thermal coefficient of expansion of fat is relatively high so allowance for this must be made in dealing with dead bodies. In human fat the mean change in density is 0.00074 per degree C, over the range of 15 to 37° C, so that, even in the living body, the density will be different in a feverish person as contrasted with the same person in hypothermia.[48] Different animal species differ somewhat in the density and thermal expansion of their body fat and in some species, notably the cow and the lamb, subcutaneous and internal fats have different densities. The density of the ether extract from muscle and brain is higher than that of the ether extract from adipose tissue.[90] All these facts must be taken into account in applying the densitometric method for the estimation of total body fat.

The Concept of "Reference Body" and of "Obesity Tissue." The non-fat portion of the body has an average density something like 1.10 gm per ml at 37° C, but there are individual variations; the value is altered by gross changes of hydration, as in edema, and it is also affected by changes in the degree of obesity. As a person grows fatter the bony mineral mass (of high density) tends to remain constant while water, connective tissue, and cells, as well as fat, tend to increase.[29,76] This follows from the nature of the adipose tissue and from the fact that many of the soft tissues of the body must make at least slight adjustments to the increase of total body size occasioned by the developing obesity. More muscle is required to carry around the added weight, blood vessels have to cover more distance, the area of the skin has to increase. These complications, how-ever, do not prevent highly useful estimates of total body fat by densitometry.

Most theoretical and practical needs for the estimation of body fat are satisfied with a relative answer. We have proposed to do this by making comparison with a "standard body," the body of a clinically healthy man aged 25 who corresponds exactly in body weight with the United States average for given height as recorded in standard height-weight tables. By definition such a body is neither obese nor emaciated, neither over-weight nor underweight. From measurements on young men selected to correspond with these height-weight requirements such a "standard" average body is found to have a density of 1.0629 gm per ml at 37° C.[98] The fat content of the "standard body" was originally estimated as 14 per cent of the total body weight.[77] Bodies with densities less than this figure are, then, relatively fat and densities above this figure refer to relatively lean bodies.

These differences can be expressed quantitatively in terms of the kind of tissue that the body tends to gain or lose when it is maintained in a state of calorie imbalance for some time. From experiments on under- and overeating to produce body weight changes of the order of 10 to 20 kg in otherwise healthy men in a period of 6 months, it appears that such weight changes involve what we have termed "obesity tissue," that is the sum of the various substances gained or lost by the body during the process of weight change. As stated, this "obesity tissue" is not pure fat, nor is it identified with adipose tissue or any other particular tissue of the body. The density of the "obesity tissue" found in our experiments averaged 0.9478 gm per ml at 37° C.[76] A given individual, then, can be considered as made of two parts, one corresponding in composition to that of the reference body and another corresponding in composition to that of "obesity tissue." In other words, a given individual can be considered as equal to the "standard body" plus or minus a certain amount of "obesity tissue."

If we let g be the proportion of the body made up by such "obesity tissue" and D the observed density of the whole body, we may write, similarly to equation number 4.

$$(5)\ g = \frac{\left(\dfrac{1.0629}{D} - 1\right)}{\left(\dfrac{1.0629}{0.9478} - 1\right)}$$

or

$$(6)\ g = (8.755/D) - 8.237$$

Suppose, for example, we observe a value of D = 1.050 in man. Then we have

$$(7)\ g = (8.755/1.050) - 8.237 = 0.101$$

and we conclude that 10.1 per cent of the body weight of this man is "obesity tissue," with 89.9 per cent of his body weight having the composition of our standard young man. A negative value for g would mean a deficiency of "obesity tissue" in comparison with the standard.

The "obesity tissue" is considered to be made up of fat, extracellular fluid and "cell residue." From measurements in experiments on men gaining weight from overeating, it appears that about 14 per cent of the gain is accounted for by extracellular fluid while the remainder is a mixture of fat and cells having an average density of 0.939 gm per ml. From the density of fat an estimate of the density of the "cells" and the determination of the extracellular fluid the composition of the obesity tissue was calculated. Our first estimate was that such obesity tissue is composed of 14 per cent extracellular fluid, 62 per cent fat and 24 per cent "cell residue."[76]

From the proportions of "standard man" and of "obesity tissue" in the body and the proportions of fat in each of these two parts, it is easy to compute the total amount of fat in the body. This will be equal to the sum of the fat in the "standard body" and in the "obesity tissue." In our example we computed that a man with a body density of 1.050 is made up by 10.1 per cent of "obesity tissue" and 89.9 per cent of "standard body." If his weight is 75 kg, his body is made of 7.58 kg (75 × 0.101) of "obesity tissue" and 67.42 kg (75 × 0.899) of "standard body." The amount of fat contributed by the "obesity tissue" is 7.58 × 0.62 = 4.70 kg, and that contributed by the "standard man" is 67.42 × 0.14 = 9.44 kg. The total amount of fat, then, is 4.70 + 9.44 = 14.14 kg or 18.85 per cent of the total body weight.

Obviously the validity of these computations depends on the validity of the values assigned to the fat content of the "standard body" and of the "obesity tissue." It was originally suggested[98] that the "standard body" of density 1.0629 contains about 14 per cent of fat, a figure accepted as within perhaps 2 per cent of the true value by several later investigators.[36,120] But, from new experiments in men changing weight, in which nitrogen balance as well as body density were determined, it appears that the true value may be nearer to 16 per cent.

We have proposed the use of a new standard of reference which we have called the "reference body" based on the analyses of the 3 human cadavers listed in Table 1–8. The density of this "reference body" was computed from the data of chemical analysis of the cadavers in Table 1–8 as described elsewhere[22] and was found to be 1.064 gm per ml at 37° C. The fat content of the "reference body" is 15.3 per cent of the total body weight. The composition and density of the "reference body" are presented in Table 1–10. The differences resulting from the substitution of the new "reference body" for the previous "standard body" are small. The important advance consists in replacing an assumed with an empirically determined fat content of the "reference body" and the corresponding increase in validity of the computation.

"Obesity tissue," as defined from the data of the experiment in men gaining weight by overeating,[76] tends to have a quite constant density of 0.9478 gm per ml at 37° C. But other data in the literature,[72,84] as well as new experiments in our laboratory, indicate that the density and composition of the "obesity tissue" gained or lost by the body are not always identical. We have attempted to provide other estimates of the composition and density of the "obesity tissue" and to correct the data of our previous experiments by using the value of 1.078 as density of the "cell residue."[22] This figure was derived, like the value for the density of the "reference body," from the data from the analyses of

Table 1-10.[22]   Weights and Volumes of the Components of 1 kg of the Reference Body (Based on the Analysis of 3 Male Cadavers), Their Densities, and the Calculated Density (d = 1.064) of the Empirically Defined "Reference Body"

Symbol	Component	Weight g	Density at 37° C g/ml	Specific Volume at 37° C ml/g	Volume at 37° C ml
A	Water	624.3	0.99371	1.0063	628.2
P	Protein	164.4	1.34	0.7463	122.7
F	Fat	153.1	0.9007*	1.1102	170.0
M_o	Bone (osseous) Mineral	47.7	2.982	0.3353	16.0
M_c	Non-osseous Mineral	10.5	3.317	0.3015	3.2
	Total	1000.0	1.064	0.9398	940.1

* 36° C

Table 1-11.[22]   Calculated Percentage Composition of "Obesity Tissue" Defined on the Basis of Weight Gain, Weight Loss, and the Difference Between Low-Density and High-Density Young Men

	Weight Gain	Weight Loss	Static Difference
Sample size	N = 10	N = 10	N = 16 and 21
Extracellular water	14	4	7
Fat	64	64	73
"Cell residue"	22	32	20
Density	0.948	0.954	0.938

the three male cadavers listed in Table 1–8. These new estimates of density and composition of the "obesity tissue" cover three different situations: weight gain, weight loss, and static weight difference. The last value applies to the difference between two groups of young men of the same age and height but differing very markedly in body weight and density. These data are presented in Table 1–11.

Formulas for the Densitometric Estimation of Body Fat. In view of the substantial variations in the composition of the "obesity tissue," it seems that no single formula is generally valid for the estimation of body fat. At present it appears that the best estimates will be obtained by using the formula which applies to the particular situation under

study. In Table 1–12 we present three formulas based on the three classes of "obesity tissue" previously discussed. The formulas based on the experiments on gain and loss of weight will be more useful in the evaluation of body composition during periods of rapid dynamic changes of body weight, while the formula based on the static differences between chronically thin and chronically obese individuals will better fit the conditions of slow changing or stable body weight.

Application of these formulas to our example of a man having a body density of 1.050 gives fat values of 20.63, 20.90 and 21.04 per cent for the formula based on the "obesity tissue" of weight gain, weight loss and static difference respectively. These values are not very different from each other, but all of

2

Table 1-12.[22] Formulas for the Estimation from Body Density (D_B), of the Amount of "Obesity Tissue" as a Fraction of Total Body Weight of the Fat Associated with the "Obesity Tissue," and of the Total Body Fat as a Fraction of Total Body Weight. The Density of the Reference Body Is 1.064, Its Fat Content 15.3% of Body Weight

Item	From Gain	From Loss	From Static Difference
Density (d_G)	0.948	0.954	0.938
Fat content of "obesity tissue" (as fraction, f_G)	0.64	0.64	0.73
"Obesity tissue," g, $=$ from body density	$\dfrac{8.696}{D_B} - 8.172$	$\dfrac{9.228}{D_B} - 8.673$	$\dfrac{7.921}{D_B} - 7.444$
Fat content, f_G, $=$ from body density	$\dfrac{5.565}{D_B} - 5.230$	$\dfrac{5.906}{D_B} - 5.551$	$\dfrac{5.782}{D_B} - 5.434$
Total body fat, f_B, $=$ from body density	$\dfrac{4.235}{D_B} - 3.827$	$\dfrac{4.494}{D_B} - 4.071$	$\dfrac{4.570}{D_B} - 4.142$

them are higher than the value of 18.85 per cent obtained by the application of the old formula illustrated on pages 13 and 14.

Body Fat from Body Water Measurements. The total amount of water in the body may be estimated on the dilution principle. An intravenous injection is made of an exactly known amount of a substance which penetrates and dissolves in all the water of the body and is not rapidly metabolized. After time is allowed for uniform distribution, a blood sample is drawn and the concentration of the test substance in the water of the blood is measured. Water labeled with isotopic hydrogen, deuterium or tritium,[113] is suitable as the test substance, but antipyrine, n-acetyl-4-aminopyrine and urea have also been used.[39,85,121] Isotopic labeled water can be used also by oral administration.[47]

Measurement of body water is useful for its own sake but it also has the advantage that it may be used to estimate the other components of the body, at least roughly. The original crude theory was that water represents a fixed fraction of the mass of the non-fat part of the body.[101] This is not precisely true even in normally hydrated bodies. In the cadavers listed in Table 1–8, the water represents a range of 69.6 to 77.9 per cent of

the fat-free mass. This range may be used to calculate limits for the proportion of fat in the body, when the total body water has been measured. Now, the total body weight (W) must be equal to the sum of the total body water (A), the total body fat (F) and the total body non-fat solids (S).

$$(8) \quad W = A + F + S$$

If we take the total body weight to be unity and represent the fractions of the different components by the corresponding lower-case letters we must have

$$(9) \quad 1 = a + f + s$$

and therefore,

$$(10) \quad f = 1 - (a + s)$$

In the preceding paragraph it was indicated that we have limits of $a = 0.696 \, (a + s)$ and $a = 0.779 \, (a + s)$. The limiting possibilities will then be

$$(11a) \quad f = 1 - a/0.696$$
$$(11b) \quad f = 1 - a/0.779$$

The application of equations 11*a* and 11*b* can be illustrated with the case of a man weighing 80 kg who is found to have a total body water mass of 45 kg, *i.e.*, a = 0.56. From equation 11*a* we have f = 0.196 and from 11*b* we have f = 0.281. The conclusion is that the man in question has a body in which from 19.6 to 28.1 per cent of the weight is made up of fat. Such a calculation is not permissible, of course, in the presence of edema or dehydration.

Body fat can also be determined from combined measurements of total body water and extracellular water. The limitations of these systems have been discussed by Keys and Brozek.[77]

Body Fat from Body Water and Densitometry. It may be suggested that a more reliable estimate of body composition would be obtained from a combination of body water and density measurements. We[77] and others have derived equations for this purpose, that of Siri[120] being as follows:

(12) f = (2.057/D) — 0.786a — 1.286

where D is the density of the whole body and f and a are the proportions of fat and of water in the body. But, as Siri pointed out, this combination really does not eliminate the uncertainty about the fundamental assumptions. The estimate of the body fat by equation 12 may have a standard deviation around ±1.7 per cent of the total body weight.[120]

Total Body Potassium in Body Composition Studies. Since potassium is present mainly in the intracellular phase, the measurement of the potassium content of the body offers a possibility for the estimation of the body cell mass. Measurement of the total potassium content of the living body has been achieved by two methods: (1) direct measurement of the gamma radiation emitted by the radioactive K 40 which occurs in a constant proportion in natural potassium, (2) measurement of the total exchangeable potassium by isotopic dilution using K 42 as a tracer.

Direct measurement of body potassium by means of its natural radioactivity was initiated by Sievert[117,118] and has been developed in this country with the introduction by Ander-

son *et al.* of the Los Alamos human counter, which makes it possible to determine the total potassium content of the body in a very short period of time.[3] The methods based on the measurement of the exchangeable potassium by isotopic dilution with K 42 are widely used at the present.[94,113,128] The available data indicate a reasonable agreement between the results obtained by the two methods,[1,34,111] although the values found by the dilution method are lower than those found by carcass analysis (Forbes and Lewis[53]). In applying the total potassium content of the body to the determination of body fat, the system is similar to that used in the determination of the fat-free body from the total water content of the body. By dividing the total amount of potassium in the body by the potassium content of 1 kg of fat-free body, the mass of fat-free body in kg can be calculated, and by subtracting the fat-free body mass from the total body weight we compute the amount of fat in the body. The problem, then, is to establish the potassium content of the fat-free body. Since the fat-free body is made up of a series of anatomical elements having different compositions it is clear that the average potassium concentration will depend on the relative proportion of these various components. The high potassium content of muscle is well known but muscle is only a part of the total fat-free body, and connective tissue and other structural materials, while having a similar degree of hydration, probably have little potassium. Interesting correlations between potassium content and fat-free cell solids ("cell residue" solids or Allen's M_3) estimated from total body water have been described and used as a basis for the estimation of body fat.[1] Anderson and Langham[4,5] have used the figure of 73 mEq of potassium/kg for the computation of the lean body mass. Forbes *et al.*[51,52] have used the figure 68.1 mEq/kg to compute the fat-free body mass. This latter figure is based on data from the analyses of four human bodies.[53] The fat-free body mass (in kg) is calculated by these authors by dividing the total body potassium (mEq) by 68.1. Burmeister and Bingert[28] in their extensive studies have calculated "cell mass" from total body potassium determinations assuming a mean potassium content of 92.5 mEq/kg of "cell mass." Fat-free body mass was calculated by these authors as 1.1 × cell mass + extracellular fluid. Extracellular fluid, in turn, was assumed to be 6.1 liters per square meter of body surface. Allen et al.[1] have shown that the total body potassium content measured by the body counter method is proportional to the body mass minus bone mineral, fat and water (this is the compartment M_3 which corresponds with our "cell residue" solids). Since the ratio K/M_3 (equivalents of potassium/kg) decreases with age and is lower in the female than in the male, the authors use a correction which takes into account the chronological age of the subject. M_3 ("cell residue" solids) for males beyond age 15 is then given by equation 13

$$(13) \quad M_3 = K/(0.354 - 0.00082\sigma)$$

in which M_3 is in kg, K in equivalents, and σ is age in years. Assuming that the ratio of M_3 to total body water and to bone mineral is constant, Allen et al.[1] estimate the amount of fat from M_3 by the following equation:

$$(14) \quad F = M - 4.964 \, M_3$$

in which F and M represent the masses of fat and of the total body respectively and M_3 the mass of the "cell residue" solids calculated from equation 13. More recently Anderson[6] has suggested a system of body partition into muscle, adipose tissue and remaining body mass as being more consistent with their data of total body potassium and total body water.

Isotopic Dilution Methods in Body Composition Studies. The determination of the composition of the human body by isotopic dilution methods has been widely used. Moore and his co-workers[86,94] have published a summary of their extensive and important work.[94] The estimation of the body cell mass depends on the measurement of the exchangeable potassium, assuming a ratio of potassium to nitrogen in the cell mass of 3 mEq of K per gm of N, and an average nitrogen content of 4 per cent (or 25 per cent of protein).

It should be noted that Moore's "Body Cell Mass" does not correspond to the "cell residue" as defined here. The estimation of the "body cell mass" assumes uniformity of potassium concentration in all the cells of the body, and the compartment so described excludes such components as connective fibers and plasma proteins that are included in the "cell residue." Final validation of this technique requires more information with direct determination of potassium. The methods of isotopic dilution have been applied by Haxhe[68] in studies on man and animals under various conditions. The changes observed by Haxhe during undernutrition are in good agreement with the data reported by others. Of particular interest are the data on the constancy of the K/N ratio in undernutrition. This finding tends to support the validity of the measurement of exchangeable potassium in the estimation of the cell mass of the body in the presence of changing nutritional status.

Subcutaneous Fat. About half of the total fat in man is in the subcutaneous layer, so measurements of subcutaneous fat may give a good index to the total fat of the body.[23,25,41,131] Unfortunately, the subcutaneous fat layer varies from place to place and the distribution is not the same in different individuals or in the same individual at different ages. For example, in young children the layer of subcutaneous fat over the triceps muscle of the arm is relatively thick, even in thin children, while the layer over the abdomen is much thinner. In adults the proportion is reversed, so data from children[108] do not apply to adults. However, sampling several sites, or even a single site in persons of a given age, may allow a useful rough estimate of the total body fatness.

Equations for the prediction of total body fat or of body density from a combination of measurements of skinfolds at different sites have been developed.[20,25,26,77,104] These show correlations between the values predicted from skinfolds and those obtained from densitometry, with coefficients of r = 0.85 to r = 0.87. This correlation means that almost 20 per cent of the variance is not accounted for by regression.

With experience, a fairly good subjective appraisal of calorie nutritional status can be made simply by digital pinching, but skinfold calipers, used as recommended by a committee of experts,[20,79] allow novice and expert alike to obtain numerical estimates of acceptable reliability.[42,77]

The skinfold should be pinched up to the point where the sides are parallel and the thickness is measured with calipers exerting a pressure of 10 gm per square mm (single jaw face area). Prolonged application of the calipers should be avoided because, after the initial deformation of the skinfold under the pressure there is a slowly progressive compression, particularly if edema is present. Advantage may be taken of this slow deformation to evaluate the presence or amount of edema.

The subcutaneous fat thickness in some parts of the body may be accurately estimated from soft-tissue roentgenograms.[60,77,123] Rather good agreement has been found between the skinfold technique and the radiographic method[26] when measuring subcutaneous fat changes. In a group of 52 middle-aged men the correlation between total body fat (from densitometry) and the thickness of the subcutaneous fat measured on roentgenograms was $r = 0.75$ and $r = 0.76$ for two sites on the arms, and $r = 0.58$ for the calf.[27] A better correlation might be expected if the sum of fat thicknesses at several sites was used.

The topographic distribution of subcutaneous fat tends to be an individual characteristic but changes in fatness induced by dietary alterations seem to be shared proportionally by all regions of the body.[23,27,41] When an obese person loses fat on a reducing diet, if the fat thickness over the triceps muscle diminishes by 10 per cent, then something like a 10 per cent reduction at other sites may be expected. This may be disappointing to reducers who hope to get thinner in some places than in others, but it does mean that simple skinfold measurements are useful for following the changes in the total fat of the body. On the other hand, the process of gaining weight after a period of dietary restriction may proceed at different rates in different places. In experiments in this laboratory it was observed that the abdominal skinfold increased at a disproportionately rapid rate.[23]

Body Composition During Growth. The process of growth and development requires energy and building material over and above the demands of ordinary maintenance and the cost of physical work. The growth of children is retarded by a restriction of food intake[78] and the growth deficit is related to the severity of the undernutrition. The rate of weight increase is more readily affected than is growth in height, but even this latter can be seriously inhibited in extreme calorie deficit.

But growth is not only a change of body size. Important changes in body composition also take place during the growth period. It has long been known[14] that the concentration of water in the body is very high in the fetus and steadily decreases during growth. During intra-uterine development total body water as a percentage of total body weight decreases from 94 to about 76 at delivery and continues to fall thereafter, with no difference between the sexes during the growing years.[56]

The change of water content of the developing body was considered by Moulton[95] as one of the basic principles in mammalian development. The other basic principle emphasized by Moulton is that fat is the great variable in the composition of the mammalian body. At a given moment of the development process the proportions of water, protein and minerals in the fat-free portion of the body become stabilized. When this stabilization is achieved the body reaches "chemical maturity." The age at which the animal reaches "chemical maturity" was considered by Moulton to be a relatively constant fraction of the total life span.

The changes in total and extracellular water in children have been studied by Friis-Hansen.[56] Total body water was determined by D_2O and extracellular water by thiosulfate. A summary of his results is presented in Table 1–13. Both total body water and extracellular water (as percentage of the total body weight) decrease as age advances, but the proportion of extracellular water decreases more than that of total body water. This is in part an expression of the increase of cell mass at the expense of extracellular fluid, in particular of the development of tissues like skeletal muscle which have a high proportion

Table 1-13. Average Percentages of the Total Body Weight Represented by Total Body Water and by Extracellular Water and the Ratio of Intracellular Water to Total Body Solids During Infancy and Childhood. Data from Friis-Hansen[56]

	0 to 11 days	11 days to ½ yr.	½ to 2 years	2 to 7 years	7 to 16 years
Total Body Water	77.6%	72.2%	59.5%	63.1%	58.4%
Extracellular Water	41.6%	33.7%	26.2%	24.7%	19.9%
Intracellular Water ÷ Total Body Solids	1.61	1.38	0.82	1.04	0.93

of intracellular water. But, in part, the age trend shown in Table 1–13 is a result of increasing body fatness. That the relative fatness of the body increases during childhood was indicated from densitometric data reported by Zook,[138] and Boyd,[16] though the methods used were unsatisfactory. Macy and Kelly[87] estimated averages of 22, 24, and 26 per cent of the body weight represented by fat in boys aged 4 to 6, 7 to 9 and 10 to 12 years, respectively, but their material was small and the calculations were based on many assumptions, including the arbitrary value of 73.2 per cent for the total water in the fat-free body. The densitometric data data obtained by Parizkova[102,103] in children 9 to 17 years of age indicate that density increases continuously in the boys, while in the girls it shows a decrease between 14 and 16 years with a slight increase at 17 to 18 years.

Mellits and Cheek[89] have reported a linear relationship between total body water and weight from infancy to young adulthood. Total body water (TW) in liters, can be predicted from body weight (WT) in kg by the following equations:

(15) TW = 1.065 + 0.603 WT (for males),

(16) TW = 1.874 + 0.493 WT (for females).

Total body water was found to be a nonlinear function of height, represented by a quadratic equation, or by two intercepting straight lines.

The increase of "cell mass" during the period of growth has been well documented by Burmeister and Bingert[28] in studies on 3,143 children using the body counter for the determination of total body potassium.

Many data have been reported in recent years on the changes of subcutaneous tissue thickness during infancy and childhood.[58,59,99,102,103,106,109,125] Maximal values are found at the end of the first year and in adolescence, with a steady increase during the adult years. The sex differences in subcutaneous tissue thickness are apparent in early childhood.

Body Composition in Old Age. With advancing years there is in adult age a progressive decrease of the cell mass of the body which has been documented by various methods. From densitometric determinations Brozek[19] estimated in men an average decrease of 0.11 kg of cell mass per year, between ages 25 and 50 years. Total body water (antipyrine space) diminishes with increasing age, without significant change of extracellular water (thiocyanate space), indicating a reduction of the "cell mass."[116] Measurements of body potassium, both by analysis of cadavers and by whole body counting, have shown progressive decrease of the total potassium content of the body. The average concentration of potassium per kg of gross body weight decreases steadily with increasing age in adult life,[1,4,96] but the potassium content per kg of fat-free body is lower in the newborn than in the adult.[51]

Recent studies are in agreement that the weight of the "cell mass" decreases continuously from early adulthood to old age. For example, Burmeister and Bingert[28] found in men an average "cell mass" of 42.5 kg at 25 to 26 years and of 34.5 kg at 65 to 70 years. There is, therefore, a mean decrease of 8 kg (about 19 per cent of the weight of the "cell mass" at 25 to 26 years) over 40 to 45 years. This result is in good agreement with the data of total body water reported by Shock *et al.*[116] These authors found a mean intracellular water volume of 28.2 liters at 20 to 29 years, and of 21.9 liters at 60 to 69 years, or a decrease of 6.3 liters. Assuming a water content of 72.7 per cent in the "cell mass," this means a reduction of "cell mass" of 8.6 kg. According to Forbes and Reina,[54] at age 65 to 70 the average man has 12 kg less lean body mass than at age 25. The corresponding figure for females is a decrease of 5 kg. It follows from the preceding data that the average man maintaining at 65 to 70 years the same body weight that he had at 25 years must have a higher proportion of body fat at his more advanced age. Because the "cell mass" represents the metabolically active compartment of the body, the continuous decrease of "cell mass" through adult life should be taken into consideration in calculating nutrient requirements and drug dosage in older persons.

CALORIE STATUS

The relationship between energy metabolism and body composition will be considered in two main aspects:

(1) The relationship between basal metabolism and body composition.

(2) The relationship between changes in body composition and changes in calorie balance.

Basal Metabolism and Body Composition. The basal metabolism is the result of energetic processes in the cells which constitute the active mass of the body; fat, extracellular fluid and bone minerals make no direct contribution to this basal metabolism. Though adipose tissue is not metabolically inert, such energy consumption as it exhibits must be attributed to the cells and not to the plain fat in it. Accordingly, it would be more reasonable to express the basal metabolic rate in units of the active tissue mass rather than in terms of the gross mass of the body or even of the popular surface area unit. In 1950 we showed that much variation, otherwise unexplained, is eliminated when basal metabolism is expressed in units of fat-free or, better, active tissue mass.[78]

For persons of given sex and age the total basal oxygen consumption is correlated to about the same extent with surface area as with the fat-free body weight.[72] The utility of the fat-free body weight as a standard of reference is clear when persons of different sex and age are compared.[10,19,36,92] For both males and females over the age range of perhaps 20 to 60 years a single value can be used to indicate the "normal" metabolic rate. The single value of 4.4 ml of oxygen per minute (or about 1.3 calories per hour) per kg of fat-free body weight can be used instead of the customary tables and graphs based on the artificial concept of surface area as the determinant of the basal metabolism.

From the foregoing it is an obvious step to suggest the converse, namely that the fat-free body mass may be estimated simply from the basal metabolism.[10,62,92] With strictly normal, healthy, young adults, this estimation is reasonably good, but more general application is questionable because of the susceptibility of the basal oxygen metabolism to hormonal and dietary influences. Obviously this estimation cannot be made if there is any suspicion of abnormality of the basal metabolic rate.

Since it appears that the basal metabolism normally is strictly proportional to the mass of "active tissue" or "cells" in the body, it follows that the basal metabolism should be closely correlated with any measure which, in turn, is highly correlated with the active cell mass. Besides the fat-free body weight, such measures are represented by the total body water and by extracellular fluid mass or volume. Without benefit of the considerations outlined above, it has been found that, indeed, basal metabolism is highly correlated with the extracellular fluid volume of the body.[35,122] A high correlation with $r = 0.896$ has been found between basal metabolism and total body potassium.[1] While the statistical correlations emphasized above are of great utility, it is essential not to lose sight of the underlying physiology.

Bray *et al.*,[18] in a study on 18 grossly obese females, reported oxygen consumption to be highly correlated with body weight and surface area, whereas the correlation was much less satisfactory with total body water and exchangeable potassium. But the measurements of oxygen consumption reported by these authors do not represent basal oxygen consumption. They correspond to the oxygen consumption over a 24-hour period calculated from the average of 6 to 11 samples of expired air taken at various intervals between 8:00 A.M. and 8:00 P.M. The patients rested for 15 to 20 minutes before each collection. The samples taken after the meals showed the increase in oxygen consumption corresponding to the specific dynamic action. It is clear that the values of oxygen consumption reported represent neither basal oxygen consumption nor total 24-hour oxygen intake.

From the foregoing discussion it might be supposed that all "cells" or all parts of the "active tissue mass" of the body have equal rates of metabolism per unit of mass. This is grossly erroneous as has been emphasized by Brozek and Grande.[21] In man, the brain and liver, together representing only about 4 per cent of the normal body mass, account for over 40 per cent of the total resting oxygen consumption, while the skeletal muscles, amounting to about 40 per cent of the body weight, contribute barely 25 per cent of the basal metabolism. These facts go far towards explaining the otherwise puzzling fact that the basal metabolism early in starvation quickly falls far more than would be predicted from a consideration of the change in total cell mass of the body.[65] Since the "active cell mass" is made up of tissues with very different metabolic rates, it is obvious that changes in the average metabolic rate of the cell mass can be produced by changes in the proportion between the various components.[62]

On the other hand, it must be considered that the metabolic rate per weight unit of cell mass varies with the partition system adopted, because the various methods used in the determination of the cell mass measure compartments of different size and composition in terms of anatomical structures. In the system of partition which has been described here, the "cell residue," by definition, contains not only the active cells of the body, but also the plasma proteins, the connective tissue fibers, etc. Consequently, the basal metabolism per weight unit of such a compartment is expected to be lower than that of a compartment defined in a more restricted way and including a higher proportion of metabolically active components. Our measurements[62] in normal young men gave values for the basal metabolism of the "cell residue" of 1.52 Calories per kg per hour (S.D. = 0.134) for a group of 13 men, and of 1.57 Calories per kg per hour (S.D. = 0.123) for another group of 12 men. The mass of the compartment was estimated by dividing the amount of intracellular water (total body water minus extracellular water) by 0.733. Ryan et al.[112] found in 14 normal men (mean age 34.9 years) a value corresponding to 1.88 Calories per kg of cell mass per hour, when cell mass was determined by dividing intracellular water by 0.70. Bernstein et al.,[13] using the same system to determine the cell mass, found in a group of young women a mean value corresponding to 2.02 Calories per kg per hour. Moore et al.[94] give values between 2.7 and 3.6 Calories per kg per hour for the "Body Cell Mass" estimated from measurements of exchangeable potassium. This seems to indicate that the compartment measured by this method is smaller in terms of mass than the "cell residue" computed from determinations of total body water and extracellular water. The interpretation of metabolic rates in terms of mass of active tissue compartments requires, then, a precise definition of the nature of the compartment measured and of the methods used. Thus, when the basal caloric production is expressed in terms of lean body mass, the values given in the literature are of the order of 1.00 to 1.17 Cal/kg/ hour.[62] It is of interest to compare these basal values with an average of 1.71 Cal/kg/ hour reported for the total energy expenditure of young men living in voluntary confinement similar to that in space cabins.[133]

The Calorie Equivalent of Weight Change. Weight loss as a consequence of negative calorie balance has been regarded largely as a reduction of the fat content of the body. Depot fat is the most important storehouse of energy in the body and represents the material preferentially used to compensate for the energy deficit due to inadequate calorie intake. This fact has been well documented in the classical literature.[63] It must be recognized, however, that the changes in body composition taking place during periods of negative energy balance are more complex than a simple loss of fat.

The most common application of information on body weight and composition is in connection with nutritional correction and control of obesity and emaciation. What is the calorie equivalent of a given amount of weight gain or loss?

The most superficial approach is to estimate that, since 1 kg of animal fat has an energy value of about 9100 Calories, therefore an accumulated nutritional deficit of 9100 Calories would be attended by a weight loss of 1 kg. This value, or the value of 9000 Calories per kg of body weight change, is still quoted from time to time, but very disparate values can be found in the medical literature. More commonly Bozenraad's data on adipose tissue[17] are misconstrued and it is concluded that 1 kg of body weight gain or loss should be the equivalent of 8000 Calories.[45,136] But adipose tissue and "obesity tissue," that is, the kind of tissue actually gained or lost when the diet is changed, are not identical in calories. Obesity tissue gained or lost in a few months, as in our experiments, would have a value between 6000 and 6500 Calories per kg if it were burned in a calorimeter.

But it by no means follows that a dietary deficit of 6000 to 6500 Calories will produce a weight loss of 1 kg. In the first place, the calorie value of the tissue lost is affected by the intensity of the calorie imbalance and the value changes as calorie imbalance continues. During the first few days on a sharply reduced diet the body tends to lose more water than fat and again, after the body has become emaciated, further reductions in body weight represent water and protein loss as well as fat. In both situations the calorie value of the lost tissue is much lower than 6000 Calories per kg. Dole and his colleagues[37] conducted well-controlled experiments on 5 obese women whose diets were alternated between excess and deficiency at 4-day intervals. The observed weight changes corresponded to averages of 2160 to 3610 Calories per kg. We have found similar values with men for the first few days of dietary restriction. Later, however, the

calorie value of the weight change rises. In one of our experiments 13 young men subsisted on a carbohydrate diet providing 1000 Calories daily while following a fixed schedule of physical activity to make the energy expenditure at the beginning of the restriction period in the order of 3200 Calories per day. The calorie equivalent of the weight lost during the first 3 days averaged 2596 Calories per kg, that of the weight lost between days 11 and 13 was 7043 Calories per kg.[23] Other data also indicate that the calorie equivalent of weight loss increases with the duration of the restriction period.[62]

Equally important is the fact that, given time, the body weight tends to reach a steady state and calorie expenditure tends to balance calorie intake, no matter what the level of the latter may be. When we changed the diet of young men from 3500 to 1500 Calories daily the weight loss was rapid at first and decreased exponentially with time until calorie equilibrium was achieved with the body weight being 25 per cent less than it had been.[130]

Much interesting information has been gathered recently in connection with the use of complete starvation as a means of reducing body weight in obese individuals. Under such circumstances the caloric value of the weight loss must be equal to the total energy expenditure, since the only source of energy available is that represented by the body tissues.[63,64] If the energy expenditure is known, the calorie equivalent of the loss can be easily calculated by dividing the total energy deficit (which in this case is equal to the energy expenditure) by the weight loss. Such computation can be made with the data reported by Consolazio et al.[31] obtained in 6 men who starved for 10 days. The average weight loss was 7.3 kg and the total energy expenditure was estimated as 25,000 Calories so the calorie equivalent of the loss is of the order of 3400 Calories per kg. This is comparable to some of the data previously reported from short-time experiments, and stresses the fact that much of the weight lost during a limited period of starvation or semi-starvation must be water.

By combining measurements of total energy expenditure and N balance it is possible to calculate the amount of fat lost during periods of starvation or food restriction.[61,62] When the energy expenditure is unknown, useful information about its level can be obtained by computing the energy value of the weight loss from its composition determined by some of the methods already discussed. This, incidentally, offers a means of checking the credibility of some data on body composition changes which, unfortunately, are frequently forgotten.[63,64] The results presented in some reports show wild disagreement between the body composition data and elementary considerations of bioenergetics. One of these reports[12] compares the effects of complete starvation and of a ketogenic diet on weight loss and body composition. The mean weight loss for 10 men for 10 days of complete starvation was 9.6 kg of which 6.2 kg were estimated as "Lean Body Mass" and 3.4 kg as fat. Simple computation using commonly accepted constants[22,63] indicates that such an average daily weight loss would have a caloric value of 3544 Calories. Accordingly, this figure should represent the energy expenditure of the subjects. This figure seems too high for starving individuals spending no energy for specific dynamic action and who, according to the authors, "had uniform moderate physical activity" in a metabolic ward. Much more incredible are the data on the same individuals when they were given a ketogenic diet (1000 Calories per day) for 10 days. They lost an average of 6.6 kg which was estimated as being made up of 0.2 kg of "Lean Body Mass" and 6.4 kg of fat. The calorie equivalent of that loss would amount to 5776 Calories per day which, added to the food intake of 1000 Calories per day, would make a total of 6776 Calories per day. The authors offer no explanation for this unbelievable increase of more than 3000 calories in the daily energy expenditure, during the period in the ketogenic diet, when, supposedly, there was no change in the level of physical activity. This example clearly indicates the need for critical examination of body composition data in the light of currently accepted principles of metabolic physiology.

Body Weight in Complete Starvation and Calorie Restriction. The paper by Thomson et al.[132] reports interesting observations about weight loss in obese individuals who fasted for long periods of time. One of the obese women fasted for 249 days and lost 34 kg or 28 per cent of her original body weight. With the exception of two patients, who had the lowest initial body weight, all the others lost substantial amounts of weight. In spite of the individual differences, the data clearly show that the average daily loss for the whole period tends to decrease with its duration. Thus the patients who starved for about 40 days showed a mean weight loss of about 0.3 per cent of their original body weight per day. The patient who starved 139 days lost weight at the rate of 0.18 per cent of the initial weight per day, and the two women who starved 236 and 249 days had mean daily weight losses of 0.15 and 0.11 per cent respectively. Similar results have been reported by Barnard et al.[8] One of the women studied fasted for 315 days and lost 66.5 kg or nearly 50 per cent of her original body weight. This corresponds to an average weight loss of about 0.15 per cent per day. Another woman starved for 74 days with a loss of about 25 per cent of her original weight and an average weight loss of 0.34 per cent per day.

These data confirm the general idea that the rate of weight loss tends to decrease as the duration of the calorie restriction increases. Even total starvation loses efficiency as a means of weight reduction, after a certain time.

No data on body composition or energy exchange were reported by Thomson et al., but some limiting calculations can be made with their data. The mean daily weight loss for 10 women on starvation treatment was 0.219 kg and, assuming that only fat was lost, this would correspond to an energy expenditure of 1970 Calories per day. On the other hand, if we assume that the tissue lost had the composition of what we have defined as "obesity tissue from static difference," the mean energy expenditure would be 1480 Calories per day. These two values give the probable limits of energy expenditure for this group of starving women. Some of the women, however, must have had extremely low energy expenditure levels, particularly in the latter part of the starvation period. The values computed from the weight loss would indicate that two of the patients (nos. 4 and 6) were not using more than an average of 800 to 1100 Calories per day.

Considerable reduction of body weight can be achieved by prolonged drastic reduction of food intake. Bortz[15] has reported the case of the 35-year-old man who lost 227 kg over a period of 723 days on a diet of 800 Calories/day. The loss corresponds to 72 per cent of his original body weight of 314 kg. The average rate of weight loss was about 0.1 per cent per day and compares with the rates observed in some of the obese women who starved for long periods. The initial maintenance calorie requirement of this patient was estimated to be of the order of 5,000 Calories/day. The estimated protein loss was 13.25 kg or about 5.8 per cent of the total weight loss. This corresponds to an average protein loss of 18 gm per day and is considerably smaller than that observed over shorter periods in starving men and in men on a 400 Calorie per day carbohydrate diet.[31,32] Allen and Musgrave[2] described the changes of body weight and body composition of obese adult men consuming a diet providing 400 Calories and 45 gm of high quality protein daily. During a mean of 49 days there was an average weight loss of 12.03 kg. It was assumed that the men were in nitrogen equilibrium and that the loss comprised essentially fat and water. From densitometric determinations it was estimated that the average fat loss was 10 kg or 83 per cent of the total weight loss. The determinations of the specific volume supported the view that the loss was indeed made up of fat and water and the calculations of total energy expenditure from the fat loss gave results in excellent agreement with previous estimates of energy expenditure for subjects with a moderate level of physical activity.[63] This interesting work seems to have achieved the desideratum of weight reduction: loss of fat without loss of protein.

The process of gaining weight, when men shift from a negative to a positive energy balance, likewise does not always give an exact picture of the excess calorie intake.

In our experiments[23] it was observed that the increase in weight was very rapid at the beginning of the refeeding period; later, in spite of continuing at the same level of excess calorie intake, no further increase of body weight was detected for some time. Since there was no doubt as to the presence of a positive energy and nitrogen balance, it seems reasonable to assume that the weight change caused by the storage of fat and protein in the body was offset by the loss of some of the water retained in excess during the first few days of refeeding. Similar observations have been reported with respect to nitrogen retention in previously underfed individuals without a corresponding increase of body weight,[33,69] and in constitutionally thin individuals.[105]

There is great variability between outpatients in regard to body weight response to dietary change, partly because of differences in activity habits, partly because the truth about dietary intakes is not always easy to discover. Obese people are not always heavy eaters, and this is true of children as well as of adults.[70] Since physical inactivity is so often at least partly responsible, we commonly advise reduction in obesity partly by reducing the diet, partly by increasing exercise. But this certainly affects the calorie equivalent of weight loss. Suppose one fat person loses 50 pounds of "obesity tissue" while another, combining exercise and reduced food, has a net loss of 50 pounds but has gained 10 pounds of muscle tissue. The former has achieved his weight loss at a cost of about 140,000 Calories; the latter has lost 60 pounds of "obesity tissue" and gained ten pounds of muscle, making a net equivalent of about 168,000 Calories. We approve more of the second person's accomplishment.

BIBLIOGRAPHY

1. Allen, Anderson, and Langham: Gerontol., 15, 348, 1960.
2. Allen and Musgrave: Am. J. Clin. Nutr., 24, 14, 1971.
3. Anderson, Schuch, Perrings, and Langham: Nucleonics, 14, 26, 1956.
4. Anderson and Langham: Science, 130, 713, 1959.
5. ———: Science, 133, 1917, 1961.

6. Anderson: Ann. New York Acad. Sci., *110*, 189, 1963.
7. Baker and Newman: Am. J. Phys. Anthropol., *15*, 601, 1957.
8. Barnard, Ford, Garnett, Mardell, and Whyman: Metabolism, *18*, 564, 1969.
9. Behnke: Harvey Lect., N.Y., *37*, 198, 1941.
10. ———: Ann. New York Acad. Sci., *56*, 1095, 1953.
11. Behnke, Feen, and Welham: J.A.M.A., *118*, 495, 1942.
12. Benoit, Martin, and Watten: Ann. Int. Med., *63*, 604, 1965.
13. Bernstein, Johnston, Ryan, Inouye and Hick: J. Appl. Physiol., *9*, 241, 1956.
14. Bezold, von: Z. wiss. Zool., *8*, 487, 1857.
15. Bortz: Am. J. Med., *47*, 325, 1969.
16. Boyd: Human Biol., *5*, 646, 1953.
17. Bozenraad: Deut. Arch. klin. Med., *103*, 120, 1911.
18. Bray, Schwartz, Rozin, and Lister: Metabolism, *19*, 418, 1970.
19. Brozek: Federation Proc., *11*, 784, 1952.
20. Brozek (ed.): *Body Measurements and Human Nutrition*, Detroit, Wayne University Press, 1956.
21. Brozek and Grande: Human Biol., *27*, 22, 1955.
22. Brozek, Grande, Anderson and Keys: Ann. New York Acad. Sci., *110*, 113, 1963.
23. Brozek, Grande, Taylor, Anderson, Buskirk, and Keys: J. Appl. Physiol., *10*, 412, 1957.
24. Brozek and Keys: Science, *112*, 788, 1950.
25. ———: Brit. J. Nutr., *5*, 194, 1951.
26. ———: Nutrit. Abst. and Rev., *20*, 247, 1951.
27. Brozek, Mori, and Keys: Science, *128*, 901, 1958.
28. Burmeister and Bingert: Klin. Wschr., *45*, 409, 1967.
29. Cheek, Schultz, Parra and Reba: Pediatric Res., *4*, 268, 1970.
30. Chen, Lee, Ko, and Shih: Mem. Fac. Med. Taiwan, Univ. Taiwan, *1*, 168, 1951.
31. Consolazio, Mataush, Johnson, Nelson, and Krzywicki: Am. J. Clin. Nutr., *20*, 672, 1967.
32. Consolazio, Mataush, Johnson, Krzywicki, Isaac, and Witt: Am. J. Clin. Nutr., *21*, 803, 1968.
33. Cook and Auken: Ann. Int. Med., *34*, 1404, 1951.
34. Corsa, Olney, Steenburg, Ball, and Moore: J. Clin. Invest., *29*, 1280, 1950.
35. Dahlstrom: Acta Physiol. Scand., *21*, Suppl. 71, 1950.
36. Döbeln, von: Acta Physiol. Scand., *37*, Suppl. 126, 1956.
37. Dole, Schwartz, Thorn, and Silver: J. Clin. Invest., *34*, 590, 1955.
38. Durnin: Proc. Nutr. Soc. (Great Britain), *20*, 52, 1961.
39. Edelman: Body water and electrolytes. In J. Brozek and A. Henschel (ed.), *Techniques for Measuring Body Composition*, Washington, D.C., National Academy of Sciences, 1961, p. 140.
40. Edholm: Proc. Nutr. Soc. (Great Britain), *20*, 71, 1961.
41. Edwards: Clin. Sci., *10*, 305, 1951.
42. ———: Voeding (Amsterdam), *16*, 57, 1955.
43. Edwards: Med. Stat. Bull. No. 2, Washington, D.C., 1943.
44. Elkinton and Danowski: *The Body Fluids*, Baltimore, The Williams & Wilkins Co., 1955, p. 26.
45. Evans: *Diseases of Metabolism*, 3rd Ed., Philadelphia, W. B. Saunders Co., 1936.
46. Falkner: Pediatrics, *29*, 467, 1962.
47. Faller, Petty, Last, Pascale, and Bond: J. Lab. & Clin. Med., *45*, 748, 1955.
48. Fidanza, Keys, and Anderson: J. Appl. Physiol., *6*, 252, 1953.
49. Fisher and Fisk: *How to Live*, New York, Funk, 1916.
50. Food and Agriculture Organization: F.A.O. Nutritional Studies, No. 15, Rome, 1957.
51. Forbes: Pediatrics, *29*, 477, 1962.
52. Forbes, Gallup, and Hursh: Science, *133*, 101, 1961.
53. Forbes and Lewis: J. Clin. Invest., *35*, 596, 1956.
54. Forbes and Reina: Metabolism, *19*, 653, 1970.
55. Forbes, Cooper, and Mitchell: J. Biol. Chem., *203*, 359, 1953.
56. Friis-Hansen: Acta Pediat., *46*, Suppl. 110, 1957.
57. Fry: J. Clin. Nutr., *1*, 453, 1953.
58. Garn: Fat Thickness and Growth Progress During Infancy. In J. Brozek (ed.): *Body Measurements and Human Nutrition*, Detroit, Wayne University Press, 1956.
59. ———: Human Biol., *29*, 337, 1957.
60. Garn and Shamir: *Methods for Research in Human Growth*, Springfield, Charles C Thomas, 1958.
61. Gilder, Cornell, Grafe, Macfarlane, Asaph, Stubenbord, Watkins, Rees, and Thorbjanarson: J. Appl. Physiol., *23*, 304, 1967.
62. Grande: Nutrition and Energy Balance in Body Composition Studies. In J. Brozek and A. Henschel (ed.); *Techniques for Measuring Body Composition*, Washington, D.C., National Academy of Sciences, 1961, p. 140.
63. ———: Ann. Int. Med., *68*, 467, 1968.
64. ———: Am. J. Clin. Nutr., *21*, 305, 1968.
65. Grande, Anderson, and Keys: J. Appl. Physiol., *12*, 230, 1958.
66. Hastings: A Manual for Physical Measurements, etc., 1902. See Hathaway, 1957.
67. Hathaway: Home Econ. Res. Report No. 2, U.S. Department of Agriculture, Washington, D.C., U.S. Government Printing Office, 1957.
68. Haxhe: La composition corporelle normale ses variations au cours de la sous-alimentation et l'hyperthyroidie, Bruxelles, Arscia, S.A., 1963.
69. Holmes, Jones, and Stanier: Brit. J. Nutr., *8*, 173, 1954.
70. Hunt, Peckos, and Fry: *Overeating, Overweight, and Obesity*, New York, National Vitamin Foundation, 1953, p. 73.
71. Johnson, Burke, and Mayer: Am. J. Clin. Nutr., *4*, 37 and 231, 1956.

72. Johnston and Bernstein: J. Lab. & Clin. Med., *45*, 109, 1955.
73. Kemsley: Ann. Eugenics, *16*, 18, 23 and 316, 1952.
74. Keys: J.A.M.A., *142*, 333, 1950.
75. ————: Am. J. Pub. Health, *43*, 1399, 1953.
76. Keys, Anderson, and Brozek: Metabolism, *4*, 427, 1955.
77. Keys and Brozek: Physiol. Rev., *33*, 245, 1953.
78. Keys, Brozek, Henschel, Mickelsen, and Taylor: *The Biology of Human Starvation*, Minneapolis, University of Minnesota Press, 1950.
79. Keys *et al.*: *Body Measurement and Human Nutrition* (J. Brozek, ed.), Detroit, Wayne University Press, 1956 and Human Biology, *28*, 1, 1956.
80. Keys, Taylor, Mickelsen, and Henschel: Science, *103*, 669, 1946.
81. Kohlrausch: Arbeitsphysiol., *2*, 23, 1930.
82. Krogman: Tabulae Biol., *20*, 1, 1941.
83. Lasker: Am. J. Phys. Anthropol., *5*, 323, 1947.
84. Ljunggren: Acta Endocrinol., Suppl. 33, 1957.
85. McCance and Widdowson: Proc. Roy. Soc. B., *138*, 115, 1950.
86. McMurray, Boling, Davis, Parker, Magnus, Ball, and Moore: Metabolism, 7, 651, 1958.
87. Macy and Kelly: Human Biol., *28*, 289, 1956.
88. Mayer: *Weight Control* (Eppright, Swanson and Iverson, eds.), Ames, Iowa, Iowa State College Press, 1955, p. 199.
89. Mellits and Cheek: Monogr. Soc. Res. Child Develop., *35*, 12, 1970.
90. Mendez, Keys, Anderson, and Grande: Metabolism, *9*, 472, 1960.
91. Metropolitan Life Insurance Co.: Statist. Bul., *23*, 6, 23 and 24, 1942.
92. Miller and Blyth: J. Appl Physiol., *5*, 73, and 311, 1952.
93. Mitchell, Hamilton, Steggerda, and Bean: J. Biol. Chem., *158*, 625, 1945.
94. Moore, Olesen, McMurray, Parker, Ball, and Boyden: *The Body Cell Mass and Its Environment*, Philadelphia, W. B. Saunders Co., 1963.
95. Moulton: J. Biol. Chem., *57*, 79, 1923.
96. Myhre and Kessler: J. Appl. Physiol., *21*, 1251, 1966.
97. Newburgh: Arch. Int. Med., *70*, 1033, 1942.
98. Newman and White: Environmental Protection Section Report No. 180, Office of the Quartermaster General, U.S. Army, Washington, D.C., 1951, p. 1.
99. Novak: Ann. New York Acad. Sci., *110*, 545, 1963.
100. Olsson and Saltin: Acta Physiol. Scand., *80*, 11, 1970.
101. Pace and Rathbun: J. Biol. Chem., *159*, 685, 1945.
102. Parizkova: Nutrition, *14*, 275, 1960.
103. ————: J. Appl. Physiol., *16*, 173, 1961.
104. Pascale, Grossman, Sloane, and Frank: *Body Measurements and Human Nutrition* (Brozek, ed.), Detroit, Wayne University Press, 1956, p. 55.
105. Passmore, Meiklejohn, Dewar, and Thow: Brit. J. Nutrit., *9*, 27, 1955.
106. Pett and Ogilvie: Human Biol., *28*, 177, 1956.

107. Randall and Monroe: Environmental Protection Branch Report No. 148, Office of the Quartermaster General, U.S. Army, Washington, D.C., 1949.
108. Reynolds: Monogr. Soc. Res. Child Develop., *15*, No. 2 (ser. No. 50), 1951.
109. Reynolds and Grote: Anat. Rec., *102*, 45, 1948.
110. Rubner: Die Gesetze des Energieverbrauchs bei der Ernaehrung, Deuticke, Leipzig and Vienna, 1902.
111. Rundo and Sagild: Nature, *175*, 774, 1955.
112. Ryan, Williams, Ansell, and Bernstein: Metabolism, *6*, 365, 1957.
113. Sagild: Scand. J. Lab. Clin. Med., *8*, 44, 1956.
114. Seltzer, Stoudt, Bell, and Mayer: Am. J. Epidemiol., *92*, 339, 1970.
115. Sheldon: *Varieties of Human Physique*, New York, Harper, 1940.
116. Shock, Watkin, Yiengst, Norris, Gaffney, Gregerman, and Falzone: J. Gerontol., *18*, 1, 1963.
117. Sievert: Arkiv. Fysik., *3*, 337, 1951.
118. ————: Strahlentherapie, *99*, 185, 1956.
119. Simonart: *La dénutrition de guerre. Etude clinique, anatomopathalogique et thérapeutique.* Brussels and Paris, Maloine, 1948.
120. Siri: *Advances in Biological and Medical Physics*, New York, Academic Press, 1956, p. 239.
121. Soberman, Brodie, Levy, Axelrod, Hollander, and Steele: J. Biol. Chem., *179*, 31, 1949.
122. Steele, Brodie, Messinger, Soberman, Berger, and Galdston: Trans. Assoc. Amer. Physicians, *57*, 214, 1949.
123. Stuart, Hill, and Shaw: Monog. Soc. Res. Child Develop. *5*, No. 3 (Serial No. 26), 1940.
124. Stuart and Meredith: Amer. J. Pub. Health, *36*, 1365, and 1373, 1946.
125. Stuart and Sobel: J. Pediat., *28*, 637, 1946.
126. Swindell, Holmes, and Robinson: Brit. J. Nutr., *22*, 667, 1968.
127. Taggart: Brit. J. Nutr., *16*, 223, 1962.
128. Talso, Miller, Cargallo, and Vasquez: Metabolism, *9*, 456, 1960.
129. Taylor, Brozek, and Keys: J. Clin. Invest., *31*, 976, 1952.
130. Taylor and Keys: Science, *112*, 215, 1950.
131. Terhederbrügge: Arch. Path. Anat. Physiol., *298*, 640, 1937.
132. Thomson, Runcie, and Miller: Lancet, *2*, 992, 1966.
133. Vanderveen: *Nutrition for long space voyages.* In Fourth International Symposium of Bioastronautics and the Exploration of Space. Editors: Roodman, Strughold and Mitchell, Brooks AFB Aerospace Medical Division (AFSC), 1968, p. 421.
134. Vierordt: *Daten und Tabellen für Mediciner und Aerzte.* Jena, Fischer, 1888.
135. Widdowson, McCance, and Spray: Clin. Sci., *10*, 113, 1951.
136. Wishnofsky: Metabolism, *1*, 554, 1952.
137. Yanagi, Hayami, Suzuki, and Nagamine: Ann. Report Nat. Inst. Nutrition, Tokyo, 1949–50, p. 1.
138. Zook: Am. J. Dis. Child., *43*, 1347, 1932.

Chapter

2A

The Proteins and Amino Acids

ANTHONY A. ALBANESE

AND

LOUISE A. ORTO

INTRODUCTION

No living matter so far discovered is devoid of protein. Indeed, it can be demonstrated that proteins play a significant role in all activities of living organisms—from viruses to man. Without exception, proteins as structural elements, or as biocatalysts, participate in every biological process at every level of biochemical organization. They are enzymes, or essential components of enzymes; they take part in many different forms in the intracellular and extracellular structure of the body; antibodies are proteins, as are a number of pituitary hormones. In combination with nucleic acids they bear inheritance factors, and small alterations in their structure may lead to disease.

Despite the multiplicity of their functions, proteins have some characteristics in common. All are constructed with a limited

Table 2A-1. **Large Protein Stores in the Body**

♂, 168.5 cm, 53.8 kg	
	gm
Total protein (N × 6.25) . .	10,006
Striated muscle	4,680
Skeleton	1,864
Skin	924
Adipose tissue	361
Estimate of blood:	
Hemoglobin	750
Albumin	250

From Forbes *et al.*[3]

assortment of building blocks—the amino acids. All are manufactured by the cells in the same way, and are in a dynamic state of breakdown and renewal. This dynamic state, so clearly expounded by Borsook[1] and Schoenheimer[2] more than 35 years ago, with its highly diverse rates of anabolism and catabolism for the different proteins and under different conditions, complicates the study of the organism as a whole.

Table 2A-1, compiled from one of the few available analyses of the human body, lists its major protein stores. The total amount of body protein is approximately 19 per cent of the fresh weight; 45 per cent of this protein is present in the muscle and 18 per cent in the skeleton, while skin and adipose tissue account for another 10 and 4 per cent respectively. Although these figures are interesting, upon closer examination they provide very little information. They would be more significant if it were known how much protein is renewed daily and what factors regulate the renewal rate.

In considering this problem, we must distinguish between the dynamic state of protein, intracellularly or extracellularly, and the regeneration of whole cells, *i.e.*, replacement of dying cells. The red blood cell may serve as a good example of this last form. Hemoglobin seems to be stable during the life span of an erythrocyte, but $\frac{1}{120}$ of our hemoglobin is renewed daily. Some cells have a very short life—as in the jejunal mucosa where most of the cells do not live longer than one day. There are indications that, once their protein is formed, it is stable for the rest of the day.[4] Such is certainly not the case in the liver, where the life span of the cell seems to be very long and the half-life of the protein mixture in the cells is not more than 4 days. Here, we may speak of a true dynamic state.

If we consider large protein masses such as collagen, which has been estimated to constitute $\frac{1}{3}$ of our body protein, approximations of renewal rate are very complex. In 1953, Neuberger et al.[5] came to the conclusion that collagen of the tendon in rats is probably metabolically inert, with a half-life of several hundred days.

Before concluding our remarks on the dynamic state of proteins, attention should be drawn to the opinion of several investigators that only a minor part of the body protein is renewed rapidly. This, however, does not imply that the participation of large deposits of proteins (e.g., muscle proteins) in the amino acid pool is small. Assuming an integrated half-life of 100 days for muscle proteins, the amount of amino acids participating daily in intermediary metabolism would be 20 gm.[6]

The initial production and continuing maintenance of body proteins depend on the dietary intake of its building stones, primarily of some specific amino acids, but also of substances from which other amino acids may be formed in the body itself. The *quantity* of the building stones of the body proteins present in the diet closely parallels its nitrogen content. It is therefore customary to express the "protein value" of food on the basis of the amount of organic nitrogen present. However, such a method, in spite of its expediency, does not take into consideration the fact that the nitrogen-containing substances of our diet serve in several roles in addition to the synthesis of body proteins.

Besides the proteins the human body contains a large variety of other nitrogenous organic substances. Included are the purines and pyrimidine bases, constituents of nucleoproteins; creatine, one of the key substances in energy transfer; choline; and many other nitrogen-containing compounds of more or less clearly recognized biologic significance.

Many of these nitrogenous substances, for instance the essential amino acids and some vitamins, must be obtained ready-made from food but others can be formed within the body from other sources. Ultimately, however, the formation of all these tissue constituents during growth and also for replacement during adult life requires the dietary supply of nitrogen-containing substances.

The biosynthesis of many amino acids, creatine, choline, and other compounds has long been postulated, but the pathways of such syntheses were more recently elucidated by following the metabolic fate of compounds tagged with isotopes.[7,8] We have learned by application of such methods that the proteins present in food are used not only for building new tissue proteins or for replacing the proteins which were destroyed by ominous "wear and tear," but also that one fraction of the dietary proteins or amino acids is utilized for the biosynthesis of other nonprotein nitrogen-containing compounds. Furthermore, dietary nitrogen, supplied not only as organic compounds but even in the form of inorganic ammonium salts, can be utilized in the synthesis of several amino acids and, therefore, some synthetic diets which do not support growth can be effectively supplemented by the addition of inorganic nitrogen sources such as ammonium salts.[9] All this indicates that the concept of "proteins in nutrition" is probably too narrow and that, in evaluations of the nutritive value of diets, not only the amino acid content, but also the presence and distribution of other nitrogen-containing compounds must be considered.

Discoveries in the field of intermediary metabolism have broken down many boundaries which separated protein, i.e., amino acid, metabolism from other fractions of the general metabolism. Nutrition research has kept pace well with these developments, but there is still some tendency in human, and especially in therapeutic, nutrition to depend on unsatisfactory methods; a tendency to apply confusing definitions and to adhere to obsolete nomenclature. These tendencies are illustrated by such practices as determining the "protein intake" indiscriminately by multiplying the nitrogen content of the diet by 6.25, or defining the protein requirement without specifying the total diet composition or the condition of the person to be fed. Another misleading habit is identification of decreased urinary nitrogen excretion with "protein anabolism."

In our subsequent discussion of the physiology of protein nutrition we will rely primarily on data collected in connection with normal mixed food intake. Without any prejudice as to whether our present Western dietary could be improved by changing the quantity or quality of protein intake, we must accept the fact that the self-selected mixed diets have been conducive to health and good development and, along with other hygienic factors and technology, have contributed to an unprecedented long life expectancy and to healthy old age.

SOURCES AND ABSORPTION OF DIETARY PROTEINS

The dietary protein intake is derived from animal and vegetable sources and the protein content of different food substances can vary considerably, as seen in Table 2A-2. Calculations based on average pre-war dietaries consumed in Western civilizations show that protein accounted for 14 per cent of the total calories and only in exceptional cases fell below 10 per cent.[10–13] Further calculations revealed that the protein in an average food intake of 2,500 calories was about 94 grams per day. Table 2A-2 also indicates that the protein content of meals prepared from natural food sources has a definite upper limit. In some instances,

Table 2A-2. Protein Content of Some Common Foods

Edible Food Substances	Calories per 100 gm	Protein per 100 gm	Protein* Calories per 100 gm Food	Protein Calories % of Total Calories
Pork meat, medium fat (cooked)	457	14.9	63.6	13.9
Beef meat, medium fat (cooked)	273	17.5	74.7	27.4
Chicken meat (total edible)	302	18.0	76.9	25.5
Fish fillet (unspecified)	132	18.8	80.1	60.7
Canned tuna (low fat)	128	28.3	120.6	95.0
Canned tuna in oil	217	27.7	118.0	54.4
Pacific sardines (canned in tomatoes)	216	17.8	76.0	35.2
Salmon, canned	173	20.2	86.3	49.9
Eggs, fresh	144	11	48.0	33.3
Eggs, dehydrated	605	47	204.9	33.9
Milk, whole	68	3.5	14.9	22.0
Skim milk, dry	360	36	153.7	42.7
Cheese, hard	341	34	145.2	42.6
Whey cheese, soft	106	14	59.8	56.4
Rice	360	6.7	25.6	7.1
Corn	356	9.3	35.5	10.0
Wheat flour (medium extraction)	350	11.7	45.6	13.0
Potatoes	70	1.7	4.65	6.7
Soybean grits	261	46	159.6	61.2
Beans, peas, dry	345	22.2	77.0	22.3
Cabbage, fresh	11	1.1	2.68	24.4
Fresh fruits (group figure)	46	0.5	1.68	3.65

* Calculated by using "The Specific Physiological Energy Factors."[10]

therapeutic diets have been recommended which contain higher quantities of protein than our normal mixed foods. In order to achieve this without increasing the total caloric intake or without consuming monotonous diets composed only of high protein foods, the mixed diets are enriched by addition of certain special-purpose foods like spray-dried egg white, skim milk powder, or any of the commercially available protein concentrates obtained from natural foods such as casein, soy protein or defatted dried lean meat.

In contrast to Western diets, food in some developing countries of the Orient and Africa, where starches, roots, vegetables and fruits are the primary staples, contains much lower quantities of proteins which are usually of poor quality.[14] The deleterious effect of such protein-deficient diets has been amply documented.[15-18]

Digestion of Proteins. Our regular food consists of more or less denatured animal or vegetable tissue which contains the protein as a constituent of its protoplasm. One part of the protein is conjugated to other substances, and the rest is usually thoroughly mixed with or closely surrounded by other substances, mainly carbohydrates and lipids. The presence of free protein is very rare in nature; an outstanding exception is egg white. Likewise natural or prepared foods contain free amino acids, as such, only in negligible quantities. The dietary proteins are macromolecular substances which are not absorbed to any considerable degree across the intestinal barrier and cannot be utilized by the body even when introduced parenterally. This means that as a rule *only* the amino acids, the smallest units of dietary proteins, can be utilized by the body as building stones for tissue protein synthesis. It has been shown that even small protein fragments such as peptides containing only few amino acids cannot be utilized by the tissues in most instances and are usually eliminated unaltered in the urine.

In contrast to these earlier results, Cannon *et al.*[18a] reported "that at least some simple peptides can be utilized parenterally in tissue protein synthesis."

Proteins are composed of a variety of different α-amino acids. These are compounds which are characterized by the presence of a terminal carboxyl and an amino group in α-position. In the protein molecule the amino acids are connected by *peptide linkages* formed between the carboxyl and amino groups of two adjacent amino acids. The digestion of food proteins to amino acids requires, besides the enzymatic cleavage of such linkages, the mechanical action of the digestive organs. In many cases, preliminary to protein cleavage, the carbohydrate or fat coating has to be broken down by these processes in order to expose the protein particles to the lytic action of gastrointestinal enzymes. The breakdown into the component amino acids occurs in the stomach and in the upper part of the intestinal tract. There the proteins are split into smaller fragments by the "proteinases" such as pepsin, trypsin, chymotrypsin, and the resulting smaller peptides are further digested by different "peptidases." Studies on the specificity of the gastrointestinal enzymes, as shown in Table 2A-3, have changed our concepts of protein digestion. The old view that large molecules are attacked first by pepsin and are consequently broken down to fragments of smaller size was based on the assumption that the peptide linkages formed between the amino and carboxyl groups of adjacent amino acids are equivalent. It was assumed that these linkages by which the amino acids are connected within the protein molecule can be attacked by any proteolytic enzyme and that the selection action of pepsin, trypsin or other enzymes is determined by the size, shape, configuration and other physicochemical properties of the protein molecule. However, more recent investigations proved that, although the peptide bonds between the different amino acids seem to be identical, their resistance to cleavage by proteolytic enzymes is different. It depends on the chemical nature of the amino acids which participate in the formation of a particular peptide bond[19] (see Table 2A-3). The polypeptide chains, the components of larger protein particles, usually have a free amino group at one end and on the other a free carboxyl group, and free polar groups seem to be necessary for the action of many

Table 2A-3. Proteolytic Enzymes

Enzyme	Produced in	Splits preferentially peptide linkages	pH-optimum
A. PROTEINASES: Attack peptide linkages in the interior of a peptide chain			
Pepsin	Stomach	In which phenylalanine or tyrosine provides amino group	1.8–2.0
Trypsin	Pancreas	In which arginine or lysine provides carboxyl group	8–9
Chymotrypsin	Pancreas	In which carboxyl group provided by tyrosine, phenylalanine, tryptophan or methionine	8–9
Cathepsin A	Tissue cells	Similar to pepsin	
Cathepsin B*		Similar to trypsin	3.5–6
Cathepsin C*		Similar to chymotrypsin	3.5–6
B. PEPTIDASES: Attack peptide linkages formed by terminal amino acids			
Carboxypeptidase	Pancreas	Next to terminal carboxyl group	7.2
Aminopeptidase	Intestines	Next to terminal amino group	7.4
Prolinase	Intestinal	Formed by proline	6.0
Prolidase	cells		

* Presence of reducing agents such as cysteine necessary for maximal activity.

proteolytic enzymes. Only proline, which contains an imino instead of an amino group, forms peptides lacking the terminal amino group. The high resistance of proline-containing peptides to enzymatic cleavage was recognized at the beginning of this century, and specific enzymes which can split such peptides have been studied and isolated.[20]

In some cases, however, the terminal amino and carboxyl groups also participate in peptide formation resulting in ring closure. Such polypeptide links are particularly resistant to enzymatic cleavage. This may explain why some antibiotics such as gramicidin or some toxins are not digested, not broken down to their constituent amino acids. Some of them, such as phalloidin, are instead absorbed unaltered, producing toxic effects within the tissues.

The pH of the surrounding medium affects the ionization of the terminal amino or carboxyl groups and this seems to be the mechanism by which the pH of the medium influences the digestibility by enzymes. The normally high acidity in the stomach provides the pH optimum for cleavage by pepsin and the low hydrogen ion concentration in the intestines produces conditions favorable for digestion by pancreatic and intestinal enzymes.

In this connection, attention is called to the studies of Linderstrøm-Lang[21] who measured the pH content of various sections of the gut. Over the first 3 hours, the pH of the gastric contents was found to be between 3 and 4, while that of the small intestine was between 6 and 8, the latter values being reached only in the ileum. In view of the rapid digestion of the protein in the upper jejunum it is surprising that these values are so far removed from the pH optima determined experimentally for isolated and purified pepsin and the pancreatic enzymes. More recently, Taylor[22] has demonstrated that gastric juice from normal subjects contains pepsin with maximum activities occurring between pH 1.6 to 2.4, and between pH 3.3 to 4.0. Measurement of proteolysis in the lower ranges of pH alone, therefore, underestimates the true extent of breakdown of which this enzyme is capable.

Other investigations indicate that, besides the classical peptide bonds, some additional linkages are also involved in shaping and stabilizing protein molecules. The β and γ

carboxyls of glutamic and aspartic acid, the non-α-amino groups of arginine or lysine, the SH groups of the sulfur-containing amino acids, and hydrogen bonds form such additional linkages within the polypeptide chain or serve as cross linkages to connect such adjacent chains.[23] All of these linkages evidently may affect enzymatic cleavage. According to recent investigations, the gastrointestinal enzymes attack not only peptides, but also some of these additional linkages present in the protein, *e.g.*, it has been demonstrated that pepsin depolymerizes protein by splitting certain cross linkages.

Some of the non-peptide linkages are split by denaturation of the protein; therefore heating or even denaturation by the high acidity in the stomach often facilitates enzymatic digestion. A well-accepted example of this effect is that of heat which, by destroying such additional linkages, uncoils the folded proteins and exposes a larger surface to enzymatic attack. It should, however, be pointed out here that excessive or prolonged heating during food preparation may sometimes form some extra linkages and thus decrease the digestibility of proteins. It was found, for instance, that toasting cereal products decreases the physiologic availability of lysine, tryptophan and other amino acids.[24,25,26]

The presence of bonds which cannot be split or can be cleaved only with difficulty by the gastrointestinal enzymes is of the highest nutritional importance. This is usually the reason why in actual feeding tests proteins do not always show the biologic values predicted on the basis of the chemically determined amino acid content after acid or alkali hydrolysis. Heating with strong acids or bases evidently can liberate amino acids from complexes which withstand the action of the digestive enzymes.[27]

The sequence of the several phases of protein digestion, such as the peptic action and the preparation of the masticated food in the stomach, the emptying of the stomach contents into the duodenum, the slow propulsion along the small intestine, and the successive action of the different proteases and peptidases in the stomach and intestine, suggests that the process of protein digestion is a well-integrated "whole." Some of the phases and the physiologic significance of these processes are only fragmentarily understood.* One of the most important problems seems to be whether the role of proteases and peptidases is solely to split dietary proteins to amino acids for absorption or whether, in addition, these enzymes fulfill some other physiologic functions. It is evident that the products of pepsin, trypsin, and erepsin digestion are different because of the selective cleavage of certain well-defined peptide linkages. It seems intriguing, therefore, to consider whether these products must fulfill some specific tasks before their terminal breakdown to absorbable amino acids. Their presence may regulate gastrointestinal motility and their lack or over-production may be responsible for some of the vaguely defined symptoms of gastrointestinal indisposition.

Pepsin, for instance, does not seem to be absolutely essential for the final digestion of proteins. Its absence need not upset intestinal digestion, as found in *achylia gastrica* where the over-all utilization of protein for maintenance of nitrogen equilibrium is not gravely disturbed. Many clinical symptoms observed in this disease suggest, however, that the products of peptic digestion may have their own specific physiologic action and there are some indications that the production of Castles intrinsic factor may be connected with the products of peptic digestion.[29]

Intestinal Absorption of Amino Acids. The amino acids liberated from the food proteins by enzymatic processes within the intestinal tract are transferred to the tissues by means of intestinal absorption. However, many of our concepts regarding these processes are still in the theoretical and elementary stages. A block schematic representation of protein utilization is given in Figure 2A–1. The combined efforts of many investigators[30] have shown that under normal conditions proteins are broken down into free amino acids and are absorbed as such into the blood. These blood amino acids are an integral part of the "metabolic amino acid

* The activating effect of some bile acids on protein digestion *in vitro* raises the question of how the bile production affects protein digestion *in vivo*.[28]

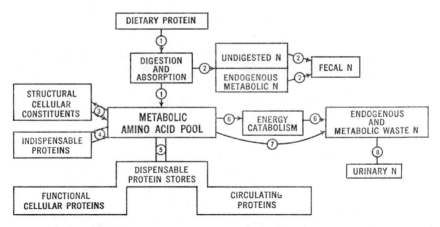

Fig. 2A-1. Schematic outline showing the general pathways of protein metabolism. (Longenecker, *Newer Methods of Nutritional Biochemistry*, courtesy of Academic Press.)

pool." Although there is always the possibility that present methods are inadequate to detect absorption of small concentrations of short chain peptides, the amount of absorption occurring in this manner would appear to be insignificant. Still to be resolved is the mechanism by which free amino acids are absorbed from the gastrointestinal tract into the blood. It had been assumed that the amino acid transfer takes place by simple diffusion, but recent studies indicate the existence of an active and selective mechanism for amino acid absorption.

After absorption, the amino acids are translocated throughout the body via the circulatory system. At this stage amino acids can enter into one of two metabolic pathways, *i.e.*, anabolism or catabolism. Anabolism is the pathway utilized to synthesize cellular protein via pathways 4 and 5. Catabolism is the reverse process involving the breakdown of body protein to amino acids (pathway 5), followed by the breakdown of the amino acids via pathway 6 with the excretion of urea, or via pathway 7 with the excretion of nitrogen-containing compounds, such as creatinine. The "dynamic equilibrium" between the two pathways is readily apparent since the "metabolic pool" is supplied with amino acids from the breakdown of tissue proteins which at this stage are indistinguishable from those contributed by dietary protein sources. Folin[31] first observed that creatinine excretion

was independent of the diet and proposed that the protein metabolism associated with creatinine production be called "endogenous protein metabolism." Also, he proposed that protein metabolism which controlled urea excretion and which was dependent upon the dietary protein be called "exogeneous protein metabolism."

Folin's general theory was quite remarkable considering the limited data available at the time. Even though his basic principles were sound and there was evidence that there are two distinct types of protein metabolism (exogenous and endogenous), further studies have shown that the two metabolic pathways are not independent of each other. The body fluids serve to transfer amino acids to be utilized in the synthesis of body proteins and other nitrogen-containing substances. From our discussion in the preceding paragraph, we are aware that these free amino acids in the body fluids are derived from exogenous and endogenous sources, thus creating a common bond between the two metabolic routes. This acid supply has been called a "metabolic pool," and it serves to establish a "dynamic equilibrium"[32] between dietary and body proteins, and between tissue proteins *per se*. Schoenheimer *et al.*[33,34] showed the reality of the dynamic state by demonstrating the rapid interchange of dietary and cellular amino acids by the use of isotopically labeled amino acids. Excellent detailed discussions of the "dynamic equilibrium" of protein metabolism have been published.[32,35-38]

The great importance of protein to the living organism is clearly manifested by the complexity of protein metabolism and the great number of physiologic functions performed by proteins (Fig. 2A-1). It is reasonable to expect many factors to influence the direction in which protein metabolism will proceed. The major influences to be considered in this connection when other necessary dietary constituents are provided in adequate amounts are (1) amino acid composition of the dietary protein, (2) dietary caloric intake, (3) dietary protein intake, and (4) the nutritional and physiologic state of the individual.

Occasionally some larger fragments like polypeptides or even proteins may also be absorbed. These larger fragments, as mentioned earlier, cannot be utilized for protein synthesis;[39,40] however, they apparently can and do lead to immunologic sensitizations and thus may be responsible for the development of allergic phenomena.* For the most part, amino acids are absorbed from the upper part of the small intestine, but other segments of the intestinal tract may participate in amino acid transfer. Using ^{35}S-labeled proteins, it was possible to show that 11 per cent of the material was taken up by the stomach wall, 60 per cent by the small intestine and 28 per cent by the colon.[41] These data suggest that both the stomach and the colon may be involved in amino acid absorption; however, all attempts to improve nitrogen equilibrium by means of rectal infusions of amino acids have thus far proved unsuccessful.

The exact mechanism involved in the absorption of amino acids is unclear. The old view that amino acids pass through the intestinal wall by simple diffusion now seems to be untenable, in view of the complexity of the factors which may alter absorption rates.[42] It has been shown that the optical isomers of amino acids are absorbed at differ-

ent rates,[43,44] in spite of the fact that the diffusion constants predicted from the identical size and shapes of the enantiomorphs should be identical. The rapid and high accumulation of labeled compounds in the mucosa cells soon after feeding isotope-labeled proteins is further evidence for an active uptake of these compounds by the cells and subsequent transfer to the circulation.[45] Furthermore, recent investigations show that the in vivo absorption of certain amino acids may be specifically inhibited by the presence of some other amino acids. For example, the presence of L-tryptophan decreases the rate of intestinal absorption of histidine in the rat, but the rate of absorption of tryptophan seems to be unaffected by the simultaneous presence of histidine.[46] In similar experiments on dogs, leucine was shown to depress the intestinal absorption of both phenylalanine and isoleucine.[47] These observations support the idea of a competition between amino acids for the selective, specific processes responsible for intestinal absorption. An uptake of L-amino acids, but not of the D-isomer, by the rat intestine against a concentration gradient not explainable by the Donnan theory has been established as further evidence for active transport.[48] In general, it would seem that the absorption of amino acids is an active function of the intestinal wall, although, owing to a limitation of methods, the mechanisms involved have not as yet been fully clarified.[42]

Such an active absorption is likewise suggested by clinical observations. Thus, it was shown that, when the functional characteristics of the intestinal wall are altered, e.g., in sprue or ulcerative colitis, intestinal absorption of amino acids is generally impaired.[49] It has frequently been observed that, after resection of large parts of the small bowel, there is a profound disturbance in the patient's capacity to absorb amino acids, but some 5 to 6 months after surgery the characteristics of the remaining bowel are so altered as to restore almost completely the total capacity for amino acid absorption. Thus there would seem to be a functional adaptation of the intestinal mucosa.

Stomach emptying, intestinal propulsion and enzymatic breakdown of the dietary pro-

* In contradistinction to this almost generally accepted view, some authors have suggested that peptides are normal products of intestinal absorption and that they, rather than amino acids, represent the "normal currency of protein metabolism."[40]

teins are normally coordinated in such a way that, even after heavy protein meals, free amino acids do not accumulate in the intestinal lumen. Amino acids are apparently absorbed at about the same rate as they are liberated from the proteins. This absorption in turn is carried out in such a way as to prevent any excessive increase in the blood amino acid concentration during protein digestion. In certain pathologic conditions, for example after total gastrectomy, this careful regulation is disturbed and there is a marked decrease in the efficiency with which dietary proteins are utilized.[50] Thus, in 6 of 14 gastrectomized patients, impairment of protein utilization with increased fecal loss of nitrogen was observed. Likewise, in only 3 of 40 patients was the normal weight restored postoperatively after elimination of the diseased stomach; in 11 of 44 cases of subtotal gastrectomy there was clear evidence of impaired protein utilization. It was assumed, on the basis of these observations that the defect was not due to a lack of peptic digestion or to the triturating function of the stomach, but was more likely due to the loss of regulated gastric emptying and its relation to properly adjusted release of amino acids.

When, because of disturbed gastrointestinal motility, difficult digestibility, or insufficient enzymatic action, proteins or peptides are incompletely digested, these, along with some of the unabsorbed amino acids, are carried into the lower sections of the intestinal tract where they are exposed to the action of the intestinal flora or are lost with the feces. Certain of the amino acids may here be decarboxylated by the intestinal microorganisms to pharmacologically active compounds, such as histamine, tyramine and tryptamine. Thus, the theory of autointoxication resulting from such bacterial action on amino acids and protein split products, once abandoned, is again being considered in relation to the development of some pathologic conditions.[51,52] Deamination of amino acids in the intestines and subsequent absorption of ammonia has been found to be responsible for the increase of the blood ammonia content in liver diseases.[51] Microbial destruction of methionine and cystine seems to lead to accumulation of abnormal S-compounds in the blood.[52]

As indicated above, the gradual, regulated enzymatic liberation of amino acid from proteins seems to be a prerequisite for the optimal utilization of dietary proteins. This is because the growth rate and the rate of protein synthesis are determined by inherent regulatory factors and cannot be accelerated by a superoptimal supply of these building stones. The amino acid sources are most efficiently utilized, therefore, when the rate of supply from the digestive tract corresponds closely to the rate of growth and synthesis. When the absorption rate is too rapid, utilization becomes less efficient. Those amino acids absorbed in excess of the requirements cannot be stored in the body for later use; the surplus is either excreted or irreversibly metabolized. These findings are clearly confirmed by experiments which demonstrate an improved utilization of proteins by adult human beings when intake and, hence absorption, are evenly distributed throughout the day by the consumption of frequent protein meals.[53] It was also found possible to achieve normal assimilation of protein after total gastrectomy by dividing and feeding the daily protein ration in ten hourly meals.

A further role of the gastrointestinal tract in handling dietary proteins has been suggested by Nasset.[54] The proteins consumed with the meals are mixed in the gastrointestinal tract with proteins present in products of the digestive organs. The author assumed therefore "that the degradation of these endogenous proteins tends to maintain an amino acid mixture of constant composition in the intestinal lumen...." This homeostatic mechanism is then responsible for the fact that even on feeding deficient proteins "the sites of protein synthesis are," at least temporarily, "offered a mixture of amino acids subject to a minimum of qualitative variations." It is hard to understand why on feeding deficient proteins those endogenous amino acids which were missing from the meal should be selectively reabsorbed. If, however, the reabsorption of endogenous amino acids is not altered, then the total of absorbed endogenous and dietary amino acids must still result in a relative deficiency of some amino acids. Investigations in children, dogs, and chickens prove that the post-absorptive increase of the blood amino acids actually reflects the deficiencies in the amino acid composition of the consumed protein.[54-57] The possible intestinal supplementation of incomplete amino acid mixtures therefore remains unproven.

The Therapeutic Use of Per Os Administered Amino Acid Preparations. The well-integrated function of the digestive organs and the consequent slow absorption of dietary amino acids present a model or pattern which must be considered in relation to therapeutic trends. The practice of administering protein hydrolysates or mixtures of amino acids in lieu of food proteins is based on the results of some investigators who have been able to maintain nitrogen equilibrium in human subjects by feeding such amino acid preparations; however, long-term feeding experiments are still lacking. On the other hand, it has been established that amino acid mixtures cannot be utilized with the same efficiency as equivalent amounts of protein. The chief reason for this decreased utilization seems to be the extremely rapid absorption of free amino acids, with consequent flooding of the tissues with amounts of amino acids which cannot be utilized so rapidly and hence must be partially wasted. A further complication arises from the disturbances which result from an increased concentration of amino acids in the intestines and in the blood.[58,59] We have already emphasized the fact that, in the course of normal protein digestion, amino acids do not accumulate; after feeding protein digests, however, abnormally high concentrations of amino acids in the intestines may produce intestinal distress and diarrhea. Due to the rapid, unregulated absorption, blood amino acid levels may increase to values which lead to nausea and vomiting. It is likely that these disturbances are responsible for the serious aversion which the patient develops towards large quantities of these hydrolysates; in any event, after a few days on such a regimen, it often becomes impossible to provide any notable fraction of the daily nitrogen requirement in the form of amino acid preparations.

The oral administration of amino acids for therapeutic purposes was based originally on a misconception concerning the digestive capacities of the human gastrointestinal tract in emaciation, disease, and after surgery. Actual feeding experiments have proven, however, that even in extreme starvation proteins can still be digested as long as food can be swallowed. It is only in the final stages of starvation that digestion is inhibited, and experiences in the western Netherlands indicated that there is no treatment available which would resuscitate such cases.[60] It was also observed that protein digests were soon rejected and vomited by the patients, and still another disadvantage was the relatively large quantity of liquid which had to be consumed along with the amino acids. When glucose was mixed with the protein hydrolysates, they were somewhat better tolerated, but, as a matter of fact, undigested skim milk-glucose mixtures were preferred by the patients who maintained their weight more effectively. The therapeutic use of protein hydrolysate in malnourished South African children provided equally disappointing results (Gillman, cf, ref. 16).

The use of protein hydrolysates was particularly recommended in cases of gastrointestinal diseases. It has been shown, however, that protein digestion and amino acid absorption in diseases like peptic ulcer, ulcerative colitis, or regional enteritis are nearly normal and the use of hydrolyzed protein in such conditions seems to be unnecessary.[61,62] All these experiments prove that the practical value of "oral" amino acid preparations has been seriously overemphasized. These preparations are most valuable dietary sources of nitrogen for short-term feeding in those cases where protein digestion is grossly disturbed or in cases of certain food allergies; but, because of their higher cost, their low palatability, and their possible noxious effects cited above, they do not seem to be generally a practical source of nitrogen. The practice of giving a fraction of the daily nitrogen requirement in the form of amino acid drinks or tablets may have its psychologic value but is obviously of little nutritional importance.

ESSENTIAL AND NONESSENTIAL AMINO ACIDS

Some of the amino acids required for protein synthesis in growth, repair and maintenance, must be supplied by the food but others may be produced by the body itself. The amino acids which have to be supplied by food are the so-called "essentials."[63,64] It should be emphasized, however, that they are not more important in metabolism or growth than the so-called "nonessentials." This distinction implies only a necessity for supply of the "essentials" from external sources. The amino acids which are essential *for man* are listed in Table 2A-4. These data indicate that the daily amino acid requirement of women seems to be somewhat lower than that of men; however no striking differences have been found. Indeed, Hegsted[64a] attempted to estimate the requirements from nitrogen-balance data on young men and women by calculating the regression

of nitrogen balance on amino acid intake and the estimated error in the intake at which nitrogen balance was achieved. These calculations indicated that the data obtained on young men and young women fall, for the most part, in the same region. Therefore, for most of the amino acids, the requirement of young men is substantially the same as that of young women.

Studies on the quantitative amino acid requirements of man began to appear in the literature of the early 1950's. The greater part of all studies were carried out primarily with young adults of college age. In more recent years, reports on the requirements of young boys, 11 to 12 years of age, and of elderly men have appeared. There is little in the literature concerning the minimum needs of children between infancy and 10 years of age or during puberty and adolescence. There is a noticeable lack of data on women of postmenopausal age and on women during pregnancy and lactation. The information that is available is often controversial, divergent, and the number of subjects studied is small. Irwin and Hegsted[64b] have recently

Table 2A-4. Comparison of Tentative Minimum Requirements of Amino Acids with Amino Acid Content of American Diets*

Amino acid	Minimum requirements[a] Women (gm/day)	Men	Amino acid content of food intakes Reynolds[b]	Futrell[c] (gm/day)	Mertz[d]	Wharton[e]
Isoleucine	0.45	0.70	4.2	2.49–5.73	0.7–4.5	2.8–3.1
Leucine	0.62	1.10	6.5	3.28–7.35	1.3–7.8	4.4–4.9
Lysine	0.50	0.80	4.0	1.7 –8.6	1.3–5.6	3.5–4.0
Methionine Cystine }	0.55	1.10	3.0	0.90–2.54	0.7–2.7	0.9–1.0
Phenylalanine Tyrosine	0.22 0.90	1.10	4.1	1.98–4.88	0.9–3.77	2.5–2.7
Threonine	0.31	0.50	2.8	1.68–3.44	0.9–3.8	2.6–2.9
Tryptophan	0.16	0.25	0.9	0.5 –1.28	—	0.4–0.5
Valine	0.65	0.80	4.2	2.85–5.39	0.8–4.9	3.1–3.4

* From Leverton in *Protein and Amino Acid Nutrition* (A. A. Albanese, Editor), courtesy of Academic Press.

[a] Values for women are from Leverton.[69]   Values for men are from Rose.[63]

[b] Reynolds *et al.*[70]

[c] Futrell *et al.*[71]

[d] Mertz *et al.*[72]

[e] Wharton *et al.*[73]

thoroughly reviewed the literature on the amino acid requirements of man.

Most of the published values were established by N-balance experiments. The requirements for maintenance of N-balance, for growth, reproduction, lactation, etc. are different.[64] If any of the essentials is missing from the diet, or is present only in inadequate quantities, then the dietary protein cannot be used for growth or maintenance even though the other amino acids are present in excess. The nonessentials lacking from the diet can be produced in the body from other sources. Their carbon skeletons arise from intermediary products of carbohydrate and fat metabolism and the amino group is transferred by the mechanisms of transamination.[65] The biogenesis of nonessential amino acids was proved by feeding ^{14}C-labeled sugar or acetic acid or by injecting $C^{14}O_2$. The ^{14}C derived necessarily from the fed sugar or fatty acid or CO_2 was incorporated into the nonessential amino acids of the milk and body proteins and the liver proteins regenerated after partial hepatectomy.[66,67,68] This proves that, in building the carbon skeleton of the nonessentials, sugar or fatty acid or CO_2 was used as a precursor. The essential amino acids, in contrast, did not contain any ^{14}C, indicating that no new formation of these amino acids from labeled precursors had occurred. Thus, the main difference between essentials and nonessentials is that the carbon skeleton of the essential amino acids cannot be formed in the animal body. The precursor of the nonessential amino acids formed in intermediary metabolism is usually the keto-analog, e.g., pyruvic acid serves as precursor for alanine, an amino group is then attached to this acid. The amino group derives either from another amino acid or from the ammonia of dietary amino compounds.[74] The transfer of the amino group from one amino acid to another is accomplished by action of the enzyme "transaminase" which is activated by the coenzyme pyridoxal phosphate. In the preparatory uptake of inorganic ammonia for the purpose of transamination, glutamic and aspartic acids seem to be the key substances (Fig. 2A-2).

It was demonstrated, after feeding ^{15}N-labeled ammonium compounds, that the essential amino acids as well as the nonessentials show uptake of [15]N. These experiments prove the important fact that most of the essential amino acids participate also in

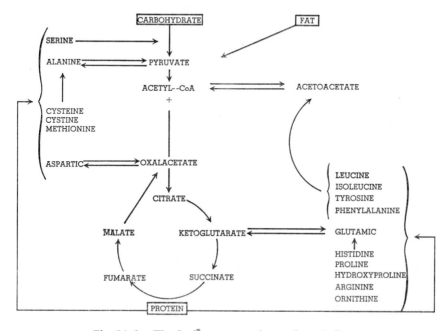

Fig. 2A-2. The final common pathway of metabolism.

the transamination reaction.[75] As further confirmation of these results, it has been shown in rat experiments that the hydroxy- or keto-analogs of the essential amino acids, with the exception of those corresponding to lysine and threonine, could actually be used for replacement of the corresponding amino acids.

According to these results, the amino acids participating in protein synthesis may be divided into three groups. In the first group belong lysine and threonine which have to be supplied in "ready-made" form. To the second group belong the other essentials which can be supplied either in the form of amino acids or in the form of their hydroxy- or keto-analogs which can be then converted to amino acids by transamination. And, finally, the nonessential amino acids which can be wholly formed from nonspecific precursors in the intermediary metabolism.

The dividing line between these groups of amino acids, however, is not sharp. Arginine, for example, which is a nonessential for the adult, cannot be formed with the necessary speed in infants; therefore, its dietary supply may be regarded as essential in early life.[76] Tyrosine, in spite of being a nonessential amino acid, does not show any ^{14}C uptake after feeding tagged sugar or acetic acid. The reason for this is that tyrosine is not newly formed in the body but derives from phenylalanine which is an essential amino acid. Tyrosine is nonessential only because it can be formed from phenylalanine; and quantitative determinations actually show that about 50 per cent of the phenylalanine requirement can be provided by tyrosine. In the biologic evaluation of amino acid mixtures or proteins it must always be remembered that a food may be satisfactory as an amino acid source even when it does not contain the necessary amounts of phenylalanine as established by the determinations of Rose, provided enough tyrosine is present. The same line of reasoning applies in the evaluation of the methionine content of proteins. Cystine present in the diet may substitute for about 30 per cent of the methionine requirement, indicating that a fraction of methionine is transformed to cystine.

For efficient protein synthesis, both the essential and nonessential amino acids must be available simultaneously and in sufficient quantities. Although the organism does not depend on dietary intake of the nonessentials, it is evident that, when their dietary supply is low, they must be produced in intermediary metabolism and be provided as free amino acids in ample quantities to secure optimal utilization of the essential amino acids. Protein synthesis, therefore, is limited not only by the supply of essential amino acids but also by the speed and efficiency with which the so-called nonessentials are made available. This phenomenon is well demonstrated by experiments in which the feeding of a mixture of essential and nonessential amino acids was more effective than feeding essentials only. The rapid availability of nonessential amino acids depends on the proper function of conversion mechanisms and it seems probable that some of the disturbances of protein formation, for instance in liver disease, may be the consequence of a failure in the formation of some nonessentials.

In the near future, the protein needs of population groups will continue to be met primarily by food sources which vary widely in protein quality and quantity. Basic information obtained by administering crystalline amino acids to human subjects, either alone or in conjunction with other food sources, should eventually elucidate some of the problems associated with the utilization of bound and free amino acids.

When foods serve as sources of dietary proteins, the relative amounts of nitrogen supplied by essential and nonessential amino acids are fixed. However, when free amino acids may be added, the sources and quantities of nitrogen can easily be manipulated. In Table 2A–5, representative foods are grouped in terms of the percentage of total nitrogen present in the essential amino acids.

Such a classification of foods is in agreement with the concept of quality based on knowledge of the limiting amino acids in each food. However, the percentage of nitrogen derived from essential amino acids is less significant when foods are combined in such a manner as to permit mutual supplementation, and particularly when free amino acids

Table 2A-5. Percentages of Total Nitrogen Supplied by the Essential Amino Acids in Certain Foods*

Total N from EAA	Foods
35% or more	Egg, human milk, cow's milk, lactalbumin, casein
34 to 30%	Meat, fish, beans, peas, soybeans, sorghum, sweet potato, spinach
29 to 25%	Lentils, oats, ragimillet, cornmeal, cottonseed meal, sesame seed meal, cashew, white potato, rice
24 to 20%	Barley, wheat flour, almond, Brazil nut, peanut
19% or less	Carrot, cassava, gelatin

* From Clark, *Newer Methods of Nutritional Biochemistry*, Vol. 2 (A. A. Albanese, editor), New York, Academic Press Inc., 1965.

are either added to foods or fed as components of experimental mixtures of purified amino acids. Examples of the foregoing include the upgrading of corn masa to the biologic value of skim milk by supplementing it with tryptophan, lysine, and isoleucine,[76b] and the improvement of wheat flour by increasing the limiting amino acids, lysine and threonine, to the levels in the FAO reference pattern.[76c] In both cases, the efficacy of the modality was measured in terms of nitrogen retention in children, and the change in quantity or percentage of nitrogen was small.

The Committee on Protein Malnutrition[76d] has pointed out that two proteins may vary in quality because of differences in the total amount of essential amino acids per unit of nitrogen in the face of similar amino acid ratios. It has suggested that for research purposes the requirements in milligrams of essential amino acids might better be expressed per gram of total essential amino acid nitrogen. Reference to essential amino acid needs in this manner would tend to minimize their unique and diverse functions and to

overlook the differences in constitution and proportion of nitrogen. Current emphasis on essential amino acid nitrogen tends to minimize the fact that amino acids function not only as necessary units for synthesis of a peptide chain, but also as integral components of the other biochemical functions. Also, it would seem that different expressions of amino acid content should be employed when a dietary protein containing essential and nonessential amino acids in fixed amounts is being evaluated than in experiments in which the quantities and proportions of these components can be modified at will.

METHODS OF PROTEIN EVALUATION

Laboratory methods have been developed which accurately reflect protein quality as applied to specific species and conditions. These have contributed greatly to the clarification of some of the problems associated with protein evaluation in man and animals. Marked differences in the nutritive value of proteins of similar amino acid content, and striking variations in the nutritive value of different samples of the same protein, impose severe limitations on the choice of a single figure as representative of nutritive value.

It seems worthwhile, therefore, to consider briefly some of the frequently used laboratory procedures now in vogue, and to point out their shortcomings and their virtues.

The Protein Efficiency Ratio (PER). This is defined as the weight gain of a growing animal, divided by its protein intake. Although it is a proximate measure of protein quality when conducted under specific conditions, it has been criticized because *only* the amount of protein consumed above maintenance is used for growth. Furthermore, the PER varies with food intake. This ratio finds use in feeding experiments with small animals, and has been employed also in infant studies.

Mitchell's Biologic Value (BV). Expressed by the formula,

$$\frac{\text{food N} - (\text{fecal N} - \text{metabolic N}) - (\text{urinary N} - \text{``endogenous'' N}) \times 100}{\text{food N} - (\text{fecal N} - \text{metabolic N})}$$

this value is obtained by means of Kjeldahl analyses of the excreta collected during non-nitrogenous but isocaloric dietary periods.[76e] More simply, it is a ratio of nitrogen retained to nitrogen absorbed. Protein quality expressed in this manner is a reflection of the percentages of absorbed nitrogen retained for growth and maintenance, but does not include a correction for incomplete absorption.

In a single index, both the BV and digestibility of a protein can be expressed by the *Net Protein Utilization (NPU)*. This product of the coefficient of digestibility and the BV represents the proportion of food nitrogen retained. Since efficiency of protein utilization is diminished when caloric intake is low or protein intake excessive, the NPU must be measured under standardized dietary conditions. Obviously, these conditions can seldom be achieved in situations of normal food intake.

In order to arrive at a relative utilization value of test proteins which would compensate for weight changes, Albanese and his associates[76f] applied the following formulas to their results with infants:

$$P = \frac{BW \times N}{1000}$$

where P = protein utilization, BW = body weight change in gm per day, and N = nitrogen retention in mg per kg per day. The coefficient of utilization of the test products, P_r, is then expressed as the numerical value of the ratio: P test protein formula, divided by P evaporated milk formula, or

$$P_r = P_{tp}/P_{em}$$

Expression of bioassay results in this manner has several advantages. It equalizes disparities between body weight changes and nitrogen retention values which often arise in infants from transpositions of body fluid compartments.[76g] Increments in nitrogenous tissue can be related directly to qualitative amino acid differences of the test nitrogenous moiety of the diets. Lastly, a simple numerical comparison of the test substance with a standard infant food, like evaporated milk, is provided.

After careful consideration of existing indices of protein utilization, Arnould[76h] has concluded that none of them provides a suitable partitioning of nitrogen needs in terms of the various physiologic functions of life.

In developing his hypothesis, this investigator measures the requirements for maintenance directly with rations containing sufficient nitrogen to assure growth. In so doing, he introduces the factor of alimentary efficiency into nitrogen utilization, a biologic property heretofore not considered. His hypothesis also explains a number of biochemical properties of amino acids which are not considered in other evaluations. It provides some clarification for the discrepancies often noted between chemical scores and biologic values. The results obtained by Arnould's method appear to be independent of the growth rate, the age, and the sex of the experimental animal, the level of protein in the ration, and the nitrogen intake. He attaches no importance whatsoever to minimum maintenance requirements because these are hardly representative of the whole need for the life processes. Although this attractive postulate may prove useful in clarifying the protein needs of experimental animals where the growth rate is of relatively short duration, application of the principle to human nutrition, where the growth rate is relatively much slower, presents a number of experimental obstacles.

Notwithstanding the premise that the nutritional quality of a protein should be established *in vivo*, reliable *in vitro* procedures for the measurement of protein quality are valuable adjuncts to biologic assessments. These procedures, which are based on chemical analyses of proteins for their essential amino acids, yield results which in many instances correlate well with biologic values. Additionally, data obtained in this manner provide an indication of the essential amino acids which limit nutritional quality, and point to the need for combining proteins or amino acids for effective supplementation of deficient or poor quality proteins.

The apparent discrepancies between *in vitro* and *in vivo* procedures seem to be due primarily to decreased digestibility and the effects of heat processing on proteins. The difficulties encountered relate to the fact that the factor of amino acid availability is not introduced. Numerous methods, including the Chemical Score of Mitchell and Block,[76i] the FAO/WHO procedure,[76j] Oser's Essential Amino Acid Index,[76k] and the enzymatic method of Melnick and his associates,[76l] have been evolved as attempts to include the "availability" component. Sheffner and his associates[76m] studied the relationship between the pattern of amino acids released by digestive enzymes and the biologic value of food proteins, and evolved an integrated index— the pepsin digest residue (PDR) amino acid index. The results obtained with this new index show good correlation with the net utilization values of the proteins studied, including those which were heat processed with various degrees of severity.

It should be pointed out that all *in vitro* methods, when used with discretion, are valuable complements to nutritional evaluation of protein quality in experimental animals. However, discrepancies often arise which introduce a disconcerting uncertainty. A comprehensive treatment of this subject may be found in an excellent review prepared by Sheffner.[76n]

Blood Ribonuclease Levels. A number of in-depth reviews which describe the advantages and disadvantages of various biochemical criteria for the evaluation of protein quality which include measurements of nitrogen balance, blood amino acids, urinary amino acids, urea and creatinine excretion, and blood protein levels have been published.[30,70a,76o,76p,76q,135] The common denominator and stimulus to these continuing efforts have been the practical inconveniences of the classical nitrogen-balance method which has long been accepted as the method of choice, despite its many and well-known biochemical shortcomings.

A new approach is now indicated by new knowledge of the biochemical relationships of tissue DNA and RNA content to protein biosynthesis.[76r] The nutritional regulation of these processes was revealed by the investigations of Munro and Clark[76s] who found that the RNA content of normal liver cells of rats varied with ingested amount of protein and amino acid profile of the protein. Subsequent

investigations by Allison and co-workers[76t] indicated that the DNA and RNA content of liver and muscle rat tissues is an intimate function not only of protein reserves in various body tissues, but also of the nutritive value of dietary proteins. In addition to these changes in tissue composition, these investigators found protein quality to be reflected in changes in ribonuclease (RNase) activity of the serum. Namely, serum RNase to serum protein ratio was highest in animals fed lysine-deficient wheat gluten (B.V. = 52), lowest in animals fed egg protein (B.V. = 100), and intermediate in the sera of animals fed casein (B.V. = 69) and cottonseed flour (B.V. = 73). Further, the positive correlation between ribonuclease activity and growth intensity of homogenates of mammalian placental tissues has been clearly demonstrated by Brody.[76u] The foregoing observations lent strong support to the hypothesis of Lang[76v] that levels of serum RNase activity might serve as criteria of the anabolic-catabolic ratio prevailing in biological organisms during the growing, mature and aging phases of the life span.

These and other reports[76w] have led to an evaluation of serum RNase levels as criteria of protein nutrition in man. To this end, nitrogen-balance data obtained in metabolic studies were correlated with parallel blood RNase measurements. The results indicate that blood RNase determinations afford a practical and useful parameter of human quantitative and qualitative protein needs and, of the effects of anabolic steroids and corticosteroids on human protein metabolism.[76x]

Typical effects of changes in protein quality and quantity on blood RNase levels and nitrogen balance are shown graphically in Figure 2A–3. The expected inverse relationship between nitrogen balance and plasma RNase is clear—namely, the postulated inverse relationship between a high plasma RNase level and marked negative nitrogen balance which was induced by the low protein-calorie intake found in Peroid I. When the protein-calorie intake was increased by choice to relatively normal levels as in Periods II, III and IV, high positive N-balances were obtained and reflected by significant de-

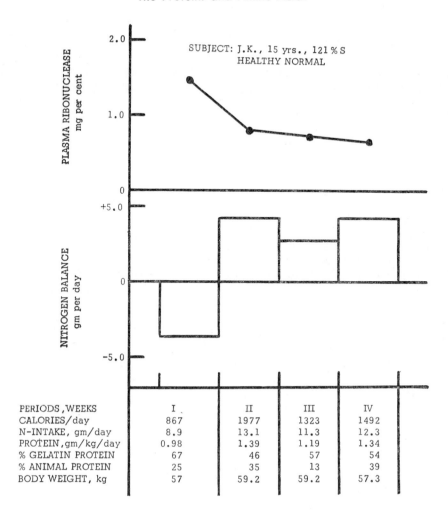

The figure contains the following axis labels and data:

PLASMA RIBONUCLEASE mg per cent (values 2.0, 1.0, 0)

SUBJECT: J.K., 15 yrs., 121% S
HEALTHY NORMAL

NITROGEN BALANCE gm per day (values +5.0, 0, -5.0)

PERIODS, WEEKS	I	II	III	IV
CALORIES/day	867	1977	1323	1492
N-INTAKE, gm/day	8.9	13.1	11.3	12.3
PROTEIN, gm/kg/day	0.98	1.39	1.19	1.34
% GELATIN PROTEIN	67	46	57	54
% ANIMAL PROTEIN	25	35	13	39
BODY WEIGHT, kg	57	59.2	59.2	57.3

Fig. 2A-3.   The relationship of plasma RNase levels to nitrogen balance in a young, healthy, normal female subject.

creases in plasma RNase activity. In reference to the purpose of these assays, it is to be noted that the high nitrogen retention in Periods II, III and IV was sustained by a protein intake which contained approximately 50 per cent gelatin—a protein well known for its deficiency of the essential amino acid, tryptophan. It would appear from these data that the nutritional defect of gelatin may be corrected by inclusion in the diet of approximately 20 per cent animal protein with a total protein intake of 1.2 gm or more per kilo per day and an adequate (25 to 30 per kilo per day) supply of calories.

These values are in good accord with recommended daily allowances for this age group.[111a]

On the basis of the foregoing observations, the usefulness of blood RNase as a criterion of the protein metabolic effects of anabolic steroids and corticosteroids was explored. The results of one such study are illustrated in Figure 2A-4. The inverse relationship between N-balance and plasma RNase levels found in previous studies occurred in these trials and is clear. Attention is called to the fact that the protein catabolic effects of 5 mg per day of prednisone in terms of nitrogen loss and plasma ribonuclease increase are far

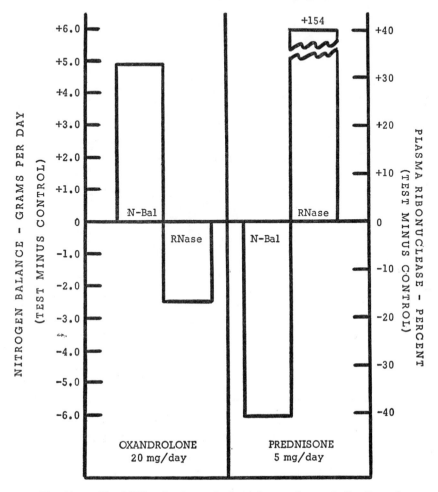

Fig. 2A-4. Blood RNase levels as criteria of the protein metabolic effects of anabolic steroids and corticosteroids.

greater than the nitrogen retention increase and plasma ribonuclease decrease induced by the administration of 20 mg per day of oxandrolone.

The results of parallel plasma RNase and nitrogen-balance measurements done systematically as a part of metabolic studies on adult male and female subjects receiving anabolic steroids and corticosteroids for a variety of clinical reasons are collected in Figure 2A–5. It is evident from these data that the RNase shifts under conditions of these substances are also inversely related to changes in N-balance.

In other words, reduced formation of body proteins frequently associated with corticosteroid therapy is accurately reflected by increases in circulating RNase. The reverse relationship obtains during anabolic steroid therapy. Application of these procedures in metabolic studies in which varying combinations of these agents were given demonstrated their usefulness in determinations of the anti-corticocatabolic activity of anabolic steroids (Figure 2A–6). It would appear from these findings that the plasma RNase measurement provides a more dynamic and convenient

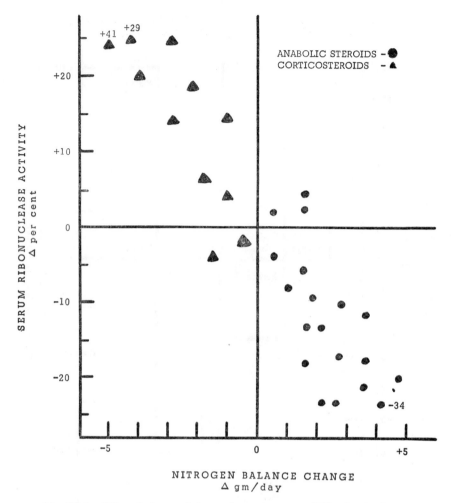

Fig. 2A-5. Effect of nitrogen-balance changes on serum RNase levels of man.

criterion of protein metabolism than the cumbersome nitrogen-balance procedure.

THE BIOLOGIC VALUE OF FOOD PROTEINS

The proteins provided by different food substances are not nutritionally equivalent. In the past the *biologic value* of a protein was determined by time- and money-consuming feeding experiments in which either growth promotion, repletion after protein depletion, or the maintenance of nitrogen equilibrium was measured. With the development of relatively simple methods for quantitative determination of amino acids in protein

hydrolysates,[77] *e.g.*, the microbiologic, enzymatic, and chromatographic methods, a "chemical scoring" of proteins has been attempted. This scoring is based on the assumption that the nutritive value of proteins depends entirely on their amino acid composition, *i.e.*, that proteins are "as good as their content of essential amino acids."

The FAO established a provisional pattern of essential amino acids[78] based on the minimum amino acid requirements determined experimentally with young adults fed purified amino acid diets. This pattern has been widely used as a basis for evaluating the quality of food proteins and protein combinations. It varies appreciably from the

Patient: Kendrick, H., Female, Age: 52 yrs., Height: 61.5 in., Weight: 89 lbs. DX: Polyneuritis

Hemoglobin, gm.%	12.5	11.7	10.9
Hematocrit, %	36.0	35.5	34.5
Sodium, mEq/L	144	140	146
Potassium, mEq/L	4.6	4.6	4.6
Chlorides, mEq/L	90	85	90
FBS, mg.%	94	92	85
BUN, mg.%	17	15	15
Thymol turbidity, units	1.6	1.9	1.7
Bilirubin, mg.%	0.5	0.4	0.3
SGOT, units	9	7	QNS
Urinary calcium, mg/day	178	103	92
" OH-proline, mg/day	5.3	7.2	5.5
" N/Creatinine ratio	13.0	9.5	9.2

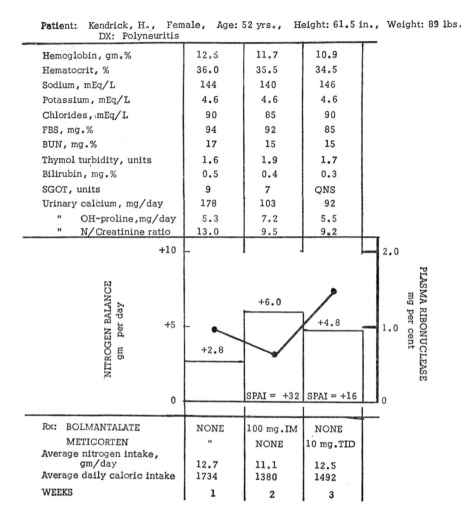

Rx: BOLMANTALATE	NONE	100 mg.IM	NONE
METICORTEN	"	NONE	10 mg.TID
Average nitrogen intake, gm/day	12.7	11.1	12.5
Average daily caloric intake	1734	1380	1492
WEEKS	1	2	3

Fig. 2A-6. The anticorticocatabolic effects of anabolic steroids in a convalescent female subject.

pattern of egg protein which has long been used as a reference standard. Before one can conclude, however, that the FAO pattern will be as effective as combinations of amino acids based on high-quality proteins like egg or milk, studies must be done with human beings to compare amino acid diets containing the FAO mixture with amino acid diets based on egg or other quality proteins. Swendseid and her associates[79] have compared the FAO pattern with that of egg protein. Kirk et al.[80] have compared it with those of milk and peanut proteins.

In the study of Swendseid and co-workers, the experimental diets provided 10 gm of nitrogen, of which 0.64 gm was supplied by low protein fruits and vegetables and 1.16 gm by a mixture of nonessential amino acids (except glycine) in the proportions of egg protein. The amount of nitrogen from essential amino acids varied in the different periods. In general, the level fed was based on the tryptophan intake, which ranged from 160 to 360 mg daily, and the proportions of the other essential amino acids were adjusted according to the FAO or the egg protein pattern. Cystine and tyrosine were considered as essential amino acids. The total nitrogen was brought to 10 gm by adding a mixture of glycine and diammonium citrate in isonitrogenous amounts. All the amino acids were supplied in the L-form.

When the daily intake of tryptophan was set at 240 mg, only one subject was in positive nitrogen balance with the FAO pattern. When the FAO pattern was fed to provide 320 mg of tryptophan, three subjects were in nitrogen balance, but one subject required the FAO mixture providing 360 mg of tryptophan before reaching a positive balance. The results were not affected by the sequence in which the amino acid mixtures were fed.

In contrast, with the egg pattern based on 240 mg of tryptophan, four of the subjects showed a higher nitrogen retention than with the FAO pattern, although they did not all reach a positive balance. In another period, whole egg protein providing 240 mg of tryptophan was substituted as the chief source of amino acids. Nitrogen retention increased in all subjects in comparison with either of the amino acid diets providing 240 mg of tryptophan. When egg protein was supplemented with essential amino acids to produce the FAO pattern, nitrogen balance decreased slightly in comparison with the period when whole egg alone provided the same tryptophan intake. These results suggest that the amino acid proportions of egg protein permit better utilization of dietary nitrogen than do the proportions of essential amino acids in the FAO pattern at the same level of tryptophan.

The requirement of young women for essential amino acid nitrogen for nitrogen balance under the test conditions ranged from 0.63 to 0.85 gm daily. This amount is considerably greater than the total of 0.48 gm daily, the figure obtained when the essential amino acids are fed at the minimum requirements (based on 160 mg of tryptophan) cited by the FAO. These values of 0.63 to 0.85 gm are still considerably lower than the values of 1.0 to 1.3 gm daily found for young men by Swendseid et al.[81] Such a difference, which appears unrelated to body weight,[78] may indicate a sex difference in the requirements for at least some of the essential amino acids.

In the study of Kirk et al.,[80] the experimental diets provided approximately 9 gm of nitrogen daily. About 0.70 gm to 0.75 gm was derived from low-protein foods in the basal diets. When essential amino acid mixtures were compared, a fixed amount of nonessential amino acids, except glycine, was also included in the diet. In the study comparing the FAO pattern and the milk protein pattern, the nonessential amino acid mixture was based on the nonessential amino acid composition of milk protein. Similarly, when the FAO pattern and the peanut pattern were compared, the nonessential amino acid mixture was based on the composition of peanut protein. The total nitrogen of all diets was brought to 9 gm by adding glycine and diammonium citrate at isonitrogenous levels. Each experimental period was preceded by a preliminary period with a diet of ordinary foods providing about 9 to 10 gm of nitrogen. This was followed by a 2- to 3-day transition period when components of the experimental diets gradually replaced the ordinary diet. Different subjects were used in the two studies.

In both studies, the essential amino acids in the FAO pattern were fed to subjects at levels based on tryptophan intakes between 120 and 240 mg daily. The tryptophan intake which supported nitrogen equilibrium was obtained for each subject although only two of the subjects were in positive nitrogen balance with this intake. The term "nitrogen equilibrium" as used in this study refers to the condition where the total nitrogen excretion is ±5 per cent of the total nitrogen intake.[82]

With the mixture patterned after milk protein or with nonfat milk solids, nitrogen retention in all subjects was greater than with the FAO pattern and, in five of six cases, nitrogen retention was better with milk solids than with the corresponding amino acid mixture. When milk solids were supplemented with essential amino acids to simulate the FAO pattern (75 per cent of the essential amino acids supplied from milk solids) and fed to each subject at the level of sulfur amino acids used with milk solids alone, nitrogen retention decreased in comparison with the retention on the milk solids.

With the amino acid mixture based on peanut protein or with peanut butter, nitrogen retention was again better than with the FAO mixture at the same level of sulfur amino acids. Nitrogen balance with peanut butter was slightly better than with the amino acid mixture based on peanut protein. Supplementation of peanut butter with essential amino acids to approximate the FAO pattern also reduced the nitrogen balance.

Both of these detailed studies again demonstrate the importance of both the proportions and the absolute amounts of essential amino acids in the diet. Despite differences in techniques, both reports suggest that the level of tryptophan in the FAO pattern may be too high, relative to some of the other amino acids. It must be remembered that several of the minimum values in the FAO pattern were determined with diets which often supplied other essential amino acids at levels above the minimum.[83,84] These circumstances may have affected utilization of the amino acid under study to produce a "minimum" value different from that which might have been obtained had all other essential amino acids been supplied at levels determined as "minimum." Another possibility with these diets is that the nonessential amino acid pattern, which was based on the food protein, may have been more favorable to utilization of the essential amino acids of the food protein than those of the FAO mixture.[85]

The essential amino acid content of common foods has been compiled by Orr and Watt.[86] This report represents a fairly good guide for designing nutritionally satisfactory meals containing proteins of different origin and chemical score.

The chemical evaluation of protein is generally in quite good agreement with the values obtained by the more complicated biologic methods.[87] In many cases, however, the actual biologic value was found to be lower than predicted on the basis of amino acid composition. The reason for this discrepancy is that not all of the amino acids present in food are necessarily physiologically available. The utilization of amino acids depends primarily on the nature of the linkages by which they are connected within the protein molecule. If these linkages are resistant to the highly specific digestive enzymes, the amino acids involved are not liberated and may be lost with the feces or destroyed by intestinal flora. Such enzyme-resistant linkages may be preformed in the protein, but they are often artifacts produced by protracted heating or storage of proteins, particularly in the presence of carbohydrates. Thus the recent trend to evaluate proteins according to their essential amino acid content has its limitations and fallacies.* A further complication in evaluation arises from the circumstance that we do not yet know how the relative concentrations of the essential amino acids and the presence of the different nonessentials influence utilization of the amino acid groups present in the protein. There is no safe way at present to establish the nutritive value of proteins other than by feeding tests. The chemical scoring can be used only in a negative sense, i.e., those proteins which do not contain some of the eight essential amino acids in proper quantities cannot be utilized as such for protein synthesis in the body.

The scoring of different foods according to the biologic value of their proteins is of much theoretical and practical importance. It has led to developing new patterns in human and animal nutrition and often can explain many forms of malnutrition in different parts of the world. It also shows the importance of selecting proteins of high biologic value when qualitative limitation is indicated by the presence of allergy or quantitative limitation is necessitated by intestinal or other diseases. It would, however, be a serious mistake to attempt to build practical human nutrition preferentially on foods containing "first class" proteins. The production of animal proteins is relatively uneconomic and their price is accordingly high.[88]

Mutual Supplementation of Dietary Proteins. Meat, fish, milk and egg proteins, due to their complete amino acid composition and good digestibility, have a high biologic value. Most of the vegetable or grain proteins are low in some essentials such as lysine, tryptophan, threonine or methionine and therefore could not promote growth satisfactorily when fed by themselves. Our meals,

* The digestibility of proteins and therefore the biologic availability of their constituent amino acids can be determined with some degree of accuracy by in vitro digestion experiments.

however, usually contain a mixture of different proteins with different amino acid composition, such as those in grains, vegetables and legumes. Furthermore, they are as a rule consumed with some meat, fish or milk proteins. It is evident that the total supply of the necessary amino acids and not the amino acid content of the single dietary proteins determines the nutritive value of the ingested meal.[89] It has been demonstrated that bouillon, containing gelatin, an incomplete protein, consumed with bread, improves the utilization of the grain protein by compensating for its low lysine content. Cereals, legumes, roots, tubers, leaves, fruits, nuts and yeasts contain proteins which, by themselves, are mostly of low biologic value. Some of them taken together, however, may supply a satisfactory amino acid mixture due to

mutual supplementation. However, effective supplementation occurs only when the deficient and supplementary proteins are fed simultaneously or within a short interval of time.[90,91] The timing in supplementation of deficient proteins represents a specific example of the importance of the time factor in protein synthesis.

The mutual supplementation of proteins has been practiced for ages but its mechanisms and importance have been recognized only recently. The Chinese, for example, consume different cereals mixed in definite proportions and in this fashion they have empirically developed meals which contain protein mixtures of high biologic value. Since proteins are not essential nutrients, as such, but serve as a source of amino acids, they may be combined to give a balanced

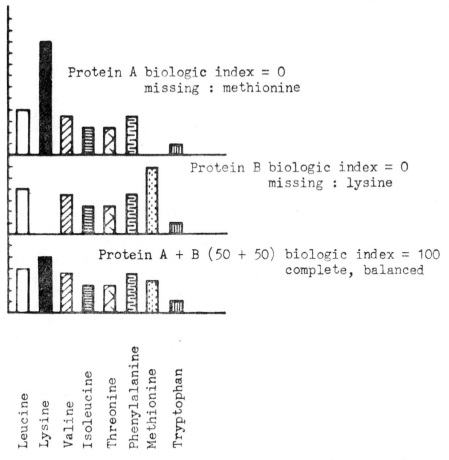

Fig. 2A-7. The principle of combination of mediocre proteins. (From Mauron.[91a])

aminogram although individually they may in fact be imbalanced. This principle is illustrated in Figure 2A–7, and it is of fundamental importance for the rational use of vegetable proteins.

The importance of the simultaneous feeding of supplementary proteins has been demonstrated *in vivo* in man. Improvement in the utilization of breakfast cereals has been shown to occur when milk proteins are fed simultaneously.[92] More recently it was reported that the complementary proteins of corn and beans, the staple food of many Central American people, are better utilized when these foods are ingested together.[93]

These findings would indicate that it is not absolutely necessary to feed *first class proteins* such as fish, meat, eggs or milk for maintenance of growth and good health. The concept of supplementation also explains why certain religious groups or even whole populations living on strictly vegetarian diets do not necessarily suffer from amino acid deficiencies. One practical implication of these findings is that when feeding proteins of low biologic value, as for instance in relief feeding or emergency diets, foods containing supplementary proteins should be fed together.

As the world supply of complete animal proteins becomes increasingly short, the economic significance of this concept is evident. In developing countries, where protein deficiencies are endemic, the production of first class meat or milk proteins, as is often suggested, may disturb the economic structure, but a well-planned vegetarian diet based on the concept of mutual supplementation would appear to be one logical solution to the protein problem.

Very important studies on the use of plant protein mixtures in child feeding have been reported by Dean. He found that certain combinations of barley, wheat, and soy protein were "nearly perfect substitutes for all the milk in the diet" in feeding children 1 to 2 years old.[94] Highly satisfactory results have been obtained also by the use of locally available plant protein mixtures in prevention and treatment of protein malnutrition, particularly kwashiorkor, in Africa and Central America.[95,96]

Supplementation of Dietary Proteins

with Synthetic Amino Acids. Another very promising trend is to improve the biologic value of the deficient protein foods by supplementation of the missing or limiting amino acids with pure synthetic compounds.[97] Methionine is already manufactured on a large scale and has proved to be of value particularly in practical supplementation of low-cost animal feeds; and great strides have been made towards the economic use of lysine and tryptophan for nutritional fortification. Fukui and his associates[97a] have studied Japanese children, 5 to 15 years of age, in urban, coastal, rural, and mountainous regions. These investigators were able to correlate physique in terms of height and weight parameters with animal protein and essential amino acid intake. Children in coastal and urban areas, where the highest intakes of animal protein prevail, were taller and heavier than their rural counterparts with medium intakes. Children in mountainous regions were the smallest in terms of physical development, due to their extremely low intakes of essential amino acids. When the diets of the children from rural and mountainous areas were supplemented with lysine, statistically significant increases were observed in height and weight. Further correction of the deficient diets in terms of lysine/tryptophan (L/T) ratios produced even more dramatic results.

The synthetic procedures currently used yield racemic compounds, and the resolution of these into optical antipodes in large-scale production is not yet economically feasible; therefore, with the exception of recently introduced synthetic L-lysine, at present only supplementation with DL-amino acids is practical. This presents a problem in the use of synthetic DL-amino acids for human nutrition.

Our natural food as well as the proteins of the human body contain only L-amino acids. In most respects the D-amino acids behave differently from their optical antipodes.[98] The peptide linkages in which D-amino acids are involved resist gastrointestinal digestion. The intestinal absorption of D-amino acids is slower and, finally, only a few of them, such as D-methionine and D-phenylalanine, can be utilized by the human organism in lieu of the natural L-forms. It seems that these two amino acids are first deaminated to the corresponding keto acids by a specific D-amino acid oxidase present in some tissues, and the keto acids are then converted by transamination to the L-amino acids. When all the essential L-amino acids are supplied with the diet, then certain D-amino acids may be utilized for synthesis of nonessential amino acids.[99]

Some of the D-amino acids are largely excreted in the urine after feeding. Most of these D-modifications enter metabolic pathways different from those followed by the L-amino acids. Their metabolism may therefore yield products with undesirable biologic activity. The fate of the D-amino acids will have to be further elucidated before practical, large scale supplementation of human food with the synthetic DL-compounds can be safely adopted.[74,100]

Comparable Nutritional Value of Animal and Vegetable Proteins.[101] It was shown in the preceding discussion that by proper selection and combination of plant proteins it is possible to devise meals which supply the necessary amino acids in satisfactory quantities. The old nutritional belief that diets containing animal proteins are necessarily superior to those composed entirely of vegetable proteins is therefore valid only with qualifications. This doctrine was originally based on several reports which showed that physical and mental development as well as health of human groups consuming foods of animal origin are generally superior to those of people adhering to strict vegetarian regimens.[102,103] Much of our thinking in this area will have to be revised, however, in the light of recent and ongoing research programs concerned with the amino acid composition and nutritional value of plant proteins and their use for the prevention and treatment of protein malnutrition in children.[104–108]

A large majority of the world's population subsists on diets predominantly of vegetable protein origin. During the past decade, food scientists have addressed themselves to the problem of overcoming protein deficiency in developing countries. The utilization of plant proteins to meet the needs will hopefully do much to alleviate the urgency of the situation. Included in this category of protein sources are: cereals and millets, legumes, nuts and oilseeds, vegetables, and leaf and grass proteins.

With regard to the essential amino acid composition of common foods of vegetable origin, the data of Orr and Watt[86] and Kuppuswamy and co-workers[104] clearly indicate that the limiting amino acids in most cereals and millets are lysine and threonine; corn is also deficient in tryptophan. Legume proteins are a good source of lysine and threonine, but are deficient in sulfur amino acids and tryptophan. In the category of nuts and oilseeds, soybean proteins are rich in lysine and threonine, but poor in methionine; sesame and sunflower seed proteins are rich in sulfur amino acids and tryptophan, but lacking in lysine. Peanut proteins are deficient in lysine, methionine, and threonine. In the vegetable class, green pea is a good source of lysine, but poor in methionine content. The green leafy vegetable proteins are generally well balanced with respect to all essential amino acids except methionine. The available data[104,108a] on the amino acid composition of protein concentrates from leaves and grasses indicate that these proteins are fairly well balanced except for methionine.

The several factors affecting the nutritive value of plant proteins include the presence of trypsin and growth inhibitors,[108b,c] amino acid deficiencies, imbalance, toxicity, and antagonism,[76d,108d,e] availability of amino acids,[108f,g] effect of heat treatment,[108h,i] and the presence of unavailable carbohydrates.[11] In spite of these shortcomings, studies carried out by a host of workers have shown that two or three plant proteins can mutually supplement each other so that the resulting mixture can have a higher nutritive value than the individual proteins. Furthermore, studies of children on vegetable diets have shown that fortification of plant proteins with limiting amino acids can substantially increase nitrogen retention.[76c,108j]

Nutritionists in various countries have developed dried milk substitutes for feeding infants, and protein supplements based on plant proteins and reinforced with essential vitamins and minerals for improving the nutritive value of the diets of preschool and school children, as well as expectant and nursing mothers.[108k-o] These substitutes have been found to be almost as effective as milk in promoting growth and improving health conditions. In view of the acute shortage of milk in developing nations, the need for large-scale production and use of dried milk substitutes and fortified plant protein supplements is at once apparent. The painstaking efforts of several research teams in Guatemala, India, Nigeria, South Africa, the Congo, Senegal, and many other areas have provided ample evidence to spearhead a multidisciplinary approach involving scientific and technical personnel in this effort to eradicate malnutrition and its sequelae of human sufferings.

PROTEIN REQUIREMENT OF MAN AND SOME FACTORS INFLUENCING IT

The study of human protein requirements has engaged the interest of scientists for scores of years. The use of different methods and various criteria has compounded the problem so that definitive requirements have not been established to the satisfaction of many. The earliest studies recorded utilized food consumption data as a basis for recommendations. Subsequently, more sophisticated metabolic studies were carried out. The literature to date is replete with investigations of other factors affecting protein requirements, such as muscular activity, stress, nitrogen reserves, protein quality, essential and nonessential nitrogen and amino acid balance and ratios. Although most age groups from premature infants through the elderly have been studied, adult men and women and premature infants are the groups studied most thoroughly. The data for adolescents and the aged are relatively scant. An excellent review has recently appeared[108p] which contains a listing and description of studies and conclusions drawn on human protein requirements.

The minimum daily protein requirement, i.e., the smallest amino acid intake which can maintain optimum growth and good health in man, can be approximated only crudely. This is because short-term investigations cannot possibly reveal late effects of insufficient protein intake, and long-term experiments, requiring strict control of the diet, cannot be performed with any semblance of accuracy on men living a normal life. In short-term experiments the balance between dietary N-intake and urinary + fecal N-excretion has frequently been studied, but this actually seems to be a rather unreliable indicator of satisfactory protein intake. The investigations of Allison[109] show that the quantities of protein necessary to maintain nitrogen equilibrium vary according to the nutritional status of the subject. When the protein stores were exhausted even small amounts of absorbed N were sufficient to produce a positive N-balance. Likewise it was found that, in patients on rice diets, nitrogen equilibrium could be maintained with small quantities of protein—quantities which would not seem to be conducive to good health.[110] These latter results do not give much information regarding daily protein requirement, but, rather, indicate the poor nutritional status of the individual.

Actually the optimal or average daily protein requirement of man would be a more important value to establish than the protein minimum. "The task to obtain this information is a formidable one,"[111] and the sum of all the present data, including the National Research Council's recommended allowances, "represent little more than intelligent guesswork as to the quantities of protein which will amply cover man's needs." Dietary calculations are usually based on the "*Recommended Dietary Allowances*" published by the National Research Council.[111a]

These protein allowances are considered to cover individual variations among most normal persons as they live in the United States under usual environmental stresses. In tables prior to 1958, the recommended protein allowance for infants was 3.5 gm per kg. The change to 2.5 gm per kg is not in our opinion considered to be based on satisfactory evidence.

The *British* committee suggests that 11 per cent of the energy allowances in adults should normally be provided by protein and during growth, pregnancy and lactation, this should be increased to 14 per cent.

The *Canadian Standard* relates protein requirement to the three-fourth power of the body weight on the assumption that protein requirement varies with body size (protein gm 2.75 $W_{Kg}^{0.75}$).

The most serious shortcomings of all these calculations are that (1) they do not take into consideration differences in the biologic value of the different food proteins; (2) they do not consider the effect of mutual supplementation of simultaneously consumed proteins; and (3) they evidently cannot take into account human variations of nutritional individuality.

In addition to the foregoing factors, injury and advanced years have been shown to have a profound effect on human protein metabolism. Cuthbertson[112] first emphasized the increase in nitrogen loss which follows injury. This observation has since been amply confirmed by numerous investigators.[113] The extent of nitrogen loss after injury is roughly proportional to the magnitude of the insult and is most marked in the previously healthy young adult male. The reaction is less in females, children, the elderly, and the malnourished. The extent and duration of the losses resulting from different trauma are

shown in Figure 2A–8. The literature reflects major differences of opinion regarding the clinical importance of this nitrogen loss and the need to treat it.

Extensive studies have shown that injury appears to produce parallel increases in nitrogen excretion and basal metabolic expenditure. The nitrogen loss of injuries has been investigated in terms of (a) the role of starvation and immobilization, (b) the possible survival value, (c) the relation to endocrine stimuli, and (d) decreased anabolism versus increased catabolism. In summary, these investigations emphasize the central role of circulating amino acids and hepatic deamination in comparing "internal" nitrogen dynamics with "external" or conventional nitrogen-balance information.

The biochemical literature contains many reports confirming the existence of definite age changes in total protein, nucleic acids and nucleoproteins associated with alterations in their biologic, physical, and chemical properties.[114]

It has been reported that modifications in the concentration of free and total amino acids take place with age and reflect marked

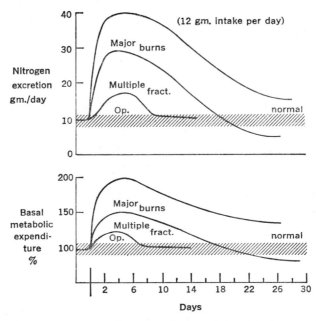

Fig. 2A-8. The approximate ranges and duration of increase in human nitrogen excretion and basal metabolic expenditure after uncomplicated elective operation (indicated as "Op."), multiple fractures, and severe burns. (Kinney,[113] *Protein Metabolism*, courtesy of Springer Verlag.)

alterations in biochemical equilibria.[115] The existence of age-induced biochemical changes finds support in a number of metabolic studies in man. Schulze[116,117] found that the minimal endogenous nitrogen excretion is lower in the aged and parallels the decreasing metabolic rate; and that proteins of animal origin are more useful than those of vegetable origin. His nitrogen-balance experiments indicated that a protein intake of 0.5 gm per kg per day maintains equilibrium in the oldster as well as in the young adult, provided the total caloric intake is adequate. A group of 36 hospitalized healthy volunteers between the ages of 60 and 92 years was fed a high-caloric, high-carbohydrate diet and the protein metabolism was estimated after a 10-day period. The results suggested that the minimum amount of protein required for nitrogen balance in the aged is equal to that required in the healthy young adult—roughly, 0.5 gm per kg per day. This requirement should be increased by a safety margin to overcome the effects of stress. Schulze felt that the oldster weighing 60 kg could take 1.0 to 1.5 gm of protein per kg per day in a mixed diet of about 2000 calories per day.

A study of the quantitative dietary needs for essential amino acids of man over 50 years of age to maintain nitrogen equilibrium was reported by Tuttle et al.[118] These studies were done with five healthy men in the age range 52 to 68 years, who were allowed to ambulate and work at hobbies, etc.,

in a metabolism ward for the period of study. The control period diet was composed of natural foods furnishing about 7 gm of nitrogen per day from good-quality protein and a caloric intake of 2014 to 2717 per day. When nitrogen equilibrium had been established the protein of the control diet was replaced by a test mixture of amino acids plus enough glycine to bring the total nitrogen intake up to 7 gm per day. The ratios of the amino acids in the test mixture were designed to approximate the composition of 18.75 gm of egg protein. Nitrogen equilibrium was achieved only when the amounts of essential amino acids in the basic mixtures were doubled. The over-all results from this investigation show that the amino acid needs of men over 50 years of age are in significant excess of the minima postulated by Rose.

These and other observations[120] point to the likelihood that the protein and amino acid needs of the aged may differ quantitatively and qualitatively from those of the young adult.

Specific Dynamic Action. The "specific dynamic action" was first described by Rubner who found that the consumption of protein-rich food raises the metabolic rate by about 12 per cent of the ingested food energy. The cause of this phenomenon has not yet been clarified in spite of many careful experiments and speculations. A new lead was offered when it was found that the consumption of incomplete proteins leads to a higher

Table 2A-6. Indispensable Amino Acid Needs of Men Over 50 Years of Age

Amino acid	Test mixture (gm)	Rose minimum (gm)	Test ±%
l-Leucine	1.72	1.10	+56
l-Isoleucine	1.28	0.70	+83
l-Lysine	1.39	0.80	+73
l-Threonine	0.77	0.50	+54
l-Tryptophan	0.38	0.25	+52
l-Valine	1.29	0.80	+61
l-Methionine	0.56	1.10	
l-Cystine	0.45	spares methionine	
l-Phenylalanine	0.96	1.10	
l-Tyrosine	0.60	spares phenylalanine	
l-Histidine	0.43	not essential	

From Higgons[119]

specific dynamic action than does consumption of complete proteins.[121] These experiments suggest that the metabolic transformation or the catabolism of those dietary amino acids which are not used for protein synthesis may be responsible for this phenomenon. The assumption that discarding amino acids present in excessive proportions is the causative factor is further supported by the finding that specific dynamic action does not seem to appear when ingested protein is used for growth and is deposited in the form of new tissue.

In calculating the protein requirement, the increment due to specific dynamic action used to be considered, to avoid possible deficits in protein supply. It should be emphasized, however, that the importance of the specific dynamic action of protein in practical nutrition seems to be highly overrated. "Practically nothing is known about it in human beings under ordinary conditions of activity and everyday living, and under normal food consumption at the usual intervals."[122] It, therefore, does not seem necessary to make special allowances for specific dynamic action in calculating the daily protein quota, since the increment of the metabolic rate is definitely *not* large enough to justify the often made assertion that a high specific dynamic action is primarily responsible for the "not fattening" or reducing effect of protein food.

In connection with diet calculations one must also consider that *physical activity* does not significantly increase the protein requirement.

Effect of Other Food Ingredients on Protein Utilization. In the foregoing sections human protein requirements were considered only with respect to amino acid composition, digestibility and some other properties of the dietary proteins themselves. Obviously, protein synthesis, growth and repair can occur only when the organism is supplied with other essential nutrients, such as vitamins and some inorganic substances. Another fact recognized as important long ago, but now too often forgotten, is that, in the absence of adequate caloric supply in the form of carbohydrates and fats, dietary amino acids cannot be utilized efficiently. This old rule, already

recognized by Voit, has gained increased significance because it has become therapeutic practice to administer protein concentrates or amino acid preparations *only* in cases where normal food intake is disturbed. This practice is based on the misconception that an adequate supply of amino acids by itself can prevent the destruction of body proteins. Another reason for the prominence of this problem was the search for satifactory survival rations in combat emergency.[123] These investigations have shown, in perfect support of earlier findings, that protein cannot be utilized for growth or maintenance nor can it prevent breakdown of tissue protein when the diet does not provide satisfactory quantities of other energy sources, such as carbohydrates and fats. This happens because the *energy requirement* of the organism has to be satisfied *first*. In starvation, in cases of restricted caloric intake, such as famine or reducing diets, the necessary energy is obtained by breakdown of tissue substances, including tissue protein. In cases where only proteins or amino acids are fed, these are metabolized into energy-yielding compounds and the nitrogen split off is excreted. It was found that, in people on severely restricted diets in general, nitrogen retention is proportional to caloric input but not proportional to the nitrogen input.[124] Most investigations seem to indicate that, unless about 50 to 60 per cent of the caloric requirement is satisfied by fat or carbohydrate, amino acids cannot be used for protein synthesis or other specific purposes. Accordingly, even the addition of 43 gm of high-grade protein, such as egg albumin, to a diet supplying a total of only 950 calories failed to improve the nitrogen balance of healthy adults over the group receiving a similar diet without protein. These results lead to the practical conclusion that proteins and amino acids should not be fed by themselves, *e.g.*, proteins "should be left out of any survival ration which provides for a daily intake of 900 calories or less."[124]

It also seems questionable whether feeding relatively large amounts of protein with severely restricted, low caloric reducing diets will protect body protein from destruction; in fact, loss of body protein on such diets has been demonstrated.[125]

In addition to their calorigenic action, carbohydrate and fat probably also have specific effects on protein metabolism.[126] Carbohydrate seems to be more effective; however, when it is provided by feeding about 150 to 200 gm of sugar, consumption of fat seems to exert an additional beneficial effect.[127,128]

The nitrogen-sparing action of sugar is most effective when it is consumed simultaneously with the protein. The timing seems to be very important, because, when glucose is fed more than four hours before or after the protein meal it loses its maximum protein-sparing action. As to the mechanisms by which carbohydrate and fat promote protein utilization apart from their calorigenic sparing action, several factors have to be considered.[129] Special attention has to be given to the retarding effect of these foods on gastro-intestinal dynamics, including gastric emptying time, secretion, motility and absorption. A prolonged digestion and protracted rate of amino acid absorption could well improve the utilization of dietary proteins. Also simultaneously fed sugar may promote protein synthesis by providing easily available precursors for rapid synthesis of some missing nonessential amino acids. Such an effect is suggested by the increased retention of ammonia, after feeding labeled ammonium citrate, when animals receive glucose, indicating that simultaneously fed sugar may expedite ammonia nitrogen utilization for amino acid synthesis.[130]

The effect of intermediary fat and carbohydrate metabolites in the metabolic phase of amino acid utilization may be very important. This has been indicated by results of experiments in man where simultaneous intravenous injection of a glucose solution considerably improved the utilization of injected amino acid mixtures.[131] Glucose also protects amino acids from breakdown. Thus, it was found that glycine given with sufficient amounts of sugar is largely retained, instead of being rapidly converted to urea.[132] It was also observed, *in vitro*, that intermediary products of fat and carbohydrate metabolism, such as lactate, pyruvate and succinate, inhibited the deamination of amino acids. Finally, carbohydrate and fat metabolites may provide some necessary links for the phosphorylation of amino acids or for other energy-consuming steps involved in the synthesis of body protein.

Effect of Excessive Amounts of Protein in Diet. The amino acid requirements are high in infancy, childhood, adolescence and during pregnancy because large amounts of proteins are newly formed in the rapidly growing tissues. Synthesis of milk proteins during lactation and growth of muscle tissue in the course of athletic training also increase the adult requirements. Similarly, replacement of lost tissue during convalescence after consumptive diseases or during rehabilitation following malnutrition requires an ample supply of dietary amino acids.

The utilization of dietary amino acids for protein synthesis is limited by the actual requirements of the body for growth and maintenance.

Protein, unlike fat, cannot be stored in appreciable quantities; therefore, dietary amino acids consumed in excess of the requirements are further metabolized, *i.e.*, after decarboxylation they enter the common mill by which carbohydrates and fats are utilized.[133] It is therefore not economical to feed relatively expensive high-protein foods in abnormally high quantities.

The question whether consumption of excessive amounts of proteins has any harmful effect cannot be answered without qualification. It is well established that Arctic explorers and other persons kept on well-controlled diets, subsisting for many years mainly on meat, do not develop any pathologic symptoms. We can, therefore, conclude that normal adults seem able to tolerate a protein intake far above actual requirements. Infants and children, particularly those not adapted to high-protein foods, do not do well on diets containing large amounts of protein.[134] It is, therefore, recommended by several authors that the protein intake be increased only gradually. This suggestion has to be considered, particularly in connection with rehabilitation diets given after malnutrition.

In addition to decreased protein efficiency, excessive ingestion of protein may lead to fluid imbalances. This circumstance arises from the fact that, whereas 350 gm of water are required for the metabolism of 100 calories of protein, approximately only 50 gm are required for the metabolism of 100 calories of either carbohydrates or fats. Thus, the consumption of protein over and above the usual levels, namely 15 per cent of the total caloric intake, can lead to increased water requirements and increased levels of end products of protein metabolism in the blood stream. These associated phenomena have been designated the protein overload effect.[135] It is obvious that the therapeutic use of high-protein diets should be carefully controlled.

The idea that excessive protein intake may lead to development of, or aggravate already existing, hypertension, or that it may cause toxic complications in pregnancy has been abandoned.[136] The assumption that protein food, due to its specific dynamic effect, may adversely influence the course of febrile diseases also proved to be false. The idea that large amounts of protein may damage the kidneys or liver has never been supported by observations in man. Even the exclusion of protein from the diet of people with developed liver or kidney damage is an obsolete practice. More recent studies have shown that diets containing ample amounts of protein very often improve the healing tendency in liver or kidney diseases. Therefore, hypertension, febrile diseases, kidney or liver ailments are no longer considered generally as contraindications to protein-rich diets. On the other hand, they should not be regarded as indications for feeding excessive amounts of protein. There is no wisdom in prolonged feeding of diets containing more protein than 20 per cent of the total caloric intake. Clinical observations suggest, and animal experiments prove, that in certain specific types of liver disturbance feeding of unduly high amounts of proteins may aggravate the disease by overtaxing liver functions involved in utilization of dietary amino acids.[137,138] It is also self-evident that in kidney diseases where there is a danger of accumulation of protein end products, with increased blood NPN, the protein intake should be restricted or even temporarily eliminated. Finally, in some cases of meta-bolic disturbances, such as cystinuria, phenylketonuria, alkaptonuria and gout, protein restriction may be of therapeutic value.[139]

FATE OF ABSORBED DIETARY AMINO ACIDS

Dynamic Equilibrium Between Tissue Proteins and Dietary Amino Acids. Amino acids absorbed in the intestines are carried with the portal blood to the liver.[140,141] Some of them are retained there to satisfy the specific requirements of this organ: the rest enter the general circulation, from which they are rapidly removed by the several tissues. This uptake, which may occur against concentration gradients as high as 1:9, seems to involve specific, selective mechanisms.[142] The liver and the kidneys are the most active in removal, while skeletal muscle is less efficient. The brain does not show any detectable uptake. The fate of the amino acids in each tissue varies according to the momentarily prevalent requirement. If enough non-protein calories are provided, the amino acids are utilized for specific purposes, such as the synthesis of proteins and of biologically active polypeptides or peptides, e.g., the synthesis of oxytocin, enzymes, glutathione or carnosine. The amino acids may also be directly transformed into other physiologically important compounds, such as epinephrine, creatine, taurine and many others.

Besides these well-recognized functions, amino acids participate in the process of "dynamic equilibrium" which exists between tissue proteins and dietary amino acids. This phenomenon was first suggested by the experiments of Schoenheimer, who showed that when labeled amino acids are fed the labels are incorporated relatively rapidly into the proteins of the different tissues. He demonstrated that tissue proteins are not rigid structures but that there is a steady "give and take" between tissue protein and dietary amino acids. This revolutionary new concept contradicted most of the earlier theories, which had assumed that tissue proteins do not regularly enter metabolism systems but are used up slowly by the daily anabolism and catabolism. According to the old theory, tissue proteins are mobilized only when the "exogenous" supply, *i.e.*, the dietary amino acid intake, is deficient. Before Schoenheimer's classic experiments, Borsook and Keighley's investigations already indicated a *continuous metabolism* of tissue proteins, even when exogenous protein supply and food intake were satisfactory.[1]

Schoenheimer and collaborators found that the rate of labeled amino acid incorporation is not equal for every tissue but depends on the life span of particular tissue proteins. Tissues containing short-lived proteins show a rapid turnover, *i.e.*, they take up and lose labeled compounds fast. That the uptake of dietary amino acids parallels the metabolic rate is indicated by the fact that fetal tissue, tumors and rejuvenating organs incorporate labeled compounds faster than do normal adult tissues. Schoenheimer's original assumption that all body proteins participate in the dynamic equilibrium has been modified by investigations which show that only about 30 per cent of human carcass protein is involved in the dynamic state, while the rest is relatively or absolutely unreactive.[143]

The ease with which labeled amino acids are incorporated into some tissue proteins forecasts a drastic revision of the current concept of the rigid structure of living protein. At present it is difficult to visualize how and why peptide bonds of preformed tissue proteins should be steadily cleaved and reformed—a process which seems to be a prerequisite for the incorporation of dietary amino acids into tissue proteins.

Biosynthesis of Proteins. Feeding experiments indicate that, for optimal protein synthesis, all constituent amino acids must be present simultaneously and in adequate quantities. If one or more of the essential amino acids are missing or are not supplied in satisfactory quantities, the rest of the amino acids, which have not been utilized for protein synthesis, are irreversibly metabolized. Excess amino acids can neither be stored in the body nor used for formation of partial building stones (plasteins) from which protein synthesis could proceed eventually. Any delay in supplementation of the missing amino acids decreases utilization so that, when 4 to 6 hours intervene between feeding the incomplete mixture and the missing

amino acids, there is detectable interference with protein synthesis.[144,145] Single-labeled amino acids disappear from the metabolic pool within 4 hours.[146]

Soon after World War II, carbon-34 became available for experimental use. This important tool allowed the biochemist to follow the course of reactions so rapid or so minute as to be otherwise immeasurable. A second significant advance was the development of cell-free *in vitro* systems capable of synthesizing specific proteins. This allowed the scientist to separate the systems, purify the fractions, and scrutinize individual steps of proteins synthesis.

With these new tools in hand, scientists soon embarked on studies designed to clarify the chemical nature and functions of the gene—defined by the classic work of Mendel as the functional unit of inheritance. Ingenious studies showed that, through the mediation of a specific chemical substance, the parent cell passes on to the daughter cell its own characteristics. In other words, the daughter cell inherits the capacity to secrete a hormone or to become a muscle fiber from "data" supplied by its parent. This "genetic information," as it is now called, was found to be in the structure of deoxyribonucleic acid (DNA).

DNA molecules are not "genes." Genes can be better described as formal entities whose roles are frequently manifested by DNA molecules (or perhaps by DNA molecules combined with special proteins).

The DNA molecule is extremely large and belongs to the general class of molecules designated as "polymers." In its natural state, DNA appears to consist of two intertwining chains (or strands) of polymers forming a long helical molecule. As is characteristic of polymers, DNA is made up of a very large number of subunit molecules called "nucleotides." Each nucleotide is composed of a purine base attached to a phosphorylated sugar.

The characteristics of every cell are determined by its proteins, particularly the enzymes. DNA contains the information, or plan, necessary for protein formation in "programmed," or code, form. Since proteins are made up of some twenty different amino acids, this code must direct the formation of protein molecules by describing specific and different sequences of these amino acids. Current evidence suggests that the sequence of nucleotides in DNA comprises the code.

Although DNA is found in the nucleus of a typical animal cell, most protein synthesis occurs in the cytoplasm. Evidence now suggests that the messenger carrying the information to the site of protein synthesis is a special type of ribonucleic acid called "messenger ribonucleic acid" (or, more simply, "messenger RNA"). RNA is a polymer very similar in structure to DNA. There are, however, two important differences: (1) RNA contains ribose (a sugar) in place of the deoxyribose of DNA, and (2) one nucleotide base is different. In RNA, uracil is present in place of its close relative, thymine, in DNA. In addition, it appears that messenger RNA may consist of only one strand. Once the information in DNA is copied in the nucleus in the form of messenger RNA, this molecule escapes from the nucleus and moves to the site of protein synthesis in the cytoplasm—that is, the ribosomes. There it acts as a template, or plan, for protein synthesis. Although the exact function of ribosomes is not clear, it is known that many of the enzymes necessary

for the final steps in protein synthesis are associated with these particles. Granting that proteins are long polymers of amino acids joined by peptide bonds, protein synthesis in the simplest case would be the polymerization of amino acids by the formation of peptide bonds. Synthesis of these bonds requires energy.[147]

In Figure 2A–9 are summarized the major steps in protein synthesis. Free amino acids within the cell may arise from one of two sources. First, they may be transported into the cell from the extracellular fluid or, second, amino acids may be synthesized by the fixation of ammonia with α-ketoglutarate to form glutamic acid, which can undergo transamination to form any of the nonessential amino acids. Intracellular amino acids are activated in a reaction requiring ATP to form amino acid adenylates, which are then bound to soluble ribonucleic acid, forming the soluble RNA-amino acid complexes. A separate and specific soluble RNA exists for each of the amino acids. In a reaction requiring guanosine triphosphate (GTP), these RNA-amino acids are transferred into the ribosomes of the microsomes where peptide bonding occurs, resulting in the formation of ribonucleoproteins. The completed protein is subsequently stripped off the

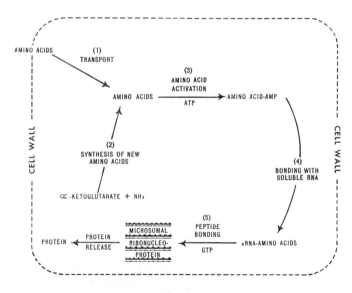

Fig. 2A-9. The mechanism of protein biosynthesis. (Wilson,[148] *Protein Metabolism,* courtesy of Springer Verlag.)

ribosome particle and released into the soluble portion of the cell.

Protein molecules used up in daily anabolic and catabolic processes have to be replaced by a synthesis which, like growth, requires the simultaneous presence of all the requisite amino acids. In a normal adult about 1.3 gm of protein is synthesized per kg of body weight per day, i.e., 91 gm for a 70-kg man.[143] The amount of protein built up for so-called adult growth, as formation of hair, nails, secretions, hormones and enzymes, is quantitatively negligible. Most of the proteins synthesized in the adult under physiologic conditions serve to replace tissue proteins actually broken down in connection with life processes. The "turnover rate" as determined with tagged amino acids indicates that the necessity for replacement varies according to the function of the different organs. Thus, the half-life of serum and liver proteins is approximately 10 days, while that of hemoglobin is 25 to 30 days, and that of muscle protein is about 185 days. Even within a given organ the turnover rate may be different for different protein fractions. The highest *rate* of protein formation has been found in the pancreas and in the intestines, *i.e.*, in organs which constantly lose newly formed proteins with their secretions.

Quantitatively, however, the most active site of protein synthesis is the liver. In addition to producing liver protein, it is also the main site of plasma albumin and fibrinogen synthesis. Serum globulin seems to be chiefly synthesized extrahepatically.

It is often assumed that plasma albumin is a transport form of protein during passage from the liver to the tissues. In experiments on the isolated mammary gland it has been shown that albumin can be used for synthesis of milk proteins, but only after degradation to amino acids.[149,150] Transfer of larger fragments, such as peptides produced by breakdown of albumin, to the newly formed milk protein does not seem to occur. It appears that plasma albumin, which has to fulfill other physiologic functions, serves only occasionally as a source of amino acids for protein synthesis.

Hoffenberg et al. used ^{131}I-labeled albumin to study 8 human subjects before and after experimental partial protein depletion and repletion. Analysis of pool sizes and turnover rates following depletion showed a marked lowering of the extravascular albumin compartment out of proportion to the fall in plasma albumin concentration and, possibly, preceding it. At the same time, albumin synthesis was greatly diminished. This pattern was constant in 7 of 8 subjects studied. Protein repletion reversed these changes.[151]

The main source of raw materials for protein formation in the tissues is the amino acids present in the tissue fluids. It has become customary to refer to the mixture of amino acids present in the different tissue fluids as the "*metabolic pool*" of amino acids, although recent experiments disprove the existence of a single homogeneous metabolic pool.

Besides synthesis of proteins, the amino acids are used for formation of smaller peptides whose biologic significance is not well understood. A list of such peptides must include *glutathione*, a tripeptide of glutamic acid, cystine, and glycine; *anserine*, containing β-alanine and histidine, and its methylated analogue *carnosine*. The major physiologic problem, *viz.*, which factors initiate and determine the extent of this peptide synthesis, is unsolved.

Metabolism of Amino Acids. The general metabolic fate of amino acids is determined by their common structural elements. A terminal carboxyl group and an amino group in the α-position* are characteristic of the amino acids naturally occurring in proteins. Proline and hydroxyproline, containing an imino group, form an exception. Due to this general structure the amino acids can participate in several bioprocesses, including peptide and protein synthesis (already discussed), deamination and decarboxylation.

Deamination. The first step on the pathway of amino acid catabolism is usually *deamination*. The basic amino group is split off and the amphoteric mono-amino acids are transformed into α-keto acids. It is an oxidative process and the elimination of two $-NH_2$ groups requires the uptake of 1 mole of oxygen. Amino acid oxidases are present in

---

* In human and animal tissues, β-alanine is present in carnosine, anserine and pantothenic acid. It may arise by decarboxylation of aspartic acid.

largest quantity in the liver and kidneys. They require flavoproteins as coenzyme. The importance of the liver in deamination has been demonstrated by the fact that, in hepatectomized animals and in acute liver atrophy in man, deamination is seriously disturbed. The deaminases or amino acid oxidases are highly specific; they act only on the L-amino acids. Although the presence of large amounts of D-amino oxidases in the organism has been established, their physiologic role has not been recognized because, under normal conditions, D-amino acids are neither taken in with the food nor produced in the body. Some amino acids require the action of specific deaminating enzymes; e.g., the existence of specific enzymes for selective deamination of glycine and glutamic acid has been demonstrated.

Urea Formation. Liberated $-NH_2$ can be utilized for production of other amino acids by transamination of their precursors. Most of it, however, goes to form urea, much of it without going through the free ammonia stage. This transport occurs in the form of glutamic or aspartic acid or their derivatives which take up the $-NH_2$ split off from amino acids.

Deamination of amino acids forms large amounts of ammonia which, if allowed to accumulate, would be highly toxic. Normally, the blood contains only 0.1 to 0.2 mg per cent of ammonia nitrogen, an amount so small that special techniques are required for its determination. A concentration of 5 mg per cent is fatal to the rabbit. The animal body detoxifies it rapidly in the liver before release into the systemic circulation. In man and other mammals detoxication is achieved largely by conversion to urea, whereas, in reptiles and birds, uric acid is formed. Considerable ammonia nitrogen may be excreted in the urine, but this is formed in the kidney and does not appreciably increase the ammonia content of the systemic blood.

In 1882, von Schroeder showed that perfusion of the dog's liver with blood containing ammonium carbonate caused the formation of urea, but no urea was produced when the liver was excluded from the circulation and the blood passed through the muscles and other organs.[152] Salaskin[153] showed that the liver forms urea when amino acids are perfused through it. Conclusive evidence that the liver is the site of urea formation was afforded by the work of Bollman et al.[154] on dogs from which the liver or kidneys, or both, had been removed. If the kidneys alone were removed, preventing excretion, the blood urea rose rapidly. If the liver was removed, and the kidneys were left intact, the blood urea fell. If both the kidneys and liver were removed, the blood urea remained constant, since urea was neither being formed nor excreted.[155]

The earliest contribution to our present knowledge of urea synthesis was made by Kossel and Dakin[156] who found that a tissue enzyme, arginase, hydrolyzed arginine to urea and ornithine.

The next step in the elucidation of urea synthesis was made in 1932 by Krebs and Henseleit.[157] These investigators, while studying urea formation from carbon dioxide and ammonia by rat liver slices surviving in vitro, found that the addition of ornithine to the incubation fluid greatly accelerated the formation of urea. Low concentrations were effective, and the amount of urea formed was out of proportion to the amount of ornithine added. Since the ornithine did not disappear from the system, and since each molecule of it stimulated the synthesis of 30 molecules of urea, it was inevitably concluded that ornithine acted as a catalyst. Krebs also found that the addition of either citrulline or arginine stimulated urea synthesis to a remarkable degree. In order to explain the catalytic effect of these compounds, Krebs proposed the series of reactions, outlined below, which are known collectively as the "ornithine cycle." Although further research has greatly elaborated Krebs' ornithine cycle and also served to integrate it with other metabolic mechanisms, its basic form remains unaltered.

The mechanism of urea synthesis was clarified greatly when Cohen and associates[158-161] developed cell-free preparations of liver tissue that would synthesize urea, and subsequently separated the preparations into a mitochondrial fraction that carried out the

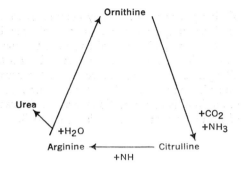

conversion of ornithine to citrulline, and a soluble protein fraction responsible for the transformation of citrulline to arginine.[162]

Beginning with Voit[163] in 1866, and through the first quarter of this century, the measurement of urea output was almost universally employed as an index of the quantity and quality of protein ingested, as well as a determinant of the effects of other foodstuffs on protein utilization.[164] The data collected in a study typical of this era are those reported by Smith[165] (Table 2A-7). It will be seen that the relationship of various nitrogen metabolites to protein intake differs quantitatively. The excretion of creatinine and uric acid remains relatively constant, whereas the output of urea and ammonia varies with intake. In these studies, Smith made no effort to establish nitrogen equilibrium but demonstrated that fecal nitrogen was relatively constant (average, 1 gm/24 hours).

More recently, Puchal and his associates[166] have found that plasma urea values appear to be inversely proportional to the gain in body weight and feed efficiency (Fig. 2A-10).

Arroyave and associates[167] have found that blood urea levels may serve not only as criteria of nutritional status in children suffering from kwashiorkor, but also as a measure of the biologic value of the repleting diet.

Further practical applications of urea levels as parameters of protein metabolism require a detailed review of the reports of San Pietro and Rittenberg[168,169] on the relationships of urea space and urea pool to protein synthesis in humans. In the development of their thesis it is assumed that, in mammals, urea is the major nitrogenous end product of protein metabolism, and that it serves no nutritive purpose. The rate of excretion of urinary urea is thus related to the rate of oxidative metabolism of the proteins whether of tissue or dietary origin.

Since urea appears to traverse all the membranes of the mammalian organism without apparent resistance, the total urea nitrogen content of the body is related to the blood urea nitrogen, as follows:

Total body urea N (mg) = 10 × blood urea N (mg/100 ml) × urea space (liters).

The size of the urea space (or pool) was measured directly with ^{15}N-labeled urea and found to be equivalent to total body water.

The kinetic interrelationships of the major nitrogenous pools of the body are assumed to be illustrated by the following scheme (Fig. 2A-11). In these calculations, let the nitro-

Table 2A-7.   Variation of Nitrogen Output as a Function of Intake in Man

Nitrogen intake (gm/day)	Urinary nitrogen (gm/day)					% of total urinary nitrogen A			
	Total A	Urea B	Am- monia C	Creati- nine D	Uric acid E	B	C	D	E
Ad libitum	12.03	10.20	0.50	0.68	0.15	83	4	6	1
0.97	2.17	0.81	0.34	0.57	0.12	37	16	16	6
0.70	1.90	0.48	0.33	0.59	0.14	24	17	30	7
0.36	1.63	0.32	0.20	0.56	0.12	20	12	34	7

(Smith, J., courtesy of J. Biol. Chem.)

gen content of the metabolic pool be P gm of nitrogen. Dietary nitrogen enters the metabolic pool at the rate of D gm of nitrogen per day. Some of the components are used for protein synthesis at the rate of S gm of nitrogen per day; another part, E_u gm of nitrogen per day, is converted to urea. The remainder of the nitrogen excreted is denoted by E_x (gm of nitrogen per day). They assume E_x to be small as compared to E_u. The total urea in the organism, U gm of nitrogen, is the urea pool. Urea enters it at the rate of E_u gm of nitrogen per day and leaves it at the same rate via the urine. Since they assume that the animal is in the stationary state, the rate of protein breakdown, R, is equal to S.

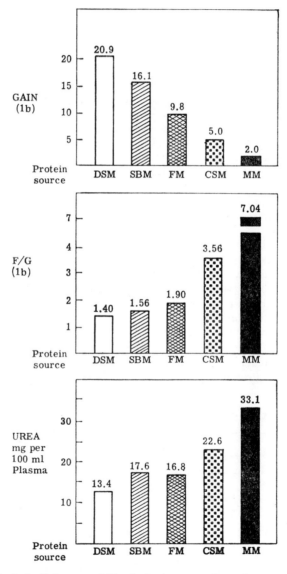

Fig. 2A-10. Growth, feed efficiency, and blood plasma urea values of young pigs fed different sources of proteins. DSM indicates dried skim milk; SBM, soybean meal; FM, fish meal; CSM, cottonseed meal; and MM, meat meal. Error mean square for testing treatment effects equals: 7.70 for total gain, 2.59 for F/G. (Puchal *et al.*, courtesy of J. Nutrition.)

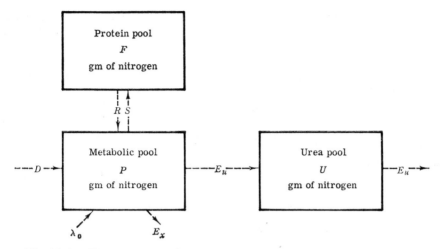

Fig. 2A-11. The kinetic interrelationships of the major nitrogen pools of the body. (San Pietro and Rittenberg, courtesy of J. Biol. Chem.)

If the total excretion of nitrogen in the urine is defined to be E_r, then

$$E_r = E_u + E_x.$$

For the stationary state,

$$D = E_r; \quad R = S$$

that is, for a subject in nitrogen balance, the rates of nitrogen intake and excretion are equal, and the rates of synthesis and breakdown of proteins are similarly equal.

The extensive isotopic data obtained by San Pietro and Rittenberg[168,169] in humans show that the size of the metabolic pool is small and may be indicated by the urinary ammonia, and that this pool is turning over at a rapid rate. These observations also suggest that the size of the urea pool is basic to an evaluation of the interrelationships between amino acids and protein metabolism.

Schimke[170] found that variations in urea excretion may be largely mediated by alterations in levels of enzymes specifically associated with urea synthesis. Starvation was associated with a five-fold increase in urea excretion, whereas a protein-free diet resulted in a 25 per cent decrease in urea excretion in comparison to rats fed a 15 per cent protein diet.

Studies of the excretion of ^{15}N-labeled urea following the administration of ^{15}N-labeled glycine revealed that growth hormone exerts very significant effects on protein metabolism. Using the method of San Pietro and Rittenberg[169] to calculate results, it was found that growth hormone increases the metabolic pool for nitrogen and the rate of protein synthesis, while the turnover rate of the pool is decreased. These results seem to be in accord with observations in the literature obtained with different techniques.[171]

Decarboxylation.[172,173] An alternate pathway of amino acid catabolism is *decarboxylation* whereby the pharmacologically inert amino acids are transformed into for the most part highly active amines. Decarboxylation itself involves splitting off CO_2 and the enzymes which perform this reaction seem to be highly specific for each amino acid. With the exception of histidine decarboxylase, all require the participation of pyridoxal phosphate as coenzyme. Decarboxylation by intestinal bacteria was recognized early and the increased formation of *putrescine* from ornithine, of *cadaverine* from lysine, *histamine* from histidine, and *tyramine* from tyrosine in the intestinal tract was often considered a sign of pathologic putrefaction leading to "intestinal autointoxication." It was shown later, however, that under normal conditions the intestinal wall and the liver can detoxicate most of the amines absorbed from the gut.

Not only the intestinal flora but also many tissues have the ability to convert amino acids into amines by decarboxylation. Thus the kidneys, and especially the liver, seem to be responsible for the formation of amines such as *tryptamine* (β-indolethylamine) from tryptophan, of *tyramine* from tyrosine, and possibly of *histamine* from histidine. The presence of large amounts of glutamic acid decarboxylase was discovered in the brain tissue. This enzyme removes only one carboxyl group from the dicarboxylic acid to produce α-amino butyric acid instead of an amine.

Another biologically important group of amines results when decarboxylation is preceded by some other metabolic changes in the original amino acid molecule. From cystic acid a cystine derivative, *taurine*, is produced by decarboxylation. Hydroxytryptophan is decarboxylated to *hydroxytryptamine*. This substance, also called "serotonin," is present in the blood and is possibly connected with the development of some types of hypertension. *Norepinephrine*, a hormone produced by the adrenal medulla, seems to be a decarboxylation product of dihydroxy-β-phenylalanine, the latter constituting an oxidation product of phenylalanine. Norepinephrine is further transformed to epinephrine, by methylation, involving the methyl group of methionine. The formation of other amines in the body, such as *ethanolamine* and *spermine*, has also been established. The large number of the so-called *biogenic amines*[174] in living organisms and their pharmacologic activity suggests that some symptoms of infectious diseases may be brought about by amines produced by the infective microorganisms. The pathogenesis of some other diseases may be associated with the action of amines produced in the disturbed intermediary metabolism.

The further metabolic fate of most of the derived compounds is closely linked to that of fats and carbohydrates. Certain of these, such as the amines, the imidazol-, the sulfur-, the indol- and the phenolic compounds, require specific enzyme systems for further metabolic changes. The keto acids produced by deamination of amino acids participate in either glycogen, fat or ketone body formation. However, the classification of amino acids as glycogenic or ketogenic substances seems to be too rigid and perhaps obsolete in the light of recent biochemical research. A thorough discussion of abnormal urinary amino acid metabolites which arise as a result of disturbances in the metabolic pathways of intermediary metabolism has been prepared by Sprince.[174a]

Transformation into Other Compounds. Besides participating in protein syntheses, the amino acids are utilized by the organism as precursors of some *hormones, vitamins, coenzymes,* and other compounds. Such so-called *"extra-protein functions"* of the amino acids can often be differentiated experimentally from the "protein function" by observing the effects after feeding a particular amino acid simultaneously with or apart from the other amino acids. Thus, tryptophan promotes niacin formation and cures niacin deficiency even when fed alone. Similarly, methionine displays its lipotropic effect even when fed apart from other amino acids.

Phenylalanine and tyrosine, which are formed by oxidation of the phenol ring in paraposition, are precursors of two types of hormonal substances. The formation of *norepinephrine* and *epinephrine* in the adrenals by decarboxylation has already been discussed. The iodination of tyrosine to *monoiodo-* and *diiodo-tyrosine* and their condensation by the thyroid cells to *thyroxine* and *triiodo-thyronine* are currently the subject of numerous investigations. *Melanin*, a dark, insoluble pigment normally present in the skin, in the hair and some other tissues, also seems to be formed from phenylalanine[175] under physiologic conditions. This process is decreased or absent in *albinism*. Abnormally large quantities of melanin are formed or accumulated in certain tumors such as *melanomas* or excreted with the urine in *melanuria*.

Phenylalanine and tyrosine may enter different metabolic pathways and several phases of these may be blocked by damage of the liver, or by hereditary gene-linked "metabolic errors," or even by some vitamin deficiencies. Impaired phenylalanine metabolism in cases of liver damage leads to *phenylketonuria*. In such cases, because of disturbed oxidation in the benzene ring, some other products of imperfect metabolism, such as phenyl-lactic acid, are also excreted. Besides disturbed oxidation, the ultimate breakdown of the ring structure is abnormal and hence *p*-hydroxy-phenylpyruvic acid is found in such urines.

Scorbutic guinea pigs and some premature children excrete similar compounds in their urines; in such instances large doses of ascorbic or folic acid may correct the metabolic disturbance. There are, however, cases where not a lack of vitamins but rather a hereditary derangement of the enzyme system is responsible for the "metabolic error"; *e.g.*, the phenylpyruvic acid excretion observed in *Folling's* disease ("oligophrenia phenylpyruvica").[176-179]

In another inborn metabolic error, *alkaptonuria*, 2-5-dihydroxy-phenylacetic acid (*homogentisic acid*) is excreted in the urine. The same compound is deposited in *ochronosis* and in some cases of *osteoarthritis*.

A versatile amino acid is *glycine*. It is a constituent of the tripeptide *glutathione;* it participates in the biosynthesis of a bile acid, *glycocholic acid;* it is utilized for the formation of *purines*, of *uric acid*, of *porphyrins*, and may be converted into other amino acids such as *serine* or *cystine*. It is conjugated with benzoic acid to *hippuric acid*. Finally, it participates via glycocyamine in the formation of *creatine*. Glycine, when administered to animals in large doses, produces toxic symptoms. This effect can be prevented by the simultaneous intake of large amounts of vitamin B_{12} and/or folic acid.

The results of intensive investigations of the biotransformation of *tryptophan* into *nicotinic* acid have shown that it involves numerous intermediary steps.[180-182] See Chapter 5, Section 7.

Studies of the urinary metabolites of the tryptophan——→ nicotinic acid pathway have led to numerous investigations to determine the enzymatic activities involved under various physiologic and pathologic conditions. Directly or indirectly, many of these observations concern problems of nutritional biochemistry.[183]

Methionine is particularly interesting because its therapeutic use in liver diseases was widely recommended as recently as a few years ago. This suggestion was based on experiments on animals in which liver damage with fat deposition was produced by inade-

quate diets. In such cases addition of methionine to the diet had a beneficial, *lipotropic* effect. Some clinical investigators, encouraged by these experiments on animals, prescribed synthetic methionine in human liver diseases. These reports, at first enthusiastic, turned out later to be not too encouraging. Methionine proved to be of little value in nutritional liver disease, such as kwashiorkor. Methionine treatment seems to give reliable results only when the liver has been damaged by a specific, experimental methionine deficiency. In fact, recent studies indicate that, in some clinical cases, methionine utilization by the damaged liver is disturbed. Methionine can be transformed to cystine and, as a methyl donor, it participates in the biosyntheses of choline, creatine, epinephrine and sarcosine; the latter being a methyl derivative of carnosine (β-alanyl-histidine). The importance of methionine in transmethylation processes, first demonstrated in Du Vigneaud's[184] important investigations, has recently been somewhat reduced. Vitamin B_{12} and folic acid promote the production and the transfer of labile methyl groups and, therefore, decrease the methionine requirement. Methionine itself can be produced in the body after feeding its methyl-free precursor, *homocystine*, and satisfactory amounts of cobalamin (B_{12}).

Aminoacidurias. After feeding protein foods, the gradual digestion and absorption so operate as to yield only a small increase in the amino acid concentration in the blood. Even on feeding or intravenous injection of amino acid solutions there is only a transitory increase in the blood amino acid concentration. However, plasma and tissues contain, in the late post-absorptive stage or in starvation, a certain amount of free amino acids. It is not yet clear whether these are merely in the state of regular transport from one tissue to another or whether they are essential homeostatic constituents. The blood amino acids are filtered or excreted in the glomeruli and are reabsorbed in a highly selective manner by the renal tubules.[185] The urine contains under normal circumstances some amino acids, both in free and in conjugated form. The total daily excretion is, on the average, 160 mg for a normal adult, *i.e.*, less

Table 2A-8. Provisional Classification of the Aminoacidurias*

I — Aminoaciduria without renal tubular defect, with raised plasma amino acid level		II — Aminoaciduria with renal tubular defect, without a raised plasma amino acid level				III — Aminoaciduria with renal tubular defect, with raised plasma amino acid level	
Acquired†	*Congenital†*	*Acquired*		*Congenital*		*Acquired*	
		With metabolic disorder	*Without metabolic disorder*	*With metabolic disorder*	*Without metabolic disorder*	*With metabolic disorder*	*Without metabolic disorder*
Liver disease	Phenylketonuria Tyrosinosis Alkaptonuria "Maple Syrup" disease	Wilson's disease Galactosemia Rickets Scurvy Nephrotic syndrome	Heavy metal poisoning (lead, cadmium, mercury, uranium, copper) Oxalic acid poisoning Lysol poisoning Burns	Fanconi syndrome Cystinosis Hartnup disease	Cystine-lysinuria	Celiac disease Adult idiopathic steatorrhea	Phosphorus poisoning

* *Chromatographic and Electrophoretic Techniques. I. Chromatography* (I. Smith, Editor) courtesy of Interscience Publishers, 1960.
† The terms "acquired" and "congenital" refer to the amino acid disorder, not to the metabolic disorder.

than 1 per cent of the total daily amino acid intake.

If the amino acid concentration in the blood increases over the threshold level, as after ingestion or rapid injections of concentrated amino acid solutions, an *alimentary* aminoaciduria develops. In mice and rats, after feeding incomplete proteins, one part of the amino acids not used for protein synthesis or for production of other specific compounds is excreted with the urine. In man, however, the amino acid content of the urine seems to be largely independent of the quality of protein present in the food.[186]

Since the kidneys are both a "clearing house" for the circulating plasma and a cellular body with a metabolism of its own, the over-all urinary picture must have a twofold interpretation. Accumulated data allow us to use this basic distinction for a classification of the pathologic aminoacidurias; in other words, we find one group of aminoacidurias that appears to be chiefly due to an overflow into the urine of raised plasma

amino acids, and another group of aminoacidurias in which a renal tubular defect interferes with the reabsorption of amino acids from the glomerular filtrate. With the scanty knowledge at our disposal, a provisional general classification must suffice; it is summarized in Table 2A–8. Prolonged inanition of a selective type that is a sequel to various forms of intestinal disease gives rise to a mixed form of aminoaciduria in which both liver dysfunction and renal tubular defect play a part.

In the lesser degrees of induced aminoaciduria only the so-called central cluster of amino acids (Fig. 2A–12) is found in significant amounts. As the aminoaciduria becomes more marked, the basic amino acids, lysine and arginine, appear as well as the sulfur-containing compounds, cystine and methionine. The other amino acids that are normally almost completely reabsorbed, such as the leucines, valine, phenylalanine, tyrosine, hydroxyproline, and proline, also appear. It is not possible to distinguish among

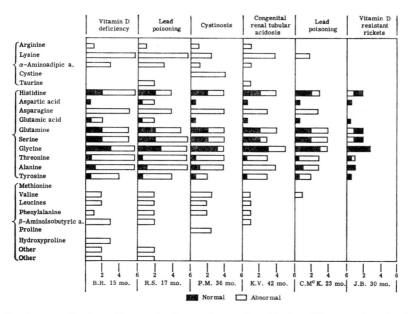

Fig. 2A-12. Pattern of amino acid excretion in acquired aminoacidurias. The excretion of each individual amino acid is indicated by the length of the bar; the solid portion represents the average normal value in children. The central cluster of amino acids includes those which are normally found in the urine. In the mild generalized aminoacidurias there is simply an increased excretion of this group. As the aminoaciduria becomes more severe, amino acids appear in the urine which are ordinarily not found in detectable amounts (Harrison, *in* Amino Acid and Protein Metabolism, Report of the Thirtieth Ross Conference on Pediatric Research [S. J. Foman, Editor].)

Table 2A-9. The Renal Tubular Failures (Nontoxic, Congenital)*

Normal function of renal tubular segment (proximal tubule)	Pathologic syndromes		Benign syndromes		
	Fanconi syndrome cystinosis	Cystine-lysinuria	Renal glycosuria	Renal glycosuria rickets	Renal aminoaciduria
REABSORPTION OF:	FAILURE TO REABSORB COMPLETELY:				
Basic amino acids	All amino acids	Basic amino acids only (cystine, lysine, arginine, ornithine)			All amino acids
Hydroxy amino acids					
Monoamino, monocarboxylic amino acids					
Glycine, creatine, phosphate	Phosphate†			Phosphate	All amino acids
Glucose	Glucose†		Glucose	Glucose	
Bicarbonate	Bicarbonate†				
Chloride					
Sodium					
Potassium	Potassium†				
Water (obligatory, isosmotic)	Water†				

* Chromatographic and Electrophoretic Techniques. I. Chromatography (I. Smith, Editor) Interscience Publishers, 1960.
† In some cases.

the various forms of induced renal amino-aciduria by the pattern of excretion of amino acids in the urine.

Some causes of induced aminoacidurias are: toxic agents, including metals and organic compounds; acquired metabolic disorders, including acidosis and hypercalcemia; adrenocortical steroidism; multiple myeloma; and deficiencies of vitamins B, C, and D. A possible common factor in the pathogenesis of the renal injury caused by heavy metals and maleic acid could be combination with active sulfhydryl groups. Maleic acid reacts with the sulfhydryl group to form thioethers and inhibits sulfhydryl-containing enzymes *in vitro.*

Some other forms of aminoaciduria and glucosuria are summarized in Table 2A–9. A benign form of aminoaciduria involving all the amino acids has been discovered to occur occasionally in adults. It appears to be a hereditarily determined deficiency and may be accompanied by glycosuria of the renal type; usually more than one member of a family is affected.

Practically all the tubular functions of the kidney may be lost either alone or in a variety of combinations predetermined by genetically operating factors, and failure of electrolyte and water metabolism are often the cause of a fatal outcome instead of the accompanying aminoaciduria, glycosuria, or rickets.

Schendel *et al.*[189] have reported data on the urinary excretion of amino acids in children with kwashiorkor during the acute phase of the illness. They found that similar results were obtained when aminoaciduria was expressed in relation to creatinine excretion, total nitrogen excretion, or percentage of intake. In pre-treatment cases, the aminoaciduria was 2.4 times the normal mean value of 14.23 mg/kg/day. Following a short period of treatment with milk, the mean excretion fell somewhat, but was still significantly greater when compared with normal control infants. The increased output of amino acids was due to increases in all 17 amino acids measured except three: methylhistidine, alanine, and, perhaps, cystine, suggesting that no specific enzyme defect so far recognized was responsible.

Edozien and associates[190] have also observed varying degrees of aminoaciduria in children between the ages of 1 to 4 years, suffering from kwashiorkor. These investigators further reported that ethanolamine and β-aminoisobutyric acid were present in the urine of untreated cases, and disappeared when an adequate diet was fed.

Some unclassified aminoacidurias and their etiologies are listed in Table 2A–10.

Aminoacidemias. Pototschnig and Pani[191] have reviewed the literature on amino acid nitrogen and free amino acids in the blood plasma of infants with kwashiorkor. In 13 normal, and 24 malnourished infants, both

Table 2A-10. Unclassified Aminoacidurias

Clinical entity	Characteristics
Pernicious anemias	Excess of taurine and occasionally an excess of one or all of the following: glycine, glutamine, histidine, serine, alanine, and β-aminoisobutyric acid
Leukemia	Normal, with slight excess of β-aminoisobutyric acid
Progressive muscular dystrophy	Severity increases with muscle loss. Pattern normal with occasional excess of threonine, valine, leucine, and arginine
Diabetes mellitus	Pattern and output vary with severity of ketosis; striking increases in the aromatic amino acids, the leucines, and lysine
Hyperparathyroidism	General increase resembling that of rickets
Hypercorticosteroidism	Unique absence of rise in arginine and histidine in urine and blood, though lysine is usually present. Not a simple action on renal tubular absorption mechanism.

Table 2A-11.   Average Concentration of Individual Plasma Amino Acids
in Normal and Malnourished Infants*

Amino acids	Normal infants		Malnourished infants		Difference (%)
	No. of cases	Leucine equivalents†	No. of cases	Leucine equivalents†	
Cystine	13	6.29	23	7.54	+20
Lysine	13	6.21	22	9.59	+54
Histidine	13	8.80	24	11.26	+28
Arginine	13	27.63	24	31.80	+15
Serine	13	6.44	24	9.18	+42
Aspartic acid	10	1.30	14	2.13	+64
Glutamic acid	13	4.25	22	6.82	+60
Glycine	13	5.34	24	8.08	+51
Threonine	13	4.27	24	6.73	+57
Alanine	13	22.17	24	29.25	+32
Tyrosine	12	2.72	22	5.75	+110
Proline	13	1.95	23	3.88	+100
Methionine	12	3.99	21	5.80	+45
Valine	13	21.09	24	25.00	+18
Phenylalanine	12	3.41	23	5.43	+59
Leucine	13	19.73	24	23.15	+17
TOTALS		145.59		191.39	+31

* From Pototschnig and Pani, Minerva Pediatr., *13*, 483, 1961.

† The concentration of all amino acids was estimated in reference to a leucine standard.

the qualitative and semiquantitative amino acid compositions of blood plasma were determined by paper chromatography (Table 2A–11). With due consideration of the limitations of the procedures employed, these investigators believe that they have demonstrated the existence of a true hyperaminoacidemia in infantile malnutrition which in varying degrees involves nearly all amino acids.

Richmond and Girdwood[192] have studied amino acid availability in control subjects and groups of patients with a variety of malabsorption disorders by means of changes in free amino acid levels and plasma α-amino nitrogen following the ingestion of casein. It was found that in the control subjects the rise in the level of free amino acids averaged 92 per cent of the fasting value, with peak values occurring ½ to 1 hour after ingestion of the casein. Except for glutamic acid, the magnitude of the rise of each amino acid was proportional to the content of that amino acid in casein. High peak values were obtained only in the postgastrectomy group and these were significantly greater for lysine, methionine and phenylalanine than in the control group.

PROTEIN ANABOLISM AND CATABOLISM

Protein *anabolism* and *catabolism* are terms widely used to indicate protein synthesis or breakdown in the organism. These terms have lost much of their exact meaning since we now know that 30 to 50 per cent of the total body protein is in steady flux; that is, under physiologic conditions, breakdown and new formation of tissue proteins are occurring simultaneously. However, it is still widely held that the intensity of the anabolic or catabolic processes can be measured by determining the net balance of the N-equilibrium. In this connection it must be remembered that "nitrogen balance is the sum of the gains and losses of N from the various compartments of the body. It is possible for an animal to be in positive N-balance and yet depleting some labile stores in protein" (Allison). An intense or torpid breakdown may well be balanced by an increased or sluggish protein synthesis or vice versa and thus may not affect the N-excretion at all. The N-excretion can be influenced by many factors so that, even in cases when N-balance is shifted decidedly to the positive or negative side, the results should be carefully evaluated. N-retention does not necessarily mean that new tissue protein is being synthesized. Thus, for instance, in myxedema after cessation of thyroid therapy N is retained, positive balance is established, but evidently the retained N has not been used for tissue-building anabolic processes but rather for a pathologic accumulation of proteinaceous material in tissue fluids.

Attempts to determine the anabolic or catabolic tendency by following the speed of uptake of labeled amino acids are of heuristic value and promising, but the conclusions arrived at by such methods are open to criticism. The main objections are discussed at other points in this chapter.

Anabolic Conditions. Total anabolism outweighs total catabolism during growth, during rehabilitation after disease or malnutrition, in the later part of pregnancy and also during physical training when new muscle tissue is formed. In such cases of N-retention a positive N-equilibrium can be easily demonstrated. There are, however, many cases where anabolism is restricted to only one or a few organs or tissues and, therefore, the protein synthesis is not reflected in a positive over-all nitrogen balance.

It is an important biologic rule that, in the formation of new tissue protein primarily for growth or repair, it is the anabolic growth or healing tendency of the cells and not the dietary supply of building stones which determines the speed and extent of protein synthesis. Growth or repair may occur in spite of an over-all negative N-balance. In such cases simultaneous catabolism induced in other organs may provide the required amino acids for the growing tissue. The first classic example was described by Miescher,[193] who found that the salmon, while migrating in fresh water to its spawning grounds, does

not consume food. The generative organs are, in spite of starvation, rapidly increasing in weight and this occurs at the expense of muscle substance which is metabolized during the migration. Other examples are pregnancy or lactation where, in cases of inadequate protein intake, body substances of the maternal organism may be broken down in order to provide building stones for the growth of the fetus or for the synthesis of milk proteins. Similar conditions can be observed during regeneration of organs which atrophied due to transient inactivity and also in wound healing. Further examples are rapidly growing tumors which obtain building blocks for protein synthesis from the breakdown of normal tissues.[194] In all these cases it is the anabolic growth, repair or healing tendency of the tissues and not the dietary supply which determines the speed of protein synthesis. Protein feeding or amino acid injection does not significantly accelerate the reparative processes in wound healing, which proceed normally, at least for a period of a few days, even when protein starvation prevails. It is evident that feeding protein improves the general condition primarily by replacing the mobilized proteins in the donor tissues.

These observations raise two interesting problems. The first one is the non-dietary source of protein utilized for promotion of growth or tissue regeneration, and the second is the identification of the signals which initiate the mobilization and transfer of tissue protein. It seems to be well established that the body does not possess protein stores containing specific "inert fractions" of body protein with the primary function of being available for such emergencies.[195] All phenomena can be satisfactorily explained by the assumption that part of the normal tissue protein can be mobilized to support growth or repair in some other organs. Liver protein seems to be particularly available as an amino acid source.[196] In dietary protein deficiency the liver loses 20 to 40 per cent of its total protein content within a few days; the remainder resists further mobilization. This does not mean, however, that the easily available liver protein represents an inert storage protein fraction. The liver is not the only organ able to furnish amino acids in case of increased need. It was shown that, after partial liver extirpation, for instance, other tissues may provide the building stones necessary for regeneration of the liver itself.

It is customary to designate the sum of the more easily available protein fraction present in many organs as "protein stores" without any prejudice to their structural specificity or physiologic importance. There is at present no way to measure how much of the total body protein can be mobilized without functional interference.

The second problem concerns the stimuli which notify the donor tissues of the prevailing amino acid demand, *i.e.*, what factors initiate or stimulate intracellular proteolysis. In this connection we have to keep in mind that protein synthesis in growth or repair is only one inseparable feature of the new formation of the whole protoplasm, and therefore the question raised above is intimately connected with the general problem of regulation of growth and repair. There are, however, many indications that hormonal[197] and nervous factors participate in protein mobilization just as they do in fat and carbohydrate mobilization. We have very little actual information about the role of nervous impulses on the deposition or mobilization of protein. Trophic disturbances involving tissue proteins are frequently observed after nerve injury.

Catabolic Conditions. When total catabolism outweighs total anabolism, body protein is broken down in excess; therefore more N is excreted with the urine than is consumed with the food, resulting in a negative N-balance. This happens when the quantity or quality of the *dietary protein* is lower than needed or the *calories* supplied with the food do not provide at least 50 to 60 per cent of the daily caloric requirement. The effect of *total starvation*[198] on nitrogen excretion has been investigated several times. One report shows that a voluntarily starving healthy woman excreted during the first few days of starvation an average of 6 to 8 gm of nitrogen, and then, in the next days, up to the twenty-sixth day, 4.26 gm, and still later 2 to 3 gm daily. It was also found that normally 90 per cent of the nitrogen is excreted in the form of urea but, during starvation, this value de-

creases to 53 to 69 per cent. This reduction was due to an increased ammonia excretion, probably the consequence of acidosis. In the Minnesota experiments with *semi-starvation* "a progressive reduction in the negativity of the nitrogen balance" was found. In patients receiving a *protein-* and *salt-free*,[199] but otherwise *high-caloric* diet (300 gm glucose plus 150 gm arachic oil = 2,550 calories), the urinary nitrogen, the urinary ammonia and the amino acid excretion fell from 6.8 gm total and 0.3 gm ammonia N, sharply at the beginning, then slowly to a minimum of 1.22 gm total nitrogen and 0.1 gm ammonia nitrogen. The progressive reduction of nitrogen excretion, as seen in starvation, semi-starvation, or on protein-free diets, occurs not only because the easily available protein fractions of the body are progressively exhausted, but probably because of adaptation to the low food intake or low protein supply.

Apart from cases where negative N-balance develops due to inadequate caloric or N-intake there are conditions in which N-excretion surpasses intake in spite of satisfactory food consumption. Such a "catabolic tendency" of the protein metabolism is predominant in some diseases, after injuries, after burns and after surgery.[200,201] In most of these cases the nitrogen excretion increases even when the protein and caloric intake are kept *abnormally high* or when protein hydrolysates have been provided *intravenously*. The urinary nitrogen:sulfur and the nitrogen: phosphorus ratios as well as the increased excretion of riboflavin indicate that it is not an inability to retain dietary nitrogen but rather an increased breakdown of tissue substance which is responsible for the highly negative nitrogen balance. In malnourished people or in depleted animals the loss of nitrogen after bone fracture either does not occur or is much smaller than in normals. We have to assume, therefore, that, during the catabolic phase, easily available protein depots are mobilized primarily; but it should be emphasized that in many cases the wastage of muscle protein is remarkable. The loss of body protein can be protracted, up to 6 weeks, after injury or surgery.[202] The time at which the nitrogen excretion reaches its maximum varies; it may be 4 to 5 days after injury or 1 to 2 days after surgery. The following example shows how large a quantity of tissue protein can be lost in this negative phase. In the 10 days following the fracture of both legs, the total nitrogen loss was found to be 137 gm. This amount represents about 7.7 per cent of the total body protein and is greater than the nitrogen content of the whole liver. Teleologic reasoning may lead to the assumption that tissue catabolism in such cases has a salutary effect, providing easily available building stones and energy for repair.[203] Results of experimental injuries in animals and the nature of the changes in carbohydrate metabolism which develop parallel with nitrogen catabolism suggest a disturbance in hormonal equilibrium as the cause of this "catabolic phase." Decreased urinary excretion of sodium, drop in the number of circulating eosinophils and increased thyroid secretion indicate, but do not establish satisfactorily, the involvement of the hypothalamus and of the pituitary-adrenal system as a direct cause of the metabolic disturbances following injury. Many clinically experienced authors seem to agree that, due to the nature of this catabolic phase, it is not advisable to enforce food intake or inject amino acids immediately after surgery.[204] Thus, for instance, only 2 out of 37 patients who had received a diet containing up to 130 gm protein and 2,100 calories per day could be brought to positive N-balance.

The human body normally has enough available protein and caloric reserves to subsist for a few days without intake of dietary proteins. In order to build up such reserves in chronically sick people, it is important to improve the nutritional status whenever possible *before* surgery. The healing tendency is not appreciably altered by early feeding or injection of nitrogen sources. After the "catabolic phase" the improvement of appetite and consumption of nutritious food, containing about 20 to 25 per cent of good protein, are important factors for early recovery.

Protein catabolism is also observed in *febrile diseases*. In fever the protein breakdown is not always directly related to the elevated body temperature or to the increased metabolic rate. It seems that the nature of the underlying disease is of impor-

tance and is similar to the catabolic phase after surgery; stimulation of the hypothalamus or some endocrine organs may influence protein metabolism.

Protein Anabolic and Catabolic Effects of Hormones. The state of the body protein reserves at the time of hormone administration may determine whether an anabolic or a catabolic response is obtained. In practice, dietary proteins are assigned a biologic value which is related to anabolic tendencies as tested in normal animals. However, some reconsideration of the biologic value of fed proteins may be necessary in endocrine deficiencies, and the need for amino acids may vary for full physiologic expression of different hormones. Further, specific nutrition may enhance hormone usefulness therapeutically.[205]

Injection of thyroxine increases nitrogen excretion; however, this effect seems to be mainly the consequence of an increased basal metabolic rate and occurs even in animals whose protein reserves have been depleted by non-protein diets consumed during the previous thirty days. The catabolic effect is not specific for the thyroid because under other conditions administration of thyroid hormone may produce anabolic effects.[206] In thyroidectomized animals or in severe hypothyroid conditions in children, thyroid hormone injections usually induce growth accompanied by positive nitrogen balance. One possible mechanism for thyroid action has been suggested on the basis of experiments with ^{15}N-labeled glycine. This hypothesis argues that small doses of thyroxine accelerate the breakdown of tissue proteins and, at the same time, reduce the rate of amino acid catabolism.[207] Before such conclusions could be accepted, it would have to be demonstrated that the same thyroid effects hold true for several other amino acids. This is especially important since glycine has certain highly specific metabolic fates, *e.g.*, participation in creatine and uric acid formation, and hence is hardly a suitable prototype for amino acids in general.

The explanation of the thyroid effect is further complicated by the fact that during accumulation of myxedema in hypothyroidism considerable amounts of nitrogen are retained. Byrom[208] assumes that the thyroid favors an adult type of a relatively protein-free extracellular fluid and that in myxedema an "infantile or atavistic" extracellular fluid containing a high protein concentration develops. This assumption is supported by the investigations of Thompson[209] who found that, in myxedematous patients, the concentration of proteins in the cerebrospinal fluid is abnormally high and is decreased by thyroid treatment. In hyperthyroidism the protein content of the liquor is low and increases with appropriate therapy.

Insulin affects protein metabolism mainly through its action on carbohydrate metabolism. In diabetes the increased glyconeogenesis involves catabolic breakdown of body proteins and, as a consequence of the abnormal sugar utilization, the protein synthesis is also disturbed. The protein "anabolic" or "negative catabolic" effect of insulin administration in diabetes is a consequence of improved carbohydrate utilization and of decreased glyconeogenesis. After insulin injection the blood amino acid concentration decreases. Furthermore, insulin increases the amino acid uptake by isolated tissues and organs of diabetic animals. These observations do not necessitate, however, the assumption that insulin has a specific effect on protein metabolism itself.[210] Insulin may facilitate protein synthesis by promoting the entry of amino acids into the cells.[211]

The retention of nitrogen as tissue protein appears to be defective in the diabetic. Chaikoff and Forker[212] have reported that the rate of nitrogen excretion is greatly increased in fasted, as well as in fed, depancreatized animals immediately after operation. It has further been reported[213] that, when insulin therapy was stopped in diabetic patients, they immediately began to lose between 4 and 8 gm of nitrogen per day. A loss of nitrogen from the body of this magnitude (25 to 50 gm of protein/day) could not be sustained for many weeks without seriously endangering the proper functioning of the tissue enzyme systems.

Whether insulin has a direct role in sparing body protein is not known, but, from the fact that phlorhizinized animals exhibit an even greater increase in protein catabolism than do depancreatized animals, it is considered

likely that the loss of nitrogen may be an indirect consequence of diminished carbohydrate utilization.[214]

Adrenal Corticoids. The compounds isolated normally from the adrenal vein may be divided into glucocorticoids, the mineral corticoids, weak androgens, progesteroids, and estrogen. The glucocorticoids include cortisol, of which 15 to 20 mg are secreted daily in adults under basal conditions, and corticosterone, of which 2 to 5 mg are secreted daily.

The most important action of glucocorticoids is gluconeogenesis. This is fundamentally a catabolic process in which there is deamination of amino acids making up the protein, with nitrogen loss and increased formation of glucose, with a rise in both liver glycogen and blood sugar. This hyperglycemic characteristic has been employed by West[215] as a criterion of the catabolic activity of natural and synthetic glucocorticoids.

The abnormal breakdown of protein results in muscle weakness and wasting and loss of bone matrix. Progressive myopathies associated with the administration of various corticosteroids have been observed clinically by Williams[216] and by Perkoff.[217] Also, Giles and associates[218] found the presence of posterior subcapsular cataracts in 37 per cent of 38 arthritic patients receiving moderate and high dosages of systemic corticosteroids for a period greater than one year. The loss of bone matrix results in resorption of calcium and calciuria, and finally in osteoporosis with spontaneous fractures.

The body protein-depleting effects of the available corticosteroids are not always counteracted by increases in food intake,[219-221] particularly when therapy at massive dosage levels is continued for prolonged periods of time. In some, but not all, instances the negative nitrogen retention effect of the corticosteroids on adults has been overcome by a protein intake upwards of 100 gm per day.[222] Corticoid-induced protein catabolism in adult males on self-selected but stable dietaries often can be significantly reduced or overcome by simultaneous administration of anabolic steroids.[223,224]

The marked decrease in protein utilization occurring in man with the administration of prednisone, prednisolone, and triamcinolone has been found to be associated with a high (25%) and consistent (P >0.01) fall in plasma lysine. Concomitant increases in plasma threonine and methionine were statistically borderline in nature.[225,226] The observed shift in free blood lysine suggested that the protein catabolic effects of these test agents might be reduced by supplements of the amino acid to the diet. The daily addition of 600 mg of L-lysine to the dietary of 8 subjects whose protein intake exceeded 88 gm of protein was associated with a complete or partial remission of protein catabolism. In 3 subjects whose protein intake was less than 70 gm per day, the nitrogen losses incident to corticoid therapy were mediated by administration of an anabolic agent, but not by the lysine supplement. Betheil and associates[227] found that administration of cortisone acetate to rats results in a rapid and striking decrease in plasma lysine and tyrosine, but an increase in phenylalanine. Alterations in amino acid patterns of the tissues were also observed. The data from the human, as well as the animal, experiments suggest that glucocorticoids influence the quantitative relationship among amino acids in plasma and tissues.

Growth Hormones. Pituitary growth hormone is distinctive in causing growth of almost all tissues and in increasing size without advancing maturation or promoting sexual development. Thyroid hormone is an important adjunct to growth and, in its absence, growth hormone is less effective.[230] In addition, the pituitary gland may secrete less growth hormone.[231]

The minimal daily dose for measurable nitrogen retention in a normal adult is approximately 2 mg, and in a pituitary dwarf 1 mg caused a positive balance lasting for several days.[236] Daily doses of the hormone, during the first week or two of administration, caused storage of nitrogen far in excess of the amount needed for rapid growth. Daily retention of 3 to 5 gm has been observed, whereas the growth of an average 9-year-old child requires about 0.25 gm of nitrogen per day.[238] It would be interesting to know the precise distribution of this rapidly accumulated nitrogen—how much ends up as structural protein, how much as enzymatic protein, how much in the synthetic machinery itself and how much as non-protein nitrogenous substances. Whether the accumulation of protein results from increased synthesis or decreased destruction of protein is not clear, but evidence of increased cellular penetration of amino acids[239] favors enhanced synthesis. It has also been shown that growth hormone increases the synthesis of protein by ribosomes isolated from the livers of hypophysectomized rats.[240]

The earliest evidence of an effect on nitrogen metabolism in man after administration of the hormone is the fall in blood urea nitrogen, probably reflecting the anabolic action, observable 6 to 24 hours after a single injection of human growth hormone.[232,238]

Human growth hormone administration increases urinary hydroxyproline excretion after 10 to 12 days. Since hydroxyproline is found almost exclusively in collagen, its urinary output may reflect bone collagen turnover and may be useful as a guide to metabolic activity of bone.[241]

Human growth hormone speeds the growth of hypopituitary dwarfs with impressive regularity. The growth rate achieved in the early months of therapy is faster than the normal rate, but diminishes with prolonged treatment. However, continued response has been observed for more than 4 years. Administration of human growth hormone has also proved useful in the correction of stature in 5 short children, 7.5 to 13 years of age.[245]

Henneman and associates[236] found that administration of human growth hormone markedly improved nitrogen retention within 3 to 6 days in 10 metabolically substandard patients (9 to 66 years).

Androgens and Anabolic Steroid Agents. The androgens have been employed for their anabolic effect. The chief deterrent to their use has been the production of androgenic effects. Consequently, there has been an intensive search for a substance which might be primarily anabolic. Of the several hundred compounds synthesized and studied in pursuit of this objective, relatively few have emerged which are available for regular clinical use. Unfortunately, animal studies can give only a partial and sometimes misleading picture of the biologic activity in man. The only therapeutically useful way to assess the anabolic value of steroids in human beings is by the nitrogen-balance method. In the interest of greater objectivity, a scoring method of the protein activity of steroids has been proposed which compensates for variations in protein intake which may be incurred in the course of the assays.[226]

The concept of the dynamic equilibrium of body constituents, as first pointed out by Schoenheimer,[75] envisions a continuous interchange at the cellular or molecular level of free amino acids with the amino acid constituents of the body proteins. Some of the factors controlling such processes are: dietary intake, membrane permeability, energy and reparation requirements, catabolism of amino acids, incorporation of amino acids into cellular protein, and hormonal balance.

The complex process of protein metabolism resulting in a net increase in the amount of body protein depends on (a) an increased rate of synthesis from precursors; (b) a decreased rate of catabolism; (c) a decreased rate of breakdown of amino acids to urea; and (d) an increased availability of precursors. A diagrammatic scheme of these processes as visualized by Engel[247] is shown in Figure 2A–13.

It is not clear from the literature which of these pathways is more important for the mediation of the protein anabolic action of the steroids. Bartlett[248] demonstrated that nitrogen retention in dogs induced by testosterone depended upon increased protein synthesis as well as on decreased breakdown of amino acids, with the nitrogen metabolic pool remaining unchanged. These findings agree with those of Gaebler and Tarnowsky[249] who reported that the decreased urinary excretion of urea accompanying testosterone treatment was not reflected in an elevated blood non-protein nitrogen.[250]

Clinical applications of these observations have been made in two studies[251,252] designed to reduce the rate of protein degradation in patients with uremia by giving them anabolic steroids in addition to the usual regimen. Using the rate of urea production as an index, on the average a 70 per cent decrease in the rate of protein catabolism occurred. This modality has the advantages of allowing the patient to receive a diet higher in protein and of hindering the breakdown of body tissues, which reduces the amount of nitrogenous waste products in the blood.[253]

The newer anabolic agents bearing advantages of low androgenicity have been em-

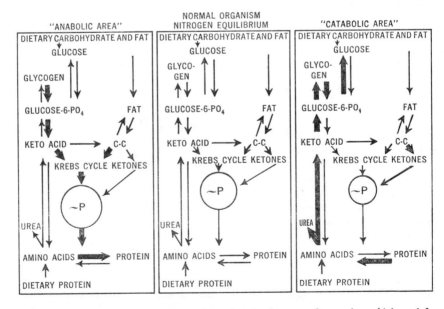

Fig. 2A-13. Diagrammatic scheme of protein metabolism in the normal organism. (Adapted from Engle. Recent Progress in Hormone Research, 6, 302, 1951.)

ployed with considerable success in a variety of other nutritional problems. Their administration to underdeveloped and underweight infants and children has been found to produce improvement in appetite and a sense of well-being, accompanied by significant gains in weight and height.[254-256] The medical management of chronically ill geriatric patients presents a number of special problems in which anabolic agents may prove useful;[257,258] in particular, protein malnutrition arising from immobilization incident to hemiplegia,[259] and corticocatabolism induced by prolonged administration of corticoids to arthritic patients.[225]

PROTEIN METABOLISM AND PHYSICAL ACTIVITY

Hypokinesis, or deconditioning, due to the lack of exercise must now be considered a major health problem. Investigations have shown that American children are less physically fit than European. These findings, and the physiologic problems of weightlessness encountered by experimental animals and men in space journeys, have revitalized interest in the nutritional aspects of the effects of physical activity.

Deitrick and associates[259a] showed that losses of body protein equivalent to $\frac{1}{2}$ to 2 pounds per week were created in healthy normal young adults immobilized and kept in bed for periods of 6 to 8 weeks. Howard and co-workers[259b] found a greater loss of body tissues in young men immobilized by fractures. In stroke patients, whose mobility was limited due to paralysis of either the right or the left side, we have observed protein losses equivalent to $1\frac{1}{2}$ to 2 pounds of muscle tissue per week. In subsequent studies it was found that protein depletion of stroke patients could be reduced in full or in part by programmed exercise and ambulation. However, the losses continued if the food intake, especially protein and calories, did not compensate for the increase in energy expenditure.

In 1917, Anderson and Lusk[259c] demonstrated that protein could be involved as an energy source only to the extent to which conditions permit the production of its metabolites, amino acids and thence glucose, to be used as calories. In fact, when calorie intake is adequate the loss of body nitrogen decreases during exercise. Although there is evidence that exercise does not increase protein requirement, a number of claims have been made for beneficial effects of supplementary protein foods during exercise. Recently, Watkin and associates[259d] concluded from careful studies that increased protein is required to maintain performance of strenuous work. They also observed that exercise led to an increased loss of nitrogen in the sweat, and concluded that this contributes significantly to increased protein requirements. The amount of nitrogen lost by perspiration depends to a large extent upon temperature of the environment, and on type and amount of work done. The protein and calorie needs of military personnel have been shown to increase tremendously with temperature, either at rest or on vigorous marches.

Measurements by Fowler and associates[259e] on trained and untrained males and females undergoing varying degrees of exercise showed that increases in serum activity levels of enzymes essential to the formation and function of body tissues were related to the previous training of the individual and the severity of exercise during a 15-minute period of test. Apparently, depending on the physiologic state of the subject, SGOT, the enzyme which has been found to increase markedly prior to and following a coronary attack, may decrease, increase, or remain unchanged in response to exercise.

Recent measurements by Albanese and his group[259f] on healthy normal young adults, before and after 20 minutes of uniform bicycle exercise, revealed marked and significant decreases in serum ribonuclease, the essential amino acids, tryptophan and phenylalanine, and the energy source, blood sugar. These changes were greater in obese or sedentary individuals. Other measurements have disclosed that serum ribonuclease increases significantly with age, twofold for each score of years beyond the age of twenty. This elevation of serum ribonuclease may well reflect the increase of sedentarianism with age, or the loss of cellular capacity for protein formation which would reduce intercellular need for ribonuclease in body fluids.

THE ROLE OF PROTEIN DEFICIENCY IN MALNUTRITION

Protein deficiency as a causative factor in human malnutrition was demonstrated by the investigations of McCay, McCarrison,[18] Boyd-Orr and Aykroyd.[102,103] Experiences collected in German and in Japanese concentration and war prisoner camps, the famous Minnesota experiments on human malnutrition, and the clinical studies on pellagra and kwashiorkor have all supplied important contributions to the understanding of protein malnutrition.[260-266]

Protein deficiency in the experimental animal can be expected to manifest itself in a great many ways because of the diverse functions of proteins in enzymatic and other vital systems. In an early publication, Kaplansky and associates[267] reported that protein deficiency in rats resulted in deranged transamination; and later, that protein synthesis was also subnormal in protein deficiency.[268] Liver slices from protein-depleted rats were incubated with pyruvic, oxalacetic, or α-ketoglutaric acids. Amino acid synthesis was generally depressed under that of control animals, particularly with regard to the conversion of pyruvate to alanine, and ketoglutarate to glutamic acid. In experiments with liver homogenates, transamination in the deficient animals was depressed an average of 30 per cent under the controls.

Effects of dietary proteins on enzymes of various tissues of experimental animals have been extensively studied. Elson[269] reported that succinoxidase activities of rat and mouse livers are reduced when protein is depleted. Beneditt and co-workers[270] found that, when rats were fed protein-deficient diets, succinoxidase decreased more rapidly than liver protein. Ross and Ely[271] found that low-protein diets resulted within 30 days in a decrease in lactic and succinic dehydrogenases in the livers of both young and adult rats.

Shirley et al.[272] found that cattle appear to differ from other species studied with respect to alteration in activity of cellular enzymes following protein depletion. They reported decreases in heart succinoxidase activity. However, in gracilis muscle, the level of succinoxidase activity increased as the dietary protein was decreased.

The specific sequelae of individual amino acid deficiencies have also been studied in animals. These investigations show, e.g., that in rats lack of arginine leads to azoospermia; insufficient methionine intake damages the liver; lack of tryptophan and some other essential amino acids leads to cataract formation. Deficiency of individual essential amino acids may also change the size and the function of some endocrine organs.[273] It has further been reported that there may be genetic differences in growth potential when chickens are placed on arginine- or lysine-deficient diets.[274] Rats fed single essential amino acid deficient diets developed pathologic lesions similar to those described in infants with kwashiorkor.[275] Continuation and further analysis of this line of research may lead to important findings on the biologic importance of the single amino acids; it may facilitate our understanding of the phenomenon called "amino acid imbalance," but it does not yet offer much toward the understanding of human malnutrition which presents itself in the form of *many* diseases producing quite *different* symptoms. This is because human malnutrition is only rarely the consequence of pure amino acid deficiency; mostly it results from protein malnutrition complicated either by low caloric intake or by the lack of such essential nutrients as vitamins and/or minerals.

Because of the participation of protein in nearly all life processes, the general symptoms of protein deficiency in man are usually quite varied and not characteristic. Early symptoms of protein deficiency are: loss of weight, stunted growth, fatigue, lack of energy, irritability, changes of temperament, decreased resistance to various damaging factors, retarded wound healing and protracted convalescence. Damages regarded by several authors as more specific consequences of protein deficiencies are: liver insufficiency, hypoproteinemia, nutritional edema and decreased resistance to infection due to impaired antibody formation. The symptoms, when developed in adults, usually can be reversed by "dietary rehabilitation," *i.e.*, by feeding palatable, high-grade, mixed food. The fast-growing, developing organism during fetal life, during infancy, or during early childhood is far more susceptible to lasting damages due to protein deficiency. Maternal malnutrition during pregnancy or lactation, or deficient protein intake after weaning, may produce permanent stigmata. Damages due to malnutrition during the early stage of development seem to be responsible for certain malformation and some chronic degenerative diseases which may become conspicuous only later in life.[276]

Insufficient amino acid supply in experimental animals leads to rapid decrease of *liver* protein; parallel with this, the resistance of the liver to toxic injuries decreases, and fatty livers may develop.[277] According to recent reports, even primary liver cancer may be produced in rats by deficient diets.[278] In spite of these experiments on animals, the role of protein deficiency in the pathogenesis of cirrhosis, primary cancer or necrosis of the human liver is still quite obscure. The important investigations of the Gilmans demonstrated that, in the malnourished *Bantus*, pellagra is usually accompanied by severe damage to the liver. These observations fail to indicate clearly, however, whether protein deficiency or some other nutritional factor is responsible for these hepatic changes.[279]

Studies of the enzyme systems of the liver in nutritional disturbances seem to be an important new field for research in liver pathology. It was found in the course of these studies that in protein deficiency the oxidase, catalase, phosphatase, arginase and cathepsin activity of the liver is decreased.[280]

It is interesting and intriguing that the activities of a number of enzymes in the bodies of a variety of animal species show a relationship to the body weight which approximates the value secured from basal metabolic rate data.[281] Histologic evidence shows that with increasing age there is a gradual reduction in the number and size of functional cells. It is thus apparent that, as living continues in the total animal, some of the cells are either unable to obtain the necessary nutrients and eliminate accumulated metabolites, or lose their capacity for maintaining essential concentration gradients between the intercellular and extracellular phases. Although there are many enzymatic processes involved in cellular metabolism, the rate of oxygen uptake offers a gross over-all estimate of metabolic activity. Studies with aging humans[282] have shown that metabolic rates decrease semi-logarithmically with advancing years. Therefore, under circumstances of a reduced metabolic rate, it is conceivable that in the older individual mild deficiencies in protein intake could have greater effects on the health and well-being than in the younger individual. These conjectures have found support in animal studies.[283]

The total quantity of circulating plasma proteins usually decreases in protein deficiency. A corresponding constriction of the total circulating plasma volume, however, may often mask the hypoproteinemia which may not be recognized if only the changes in plasma protein concentration are investigated. The different protein fractions do not participate equally in the loss of total plasma protein: the albumin decreases much faster than the globulin, probably as a sign of early liver damage.

It was generally assumed earlier that hypoproteinemia develops in malnutrition because there are not enough amino acids available for satisfactory plasma protein synthesis. A review of the more recent pertinent literature, however, supports the contention that hypoproteinemia in malnutrition represents primarily a defect of the regulation which maintains the plasma proteins at physiologic levels. Attributing it to a single factor, *viz.* the lack of available essential amino acids, does not facilitate the understanding of this basic disturbance. It is also more and more evident that there is not such a close connection between loss of body proteins and development of hypoproteinemia as was assumed earlier. During rehabilitation, plasma proteins are resynthesized preferentially and their production may start at the time when the nitrogen equilibrium is still negative.

Another symptom which may develop during protein deficiency is *anemia*. Experiments on animals and clinical investigations indicate that the body protects the amount of circulating hemoglobin even more carefully than that of the other plasma proteins. Hemoglobin may therefore be regenerated even during the development of hypoprotein-emia.[284-286]

A much discussed sign of human mal-nutrition is *edema*.[287,288] It was assumed for many decades that edema in starvation is the direct consequence of decreased intravascular osmotic pressure which develops when the plasma albumin concentration decreases. Recent investigations showed, however, that there is no lower limit of blood protein con-centration at which edema necessarily has to develop. The extension of the sodium space and the increase of the extracellular fluid, with the appearance of pitting edema, seem to be a consequence of disturbances in the regulation of water balance. Altered hor-monal functions, *e.g.*, production of anti-diuretic substances, seem to be the causative factors in emergence of edema, and not only the disturbance of intra- or extravascular osmotic equilibrium as was assumed earlier on the basis of Starling's classic investigations.

Decreased resistance to infectious diseases as a consequence of famine and malnutrition has been observed by several authors. The re-sults of animal experiments of Cannon and collaborators led to the assumption that protein deficiency, which interferes with the normal production of antibodies, may be the direct cause for this decreased resistance. The data of these authors have been con-firmed by experiments in guinea pigs and rabbits where restricted feeding depressed the serologic responses to antigenic stimuli. Some authors, however, were not able to support Cannon's contention because they found no difference in immune responses to bacterial infection and in secondary antigenic stimulation between normal and protein-starved rats.[289]

Experiences in man led similarly to equivocal results. A recent report indicates that there is no significant difference in the ability of kwashiorkor and non-kwashiorkor children to produce antibodies in response to typhoid antigen.[290] However, Scrimshaw's comprehensive review of the interaction be-tween nutrition and infection strongly sug-gests that a definite cause-effect relationship exists.[291] Some authors found that diphtheria antibody formation was normal in people who

lost as much as 40 per cent of their weight by malnutrition.[292] In "Studies of Under-nutrition" in Wuppertal the response of a group of 57 undernourished persons to anti-genic stimuli proved to be significantly less than that of a normal control group of 16 subjects. Wohl and his associates[293] have found a reduction in antibody response in 102 patients with hypoproteinemia resulting from a variety of diseases, including diabetes. It is significant that the H-agglutinin titer after 3 injections with typhoid was markedly improved in some patients receiving protein supplements. Grafe[294] reported that in Germany during the famine period following World War II, the incidence of infectious diseases increased only slightly but a particu-lar increase in tuberculosis was observed. The author expressed the opinion, however, that it was not the protein in the restricted German diet which was the responsible factor.

A remarkable but still insufficiently studied late effect of protracted malnutrition is the "lipophile dystrophy."[295] This disturbance was observed in the early phases of rehabilita-tion during which no N was retained in spite of satisfactory protein and caloric intake. This disturbance is different from that observed during the "catabolic phase" following injury, because in "lipophile dys-trophy" large amounts of fat are accumu-lated due to positive caloric balance and only the N-retention, the protein synthesis, is disturbed. It seems that damage to the endocrine system suffered during malnutri-tion may be responsible for this syndrome.

It was stated by Osborne and Mendel[296] about 55 years ago that "the tissues either form a typical protoplasmic product or none at all." This observation has since been confirmed repeatedly. In absence of some amino acids no incomplete proteins—those missing some building stones—are formed, and protein synthesis ceases completely.

The somewhat dogmatic statement made by these masters of nutritional science is, however, valid for *physiologic* conditions only. Modern analytical methods led to the discovery that abnormal proteins may be formed in the tissues under pathologic con-ditions. Such are the hemoglobin formed in sickle cell anemia[297] or cases of "paraproteinemia," where abnormal proteins are found in the blood plasma.[298-300]

These important results opened an entirely new field not only in the biochemistry of proteins, but also in chemical pathology.

BIBLIOGRAPHY

1. Borsook and Keighley: Proc. Royal Soc., London, Biol. Sci., *118*, 488, 1935.
2. Schoenheimer, Ratner, and Rittenberg: J. Biol. Chem., *130*, 703, 1939.
3. Forbes, Cooper, and Mitchell: J. Biol. Chem., *203*, 359, 1953.
4. Lipkin and Quastler: J. Clin. Invest., *41*, 646, 1962.
5. Neuberger and Slack: Biochem. J., *53*, 47, 1953.
6. Querido: in *Protein Metabolism* (F. Gross, editor), Berlin, Springer Verlag, pp. 1-7, 1962.
7. Meister: *Amino Acids: Biochemistry and Physiology of Nutrition*, Vol. I, p. 103 (Bourne and Kidder, editors), New York, Academic Press, 1953.
8. Bach: *The Metabolism of Protein Constituents in the Mammalian Body*, Oxford, Clarendon Press, 1952. Fruton and Simmonds: *General Biochemistry*, New York, Wiley, 1953.
9. Rose, Smith, Womack, and Shane: J. Biol. Chem., *181*, 307, 1949.
10. *Consumption of Food in the United States, 1909-52*, U.S. Dept. of Agriculture, Washington, D.C., 1953.
11. McCance and Widdowson: *The Chemical Composition of Foods*, London, H. M. Stationery Office, 1946.
12. *Food Composition Tables for International Use*, Food Agricult. Organization, Washington, D.C., 1949.
13. *Composition of Foods Used in Far Eastern Countries*, U.S. Department of Agriculture, 1952. Composition of Foods, Agr. Handbook No. 8, U.S. Dept. Agr.
14. Nicholls: *Tropical Nutrition and Dietetics*, 3rd Ed., London, Baillière, Tindall & Cox, 1951.
15. Keys, Brozek, Henschel, Mickelsen, and Taylor: *The Biology of Human Starvation*, Minneapolis, The University of Minnesota Press, 1950.
16. Gillman and Gillman: *Perspectives in Human Malnutrition*, New York, Grune & Stratton, p. 187, 1951.
17. deCastro: *The Geography of Hunger*, Boston, Little, Brown & Co., 1952.
18. McCarrison: *Nutrition and Health*, London, Faber & Faber, Ltd., 1943.
18a. Cannon, Frazier, and Hughes: Science, *119*, 578, 1954.
19. Bergmann and Fruton: *Advances in Enzymology*, Vol. 1, New York, Interscience Publishers, Inc., 1941.
20. Smith: Adv. in Enzymology, *13*, 191, 1951.
21. Linderstrøm-Lang, K. U.: Lane Medical Lectures, Stanford Univ., 1952.
22. Taylor, W. H.: Biochem. J., *71*, 73, 1959.
23. Haurowitz: *Chemistry and Biology of Proteins*, New York, Academic Press, Inc., 1950.
24. Morgan: J. Biol. Chem., *90*, 771, 1931.
25. Rice and Beuk: Adv. in Food Res. IV: *233*, New York, Academic Press, 1953.
26. Frazier, Cannon, and Hughes: Food Research, *18*, 91, 1953.
27 Geiger, Courtney, and Geiger: Arch. Biochem. & Biophysics, *41*, 74, 1952.
28. Christensen: Gastroenterology, *18*, 235, 1951.
29. Ellenbogen: in *Newer Methods of Nutritiona Biochemistry* (A. A. Albanese, editor), New York, Academic Press, pp. 235-287, 1963.
30. Longenecker: in *Newer Methods of Nutritional Biochemistry* (A. A. Albanese, editor), New York, Academic Press, pp. 113-144, 1963.
31. Folin: Am. J. Physiol., *13*, 117, 1905.
32. Whipple: Hemoglobin, *Plasma Protein and Cell Protein*, Springfield, Charles C Thomas, 1948.
33. Schoenheimer: in *Dynamic State of Body Constituents* (H. T. Clarke, editor) Cambridge, Harvard Univ. Press, 1942.
34. Bloch, Schoenheimer, and Rittenberg: J. Biol. Chem., *138*, 155, 1941.
35. Allison and Fitzpatrick. *Dietary Proteins in Health and Disease*, Springfield, Charles C Thomas, 1960.
36. Allison: Physiol. Revs., *35*, 664, 1955.
37. ———: in *Protein and Amino Acid Nutrition* (A. A. Albanese, editor), New York, Academic Press, pp. 97-116, 1959.
38. Bender: J. Sci. Food Agric., *5*, 305, 1954.
39. Christensen: J. Nutrition, *42*, 189, 1950.
40. Fisher: *Protein Metabolism*, p. 18, London, Methuen and Co., 1954.
41. Schlussel and Sunder-Plassmann: Klin. Wochschr., *31*, 545, 1953.
42. Suda and Ueda: in *Newer Methods of Nutritional Biochemistry* (A. A. Albanese, editor), New York, Academic Press, pp. 145-157, 1963.
43. Gibson and Wiseman: Biochem. J., *48*, 426, 1951.
44. Schofield and Lewis: J. Biol. Chem., *168*, 439, 1947.
45. Althausen, *et al.*: Gastroenterology, *16*, 126, 1950.
46. Pinsky and Geiger: Proc. Soc. Exper. Biol. & Med., *81*, 55, 1952.
47. Orten, VanBuren, and Johnston: Fed. Proc., *11*, 452, 1952.
48. Agar, Hird, and Sidhu: J. Physiol., *121*, 255, 1953.
49. Zetzel, Banks, and Sagall: Am. J. Digest Dis., *9*, 350, 1942.
50. Everson: Inter. Abst. Surg., *95*, 209, 1952.
51. McDermott, Adams, and Riddell: Proc. Soc. Exper. Biol. & Med., *88*, 880, 1955.
52. Challenger and Walshe: Lancet, *1*, 1239, 1955.
53. Brain and Stammers: Lancet, *1*, 1137, 1951.
54. Nasset: J.A.M.A., *164*, 172, 1957.
55. Schreier: J. Pediatrics, *46*, 86, 1955.
56. Denton and Elvehjem: J. Biol. Chem., *206*, 449, 1954.

57. Charkey, Manning, Kano, Gassner, Hopwood and Madsen: Poultry Sci., *32*, 639, 1953.
58. Rhoads: Inter. Abst. Surg., *94*, 417, 1952.
59. Nasset: J. Nutrition, *61*, 555, 1957.
60. *Malnutrition and Starvation in Western Netherlands*, The Hague General State Printing Office, 1948.
61. Kirsner, Brandt, and Sheffner: J. Am. Diet. Assoc., *29*, 1103, 1953.
62. Cuthbertson: Ann. Rev. Med., *4*, 135, 1953.
63. Rose: Fed. Proc., *8*, 546, 1949.
64. Reynolds: Am. J. Clin. Nutr., *6*, 439, 1958.
64a.Hegsted: Fed. Proc., *22*, 1424, 1963.
64b.Irwin and Hegsted: J. Nutrition, *101*, 539, 1971.
65. Braunstein: Adv. Protein Chem., *3*, 1, 1947.
66. Black, Kleiber, and Smith: J. Biol. Chem., *197*, 365, 1952.
67. Geiger and Wick: Arch. f. Exp. Path. u. Pharm., *219*, 518, 1953.
68. Steele: J. Biol. Chem., *198*, 237, 1952.
69. Leverton: in *Protein and Amino Acid Nutrition* (A. A. Albanese, editor), New York, Academic Press, pp. 477–506, 1959.
70. Reynolds, Futrell, and Baumann: J. Am. Dietet. Assoc., *29*, 359, 1953.
71. Futrell, Lutz, Reynolds, and Baumann: J. Nutrition, *46*, 299, 1952.
72. Mertz, Baxter, Jackson, Roderuck, and Weis: J. Nutrition, *46*, 313, 1952.
73. Wharton, Tyrrell, and Patton: J. Am. Dietet. Assoc., *29*, 573, 1953.
74. Frost: in *Protein and Amino Acid Nutrition* (A. A. Albanese, editor), New York, Academic Press, pp. 225–279, 1959.
75. Schoenheimer: *The Dynamic State of Body Constituents* (H. T. Clarke, editor), Cambridge, Harvard Univ. Press, 2nd edition, 1946.
76. Albanese: *The Protein and Amino Acid Requirements of Man; Protein and Amino Acid Requirements of Mammals* (A. A. Albanese, editor), New York, Academic Press, p. 116, 1950.
76a.Clark: in *Newer Methods of Nutritional Biochemistry* (A. A. Albanese, editor), Vol. 2, New York, Academic Press, pp. 123–159, 1965.
76b.Scrimshaw, Bressani, Behar, and Viteri: J. Nutrition, *66*, 485, 1958.
76c.Bressani, Wilson, Behar, and Scrimshaw: J. Nutrition, *70*, 176, 1960.
76d.*National Academy of Sciences, National Research Council Publ. 1100*, Committee on Protein Malnutrition, Washington, D.C., 1963.
76e.Mitchell: J. Boll. Chem., *58*, 873, 1924.
76f.Albanese, Higgons, Hyde, and Orto: Am. J. Clin. Nutrition, *4*, 161, 1956.
76g.Albanese, Holt, Irby, Snyderman, and Lein: Bull. Johns Hopkins Hosp., *80*, 149, 1947.
76h.Arnould: *L'Utilisation des Proteines Pour la Croissance*, Louvain, Belgium, University of Louvain. Doctoral Dissertation, Jan. 1961.
76i.Mitchell and Block: J. Biol. Chem., *163*, 599, 1946.
76j.*Protein Requirements, Report of a Joint FAO/WHO Expert Group*. World Health Organization Technical Report Series 301, 1965.
76k.Oser: in *Protein and Amino Acid Nutrition* (A. A. Albanese, editor), New York, Academic Press, pp. 281–295, 1959.
76l. Melnick, Oser, and Weiss: Science, *103*, 326, 1946.
76m.Sheffner, Eckfeldt, and Spector: J. Nutrition, *60*, 105, 1956.
76n.Sheffner: in *Newer Methods of Nutritional Biochemistry* (A. A. Albanese, editor), Vol. 3, New York, Academic Press, 1967.
76a.Fisher: in *Newer Methods of Nutritional Biochemistry*, Vol. 3, New York, Academic Press, pp. 101–124, 1967.
76p.Kiriyama: in *Newer Methods of Nutritional Biochemistry*, Vol. 4, New York, Academic Press, pp. 37–78, 1970.
76q.Berry: in *Newer Methods of Nutritional Biochemistry*, Vol. 4, New York, Academic Press, pp. 79–122, 1970.
76r.Young, and Alexis: J. Nutrition, *96*, 255, 1968.
76s.Munro, and Clark: Proc. Nutr. Soc., *19*, 55, 1960.
76t.Allison, Wannemacher, Banks, Wunner, and Gomez-Brenes: J. Nutrition, *78*, 333, 1962.
76u.Brody: Biochem. Biophys. Acta, *24*, 502, 1957.
76v.Lang: J. Geront., *22*, 53, 1967.
76w.Medvedev: Uspekhi Souremenoy Biologii, *51*, 299, 1961.
76x.Albanese, Orto, Zavattaro, and De Carlo: Nutrition Reports International, *4*, 151, 1971.
77. Tristram: Adv. Protein Chem., *5*, 83, 1949.
78. *Protein Requirements FAO Nutritional Studies No. 16.* FAO of the United Nations, Rome, 1957.
79. Swendseid, Harris, and Tuttle: J. Nutrition, *77*, 391, 1962.
80. Kirk, Metheny, and Reynolds: J. Nutrition, *77*, 448, 1962.
81. Swendseid, Watts, Harris, and Tuttle: J. Nutrition, *75*, 295, 1961.
82. Leverton, Gram, Chaloupka, Brodovsky, and Mitchell: J. Nutrition, *58*, 59, 1956.
83. Leverton and Steel: J. Nutrition, *78*, 10, 1962.
84. Rose: Nutrition Abstr. & Revs., *27*, 631, 1957.
85. Snyderman, Holt, Dancis, Roitman, Boyer and Balis: J. Nutrition, *78*, 57, 1962.
86. Orr and Watt: *Amino Acid Content of Foods: Home Economics Research Report No. 4*, Washington, U.S. Dept. of Agriculture, 1957.
87. Block and Mitchell: Nutr. Abst. Rev., *16*, 249, 1946–47.
88. Brown: *The Challenge of Man's Future*, New York, Viking Press, 1954.
89. Jansen: J. Nutrition, *76*, Suppl. 1, 1962.
90. Geiger: J. Nutr., *36*, 813, 1948.
91. Henry and Kon: J. Dairy Res., *14*, 330, 1946.
91a.Mauron: in *Proceedings VIIth International Congress of Nutrition*, Ad hoc Commission of the Research Council for Food, Agriculture and Forestry, Hamburg, Germany, Aug. 5, 1966.
92. Leverton, Gram, and Chaloupka: J. Nutrition, *44*, 537, 1951.
93. Harris and Malaspina: Abst. in Food Tech., *5*, No. 5, May, 1953.

94. Dean: *Medical Research Council Special Report Series 279*, London, H. M. P., 1953.
95. ———: *Protein Malnutrition* (Proc. Conf. Jamaica), p. 195, Cambridge, University Press, 1955.
96. Scrimshaw: *Amino Acid Malnutrition*, p. 28, Rutgers Univ. Press, 1957.
97. Flodin: Agr. & Food Chem., *1*, 222, 1953.
97a.Fukui, Fukui, Sasaki, and Murakami: Tokushima J. Exper. Med., *8*, 1, 1961.
98. Phillips and Berg: J. Nutr., *53*, 481, 1954.
99. Berg: Physiol. Rev., *33*, 145, 1953.
100. Neuberger: Biochem. Soc. Symposia, *1*, 20, 1948.
101. British Nutritional Society: Brit. J. Nutr., *5*, 243, 1951.
102. Aykroyd: *Human Nutrition and Diet*, London, 1937.
103. Orr: Sci. American, *183*, No. 2, 1950.
104. Kuppuswamy, Srinivasan, and Subrahmanyan: *Protein in Foods*, Spl. Rep. Series No. 33, Indian Council of Medical Research, New Delhi, 1958.
105. Patwardhan and Ramachandran: Science and Culture, *25*, 401, 1960.
106. *Meeting Protein Needs of Infants and Preschool Children*, Food and Nutrition Board Publ. 843, National Academy of Sciences, National Research Council, Washington, D.C., 1961.
107. Behar, Bressani, and Scrimshaw: in *World Review of Nutrition and Dietetics*, Vol. 1 (C. H. Bourne, editor), London, Pitman Publishing Co., p. 77, 1959.
108. Parpia, Narayanarao, Rajagopalan, and Swaminathan: J. Nutrition & Dietet., *1*, 114, 1964.
108a.Gerloff, Lima, and Stahmann: J. Agric. Food Chem., *13*, 139, 1965.
108b.Liener: Am. J. Clin. Nutrition, *11*, 281, 1962.
108c.Venkatrao, Leela, Swaminathan, and Parpia: J. Nutrition & Dietet., *1*, 304, 1964.
108d.Munaver and Harper: J. Nutrition, *69*, 58, 1959.
108e.Jones: Federation Proc., *21*, 1, 1962.
108f.Guthneck, Bennett, and Schweigert: J. Nutrition, *49*, 289, 1953.
108g.Schweigert and Guthneck: J. Nutrition, *54*, 333, 1954.
108h.Liener: in *Nutritional Evaluation of Food Processing* (Harris and Von Loesecke, editors), New York, John Wiley & Sons, p. 231, 1960.
108i.Liener: in *Processed Plant Protein Foods* (A. M. Altschul, editor), London, Academic Press, p. 79, 1958.
108j.Barness, Kaye, and Valyasevi: Am. J. Clin. Nutrition, *9*, 331, 1961.
108k.Guggenheim and Szmelcman: in *7th Intern. Congr. Nutrition Symposium on Vegetables as Protein Sources for Infants*, Hamburg, Germany, August 5, 1966.
108l.McLaren, Asfour, Cowan, Pellett, and Tannous: ibid loc.
108m.Parthasarathy, Doraiswamy, Tasker, Narayanarao, and Swaminathan: J. Nutrition & Dietet., *1*, 285, 1964.
108n.Behar, Viteri, Bressani, Arroyave, Squibb, and Scrimshaw: Ann. New York Acad. Sciences, *69*, 954, 1958.
108o.Truswell and Brock: South African Med. J., *35*, 98, 1959.
108p.Irwin and Hegsted: J. Nutrition, *101*, 385, 1971.
109. Allison: Fed. Proc., *10*, 676, 1951.
110. Watkin, Froeb, Hatch, and Gutman: Am. J. Med., *9*, 485, 1950.
111. Report of the Committee on Nutrition, British Medical Assoc., London, 1950.
111a.*Recommended Daily Dietary Allowances, Revised 1963*, Food and Nutrition Board, National Academy of Sciences—National Research Council, Washington, D.C.
112. Cuthbertson: Quart. J. Med., *1*, 233, 1932.
113. Kinney: in *Protein Metabolism* (F. Gross, editor), Berlin, Springer Verlag, pp. 275–296, 1962.
113a.Schreier and Karch: Lang. Arch. u. Dtsch. Z. Chir., *280*, 516, 1955.
114. Medvedev: in *Biological Aspects of Aging* (N. W. Shock, editor), New York, Columbia Univ. Press, pp. 255–266, 1962.
115. Oeriu and Tanase: in *Biological Aspects of Aging* (N. W. Shock, editor), New York, Columbia Univ. Press, pp. 281–288, 1962.
116. Schulze: Z. Altersforsch., *8*, 64, 1954.
117. Schulze: In *Old Age in the Modern World*, London, E. & S. Livingstone, pp. 122–127, 1955.
118. Tuttle, Swendseid, Mulcare, Griffith, and Bassett: Metabolism, *6*, 564, 1957.
119. Higgons: in *Protein and Amino Acid Nutrition* (A. A. Albanese, editor), New York, Academic Press, pp. 507–552, 1959.
120. Albanese, Higgons, Orto, and Zavattaro: Geriatrics, *12*, 465, 1957.
121. Anderson and Nasset: J. Nutr., *36*, 703, 1948.
122. Hawkins: Science, *116*, 19, 1952.
123. Gamble: Harvey Lectures, *42*, 247, 1947.
124. Quinn, Kleeman, Bass, and Henschel: Report 201, Office of the Quartermaster General (March), 1953.
125. Keys and Brozek: Physiol. Rev., *33*, 245, 1953.
126. Munro: Physiol. Rev., *31*, 449, 1951.
127. Swanson: Fed. Proc., *10*, 660, 1951.
128. Schwimmer and McGavack: New York State J. Med., *48*, 1797, 1948.
129. Geiger: Fed. Proc., *10*, 670, 1951.
130. Hoberman and Graff: J. Biol. Chem., *186*, 373, 1950.
131. Elman: J. Clin. Nutr., *1*, 287, 1953.
132. Handler, Kamin, and Harris: J. Biol. Chem., *179*, 283, 1949.
133. Peters: Yale J. Biol. & Med., *24*, 48, 1951.
134. Lanman: *Infant Nutrition*, p. 34, Sugar Research Foundation, New York, 1952.
135. Albanese and Orto: in *Newer Methods of Nutritional Biochemistry* (A. A. Albanese, editor), New York, Academic Press, pp. 1–112, 1963.
136. Wilhelmj, McDonough, and McCarthy: Am. J. Dig. Dis., *20*, 117, 1953.
137. Rappaport, MacDonald, and Borowy: Surg., Gynec. & Obst., *97*, 748, 1953.

138. McDermott, Jr. and Adams: J. Clin. Invest., *33*, 1, 1954.
139. Borst: Lancet, *1*, 824, 1948.
140. Dent and Schilling: Biochem. J., *44*, 318, 1949.
141. Denton and Elvehjem: J. Biol. Chem., *206*, 455, 1954.
142. Awapara and Marvin: J. Biol. Chem., *178*, 691, 1949.
143. Sprinson and Rittenberg: J. Biol. Chem., *180*, 715, 1949.
144. Geiger: Science, *111*, 594, 1950.
145. Cannon: *Recent Advances in Nutrition*, University of Kansas Press, 1950.
146. King: Fed. Proc., *22*, 1115, 1963.
147. *The Synthesis of Protein* (J. P. Burnett, editor), based on an exhibit of Eli Lilly and Company, Annual Meeting of the American Medical Association, Atlantic City, June, 1963.
148. Wilson: in *Protein Metabolism* (F. Gross, editor), Berlin, Springer Verlag, pp. 26–40, 1962.
149. Abdou and Tarver: J. Biol. Chem., *190*, 781, 1951.
150. Askonas, Campbell, and Work: Biochem. J., *56*, V, 1954.
151. Hoffenberg, Saunders, Linder, Black, and Brock: in *Protein Metabolism* (F. Gross, editor), Berlin, Springer Verlag, pp. 314–325, 1962.
152. Schroeder: Arch. Exptl. Pathol. Pharmakol., *15*, 364, 1882.
153. Salaskin: Z. Physiol. Chem., *25*, 128, 1898.
154. Bollman, Mann, and Magath: Am. J. Physiol., *64*, 371, 1924.
155. West and Todd: *Textbook of Biochemistry*, 2nd edition, New York, Macmillan, 1957.
156. Kossel and Dakin: Ztschr. f. Physiol. Chem., *41*, 321, 1904.
157. Krebs and Henseleit: Ztschr. f. Physiol. Chem., *210*, 33, 1932.
158. Cohen and Hayano: J. Biol. Chem., *166*, 239, 1946.
159. ———: J. Biol. Chem., *166*, 251, 1946.
160. ———: J. Biol. Chem., *170*, 687, 1947.
161. ———: J. Biol. Chem., *172*, 405, 1948.
162. Salter: in *Diseases of Metabolism* (G. G. Duncan, editor), 4th edition, Philadelphia, W. B. Saunders, pp. 1–65, 1959.
163. Voit: Z. Biol., *2*, 307, 1866.
164. Lusk: *Science of Nutrition*, 4th edition, Philadelphia, W. B. Saunders, pp. 352–357, 1928.
165. Smith: J. Biol. Chem., *68*, 15, 1926.
166. Puchal, Hays, Speer, Jones, and Catron: J. Nutrition, *76*, 11, 1962.
167. Arroyave: Personal communication.
168. San Pietro and Rittenberg: J. Biol. Chem., *201*, 445, 1953.
169. ———: J. Biol. Chem., *201*, 457, 1953.
170. Schimke: J. Biol. Chem., *237*, 1921, 1962.
171. Haak, Kassenaar, and Querido: in *Protein Metabolism* (F. Gross, editor), Berlin, Springer Verlag, pp. 150–160, 1962.
172. Gale: Adv. in Enzymol., *6*, 1, 1946.
173. Werle: Ztft. f. Vitamin Hormon und Fermentforschg, *1*, 504, 1948.

174. Guggenheim: *Die biogenen Amine*, Basel, Karger, 1940.
174a. Sprince: in *Newer Methods of Nutritional Biochemistry* (A. A. Albanese, editor), Vol. 2, New York, Academic Press, pp. 161–248, 1965.
175. Kertesz: Bull. de la Soc. de Chimie Biologique, *35*, 1157, 1953.
176. Schreier: Klin. Woch., *31*, 729, 1953.
177. Boscott and Bickel: Biochem. J., *56*, I, 1954.
178. Bickel, Gerrard, and Hickmans: Lancet, *2*, 812, 1953.
179. Nitowsky, Govan, and Gordon: Am. J. Dis. Child., *85*, 462, 1953.
180. Goldsmith, Sarett, Register, and Gibbens: J. Clin. Invest., *31*, 533, 1952.
181. Sarett and Goldsmith: J. Biol. Chem., *167*, 293, 1947.
182. ———: J. Biol. Chem., *177*, 461, 1949.
183. Chiancone: in *Newer Methods of Nutritional Biochemistry* (A. A. Albanese, editor), Vol. 2, New York, Academic Press, pp. 249–284, 1965.
184. Du Vigneaud: *A Trail of Research*, Ithaca, Cornell Univ. Press, 1952.
185. Goettsch, Lyttle, Grim, and Dunbar: Am. J. Physiol., *140*, 688, 1943.
186. Nasset and Tully: J. Nutr., *44*, 477, 1951.
187. *Chromatographic and Electrophoretic Techniques. I. Chromatography* (I. Smith, editor), 2nd edition, New York, Interscience Publishers, 1960.
188. Harrison: in *Amino Acid and Protein Metabolism*, Report of the Thirtieth Ross Conference on Pediatric Research (S. J. Fomon, editor), Columbus, Ross Laboratories, p. 89, 1959.
189. Schendel, Antonis, and Hansen: Pediatrics, *23*, 662, 1959.
190. Edozien, Phillips, and Collis: Lancet, *1*, 615, 1960.
191. Pototschnig and Pani: Minerva Pediat., *13*, 483, 1961.
192. Richmond and Girdwood: Clin. Sci., *22*, 301, 1962.
193. Miescher: *Die Histochemischen und Physiologischen Arbeiten*, Vogel, Leipzig, 1897.
194. Tannenbaum and Silverstone: Adv. Cancer Res., *1*, 452, 1953.
195. Madden and Clay: J. Exp. Med., *82*, 65, 1945.
196. Kosterlitz and Campbell: Nutr. Abstr. & Rev., *15*, 1, 1945.
197. Wennecker and Sussmann: Proc. Soc. Exper. Biol. & Med., *76*, 683, 1951.
198. Vollmer and Berning: Ztft. ges. exp. Med., *118*, 604, 1952.
199. Lowe: Clin. Sci., *12*, 57, 1953.
200. Moore and Ball: *Metabolic Response to Surgery*, Springfield, Charles C Thomas, 1952.
201. Cuthbertson: Brit. Med. Bull., *10*, 33, 1954.
202. O'Connell and Gardner: J.A.M.A., *153*, 706, 1953.
203. Needham: *Regeneration and Wound Healing*, London, Methuen & Co., 1952.
204. Rhoads: Fed. Proc., *11*, 659, 1952.
205. Leatham: *Protein Metabolism* (F. Gross, editor), Berlin, Springer Verlag, pp. 202–221, 1962.

206. Deuel, Sandiford, Sandiford, and Boothby: J. Biol. Chem., 76, 407, 1928.
207. Hoberman and Graff: Yale J. Biol. & Med., 23, 195, 1950.
208. Byrom: Clin. Sci., 1, 272, 1934.
209. Thompson: J. Clin. Endocrin. & Metab., 13, 457, 1953.
210. Lukens: Influence of Insulin on Protein Metabolism, 19th Int. Physiol. Congress, Montreal, 1953, p. 12.
211. Kipnis and Noall: Bioch. biophys. Acta Amst., 27, 226, 1958.
212. Chaikoff and Forker: Endocrinology, 46, 319, 1950.
213. Atchley, Loeb, Richards, Benedict, and Driscoll: J. Clin. Invest., 12, 297, 1933.
214. Russell: in A Textbook of Physiology (J. F. Fulton, editor), 17th edition, Philadelphia, W. B. Saunders, pp. 1153–1165, 1955.
215. West: Diabetes, 8, 22, 1959.
216. Williams and Bond: Lancet, 2, 698, 1959.
217. Perkoff, Silber, Tyler, Cartwright, and Wintrobe: Am. J. Med., 26, 891, 1959.
218. Giles, Mason, Duff, and McLean: J. Am. Med. Assoc., 182, 719, 1962.
219. Reifenstein and Albright: J. Clin. Invest., 26, 24, 1947.
220. Knox and Auerbach: J. Biol. Chem., 214, 307, 1955.
221. Goldstein, Stella, and Knox: J. Biol. Chem., 237, 1723, 1962.
222. Ginoulhiac: Acta Vitamin, 13, 149, 1959.
223. Albanese: Unpublished data.
224. Ford: Corticocatabolism, Scientific Exhibit, Annual Meeting, Am. Med. Assoc., Atlantic City, N. J., June, 1963.
225. Albanese, Lorenze, and Orto: N.Y. State J. Med., 61, 3998, 1961.
226. ———: N.Y. State J. Med., 62, 1607, 1962.
227. Betheil, Feigelson, and Feigelson: Federation Proc., 22, 408, 1963.
228. Li: Federation Proc., 16, 775, 1957.
229. Beck, McGarry, Dyrenfurth, and Venning: Science, 125, 884, 1957.
230. Scow: Am. J. Physiol., 196, 859, 1959.
231. Solomon and Greep: Endocrinology, 65, 158, 1959.
232. Pearson, Lipsett, Greenberg, and Ray: Effects of Human Growth Hormone in Hypophysectomized Patients, presented at the 39th Annual Meeting of the Endocrine Society, New York City, May-June, 1957.
233. Bergenstal, Lubs, Hallman, Patten, Levine, and Li: J. Lab. & Clin. Med., 50, 791, 1957.
234. Beck, McGarry, Dyrenfurth, and Venning: Ann. Intern. Med., 49, 1090, 1958.
235. Ikkos, Luft, and Gemzell: Lancet, 1, 720, 1958.
236. Henneman, Forbes, Moldawer, Dempsey, and Carroll: J. Clin. Invest., 39, 1223, 1960.
237. Shepard, Nielsen, Johnson, and Bernstein: J. Dis. Child., 99, 74, 1960.
238. Raben: Recent Progress in Hormone Research, 15, 71, 1959.
239. Kostyo and Knobil: Endocrinology, 65, 525, 1959.
240. Korner: Biochem. J., 81, 292, 1961.
241. Dull and Henneman: New England J. Med., 268, 132, 1963.
242. Dole: J. Clin. Invest., 35, 150, 1956.
243. Gordon and Cherkes: J. Clin. Invest., 35, 206, 1956.
244. Monckeberg, Donoso, Oxman, Pak, and Meneghello: Pediatrics, 31, 58, 1963.
245. Raben: New England J. Med., 266, 31, 1962.
246. Kochakian and Murlin: J. Nutrition, 10, 437, 1935.
247. Engel: Recent Progress in Hormone Research, 6, 302, 1951.
248. Bartlett: Endocrinology, 52, 272, 1953.
249. Gaebler and Tarnowski: Endocrinology, 33, 317, 1943.
250. Tainter, Arnold, Beyler, Potts, and Roth: Anabolic Steroids in the Management of the Diabetic Patient, presented at the Texas Diabetes Assoc., Texas Med. Assoc. Annual Session, Dallas, April, 1963.
251. McCracken and Parson: Lancet, 2, 885, 1958.
252. Gjorp and Thaysen: Lancet, 2, 889, 1958.
253. Editorial: Anabolic Steroids and Uremia, Nutrition Revs., 17, 72, 1959.
254. Collective Study, Dept. of Medical Research, Winthrop Labs., New York, 1962.
255. Bierich: Acta Endocrinol. (KBH) Suppl., 63, 89, 1962.
256. Scharer, Habich, and Prader: Helv. Med. Acta, 27, Fasc. 5/6, 530, 1960.
257. Glas and Lansing: J. Am. Geriat. Soc., 10, 509, 1962.
258. van Wayjen and Butze: Acta Endocrinol., 39, suppl. 63, 1, 1962.
259. Albanese, Lorenze, and Orto: N.Y. State J. Med., 63, 80, 1963.
259a. Deitrick, Whedon, and Schorr: Am. J. Med., 4, 3, 1948.
259b. Howard, Parson, Stein, Eisenberg, and Reidt: Bull. Johns Hopkins Hosp., 75, 156, 1944.
249c. Anderson and Lusk: J. Biol. Chem., 32, 421, 1917.
259d. Watkin, Das, and McCarthy: Federation Proc., 23, 399, 1964.
259e. Fowler, Chowdhury, Pearson, Gardner, and Bratton: J. Applied Physiol., 17, 943, 1962.
259f. Albanese: Effect of Exercise on Nutritional Requirements. Presented at Gordon Research Food and Nutrition Conference, New London, New Hampshire, July 18–22, 1966.
260. Studies of Undernutrition, Wuppertal, 1946–9, Med. Res. Council Special Report, Ser. No. 275, London, 1951.
261. Brock and Autret: Kwashiorkor in Africa, F. A. O. Report, Rome, 1952.
262. Pollack and Halpern: Adv. Protein Chem., 6, 383, 1951.
263. Davies: Ann. Rev. Med., 3, 99, 1952.
264. Autret and Behar: Sindrome Policarencial Infantil (Kwashiorkor) and its Prevention in Central America, Rome, FAO, 1954.

265. Frenk: Federation Proc., *20*, 96–102, 1961.
266. Waterlow and Scrimshaw: *The Concept of Kwashiorkor from a Public Health Point of View*, Bull. World Health Organization, *16*, 458, 1957.
267. Kaplansky, Berezovskaya, and Schmerling: Biokhimiya, *10*, 401, 1945.
268. Berezovskaya and Smirnova: Biokhimiya, *21*, 457, 1956.
269. Elson: Biochem. J., *41*, 21, 1947.
270. Beneditt, Steffee, Gill, and Johnston: Fed. Proc., *8*, 350, 1949.
271. Ross and Ely: J. Franklin Inst., *258*, 241, 1951.
272. Shirley, Bedrak, Warnick, Hentges, and Davis: J. Nutrition, *67*, 159, 1959.
273. Samuels: *Effect of Protein and Amino Acids of the Diet on Endocrine System, Protein, Metabolism and Hormones*, Rutgers Univ. Press, 1953.
274. Griminger and Fisher: Proc. Soc. Exper. Biol. & Med., *111*, 754, 1962.
275. Sidransky and Rechcigl: J. Nutrition, *78*, 269, 1962.
276. Oomen: Nutr. Rev., *12*, 33, 1954.
277. Gyorgy and Goldblatt: J. Exp. Med., *89*, 245, 1949.
278. Berman: *Primary Carcinoma of the Liver*, London, H. K. Lewis & Co., 1951.
279. Kalk: Deutsche Med. Wochenshcr., *75*, 225, 1950.
280. Allison: J. Agr. Food Chem., *1*, 71, 1953.
281. Brody: *Bioenergetics and Growth*, New York, Reinhold Publishing Corp., p. 76, 1945.
282. Shock, Watkin, and Viengst: in *Old Age in the Modern World*, E. & S. Livingstone, London, pp. 127–137, 1955.
283. Ashida: in *Newer Methods of Nutritional Biochemistry* (A. A. Albanese, editor), New York, Academic Press, pp. 159–184, 1963.
284. Whipple: Pasteur Lecture, Proc. Inst. Med. Chicago, *14*, 2, 1942.
285. Davies: Brit. Med. J., *1*, 45, 1945.
286. Drabkin: Physiol. Rev., *31*, 345, 1951.
287. Bansi: *Das Hungerodem*, Stuttgart, F. Enke, 1949.
288. McCance: *Hunger Oedema, Studies of Undernutrition*, Wuppertal.
289. Metcoff: Am. J. Public Health, *39*, 862, 1949.
290. Pretorius and deVilliers: Am. J. Clin. Nutr., *10*, 379, 1962.
291. Scrimshaw, Taylor, and Gordon: Am. J. Med. Sci., *237*, 367, 1959.
292. Balch: J. Immunol., *64*, 397, 1950.
293. Wohl, Reinhold, and Rose: Arch. Int. Med., *83*, 402, 1949.
294. Grafe: Deutsche Med. Wchschft., *75*, 441, 1950.
295. Bansi: Med. Klin., *42*, 397, 1947.
296. Osborne and Mendel: J. Biol. Chem., *17*, 325, 1914.
297. Pauling, Itano, Singer, and Wells: Science, *110*, 543, 1949.
298. Waldenstrom: Adv. Inter. Med., *5*, 398, 1952.
299. Schreier: Bioch. Ztft., *321*, 528, 1951.
300. Putnam and Stelos: J. Biol. Chem., *203*, 347, 1953.

Chapter

2B

Abnormalities in Serum Protein Metabolism and Amino Acid Effects[*]

Marcus A. Rothschild,

Murray Oratz,

and

Sidney S. Schreiber

ABNORMALITIES IN SERUM PROTEIN METABOLISM

Mechanism of Serum Protein Production. The liver is the major site of serum protein synthesis except for the immunoglobulins. Within the hepatocyte there exists a specific assembly line for the production and transport of serum proteins. The messenger RNA's for serum proteins are more or less saturated with ribosomes. These ribosomes contain RNA and protein, and act as the "read out" mechanisms for the mRNA. Ribosomes are composed of two subunits; the smaller subunit (40 S) is attached to mRNA while the larger (60 S) is anchored to the microtubular structure — the endoplasmic reticulum. The growing serum protein molecule starts at the interphase between the two subunits, travels down through the center of the larger unit and then moves along the endoplasmic reticulum until it is extruded at the cell surface via the Golgi apparatus.[1-3] Many factors affect this system directly or indirectly. The end result of this synthetic system is the release of these proteins into the plasma, while the plasma level represents only the complex end result of synthesis, degradation and distribution (Table 2B–1).

* Supported in part by the U.S. Public Health Service Grant AM 02489

Lymphocytes, spleen cells, plasma cells and, in the case of immunoglobulin A, mucosal cells are the site of synthesis of the immunoglobulins. In germ-free animals the levels of these serum proteins are very low and the only known stimulus to their production is an appropriate antigenic stimulus. The transport of these serum proteins from their subcellular site of origin, the polysome, probably follows the same course as outlined for albumin.[4]

Nutrition. In malnutrition, regardless of the cause, the basic assembly line for protein synthesis is disrupted within the liver. Albumin synthesis is rapidly slowed, and a fast for as short a period as 12 to 24 hours reduces albumin synthesis by at least one third. Initially there is a rapid loss of hepatic RNA and protein—which, after about 48 hours, slows. However, even with this slow rate of loss, cellular synthesis of these organelles is slowed further.[6] The amino acid supply for continued protein synthesis in fasting is nearly completely drawn from recycling hepatic amino acids.[5-10] If the malnutrition continues, albumin production may fall to values $\frac{1}{5}$ of the normal average value of 200 mg/kg/day. The effects of malnutrition on gamma globulin synthesis are not as clear cut, perhaps because this condition is frequently associated with infectious processes and the serum gamma globulin values are not de-

89

Table 2B-1.   Normal Values for Serum Protein Levels and Synthesis Rates

Serum Protein	Site(s) of Synthesis	Normal Serum Levels mg/100 ml	Synthetic Rate mg/kg/d
Albumin	Liver	3500–4500	150–200
Prealbumin	Liver	28–35	—
α_1 Lipoprotein (High density)	Liver	37–117	10–20 (peptide)
Orosomucoid	Liver	75–100	—
Haptoglobulin	Liver	30–190	10–25
Ceruloplasmin	Liver	27–39	2–5
α_2 Macroglobulin	?	220–380	—
α_2 Lipoproteins (Low density)	Liver G.I. tract	150–230	—
β Lipoprotein (Low density)	Liver	280–440	12–18 (peptide)
Transferrin	Liver ? spleen	200–320	6–25
Fibrinogen	Liver	200–600	30–40
IgG	Lymphocytes, spleen plasma cells	11–1200	20–30
IgM	Lymphocytes spleen	78–93	5–6
IgA	Lymphocytes mucosa	250	20–30
IgD	Lymphocytes	0.3–30	0.4
IgE	Lymphocytes	0.05	0.017

Reprinted in part from Table II, page 178 from H. E. Schultze, and J. F. Heremans, *Molecular Biology of Human Proteins*. New York, Elsevier Publishing Co., 1966 with permission.

pressed.   In malnutrition and protein-deficient states gamma globulin is capable of marked increments, even though albumin production cannot increase.[7–12]   The average synthetic rate for gamma globulin was 163/mg/kg/day in patients with kwashiorkor who were chronically infected and 51 mg/kg/day in "control" non-infected patients with this same disease.[7]   Altered fibrinogen synthesis does not appear to be of significance in malnutrition and malnutrition does not limit the stimulus to fibrinogen synthesis which follows intercurrent infections.   However, employing the isolated perfused liver derived from a donor rat which had been fasted for 6 days, the synthesis of fibrinogen, α_1 acid glycoprotein, α_2 acute phase globulin, haptoglobulin, in addition to albumin, occurred at a much reduced rate.[13]   The effects of altered nutrition *in vivo* on the myriad of other serum proteins are not known, but, clinically, the alteration is primarily in the albumin fraction.   As the serum albumin level falls, albumin degradation decreases, compensating in part for the depressed synthetic rate.[5,14]   Realimentation does not alter degradation but synthesis is rapidly stimulated and the serum albumin level rises once the extravascular albumin pool has been replaced.

Hormonal Influences. The effects of thyroid hormone and cortisone on albumin, globulin, and fibrinogen metabolism have been carefully studied.[15-23] In hyperthyroid patients or in patients receiving large doses of exogenous thyroid, both albumin synthesis and degradation are increased and there is no significant alteration in the serum protein level.[19] Gamma globulin turnover also increases and thus the demand for an adequate supply of amino acids is increased.[15] In hypothyroidism, albumin synthesis is slowed and there is a shift of albumin from the intravascular pool to extra plasma sites.[19] Some lowering of the plasma level may occur. Fibrinogen degradation and probably synthesis are also quantitatively affected by thyroid hormone level.[23] In situations where both malnutrition and decreased thyroid function are present, such as during acclimatization to heat, fibrinogen metabolism is slowed.[24,25]

Cortisone acetate, while considered to be antianabolic, exerts a strong anabolic effect on the visceral organs and stimulates albumin synthesis.[18,26,27] Within the liver there is a marked increase in nitrogen deposition and amino acids and a stimulus to RNA synthesis occurs, thus more than one factor is present to account for the increase in albumin synthesis. Both albumin and gamma globulin degradation are enhanced with high doses of steroids and gamma globulin synthesis may be lowered.[4,29] However, in both health and disease, excess cortisone acetate fails to stimulate fibrinogen synthesis, indicating that the effects of steroid hormones are not generalized and that fibrinogen synthesis is not responsive to the same stimuli as albumin.[22] Cortisone is necessary for the production of other acute phase proteins however, for injury alone without the availability of cortisone fails to stimulate these proteins which are so intimately related to injury.[30-32] Insulin promotes the synthesis of serum albumin *in vitro* but the clinical state of diabetes is not characterized by hypoalbuminemia or low albumin synthesis.[16] The transport of albumin through the capillary membrane is speeded in diabetes.[33]

Growth hormone is necessary for continued function of the hepatocyte in terms of plasma protein synthesis but the mechanism of its action is unknown.[34] Hypophysectomy lowers albumin synthesis and α_1 globulin is also lowered, but the other serum proteins are affected minimally. The addition of growth hormone stimulates albumin synthesis, possibly by stimulating mRNA and rRNA synthesis. Likewise insulin appears necessary to maintain adequate synthetic rates of the serum proteins, perhaps via similar RNA mechanisms.[34-37]

Environment. Few studies have been conducted in different environments but our expanding horizons make this a more and more important field. During acclimatization to heat, albumin and fibrinogen metabolism are rapidly lowered. In higher altitudes, albumin degradation appears to be stimulated but data on other proteins are not available. In tropical climates the gamma globulin levels are elevated and a slight depression in serum albumin has been found. In all of these stressful situations, changes in hormonal balance and nutrition may play the dominant regulatory role.[24,25,38]

Stress. The plasma levels of the serum proteins may change greatly following stress and trauma (Table 2B-2), with the acute phase proteins showing an increase and albumin decreasing.[38-45] Severe injury, surgical intervention, cancer and coronary thrombosis are varied types of stress, yet the serum protein pattern changes in a predictable fashion with early rises in α_1 and α_2 globulin, transferrin, and fibrinogen. The series of events within the liver following injury are an increased synthesis of RNA followed by more aggregated polysomes and an increased ability of this system to make protein. Albumin is not usually one of these proteins and albumin levels usually are depressed. Gamma globulin levels and synthesis will vary with the degree of associated infection. The response of some serum proteins to stress is mediated by hormonal levels: new RNA synthesis by the liver cell is stimulated by growth hormone and by insulin, and the levels of these hormones are altered in any stressful situation.[34-37]

The changes in the serum proteins are

Table 2B-2.   Proteins of Human Plasma Showing Altered Concentration after Trauma

Concentration Proteins		Concentration in Plasma (% of preoperative values)
Increased	Fibrinogen	>200
	Haptoglobin	206
	Orosomucoid	>200
	C-Reactive protein	>200
	α_1-Antitrypsin	>200
	Slow β-Globulin	173
	Inter α-globulin	189
	Complement C'3	122
	Ceruloplasmin	124
	Easily precipitable glycoprotein	140
Unchanged	More than 30 other proteins	
Decreased	Thyroxine binding prealbumin	69
	α-Lipoprotein	—
	β-Lipoprotein	77
	Transferrin	78
	Albumin	80

All the patients had undergone minor surgery 8 hours or more before the second blood sample was taken. (Reprinted from Gordon, A. H. in *Plasma Protein Metabolism*, Eds. M. A. Rothschild, and T. A. Waldmann: New York, Academic Press, 1970 with permission.)

most marked in severe burns. The three main classes of immunoglobulins IgM, IgG, and IgA all appear to undergo the same reaction. Data on IgD and IgE are not available. Initially there is a decrease in the serum levels, followed by significant increases, reaching peaks between 10 days and 3 weeks after the burn. In severely burned patients who later die in sepsis, the immunoglobulins do not show this marked increase. Intravenously injected labeled gamma globulin leaves the vascular bed within 48 hours, due to losses though the burned areas in addition to excessive degradation. The changes in serum albumin are even more drastic. Since the skin is the major site of extravascular albumin,[46] the patient with the severe burn has not only lost albumin through the injured urea, but also has lost the major extravascular pool to replace these plasma losses. Further albumin synthesis is depressed and a marked shift of albumin from plasma to extraplasma sites, secondary to an increase in capillary permeability, occurs. Fibrinogen synthesis and catabolism are both increased during the first 2 weeks after the severe burn, resulting in higher plasma levels. The stimulus to this increase in synthesis is not known.

Many undefined mechanisms appear responsible for the diverse reactions of the serum proteins to stress. Altered hormonal levels, infection, a tissue injury factor and the nutritional state all play important roles. It has been postulated that disruption of lysosomes may be the specific event common to trauma, with either the lysosomal enzymes acting as specific stimulators or more likely lysing specific inhibitors, permitting excessive synthesis.[40,42] It is interesting to speculate that these varied reactions of the liver in synthesizing proteins at different rates may be due to specialization within the liver such that, while most of the liver cells have the potential for all protein synthesis, specific cells are repressed from expressing this capacity in acute stress.

Cirrhosis. The level of serum albumin has long been considered to be the index of the liver's albumin-synthesizing capacity and, in liver disease, hypoalbuminemia is a common finding. However in many patients, particularly those with ascites, the exchangeable albumin pool is not depressed.[47-53] In 14 of 19 patients with portal cirrhosis and ascites from alcoholism who were studied after hospitalization, albumin synthesis was found to be normal or elevated. Thus, once the acute effects of alcohol were removed, and the patients given an adequate diet, albumin synthesis was capable of significant increments. Fibrinogen synthesis has not been found to be impaired in cirrhosis of the liver and, while albumin synthesis may be stimulated by cortisone in cirrhotic subjects, fibrinogen synthesis is not affected. Gamma globulin levels are frequently elevated in liver disease and in fact the depression of the serum albumin level may represent a colloid osmotic effect produced by the elevated gamma globulin, which interferes with or inhibits albumin synthesis.

The pattern of serum protein metabolism in cirrhosis is most complicated because of the interplay of toxic or infectious agents, malnutrition, hormonal imbalance and altered distribution of the serum proteins. Suffice it to say that each of these aspects should be studied in an attempt to provide the optimum conditions for the decreased liver to function.[54-56]

Renal Disease. Proteinuria is the prime factor in altering the serum protein pattern in patients with renal disease. When the patient first develops proteinuria, the serum protein levels are normal and losses into the urine must be massive. Thereafter, as the serum levels fall, loss decreases and degradation decreases, perhaps as an attempt to compensate for renal losses.[57-63] It is surprising that hepatic albumin synthesis does not always increase to compensate for these renal losses, for the capacity of the liver cell to produce albumin in nephrotic states is tremendous. Clinically this reserve capacity is not utilized. However, this lack of increased synthesis may be protective. If the dietary nitrogen is increased then, in nephrotic subjects, the increased albumin synthesis would result in greater urinary losses. Normally a small amount of albumin is filtered through the glomeruli, reabsorbed by the tubules and degraded within tubular cells. This catabolism is negligible during health but, during albuminuric states, this form of catabolism is significant. Urinary globulin loss may

also be significant. IgA and IgG are lost to a larger degree than IgM. In glomerular disease, the hypogammaglobulinemia and increased rate of loss of IgG from the plasma are related primarily to loss of this protein into the urine.[4] However, increased catabolism by the functioning tubular cells is also a factor. In diseases such as the Fanconi syndrome, cystinosis, cadmium or heavy metal toxicity, where tubular disease predominates, loss of small molecular protein into the urine predominates. These proteins which are filtered are simply not reabsorbed and are not subject to tubular degradation with conservation of amino acids. It has been shown that the metabolism of many serum proteins small enough to pass through the basement membrane is subject to a renal catabolic system. In tubular disease the overall loss from the body is increased but degradation is decreased, as with the albumin molecule. In more chronic renal disease with uremia, the survival of those smaller proteins may even be prolonged since there is less renal tissue capable of functioning catabolically.

Gastrointestinal Disorders. All the serum proteins are present on the mucosal surface of the gut[64,65] and the gastrointestinal tract has been considered to play many different roles in the catabolism of serum protein.[66-82] Initial estimates of the fraction of total albumin and gamma globulin catabolism occurring in the gastrointestinal tract varied from 10 to 70 per cent. Most of these studies employed small segments of bowel and studies were conducted for short periods of time, thus the potential errors were considerable. The problem of studying *in vivo* intestinal degradation relates to the fact that undenatured protein tracers are not available, with the possible exception of copper-labeled ceruloplasmin. The use of polyvinylpyrrolidone or iron-labeled dextran to study protein losses into the gut is, of course, subject to question, because these substances are not proteins. Chromium-labeled albumin, which is the most commonly employed tracer, is relatively degraded during labeling and rapid losses from the plasma occur early. However, following 4 or 5 days of injection, the remaining chromium-labeled albumin behaves more like iodinated albumin. When both of these tracers are used (^{125}I albumin and ^{51}Cr albumin) the total degradation rate may be determined from the iodine tag and the stool clearance from the chromium label. Employing this exacting technique, the absolute fecal "catabolic rate" accounts for no more than 5 to 10 per cent of total albumin degradation in normal subjects.

Since the serum proteins have been found on the mucosal serum of the gut from the mouth to the intestinal tract and in the bile,[30] some protein degradation should be expected. Pathologically there are two main conditions leading to loss of more protein into the intestinal tract. One relates to increased lymphatic pressure leading to loss of lymph into the gut. Intestinal lymphangiectasis, constrictive pericarditis, Whipple's disease and involvement of the abdominal lymph nodes by widespread infection or tumor are examples of this type. The second mechanism is related inflammatory bowel disease with altered mucosa, as in hypertrophic gastritis, colitis and ileitis. In these conditions there is bulk loss of the plasma proteins and the absolute degradation rate of gamma globulin and albumin (those proteins that have been studied extensively) is elevated. The contribution of the intestinal tract to the total elevated degradation and loss may be 50 per cent or more. Usually, endogenous degradation is decreased compensatorily. However, hypoproteinemia, which is associated with these conditions, cannot be related to the degradation alone, for the capacity to produce serum proteins should far exceed the increased losses. Thus, at the heart of the disorders are relative decreased synthetic rates. These in turn may be significantly influenced by the specific nutrition or amino acid deficiencies which may characterize the specific gastrointestinal disorder. Thus, in essence, the intestinal tract is a potential degradative site leading in disease states to hypoproteinemia which, in turn, is related primarily to defective protein production. Nutrition is certainly a most important factor in maintaining serum protein levels in these diseases (Tables 2B-3 and 4).

AMINO ACID ABNORMALITIES

The plasma free amino acid pool represents less than 1 to 5 per cent of the total amino acid pool in the body and, thus, it is immediately clear that changes in the plasma amino acid levels may have no bearing or biochemical implications at the site of protein synthesis in the tissues. The plasma, liver and kidney contain less than 10 to 15 per

Table 2B-3.   Disorders of Immunoglobulin Synthesis

I. Deficiency of all immunoglobulin classes
  A. Autosomal recessive lymphopenic agammaglobulinemia (Swiss-type agammaglobulinemia)
  B. Sex-linked recessive lymphopenic agammaglobulinemia (thymic alymphoplasia)
  C. Sex-linked agammaglobulinemia (Bruton-type agammaglobulinemia)
  D. Primary immunoglobulin deficiency
      1. Acquired agammaglobulinemia
      2. Congenital agammaglobulinemia (sporadic, nonsex-linked)
  E. Secondary immunoglobulin deficiency-chronic lymphocytic leukemia
  F. Acquired agammaglobulinemia with thymoma

II. Selectic immunoglobulin deficiencies
  A. Lymphopenic immune deficiency with dysgammaglobulinemia
  B. Dysgammaglobulinemia Type I—↑IgM, ↓IgG, ↓IgA
  C. Other dysgammaglobulinemias with varying immunoglobulin patterns
  D. Ataxia telangiectasia
  E. Isolated absence of IgA associated with malabsorption
  F. Asymptomatic absence of IgA

Reprinted from Strober, W., Blaese, R. M., and Waldmann, T. A. in *Plasma Protein Metabolism*, Eds. M. A. Rothschild, and T. A. Waldmann: New York, Academic Press, 1970 with permission.

Table 2B-4. Disorders of Immunoglobulin Catabolism

I. Hypercatabolism
  A. Excessive loss of immunoglobulins
    1. Nephrotic syndrome
    2. Protein-losing gastroenteropathy
  B. Endogenous hypercatabolism
    1. Hypercatabolism affecting a single immunoglobulin
      a. Myotonic dystrophy-hypercatabolism of IgG
      b. Dysgammaglobulinemia and anti-immunoglobulin antibodies
    2. Hypercatabolism affecting more than one immunoglobulin (as well as other serum proteins)
      a. Wiskott-Aldrich syndrome
      b. Familial hypercatabolic hypoproteinemia
      c. Hypermetabolic states
      d. Nephrotic syndrome

II. Hypocatabolism-nephron loss disease with decreased endogenous catabolism of L-chains and other low molecular weight serum proteins

III. Abnormal pathway of metabolism-renal tubular disease with ↑ protein excretion and ↓ endogenous catabolism of protein

Reprinted from Strober, W., Blaese, R. M., and Waldmann, T. A. in *Plasma Protein Metabolism*, Eds., M. A. Rothschild, and T. A. Waldmann: New York, Academic Press, 1970 with permission.

cent of the pool, while muscle and intestine make up the mass of the available amino acid stores.

There are specific transport systems for groups of amino acids, specific permeabilities of different tissues and specific interrelationships between one amino acid and another in terms of competition for entrance into the cell.

The period of time an absorbed amino acid remains in the plasma is short and equilibrium with the various extracellular spaces probably requires only minutes or less.[84,85] However, penetration into cells is a much longer process and, in fact, there may even be rather marked cellular compartmentalization as well. The levels in the plasma represent the net result of three metabolic pathways, protein synthesis and degradation, and synthesis of intermediate compounds. Further, the type of protein digested, the metabolic state of the body, the prior nutritional state and the degree of stress all are interrelated.[83]

Thus, the plasma amino acid level cannot be taken as a true guide to what may be happening to protein synthesis. For example, as fasting proceeds the amino acids available for protein synthesis within the liver cell are derived mainly from recirculation of the intracellular pool (derived from degradation) rather than from exogenous sources.[86] In malnutrition, in cirrhosis or in renal disease different patterns of amino acid changes in the plasma have been observed.[87-94]

Munro has recently reviewed the factors involved in the regulation of the free amino acid pool and the effects of these changes on protein synthesis, but there are few data on the influence of specific amino acid deficiencies on serum protein synthesis.[83] In general, different effects would be expected when the experimental or clinical states change from an acute to an "in balance" to a chronic deficiency; or from an *in vitro* study to an *in vivo* situation, where hormonal changes and muscle pools are present. Thus, the interpretation of specific effects of different amino acids is most difficult. In chronic diseases characterized by malnutrition, such as marasmus and kwashiorkor, the plasma levels of amino acids are usually depressed, with arginine, leucine and valine usually being the lowest. In chronic uremia, no marked alteration occurs. In chronic liver disease, leucine, valine, and isoleucine values are usually depressed, with an elevation in methionine frequently reported. It is not possible to arrive at any specific interpretation from the available *in vivo* data, except to arrive at specific limits in terms of growth of the whole organism, or of the limiting amino acid in a diet. Marked variations occur in the basic requirements.[95]

Following the intake of food, the liver is rapidly bathed with blood high in amino acid content. About one half of these amino acids probably undergo rapid degradation—much of the remainder is incorporated into new protein and a small but variable fraction reaches the systemic circulation. During fasting, the cellular recycling of intracellular hepatic amino acids from degradation to synthesis provides most of the hepatic free amino acids.[85] Thereafter, peripheral protein degradation in muscle tissue provides the amino acids for other protein synthesis. An adequate supply of all amino acids is needed and an imbalance causes changes in growth rate, decreased protein synthesis and alterations in levels of other amino acids. Usually this imbalance will not be eaten and, thus, the effects of starvation occur first. For example, a threonine-deficient diet results in elevations of all free amino acids in intestine and in liver, a depression in threonine, histidine, serine, glutamine in muscle, and increases in valine and lysine in plasma. On the other hand, force feeding of this diet results in reaggregation of the hepatic polysomal system, with an increase in protein synthesis by this subcellular system.[96] Further, in fasting there is a marked disaggregation of the hepatic polysome which may be reaggregated by an excess of tryptophan.[96] Yet *in vivo* reaggregation can also be caused by a diet devoid of tryptophan, probably secondary to a release of muscle amino acids.[97] To complicate this picture even more there is the problem of an *in vivo* diurnal variation in the plasma amino acid level which is dependent on the spacing of food intake but not necessarily on dietary imbalance.[98]

Specific model systems, where only a single permutation is made, are needed for each protein and probably for each amino acid before the clear definition of cause and effect can be outlined. Specific examples of such actions are available, however.[91-93] Tryp-

tophan is essential for the maintenance of the aggregated polysome in liver[96] and in brain[100] and stimulation to both mRNA[101] and rRNA synthesis has been reported. Lysine and valine are required for ribosome subunit synthesis.[99] Excess phenylalanine results in disaggregation of brain polysomes.[100] Tryptophan, in the isolated perfused liver, stimulates albumin synthesis.[102] At the moment, no single amino acid abnormality can be isolated as influencing protein synthesis *in vivo* though it is tempting to speculate that this is the ultimate control mechanism.

The specific effects of diet, stress, hormones, environment and disease on plasma proteins with specific functions are not well studied. Lipid intake influences the synthesis of the various classes of lipoproteins. Yet the relationship between lipid intake and the synthesis of protein fractions is not clarified. Likewise, the proteins involved in clotting, hemoglobin transport, iron transport and heavy metal transport may have their synthetic rates regulated by feedback mechanisms related to their specific functions.

Until unique systems are available for the study of each of these proteins, the specific effects of the various amino acids must remain in the realm of speculation.

BIBLIOGRAPHY

1. Munro: Regulation mechanism, in protein metabolism in *Mammalian Protein Metabolism*, Ed., H. Munro, New York, Academic Press, Vol. 4, p. 3, 1970.
2. Peters, Fleischer, and Fleischer: J. Biol. Chem., *240*, 216, 1971.
3. Schultze and Heremans: *Molecular Biology of Human Proteins*, New York, Elsevier Publ. Co., Sect. III, 321–518, 1966.
4. Waldmann and Strober: Prog. In Allergy, *13*, 1, 1969.
5. Rothschild, Oratz, and Schreiber: Factors regulating serum protein metabolism, in *Protides of the Biologic Fluids*, Ed., H. Peeters, New York, Elsevier Publ. Co., Vol. 14, p. 267, 1967.
6. Enwonwu, and Munro: Arch. of Biochem. and Biophy., *138*, 532, 1970.
7. Cohen, and Hansen: Clin. Sc., *23*, 351, 1962.
8. Waterlow: Lancet, 2, 7578, 1968.
9. Hoffenberg, Black, and Brock: J. Clin. Invest., *45*, 143, 1966.
10. Freeman and Gordon: Clin. Sc., *26*, 17, 1964.
11. Rothschild, Oratz, Mongelli, and Schreiber: J. Clin. Invest., *47*, 2591, 1968.

12. Viteri, Behar, Arroyave, and Scrimshaw: Clinical Aspects of Protein Malnutrition, in *Mammalian Protein Metabolism*. Ed. H. N. Munro, New York, Academic Press, Vol. II, p. 523, 1964.
13. John and Miller: J. Biol. Chem., *244*, 6134, 1969.
14. Kirsch, Frith, Black, and Hoffenberg: Nature, *217*, 578, 1968.
15. Farthing, Gerwing, and Shewell: J. Endo., *21*, 83, 1960.
16. Balegno and Neuhaus: Life Sc., *9*, 1039, 1970.
17. Jefferson and Korner: Biochem. J., *104*, 826, 1967.
18. Rothschild, Schreiber, Oratz and McGee: J. Clin. Invest., *37*, 1229, 1958.
19. Rothschild, Bauman, Yalow and Berson: J. Clin. Invest., *36*, 422, 1957.
20. Ulrich, Turner and Li: J. Biol. Chem., *209*, 117, 1954.
21. Wagle: Arch. of Biochem. and Biophy., *102*, 373, 1963.
22. Cain, Mayer, and Jones: J. Clin. Invest., *42*, 2178, 1970.
23. Regoeczi: Abnormal Fibrinogen Metabolism, in *Plasma Protein Metabolism*, Eds. M. A. Rothschild and T. A. Waldmann, New York, Academic Press, p. 459, 1970.
24. Oratz, Walker, Schreiber, Gross and Rothschild: Am. J. Physiol., *213*, 1341, 1967.
25. Curtain, Gajdusek, Kidsos, Gorman, Champness and Rodrique: Am. J. Trop. Med. Hyg., *14*, 678, 1965.
26. Silber, and Porta: Endrin., *52*, 518, 1953.
27. Kochakian and Robertson: J. Biol. Chem., *190*, 481, 1951.
28. Manchester: Sites of hormonal regulation of protein metabolism, in *Mammalian Protein Metabolism*, Vol. IV, Ed. H. Munro, New York, Academic Press, 229, 1970.
29. Levy and Waldmann: J. Clin. Invest., *49*, 1679, 1970.
30. Neuhaus, Balegno and Chandler: Am. J. Physiol., *211*, 151, 1966.
31. Sarcione: Regulation of plasma Alpha₂ (acute phase) globulin synthesis in rat liver, in *Plasma Protein Metabolism*. Eds., M. A. Rothschild and T. A. Waldmann. New York, Academic Press, 1970.
32. Gordon: Effects of trauma and partial hepatectomy on the rates of synthesis of plasma proteins by the liver, in *Plasma Protein Metabolism*, Eds., M. A. Rothschild, and T. A. Waldmann, New York, Academic Press, 351, 1970.
33. Ismael, Khalifa, and Madwar: Lancet, *2*, 810, 1965.
34. Jefferson and Korner: Biochem. J., *104*, 826, 1967.
35. Enerback, Lundin and Mellgren: Acta Endo., *32*, 552, 1959.
36. Brewer, Foster and Sells: J. Biol. Chem., *244*, 1389, 1969.
37. Garren, Richardson, and Crocco: J. Biol. Chem., *242*, 650, 1967.
38. Surks: J. Clin. Invest., *45*, 1442, 1966.
39. Birke: Regulation of protein metabolism in burns, in *Plasma Protein Metabolism*, Eds. M. A. Rothschild, and T. A. Waldmann, New York, Academic Press, 415, 1970.
40. Koj and Allison: Folia Biologica, *17*, 37, 1969.
41. Birke, Liljedlahl, Plantin and Reizenstein: Acta Clin. Scand., *134*, 27, 1967.
42. Koj and McFarlane: Biochem. J., *108*, 137, 1968.
43. Kukral, Zeinch, Dobryszycka, Pollitt and Stone: N. Clin. Sc., *36*, 221, 1969.
44. Davies, Ricketts, and Bull: Clin. Sc., *23*, 411, 1962.
45. Krauss, Schrott and Sarcione: Am. J. Med. Sci., *252*, 84, 1966.
46. Rothschild, Bauman, Yalow and Berson: J. Clin. Invest., *34*, 1354, 1955.
47. Post and Patek: Arch. Int. Med., *69*, 67, 83, 1942.
48. Sterling: J. Clin. Invest., *30*, 1228, 1951.
49. Wikinson and Mendenhall: Clin. Sc., *25*, 281, 1963.
50. Hasch, Jarnum and Tygestrup: Acta Med. Scand., *182*, 83, 1967.
51. Dykes: Clin. Sc., *34*, 161, 1968.
52. Berson and Yalow: J. Clin. Invest., *33*, 377, 1954.
53. Rothschild, Oratz, Zimmon, Schreiber, Weiner and Van Caneghem: J. Clin. Invest., *48*, 344, 1969.
54. Rothschild, Oratz and Schreiber: Scand. J. Gastro. Suppl., *7*, 17, 1970.
55. Peterson: J. Clin. Invest., *39*, 230, 1960.
56. Cavalieri and Searle: J. Clin. Invest., *45*, 939, 1966.
57. Bauman, Rothschild, Yalow and Berson: J. Clin. Invest., *34*, 1359, 1955.
58. Jensen, Rossing, Andersen and Jarnum: Clin. Sc., *33*, 445, 1967.
59. Gitlin, Janeway and Fan: J. Clin. Invest., *35*, 44, 1956.
60. Katz: J. Lab. Clin. Med., *53*, 486, 1959.
61. Katz, Benorris and Sellers: J. Lab. Clin. Med., *62*, 910, 1963.
62. Marsh and Drabkin: J. Biol. Chem., *230*, 1063, 1958.
63. ———: J. Biol. Chem., *230*, 1073, 1958.
64. Horowitz and Hollander: J. Biol. Chem., *236*, 770, 1961.
65. Tarver, Armstrong, Debro and Margen: Ann. N.Y. Acad. Sc., *94*, 23, 1961.
66. Gullberg and Olhagen: Nature, *184*, 1848, 1950.
67. Holman, Nickel and Sleisenger: Am. J. Med., *27*, 963, 1959.
68. Weterfors: Acta Med. Scand., Suppl., *430*, 177, 1, 1965.
69. Waldmann: Gastroenterology, *5*, 422, 1966.
70. Kerr, Dubois and Holt: J. Clin. Invest., *46*, 2064, 1967.
71. Andersen and Jarnum: Lancet, *1*, 1060, 1966.
72. Dawson, Williams and Williams: Brit. Med. J., *2*, 667, 1961.

73. Laster, Waldmann, Fenester and Singleton: J. Clin. Invest., *45*, 637, 1966.
74. Waldmann and Schwab: J. Clin. Invest., *44*, 1523, 1965.
75. Rothschild, Oratz and Schreiber: Am. J. Digest. Dis., *14*, 711, 1969.
76. Sternlieb, Morell, Wochner, Aisen and Waldmann: Proc. Physiol. and Pathophysiol. of Plasma Prot. Met. 3rd. Symposium. H. Huber, Berne, p. 34, 1964.
77. Franks, Edwards, Lackey and Fitzgerald: J. Gen. Physiol., *46*, 415; 427, 1963.
78. Wilkinson, Pinto and Senior: New Eng. J. Med., *273*, 1178, 1965.
79. Jeffries, Holman and Sleisenger: New Eng. J. Med., *266*, 652, 1962.
80. Hardwicke, Rankin, Baker and Preisig: Clin. Sc., *26*, 509, 1964.
81. Wochner, Weissman, Waldmann, Houston and Berlin: J. Clin. Invest., *47*, 971, 1968.
82. Jeejeebhoy, Samuel, Singh, Nadkarni, Desai, Borkari and Mani: Gastro., *56*, 252, 1969.
83. Munro: Free amino acid pools and their role in regulation, in *Mammalian Protein Metabolism*, Vol. 4 Ed. H. N. Munro, New York, Academic Press, p. 299, 1970.
84. Hider, Fern and London: Biochem. J., *121*, 817, 1971.
85. Kinnis, Reiss and Helmreich: Biochem. and Biophy. Acta, *51*, 519, 1961.
86. Gan and Jeffay: Biochem. Biophy. Acta, *148*, 448, 1967.
87. Waterlow and Stephen: Clin. Sc., *35*, 287, 1968.
88. Walshe: Quart. J. Med., *88*, 483, 1953.
89. Iber, Rosen, Levenson and Chalmers: J. Lab. Clin. Med., *50*, 417, 1957.
90. Wu, Bollman and Butt: J. Clin. Invest., *34*, 845, 1955.
91. Iob, Coon and Sloan: J. Surg. Res., *7*, 41, 1967.
92. ————: Surg. Res., *6*, 233, 1966.
93. Ness, Takahashi and Lee: J. Clin. Endo. and Met., *85*, 1166, 1969.
94. Rubini and Gordon: Nephron, *5*, 339, 1968.
95. Irwin and Hegsted: J. Nutrition, *101*, 539, 1971.
96. Staehlin, Verney and Sidransky: Biochem. Biophy. Acta, *145*, 105, 1967.
97. Sidransky and Verney: Proc. Soc. Exp. Biol. and Med., *135*, 618, 1970.
98. Wurtman: Diurnal rhythms, in *Mammalian Protein Metabolism* Vol. 4. Ed. H. N. Munro, New York, Academic Press, 445, 1970.
99. Madin: Nature, *224*, 1203, 1969.
100. Aoki and Siegil: Science, *168*, 130, 1970.
101. Vesely and Cihak: Biochem. Biophy. Acta, *204*, 614, 1970.
102. Rothschild, Oratz, Mongelli, Fishman and Schreiber: Am. J. Nutrition, *98*, 395, 1969.

Chapter

3

Carbohydrates

RACHMIEL LEVINE

Before the development of the modern food processing and distributing industry (and, at present, in those parts of the world which have not undergone that development), the proportion of carbohydrate in the diet of any region was largely governed by the local flora and fauna. Even now the proportionate intake of carbohydrate is high in tropical countries, where vegetation is luxurious and the climate leads to rapid spoilage of meat products. On the other hand, the inhabitants of the Far North have always lived on a diet consisting chiefly of meat and fish. Adequate nutrition is possible at both dietary extremes, if the need for calories, essential food factors, vitamins, and minerals is met.[1-4]

Though there has been some change during the past 70 years in the food sources from which the carbohydrates are derived, the proportion of carbohydrate in the dietary of the United States has remained at about 50 per cent of the total caloric intake. Since certain foods high in carbohydrate content are relatively inexpensive, the proportion of carbohydrate in the diet has been greater at lower economic levels than in the more prosperous groups of the population. The poorer nutritional status of the lowest income groups, however, is not so much a reflection of their high carbohydrate intake as it is a result of the particular foods from which they derive their carbohydrates. The highly refined grains and sugars, developed commercially largely because of their resistance to spoilage, are the cheapest sources of calories generally available. But they have been deprived of most of the protective elements with which

they are naturally endowed; hence a *casually selected* high-carbohydrate diet is likely to be poor in the essential amino acids, vitamins, and minerals.[5]

THE CARBOHYDRATES IN FOODS

The carbohydrates in the ordinary American diet, the food sources from which they are derived, and the quantitative importance of each in the total intake are indicated in Table 3-1.

DIGESTION AND ABSORPTION OF CARBOHYDRATES

Digestion.[7] The digestion of carbohydrates starts in the oral cavity. Here the secretion of the parotid gland, which contains an amylase (ptyalin), is mixed with the food and begins the conversion of starch, glycogen, and dextrins into maltose. This digestion continues in the stomach until the hydrochloric acid secreted there destroys the amylase activity and substitutes acid hydrolysis for enzymatic splitting. If continued long enough, the acid hydrolysis could reduce all the digestible carbohydrates to the monosaccharide stage. The stomach usually empties itself, however, before this can occur; the digestion of carbohydrate is then taken up by the enzymes of the small intestine, which operate in the more alkaline medium which prevails there. The enzymes in the small intestine are amylases secreted by the pancreas, and amylases, maltase, sucrase, and lactase secreted by the wall of the small

Table 3-1. Types and Sources of Carbohydrates in the American Dietary
(Food and Life, Yearbook of Agriculture[6])

Carbohydrates	*Approx. % of Total CHO Intake	Chief Food Sources	End Products of Digestion	Remarks
Polysaccharides				
(a) Indigestible:				
1. Celluloses and Hemicelluloses	3	Stalks and leaves of vegetables, outer covering of seeds	0	May be partially split to glucose by bacterial action in large bowel.
2. Pectins		Fruits	0	Chemical hydrolysis yields galactose and arabinose. Digestion incomplete, further splitting by bacteria may occur in large bowel.
(b) Partially digestible:				
1. Inulin		Jerusalem artichokes, onions, garlic	Fructose	
2. Galactogens	2	Snails	Galactose	
3. Mannosans		Legumes	Mannose	
4. Raffinose		Sugar beets	Glucose, Fractose and Galactose	
5. Pentosans		Fruits and gums	Pentoses	
(c) Digestible:				
1. Starch and Dextrins	50	Grains, vegetables (especially tubers and legumes)	Glucose	The most important group quantitatively. Usually accompanied by some maltose.
2. Glycogen	negligible	Meat products and seafood	Glucose	

				Remarks
Disaccharides				
1. Sucrose	25	Cane and beet sugars, molasses, maple syrup	Glucose and Fructose	In fruits and vegetables, the contents of glucose and fructose depend on species, ripeness and state of preservation.
2. Lactose	10	Milk and milk products	Glucose and Galactose	
3. Maltose	negligible	Malt products	Glucose	
Monosaccharides				
(a) Hexoses:				
1. Glucose	5	Fruits, honey, corn syrup	Glucose	
2. Fructose	5	Fruits, honey	Fructose	
3. Galactose	0	0	Galacotse	These monosaccharides do not occur in free form in foods (see under lactose and mannosans).
4. Mannose	0	0	Mannose	
(b) Pentoses:				
1. Ribose	0	0	Ribose	These monosaccharides do not occur in free form in foods. They are derived from pentosans of fruits and from the nucleic acids of meat products and seafood.
2. Xylose	0	0	Xylose	
3. Arabinose	0	0	Arabinose	

* Calculated from the average dietary of the middle-income group in the United States.

bowel. All these enzymes are capable of splitting the particular sugars which they attack to the monosaccharide stage.

We have accounted for the digestion of starch, dextrins, glycogen, and the disaccharides. Sugars ingested as monosaccharides do not require digestion. All the remaining carbohydrates pass through the stomach and small intestine unchanged. In the large bowel, they are subjected to the enzymatic influence of the profuse bacterial flora normal there and may to some extent be broken down to monosaccharides. It is possible that minor amounts of carbohydrate are made available in this manner for absorption into the blood stream (see Fig. 3–1).

Absorption. The monosaccharides ingested as such or arising from the digestion of carbohydrates are almost completely absorbed in the small intestine. Small amounts may be absorbed from the stomach. The portion of the epithelial cell lining the mucosa in contact with the lumen of the intestine is the so-called brush border. It is a specialized area containing the enzymes which split disaccharides (lactase, sucrase, etc.) and the machinery for the absorption of the monosaccharides. Glucose (as well as galactose, d-xylose, etc.) enter through the cell membrane by attachment to a specific "carrier" molecule which transports the sugar molecules across the membrane. This type of carrier-mediated process operates in most animal cells and can account for a transport from a region of higher to a region of lower concentration until equilibrium is reached. However, intestinal absorption occurs against a gradient. The sugar "accumulates" intracellularly and then diffuses to the serosal side and enters the blood stream. This uphill transport occurs because the same "carrier" also attaches to Na^+. Since a respiring cell constantly "pumps" Na^+ out of the interior, the concentration of Na^+ intracellularly is kept low. The joint sugar-Na^+ carrier moves inward so long as the combined sugar and Na^+ concentration in the cell is lower than in the lumen. Hence intracellular sugar concentration rises but is continuously being depleted by removal into the portal blood. Hence sugar absorption

goes on even when the intra-intestinal sugar concentration is low, as long as Na^+ is present.[8–12] Fructose seems to be absorbed by a different mechanism.[12] Some of the glucose entering the epithelium is utilized there to provide cell energy, the proportion so used varying with the animal species.

Rate of Absorption of Monosaccharides. The actual rates of absorption of the three common monosaccharides vary widely. It has been shown in rats, for example, that, if the rate for glucose is represented as 100, that for galactose will be 110, for fructose 43, but for mannose and the pentoses only 9.[13] There are few reliable data on the absolute rates at which the various monosaccharides can be absorbed from the gastrointestinal tract of the human being under normal circumstances. The best available evidence, the work of Groen,[14] indicates that the rate of absorption of glucose from a 50 cm length of jejunum is about 8.0 gm per hour, that for galactose about 9.5 gm per hour, and that for fructose about 5 gm per hour. These rates are for concentrations of sugar of 10 per cent and above. Below 10 per cent, the rate of absorption varies directly with the concentration.

Factors Influencing Absorption. From a practical standpoint, the figures quoted above may have little relation to the rate at which a monosaccharide enters the blood stream when it is eaten as such or arises from the processes of digestion under the usual conditions of feeding. In the latter case, the time elapsing before it is absorbed from the gastrointestinal tract will be governed largely by (1) the rate at which it enters the small intestine and (2) the mixture of foods in the small intestine at the time of absorption. The rate at which the sugar arrives at the small intestine depends largely on the motility of the stomach and the control of the duodenal sphincter, which can be affected by such various phenomena as hunger, emotion, local irritation (including that induced by condiments) and the composition and consistency of the food mass after mastication.[7] The food mixture in the small intestine affects the rate of absorption by reason of the competition of the various constituents in the mixture for the absorbing surface of the mucosa and, in the case of monosaccharides specifically absorbed,

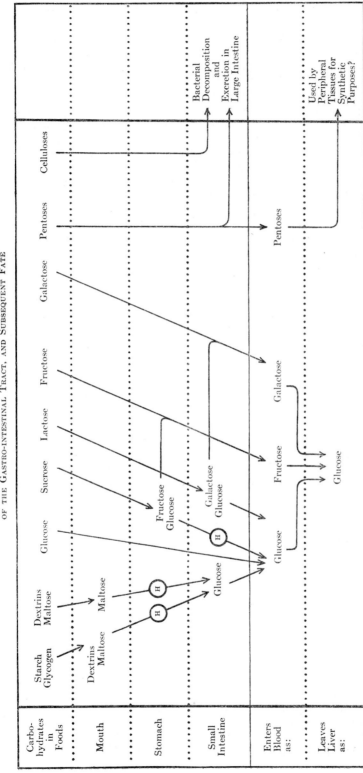

PRODUCTS OF CARBOHYDRATE DIGESTION AT VARIOUS LEVELS
OF THE GASTRO-INTESTINAL TRACT, AND SUBSEQUENT FATE

Ⓗ indicates that the same products as at the preceding level continue to appear.

Fig. 3-1.

by competition for the available transport systems.

Other factors which influence the amount of carbohydrate absorbed in a given individual at a particular time are: (1) the normality of the mucous membrane of the small intestine and the length of time during which the carbohydrate is in contact with it; (2) endocrine function, particularly that of the anterior pituitary gland,[15] the thyroid[15] and the adrenal cortex,[16] and (3) the adequacy of vitamin intake, especially that of the B complex.[17]

Since the absorption of the important end products of carbohydrate digestion requires chemical activity by the mucous membrane, it is obvious that any abnormality of the mucosal cells might interfere with carbohydrate absorption. Enteritis (inflammation) is a not uncommon disturbance of this kind. Celiac disease may represent a more obscure disturbance of a similar nature. Defects and malfunction of the brush border of the intestinal epithelium may be expected to cause a variety of disorders associated with intolerance to disaccharides and to monosaccharides. Such is the case[18-20] and it seems entirely consonant with the present concepts of the sites and mechanisms of digestion and absorption. Even when the mucosa is normal, however, an excessive rate of movement of the carbohydrate along the gastrointestinal tract accompanying diarrheas of various origins may hurry a portion of the ingested carbohydrate into the large bowel before it can be absorbed.

Normal absorption of carbohydrate does not occur if there is an anterior pituitary deficiency. This probably depends for the most part upon the secondary hypofunction of the thyroid gland, for the same result may be obtained after removal of the thyroid gland when the hypophysis is intact. Furthermore, the defect in absorption accompanying hypopituitarism may be relieved by the administration of thyroid extract.[15] Indeed, Althausen and his co-workers[21] have attempted to make use of this phenomenon as a clinical test of the state of activity of the thyroid gland. They administer a standard amount of galactose by mouth, follow the rise of galactose concentration in the blood, and

use the rate of the latter as a criterion of thyroid function.

The adrenal cortex influences carbohydrate absorption through its regulation of the sodium chloride exchange in the body.[11] The absorption of carbohydrate from the intestine is subnormal in adrenal cortical deficiency, but can be restored to normal without the use of adrenal cortical extracts if the sodium chloride of the blood is raised to normal levels by adequate salt intake.[16]

Insulin, which has such an important influence on other aspects of carbohydrate metabolism, is without apparent effect upon the absorptive capacity of the intestinal mucous membrane.

THE DISTRIBUTION OF CARBOHYDRATE IN THE BODY: ITS FUNCTIONS AND USES

In order to understand the distribution of carbohydrate in the body and to appreciate its particular functions and uses, it is necessary first to consider the relation of carbohydrate metabolism to that of the other two major foodstuffs, fat and protein.

Carbohydrates, Proteins and Fats. Protein constitutes 75 per cent of the dry weight of the soft tissues of the body. In view of the protein nature of the tissue enzymes, it is a fair generalization to say that the proteins, together with the hormones, vitamins, and minerals, constitute the metabolic machinery of the body. In emergencies, a certain amount of the protein machinery can be broken down and converted into fuel. The amount of body protein available for this purpose at any one time, however, is strictly limited, as is also the period of survival possible when the body has exhausted its fat stores and is forced to depend upon endogenous protein alone.[22]

Fat differs from protein in that it can be stored in practically unlimited quantities. It is deposited chiefly within specialized cells of connective tissue and does not become an integral part of the working organs of the body. When food intake is inadequate to supply the caloric needs of the organism, sufficient fat is mobilized to make up the caloric deficit. In this way, practically the entire fat store of the body can be depleted without detriment to health. Whatever harm accompanies extreme emaciation can be explained by specific deficiencies in the protective food factors incidental to the general restriction in food intake and by the loss of certain secondary structural functions of fat having to do with heat insulation and the architectural cushioning of organs. Fat is, therefore, primarily a fuel storage material. When food is ingested in excess of caloric expenditure (whether taken in the form of carbohydrate, protein or fat), the equivalent of the excess calories is deposited as fat in the adipose tissues.

Carbohydrate resembles fat in that it is a fuel material but differs from it in that it is an indispensable one. Certain tissues of the body constantly require and use carbohydrate under all physiologic conditions.[23] Even a temporary fall in the blood sugar below certain critical levels is accompanied by serious disability. Nevertheless, the amount of carbohydrate in the body at any one time is very small. This amount, if not replaced as used, would sustain life for only a portion of one day. Table 3–2 compares the total effective carbohydrate content of a hypothetic average normal man with his caloric requirement.

From this it is clear that, unless large amounts of carbohydrate are regularly ingested, the carbohydrate needs of the body must be met by the conversion of other foodstuffs into carbohydrate. It is an active fuel of the body; it is stored only in small quantities and is taken in or made as required.

Carbohydrate Distribution. The available carbohydrate of the body is largely present in the form of glycogen in the skeletal, cardiac, and smooth muscles. In these motor tissues it serves as an emergency reserve of fuel which can be mobilized more rapidly than glucose can reach them through the regular channels. Most of the remaining carbohydrate in the body is found in the manufacturing and distributing system, namely, in the liver as glycogen and in the blood and extracellular fluids as glucose. Relatively small amounts of glycogen are also found in practically all other organs and tissues of the body.

The reason the greater part of the body carbohydrate is present as glycogen (the polymerized storage form of glucose) is that all the hexoses which result from the digestion of carbohydrate in the intestine, and are absorbed into the blood stream, are converted into glucose. This occurs largely, but perhaps not entirely, in the liver.[24,25] Similarly, in the post-absorptive state or during fasting, when the liver must supply sugar to the blood from the body's own resources, glucose is the carbohydrate it manufactures from amino acids and the glycerol of fat. Nevertheless, there are other forms of carbohydrate in most tissues and organs. Among these are special-purpose carbohydrates, substances presumably not used as fuel, for example, the galactose in the galactolipins of

Table 3-2. Caloric Equivalent of Carbohydrate Content of Normal Man

Body Weight: 70 kg Liver Weight: 1800 gm Muscle Mass: 35 kg Volume of Blood and Extracellular Fluids: 21 liters.

	Percentage	gm
Muscle glycogen	0.70	245
Liver glycogen	6.00	108
Blood and extracellular fluid sugar	0.08	17

Total body carbohydrate	370 gm
Caloric equivalent (370 × 4.1)	1517 calories
Caloric requirement (Sedentary occupation)	2800 calories per 24 hours or 116.7 calories per hour

Total body carbohydrate could supply caloric needs for $\left(\dfrac{1517}{116.7}\right)$ ....13 hours

Table 3-3.   The Distribution of Carbohydrate in Various Tissues of Rat, Dog and Man[*]

Tissue	Rat Glycogen, Percentage	Rat Glucose, mg Percentage	Dog Glycogen, Percentage	Dog Glucose, mg Percentage	Man Glycogen, Percentage	Man Glucose, mg Percentage
Skeletal muscle	0.81–1.06[28]	50–70	0.55[30]	40–60	0.4–0.6[31]	....
Liver	2.5–8.3[28]	....	6.10[30]	....	1.5–6.0[32]	....
Heart . . .	0.3–0.6[30]	....	0.47[30]	....	....	....
Kidney . . .	....	....	0.15[30]	....	0.4[32]	....
Brain	0.08[29]	....	0.1[29]	57[29]	....	....
Skin	....	77[33]	0.08[33]	71[33]	0.08[33]	60–82[33]
Blood and Extracellular Fluids	....	90–129[28]	....	60–80	....	60–90

[*] The figures represent ranges found on a mixed diet.

nervous tissues,[26] the pentoses associated with the nucleoproteins, and the sugars of the widely distributed glycoproteins.[26] And, during lactation, lactose is made in the breast and is present in the secreted milk. Finally, there are a number of such degradation products of glucose as the hexose and triose phosphates,[27] which are caught in transit as the glucose is utilized.

Table 3–3 summarizes the distribution of the quantitatively important forms of carbohydrate in man and in certain laboratory animals. To some extent, we must rely on the data obtained from experiments with animals to interpret the relatively meager data available for human beings. This is because both glucose and glycogen (especially the latter) are labile substances when present in the tissues and few opportunities to obtain human tissues under the proper conditions for accurate analysis present themselves. However, the close agreement of the reliable data which we do have for human beings with those obtained from experiments with animals increases their significance.

The Fuel of Muscular Exercise. In an exhaustive review of the subject in 1942 Gemmill[34] has aptly reviewed the situation with regard to the fuel of muscular exercise as follows:

From the survey of the literature it is obvious that the use of carbohydrate is of primary importance as a fuel for muscular exercise in man. The evidence comes from the slight increase in efficiency on a carbohydrate diet, the prolongation of muscular effort when carbohydrate is ingested, the fall in blood sugar during long continued muscular exercise and the production of lactate at the beginning of exercise and during severe exercise. The evidence that protein is used during exercise indicates that it is of secondary importance, probably to supply carbohydrate or carbohydrate intermediates. The results of experiments on fat utilization during muscular work have demonstrated that this substance is used indirectly. There is no experimental evidence at the present time for the direct utilization of fat by mammalian muscle. However, the indirect utilization of protein or fat must be an efficient process, since the exclusive feeding of these substances to man does not have a marked effect on muscular efficiency during short periods of exercise.[34]

However, since Gemmill's review was written, evidence has been brought forward to indicate that fatty acids can be oxidized by the liverless animal[35] and by muscle extracts *in vitro*.[36,37a] But whether this occurs in intact muscle, or to what extent it occurs in relation to the total caloric expenditure, has not been determined. As a matter of fact, the work on the whole animal was done under resting conditions, so that the peripheral oxidation of fat observed may have no bearing as regards the fuel of muscular exercise. Hence is still necessary to conclude that carbohydrate is the major fuel of muscular exercise.

The significance of this from the standpoint

of nutrition is obvious. If carbohydrate is not available as such in the diet, it must, in order to satisfy the fuel requirements of the active tissues, be made by the body from those foodstuffs present in the diet. The eating of adequate amounts of carbohydrate therefore spares the body the work of making its fuel. As fuel, carbohydrate is naturally more important when the body engages in moderate or severe muscular exertion than it is when the body is at rest. The great demand for fuel accompanying muscular exercise may rapidly exhaust the carbohydrate stores. This is evidenced by a decrease in the glycogen content of the liver and the muscles; if the exertion is sufficiently severe and prolonged, it may result in an abnormal lowering of the blood sugar level. These phenomena are accompanied by increased breakdown of body protein (reflected in an increased excretion of nitrogen in the urine) and accelerated breakdown of body fat (reflected in a rise in the level of ketone bodies in blood and urine). When violent exercise is preceded or accompanied by a large intake of carbohydrate, the body, on the basis of calories expended per unit of oxygen intake, works somewhat more efficiently. And there is a minimum increase in nitrogen excretion and ketone formation. This effect

of carbohydrate is an example of its protein-sparing and antiketogenic action.

The Efficiency of Carbohydrate as a Fuel. It has just been said above that carbohydrate is a more efficient fuel for muscular exercise than either protein or fat. This does not imply that portions of the protein or fat molecules are wasted when they are so used. It means that protein and fat molecules, when used as fuel, yield less than their total caloric value in the form which can be used by muscle. The remainder is used for the conversion of these molecules into suitable fuel. This conversion occurs in the liver and in adipose tissue which supply the other organs with fuel by way of the blood stream.

Since the amount of glycogen present in the muscle at any one time is sufficient for only short periods of work, the carbohydrate used by the muscle must eventually come from the blood sugar. The glycogen within the muscle cells may be reasonably supposed to serve best in emergencies, when the muscle is unable to draw sugar from the blood as quickly as needed. But, as a matter of fact, glycogen is more than a conveniently packaged form of carbohydrate lying on the pantry shelf. It is known that more energy is derivable from a certain amount of glycogen than from an equivalent amount of blood

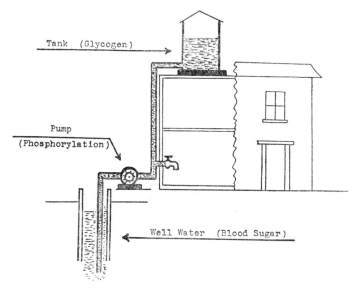

Fig. 3-2.

sugar. Since it requires a certain amount of energy to bring the blood sugar into the metabolic system of the muscle (as hexose-6-phosphate), all the energy inherent in the glucose is not available for useful work. On the other hand, the breakdown of glycogen to the same stage does not require energy input; hence all its inherent energy is quickly made available. This is not to say that one gets something for nothing from glycogen; it requires some energy to build up the glycogen in the first place. But this energy is expended during a quiescent period when plenty of it is available. The situation is analogous to that portrayed in Figure 3–2.[37b]

Here the water in the well represents the blood sugar, the pump stands for the phosphorylating mechanisms, and the tank on the roof represents the glycogen store. It is readily understandable that, when the tank contains stored water, the tap can deliver a rate of flow far beyond the rate capacity of the pump. The water stored during periods when the tap is closed is at a higher level than the original source of the water and, therefore, stores some of the energy applied by the pump. This potential energy is released when the tap is opened. Too great an outflow from the tap will, of course, exhaust the stored water and reduce the rate of flow from the tap to the rate at which the pump is capable of operating. A similar condition obtains in muscle when excessive rates of work over prolonged periods are attempted.

The application of these physiologic facts to clinical phenomena is exemplified by the greater stores of glycogen and of phosphate esters found in the muscles of animals which have been trained to perform prolonged work.[38] This probably also applies to the physical abilities of manual laborers and of athletes. Conversely, the characteristically low muscle glycogen level found in poorly controlled diabetic patients and in hyperthyroid individuals is accompanied by muscular weakness. The importance of an available glycogen store for muscular work is demonstrated by the pathologic fatigue and exhaustion experienced by patients who suffer from a form of glycogen storage disease

known as the McArdle syndrome.[39] The virtual absence of muscle phosphorylase in this disorder prevents the use of glycogen as a fuel and can be alleviated only by rest or the continual infusion of glucose.

Special Functions of Carbohydrate in the Liver. In the liver, aside from its use as fuel, carbohydrate has protective and detoxifying action and a regulating influence on protein and fat metabolism.

The liver of a well-fed normal animal contains a higher percentage of glycogen than any other of that animal's tissues. It is known that such a liver is more resistant to various types of noxious agents than one which has been deprived of its glycogen by starvation or disease. This has been shown in animals for such various types of poisons as carbon tetrachloride,[40] alcohol[41] and arsenic[42] and, in human beings, for a variety of diseases accompanied by toxemias of bacterial origin.[43,44] The defenses of the liver against toxic agents are of great importance to the body as a whole, for one of the chief functions of the liver is to remove or destroy such agents (toxins) before they reach other vital tissues which are not equipped to deal with them. For this reason, the maintenance of a high glycogen level in the liver is essential to the health of the whole organism.

More definite knowledge is available of the role of carbohydrate in specific chemical reactions which transform certain poisons into relatively innocuous substances. One such mechanism is the conjugation of glycuronic acid derived from carbohydrate with chemical substances which possess a phenolic hydroxyl group.[45] Indeed this mechanism is one of the means by which the body regulates its steroid hormone metabolism and protects itself from the harm which might result from an excess of the sex hormones.[46] It is also possible that carcinogenic substances of the steroid type may be disposed of in the same manner. Another hepatic detoxifying mechanism is the acetylation of such substances as p-aminobenzoic acid[47] and sulfanilamide.[48] In this type of conjugation, the acetyl groups are derived from carbohydrate, probably through pyruvate and acetyl phosphate. The rates of glycuronate formation and of acetylation have been shown to depend directly upon the concentration of carbohydrate in the liver.[48,49]

The protein-sparing action of carbohydrate has already been mentioned. This action occurs partly in the liver, for that is the organ primarily responsible for the deamination of amino acids. Up to the point of deamination, the fate of amino acids in metabolism is not finally determined. They may be used as building blocks from which to form proteins for the repair or growth of tissues, or they may be broken down for use as fuel. Once deamination has occurred, the amino acids are divorced from protein metabolism. The amino group is converted to urea and excreted; the non-nitrogenous fraction is either used as a source of energy or is converted to carbohydrate or fat. The rate of deamination in the liver decreases as the available carbohydrate increases.[50] An ample supply of carbohydrate thus conserves the products of protein breakdown in a form which may be used by the body to build or maintain its own protein structure. To put it in another way, a minimal intake of protein, adequate for the body's needs when taken together with good amounts of carbohydrate, may become inadequate when the carbohydrate intake is insufficient.[51]

The availability of carbohydrate to the liver also determines how much fat will be broken down by it. There is no direct index of the rate of fat metabolism in the liver, for, unlike protein metabolism, it is not accompanied by the excretion of a characteristic end product in the urine. However, it happens that fatty acids in excess are not completely metabolized by the liver and that β-hydroxybutyric and acetoacetic acids accumulate.[52,53,54] These ketone bodies go to the peripheral tissues for complete oxidation. Ordinarily, the rate of fat breakdown and ketone body formation is such that the ketone bodies are promptly disposed of by the peripheral tissues. But when fatty acid breakdown becomes excessively rapid and the rate of ketone formation in the liver begins to exceed the rate of disposal by the peripheral tissues, accumulation of the ketone bodies begins to occur in the blood and excretion of them in the urine (ketosis). Under these circumstances, in an otherwise normal animal, the administration of carbohydrate causes a prompt disappearance of the ketone bodies (antiketogenic action). Carbohydrate intake by the adipose tissues inhibits their output of fatty acids, which are the raw material for ketone production.[55] Together with its protein-sparing action, the antiketogenic action of carbohydrate serves to regulate the proportion of the different foodstuffs prepared by the liver for use as fuel in the peripheral tissues.

In discussing the special functions of carbohydrate in the liver, we have referred both to the glycogen content of that organ and to the "availability" of carbohydrate to it. These terms may or may not be synonymous. In any case, the glycogen content of the liver is a good index of the amount of carbohydrate available to the hepatic cells; and from a nutritional standpoint it is important to remember that carbohydrate is the foodstuff which leads to the highest levels of liver glycogen. Fairly good glycogen stores in the liver can be obtained when protein is predominant in the diet, but a high-fat diet results in a liver poor in glycogen. The medical uses of the high-carbohydrate diet or of the intravenous administration of dextrose solution are directed towards the protection of the liver by insuring the build up of rich glycogen stores.[43] Protein has been used with the same ultimate purpose in mind, but it is less effective, probably because its effectiveness is in proportion to its convertibility into sugar.

In attempting to drive the hepatic glycogen stores upward at a maximal rate for therapeutic purposes, physicians have often attempted to reinforce the effect of high-carbohydrate intake by the simultaneous administration of insulin. This is not the place to discuss the physiologic action of this hormone, but it is important to note that the administration of insulin with carbohydrate to the nondiabetic organism actually results in a lower liver glycogen level than does administration of the same amount of carbohydrate without insulin.[56] This is because insulin also influences the intake of glucose and the deposition of glycogen in the skeletal muscles. The bulk of these muscles, much greater than that of the liver, serves to draw off most of the administered carbohydrate; hence the liver is deprived of glycogen which might otherwise be deposited in it.

Carbohydrate and the Heart. The previous discussion of carbohydrate as the most efficient fuel for muscular exercise and of the muscle glycogen as an important emergency source of contractile energy applies in even greater measure to cardiac muscle than it does to skeletal muscle. The latter can in some measure accommodate itself to a decreased supply of carbohydrate by decreasing its work. The heart cannot stop to rest. A temporary reduction in the supply of sugar to the normal heart (as in induced attacks of hypoglycemia) has little apparent effect on the organ, although a definite change in the electrocardiogram may be noted.[57] The apparent lack of influence of hypoglycemia on the heart may be due to the normally good glycogen stores to be found there. But in the heart which has been damaged by disease and in which the initial glycogen stores are poor, hypoglycemia may precipitate stenocardia. This has been noted in diabetic[58] as well as in nondiabetic cardiac patients; both, it has also been observed, are likely to do better when the blood sugar is somewhat elevated, even above the normal range. High-carbohydrate therapy has been successfully used on this basis.[59] The cardiac glycogen level is regulated in part by the anterior pituitary. Because of this influence cardiac glycogen rises during fasting and after pancreatectomy or phlorhizination.[60]

The Indispensability of Carbohydrate to the Central Nervous System. Of all the organs and tissues in the body the central nervous system is most dependent upon the minute-by-minute supply of glucose from the blood. In the discussion of carbohydrate as fuel for muscular exercise, it was stated that carbohydrate could be used directly, protein and fat only indirectly. With regard to the central nervous system, it has been well established that under normal conditions of feeding, carbohydrate is the principal fuel.[61] And the need of nerve tissue for glucose is even more specific than this statement would indicate. It is true that, when slices of brain tissue are studied *in vitro* with regard to their ability to maintain respiration at the expense of various substrates, a number of degradation products of glucose will serve as well or better than glucose.[61] But, none of these intermediates has been shown to have any ameliorating effect upon the hypoglycemic symptoms caused by lowering the blood sugar level *in vivo*.[62] In other words, glucose as such has a specific influence and is indispensable for the maintenance of the functional integrity of the nerve tissue. When the level of blood sugar is lowered in a living organism, tissues having ample stores of glycogen may use these to tide them over the lean period. Nervous tissue has little glycogen, and it is doubtful whether that little can be mobilized for use in emergencies. The glycogen content of nervous tissue remains more or less constant under most conditions, including hyperglycemia and hypoglycemia, and may be largely an integral part of the nerve structure.[29] The unavailability of the glycogen present in the nerve cells for metabolic use is evidenced by the dramatically rapid development of hypoglycemic symptoms when the blood sugar level is lowered. During a prolonged fast (3 weeks or over) the cells of the central nervous system seem to be able to adapt their metabolic apparatus to utilize the ketone bodies in place of glucose and derive functional energy from these metabolites.[63] This is a most interesting finding, which, however, has no bearing upon the indispensability of glucose for the CNS under normal circumstances of everyday life.

The susceptibility of the central nervous system to hypoglycemic shock has been utilized in the treatment of schizophrenia and other nervous disorders. The hypoglycemia has been produced by the administration of large doses of insulin, and the earlier advocates of the method spoke of the possible favorable effect of the hormone on the metabolism of the brain. It is now evident that insulin produces its results by lowering the blood sugar level as it forces the sugar into the peripheral tissues, largely the muscles. By this means the central nervous system is deprived of its indispensable substrate and suffers true shock or damage, which does not differ very much in either its mechanism or its results from the type of shock caused by asphyxia. Indeed the latter, in one form or another, has also been used as a method of treatment. That the insulin shock treatment is correctly named and does not have a favorable influence on metabolism is also shown by the fact that prolonged hypoglycemia results in histologically demonstrable and functionally irreversible damage to brain tissue.[64]

THE RELATIONS OF CARBOHYDRATE TO OTHER NUTRIENTS IN THE BODY

The Transformation of Carbohydrate into Fat. In the previous discussion of fat as a fuel storage material, it was pointed out that, when food in excess of caloric expenditure is ingested (whether in the form of carbohydrate, protein, or fat), the equivalent of the excess calories is deposited as fat in the adipose tissues. With this in mind, it is, strictly speaking, incorrect to label any of the foodstuffs as being particularly "fattening." Any one of them may be so if taken in sufficient quantities. But, because of its proportion in the diet, its lower cost, and its use in confections, carbohydrate is quantitatively the most important precursor of fat.

It had been thought previously that the transformation of carbohydrate into fat occurs exclusively in the liver. Apparently this is not so; for, using ^{14}C-labeled glucose, Chaikoff et al.[65] showed that the liverless animal could perform that transformation. The degree to which the liver or the adipose tissue is the main site of fat synthesis seems to vary with the animal species. In the rat the adipose tissue is the principal site of lipogenesis while in other species, including man, the evidence favors the view that the liver is an important locus of fat formation. The triglycerides are then transported to the fat cells where they are stored.[66]

The fat which arises from carbohydrate in the body is the so-called "hard" fat, composed in the main of the highly saturated palmitic and stearic acids. This is probably of more concern to stock raisers than to human nutritionists. The former have long known that they could control the physical qualities of the fat in meats by varying the proportions of carbohydrate and oils in the diet of their animals. Of course, carbohydrate cannot be substituted completely for fat in the diet, since it does not carry with it the essential fatty acids and the fat-soluble vitamins, which cannot be manufactured by the body.

The chemical pathway which glucose follows on its way to fat is quite well understood. It was long known that thiamin (vitamin B_1) was necessary for the formation of fat from carbohydrate.[67] Since thiamin is known to be a necessary coenzyme in the reactions of pyruvic acid, a possible route for the initial steps of carbohydrate to fat is thus outlined. The carbohydrate is degraded to pyruvic acid, which in turn forms acetyl CoA. The further growth of the fatty acid chain (by one pathway) occurs in a reverse manner to that which has been described for its breakdown. According to the best hypothesis, the latter process involves the successive splitting off of 2-carbon atom fragments as acetic acid.[52,68] The reverse of this process in fat formation would demand the successive appearance of fatty acids composed of 4-, 6-, 8-, 10-, 12-, 14-, and 16-carbon atoms. While this has not been demonstrated for adipose tissue, it is suggestive that all these stages of fat formation are found in an organ which is a very active fat-builder, namely, the lactating breast.[69] More recent evidence[70] indicates that a major pathway of lipogenesis is the formation, from acetyl CoA, of the 3-carbon malonyl CoA. The 16-carbon fatty acid is formed according to the following equation.

$$7 \text{ Malonyl·CoA} + 1 \text{ Acetyl·CoA} \longrightarrow 1 \text{ Palmityl·CoA} + 7 \text{ CO}_2$$

Carbohydrate and Protein Metabolism. Earlier writers on metabolism have talked somewhat loosely of the formation of protein from carbohydrate. Strictly speaking, such a transformation is impossible for the amino groups which characterize the building stones of proteins must be derived from amino acids or proteins ingested as such. What can and does occur is the exchange of the amino group of an amino acid with the keto group of a keto acid derived from carbohydrate, a process known as transamination.[71,72] In this process, the carbon residue of the amino acid reverts to a carbohydrate intermediate, so that there is no quantitative increase in the amount of protein precursor resulting from the reaction. What the body gains from the interchange is the ability to transform an amino acid it has in excess into another it needs. For example, by exchange with α-ketoglutarate, alanine may be transformed to glutamic acid with pyruvic acid as the by-product, as follows:

dromes which have been described are, therefore, merely the most obvious manifestations, those occurring in the tissues and organs which suffer most acutely and are most easily accessible for purposes of examination. Consideration of Figure 3–3 also shows the fallacy of regarding any single factor of the B complex as more important than another, for the normal chain of events can be broken by a lack of any one of them. For this reason, and until we have isolated and know the precise

$$COOH—CH_2—CH_2—CO—COOH + CH_3—CHNH_2—COOH \rightleftarrows$$
$$COOH—CH_2—CH_2—CHNH_2—COOH + CH_3—CO—COOH$$

The Vitamin B Complex in Carbohydrate Nutrition. It is known that the vitamin B complex plays an integral part in carbohydrate metabolism and that the need for this group of vitamins depends upon the amount of carbohydrate eaten. Why was knowledge of its existence not acquired much earlier in human experience, and why did the race not suffer from lack of that knowledge? The answer to these questions is that it was only in comparatively recent times that the natural union between the vitamin B complex and carbohydrate, a union existing in whole grain and plants, was broken by the industrial processing of foods. Before this occurred, the supply of the B vitamins was automatically adjusted to the amount of carbohydrate eaten; the occurrence of vitamin B deficiency with its consequent disturbance in nutrition is, therefore, a comparatively recent development in the Western World. In the Orient, the earlier large-scale introduction of polished rice led to the first known instances of vitamin B deficiency (beriberi) and, indeed, to the first recognition of the existence of this group of vitamins.

Figure 3–3 outlines the known steps in the breakdown of carbohydrate and indicates the points at which the coenzymes derived from the B-group of vitamins play essential roles. The role of various minerals in carbohydrate metabolism is similarly indicated.

Since the breakdown of carbohydrate is essentially similar in all tissues and organs, it follows that a vitamin B deficiency will impair carbohydrate metabolism in every structure of the body. The clinical syn-

function and optimal proportion of each component part of the B complex, a source containing all the factors remains the best protective dietary supplement with which to avoid the evils of modern food refinement.

The Utilization of Simple Sugars other than Glucose. In the previous section on the distribution of carbohydrate in the body, it was pointed out that all the hexoses absorbed from the gastrointestinal tract are converted into either glucose or glycogen. This conversion, which takes place largely in the liver, is ordinarily so efficient that there is little need to consider any other fate which sugars like fructose and galactose may undergo. However, under special circumstances, as when the function of the liver is impaired or these sugars enter the blood in overwhelming quantities, there occur interesting anomalies of carbohydrate nutrition which deserve some brief mention. Lactose is also of interest here for, during lactation, it is formed in large quantities by the breast of the female; at that time, too, it may appear in the blood and the urine. The pentoses are sometimes involved in an hereditary anomaly of metabolism.

Fructose. Though the conversion of fructose to glucose occurs largely in the liver, there is some evidence that it may take place to a smaller extent in the intestinal mucosa and the kidney.[24,73] The hexokinases of certain tissues (muscle, brain) can catalyze the formation of fructose-6-phosphate from fructose. Other tissues (especially liver) contain a specific fructokinase which leads to the formation of fructose-1-phosphate which

POINTS OF ACTION OF VITAMINS AND MINERALS IN CARBOHYDRATE METABOLISM

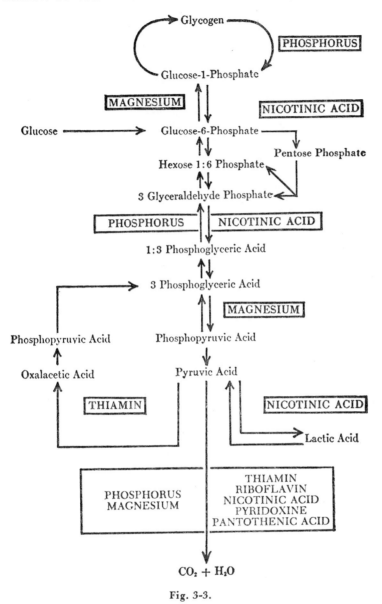

Fig. 3-3.

in turn is split to trioses. The trioses may be transformed to pyruvic and lactic acids or re-synthesized to fructose diphosphate. This ester proceeds, by reversal of the glycolytic steps, to glycogen, or to free glucose by the action of glucose-6-phosphatase.[74] Hence when fructose appears in excess in the blood it is accompanied by a rise in lactic acid.[75]

When any of the foregoing hepatic mechanisms are impaired, either by liver disease or by an hereditary anomaly known as essential fructosuria, there is difficulty in disposing of the fructose taken in through the gastrointestinal tract and it accumulates as such in the blood. And since it is a substance which is not held back by the kidney as efficiently as is glucose, it appears in the urine in abnormal quantities. Fructose is a reducing sugar not distinguishable from glucose by the routine chemical tests. From the medical standpoint, therefore, it is important not to confuse fructosuria with diabetes mellitus. In certain types of fructose intolerance, the blood glucose value falls to levels which may cause symptoms of hypoglycemia.[76]

Lactose and Galactose. Lactose is split into glucose and galactose in the process of digestion. It may, therefore, be considered together with the galactose ingested as such. However, from a nutritional standpoint, the presence of lactose in milk and milk products renders it much more important than galactose.

There is good evidence that galactose is converted to glucose by the liver by first undergoing a phosphorylation. The galactose-1-phosphate reacts with uridine-diphosphoglucose (UDPG) to form uridine-diphosphogalactose (UDPGal). The enzyme catalyzing this transformation is called uridyl transferase and is the system which is found deficient in galactosemia.[77] The morphological and clinical abnormalities of galactosemia are due to the intracellular accumulation of galactose-1-phosphate, especially in the CNS and the liver. The lactating breast manufactures lactose and presumably has galactose available for the purpose,[78] but it is not known whether all the galactose is made in the breast or whether some of it originates in the liver and is transported to the breast. Since both lactose and galactose may be found in the blood and urine of lactating females, the mere presence of these abnormal constituents does not give any indication of their site of origin. As with fructose, it is of importance medically to distinguish between galactosuria, lactosuria, and glucosuria.

Pentoses. In contrast to the hexoses, which are important energy materials, the 5-carbon atom sugars are much more important as part of the machinery of the body. Pentoses are incorporated in at least one vitamin (riboflavin), several tissue coenzymes (diphosphopyridine nucleotide, triphosphopyridine nucleotide, alloxazine adenine dinucleotide), and all the nucleoproteins. However, when pentoses as such are ingested, they are not utilized but are eliminated, more or less quantitatively, in the urine and feces. It is possible that the pentoses which are eaten in combined form as part of natural food constituents (riboflavin and the nucleotides, for example) do contribute to the pentose content of the tissues. It is known that the body is able to synthesize pentoses for itself—from glucose by way of the pentose shunt and from glucuronic acid.[79] The hereditary anomaly known as "essential pentosuria" consists of the urinary excretion of l-xylose which gives a positive reduction test for "sugar." Hence pentosurics are often mistaken for cases of diabetes. Normally the body makes glucuronic acid from glucose especially in the liver. The bulk of this sugar acid is used to form glucuronides which are excreted. Any remaining glucuronic acid is ordinarily remade into glucose as follows:

Glucuronic → Gulonic → *l-xylose* → xylitol → d-xylose → d-xylosephosphate → glucose-6-P, etc.

In the pentosuric the enzyme system operating on l-xylose→xylitol is defective. Hence the pentose accumulates and is excreted. Fortunately this is a harmless biochemical error, which may, however, lead to a wrong diagnosis.[80]

SUMMARY

We must take cognizance of the human failing whereby the very act of examining a subject in great detail tends to exaggerate its importance. We have seen that carbohydrate, not only is the primary fuel of the body, but also is involved in important portions of its functional machinery. The carbohydrate stores, though relatively small in comparison with those of fat, play a protective role in some of the most vital organs. They may be of the utmost importance when a ready source of energy is required to enable the organism as a whole to cope with an emergency. Despite all this, however, the evolutionary processes have resulted in so flexible a metabolic system that the higher mammals and man can get along very nicely when little or no carbohydrate is available. Under these circumstances, the body makes its own carbohydrate fuel from noncarbohydrate materials. But this is a wasteful process because some energy must be used for the conversions and there is more wear and tear on the metabolic machinery.

If, with the foregoing considerations in mind, we could divorce ourselves from previous dietary experience and construct an ideal adult diet, we would choose the following: (1) protein sufficient in quantity and quality to repair the protein machinery from day to day—and a little more, to be on the safe side (and of course a sufficiency of all the vitamins and minerals); (2) enough fat to carry the essential fatty acids and fat-soluble vitamins and make it unnecessary to eat too large a bulk of other food; (3) enough carbohydrate to supply all the rest of the calories necessary to maintain weight. The diet outlined is a fair approximation of that which the human race has actually adopted on the basis of experience in those fortunate parts of the world where food resources are rich and the choice is not limited.

BIBLIOGRAPHY

1. Heinbecker: J. Biol. Chem., *80*, 461, 1928.
2. Tolstoi: J. Biol. Chem., *83*, 753, 1929.
3. Chwalibogowski: Acta Paediat., *22*, 110, 1938.
4. Follis and Straight: Bull. Johns Hopkins Hosp., *72*, 39, 1943.
5. Food and Life, Yearbook of Agriculture, Department of Agriculture, United States Government Printing Office, 1939, pp. 323 ff.
6. Food and Life, Yearbook of Agriculture, pp. 110, 152–157, 305. (5).
7. Cantarow and Schepartz: *Biochemistry* (Chapter 8), 3rd Ed., Philadelphia, W. B. Saunders Co., 1962.
8. Crane and Krane: Bioch. Bioph. Acta, *20*, 568, 1956.
9. Wilson: J. Biol. Chem., *222*, 751, 1956.
10. Fridhandler and Quastel: Arch. Bioch., *56*, 412, 1955.
11. Crane: Physiol. Rev., *40*, 789, 1960.
12. Crane: *Handbook of Physiology*—subsection, Alimentary Canal, Vol. I, Am. Physiol. Soc., 1967.
13. Cori: J. Biol. Chem., *66*, 691, 1925.
14. Groen: J. Clin. Investigation, *16*, 245, 1937.
15. Russell: Am. J. Physiol., *122*, 547, 1938.
16. Althausen, Anderson, and Stockholm: Proc. Soc. Exper. Biol. & Med., *40*, 342, 1939.
17. Reder and Gallup: Proc. Oklahoma Acad. Sci., *15*, 58, 1935.
18. **Crane: Gastroenterology, *50*, 254, 1966.**
19. Alpers and Isselbacher: Adv. Metab. Disorders, *4*, 75, 1970.
20. Lindquist and Meeuwisse: Acta Pediatrica, *51*, 674, 1962.
21. Althausen and Wever: J. Clin. Investigation, *16*, 257, 1937.
22. Lusk: *The Science of Nutrition*, 4 Ed., Philadelphia, W. B. Saunders Co., 1928, p. 75 ff.
23. Soskin: Physiol. Rev., *21*, 140, 1941.
24. Bollmann and Mann: Am. J. Physiol., *96*, 683, 1931.
25. Bollman, Mann, and Power: Am. J. Physiol., *111*, 483, 1935.
26. Peters and Van Slyke: *Quantitative Clinical Chemistry*, Baltimore, The Williams & Wilkins Co., 1931, Vol. 1, p. 222.
27. Meyerhoff: Biological Symposia, *5*, 141, 1941.
28. Guest: J. Nutrition, *22*, 205, 1941.
29. Kerr and Ghantus: J. Biol. Chem., *116*, 9, 1936.
30. Lusk: *The Science of Nutrition*, pp. 319–325 (20).
31. Moscati: Beitr. z. Chem. und Physiol., *10*, 337, 1908.
32. Popper and Wozasek: Virchows Arch. f. path. Anat., *279*, 819, 1931.
33. Cornbleet: Arch. Dermat. & Syph., *41*, 193, 1940.
34. Gemmill: Physiol. Rev., *22*, 32, 1942.
35. Goldman, Chaikoff, Reinhardt, Entenman, and Dauben: J. Biol. Chem., *186*, 718, 1950.
36. Lehninger: J. Biol. Chem., *165*, 131, 1946.
37a. Weinhouse, Millington, and Volk: J. Biol. Chem., *185*, 191, 1950.
37b. Soskin: Arch. Int. Med., *71*, 219, 1943.
38. Palladin: Bull. Soc. Chim. Biol., *13*, 13, 1931.
39. Schneid, R. and Mahler, R.: J. Clin. Invest., *38*, 1040, 1959.
40. Bollman: Arch. Path., *29*, 732, 1940.
41. Holmes: Physiol. Rev., *19*, 439, 1939.
42. Glahn, Flinn, and Keim: Arch. Path., *25*, 488, 1938.
43. Soskin, Allweiss, and Mirsky: Arch. Int. Med., *56*, 927, 1935.
44. Soskin and Hyman: Arch. Int. Med., *64*, 1265, 1939.
45. Young: Physiol. Rev., *19*, 323, 1939.
46. Heller: Endocrinology, *26*, 619, 1940.
47. Harrow, Power, and Sherwin: Proc. Soc. Exp. Biol. & Med., *24*, 422, 1936–37.
48. Klein and Harris: J. Biol. Chem., *124*, 613, 1938.
49. Lipschitz and Bueding: J. Biol. Chem., *129*, 333, 1939.
50. Krebs and Henseleit: Ztsch. f. Physiol. Chem., *210*, 33, 1932.
51. Thomas: Arch. f. Physiol., *22*, 249, 1910 (Suppl.).
52. Soskin and Levine: Arch. Int. Med., *68*, 674, 1941.
53. Stadie: Ann. Int. Med., *15*, 783, 1941.
54. Mackay: J. Clin. Endocr., *3*, 101, 1943.
55. Dole, V. P. in Page, I. H. (ed): *Chemistry of Lipids as Related to Atherosclerosis*. Springfield, Charles C Thomas, 1958, p. 189.
56. Bridge: Bull. Johns Hopkins Hosp., *62*, 408, 1938.

57. Soskin, Katz, and Frisch: Ann. Int. Med., *8*, 900, 1935.
58. Soskin, Katz, Strouse, and Rubinfeld: Arch. Int. Med., *51*, 122, 1933.
59. White: *Heart Disease*, 2nd Ed., New York, The Macmillan Co., 1937, p. 285.
60. Russell and Bloom: Endocrinology, *58*, 83, 1956.
61. Quastel: Physiol. Rev., *19*, 422, 1939.
62. Jensen: *Insulin: Its Chemistry and Physiology*, London, Oxford Univ. Press, 1938.
63. Owen, Morgan, Kemp, Sullivan, Herrera and Cahill: J. Clin. Invest., *46*, 1589, 1967.
64. Lawrence, Meyer, and Nevin: Quart. J. Med., *11*, 181, 1942.
65. Chernick, Masoro, and Chaikoff: Proc. Soc. Exper. Biol. & Med., *73*, 348, 1950.
66. Jeanrenaud: Ergebn. Physiol., *60*, 57, 1968.
67. Longenecker, Gavin, and McHenry: J. Biol. Chem., *134*, 693, 1940.
68. MacKay, Barnes, Carne, and Wick: J. Biol. Chem., *135*, 157, 1940.
69. Best and Taylor: *The Physiological Basis of Medical Practice*, Baltimore, Williams & Wilkins Co., 1939, pp. 1238 ff.
70. Langdon and Phillips: Ann. Rev. Bioch., *30*, 189, 1961.
71. Braunstein and Kritzman: Enzymologia, *2*, 129, 1937.
72. Cohen: *Transamination in Symposium on Respiratory Enzymes*, Madison, University of Wisconsin Press, 1942, p. 210.
73. Reinecke: Am. J. Physiol., *136*, 167, 1942.
74. Hers: Arch. internat. de physiol., *61*, 426, 1953.
75. Lundsgaard: Bull. Johns Hopkins Hosp., *63*, 90, 1938.
76. Kalckar, Anderson and Isselbacher: Bioch. Biophys. Acta, *20*, 262, 1956.
77. Froesch, Prader, Labhart, Stuber, and Wolf: Schweiz. Med. Wchschr., *87*, 1168, 1957.
78. Petersen: J. Dairy Sci., *25*, 71, 1942.
79. Enklewitz and Lasker: J. Biol. Chem., *110*, 443, 1935.
80. Touster, O.: Biochim. Biophys. Acta, *25*, 196, 1957.

Chapter

4

Fats and Other Lipids

ROSLYN B. ALFIN-SLATER

AND

LILLA AFTERGOOD

Lipids are a heterogeneous group of biologically important compounds which are classified together because of their similar solubility in organic solvents, *e.g.* acetone, ethyl ether, petroleum ether, and chloroform. Also, usually in their molecular structure there is a fatty acid or fatty acid derivative. Fats are the most concentrated form of energy available to the body providing approximately 9 Kcalories/gm fat. All tissues of the body, except the central nervous system, are able to utilize fatty acids as a source of energy.

LIPID CLASSIFICATION

Fats are of both animal and vegetable origin and, in foods, consist primarily of triglycerides. Triglycerides are composed of 1 molecule of glycerol and 3 fatty acid molecules, which can be the same or different. The physical state of triglycerides depends on the chain length and degree of unsaturation of their fatty acid components—the more unsaturated the fatty acids and the shorter the chain length, the lower the melting point of the fat. In edible fats or oils the fatty acids are usually of either 16 or 18 carbon atoms and may be saturated, unsaturated or polyunsaturated. Animal fats also contain cholesterol, either free or combined with a fatty acid as a cholesterol ester. Cholesterol is a compound of physiological importance, which acts as a structural element in the cell

wall and is an intermediary in the synthesis of many physiologically active steroids and hormones in the body. Vegetable oils have no cholesterol but contain plant sterols which are poorly absorbed by the animal body and, in fact, interfere with the absorption of cholesterol. Edible fats also contain small amounts of phospholipids which are important emulsifying agents and are essential for the proper digestion of fats, in general.

Lipids may be classified according to the following abbreviated scheme:

1. Triglycerides (neutral fats). These are glycerol esters of fatty acids.

2. Phosphatides (phospholipids). These are compounds that contain phosphate, fatty acids, glycerol and a nitrogenous compound. There are various classes of phospholipids depending on the particular nitrogen-containing compound and fatty acid residues. For example, lecithin is composed of glycerol, 2 fatty acids (usually one unsaturated), phosphate and choline.

3. Sphingolipids contain a fatty acid, phosphate, choline and an amino alcohol, sphingosine.

4. Glycolipids are composed of a carbohydrate, a fatty acid, and an amino alcohol. Cerebrosides, which occur largely in the brain, may also be classified as glycolipids.

5. Steroids and sterols are high molecular weight compounds with a characteristic cyclopentanophenanthrene nucleus. The sterols contain a free hydroxyl group and

can be considered as high molecular weight alcohols. These would include cholesterol and the plant sterols, *e.g.*, sitosterol.

6. Waxes are esters of fatty acids with alcohols other than glycerol.

7. The fat-soluble vitamins A, D, E, and K are also classified as lipids but these will be discussed in separate chapters.

In this chapter we shall review: (1) digestion and absorption of the three major lipid classes, triglycerides, phospholipids, and cholesterol and its esters, and factors which affect or interfere with absorption, (2) transport of lipids between lymph and tissues, (3) lipid composition of various organs, (4) biosynthesis of lipids, (5) metabolism of cholesterol and the essential fatty acids, and (6) the importance of fat in the diet.

PROPERTIES OF FATS

Fats will combine with iodine and with other halogens in proportion to the number of the double bonds. The so-called "iodine number" or "iodine value" (I.V.) is a constant which gives information as to the degree of unsaturation of fats. Thus, coconut oil, composed largely of saturated fatty acids, has an iodine number of only 8 to 10. Butter fat has an I.V. ranging from 26 to 38, while linseed oil has the exceedingly high I.V. of 177 to 209. Iodine values for common vegetable fats are as follows: corn oil, 115 to 124; cottonseed oil, 105 to 115; olive oil, 79 to 90; peanut oil, 85 to 100; and soybean oil, 130 to 138. In contrast with these values, typical animal fats have the following iodine numbers: lard, 50 to 65; beef tallow, 35 to 45; and mutton tallow, 32 to 45.

The unsaturated bonds can be saturated with hydrogen when the fats are subjected to a fairly high temperature in the presence of hydrogen gas together with finely divided nickel, which acts as a catalyst in bringing about the combination of hydrogen with the unsaturated linkages. By means of this process, called hydrogenation, oils, liquid at ordinary temperatures, can be converted to fats, which are ordinarily solid. The extent to which the melting point may be increased depends upon the completeness of hydrogenation. On complete hydrogenation, most of the common animal and vegetable fats reach a maximum melting point of 65° C (194° F), which approximates the melting point of tristearin.

Hydrogenation is widely employed for converting liquid oils into solid fats in the manufacture of shortenings and margarines. Two processes are available for the preparation of these hydrogenated fats, *i.e.*, either the partial hydrogenation of the total fat to the desired melting point (35° to 48° C) resulting in the formation of isomers of the naturally occurring fatty acids, or the complete hydrogenation of a portion of the fat, which is then mixed with a sufficient amount of the unhydrogenated oil to give a blended fat with an appropriate melting point.[1]

The double bonds of fats are especially vulnerable to oxidation. The addition of oxygen may take place at such linkages, with the formation of oxides and peroxides, which eventually give rise to shorter chain acids and aldehydes. These peroxides are powerful oxidizing agents, and they may destroy important vitamins present in the fats. This is probably one of the reasons for the harmful nutritional effect of rancid fats. However, the spontaneous autooxidation of unsaturated fats is markedly inhibited by the presence of natural antioxidants in the fat. The most important of these, which are widely distributed in vegetable oils, are the tocopherols (vitamins E). δ-Tocopherol is the most powerful antioxidant, while γ-, β-, and α-tocopherol have decreasing potencies as antioxidants. The vitamin E effect is exactly opposite, α-tocopherol being the most active and δ-tocopherol the least active form of the vitamin.

In addition to the tocopherols, a number of other compounds have been found to possess antioxidant properties; these are now widely employed in prolonging the shelf life of foods. The commonest of these are NDGA (nor-di-hydroguaiaretic acid), gum guaiac, propyl gallate and gallic acid, butyl-hydroxyanisole (BHA), butyl-hydroxytoluene (BHT), and ascorbic acid.

A second location at which all fats and oils are vulnerable is at the ester linkages where the fatty acids are combined with the alcohol groups of glycerol. The fat molecules may be readily ruptured at these ester linkages by heating with sodium hydroxide or with potassium hydroxide. Under such conditions, glycerol is released and the fatty acids are transformed to water-soluble soaps. The saponification of fats, when performed under standardized conditions, can be used as an index of the average molecular weight of the fatty acids present in the fat. The saponification number is defined as milligrams of potassium hydroxide required to saponify 1 gm of fat.

Ordinarily saponification requires heat and strong alkali, but it can also be effected at body temperature under physiologic conditions by enzymes present in the secretions of the gastrointestinal tract. The hydrolysis of fats is an important phenomenon, not only in the digestion and absorption of fats and oils, but also in their preservation. One of the common reactions which leads to the spoilage of fats is so-called hydrolytic rancidity. This is particularly well recognized in the case of rancid butter, in which the presence of free butyric acid produced in this manner is responsible for the development of the unpleasant odor and flavor associated with stale butter.

DIGESTION AND ABSORPTION OF TRIGLYCERIDES

Most of the fat we ingest is in the form of triglycerides. Food also contains some phospholipid, cholesterol and its esters, and the fat-soluble vitamins. The total fat intake ranges from 25 to 150 gm per day, or about 40 per cent of the total daily caloric intake for many Americans. Although the glycerol component is constant in structure, the fatty acids may be long or short chain, and saturated or unsaturated. Unsaturated fatty acids may contain one, two, three or even more double bonds, and these fatty acids may be attached to the different carbon atoms of the glycerol molecule. The fatty acids comprising the triglycerides may be all the same or may be mixtures of two or three different fatty acids. All these variables exert an influence on the extent of digestibility, the efficiency of absorption and, in general, the subsequent fate of the molecule.

In 1936, Verzár and McDougall[2] postulated that in order for lipids to be absorbed, complete hydrolysis of triglycerides to fatty acids and glycerol was necessary. Approximately 10 years later, Frazer[3] proposed the "partition" theory wherein he suggested that, although some fat was absorbed in the form of free fatty acids which then entered the portal system, other fat could be absorbed without prior hydrolysis, as minute micelles, in conjunction with bile salts and fatty acids, through holes in the intestinal brush border, provided that the particles were less than 0.5 μ in diameter. This unhydrolyzed triglyceride would then appear in the lymphatic system. The current view of fat digestion and absorption is a combination and modification of these theories.

The digestion and absorption of fat occur in the small intestine. No digestive changes take place in the mouth. However, the process of chewing yields a certain amount of separation of nutrients by virtue of the action of salivary amylase on the carbohydrate moiety of the ingested food mixture. Further mechanical separation of the fatty material from the other nutrients occurs in the stomach. In addition, in the stomach proteolytic enzymes act on the proteins, the amylases continue to catalyze hydrolysis of carbohydrates and, as a result, most of the fat is freed from the food mixture as a coarse emulsion. There is some evidence that a limited amount of lipolysis occurs in the stomach. It is doubtful that this is a result of the presence of gastric lipases; more probably it is due to the regurgitation of pancreatic lipase (glycerol ester hydrolase) via the small intestine into the stomach.[4] However, some hydrolysis of medium-chain triglycerides (*i.e.* those with fatty acids with 6 to 12 carbon atoms) has been observed in rat stomach even though pancreatic enzymes were excluded by prolonged diversion of the pancreatic flow.[5]

The fat emulsion then enters the distal duodenum in small regulated portions. The time at which this occurs depends on the amount of fat present in the food mixture; the more fat the longer the food stays in the stomach. In the duodenum the fat emulsion is mixed with bile and pancreatic lipase. Pancreatic lipase is the principal enzyme concerned with fat lipolysis in the intestine. Pancreatic lipase attacks the triglyceride molecules specifically and sequentially at the 1 and 3 positions forming first the 1,2-diglycerides and liberating one fatty acid, and thereafter the 2-monoglyceride and another fatty acid molecule.[6,7] The rate of hydrolysis of triglycerides by pancreatic lipase is dependent on the chain length. Unsaturated fatty acids are hydrolyzed more rapidly than are saturated fatty acids.[8]

The present concept of digestion and absorption is that approximately 40 to 50 per cent of the triglyceride is completely hydrolyzed to glycerol and fatty acids prior to absorption; 40 to 50 per cent of the fat is partially hydrolyzed to monoglycerides, and approximately 10 per cent of the ingested lipid remains as triglyceride or as diglyceride.[9] In some instances, as much as 80 per cent of dietary triglyceride is absorbed as the 2-monoglyceride.[11] The absorption of the 2-monoglyceride appears to be the major route of fat absorption in man under normal conditions.[10] Monoglycerides have been shown to be relatively resistant to further attack by pancreatic lipase.[12] The monoglycerides, predominantly as the 2-monoglycerides, enter the mucosal cell and are absorbed as such.

The free fatty acids and the 2-monoglycerides combine with conjugated bile salts to form a microemulsion which facilitates the entrance of the fat into the mucosa. Partial isomerization of the 2-monoglyceride may take place at this time, as well as some further hydrolysis to glycerol and fatty acid, catalyzed by a monoglyceride lipase present in the microsomal fraction of the mucosa.[13] After absorption the fatty acids with chain lengths shorter than 12 carbon atoms are transported directly to the liver via the portal vein without reesterification.[14] The water-soluble glycerol is quickly absorbed by passive transport. The conjugated bile salts which are essential for the microemulsion or micelle formation are not absorbed through the mucosa with the fatty acids and monoglycerides; they reenter the lumen in the distal small bowel and are recirculated through the liver and bile back to the intestine.[15] The bile acid pool is cycled several times daily

through the intestine and liver and a relatively small amount of bile acid is synthesized de novo each day to replace that which escapes absorption and which is excreted as acidic steroids.[16] The most significant role of bile salts in fat absorption is that of the solubilization of lipids. Solubilization is necessary for the optimal rates of transfer of fatty acids and monoglycerides from the lumen to the absorptive cell. The effect of bile salts on the metabolism of the absorptive cell is still uncertain.[17]

As the longer-chain fatty acids are absorbed they are reesterified. The first step in this process is the activation of the fatty acids to form the acyl-CoA derivatives, in the presence of the energy supplier, ATP, and with the help of a very active, long-chain fatty acid thiokinase in the mucosa which requires CoA, ATP and Mg^{++} as cofactors. A similar enzyme occurs in liver and in adipose tissue.[18] The fatty acyl-CoA then reacts with L-α-glycerophosphate, formed from glycerol via a glycerokinase and ATP,[19] to yield monoglyceride phosphate or lysophosphatidic acid. Lysophosphatidic acid then adds on another fatty acyl-CoA to form diglyceride phosphate or phosphatidic acid. The phosphate group is then removed by the action of a phosphatidic acid phosphatase,[20] which is quite active in the intestinal mucosa, to form the diglyceride. The diglyceride then adds on a third fatty acyl-CoA forming the triglyceride molecule. Kennedy[21] has shown that in the liver L-α-glycerophosphate is the immediate precursor for glyceride-glycerol. Glucose is also a good precursor of L-α-glycerophosphate. Both the glycolytic and oxidative pathways of glucose metabolism are active in the gut mucosa and it is probable that both pathways are involved in the conversion of glucose to L-α-glycerophosphate.

The enzymes which re-form the long-chain triglyceride molecule exhibit a low specificity toward the medium length fatty acids.[18] Since an extensive hydrolysis of these medium-chain triglycerides is effected by a specific intestinal lipase, the medium-chain fatty acids are transported across the mucosal cell into the portal blood as free acids.[22]

One of the now disproved theories of fat absorption involved the engulfing by mucosal cells of minute, unhydrolyzed fat particles by a process called pinocytosis. Recent electron microscope studies have ruled out the absorption of triglycerides through pinocytosis as a major pathway.[23]

DIGESTION AND ABSORPTION OF OTHER LIPIDS

Although most fats contain triglycerides as their major component, other lipid substances are present in small amounts. These comprise chiefly phospholipids and the non-saponifiable fraction—the sterols, the tocopherols, the carotenoids and, in some cases, vitamins A and D.

Phospholipids. Crude fats contain phospholipids but these are largely removed in the refining processes. However, other foods do contain a phospholipid component. Artom and Swanson[24] using ^{32}P-labeled lecithin have shown that some of the chyle lecithin is derived from phospholipid absorbed from the gastrointestinal tract without prior hydrolysis into its components: glycerol, phosphate, choline and fatty acids. Blomstrand[25] confirmed the fact that some unhydrolyzed phosphatides may be absorbed by the mucosal cells although usually there is rather extensive hydrolysis of the phospholipids. At least one third of the dietary lecithin is incorporated into the chylomicron lecithin.[26] Lecithin in the intestine is hydrolyzed to α-acyl-lysolecithin and is absorbed as such. In the mucosal cell, the lysolecithin is acylated to form lecithin. It has been suggested that the rest of the chylomicron lecithin arises from three sources, serum lysolecithin, lecithin from bile, and lecithin synthesized de novo in the intestinal mucosal cell. Frazer[27] has suggested that lecithin actually enhances fat absorption by stabilizing the fat particles prior to transport via the intestine. It has been proposed that phospholipids provide a link between the glyceride and outer protein layer in the formation of the chylomicrons.[28]

Cholesterol. The daily ingestion of cholesterol in Western society varies from 0.2 to 2 gm.[29] Cholesterol occurs in foods in the unesterified form as well as esterified to fatty acids. Esterified cholesterol is hydrolyzed in the intestinal lumen by means of a pancreatic cholesterol esterase to free cholesterol and fatty acids; it appears that only free cholesterol is absorbed by the intestine.[30] In the mucosa cholesterol mixes with a pool of free cholesterol of endogenous origin.[31] Here, most of cholesterol is esterified with fatty acids, after which the free (30 per cent) and esterified (70 per cent) cholesterol, together with triglycerides and phospholipids, pass into the lymph in the form of chylomicrons.[32,33] Cholesterol absorption is enhanced by the presence of dietary fat. Sylven and Borgström[34] recently reported that the amount of cholesterol absorbed which appeared in the lymph was directly proportional to the chain length of the carrier triglycerides; with increasing chain length of the triglyceride fatty acids the amount of cholesterol which appeared in the lymph was also increased. It has been suggested that dietary fat improves cholesterol absorption by stimulating the flow of bile and also by providing the fatty acids with which cholesterol is esterified.[35] Both cholesterol esterases and bile salts are important in cholesterol absorption. Siperstein and co-workers[36] have concluded that bile is essential for the passage of cholesterol from the intestinal lumen to the lymph. Swell and co-workers[31] feel that bile acts as a cofactor for cholesterol esterase.

The peak of cholesterol absorption takes place in approximately 6 to 9 hours.[37] The absorption of cholesterol from food is not complete. It has been estimated that only 50 per cent of the cholesterol ingested is absorbed[38] but this occurred when 5 gm of cholesterol were fed with 100 gm of olive oil. In other studies where 60 mg of cholesterol in a diet containing 40 per cent fat were fed to normal young adults of both sexes, it was found that 79 per cent of the cholesterol was absorbed.[39] The absorption of cholesterol was found to depend on the size of the dose; with increasing amounts fed, the percentage absorbed decreased although the actual amount absorbed increased. Ivy and co-workers[40] observed that in 11 subjects fed a low fat diet, the total capacity of the intestine to absorb cholesterol was 2 gm daily of exogenous cholesterol plus 0.98 gm of endogenously synthesized cholesterol. More recently the question of cholesterol absorption was investigated by Wilson and Lindsey[41] using balance studies in a so-called "steady state" condition. They confirmed the limited ability of the human to absorb cholesterol and have reported a maximum absorption in man of approximately 300 mg of exogenous cholesterol per day. Borgström,[42] however, using "non-steady state" conditions reported that the total amount of cholesterol absorbed was proportional to the amount fed; in his experiments as much as 1.8 gm cholesterol per day was absorbed. Bloomfield[43] found that cholesterol was better absorbed when fed with safflower oil than with butter. Unsaturated fatty acid esters of cholesterol seem to be better absorbed than are the medium- and long-chain saturated fatty acid esters. Aftergood et al.[44] found that cholesterol absorption in rats was essentially the same (approximately 50 per cent) regardless of whether cholesterol was fed with a saturated fat (lard) or an unsaturated fat (cottonseed oil). Undoubtedly there are many factors which affect the absorption of cholesterol, e.g. the amount of the cholesterol fed at one time, the frequency of its ingestion, the type of dietary fat fed concomitantly, the age of the subject, previous dietary history, and genetic factors.[30,32]

Sterols other than cholesterol are not well absorbed. In fact certain plant sterols, e.g. β-sitosterol, are not only poorly absorbed themselves but they also interfere with the absorption of cholesterol.[45,46] This may be due to competition for the enzyme, cholesterol esterase.[47] This property has led to use of plant sterol emulsions as a therapeutic tool in reducing hypercholesterolemia.

Undoubtedly foods contain many other lipids which are present in minor amounts but which may play important metabolic and physiological roles. Information on these components is scarce at the present time.

These minor lipids may include sterol glucosides, mono- and digalactosyl-glycerides, sulfolipids, fatty acids with triple bonds rather than the double bonds which occur more frequently and cyclopropenoid fatty acids.[48]

Cyclopropenoid fatty acids, e.g. sterculic and malvalic acids, occur in small amounts in cottonseed oil.[49]

Thus, through a process of hydrolysis and subsequent resynthesis, dietary lipids, insoluble in water, are being transferred from food via an aqueous medium through the intestine into the blood. In addition, resynthesized lipids are of a composition and configuration suitable for the next step in their metabolism.

FACTORS AFFECTING FAT ABSORPTION

Digestibility. Although all edible fats are practically completely digested and utilized, the rate at which they are utilized may differ considerably. Fats which are absorbed slowly seem to be as well utilized when they are given in small quantities as are fats which are rapidly absorbed. When a slowly absorbed fat is fed in large doses, a considerable amount may be lost to the feces. As far as its nutritional value is concerned, it does not seem to matter whether the fat is absorbed slowly or rapidly. Fat which is more quickly absorbed is more rapidly available to the tissues and is less likely to produce digestive upsets; fats which are more slowly absorbed and remain in the gastrointestinal tract for a longer period of time extend the period of satiety after a meal and are less of a "burden" on the fat transport systems. They produce a sustained but lower lipemia over a long period of time rather than sudden large hyperlipemias which occur when rapidly absorbed fats are ingested.

In general, both animal and vegetable fats are practically completely utilized. Their coefficient of digestibility (or per cent digestibility) is calculated by the general formula:

$$\frac{\text{Fat ingested} - \text{fat excreted (corrected for metabolic fat)}}{\text{Fat ingested}} \times 100 = \% \text{ Digestibility}$$

Ordinarily, this is approximately 95 per cent. Calloway and Kurtz[50] studied the digestibility of a number of natural edible fats (coconut oil, butter fat, soybean oil, corn oil, lard and cottonseed oil) and found that they were all practically completely digested. In studies with butter fat, butter oil, cod liver oil, corn oil, lard and two shortenings, Steenbock et al.[51] showed that these lipid substances were all absorbed to the same extent, with the maximum absorption occurring after 6 to 8 hours. The per cent fat absorbed after 2 hours varied from 24 to 41 per cent; after 4 hours, 53 to 71 per cent; after 6 hours, 68 to 86 per cent; and after 12 hours, 97 to 99 per cent.

The rate of absorption of hydrogenated fats is comparable to that of natural fats of the same melting point and approximate fatty acid composition. Since the rate of absorption is influenced primarily by melting point, fats having a high content of stearic acid (e.g. completely hydrogenated fats like hydrogenated lard and hydrogenated cottonseed oil with melting points of 54° and 55° C) have a lower digestibility and a slow rate of absorption. However, in fats containing mixed triglycerides into which stearic acid is incorporated along with unsaturated fatty acids, the digestibility is not impaired. Also, it has been reported that the absorption of tristearin in the rat is improved by the concomitant feeding of triolein, which possibly increases its solubility in the bile.[52]

Amount of Fat Consumed. The rate at which fat leaves the intestine is at first increased when larger amounts are present; with large amounts, the percentage of fat absorbed is decreased since some is lost to the feces before it can be absorbed by the intestinal mucosa.

Age of Subject. It has been shown by several investigators that infants under 1 year of age absorb fat inefficiently.[53,54] Also, fat is more slowly absorbed and metabolized in aged individuals than in younger adults.[55]

Emulsifying Agents. Emulsifying agents like lecithin and Tween 80 can increase the digestibility of a poorly absorbed fat and can also increase the *rate* of absorption of fats which are well digested and absorbed.[56] For example, Tween 80 (polyoxy-ethylene-sorbitan-monooleate) was able to increase fat absorption in patients with sprue (a disease in which fat is poorly absorbed) and in those suffering from certain pancreatic disorders.[57,58] However, more definitive therapy is recommended.

Fatty Acid Composition of Triglyceride Molecule. In general, short-chain fatty acid triglycerides are absorbed faster than longer-chain fatty acid triglycerides, with triacetin and tributyrin absorbed more rapidly than tricaproin and tricaprylin.[59] Triglycerides with odd-chain fatty acids are absorbed more slowly than even-chain fatty acid triglycerides.[60] It has been shown that triglycerides with palmitic acid on position 2 are better absorbed than are fats with palmitic acid on other positions, or with other fatty acids on position 2. Tomarelli and associates[61] and Filer and co-workers[62] have reported that the absorption of fats is affected adversely when palmitic and/or stearic acids appear in the 1,3 positions of the triglyceride molecule.

Overheating of Fats. Although the heating of fats to temperatures ordinarily employed for frying and cooking (205° to 210° C) neither changes the digestibility of the fat nor produces toxic substances,[63–65] when fats are heated in air at high temperatures (over 250° C), changes in many of the physical and chemical characteristics of the fat are observed. Viscosity is increased, iodine value is decreased, and digestibility is reduced. This was shown in studies by Lassen and co-workers[66] when they noted a progressive decrease in digestibility with increasing exposure of the fat to heat.

Calcium. The relationship between calcium and fat metabolism has been recognized for many years. It has been reported by Harkins et al.[67] that, in conditions of lipid malabsorption due to a *deficiency* of bile salts, calcium absorption was decreased. Further interrelationships between calcium and fat as concerns the absorption of these two nutrients have been shown with experiments on animals; the absorption of calcium requires the presence of fat in the diet although at very high levels of fat, especially those with the higher melting points, the absorption of calcium is depressed.[68] Similarly, for optimal absorption of fat, some calcium is required, although at high calcium levels there is a decreased absorption of fats,[69] especially those with high melting points, *e.g.* those containing lauric, myristic, palmitic and stearic acids in their triglycerides. The digestibility of fats with a high concentration of unsaturated fatty acids, *e.g.* oleic and linoleic acids, is not affected by the presence of calcium.[70] In fact, triglycerides containing oleic acid enhance calcium absorption.[71]

The mechanism for the action by which calcium interferes with the absorption of saturated fats seems to be the formation of poorly absorbed calcium salts of these saturated fatty acids. It was reported that the proportion of calcium lost in the feces, or the amount of fatty acid which is not absorbed because it is excreted as the calcium soap, depends on the type of fat in the diet.[72] In rats, fecal fatty acids become progressively more saturated as the calcium content of the diet is increased.[73] In infants ingesting fat other than human milk fat, both calcium and saturated fatty acids of long-chain length are lost in the stool.[74] On the other hand, Gorman *et al.*[75] reported that the apparent digestibility of fat and the amount of fecal fat were not influenced by low to moderate levels of calcium and protein.

Malabsorption of Fats

Bile Salts and Pancreatic Lipase. Lipid malabsorption may occur for a variety of reasons. As noted above the process of converting the triglycerides in foods to the triglycerides appearing in chylomicrons involves many steps. It is not surprising to learn that interference with the supply of any of the participating factors may adversely affect fat absorption.[20] The two major compounds involved in digestion and absorption of fats are bile salts and pancreatic lipase.

Bile salts are essential not only for the absorption of neutral fat, but also for the absorption of other lipids from the intestinal tract. They act as detergents aiding in the emulsification of fat within the lumen of the intestine. They form micellar particles with fat and/or with the digestion products of fat and transport these micelles to the intestinal mucosa where the products of fat digestion are absorbed. Bile salts are synthesized by the liver from cholesterol; the most common bile

salts found in mammals are the glycine and taurine derivatives of cholic acid and chenodeoxycholic acid. Bile salts are secreted in rather large quantities. In man, approximately 30 gm are excreted each day; this is approximately 6 times the amount in the body pool and is much larger than can be accounted for by normal biosynthesis. This large amount of available bile salts is made possible by its absorption from the intestine, transport to the liver and resecretion by the liver into the ileum of the intestine. This process is called enterohepatic circulation.

It is obvious that any interference with bile salt production, transport, absorption and storage will interfere with the absorption of fat. A decreased supply of bile salts in the intestine may be a result of the inability of the liver to synthesize bile salts or to effect the conjugation of bile salts with glycine or taurine. When unconjugated bile products are secreted they can interfere with micellar formation and therefore also with the uptake of lipids by the mucosa. An obstruction in the bile duct can prevent the bile from flowing into the intestine. Also, an impairment in the enterohepatic circulation due to poor absorption of bile salts from the ileum and subsequent losses in the feces may account for an insufficient supply of bile salts and hence decreased fat absorption. Clinical aspects of this problem are discussed in other chapters.

Pancreatic lipase, which is the most important enzyme for fat lipolysis, may be in short supply if there is an inflammation or tumor of the pancreas. The disease, cystic fibrosis,[76] also results in a deficiency of pancreatic enzymes causing impaired fat lipolysis and absorption and a subsequent excessive loss of fat through the feces. The treatment of pancreatic insufficiency is discussed in another chapter.

Intestinal Mucosa. Any defects in the structure or metabolism of the cells of the intestinal mucosa may have an inhibitory effect on fat absorption[18,77,78] as well as on the absorption of other nutrients. This topic is considered in detail in other chapters.

Protein and Lipoprotein Formation. Since protein is a necessary component of lipoproteins and chylomicrons, inhibition of protein and lipoprotein synthesis would interfere with chylomicron formation and would therefore prevent the movement of triglyceride into the lymphatics. Isselbacher and Budz have shown that the normal intestinal mucosa can synthesize protein and lipoproteins.[79] It has also been demonstrated that substances which inhibit protein synthesis, e.g. puromycin, acetoxycycloheximide, ethionine, and carbon tetrachloride, cause a postprandial accumulation of triglyceride in the intestinal mucosa and a depressed serum trigylceride level.[80,81] A genetic disease in which there is a deficiency of β-lipoproteins (a-beta-lipoproteinemia) is also associated with impaired fat metabolism; here, also, there is interference with the movement of lipid from the intestinal mucosa into the lymph.[82] In many disorders of fat absorption, triglycerides of medium-chain-length fatty acids are better absorbed than are the fats composed of long-chain fatty acids,[83] since the shorter-chain fatty acid triglycerides are absorbed directly into the portal circulation.

FAT TRANSPORT FROM LYMPH TO TISSUES

Chylomicron Formation. The triglycerides synthesized in the mucosa from dietary fatty acids appear in the lymph as chylomicrons. These are complex compounds containing triglycerides, phospholipid, cholesterol and its esters, and protein.[84,85] Protein, free cholesterol and phospholipid (lecithin) form an outer coating for the triglyceride.[86]

Chylomicrons are made in the smooth endoplasmic reticulum of the mucosal cell. Although the amount of protein in the chylomicron particle is very small (0.2 to 0.5 per cent),[87] it is essential for chylomicron formation. There is some indication that the protein for the chylomicron is synthesized by the gut.[88] After their formation the chylomicrons are discharged into the intercellular space and appear in the lacteals, from which they are collected into the thoracic duct; they finally enter the blood system through the subclavian vein.[89] The presence of large amounts of chylomicrons in blood makes the plasma milky (lipemic) in appearance. The half-life of the circulating chylomicron constituents is of the order of a few minutes.[90]

Nature of Fatty Acids in Lymph Triglycerides. It is now believed that practically all of the triglycerides (with the exception of the very small amount of fatty acids of short- and medium-chain glycerides which may be present in food and which are absorbed directly into the portal circulation), and other lipids as well, enter the lymph from the intestine on their way to the liver and to other tissues. Although most of the fatty acids in chylomicron triglycerides are derived from the diet,[91] endogenous fatty acids may be incorporated in significant amounts since the mucosal cell cannot distinguish between fatty acids from dietary fat, from circulating free fatty acids, or from lipogenesis. The fatty acid composition of the dietary fat also influences to some degree the fatty acid composition of the chylomicron cholesterol ester and to a lesser degree the composition of the chylomicron phospholipids.[28] Medium-chain-length triglycerides have been found to induce the highest cholesterol content in chylomicrons.[92]

Lipoprotein Lipase and Chylomicron Hydrolysis. The triglycerides of chylomicrons are quickly hydrolyzed by the lipoprotein lipase, also known as the clearing factor.[93] Serum albumin, which serves as an acceptor for the fatty acids formed by the action of the enzyme on the triglycerides, is required for its activity. The fatty acid-albumin complex acts as a dispersing agent for residual glycerides which now may be more easily assimilated by the tissues.[94] Blood heparin levels have been found to be related to the activity of the clearing factor and to the lipemia.[95] A lack of sufficient endogenous heparin has been shown to be the cause of hyperlipemia.[96] It has been suggested that liver contains an inhibitor of lipoprotein lipase which is counteracted by the addition of large amounts of heparin.[97] Lipoprotein lipase is more or less specific for intact chylomicrons; free cholesterol exerts an inhibitory action.[98] No lipoprotein lipase activity has been found in the liver but it is present in the extracts of heart and adipose tissue. Less lipoprotein lipase activity has been found in the adipose tissue of rats fed saturated fats than in those fed polyunsaturated fatty acids.[99]

Lipoproteins. Lipids are ubiquitous components of cells and tissues. Since they are not sufficiently polar to circulate freely in an aqueous medium such as plasma, they are dependent for mobility on combination with a carrier protein to form lipoproteins which confers the necessary solubility to allow their distribution in body fluids.[100] The classification of lipoproteins is based on the method of isolation, *i.e.* ultracentrifugal separation or electrophoresis. The differentiation, based on density versus electrophoretic mobility, is comparable in most instances and very often these classifications are used interchangeably. Thus very low density lipoproteins (VLDL) were found to be identical with the pre-β fraction (density range 0.95 to 1.006 gm/ml); the low density lipoproteins (LDL) correspond to the β-fraction (1.006 to 1.063 gm/ml) and the high density lipoproteins (HDL) correspond to the α-fraction as is seen on paper electrophoresis (1.063 to 1.21 gm/ml).[101] Chylomicrons which contain a small amount of protein and large amounts of triglyceride may be considered a borderline group of lipoproteins of a particularly low density. Information concerning the functional significance of lipoproteins has accumulated in recent years.[102–106]

The major classes of human plasma lipoproteins, their lipid composition, pathologic disorders and treatment are considered in another chapter.

PLASMA LIPIDS

Triglycerides are the most variable component of the plasma lipids. They range between 10 to 200 mg/100 ml plasma depending on individual variation, and time elapsed after ingestion of a fat-containing meal. The peak of absorption of lipid and therefore the time of maximum lipemia is usually 4 to 6 hours following the meal. Most of the triglyceride is carried in the LDL and VLDL fractions.

Plasma FFA are derived from adipose tissue, are bound to albumin and lipoproteins, and are characterized by a rapid turnover. Depending on the nutritional status of the animal, their concentration ranges between 0.3 to 0.5 mEq/liter; the higher values occur in the fasting or malnourished animal.

Phospholipids are less variable, although they are present at a rather high level, *i.e.* 50 per cent of plasma lipids. Most of the phospholipid occurs as lecithin, and it is carried primarily in the HDL and LDL fractions. Phospholipids, in association with the protein moiety, may serve as the structural elements of the circulating lipoproteins, whereas cholesterol and triglycerides are probably the lipids which are transported.

Cholesterol is carried primarily by the LDL. Total serum cholesterol in the average adult man ranges from 140 to 260 mg/100 ml plasma. About 70 per cent occurs as cholesterol esterified with fatty acids. The serum cholesterol level varies with race, age, sex and diet and probably is under genetic control. Serum cholesterol levels have been intensively and extensively investigated because of their probable association with the disease, atherosclerosis.

TISSUE LIPIDS AND METABOLISM

Erythrocytes. The erythrocytes differ markedly in composition from the blood plasma. Erythrocyte lipids are composed mainly of free cholesterol and phospholipids. Less than 3 per cent of total erythrocyte fatty acids occur in defined lipids other than phospholipids. The concentration of phospholipids in red cells is approximately double that in plasma, and the proportion of phospholipids which occurs in red cells is also different from that in plasma. For example, 35 per cent of the total phosphatides in erythrocytes are lecithins, whereas lecithin comprises 75 per cent of the plasma phospholipids; ethanolamine phosphoglycerides comprise 30 per cent of total phosphatides in erythrocytes and 5 per cent in plasma; serine phosphoglycerides comprise 10 per cent of erythrocyte phosphatides but are not present in plasma. Plasmalogens make up 20 per cent of the total red cell phosphatides but only 3 to 5 per cent of plasma phosphatides. Of the fatty acids in the erythrocyte phospholipids, about 50 per cent are unsaturated, whereas in plasma neutral lipids, the unsaturated fatty acids constitute 65 to 75 per cent of the total.[107] It has been shown that the fatty acid pattern of human erythrocyte phospholipids can be altered by diet.[108] In the case of cholesterol, the quantity is somewhat lower in the cells than in the plasma. Whereas cholesterol esters were found to comprise approximately 70 per cent of the total plasma cholesterol, the concentration in red cells has been reported to be from 0 to 20 per cent.[109]

Leukocytes have a higher proportion of total lipids than either plasma or red blood cells. Leukocytes also contain an appreciable amount of neutral fat.[110]

Cell Membranes. It has been recognized that lipids, phospholipids in particular, perform a basic role in the structure and function of biological membranes, at intercellular surfaces as well as at intracellular surfaces, such as those of mitochondria.[111] The essentiality of lipid has been established for the electron transfer process[112] as well as for the activities of many enzymes.[113] The general role of phospholipid appears to be in the control of membrane formation. The lipid structure of the plasma membranes serves as a barrier for the diffusion of various substances across the cell wall.

Even though lipids and protein are the major components of the cell membrane, its chemical composition varies.[114] The lipid/protein ratio of myelin is 3 whereas most other membranes have ratios of about 0.5. Myelin has large amounts of glycosyl ceramides, the erythrocyte plasma membrane and myelin contain large quantities of sphingolipid, whereas microsomal and mitochondrial membranes have almost none; at the same time these are rich in phospho-

mammalian organs have characteristic lipid profiles.

Liver. The liver is the major site of lipid metabolism. Most of the triglyceride circulating in the blood is initially removed by the liver.[115] Here it undergoes a variety of energy-producing and energy-consuming processes, the two most important being fatty acid oxidation and fatty acid synthesis. Fatty acids become available for oxidation in the liver through three sources: (1) synthesis in the liver from dietary carbohydrate when provided in excess of need, (2) hydrolysis of the chylomicron triglyceride derived from dietary fat, and (3) mobilization of free fatty acids from adipose tissue via an albumin complex in the blood.

The usual disposition of free fatty acids is conversion to triglyceride. There are various factors which regulate the amount of triglyceride which is stored in the liver. One of the processes by which excess triglyceride is removed is through the oxidation of the triglyceride fatty acids to CO_2 and H_2O preceded by lipolysis of the triglyceride to free fatty acids + glycerol.

Fatty Acid Oxidation. Fatty acid oxidation is an energy-producing process which proceeds in a stepwise fashion through successive β-oxidations. The enzymes required for the oxidative reactions are contained in the mitochondria of the cell and the energy which is produced is stored as high-energy compounds such as ATP. The reaction sequence by which fatty acids are oxidized is such that 2-carbon units are successively split off.[116] In this way the complete oxidation of palmitic acid releases ultimately 2500 Kcal.[117]

The first step in the sequence is the activation of palmitic acid with the formation of the CoA-thioester:

$$\text{Fatty acid} + \text{CoASH} + \text{ATP} \xrightarrow[\text{Mg}^{++}]{\text{thiokinase}} \text{fatty acyl-CoA} + \text{AMP} + \text{PP}$$

glycerides. Cardiolipin is present exclusively in mitochondrial membranes.

In addition to these subcellular differences in lipid composition, many studies of a variety of tissues indicate that many of the

There are three different thiokinases which are specific for different chain length fatty acids. The second step is an α,β-dehydrogenation of the fatty acyl-CoA catalyzed by acyldehydrogenases. Here, too, three enzymes with chain length specificity have been isolated. The resulting compound is trans-

$$R\text{-}CH \doteqdot CH\text{-}\overset{\overset{\displaystyle O}{\|}}{C}\text{-}SCoA$$

and a reduced acceptor, $FADH_2$ (flavin adenine dinucleotide), which transfers the electrons through another flavoprotein to the cytochrome b of the mitochondrial electron transport system. The third step is the hydration of the α,β-unsaturated fatty acyl-CoA by the enzyme, enoyl-CoA hydrase, with the production of the L-(+)-hydroxyacyl-CoA derivative. This compound is then oxidized in the fourth step by a β-hydroxy-acyl dehydrogenase to beta-ketoacyl-CoA. The electrons are transferred to

to CO_2 and H_2O by extrahepatic tissues or may be excreted in the urine.

For the oxidation of unsaturated fatty acids two additional enzymes, an isomerase and an epimerase, are necessary; these also are located in the mitochondria. The rates of oxidation for both saturated and polyunsaturated fatty acids have been found to be the same.[120]

Fatty acids can also undergo other types of oxidative processes. Mead and Levis,[121] on the basis of analysis of the radioactivity in C_{23} acids of brain cerebrosides, have proposed a theory of α-oxidation of long-chain fatty acids in brain through the α-hydroxy acids as follows:

$$R\text{---}CH_2\text{---}COOH \rightarrow R\text{---}\overset{\overset{\displaystyle OH}{|}}{C}H\text{---}COOH \rightarrow R\text{---}COOH$$

NAD^+ (nicotinamide adenine dinucleotide). The last step is the thiolytic cleavage of the β-ketoacyl-CoA by a thiolase to form a fatty acyl-CoA with two less carbon atoms than the original and one molecule of acetyl-CoA. The equilibrium constant for this reaction favors acetyl-CoA formation:

Fulco and Mead[122] have shown that α-hydroxy acids are formed by direct hydroxylation of preformed, unsubstituted long-chain fatty acids. Alpha-oxidation is catalyzed by enzymes located in the microsomes.[123]

Carnitine (β-hydroxy-α-trimethylammonium butyrate), found in skeletal muscle and

$$R\text{---}\overset{\overset{\displaystyle O}{\|}}{C}\text{---}CH_2\text{---}\overset{\overset{\displaystyle O}{\|}}{C}\text{---}SCoA + CoASH \rightarrow R\text{---}\overset{\overset{\displaystyle O}{\|}}{C}\text{---}SCoA + CH_3\text{---}\overset{\overset{\displaystyle O}{\|}}{C}\text{---}SCoA$$

The resulting fatty acyl-CoA is now ready for another passage through the oxidation cycle[118,119] until it is completely degraded to acetyl-CoA's.

Acetyl-CoA is normally oxidized to CO_2 and H_2O via the citric acid cycle. In starvation or in uncorrected diabetes, considerable amounts of acetyl-CoA accumulate because of impaired citric acid cycle activity. These acetyl-CoA's condense to form ketone bodies, i.e. acetoacetate, β-hydroxybutyrate and acetone. An excessive amount of these compounds produces the condition called ketosis. The condensation of two acetyl-CoA's releases coenzyme A which is then available for activation of fatty acids for further oxidation. Ketone bodies either may be further oxidized

probably in other tissues as well, has been reported to stimulate long-chain fatty acid oxidation in liver slices and homogenates[124] as well as in mitochondrial preparations.[125,126] Apparently the stimulation of fatty acid oxidation is mediated via acylcarnitine formation. It has been suggested that acylcarnitine derivatives may function as carriers of acyl groups from extramitochondrial to intramitochondrial coenzyme A. In the absence of carnitine, transport of acyl-CoA to the fatty acid oxidizing system seems to be rate limiting.

Fatty Acid Synthesis. When the mechanism of the β-oxidation of fatty acids became elucidated it was assumed that fatty acid synthesis occurred by the reversal of the β-oxidation pathway. However, as a result of extensive studies involving liver, adipose tissue, mammary gland,[127] yeast[128] and *E. coli*[129] systems, it has been established that there are three systems responsible for fatty acid synthesis. These are (1) the cytoplasmic, the *de novo* or palmitate-synthesizing system; (2) the mitochondrial, concerned with the elongation of available fatty acids and (3) the microsomal, also concerned with elongation, but particularly involved in the synthesis of the unsaturated fatty acids.

In the cytoplasm, fatty acids of 16 or 18 C are built sequentially from two carbon fragments. The first step is the carboxylation of acetyl-CoA to malonyl-CoA[130] by acetyl-CoA carboxylase which has biotin as its prosthetic group:

ducing palmitic and stearic acids. However since the organism apparently needs longer-chain fatty acids as well, two other systems are operative to elongate these endogenously synthesized fatty acids and fatty acids derived from the diet. In the mitochondria, acetyl-CoA is the two carbon donor and both NADH and NADPH (reduced nicotinamide adenine dinucleotide phosphate) are required.[133] The system elongates fatty acids of chain lengths C_{10}-C_{22} at different rates, with unsaturated fatty acids being elongated at a faster rate than their saturated homologs. This is essentially the reverse of the β-oxidation pathway except that the acyl dehydrogenase is replaced by an enzyme which catalyzes the reduction of trans-α,β-unsaturated acyl-CoA by NADPH.

$$ATP + HCO_3^- + CH_3-\overset{O}{\overset{\|}{C}}-SCoA \rightarrow ADP + PP + {}^-O-\overset{O}{\overset{\|}{C}}-CH_2-\overset{O}{\overset{\|}{C}}-SCoA$$

The second step is the conversion of malonyl-CoA to palmitate. This is catalyzed by a group of enzymes, the fatty acid synthetases. Protein-bound acyl derivatives have been postulated as intermediates.[131] The following reaction sequence has been established. During the condensation of acetyl-CoA and malonyl-CoA, a simultaneous decarboxylation takes place forming acetoacetyl-S-enzyme. The intermediates remain bound covalently to the protein by thioester linkages. Then acetoacetyl-S-enzyme is reduced by NADPH to D-(−)-β-hydroxy-butyryl-S-enzyme and dehydrated to trans-2-butenoyl-S-enzyme. The resulting α,β-unsaturated fatty acyl-S-enzyme is reduced by a second NADPH. Electron transfer is mediated by FMNH₂ (reduced flavin mononucleotide). Seven passages through this reaction yield palmitic acid according to the following equation:

Microsomes contain an enzyme system which catalyzes the elongation of fatty acyl-CoA to longer-chain acids in the presence of malonyl-CoA and NADPH.[134] Acetyl-CoA is inactive in this system and NADPH is the preferred electron donor. Saturated fatty acids of C_{10}-C_{16} are elongated at faster rates than are other saturated acids; however, the more unsaturated the fatty acid the faster is its rate of elongation. In all probabilities this system is the one responsible for the synthesis of arachidonic acid from linoleic acid.

The desaturation of fatty acids, *e.g.* production of oleic acid from stearic acid, is catalyzed by an enzyme system found in the microsomal fraction of the cell. NADH is the preferred electron donor. Microsomal enzymes also catalyze the desaturation of monoenoic to dienoic acids[135] but not to the essential dienoic acid, linoleic acid. Since animals have lost the ability to synthesize linoleic

$$CH_3-\overset{O}{\overset{\|}{C}}-SCoA + 7HO-\overset{O}{\overset{\|}{C}}-CH_2-\overset{O}{\overset{\|}{C}}-SCoA + 14H^+ \rightarrow CH_3-(CH_2)_{14}-\overset{O}{\overset{\|}{C}}-OH + 7CO_2 + 8 CoASH + 14NADP^+ + 6H_2O$$

Many tissues other than liver including adipose tissue itself[133] are capable of fatty acid biosynthesis.

The cytoplasmic system is efficient in pro-

acid they have to depend on dietary sources for an adequate supply of this essential fatty acid. However, linoleic acid can also be metabolized through sequences of desaturation and elongation yielding arachidonic acid and the longer-chain PUFA (polyunsaturated fatty acids).

Lipid Accumulation. Because of its activity in all aspects of lipid metabolism, a multiplicity of conditions are possible in which an accumulation of triglycerides occurs in the liver. The general mechanisms responsible may be an increased synthesis of triglycerides, a decreased oxidation of triglyceride fatty acids, an increased uptake of triglycerides or fatty acids from the blood, a decreased secretion of triglycerides by the liver or a combination of these factors.[136] Fatty livers produced by starvation, diabetes or the administration of anterior pituitary hormones are due to an increased mobilization of fatty acids from adipose tissue.[137] The involvement of choline and sulfur-containing amino acids in the production of fatty liver is not quite well understood, although it is thought that decreased phospholipid synthesis resulting from a choline deficiency may be involved in this impaired lipid removal from the liver.[138] The administration of ethionine, which interferes with lipoprotein synthesis, also may be responsible for neutral fat accumulation.[139] Poisons, like CCl_4,[140] and drugs, like puromycin, produce fatty livers together with a decreased plasma lipoprotein level.[141] Orotic acid which interferes with the normal formation of hepatic nucleotides causes fatty livers accompanied by low plasma lipoproteins.[142] A fatty liver can result in man from acute or chronic ethanol ingestion.[143] Liver injury is commonly produced when ethanol is ingested in conjunction with deficient, low-fat diets. A diet with 25 per cent of calories as fat appears to be optimal for minimizing the steatogenic effects of ethanol.[144] Fatty livers may also be attributable to a deficiency of essential fatty acids, probably due in part to a depressed phospholipid synthesis. An abnormal accumulation of cholesterol also occurs in essential fatty acid deficiency.[145]

Adipose Tissue. The final site of deposition of dietary fatty acids in excess of calorie requirement as well as the major source of triglyceride reserves in the body is adipose tissue. It is assumed that lipoprotein lipase, which is bound to the surface of the capillary endothelium in adipose tissue, catalyzes the hydrolysis of the chylomicron triglycerides to free fatty acids and glycerol.[146] The glycerol produced is released by adipose tissue rather than being utilized for resynthesis of triglycerides since the enzyme, glycerol kinase, is not present in adipose tissue.[147]

Upon entering the adipose tissue cell, the free fatty acids are converted to fatty acyl-CoA, which reacts with L-α-glycerophosphate (formed from glucose) to form phosphatidic acid, which, in turn, is converted to triglyceride by an enzyme system utilizing still another fatty acyl-CoA molecule. Therefore when the animal is ingesting carbohydrates along with fat, adipose tissue plays a greater role relative to liver in processing chylomicron triglycerides than when the diet contains only fat.[148] The correlation between the fat-induced hyperlipemia and the tissue level of lipoprotein lipase provides supportive evidence for the functioning of lipoprotein lipase in the uptake of chylomicron triglyceride by the tissues. However, the exchange of triglyceride fatty acids of the plasma with those of the liver is much more rapid than any net uptake by adipose tissue.[149] Thus, most of the triglycerides appearing in adipose tissue have previously gone through resynthesis in the liver and have lost most of their original identity.

A reciprocal regulation of lipoprotein lipase activity has been established in rat adipocytes.[150] Cyclic AMP (adenosine-3′,5′-monophosphate) activates hormone-sensitive lipase resulting in the production of free fatty acids. In the presence of glucose and insulin some of the free fatty acids are reesterified to triglycerides leading to an increased consumption of ATP, hence to a decrease in protein synthesis and consequent reduction in lipase activity.

Adipose tissue is important as source of energy in the newborn and in infancy.[151] The lipid content of adipose tissue accounts for 40 per cent of the weight of the newborn and increases with increasing age to 75 per cent in the adult.[152] Age has a major influence on the fatty acid composition of superficial depot fat of childhood.[153] Linoleic acid appears to be high in the infant, and thereafter diminishes. No sex differences were found at the early stages of development; however, some differences in fatty acids, *i.e.* lower oleic and higher stearic acid content, have been reported in normal adult males as compared with normal adult females.[154] Inhabitants of the U.S. have higher levels of myristic, palmitic, stearic and oleic acids and lower levels of palmitoleic, linoleic and linolenic acids in adipose tissue than their Japanese counterparts. In addition, linoleic acid seems to decrease with age in the U.S. population, whereas the Japanese have a higher content of polyunsaturated acids and no correlation with age.[155]

Hirsch and Han[156] have investigated the effects of age, food restriction and hyperphagia on adipose cellularity in rats. They have established that the number of adipose tissue cells in the normal rat increases up to 15 weeks of age. Subsequently, however, the increase in adipose depot size occurs solely through an increase in cell size, *i.e.* the amount of lipid per cell. While food deprivation during the first 3 weeks of life leads to a reduction in cell number, as well as in cell size, at a later age, starvation has no effect on cell number.[157]

Obesity has been defined[158] as that bodily state in which there is excessive accumulation of fat in both the relative and the absolute sense. It has been suggested[159] that it occurs as the result of substrate excess, when food intake exceeds the rate at which foodstuffs are combusted, and also when there is an enhanced insulin activity.

The composition of fat in the fat depots is sensitive to dietary unsaturated fatty acids. The proportion of linoleic and linolenic acids present is a function of their content in the diet. Changes in fatty acid patterns in adipose tissue induced by the diet appear slowly over a period of months.[160] In men fed an unsaturated fat diet for prolonged periods, the linoleic acid content of adipose tissue rose from 11 per cent of the total fatty acids to 32 per cent after 5 years.[161] When animals are exposed to a cold temperature they deposit more liquid fats with a lower melting point and a higher iodine number than when exposed to warmer climates.[162]

Adipose tissue triglycerides are released as their hydrolyzed products, *i.e.* fatty acids and glycerol. The rate of fatty acid release from stored adipose tissue triglycerides during periods of caloric deficiency and stress is determined by the relative rates of hydrolysis of these triglycerides, of reesterification of fatty acids, and of transport of fatty acids from the cell where they can combine with albumin.[163] Free fatty acids from adipose tissue are utilized in many organs and supply a considerable portion of the metabolic energy of heart and skeletal muscle.[164] The liver utilizes large quantities of free fatty acids which it removes from the circulation.

Because of a high rate of hormone-sensitive triglyceride lipase activity and a low rate of triglyceride biosynthesis in the adipose tissue, fat mobilization occurs at high rates in fasting mammals; very little fat mobilization occurs in fed animals. Catecholamines play a well-defined role in fat mobilization from adipose tissue.[165] They activate lipases by increasing the concentration of cyclic AMP in adipose tissue cells. Tissues of mammals contain compounds called prostaglandins which can modify fat mobilization. These are biosynthesized from the essential fatty acids and will be discussed later.

Gonadal Lipids. The importance of lipids in gonadal function became apparent when male and female rats placed on essential fatty acid-deficient diets exhibited impaired reproductive performance. Analyses of rat testes reveal that 80 per cent of the lipid occurs as phospholipid,[166] predominantly phosphatidyl choline. The major saturated fatty acid of the phospholipid fraction is palmitic, whereas arachidonic acid is the major polyenoic acid. The highly unsaturated fatty acid, docosapentaenoic, is also present in considerable quantity. The high concentration of this 22 carbon polyenoic fatty acid is characteristic of testis tissue in a variety of mammals[167] and seems to be correlated with spermatogenesis and maturation of sperm. A decrease in essential fatty acid content in testes with age corresponds with the involution of the active tissue.[168] Polyenoic fatty acids appear to be functionally important in gonadal tissue, in general, since it has been reported that a high content of PUFA derived from linoleic acid is a characteristic of Graafian follicle in beef and pork.[169]

Rat testes also contain small quantities of triglycerides and cholesterol; most of the cholesterol is unesterified (96 per cent).[166] However in ovaries, approximately 70 per cent of the cholesterol is esterified.[170,171] The cholesterol content in the ovary has been shown to fluctuate with the estrous cycle in the rat.[172] Cholesterol ester depletion occurs simultaneously with steroid hormone secretion in both adrenal and ovarian tissue,[173] resulting from the conversion of cholesterol to pregnenolone. In general, there is a rapid turnover of ovarian cholesterol.[174,175] Ovaries also contain rather high levels of PUFA, e.g. arachidonic and docosatetraenoic acids.[176]

Adrenal Lipids. The adrenal cortex is rich in cholesterol, particularly in cholesterol esters.[177] The cholesterol concentration, particularly cholesteryl arachidonate, is easily decreased by stresses such as infection,[178] and by hormone treatment.[179,180] Cholesterol is an obligatory precursor in the biosynthetic pathway of adrenocortical steroids.[181] The apparent selectivity in depletion of cholesteryl esters is probably due to differences in their rates of hydrolysis.[182] Adrenals are among the most active of the tissues capable of removing cholesteryl esters from plasma;[183,184] here these cholesterol esters have a rapid turnover rate.[175]

Recently Takayasu et al.[185] compared the fatty acid composition of human and rat adrenal lipids. The adrenal phospholipid contained about 20 per cent arachidonate in man and about 40 per cent in rats. The docosatetraenoic acid content was also particularly high in the rat and also was a major component in human adrenal cholesterol esters. The type of fatty acids incorporated into the cholesterol ester fraction can be influenced by the fatty acid composition of dietary lipids.[186]

Brain. Brain tissue is particularly rich in lipids. Brain lipids are formed to a large extent before, or immediately after, birth and are then considered to be relatively stable from a metabolic point of view. However, a reduced deposition of brain lipids as well as an alteration in the fatty acid portion of the phospholipid molecules was reported when essential fatty acid deficiency was induced early in experimental animals.[187]

Fatty acid chain elongation is closely related to myelination.[188] Myelin contains high levels of galactolipids, plasmalogens and cholesterol.[189] Seventy per cent of total rat brain cholesterol is contained in myelin as is practically all of the cerebroside, most of the phosphatidyl ethanolamine, and 70 per cent of total sulphatides and sphingomyelin.[190] A reduced rate of growth (due to malnutrition) causes a delay in the accumulation of lipids in myelin. Myelin composition is fixed and a deficiency of one of the lipid components limits the assembly of the whole lipid portion of the membrane.[191]

Apparently dietary fatty acids can influence the composition of brain fatty acids.[192] Dhopeshwarkar and Mead[193,194] have shown that palmitate and oleate can penetrate the brain tissue lipids without prior degradation by β-oxidation to acetate. These workers[195] have also observed that elongation of fatty acids is more pronounced in the adult brain than in weanling rats. It has been postulated that rat brain may require different amounts of essential fatty acids during aging.[196] A large group of even- and odd-numbered α-hydroxy-fatty acids with 20 to 26 C atoms occurs in brain cerebrosides.[122]

Cholesterol is present in brain primarily unesterified. During myelination the concentration of esterified cholesterol never exceeds 2 per cent[197] and later it constitutes only 0.1 to 0.2 per cent of the total cholesterol. After completion of the myelination process cholesteryl arachidonate is the major ester. During early development large amounts of desmosterol are found in rat brain but they later disappear.[198] Possibly both cholesterol esters and desmosterol may have important roles in sterol synthesis and metabolism during development, differentiation, and myelination. In the adult brain, the turnover of brain cholesterol is considerably slower than it is in other tissues.

CHOLESTEROL METABOLISM

Cholesterol is an integral part of cell structure and is synthesized in most tissues, with the possible exception of adult brain. Liver is probably the most active site of cholesterolgenesis, although, in man, the extrahepatic tissues biosynthesize more cholesterol than does the liver.[199] In man no more than 40 per cent of circulating cholesterol is derived from the diet even when high cholesterol diets are consumed.[200] There is a difference in the dietary regulation of cholesterol synthesis between the liver and extrahepatic tissues and between animals and man. In rats and other animals, a negative feedback mechanism operates and therefore feeding cholesterol to animals produces a marked suppression of hepatic cholesterol synthesis; however no significant changes are induced in the gastrointestinal tract. In man, exogenous cholesterol does not suppress cholesterol-genesis in extrahepatic tissues and there is still some controversy as to the effect on liver; the existence of a negative feedback control is indeed questionable.[201,199] The rate of cholesterol synthesis in the human intestine may approximate that of cholesterolgenesis in the human liver.[32] The concentration of bile may be involved in controlling cholesterol synthesis in the intestine.

The entire cholesterol molecule is biosynthesized from acetyl groups. The complete chemical synthesis of cholesterol and squalene from labeled precursors followed by complete chemical degradation[202,203] made it possible to identify the origin of each carbon atom of the molecule.

Cholesterol biosynthesis may be considered as a sequence of reactions as follows: (1) the conversion of acetyl-CoA to mevalonic acid, (2) the conversion of mevalonic acid through geraniol and farnesol to squalene, (3) the cyclization of squalene to form lanosterol, and (4) the conversion of lanosterol to cholesterol. One of the important metabolic sites at which cholesterol synthesis is regulated has been demonstrated by Gould and Popják[204] to be the reduction of β-hydroxy-β-methyl-glutaryl-CoA to mevalonate. Other studies[205] have suggested that additional sites beyond the mevalonate stage might also be inhibited by starvation, by high cholesterol diets and by drugs.

Although liver has been considered to be the major source of plasma cholesterol esters,[206] more recent studies suggest that they may originate in both the liver and plasma.[207] Whereas cholesteryl arachidonate is the major ester in rat plasma, cholesteryl oleate predominates in the liver unless the diet contains very high proportions of other fatty acids.[208] Presumably only some types of cholesterol esters are secreted into plasma in the rat but the nature of this selective process is unknown.

The metabolism of cholesterol esters is considerably different in man from that which occurs in the rat. The cholesterol esters of LD and HD lipoproteins are similar,[209] with cholesteryl linoleate the most abundant of the esters. Human liver, however, contains mostly saturated esters.

About two thirds of the cholesterol esters are carried in the LD lipoproteins where the greatest turnover occurs. The turnover of the cholesterol esters in the different lipoproteins is similar in normocholesterolemic and hypercholesterolemic subjects and is not altered by dietary changes despite marked changes in the composition of the cholesterol esters.[210] The possible mechanisms that regulate plasma cholesterol ester turnover have been reviewed by Goodman.[30]

It is likely that in man most of the cholesterol esters in plasma are formed as a result of the activity of the LCAT (lecithin-cholesterol-acyl transferase) enzyme.[211] In the rat this enzyme is responsible primarily for the formation of cholesterol esters in the HDL fraction.[199,212] This enzyme shows some specificity for certain fatty acids, acting primarily in the transfer of linoleic acid in human plasma and arachidonic acid in rat plasma from the 2-position of lecithin to free cholesterol to form the cholesterol ester. Apparently this esterification is followed by a transfer of esterified cholesterol from HDL to VLDL in exchange for triglycerides.[213] In the rat the activity of the plasma-esterifying system has been shown to be increased during starvation,[214] in diabetes, after the ingestion of ethanol[215] and after treatment with female sex hormones.[170] The composition and distribution of plasma lipoproteins may influence the activity of the LCAT enzyme. HD lipoprotein promotes this transesterification reaction by acting as an acceptor of the lysolecithin produced during the reaction.[216] There is a possibility that cholesterol ester turnover represents transport of cholesterol from tissues which synthesize cholesterol to the liver which is the major site of cholesterol catabolism. A hereditary deficiency of LCAT has been reported[217] with interesting biochemical manifestations, e.g. hypercholesterolemia with less than 10 per cent of esterified cholesterol (normal is approximately 30 per cent), high lecithin and low lysolecithin concentration in plasma, and a cholesterol ester composition which resembles neither normal hepatic cholesterol esters nor plasma cholesterol esters and therefore is probably derived from the intestine.

Plasma cholesterol levels can be influenced by diet. Alfin-Slater et al.[145] described the relationship between essential fatty acids and plasma cholesterol in rats, and, as early as 1952, Kinsell et al.[218] described the cholesterol-lowering effect of PUFA in humans. The mechanisms by which this is effected are still not clear. Some studies demonstrate a concomitant increase in fecal sterol excretion or turnover with PUFA diets,[219,220] whereas other studies are not in agreement with these results.[221,222] Plant sterols which are poorly absorbed also decrease the absorption of dietary and endogenous cholesterol.[46] Saturated and unsaturated fatty acids are incorporated into plasma cholesterol esters more readily when they are derived from endogenous synthesis rather than from the diet.[209]

A major pathway for the degradation of cholesterol in mammals is the conversion of cholesterol to bile salts. This process occurs exclusively in the liver.[223] The chemical changes taking place involve the conversion of the isooctyl side chain of cholesterol to a five-carbon monocarboxylic acid side chain, the inversion of β-oriented OH at C_3 to α-orientation, the reduction of unsaturation at C_5 and the addition of one or more OH groups at C_7 or C_{12}.[224] The enzymes required for bile acid formation have been found in both the mitochondrial and microsomal regions of liver cell. The microsomes contain enzymes that catalyze the conjugation of bile acids with either glycine or taurine to form conjugated bile salts. It is estimated that about 0.8 gm of cholesterol is degraded to bile acids daily. In human bile the principal bile acids are cholic, chenodeoxycholic and deoxycholic acids.[225]

The formation of bile acids by the liver is under negative feedback control, i.e. the bile acids returning to the liver following absorption from the intestine inhibit the synthesis by liver of new bile acids.[226]

Another important aspect of the metabolism of cholesterol is its conversion to steroid hormones. In the adrenals, cholesterol (perhaps as the sulfate[227]) is the precursor of pregnenolone[228] which is the precursor for progesterone, testosterone and estrogens. Cholesterol is also the precursor of adrenocortical steroids such as aldosterone, cortisol, and of vitamin D through irradiation of 7-dehydrocholesterol in the skin.

ESSENTIAL FATTY ACIDS (EFA)

In recent years several rather comprehensive reviews on EFA have appeared.[229-231] Research in this area has been quite extensive and very rewarding but much still remains to be elucidated.

EFA are those fatty acids that either cannot be biosynthesized or are synthesized in inadequate amounts by animals that require these nutrients for growth, maintenance and proper functioning of many physiological processes. It has been recognized that many fatty acids have essential fatty acid activity but the three most important are linoleic (18:2, cis-9,12-octadecadienoic) linolenic (18:3, cis-9,12,15-octadecatrienoic); and arachidonic acids (20:4, cis-5,8,11,14-eicosatetraenoic); these vary in activity in alleviating symptoms of EFA deficiency. Various deficiency symptoms have been observed in many animal species in response to feeding diets low in or free from EFA: in chickens, low fertility and hatchability; in rabbits, diminished growth and loss of hair; in fish, changes in dermal pigmentation; in rats, loss of weight, eczematous dermatitis, impairment of reproduction, changes in cell membrane function, and changes in enzymatic activity along with characteristic changes in FA composition of tissue lipids. In general, EFA deficiency is associated with decreased concentrations of dienoic, tetraenoic, pentaenoic and hexaenoic acids and increased concentrations of monoenoic and trienoic acids. A diagnostic approach for the assessment of EFA deficiency has been suggested using the ratio of the concentrations of triene to tetraene fatty acids in plasma and tissues; values over 0.4 indicate an EFA deficiency.[232] Some of the deficiency symptoms, such as dry and scaly skin and poor gain in weight, have been observed in human infants fed diets low in polyunsaturated fatty acids.[233] In the rat, feeding cholesterol in the absence of fat causes EFA deficiency symptoms to appear earlier.[234] It is thought that cholesterol may inhibit the formation of arachidonic acid (which is probably the active form of the essential fatty acids) from linoleic acid.[235] On the other hand, the rate of conversion of linoleate to arachidonate and the synthesis of phospholipids is greater in livers of EFA-deficient rats than in the controls.[236] Feeding adequate amounts of arachidonate to EFA-deficient rats cures all deficiency symptoms although the linoleic acid tissue content remains at a level similar to that in EFA-deficient animals.[237]

EFA may be necessary for the efficient transport and metabolism of cholesterol since it has been reported that in the absence of fat in the diet, abnormally large amounts of cholesterol, triglycerides, and phospholipds[145,236] accumulate in the liver. EFA's undergo chain lengthening and desaturation in the body; linoleate forms arachidonate, and linolenate yields the more highly polyunsaturated fatty acids. It has been suggested[238] that linoleate and linolenate compete for a common system of enzymes for elongation and for conversion to their more highly unsaturated derivatives. For any given chain length, the more unsaturated fatty acid has the greater affinity for the enzyme system. Oleate and linoleate also compete as substrates for the enzymes involved in the transformation of linoleic to arachidonic acid.[239] According to Nervi and Brenner[240] this competitive inhibition may occur at all stages, i.e. at desaturation, elongation and esterification. Saturated fatty acids also interfere with the metabolism of EFA since in some instances an enhanced utilization of residual EFA occurs in animals

receiving the essential fatty acid-deficient diet together with saturated fatty acids.[241]

There appears to be a sex difference in EFA requirement. Female rats have 1.3 to 1.6 times more polyenoic acid in tissues than do males.[242] Estrogenic hormones seem to exert a sparing effect on PUFA in the plasma and liver of rats.[243] Although the optimum requirement of EFA for the male rat is approximately 1.3 per cent of calories, that for female rats is approximately 0.5 per cent.[242] Similar differences in EFA requirement have been observed in other animal species as well.[244,245]

EFA deficiency results in alterations in cell membranes. It is probable that the change in the fatty acid composition of phospholipids of the membrane is the primary lesion of EFA deficiency.[246] One of the biochemical criteria for EFA deficiency is the effect on mitochondrial permeability;[247] liver mitochondria prepared from EFA-deficient rats evidently have altered permeability since they swell rapidly in vitro, and possibly in vivo as well, under conditions that preserve the shape and size of normal mitochondria.[248] It has been shown[249] that mitochondria prepared from livers of EFA-deficient rats oxidize substrates of the citric acid cycle more rapidly than do normal mitochondria. At the same time less high-energy phosphate is formed.[250] This uncoupled phosphorylation might thus explain the increased metabolic rate, the high endogenous respiration and the elevated cytochrome oxidase activity[231] seen in the EFA-deficient animal.

It is known that it is difficult to deplete adult animals of essential fatty acids because of their large reservoir of linoleate in adipose tissue. Even prolonged feeding of a deficient diet may not produce deficiency symptoms, although Collins and Sinclair[251] have produced an EFA deficiency in patients through parenteral feeding of saturated fat. Essential fatty acid deficiency symptoms have been produced in adult rats by feeding a fat-free diet in restricted amounts until they weighed one half of their original weight, and then by feeding the fat-free diet ad libitum.[252] It is in young growing animals that the essential fatty deficiency is produced in the shortest length of time.[253] It is now established that essential fatty acids are required by the human infant.[233]

Further recognition of the importance of essential fatty acids in nutrition has recently been demonstrated by the fact that EFA are precursors for the hormone-like substances called prostaglandins.[254]

PROSTAGLANDINS

About 40 years ago, Goldblatt[255] and von Euler[256] independently discovered that seminal fluid and extracts of vesicular glands contained a lipid fraction with potent vasodepressor activity which was also able to stimulate smooth muscle. In 1960 Bergström and Sjövall[257] crystallized from many kilograms of sheep vesicular glands an active principle which they named prostaglandin E_1 (PGE$_1$). Three years later, Bergström and co-workers[258] established the structure of PGE$_1$ and also of a series of structurally related compounds.

To date there have been dozens of different, naturally occurring prostaglandins isolated, all of which are derivatives of prostanoic acid (C20-cyclopentanoic acid) and which appear to be widely distributed in animal tissues.[259] Four series of natural prostaglandins have been described, designated by the letters E, F, A, and B, corresponding to differences in the ring structure and variations in degree of unsaturation of the side chain.

In 1964, two groups of investigators, Van Dorp et al.[260] and Bergström et al.,[261] reported that prostaglandins could be synthesized from polyunsaturated fatty acids. The conversion involved a ring closure (Fig. 4–1). A competition between unsaturated fatty acids was observed in PG formation, i.e. linolenic acid was found to compete irreversibly with arachidonic acid for PG synthetase.[262] Although prostaglandins can be formed from a variety of polyunsaturated fatty acids, Van Dorp and co-workers[260,263] found that biologically active prostaglandins

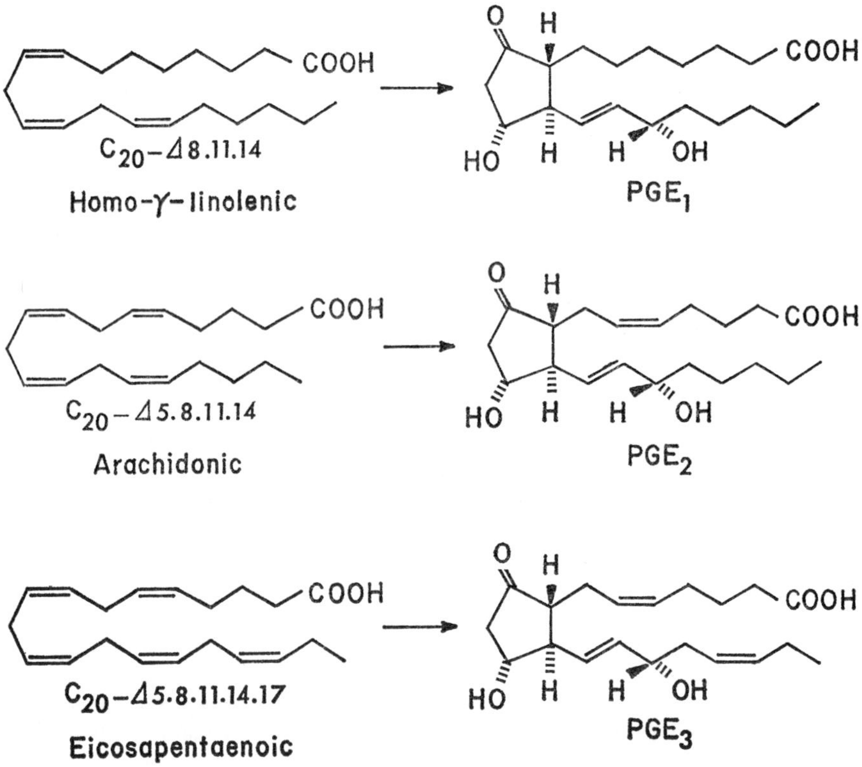

Fig. 4-1. Formation of prostaglandins from unsaturated fatty acids.

are formed only from those unsaturated fatty acids which have appreciable EFA activity; therefore, these workers postulated that the sole essential function of the EFA was as precursors for prostaglandin formation. However, attempts to cure EFA deficiency in rats by oral or intravenous administration of prostaglandins have been unsuccessful. It is possible, of course, that the administered prostaglandins did not reach the location where they were needed, and it is also possible that there is a difference between administered prostaglandin and prostaglandins formed in situ. However, this is the first time since the discovery of essential fatty acids that the role of EFA as precursors for other physiologically active metabolites has been studied.

The functions of prostaglandins in animal metabolism are many and varied. Since the highest concentrations of prostaglandin activity are found in accessory reproductive tissues and in semen, it was originally proposed that prostaglandins played a role in reproduction either by causing vasodilation, facilitating ejaculation, or contributing to sperm viability and transport.[264] It has been proposed that in man the seminal prostaglandins inhibit uterine motility thus facilitating the meeting of sperm and ovum. Although prostaglandins aid in conception, they can also be used in inducing labor and promoting abortion.[265]

Prostaglandins are extremely potent. A few nanograms (1×10^{-9} gm) cause contraction of smooth muscle. In vivo, a microgram per kilogram causes a significant drop in blood pressure. Prostaglandins affect heart rate. They are normal constituents of the brain in many species of animals and probably act as transmitters at central nervous synapses.

The prostaglandins are not equally potent nor do they all act in a similar fashion. For example, while PGE_1 and PGE_2 are powerful vasodilators, $PGF_{2\alpha}$ is a vasopressor in dogs and rats.[266] Qualitative differences have been noted between PGE, $PGF_{2\alpha}$ and PGA_1 and quantitative differences have been found between PGE_1 and PGE_2. PGE_1 is a potent inhibitor of lipolysis. In some respects it behaves like a competitive inhibitor of hormones that increase lipolysis.[267] The hormones activate the enzyme system, adenyl

cyclase, which catalyzes the formation of cyclic AMP from ATP. The antilipolytic action of PGE_1 probably results from the inhibition of adenyl cyclase.[268] Usually less lipolysis takes place in adipose tissue of PUFA-fed rats than in the adipose tissue of rats fed saturated fats, which is probably due to the conversion of PUFA to PG.[269]

Even low concentrations of PG inhibit stimulated lipolysis efficiently. In adipose tissue of EFA-deficient animals, however, there is a decreased release of PGE_2 resulting in an increase in lipolysis and also a pronounced inhibition of stimulated lipolysis by administered PGE_2.[270]

It has been established that PGE_1 prevents the development of, as well as aids in the disappearance of, aggregates of platelets.[271] This fact, together with the known effects of prostaglandins on blood pressure and vasodilation, may indicate a possible therapeutic use in cardiovascular disease.

BIBLIOGRAPHY

1. Melnick and Luckman: U.S. Patent 2 955 039, 1960.
2. Verzár and McDougall: *Absorption from the Intestine*, London, Longmans, Green & Co., 1936.
3. Frazer: Physiol. Rev., *26*, 103, 1946.
4. Borgström: Absorption of triglycerides, In *Lipid Transport* (Meng, ed.), Springfield, Charles C Thomas, p. 15, 1964.
5. Clark, Brouse and Holt: Gastroenterology, *56*, 214, 1969.
6. Borgström and Hoffmann: Hydrolysis of micellar solutions of long chain monoglycerides by pancreatic lipase. In *Biochemical Problems of Lipids* (Frazer, ed.), Amsterdam, Elsevier, 1963.
7. Desnuelle and Savary: J. Lipid Res., *4*, 369, 1963.
8. Hoffmann and Borgström: Biochim. Biophys. Acta, *70*, 317, 1965.
9. Mattson and Volpenheim: J. Biol. Chem., *237*, 53, 1962.
10. Kayden, Senior and Mattson: J. Clin. Invest., *46*, 1695, 1967.
11. Raghavan and Ganguly: Biochem. J., *113*, 81, 1969.
12. Desneulle, Naudet and Rouzier: Biochim. Biophys. Acta, *2*, 561, 1948.
13. Senior and Isselbacher: Biochem. Biophys. Res. Commun., *6*, 274, 1961.
14. Kiyasu, Bloom and Chaikoff: J. Biol. Chem., *199*, 415, 1952.
15. Weiner and Lack: Amer. J. Physiol., *202*, 155, 1962.

16. Dietschy: J. Lipid Res., *9*, 297, 1968.
17. Simmonds: Amer. J. Clin. Nutr., *22*, 266, 1969.
18. Dawson and Isselbacher: J. Clin. Invest., *39*, 150, 1960.
19. Haessler and Isselbacher: Biochim. Biophys. Acta, *73*, 427, 1963.
20. Isselbacher: Fed. Proc., *26*, 1420, 1967.
21. Kennedy: J. Biol. Chem., *201*, 399, 1953.
22. Bennett and Holt: J. Clin. Invest., *47*, 612, 1968.
23. McKay, Kaunitz, Csavassy and Johnson: Metabolism, *16*, 111, 1967.
24. Artom and Swanson: J. Biol. Chem., *175*, 871, 1948.
25. Blomstrand: Acta Physiol. Scand., *34*, 147, 1955.
26. Stein and Stein: Biochim. Biophys. Acta, *116*, 95, 1966.
27. Frazer: Brit. Med. Bull., *14*, 212, 1958.
28. Schlierf, Falor, Wood, Lee, and Kinsell: Amer. J. Clin. Nutr., *22*, 79, 1969.
29. Keys: In *World Trends in Cardiology: Cardiovascular Epidemiology* (Keys and White, Eds.) vol. 1. New York, Harper & Row, p. 165, 1965.
30. Goodman: Physiol. Rev., *45*, 747, 1965.
31. Swell, Trout, Hopper, Field, and Treadwell: Ann. N.Y. Acad. Sci., *72*, 813, 1959.
32. Dietschy and Wilson: New Eng. J. Med., *282*, 1179, 1970.
33. Feldman and Henderson: Biochim. Biophys. Acta, *193*, 221, 1969.
34. Sylven and Borgström: J. Lipid Res., *10*, 351, 1969.
35. Swell, Flick, Field, and Treadwell: Amer. J. Physiol., *180*, 124, 1955.
36. Siperstein, Chaikoff, and Reinhardt: J. Biol. Chem., *189*, 111, 1952.
37. Blomstrand and Ahrens: J. Biol. Chem., *233*, 327, 1958.
38. Bürger and Winterseel: Z. Physiol. Chem., *181*, 255, 1929.
39. Cheng and Stanley: J. Clin. Invest., *35*, 696, 1956.
40. Ivy, Karvinen, Lin, and Ivy: J. Appl. Physiol., *11*, 1, 1957.
41. Wilson and Lindsey: J. Clin. Invest., *44*, 1805, 1965.
42. Borgström: In *Proc. 1967 Deuel Conference on Lipids* (Cowgill and Kinsell, eds.) p. 63, Washington, D.C., U.S. Gov. Printing Office, 1967.
43. Bloomfield: J. Lab. Clin. Med., *64*, 613, 1964.
44. Aftergood, Deuel, and Alfin-Slater: J. Nutr., *62*, 129, 1957.
45. Alfin-Slater, Wells, Aftergood, Melnick and Deuel: Circ. Res., *2*, 471, 1954.
46. Grundy, Ahrens, and Davignon: J. Lipid Res., *10*, 304, 1969.
47. Ivy, Lin, and Karvinen: Amer. J. Physiol., *183*, 79, 1955.
48. Mattson: Fate of dietary lipids, In *Proc. 1967 Deuel Conference on Lipids*, (Cowgill and Kinsell, eds.) p. 1, Washington, D.C., U.S. Gov. Printing Office, 1967.

49. Carter and Frampton: Chem. Rev., *64*, 497, 1964.
50. Calloway and Kurtz: Food Res., *21*, 621, 1956.
51. Steenbock, Irwin, and Weber: J. Nutr., *12*, 103, 1936.
52. Hamilton, Webb, and Dawson: Biochim. Biophys. Acta, *176*, 27, 1969.
53. Sobel, Besman, and Kramer: Amer. J. Dis. Child., *77*, 576, 1949.
54. Tidwell, Holt, Farrow, and Neale: J. Pediat., *6*, 481, 1935.
55. Becker, Meyer, and Necheles: Gastroenterology, *14*, 80, 1950.
56. Augur, Rollman, and Deuel: J. Nutr., *33*, 177, 1947.
57. Jones, Culver, Drummey, and Ryan: Ann. Int. Med., *29*, 1, 1948.
58. Wollaeger, Comfort, Weir, and Osterberg: Gastroenterology, *6*, 93, 1946.
59. Deuel and Hallman: J. Nutr., *20*, 227, 1940.
60. Deuel, Hallman, and Reifman: J. Nutr., *21*, 373, 1941.
61. Tomarelli, Meyer, Waeber and Bernhart: J. Nutr., *95*, 583, 1968.
62. Filer, Mattson, and Fomon: J. Nutr., *99*, 293, 1969.
63. Alfin-Slater, Auerbach and Aftergood: J. Amer. Oil Chem. Soc., *36*, 638, 1959.
64. Nolen, Alexander and Artman: J. Nutr., *93*, 337, 1967.
65. Alfin-Slater, Morris, Aftergood and Melnick: J. Amer. Oil Chem. Soc., *46*, 657, 1969.
66. Lassen, Bacon, and Dunn: Arch. Biochem., *23*, 1, 1949.
67. Harkins, Hagerman, and Sarett: J. Nutr., *87*, 85, 1965.
68. Nicolaysen, Eeg-Larsen, and Malm: Physiol. Rev., *33*, 424, 1953.
69. Werner, and Lutwak: Fed. Proc., *22*, 553, 1963.
70. Cheng, Morehouse, and Deuel: J. Nutr., *37*, 237, 1949.
71. Young and Garrett: J. Nutr., *81*, 321, 1963.
72. Steggerda and Mitchell: J. Nutr., *45*, 201, 1951.
73. Fleischman, Yacowitz, Hayton, and Bierenbaum: J. Nutr., *88*, 255, 1966.
74. Williams, Rose, Morrow, Sloan and Barnes: Amer. J. Clin. Nutr., *23*, 1322, 1970.
75. Gorman, Ritchey, Abernathy, and Korslund: J. Amer. Diet. Ass., *57*, 513, 1970.
76. Fernandez, van de Kamer, and Weijers: J. Clin. Invest., *41*, 488, 1962.
77. Holt and Clark: Amer. J. Clin. Nutr., *22*, 279, 1969.
78. Brice, Owen, and Tyor: Gastroenterology, *48*, 584, 1965.
79. Isselbacher, and Budz: Nature, *200*, 364, 1963.
80. Sabesin and Isselbacher: Science, *147*, 1149, 1965.
81. Hyams, Sabesin, Greenberger, and Isselbacher: Biochim. Biophys. Acta, *125*, 166, 1966.
82. Levy, Fredrickson, and Laster: J. Clin. Invest., *45*, 531, 1966.
83. Holt, Hashim, and Van Itallie: Amer. J. Gastroenterol., *43*, 549, 1965.

84. Laurell: Acta Physiol. Scand., *30*, 289, 1953.
85. Bragdon, Havel, and Boyle: J. Lab. Clin. Med., *48*, 36, 1956.
86. Zilversmit: Fed. Proc., *26*, 1599, 1967.
87. Bragdon: Arch. Biochem. Biophys., *75*, 528, 1956.
88. Rodbell, Fredrickson, and Ono: J. Biol. Chem., *234*, 567, 1959.
89. Dole and Hamlin: Physiol. Rev., *42*, 674, 1962.
90. Nestel, Havel, and Bezman: J. Clin. Invest., *41*, 1915, 1962.
91. Kayden, Karmen, and Dumont: J. Clin. Invest., *42*, 1373, 1963.
92. Sylven: Acta Physiol. Scand., *79*, 516, 1970.
93. Levy: Rev. Canad. Biol., *17*, 1, 1958.
94. Redgrave: J. Clin. Invest., *49*, 465, 1970.
95. Engelberg: Acta Med. Scand., *151*, 161, 1955.
96. Engelberg: Amer. J. Clin. Nutr., *8*, 21, 1960.
97. Felts and Mayes: Nature, *214*, 620, 1967.
98. Fielding: Biochim. Biophys. Acta, *218*, 221, 1970.
99. Nestel, Carroll, and Havenstein: Metabolism, *9*, 1, 1970.
100. Fredrickson, Levy, and Lees: New Eng. J. Med., *276*, 34, 1967.
101. Schumaker and Adams: Ann. Rev. Biochem., *38*, 113, 1969.
102. Walton: J. Atheroscler. Res., *7*, 533, 1967.
103. Nichols: Proc. Nat. Acad. Sci., *64*, 1128, 1969.
104. Gofman and Tandy: In *Atherosclerotic Vascular Disease* (Brest and Moyer, Eds.), New York, Appleton-Century-Crofts. p. 162, 1967.
105. Windmueller and Spaeth: Arch. Biochem. Biophys., *122*, 362, 1967.
106. Fredrickson: Proc. Nat. Acad. Sci., *64*, 1138, 1969.
107. Farquhar: Biochim. Biophys. Acta, *60*, 80, 1962.
108. Farquhar and Ahrens: J. Clin. Invest., *42*, 675, 1963.
109. Sperry: J. Biol. Chem., *111*, 467, 1935.
110. Boyd: J. Biol. Chem., *101*, 323, 1933.
111. Green and Tzagoloff: J. Lipid Res., *7*, 587, 1966.
112. Tzagoloff and MacLennan: Biochim. Biophys. Acta, *99*, 476, 1965.
113. Sekuzu, Jurtshuk, and Green: J. Biol. Chem., *238*, 975, 1963.
114. Korn: Science, *153*, 1491, 1966.
115. Stein and Shapiro: J. Lipid Res., *1*, 326, 1960.
116. Lynen: Harvey Lect., *48*, 210, 1952.
117. Krebs and Lowenstein: In *Metabolic Pathways. I* (Greenberg, ed.), New York, Academic Press, p. 192, 1960.
118. Wakil: Fatty acid metabolism, In *Lipid Metabolism* (Wakil, S. J., Ed.), New York, Academic Press, p. 1, 1970.
119. Stoffel: The chemistry of mammalian lipids, In *Lipids and Lipidoses* (Schettler, Ed.), New York, Springer-Verlag, p. 1, 1967.
120. Stoffel and Schiefer: Z. Physiol. Chem., *341*, 84, 1965.
121. Mead and Levis: Biochem. Biophys. Res. Commun., *9*, 231, 1962.
122. Fulco and Mead: J. Biol. Chem., *236*, 2416, 1961.
123. Fulco: J. Biol. Chem., *242*, 3608, 1967.
124. Fritz: Acta Physiol. Scand., *34*, 367, 1955.
125. Fritz: Amer. J. Physiol., *197*, 297, 1959.
126. Fritz and Yue: J. Lipid Res., *4*, 279, 1963.
127. Wakil: Biochim. Biophys. Acta, *34*, 227, 1959.
128. Lynen: In *Organizational Biosynthesis* (Vogel, Ed.), New York, Academic Press, p. 243, 1967.
129. Wakil, Pugh, and Sauer: Proc. Nat. Acad. Sci., *52*, 106, 1964.
130. Wakil and Gibson: Biochim. Biophys. Acta, *41*, 122, 1960.
131. Lynen: Fed. Proc., *20*, 941, 1961.
132. Cahill, Jeanrenaud, Leboeuf, and Renold: Ann. N.Y. Acad. Sci., *82*, 403, 1959.
133. Wakil: J. Lipid Res., *2*, 1, 1961.
134. Mohrhauer, Christiansen, Gan, Deubig and Holman: J. Biol. Chem., *242*, 4507, 1967.
135. Holloway, Peluffo and Wakil: Biochem. Biophys. Res. Commun., *12*, 300, 1963.
136. Shapiro: Biochemistry of triglycerides, In *Lipids and Lipidoses*, (Schettler, Ed.), New York, Springer-Verlag, p. 40, 1967.
137. Stetten and Salcedo: J. Biol. Chem., *156*, 27, 1944.
138. Day and Levy: Biochem. Med., *3*, 177, 1969.
139. Olivecrona: Acta Physiol. Scand., *54*, 287, 1962.
140. Aiyar, Fatterpaker, and Sreenivasan: Biochem. J., *90*, 558, 1964.
141. Robinson and Seakins: Biochim. Biophys. Acta, *62*, 163, 1962.
142. Creasey, Hankins, and Handschumaker: J. Biol. Chem., *236*, 2064, 1961.
143. Lieber and Rubin: Amer. J. Med., *44*, 200, 1968.
144. Lieber and DeCarli: Amer. J. Clin. Nutr., *23*, 474, 1970.
145. Alfin-Slater, Aftergood, Wells, and Deuel: Arch. Biochem. Biophys., *52*, 180, 1954.
146. Bezman, Felts, and Havel: J. Lipid Res., *3*, 427, 1963.
147. Ball: Ann. N.Y. Acad. Sci., *131*, 225, 1965.
148. Bragdon and Gordon: J. Clin. Invest., *37*, 574, 1958.
149. Carlson and Ekeland: J. Clin. Invest., *42*, 714, 1963.
150. Patten: J. Biol. Chem., *245*, 5577, 1970.
151. Shiff, Stern and Leduc: Pediatrics, *37*, 577, 1966.
152. Baker: Amer. J. Clin. Nutr., *22*, 829, 1969.
153. Birkbeck: Acta Pediat. Scand., *59*, 505, 1970.
154. Heffernan: Amer. J. Clin. Nutr., *15*, 5, 1964.
155. Insull, Lang, Hsi and Yoshimura: J. Clin. Invest., *48*, 1313, 1969.
156. Hirsch and Han: J. Lipid Res., *10*, 77, 1969.
157. Knittle and Hirsch: J. Clin. Invest., *47*, 2091, 1968.
158. Newburgh: Physiol. Rev., *24*, 18, 1944.
159. Rabinovitz: Ann. Rev. Med., *21*, 241, 1970.
160. Hirsch, Farquhar, Ahrens, Peterson, and Stoffel: Amer. J. Clin. Nutr., *8*, 499, 1960.

161. Dayton, Hashimoto, Dixon, and Pearce: J. Lipid Res., 7, 103, 1966.
162. Williams and Platner: Amer. J. Physiol., 212, 167, 1967.
163. Baldwin: Fed. Proc., 29, 1277, 1970.
164. Fredrickson and Gordon: Physiol. Rev., 38, 585, 1958.
165. Sdrobici, Bonaparte, Pieptea, and Sapatino: Nutr. Dieta, 9, 271, 1967.
166. Oshima and Carpenter: Biochim. Biophys. Acta, 152, 479, 1968.
167. Bieri and Prival: Comp. Biochem. Physiol., 15, 275, 1965.
168. Turchetto, Martinelli and Weiss: Life Sci., 8, 271, 1969.
169. Holman and Hofstetter: J. Amer. Oil. Chem. Soc., 42, 540, 1965.
170. Aftergood, Hernandez, and Alfin-Slater: J. Lipid Res., 9, 447, 1968.
171. Herbst: Endocrinology, 81, 54, 1967.
172. Clark and Zarrow: Acta Endocrinol., 56, 445, 1967.
173. Behrman and Armstrong: Endocrinology, 85, 474, 1969.
174. Behrman, Armstrong, and Greep: Canad. J. Biochem., 48, 881, 1970.
175. Aftergood and Alfin-Slater: Effect of an oral contraceptive steroid mixture on some aspects of lipid metabolism in the rat. In *Metabolic Effects of Gonadal Hormones and Contraceptive Steroids*, (Salhanick, Ed.), New York, Plenum Press, p. 265, 1969.
176. Arai and Rennels: Tex. Rep. Biol. Med., 25, 509, 1967.
177. Moses, Davis, Rosenthal, and Garren: Science, 163, 1203, 1969.
178. Adams and Baxter: Arch. Pathol., 48, 13, 1949.
179. Riley: Biochem. J., 87, 500, 1963.
180. Aftergood and Alfin-Slater: J. Lipid Res., 12, 306, 1971.
181. Krum, Morris, and Bennett: Endocrinology, 74, 543, 1967.
182. Gidez and Feller: J. Lipid Res., 10, 656, 1969.
183. Brot, Lossow, and Chaikoff: J. Lipid Res., 5, 63, 1964.
184. Borkowski, Levin, Delcroix, and Klastersky: J. Appl. Physiol., 28, 42, 1970.
185. Takayasu, Okuda, and Yoshikawa: Lipids, 5, 743, 1970.
186. Egwin and Sgoutas: J. Nutr., 101, 315, 1971.
187. Galli, White, and Paoletti: J. Neurochem., 17, 347, 1970.
188. Aeberhard, Grippo, and Menkes: Pediat. Res., 3, 590, 1969.
189. Geison and Weisman: J. Nutr., 100, 315, 1970.
190. Winick: J. Pediat., 74, 667, 1969.
191. Smith, Hasinoff and Fumagalli: Lipids, 5, 665, 1969.
192. Rathbone: Biochem. J., 97, 620, 1965.
193. Dhopeshwarkar and Mead: Biochim. Biophys. Acta, 187, 461, 1969.
194. Dhopeshwarkar and Mead: Biochim. Biophys. Acta, 210, 250, 1970.
195. Dhopeshwarkar, Maier and Mead: Biochim. Biophys. Acta, 187, 6, 1969.
196. Turchetto and Barri: Nutr. Dieta, 11, 34, 1968.
197. Alling and Svennerholm: J. Neurochem., 16, 751, 1969.
198. Banik and Davison: J. Neurochem., 14, 594, 1967.
199. Nestel: Adv. Lipid Res., 8, 1, 1970.
200. Grundy and Ahrens: J. Lipid Res., 10, 91, 1969.
201. Miettinen: Ann. Clin. Res., 2, 300, 1970.
202. Cornforth, Gore and Popják: Biochim. J., 65, 94, 1957.
203. Cornforth and Popják: Biochim. J., 58, 403, 1954.
204. Gould and Popják: Biochim. J., 66, 51p, 1957.
205. Gould and Swyryd: J. Lipid Res., 7, 698, 1966.
206. Friedman and Byers: J. Clin. Invest., 34, 1369, 1955.
207. Gidez, Roheim, and Eder: J. Lipid Res., 8, 7, 1967.
208. Morin, Bernick, Mead, and Alfin-Slater: J. Lipid Res., 3, 432, 1962.
209. Nestel, and Couzens: J. Lipid Res., 7, 487, 1966.
210. Nestel, Couzens, and Hirsch: J. Lab. Clin. Med., 66, 582, 1965.
211. Glomset: J. Lipid Res., 9, 155, 1968.
212. Glomset, Janssen, Kennedy, and Dobbins: J. Lipid Res., 7, 69, 1966.
213. Nichols and Smith: J. Lipid Res., 6, 206, 1965.
214. Swell and Law: Proc. Soc. Exp. Biol. Med., 129, 363, 1968.
215. Wells: Fed. Proc., 28, 447, 1969.
216. Glomset: Biochim. Biophys. Acta, 65, 128, 1962.
217. Gjone and Norum: Acta Med. Scand., 183, 107, 1968.
218. Kinsell, Partridge, Boling, Margen and Michaels: J. Clin. Endocrinol., 12, 909, 1952.
219. Connor, Witiak, Stone, and Armstrong: J. Clin. Invest., 48, 1363, 1969.
220. Wood, Shioda and Kinsell: Lancet, 2, 604, 1966.
221. Hellström and Lindstedt: Amer. J. Clin. Nutr., 18, 46, 1966.
222. Avigan and Steinberg: J. Clin. Invest., 44, 1845, 1965.
223. Harold, Felts, and Chaikoff: Amer. J. Physiol., 183, 459, 1955.
224. Holloway: Steroid metabolism. In *Lipid Metabolism* (Wakil, ed.), New York, Academic Press, p. 371, 1970.
225. Kritchevsky: Biochemistry of steroids. In *Lipids and Lipidoses*, (Schettler, ed.), New York, Springer-Verlag, p. 66, 1967.
226. Whitehouse and Staple: Proc. Soc. Exp. Biol. Med., 101, 439, 1959.
227. Roberts, Bandi, Calvin, Drucker, and Lieberman: J. Amer. Chem. Soc., 86, 958, 1964.
228. Constantopoulos and Tchen: J. Biol. Chem., 236, 65, 1961.
229. Alfin-Slater and Aftergood: Physiol. Rev., 48, 758, 1968.

230. Guarnieri and Johnson: Adv. Lipid Res., *8*, 115, 1970.
231. Holman: Prog. Chem. Fats, *9*, 275, 1968.
232. Holman: J. Nutr., *70*, 405, 1960.
233. Hansen, Wiese, Boelsche, Haggard, Adam, and Davis: Pediatrics, *31*, 171, 1963.
234. Takasugi and Imai: J. Biochem., *60*, 191, 1966.
235. Aftergood and Alfin-Slater: J. Lipid Res., *8*, 126, 1967.
236. Fukazawa, Privett, and Takahashi: Lipids, *6*, 388, 1971.
237. Rahm and Holman: J. Nutr. *84*, 149, 1964.
238. Holman and Mohrhauer: Acta Chem. Scand., *17*, S84, 1963.
239. Dhopeshwarkar and Mead: J. Amer. Oil Chem. Soc., *38*, 297, 1961.
240. Nervi and Brenner: Acta Physiol. Latinoamer., *15*, 308, 1965.
241. Alfin-Slater, Morris, Hansen, and Proctor: J. Nutr., *87*, 168, 1965.
242. Pudelkiewicz, Seufert, and Holman: J. Nutr., *94*, 138, 1968.
243. Aftergood and Alfin-Slater: J. Lipid Res., *6*, 287, 1965.
244. Sewell and McDowell: J. Nutr., *89*, 64, 1966.
245. Reid, Bieri, Plock and Andrews: J. Nutr., *82*, 401, 1964.
246. Sinclair: EFA. In *Lipid Pharmacology* (Paoletti, ed.), New York, Academic Press, p. 237, 1964.
247. Decker and Mertz: J. Nutr., *91*, 324, 1967.
248. Smithson: Anat. Rec., *157*, 324, 1967.
249. Kunkel and Williams: J. Biol. Chem., *189*, 755, 1951.
250. Klein and Johnson: J. Biol. Chem., *211*, 103, 1954.
251. Collins and Sinclair: Australian Bioch. Soc. Proc., *2*, 19, 1969.
252. Barki, Nath, Hart, and Elvehjem: Proc. Soc. Exp. Biol. Med., *66*, 474, 1947.
253. Nørby: Brit. J. Nutr., *19*, 209, 1965.
254. Kupiecki and Weeks: Fed. Proc., *25*, 719, 1966.
255. Goldblatt: J. Physiol., *84*, 208, 1935.
256. von Euler: Arch. Exp. Pathol. Pharmakol., *175*, 78, 1934.
257. Bergström and Sjövall: Acta Chem. Scand., *14*, 1701, 1960.
258. Bergström, Ryhage, Samuelsson, and Sjövall: J. Biol. Chem., *238*, 3555, 1963.
259. Horton: Physiol. Rev., *49*, 133, 1969.
260. Van Dorp, Beerthuis, Nugteren, and Vonkeman: Biochim. Biophys. Acta, *90*, 204, 1964.
261. Bergström, Danielsson, and Samuelsson: Biochim. Biophys. Acta, *90*, 207, 1964.
262. Pace-Asciak and Wolfe: Biochim. Biophys. Acta, *152*, 784, 1968.
263. Van Dorp, Beerthuis, Nugteren, and Vonkeman: Nature, *203*, 839, 1964.
264. Patel: Ann. Intern, Med., *73*, 483, 1970.
265. Kaufman, Freeman, and Mishell: Contraception, *3*, 121, 1971.
266. Weeks: Circ. Res., *24*, Suppl. 1, 1–123, 1969.
267. Stock and Westermann: Life Sci., *5*, 1667, 1966.
268. Bergström and Samuelsson: Endeavour, *27*, 109, 1968.
269. Pawar and Tidwell: Biochim. Biophys. Acta, *164*, 167, 1968.
270. Christ and Nugteren: Biochim. Biophys. Acta, *218*, 296, 1970.
271. Thomasson: Nutr. Dieta, *11*, 228, 1969.

Chapter

5

The Vitamins

Section A   Vitamin A and Carotene[*]

OSWALD A. ROELS

AND

NAN S. T. LUI

HISTORY

Man's earliest knowledge of vitamin A resulted from disease symptoms caused by its absence. One of the first symptoms of vitamin A deficiency is night blindness. Its nutritional cure has been known for thousands of years. Eber's Papyrus, an ancient Egyptian medical treatise of about 1500 B.C., recommends eating roast ox-liver, or the liver of black cocks, to cure it. The famous Greek philosopher, Hippocrates, prescribed raw ox-liver for the cure of night blindness. One of us found in 1955 that medicine-men in Ruanda-Urundi (Central Africa) prescribed chicken liver to cure night-blindness.

In the early part of the 20th century, McCollum and his colleagues at the University of Wisconsin, and Osborne and Mendel at Yale University were interested in the mysterious ingredients present in natural foods, which were essential to supplement diets of purified proteins, carbohydrates, fats and minerals to support life and growth. In 1915, McCollum and Davis[1] described "fat-soluble A", a growth-promoting factor isolated from animal fats and fish oils. Animals fed a diet consisting mainly of polished rice, casein and minerals did not develop normally unless this factor was added. Drum-

* Lamont-Doherty Geological Observatory Contribution No. 1824

mond[2] suggested later that the "fat-soluble factor A" should be named vitamin A. Vitamin A deficiency was also shown to be responsible for xerophthalmia[3] and certain forms of night blindness.[4] In the meantime, vitamin A activity had also been found in plant material. Steenbock et al.[5,6] found that vitamin A activity was associated with the yellow carotenes present in plants.

In a now classical paper, Bloch[7] demonstrated clearly that the widespread occurrence of xerophthalmia among children in Denmark could be prevented by feeding them butterfat or cod-liver oil. He also proved that the disease could not be attributed to the absence of fat, as such, because children receiving margarine or pork-fat suffered severely from xerophthalmia. He had earlier stressed the inhibition of growth and the increased susceptibility to infection in children suffering from xerophthalmia and its accompanying night blindness. Bloch terminated the paper which he read before the World Dairy Congress, Washington, D.C., October 3, 1923, with the following statement:

What I have said here and proved to you, testifies to the enormous importance of milk as food for the child. No other article can replace milk. Absence of milk from the diet or the inclusion of unfavorably modified milk is the origin of most serious diseases. By ordering milk, and especially cream and butter, not only is this terrible eye disease cured—which I believe will be discovered in every country when it is looked for—but these dairy products are of the greatest importance for growth and development and for the cure of our greatest infectious diseases.

Moore[8] demonstrated that the carotenes were structurally related to vitamin A and were converted *in vivo* to the vitamin. Thus, the provitamin status of β-carotene and certain other carotenoids was established.

The structural formulae of vitamin A and β-carotene were first proposed by Karrer *et al.*, in 1930–1931.[9,10] Isler and his colleagues synthesized the first pure vitamin A in 1947.[11] Three years later, Karrer *et al.*[12] and Inhoffen *et al.*[13] reported the synthesis of β-carotene. Both retinol and β-carotene

are now synthesized by the ton in the pharmaceutical industry.

STRUCTURE OF COMPOUNDS WITH VITAMIN A ACTIVITY

The term "vitamin A" is now used to designate several biologically-active compounds.

Retinol, 3-dehydro-retinol and their Esters. Retinol (vitamin A₁) and 3-dehydro-retinol (vitamin A₂) are alcohols with the structures[9,10] shown in Figure 5A–1.

Vitamin A exists naturally in several isomeric forms. This is a *cis-trans* isomerism resulting from configurational differences at the double bonds in the side chain, illustrated in Figure 5A–2.

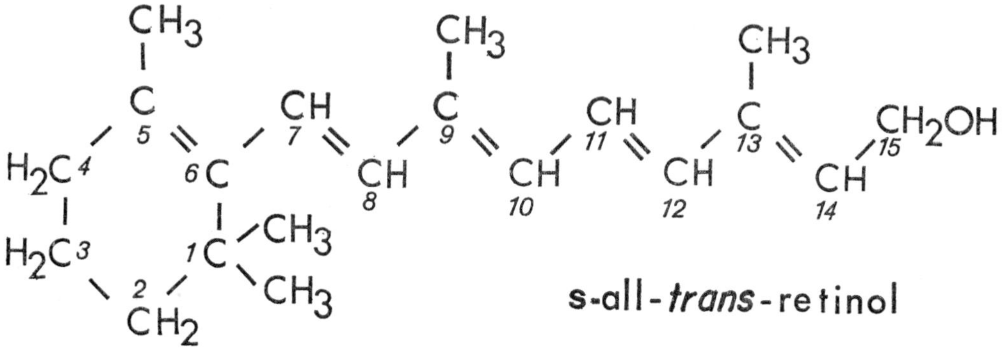

s-all-*trans*-retinol

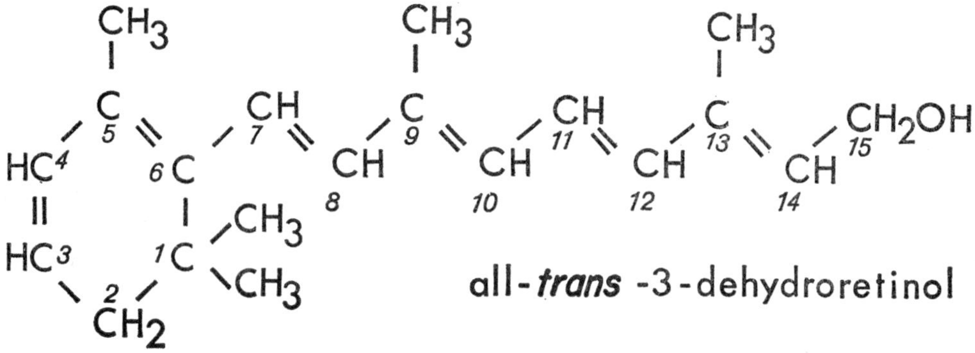

all-*trans*-3-dehydroretinol

Fig. 5A-1

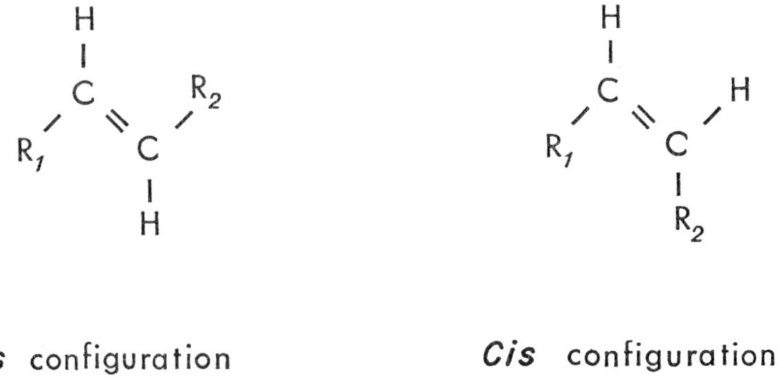

Trans configuration   Cis configuration

Fig. 5A-2. *Cis-trans* isomerism.

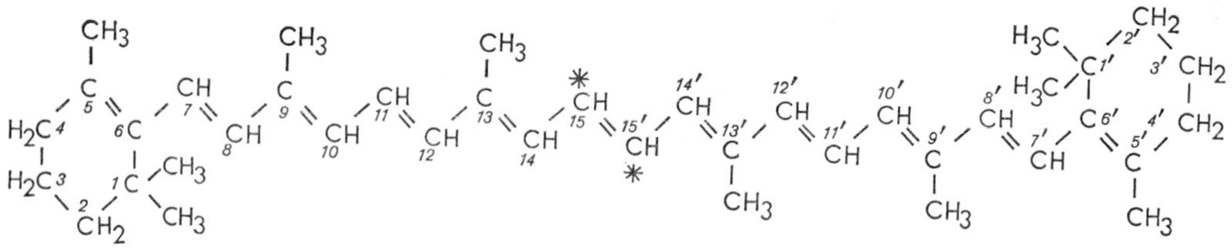

Fig. 5A-3. *β*-carotene.

The major naturally-occurring form of vitamin A is the all-*trans* isomer. Neo-vitamin A (13-*cis*) has about 85 per cent of the potency of the all-*trans* form, and the 11-*cis* isomer (neo-b) has 75 per cent of the biological activity of the all-*trans* isomer.[14] 3-Dehydroretinol has only about half the biological activity of retinol[15] and also exists in various isomeric forms. Vitamin A esters

$$(R-CH_2O-\overset{\overset{\textstyle O}{\|}}{C}-R',$$

where R' is the hydrocarbon chain of the esterifying fatty acid) appear to be the storage form of vitamin A in animal tissues. Reti[16] found that vitamin A was present mainly in the ester form in the liver of various fish, birds and mammals. In mammals, the stored retinyl ester is hydrolyzed by a liver enzyme; free retinol then travels via the blood stream to the tissue where a metabolic requirement exists.[17]

Retinal and Retinoic Acid. Retinal (RCHO) is the aldehyde corresponding to retinol. It is the active form of vitamin A in vision[18] and also fulfills certain other functions of vitamin A.[19] Retinoic acid (RCOOH) is the acid corresponding to retinol. It can

support growth of vitamin A-deficient animals, but cannot prevent blindness.[20] Retinal and retinoic acid also exist in *cis-trans* isomeric forms. The structural formulae of retinal and retinoic acid differ only from that of retinol, shown in Figure 5A–1, by having another functional group on carbon atom 15.

Carotenoids With Provitamin A Activity. Among the commonly occurring carotenoids, such as *α*-carotene, *β*-carotene, *γ*-carotene and lycopene, *β*-carotene is the most important provitamin A. *β*-carotene is a symmetrical molecule containing two *β*-ionone rings connected by a conjugated chain. It has the structure shown in Figure 5A–3.

In *α*-carotene and *γ*-carotene, one of the *β*-ionone rings is replaced by the structures shown in Figure 5A–4.

The remainder of the molecules are identical.[21,22] The biopotency of *α*- and *γ*-carotene is about half that of *β*-carotene.[23,24] The biological activity of these carotenoids with provitamin A activity results from their conversion to vitamin A by the organism.[8] The mechanism of this reaction is oxygenation at carbon atoms 15 and 15' (marked * in figure

5A–3) and subsequent splitting of the molecule at that point.[25]

GENERAL CHEMICAL PROPERTIES OF VITAMIN A AND THE PROVITAMINS A

Vitamin A. Retinol melts at 63 to 64°C and has an absorption maximum in ethanol at 324 to 325 nm with an $E_{1cm}^{1\%} = 1832$.[26] The vitamin is soluble in fats and in all the usual organic solvents. It is insoluble in water, but may be dispersed in the aqueous phase by emulsification or by attachment to proteins.[26,27] Retinol and its esters have a yellowish-green fluorescence. The fluorescence of retinyl esters in alcoholic solution increases rapidly followed by destruction.[28] In the absence of antioxidants, vitamin A is very unstable in oxygen: the oxidation products are ill-defined.[29]

Oxidation. Potassium permanganate oxidation of retinol yields retinal.[30] This has led to the use of manganese dioxide as an oxidant to convert allylic alcohols into the corresponding aldehydes.[31] A petroleum ether solution of retinol, left in the dark at room temperature in the presence of manganese dioxide, yields retinal.

Reduction. Lithium aluminum hydride reduces vitamin A aldehydes, acids and acid esters to the corresponding retinol homolog.[32] Sodium or potassium borohydride has the same effect.[33]

Isomerization. Retinal is isomerized by exposure to light. Each isomer gives a steady-state mixture of all possible isomers with the all-*trans* retinal always dominant.[33,34] Thermal isomerization of aqueous solutions also occurs.[33,34]

Instability Towards Acids. Vitamin A is extremely sensitive towards acids; they can cause rearrangement of the double bonds and dehydration.[35,36]

Color Reactions. Acidic reagents give transient blue color reactions with vitamin A. These tests are useful for qualitative or comparative measurements. The purple color obtained with sulfuric acid was one of the first methods used to identify vitamin A in liver oils.[27] Later, arsenic trichloride and the Carr-Price reagent (antimony trichloride in chloroform) were used.[37] More recently, other Lewis acids such as trifluoroacetic acid have been used for the quantitative determination of the vitamin.[38]

Provitamins A. β-Carotene melts at 181 to 182°C. In petroleum ether, all-*trans* β-carotene has absorption maxima at 453, 481 and 273 nm.[39] Pure synthetic, crystalline all-*trans* β-carotene, after drying in a high-vacuum drying pistol, should give an $E_{1cm}^{1\%}$ value of 2,518 at 451 nm in *n*-hexane. It should have absorption maxima in the same solvent at 451 nm and 479 nm and an absorption minimum at 468 nm.[40] β-Carotene is readily soluble in carbon disulfide,

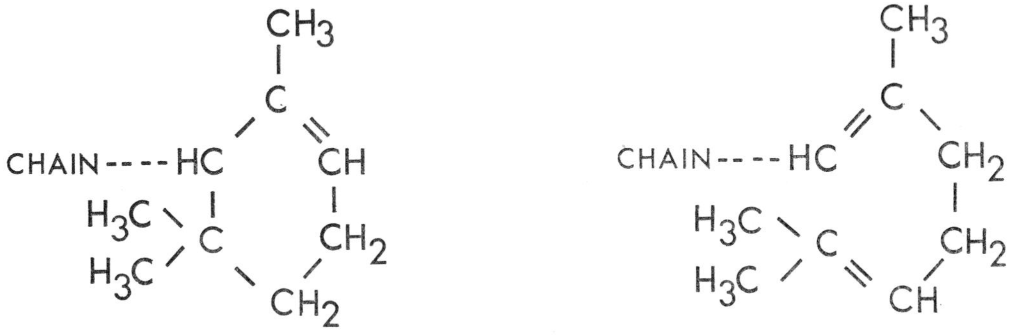

α-carotene

γ-carotene

Fig. 5A-4.

chloroform and benzene. It is almost insoluble in ethanol and methanol. The carotenes take up oxygen rapidly when exposed to air, giving colorless products. This destruction by oxygen is accelerated by light.[41] Like most other carotenoids, carotene produces colors with various reagents, including sulfuric acid and nitric acid.[42] With antimony trichloride, carotene yields a blue color as does vitamin A. The reaction is less rapid, however, and two absorption maxima occur at 490 nm[42] and 1020 nm,[43] against 620 nm for vitamin A. *Cis-trans* isomerism occurs in carotenoids.[44] It may be induced by refluxing the pigment in a solvent, by illumination, by treatment with acids or iodine, or by melting the crystals.[44]

THE DETERMINATION OF VITAMIN A AND ITS PROVITAMINS

Vitamin A and its related compounds can be measured by biological, physical and chemical methods.

Physical Methods. The principal physical assays of vitamin A are based on the characteristic light absorption of vitamin A and of the provitamin A compounds. Retinol and its related compounds show maximum absorption in the near-ultraviolet.[26] The provitamins show maximum absorption near 460 nm.[39,44] The extinction coefficients of various vitamin A and provitamin A compounds have been carefully determined by different laboratories. Thus, by measuring the extinction at the absorption maximum, the quantity of vitamin A or provitamin A compound in a solution can be calculated. Irrelevant absorption, caused by contaminants, often results in high extinction values for vitamin A at its maximum absorption. To obviate this, Morton and Stubbs[45] introduced a correction procedure which assumes that the absorption curve of the substances responsible for the irrelevant absorption is approximately linear at wavelengths near and on either side of the absorption maximum of vitamin A. Cama *et al.*[46] have investigated this for retinol and retinyl acetate and arrived at different 'fixative points' in different solvents and have given the correction formula in each case. According to these authors,

the fixative points for retinol in cyclohexane are E_1 (312.5 nm), E_2 (326.5 nm) and E_3 (336.7 nm). The suggested correction formula is

$$E(\text{corr.}) = 7(E_2 - 0.442\ E_1 - 0.578\ E_3).$$

Recently, the Vitamin Division of the International Union of Pure and Applied Chemistry[47] has suggested that oil samples should be purified by chromatography if the irrelevant absorption maximum of the unsaponifiable fraction in isopropanol is outside the region 323 to 327 nm, or when E300nm/E325nm is greater than 0.73.

The fluorescence of vitamin A has been most successfully exploited by Popper and his associates for the detection of the vitamin in tissue sections and to study the distribution of the vitamin in the animal body.[48] Fujita and Aoyama[49] described a quantitative fluorimetric assay of total vitamin A (retinyl ester plus retinol) in the unsaponifiable matter of various oils; however, carotene and vitamin D interfered with the assay under the experimental conditions described.

Dunagin and Olson[50] have recently succeeded in quantitatively separating retinol and some of its derivatives by gas/liquid chromatography.

Other methods such as infrared spectrophotometry[51] and nuclear magnetic resonance[52] and mass spectroscopy[53] have been used for the identification of stereoisomers of retinol.

Chemical Methods. A number of colorimetric assays are based on color reactions produced by retinol and related compounds with a variety of reagents. Several Lewis acids (trifluoroacetic acid, perchloric acid, stannic chloride, boron trifluoride, antimony trichloride) and glycerol dichlorohydrin produce colored products with vitamin A.[54] These color reactions have been used for the quantitative and qualitative determination of vitamin A. The Carr-Price test[37,55] is one of the most widely used color reactions for vitamin A determination. In the test, vitamin A reacts with antimony trichloride in chloroform, giving rise to a blue color with its absorption maximum at 620 nm, $E_{1cm}^{1\%} = 4800$.

More recently, Neeld and Pearson[38] have introduced a far superior new colorimetric procedure for the assay of vitamin A, based on the blue color produced by trifluoroacetic acid with vitamin A. This procedure can also be used to determine retinyl esters, retinal and retinoic acid.[54] The concentration of these forms of vitamin A can be determined by comparing the molar absorptivities to that of vitamin A at the appropriate wavelengths. The major advantage of the trifluoroacetic acid method is that the color is more stable and less susceptible to interference by traces of moisture than the Carr-Price method.

Bioassay Procedures. The various forms of vitamin A and provitamin A have a number of common physiological effects in the animal body. But the various vitamin A compounds differ chemically, and there are marked differences in their biological potencies. The definitive assay for vitamin A activity is based upon its biological activity. The three bioassays generally used will be discussed below and are described in great detail by Bliss and Roels in *The Vitamins*, Vol. VI (György and Pearson, Eds.), 2nd ed., New York, Academic Press, pp. 197–210, 1967.

The Growth Assay. Young rats are depleted of vitamin A stores until they no longer grow on the vitamin A-free test diet. Different individuals are then fed graded doses of vitamin A or of the compound in which vitamin A is to be determined under standardized conditions, and the gain in weight during the test period is related to the logarithm of the dose. Generally males are used since there is a sexual difference in response to the vitamin A deficiency. Because litter-mates grow at more nearly the same rate than rats from different litters, the segregation of litter differences in setting up an assay can increase its precision materially. Coward[56] has used statistical methods to calculate the vitamin A activity of the unknown in International Units. One International Unit of vitamin A corresponds to 0.6 µg of β-carotene and to 0.3 µg of retinol. Most workers agree that, under the conditions most commonly pertaining in biological

testing, these two units have virtually the same activity.

The Vaginal Smear Assay. This method is based on an early symptom of vitamin A deficiency in the female rat, *i.e.*, the interruption of the normal estrous cycle with the persistence of cornified cells in vaginal smears. Administration of vitamin A or of vitamin A-containing compounds leads to quick return of the normal smear. Pugsley and his collaborators[57] have developed a quantitative method from this relationship, which has several advantages over the growth assay in both precision and efficiency. Ovariectomized rats are used to ensure against misinterpreting the response, which is then highly specific for vitamin A. In the range of about 25 to 150 I.U. (the total amount of vitamin A administered over a period of 2 to 3 successive days), the response can be plotted linearly against the log dose of vitamin A.

The Liver Storage Assay. This method, originally devised by Guggenheim and Koch[58] is based on the assimilation and liver storage of vitamin A by the depleted rat. The vitamin A content of the liver is directly proportional to the ingested dose over a range of 500 to 10,000 I.U. (total amount of vitamin A administered over a period of 2 to 3 days).

THE OCCURRENCE OF VITAMIN A IN FOODS

The carotenoid pigments are widely distributed in plant and animal tissues. They are characterized by their typical red, yellow and orange colors. Since many of them have no vitamin A activity, the occurrence of a pigmented carotenoid in food should not necessarily be taken as an indication of its value as a source of provitamin A.

Xanthophyll and lycopene are among the most frequently occurring carotenoid pigments and have no vitamin A activity whatsoever. Thus, chromatographic separation of different carotenoid pigments, identification of each compound with provitamin A activity, and determination of its biological activity are necessary to correctly establish the provitamin A content of foodstuffs.[59]

Fruits contain varying, but generally low, amounts of carotenoids. Cereals and cereal foods in general do not contain carotenoids or preformed vitamin A. The only exception to this is the soybean, which contains traces of carotene. Among the vegetable oils, the richest source of provitamin A is palm oil (the oil extracted from the fruit coat of *Elaeis guineensis*). The provitamin A activity of the red palm oil from ripe fruits varies from 65,000 to 113,000 International Units of provitamin A activity per 100 grams oil.[60]

Preformed vitamin A is found almost exclusively in animals. Human and animal organisms tend to concentrate most of the vitamin A in the liver where it appears to be stored. Other significant pools of the vitamin A are found in the kidney, milk and blood plasma. Milk products and eggs are usually rich sources of vitamin A. In skim-milk and skim-milk products, practically all carotenoids and preformed vitamin A have been removed together with the fat. Among the meats, pork, beef, chicken, lamb, rabbit, turkey and veal contain only traces of vitamin A. Fish liver oils are generally extremely rich sources of the vitamin. The vitamin A content of fish liver oil varies over a wide range. The highest value was found in red Steenbras, which contained up to 1,130,000 International Units of vitamin A per gram oil.[61]

Extensive data on vitamin A activity of raw, processed and prepared foods were published in 1950 and 1966 by Watt and Merrill of the Bureau of Human Nutrition and Home Economics of the United States Department of Agriculture.[62] In these handbooks, vitamin A values, expressed as International Units, are listed for 751 different foodstuffs.

GENERAL METABOLISM OF VITAMIN A AND THE PROVITAMINS A

Absorption. *Carotenoids.* In most mammals, most of the ingested provitamin A is converted to vitamin A in the intestinal wall. There is, however, a great deal of species specificity in the ability of different mammals to absorb dietary carotenoids. Man and the bovine can absorb both vitamin A and the carotenoids, and convert carotenoids with provitamin A activity to the vitamin. In contrast, the rat and the pig do not absorb

significant amounts of carotenoid pigments. However, they can convert provitamin A to the vitamin in the gut.[63] The small intestine is the most important organ involved in the conversion of provitamin to the vitamin, although other tissues are also capable of carrying out this process.[64,65] The carotene cleavage enzyme (β-carotene 15,15'-oxygenase) has been demonstrated in rat intestine, liver and kidney. The reaction catalyzed by the enzyme requires oxygen. The initial and sole product which has been identified is retinal.[66] Two moles of retinal are formed for each mole of β-carotene consumed.[67] A number of factors affect the absorption of the provitamin A from the intestine. The absorption of dietary carotenoids is significantly hampered when the diet is unusually low in fat.[68] The quality of fat also influences the absorption of dietary provitamin A from the intestinal tract. The amount of carotene absorbed from raw carrots is highest when low molecular weight fatty acids are given, and the percentage of absorbed carotenoids falls as the chain length of the fatty acids increases.[69] Conjugated bile acids with one free hydroxyl group have a stimulating effect on carotene absorption and on cleavage of the carotene molecule in the intestines of the chick, the hamster, the rat and the rabbit.[70]

Vitamin A. The major dietary form of vitamin A is all-*trans* retinyl ester. In the upper intestine, the ester is hydrolyzed by pancreatic retinyl ester hydrolase and is absorbed into the intestinal cells in micellar form. Retinol from dietary sources or resulting from the hydrolysis of dietary retinyl ester, passes the mucosal cell wall, and is mainly esterified and incorporated into chylomicrons,[71,72] but a small portion may be oxidized to retinal and further to retinoic acid.[73,74] Other derivatives of retinol are also readily absorbed: retinal is absorbed as such and is mainly reduced and converted to retinyl ester within the mucosa,[75] although a portion is converted to retinoic acid.[74] Retinoic acid, when administered as a sodium salt in the diet, is absorbed as such.[76]

Transport. Retinyl esters in chylomicrons formed in the intestinal mucosal cells travel through the lymphatic system, via the thoracic duct, to the blood stream, and are stored in the liver. Stored retinyl ester is hydrolyzed there by a liver enzyme,[77] and free retinol then travels via the blood stream to the tissue where a metabolic requirement exists. Only 10 to 17 per cent of the vitamin A content of the blood in normal human subjects in the fasting state is in the ester form. However, in the post-absorptive state after vitamin A intake, the percentage of the ester in the circulating blood increases rapidly as a result of the vitamin A ester arriving in the blood stream from the gut via the lymphatic system.[78] The blood level of vitamin A is independent of the liver reserves: as long as there are very small reserves of vitamin A present in the liver, the blood level remains normal. As soon as the liver is depleted of its vitamin A reserves, the blood vitamin A level falls rapidly.[79] In human blood, the newly absorbed vitamin A ester occurs mainly in the Sf 10 to 100 lipoprotein fraction of the blood stream. Twenty per cent of the free retinol present in serum is associated with Sf 3 to 9 serum lipoprotein fraction, which also carries about 80 per cent of the β-carotene and lycopene in human serum. The major portion of retinol is transported by the high density plasma protein fraction.[80] Recently, it has been shown that retinol circulates in human plasma bound to a specific transport protein, retinol binding protein (RBP). The purified RBP has a molecular weight of 21,000. There seems to be one binding site for one molecule of retinol per molecule of RBP. In plasma, RBP circulates as a complex together with another larger protein with pre-albumin mobility. On electrophoresis, pre-albumin and RBP complex with each other in 1:1 molar ratio.[81]

Storage. In 1931 Moore did the first quantitative determinations of vitamin A in rat tissues using the Carr-Price reaction.[82] He found that the liver contained large amounts of the vitamin, whereas traces were found in the intraperitoneal fat, kidney and lung. When rats are given very large doses of vitamin A, the vitamin can be found in appreciable amounts in the adrenals, and traces are found in the pancreas, thymus and spleen. This distribution of vitamin A throughout the body is typical for many mammals. In birds and fish, the liver is usually also the most important site of storage. However, certain sea birds have stomach oils which are very rich in vitamin A and some fish have extraordinarily high amounts of vitamin A in the intestinal wall. In some types of shrimp, the eyes contain practically the entire body reserve of the vitamin.[83] Generally speaking, carotenoids are more evenly distributed throughout the body of these animal species which have carotenoids. Frequently, carotenoids are concentrated in depot fat. The ovaries of animals with yellow body fat sometimes contain high quantities of carotenoids concentrated in the *corpora lutea* and in the *corpora rubra*.[84] Vitamin A in cod liver oil is present mainly in the ester form.[85] In rat liver, small amounts of vitamin A alcohol are always present but retinyl palmitate is the dominant storage form.[86] Vitamin A alcohol is stored in the parenchymal cells of the liver; whereas vitamin A ester is stored in the Kupfer cells.[87]

Catabolism. Within the liver, retinol may be conjugated with uridine diphosphoglucuronic acid to form its O-glucosiduronate, or may be oxidized to retinal and then to retinoic acid.[88,89] Retinoic acid also forms a glucuronide in the liver, and these glucuronides, together with a small amount of free retinoic acid are excreted efficiently into the bile.[88,90,91] Retinoic acid may also be decarboxylated in the liver to a series of yet undefined products, or might possibly lose a two-carbon fragment from the terminal portion of the side chain which is subsequently oxidized to CO_2.[92] In the eye, retinol derived from the blood is oxidized to retinal before its isomerization and combination with opsin (described below).[93] The oxidation of retinol to retinal and then to retinoic acid also occurs in the kidney[94] and in the intestine.[73]

Excretion. The vitamin A glucuronides in the bile are partially re-absorbed in the gut and transported back to the liver, in an enterohepatic circulation.[95] Most of the biliary glucuronides of vitamin A, however, seem to be hydrolyzed in the gut, apparently by β-glucuronidase of enteric bacteria. They are then excreted in the feces as a mixture of free retinoic acid, possibly free retinal, the intact glucuronides, and some other un-identified products.[92,96] The kidney also excretes an appreciable amount of an ingested dose of retinoic acid in different forms, including the glucuronide and other unidentified compounds.[97]

ROLE OF VITAMIN A IN BIOCHEMICAL SYSTEMS

Function of Vitamin A in Vision. George Wald was awarded the Nobel Prize for Medicine in 1967 for his discovery of the biochemical role of vitamin A in the visual system.

The retina of the eye of most vertebrates contains two distinct photoreceptor systems: the cones are concerned with acute perception and the rods are involved with vision in dim light. The photosensitive pigment of the rods is called rhodopsin and is a combination of retinal and a protein, opsin. The photoreceptor of cones contains the same chromophore (retinal) but the protein moiety is different from that in rods and is called iodopsin. The chromophore of the visual pigments in rods and cones of most vertebrates is retinal. 3-Dehydroretinal fulfills the same function in fresh-water fish and certain amphibians.[98,99] In the eye, retinol can be oxidized to retinal. The reaction is catalyzed by an alcohol dehydrogenase with nicotinamide-adenine-dinucleotide as coenzyme.[100] In rhodopsin, retinal is in the 11-*cis* form. After absorbing quanta of light, the 11-*cis* retinal of rhodopsin is isomerized, and the pigment is subsequently hydrolyzed to the protein (opsin) and all-*trans* retinal. The energy exchange in this process causes potential differences, producing a nervous excitation transmitted via the optic nerves to the brain, resulting in visual sensations. In the dark, some of the all-*trans* retinal is isomerized by retinal isomerase of the eye tissue to the 11-*cis* isomer, which then combines with opsin to regenerate rhodopsin.[101] More recently, Brown and Wald have shown that a similar mechanism operates at high light intensities and enables us to see different colors.[102]

The binding between retinal and opsin is believed to be a Schiff-base type of linkage formed by the condensation of the aldehyde group of retinal with the ε-amino group of lysine in opsin.[103] Other studies suggest that retinal may link to lysine or cysteine of opsin by a substituted aldiminic linkage.[104] Recent experimental results indicate that retinal may be bound to phosphatidylethanolamine of the lipid-opsin complex prior to photolysis; it is transferred from there to a lysine ε-amino group of opsin in the process of photolysis.[105]

Function of Vitamin A Outside the Visual Cycle. *Effect on Major Metabolic Pathways.* Vitamin A deficiency does not disturb the tricarboxylic acid cycle[106] in carbohydrate metabolism. However, glycogen biosynthesis from acetate, lactate, and glycerol appears to be slowed down and can be reversed by cortisone administration.[107]

Interaction between vitamin A compounds and other members of the lipid class has also been studied extensively. Vitamin A metabolism is linked with that of coenzyme Q, vitamin E, vitamin D, the sterols, and the biosynthesis of squalene. Interaction of vitamins A and E seems to be important in regulating stability of biological membranes.[108] Ubiquinone (coenzyme Q) increases in the liver of vitamin A-deficient rats.[109] Vitamin A deficiency increases the biosynthesis of squalene and of ubiquinone in rat liver and reduces cholesterol formation.[110]

The utilization of liver vitamin A stores is directly proportional to protein intake when animals are fed a diet low in the vitamin. Low protein diets retard the onset of deficiency symptoms. Conversely, increased protein intake will rapidly deplete liver reserves of vitamin A.[111] Vitamin A also influences synthesis of both serum and muscle proteins.[112,113] Glycoprotein synthesis in the intestinal mucosa is impaired in vitamin A deficiency: by using a cell-free protein synthesis system, it was found that this lesion was located in the pH 5 fraction. In studying the role of vitamin A in the biosynthesis of glycopeptides, it was found that vitamin A was needed for carrying mono- or oligo-saccharide units to an acceptor site for the biosynthesis of glycoproteins situated in the cell membrane.[114]

Effect on Cell Membranes. Vitamin A-deficient animals do not only become blind, but die. Many physiological functions are affected by vitamin A and a large number of pathological lesions appear in vitamin A-deficient animals.[115] Vitamin A must therefore perform a very essential metabolic function common to many biochemical systems and to diverse tissues in living animals. In the past few years, an increasing amount of evidence has pointed towards a probable function of vitamin A in regulating membrane structure and function. Liver lysosomes of vitamin A-deficient rats are labilized.[116,117] Normal vitamin A concentration ensures optimum stability of these lysosomes. Large doses of the vitamin labilize the lysosomal membrane *in vivo* as well as *in vitro*.[118] The structure and stability of erythrocyte membranes are also markedly altered in vitamin A-deficient rats.[119,120] More recently, it has been demonstrated that vitamin A is associated with several purified biological membranes. In rat kidney endoplasmic reticulum, the major forms of vitamin A compounds appear to be retinol and retinoic acid.[121]

THE PATHOLOGY OF VITAMIN A DEFICIENCY AND EXCESS

Hypovitaminosis-A. Vitamin A deficiency causes many lesions; its earliest symptom is a failure of the retina to obtain adequate supplies of vitamin A aldehyde for the formation of rhodopsin, resulting in night blindness. This lesion is fully reversible, but may rapidly be followed by structural changes in the retina as a secondary complication.[122] Thus, the first symptoms of vitamin A deficiency are night blindness and xerosis (drying) of the conjunctiva. If deficiency continues, xerosis of the cornea appears, followed by corneal distortion. The loss of continuity of the surface epithelium with formation of a noninflammatory "ulcer" and infiltration of the stroma leads to softening of the cornea, perforation, and iris prolapse. In untreated cases, the corneal structure melts rapidly into a gelatinous mass. Endophthalmitis frequently supervenes secondarily. These advanced changes are known as keratomalacia. Keratomalacia, particularly in infants and young children, is an acute process and may occur rapidly, before the more chronic changes of xerosis occur. The severity of the lesions and rapidity with which they occur are, in general, inversely proportional to age.[123,124] Blindness due to vitamin A deficiency is most frequently caused by loss of the lens through perforation of the cornea. It is therefore not directly related to the biochemical function of vitamin A in the visual cycle, but to the function of the vitamin in general metabolism which is not clearly understood to date.

Xerosis also occurs throughout the body and can be a prolific source of secondary lesions, such as infections and pathological calcification. The general tendency of xerosis is to replace columnar epithelia in many sites by thick layers of horny, stratified epithelium. This change is often described as a metaplasia, implying that the tissues have changed in form. The term keratinization, implying that the membrane becomes horny, is also used.[125,126] Nerve lesions and increased pressure in the cerebrospinal fluid may accompany the bony changes or may develop independently.[127,128] Numerous anatomical deformities can occur in the fetus resulting from vitamin A deficiency in the maternal diet.[129]

Frequently, vitamin A deficiency is associated with protein malnutrition. Patients with kwashiorkor usually have very low serum vitamin A levels. When adequate dietary proteins are given, their serum vitamin A rises without administration of vitamin A, provided the patients have sufficient liver reserves of the vitamin. Adequate serum proteins are necessary to mobilize vitamin A from the liver into the blood stream. The situation is different in patients with kwashiorkor whose liver vitamin A reserves are low to start with. When dietary protein supplements are given to these patients, their vitamin A requirement increases, and mobilizes the last reserves of the vitamin from the liver, thus precipitating vitamin A deficiency. These observations show the importance of supplementing protein with vitamin A to protein-deficient patients.[130]

A special word of caution is necessary here. Oomen et al.[131] report that there have been epidemic outbreaks of vitamin A deficiency coinciding with the distribution of skim milk by the United Nations Children's Fund (UNICEF) in Brazil. This was attributed to the fact that vitamin A capsules, which were distributed with the milk, were not given to the children for various reasons such as the following: the children did not like them, the parents took the capsules and gave only the milk to the children, or the parents sold the capsules to make a little money. It is obvious that the milk could not have caused the eye lesions, whereas the lack of vitamin A might have done so. Parents were told that if they did not give the vitamin A capsules with the milk, their children might lose their sight, particularly when milk was the only food they received. This obviously stresses the enormous importance of supplementing skim milk with vitamin A. It was not until the fall of 1968 that nonfat dry milk used in the food donation programs in the United States was fortified with vitamin A.

Hypervitaminosis-A. There are several reports in the literature of acute hypervitaminosis-A in infants due to single, massive doses of vitamin A. The main manifestations of toxicity are transient hydrocephalus and vomiting.[132] Outbreaks of acute vitamin A intoxication have been noted in Arctic explorers who ingested large quantities of polar bear liver.

Chronic hypervitaminosis A in adults has occurred most frequently in patients who received large doses (20 to 30 times RDA) of this vitamin as treatment for dermatological conditions, and who continued subsequent intake without medical supervision. It has also been reported in food faddists[133] who included large doses of vitamin preparations in their daily dietary regimens. In patients with chronic hypervitaminosis A, fatigue, malaise, and lethargy are common complaints, usually accompanied by abdominal discomfort, bone or joint pain or both, severe, throbbing headaches, insomnia and restlessness, night sweats, loss of body hair or brittle nails or both. Constipation, irregular menses, and emotional lability have been reported. Physical examination usually reveals dry, scaly, rough skin, peripheral edema, and mouth fissures. Exophthalmus is also common.[134,135]

Hypercarotenosis. Massive doses of carotene are not converted to vitamin A rapidly enough to induce vitamin A toxicity, but excess carotene accumulates in the body. Isolated cases of hypercarotenosis have been reported, resulting from grossly excessive intakes of vegetables with carotenoid content, especially carrots. In contrast to vitamin A, excessive intakes of carotenoids do not produce clinical symptoms other than yellow skin, which disappears when ingestion of carotenoids is discontinued.[135]

VITAMIN A REQUIREMENTS OF MAN AND ANIMALS

The Food and Nutrition Board of the U.S. National Academy of Sciences—National Research Council states:

In the United States, the usual foods available are estimated to provide about 7,500 I.U. of vitamin A per day: about 3,500 I.U. derived from vegetables and fruits; 2,000 I.U. from fats, oils, and dairy products; and 2,000 I.U. from meat, fish, and eggs. Thus, about one-half of the apparent vitamin A intake is in the form of the provitamin.

For the reference man and woman, the RDA is set at 5,000 I.U. of vitamin A. For practical purposes, within the United States, it is not considered to be necessary to further adjust the RDA of 5,000 I.U. for variations in the proportions of preformed vitamin A and provitamin A in the diet.

Since few studies have been conducted on the vitamin A requirement of human infants, the RDA for this age group is deduced from the fact that human milk apparently supplies adequate vitamin A for good health during the first year of life. Human milk has a vitamin A content of 170 I.U./100 ml. Assuming consumption of approximately 850 ml of human milk, the infant would receive about 1,500 I.U. and this is taken as the RDA.

Investigations are needed to establish the requirements for vitamin A during childhood, adolescence, and other periods when growth spurts normally occur. In their absence, only interpolated estimates of allowances can be made for boys and girls of different ages, based on average body weights, plus additional arbitrary amounts to satisfy growth needs.

About 1,000 I.U./day additional vitamin A should be provided during the latter two-thirds of pregnancy, since the nutritional well-being of the rapidly growing fetus is dependent on the mother's intake of this vitamin. To help ensure the nursing infant ample amounts of vitamin A, an additional 3,000 I.U. is recommended during lactation.

Doses as low as 18,500 I.U. of a water-dispersed vitamin A–D preparation daily for one to three months are reported to be toxic for infants three to six months of age.[136]

The vitamin A requirements may be modified by age, growth, caloric intake, physical expenditure and special needs during pregnancy and lactation. The recommended daily dietary allowances of vitamin A in I.U. are as follows: adults 5,000; pregnancy (latter half) 6,000; lactation 8,000; infants to 1 year 1,500; children 1 to 3 years 2,000; 3 to 6 years 2,500; 6 to 9 years 3,500; 9 to 12 years 4,500; 12 to 20 years 5,000.[136]

Extensive studies of the vitamin A requirements of rats and farm animals have been undertaken. About 2 I.U. of either vitamin A or β-carotene are required to restore growth in young rats deficient in the vitamin. Much larger doses, however, are necessary to allow maximum longevity (100 I.U. per rat daily) or storage of the vitamin in the liver (30 I.U. per rat daily).[137] For beef cattle, the *National Research Council* recommended a daily allowance of 22 I.U. of vitamin A (alcohol) per kg body weight or 220 I.U. of carotene per kg body weight. For growing pigs, an allowance of 150 I.U. of carotene per kg body weight was recommended, to be increased to 200 I.U. in pregnancy and to 330 I.U. during lactation.[138]

An important study of the vitamin A requirement of adults was undertaken from 1942 through 1944 in Sheffield, England by the Medical Research Council.[139] It was found that 1,300 International Units (I.U.) of retinol daily was the minimum protective dose. To provide a margin of safety and to allow for individual variations in vitamin A requirement, the investigators recommended a daily dose of 2,500 I.U. for adults. Based on the same study, the minimum protective dose of β-carotene is about 1,500 I.U. daily, and 3,000 I.U. is adequate to cover individual variations and to provide a margin of safety based on the supposition that 100% of the β-carotene is biologically available. It should be noted, however, that several studies on carotene absorption in man have indicated a relatively low efficiency of absorption of carotene from various sources. For this reason, it was recommended that the adult daily requirement for carotene be put at 7,500 I.U. This figure would be roughly representative of the efficiency of absorption of carotene from various dietary sources. The authors of the Sheffield study warned that their figures for vitamin A and carotene requirement should be used with discretion, since their data were based on deprivation and cure of healthy men between the ages of 20 and 30 years.

NORMAL SERUM LEVELS AND LIVER RESERVES OF VITAMIN A IN MAN

Moore[140] has discussed the vitamin A status in normal health and in experimental deficiency in man at great length in his standard work on vitamin A. He reports that liver vitamin A reserves were determined in accidentally killed humans in Britain, Holland, South Africa, China, Norway, Sweden and Scotland. He has also reviewed a wide variety of serum vitamin A and serum carotene levels in humans measured in studies undertaken in the United States, Great Britain, South Africa and Norway. The grand average of these studies indicates a serum vitamin A level of approximately 40 μg/100 ml for these human populations. The corresponding serum carotenoid level was 137 μg/100 ml. Much wider ranges for liver vitamin A reserves determined on victims of accidental death are reported with the averages from different countries ranging from 24 μg/g liver for China to 191 μg vitamin A per gram liver for Scotland.

It was found in a recent study on Canadians,[141,142] that the liver vitamin A stores of 15 to 32 per cent of subjects examined on autopsy were less than 40 μg/gm of liver; however, many of these specimens were obtained from diseased subjects. A study on autopsy material from Canadians who died in accidents revealed that one group of accidental death victims had higher liver vitamin A reserves than those who died from diseases, whereas, another group of accidental death victims had values very similar to those who died from disease.

A recent study reported the vitamin A liver stores of accident victims in New York City.[143] For 101 human livers, the mean vitamin A content was 126 μg/gm wet tissue with a range of 7 to 668 μg and a median of 66 μg. Post-mortem blood samples were obtained from 50 of the subjects and the main serum vitamin A level was found to be 49 ± 16 μg/100 ml serum with a carotene value of 113 ± 51 μg/100 ml of serum.

In a recent study undertaken in West Germany on a well-fed population, the average serum vitamin A content was found to be 52.7 ± 13.2 μg/100 ml for 165 males and 50.5 ± 12.7 μg vitamin A per 100 ml serum for 216 females. The corresponding carotene concentrations were 85.6 ± 28.6 μg/100 ml for the males and 94.0 ± 34.3 μg/100 ml for the females; some age trends were noticeable.[144]

It should be stressed here that serum levels do not reflect liver reserves of vitamin A in experimental animals, except after almost complete exhaustion of the liver reserves. At that stage, serum vitamin A levels fall rapidly. Low serum levels of vitamin A are therefore often, but not always, an indication of vitamin A deficiency: dangerously low liver reserves may occur simultaneously with near normal blood levels of the vitamin.

Levels below 20 μg/100 ml serum are certainly on the low side and levels below 10 μg/100 ml serum are very low indeed and more than likely indicative of serious vitamin A deficiency.

Serum carotene levels are much more variable than those of vitamin A: the serum carotene levels directly reflect dietary intakes of carotenoids. Extremely high levels of carotene can be found in populations consuming carotene-rich diets such as red palm oil.

Studies of the liver reserves of patients who died from various diseases have indicated ranges lower than those found in cases of accidental death. Moreover, the loss of vitamin A reserves is greater in some diseases than in other. For example, the loss in appendicitis appears to be about 50 per cent, in pneumonia 70 per cent, and in chronic nephritis 89 per cent. In the last two diseases these losses are due, at least partially, to excretion of the vitamin in the urine. In chronic and incurable diseases the situation may be complicated by failure in the absorption or metabolism of the vitamin. Usually this abnormality may have little effect on the course of the disease, but the possibility of aggravation of the main lesion by superimposed hypovitaminosis-A should be borne in mind. The administration of the vitamin seems advisable, provided it causes no digestive disturbance.[145]

Massive vitamin A therapy has been used in the treatment of premenstrual tension[146] and certain skin diseases.[147] Serious poisoning often results from treatment with vitamin A beyond upper limits of tolerance. Doses of 200,000 I.U. daily may cause chronic hypervitaminosis-A if continued over prolonged periods. Single doses of 2,000,000 I. U. may induce acute hypervitaminosis-A.

The materials available for the prevention and cure of vitamin A deficiency include vitamin A-containing foods, fish-liver oils, concentrates derived from them, preparations of carotene in oil, and synthetic forms of vitamin A, made available as the palmitate, stearate or acetate ester and in the alcohol form. Retinyl palmitate now sells at approximately five U.S. cents for 1,000,000 I.U. wholesale.

VITAMIN A THERAPY

Night blindness and the milder conjunctival changes respond well to 30,000 I.U. of vitamin A daily for a few days, given as cod or halibut liver oil.[148] Corneal damage must be treated as an emergency; a dose causing a rapid increase in the level of vitamin A in the blood plasma seems to be necessary. Since the adult liver can absorb at least 500,000 I.U., doses of the vitamin should be so adjusted as to make this amount available during the first few days of treatment. Children should be given smaller doses.[149]

In most patients, oral treatment is decidedly more effective than parenteral. When lesions of the gastrointestinal tract are involved, however, the administration of the vitamin by injection may be necessary. If so, an aqueous dispersion of the vitamin should be used.[148] Intramuscular injections of oily solutions of the vitamin are practically useless.

VITAMIN A IN DISEASES OTHER THAN THOSE DUE TO ITS DEFICIENCY AND EXCESS

Moore[140] has made an extensive survey of the literature concerning vitamin A status in patients with diseases not attributed to vitamin A deficiency. Cancer, tuberculosis, and chronic infections, particularly pneumonia, chronic nephritis, urinary tract infections, and prostate diseases may cause massive urinary excretion of vitamin A. Since it has been claimed that urinary excretion of vitamin A in patients is highly selective, no carotenoids or other lipids appear in the urine simultaneously with vitamin A.

There is a high incidence of respiratory infections, gastroenteritis, measles, and other infectious diseases among children suffering from xerophthalmia. It remains to be seen whether in these cases, generally occurring in areas where marasmus or kwashiorkor are endemic, severe vitamin A deficiency results from infectious disease or vice versa, whether the greater susceptibility to infectious disease was caused by vitamin A deficiency or by lowered reserves of the vitamin.

Attention should be given to vitamin A status in patients with diseases in which fat absorption is defective. Serum vitamin A levels are depressed in patients with celiac disease, sprue, obstructive jaundice, cystic fibrosis, and in giardiasis. In general, serum vitamin A levels decrease in pyrexia. This has been noticed particularly in children with rheumatic fever. In patients with infectious hepatitis, plasma levels of vitamin A are found to be low; in this disease, both pyrexia and a hepatic reaction are involved and, therefore, this lowering of vitamin A levels is, perhaps, to be expected. Cirrhosis of the liver usually results in extremely low, and sometimes completely absent, reserves of vitamin A in the liver.

BIBLIOGRAPHY

1. McCollum and Davis: J. Biol. Chem., 23, 181, 1915.
2. Drummond: Biochem. J., 14, 660, 1920.
3. McCollum and Simmonds: J. Biol. Chem., 32, 181, 1917.
4. Fridericia and Holm: Am. J. Physiol., 73, 63, 1925.
5. Steenbock and Boutwell: J. Biol. Chem., 41, 163, 1920.
6. Steenbock and Sell: J. Biol. Chem., 51, 63, 1922.
7. Bloch: J. Dairy Sci., 7, 1, 1924.
8. Moore: Biochem. J., 24, 692, 1930.
9. Karrer, Helfenstein, Wehrli and Wettstein: Helv. Chim. Acta, 13, 1084, 1930.
10. Karrer, Morf and Schöpp: Helv. Chim. Acta, 14, 1036 and 1431, 1931.
11. Isler, Huber, Ronco and Kofler: Helv. Chim. Acta, 30, 1911, 1947.
12. Karrer and Eugster: Helv. Chim. Acta, 33, 1172, 1950.
13. Inhoffen, Bohlmann, Bartram, Rummert and Pommer: Ann. Chem., 570, 54, 1950.
14. Harris, Ames and Brinkman: J. Amer. Chem. Soc., 73, 1252, 1951.
15. Shantz: Science, 108, 417, 1948.
16. Reti: Compt. Rend. Soc. Biol., 120, 577, 1935.
17. Ganguly: Vitamins Hormones, 18, 387, 1960.
18. Wald: Vitamins Hormones, 18, 417, 1960.
19. Ames: Ann. Rev. Biochem., 27, 371, 1958.
20. Dowling and Wald: Vitamins Hormones, 18, 387, 1960.
21. Karrer, Morf and Walker: Helv. Chim. Acta, 16, 975, 1933.
22. Winterstein: Z. Physiol. Chem., 215, 51, 1933.
23. Deuel, Sumner, Johnston, Polgár and Zechmeister: Arch. Biochem., 6, 157, 1945.
24. Zechmeister, Pinckard, Greenberg, Straub, Fukui and Deuel, Jr.: Arch. Biochem., 23, 242, 1949.
25. Olson: J. Biol. Chem., 236, 349, 1961.
26. Boldingh, Cama, Collins, Morton, Gridgeman, Isler, Kofler, Taylor, Wieland and Bradbury: Nature, 168, 598, 1951.
27. Drummond and Watson: Analyst, 47, 341, 1922.
28. Sobotka, Kann and Loewenstein: J. Am. Chem. Soc., 65, 1959, 1943.
29. Embree and Shantz: J. Am. Chem. Soc., 65, 906, 1943.
30. Morton: Nature, 153, 69, 1944.
31. Ball, Goodwin and Morton: Biochem. J., 42, 516, 1948.
32. Robeson, Cawley, Weisler, Stern, Eddinger and Chechak: J. Am. Chem. Soc., 77, 4111, 1955.
33. Brown and Wald: J. Biol. Chem., 222, 865, 1956.
34. Wald, Brown, Hubbard, and Oroshnik: Proc. Natl. Acad. Sci. U.S., 41, 438, 1955.
35. Beutel, Hinkley and Pollak: J. Am. Chem. Soc., 77, 5166, 1955.
36. Barnholdt: Acta Chem. Scand., 11, 909, 1957.
37. Carr and Price: Biochem. J., 20, 497, 1926.
38. Neeld and Pearson: J. Nutr., 79, 454, 1963.

39. Zechmeister and Polgár: J. Am. Chem. Soc., *65*, 1522, 1943.
40. Bickoff, White, Bevenue and Williams: J. Assoc. Offic. Agr. Chemists., *31*, 633, 1948.
41. Baur: Helv. Chim. Acta, *19*, 1210, 1936.
42. Karrer and Jucker: *Carotenoids*, Amsterdam, Elsevier Publ. Co., pp. 126, 150, 161, 1950.
43. Collins: Nature, *165*, 817, 1950.
44. Zechmeister: *Cis-Trans Isomeric Carotenoids, Vitamin A and Arylpolyenes*, Vienna, Springer-Verlag, 1962.
45. Morton and Stubbs: Analyst, *71*, 348, 1946.
46. Cama, Collins and Morton: Biochem J., *50*, 48, 1951.
47. Brunius: Nature, *181*, 395, 1958.
48. Popper: Physiol. Rev., *24*, 205, 1944.
49. Fujita and Aoyama: J. Biochem. (Tokyo), *38*, 271, 1951.
50. Dunagin and Olson: Anal. Chem., *36*, 756, 1964.
51. Brown, Blum and Stern: Nature, *184*, 1377, 1959.
52. Von Planta, unpublished data, quoted in Kofler and Rubin: Vitamins Hormones, *18*, 315, 1960.
53. Bliss and György: *Vitamin Methods*, (György, Ed.), Vol. 2, New York, Academic Press, pp. 45–275, 1951.
54. Dugan, Frigerio and Siebert: Anal. Chem., *36*, 114, 1964.
55. Roels and Trout: Am. J. Clin. Nutr., *1*, 197, 1959.
56. Coward: *The Biological Standardisation of Vitamins*, 2nd ed., London, Baillière, Tindall & Cox, p. 23, 1947.
57. Pugsley, Wills and Crandall: J. Nutr., *28*, 365–379, 1944.
58. Guggenheim and Koch: Biochem. J., *38*, 256, 1944.
59. Booth: *Carotene, Its Determination in Biological Materials*, Cambridge, England, Heffer, 1957.
60. Hunter and Scott: Biochem. J., *38*, 211, 1944.
61. Rapsan, Schwartz and Van Rensburg: J. Soc. Chem. Ind. (London), *65*, 61, 1945.
62. Watt and Merrill: U.S. Dept. Agr., Agr. Handbook 8, 1950, 1966.
63. Thompson, Brande, Coates, Cowie, Ganguly and Kon: Brit. J. Nutr., *4*, 398, 1950.
64. Bieri and Pollard: Brit. J. Nutr., *8*, 32, 1954.
65. Zachman and Olson: J. Biol. Chem., *238*, 541, 1963.
66. Olson and Hayaishi: Proc. Natl. Acad. Sci., *54*, 1364, 1965.
67. Goodman, Huang, Kanai, and Shiratori: J. Biol. Chem., *242*, 3543, 1967.
68. Roels, Trout and Dujacquier: J. Nutr., *65*, 115, 1958.
69. Brown and Bloor: J. Nutr., *29*, 349, 1945.
70. Olson: Fed. Proc., *21*, 473, 1962.
71. Mahadevan, Seshadri-Sastry and Ganguly: Biochem. J., 88, 531, 1963.
72. Mahadevan, Seshadri-Sastry and Ganguly: Biochem. J., *88*, 534, 1963.
73. Huang and Goodman: J. Biol. Chem., *240*, 2839, 1965.
74. Fidge, Shiratori, Ganguly and Goodman: J. Lipid Res., *9*, 103, 1968.
75. Deshmuk, Murthy, Mahadevan and Ganguly: Biochem. J., *96*, 377, 1965.
76. Deshmuk, Malathi, Subba-Rao and Ganguly: Indian J. Biochem., *1*, 164, 1964.
77. Mahadevan, Ayyoub and Roels: J. Biol. Chem., *241*, 57, 1966.
78. Hoch and Hoch: Brit. J. Exptl. Pathol., *27*, 316, 1946.
79. Dowling and Wald: Proc. Natl. Acad. Sci. U.S., *44*, 648, 1958.
80. Krinsky, Cornwell and Oncley: Arch. Biochem. Biophys., *73*, 233, 1958.
81. Kanai, Raz and Goodman: J. Clin. Invest., *47*, 2025, 1968.
82. Moore: Biochem. J., *25*, 275, 1931.
83. Moore: *Vitamin A*, Amsterdam, Elsevier Publ. Col, p. 212, 1957.
84. Kuhn and Brockmann: Z. Physiol. Chem., *206*, 41, 1932.
85. Bacharach and Smith: Quart. J. Pharm., *1*, 539, 1928.
86. Gray and Cawley: J. Nutr., *23*, 301, 1942.
87. Krishnamurthy and Ganguly: Nature, *177*, 575, 1956.
88. Lippel and Olson: J. Lipid. Res., *9*, 168, 1968.
89. Mahadevan, Murthy and Ganguly: Biochem. J., *85*, 326, 1962.
90. Dunagin, Meadows and Olson: Science, *148*, 86, 1965.
91. Dunagin, Zachman and Olson: Biochim. Biophys. Acta, *124*, 71, 1966.
92. De Luca and Roberts: Am. J. Clin. Nutr., *22*, 945, 1969.
93. Wald: Vitamins Hormones, *18*, 417, 1960.
94. Kleiner-Bossaler and De Luca: Arch. Biochem. Biophys., *142*, 371, 1971.
95. Zachman, Dunagin and Olson: J. Lipid. Res., *2*, 3, 1966.
96. Natu and Olson: J. Nutr., *93*, 461, 1967.
97. Sundaresan and Therriault: Biochim. Biophys. Acta, *158*, 92, 1968.
98. Wald: Vitamins Hormones, *1*, 195, 1943.
99. Wald, Brown, and Smith: Science, *118*, 505, 1953.
100. Wald and Hubbard: Proc. Natl. Acad. Sci. U.S., *36*, 92, 1950.
101. Hubbard and Colman: Science, *130*, 977, 1959.
102. Brown and Wald: Nature, *200*, 37, 1963.
103. Ball, Collins Dabi and Morton: Biochem. J., *45*, 304, 1949.
104. Heller: Biochemistry, *7*, 2914, 1968.
105. Kimble, Poincelot and Abrahamson: Biochemistry, *9*, 1817, 1970.
106. Wolf, Lane and Johnson: J. Biol. Chem., *225*, 995, 1957.
107. Johnson and Wolf: Vitamins Hormones, *18*, 465, 1960.
108. Roels, Trout and Guha: Biochem. J., *97*, 353, 1965.

109. Lowe, Morton and Harrison: Nature, 172, 716, 1953.
110. Wiss and Gloor: Vitamins Hormones, 18, 485, 1960.
111. McLaren: Brit. J. Ophthalmol., 43, 234, 1959.
112. Vakil, Roels and Trout: Brit. J. Nutr., 18, 217, 1964.
113. Moore: Vitamins Hormones, 18, 431, 1960.
114. De Luca and Wolf: Internat. J. Vit. Res., 40, 284, 1970.
115. Moore: *Vitamin A*, New York, Elsevier Publ. Co., pp. 296–297, 1957.
116. Roxas, Sessa, Trout, Guha and Roels: Fed. Proc., 23, 293, 1964.
117. Roels, Trout and Guha: Biochem. J., 93, 23, 1964.
118. Roels: *The Vitamins*, (Sebrell and Harris, Ed.), 2nd ed., Vol. 1, New York, Academic Press, pp. 193–204, 1967.
119. Anderson, Pfister and Roels: Nature, 213, 47, 1967.
120. Roels, Anderson, Lui, Shah and Trout.: Am. J. Clin. Nutr., 22, 1020, 1969.
121. Mack, Lui, Anderson and Roels: To be published.
122. Dowling and Wald: Proc. Natl. Acad. Sci. U.S., 44, 648, 1958.
123. McLaren, Oomen, and Escapini: Bull. World Health Organ., 34, 357, 1966.
124. Paton and McLaren: Am. J. Ophthalmol., 50, 568, 1960.
125. Wolbach: Vitamins, 1, 106, 1954.
126. Pillat: Arch. Ophthalmol., 2, 256, 1929.
127. Coetzer: Biochem. J., 45, 628, 1949.
128. Mellanby: Proc. Roy. Soc., B132, 28, 1944.
129. Mason: Am. J. Anat., 57, 303, 1935.
130. Arroyave, Wilson and Mendez: Amer. J. Clin. Nutr., 9, 180, 1961.
131. Oomen, McLaren and Escapini: Trop. Geograph. Med., 16, 271, 1964.
132. Lindhard: Medd. Groenland, 41, 461, 1913.
133. Bergen and Roels: Am. J. Clin. Nutr., 16, 265, 1965.
134. Gerber, Raeb and Sobel: Am. J. Med., 16, 729, 1954.
135. Josephs: Am. J. Dis. Child., 67, 33, 1944.
136. National Academy of Sciences—National Research Council, Food and Nutrition Board, *Recommended Dietary Allowances*, Publ. 1694, 7th edition, Washington, D.C., 1968.
137. Moore: *Vitamin A*, Amsterdam, Elsevier Publ. Co., p. 228, 1957.
138. National Academy of Sciences—National Research Council, *Recommended Nutrient Allowances for Farm Animals*, Washington, D.C., 1944, 1949, 1950.
139. Hume and Krebs: Med. Res. Counc. Spec. Rep. Ser. No. 264, London, 1949.
140. Moore: *Vitamin A*, Amsterdam, Elsevier Publ. Co., pp. 355–374, 1957.
141. Hoppner, Phillips, Erdsdy, Murray, and Perrin: Can. Med. Assoc. J., 101, 84, 1969.
142. Hoppner, Phillips, Murray and Campbell: Can. Med. Assoc. J., 99, 983, 1968.
143. Underwood, Siegel, Weisell and Dolinski: Amer. J. Clin. Nutr., 23, 1037, 1970.
144. Kasper: Internat. Z. Vit. Forschung., 38, 142, 1968.
145. Moore: Biochem. J., 31, 155, 1937.
146. Argonz and Abinzano: J. Clin. Endocrinol., 10, 1579, 1950.
147. Leitner and Moore: Lancet, 251, 262, 1946.
148. McLaren: Trans. Roy. Soc. Trop. Med. Hyg., 60, 436, 1966.
149. Moore: In *The Vitamins*, (Sebrell and Harris, Eds.) 2nd Ed., Vol. 1, New York, Academic Press, p. 283, 1967.

Chapter

5

Section B   Vitamin D*

J. L. OMDAHL†

AND

H. F. DeLuca

BACKGROUND

The disease rickets appears to have been evident in ancient times, possibly resulting from advances in urbanization.[1] Bardsley, in 1807, wrote about the effective use of cod liver oil in the treatment of osteomalacia,[2] while Palm,[3] in 1890, suggested that sunlight possessed antirachitic action.   In 1919 Sir Edward Mellanby succeeded in producing the disease in experimental animals and found it could be prevented by the administration of cod liver oil.[4] McCollum and associates[5] found that the antirachitic factor in cod liver oil was stable to heat and aeration; thereby differing from the previously discovered vitamin A.   McCollum named the factor vitamin D.[6] The elegant work of Steenbock and associates[7,8] demonstrated that antirachitic activity could be produced in food and animals by ultraviolet irradiation. This discovery aided in the eventual identification of vitamin D_2[9,10] and eliminated rickets as a major medical problem.

A distinct time lag exists between administration of vitamin D to deficient animals and detection of a physiological response (e.g. enhanced intestinal calcium absorption). The conversion of vitamin D to active metabolites and the stimulation of protein synthesis and/or assembly constitute the main events occurring during this time period.

* Supported by a grant from the U.S.P.H.S. No. AM-14881 and the Steenbock Research Fund.
† Recipient of an NIH Postdoctoral Fellowship, No. 5-FO2-AM43354–02.

In view of these recent findings it is interesting that by current definitions vitamin D can be considered both a vitamin and a hormone. Vitamin D is an organic compound which acts as a micronutrient and whose ingestion is required by most urban populations in the United States (i.e. acts as a vitamin). However, there is no need for vitamin D supplementation in people who are able to meet their vitamin need through the sunlight activation of 7-dehydrocholesterol in the skin. The vitamin D thus produced is metabolized to an active form(s) which then acts on distinct target tissue with feedback control occurring at the site of active metabolite synthesis. In this latter case, vitamin D acts as a hormone.

VITAMIN D CHEMISTRY

The D vitamins are characteristically found in the sterol fraction of biological extracts. Vitamins D_2 and D_3, the more common forms of the vitamin, are derived from ergosterol and cholesterol, respectively, and are therefore named ergocalciferol and cholecalciferol (Fig. 5B–1).

The triene structure of vitamin D gives a characteristic absorption band at 265 nm with an absorption minimum at 228 nm. Vitamin D is fairly stable and soluble in several organic solvents, although care should be taken to store solutions of the vitamin under nitrogen at −20° C. The main problem is the ease of oxidation of the triene system.

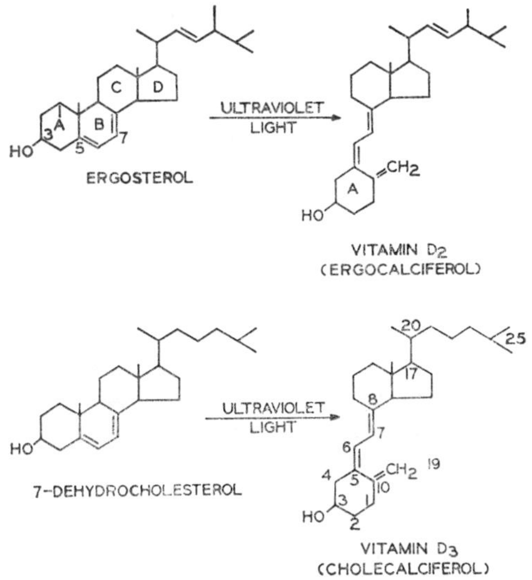

Fig. 5B-1. Formation of vitamin D_2 and vitamin D_3 from treatment of ergosterol and 7-dehydrocholesterol with ultraviolet light.

Often α-tocopherol can be used to help stabilize but it is best to exclude oxygen. Aqueous suspensions are particularly unstable because of dissolved oxygen. Oil or propylene glycol solutions of the vitamin, however, are quite stable.

Chemical alteration of existing functional groups or double bonds results in a product with decreased antirachitic activity. Vitamin D_4 is produced by the reduction of the 22,23 double bond in vitamin D_2 and is only $\frac{1}{2}$ to $\frac{3}{4}$ as active as the parent vitamin. Substitution of a Cl,Br[11] or a mercaptan[12] group for the 3-OH function results in loss of activity. Reduction of the methylene group on ring A and rotation of the ring 180° results in dihydrotachysterol (present in solutions of AT-10), a compound which is less active than the parent vitamin at low doses but of therapeutic value for hypoparathyroid patients when given at a pharmacological level.[13]

BIOLOGICAL ASSAY

Only a small amount of vitamin D is required (e.g. 1 IU in the rat, where 1 mg = 40,000 IU) to elicit a physiological response. Although advances have been made concerning the chemical detection of vitamin D,[14] the most sensitive methods still involve in vivo biological assays.

The rat line test[15] remains the method of choice. A single dose of standard vitamin D will promote calcification in the epiphyseal plate of the rachitic rat. Silver nitrate (1.5 per cent w/v) staining of sectioned bone is used for visual detection of new calcification which increases as a function of the dose of vitamin D.

Per cent bone ash is also used in chicks and rats as an assay for vitamin D. The bone ash content of tibia is determined after feeding chicks a rachitogenic diet and standard doses of vitamin D for 21 days.[16] Increase in bone ash is correlated to the dose of vitamin D. The chick bone ash method is the primary method used for vitamin D_3. To differentiate between vitamins D_2 and D_3 an efficacy ratio of rat to chick response is used. Chicks give a response to D_3 which is tenfold greater than to vitamin D_2 while rats respond equally well to both compounds.

VITAMIN D ABSORPTION AND EXCRETION

Vitamin D is absorbed with food fats, therefore, inhibition of normal fat absorption (steatorrhea) results in a diminished absorption of ingested vitamin D. Patients with chronic pancreatitis, celiac disease and biliary obstruction were found to malabsorb ^{3}H-vitamin D_3.[17] Absorption occurs in the jejunum and/or ileum. Bile is essential[18,19] with the majority of an absorbed dose of vitamin D present in the chylomicrons of the lymphatic system.[17] Vitamin D concentrates rapidly in the liver where it is hydroxylated to 25-hydroxycholecalciferol (25-HCC).[20] The movement of vitamin D and its metabolites from the plasma chylomicrons and lipoproteins appears to occur in the liver by transfer to an α_1-globulin fraction which acts as a carrier for the vitamin.[21]

Bile appears to be the major pathway of vitamin D metabolite excretion. Patients having biliary fistulas excrete little radioactivity from a dose of ^{3}H-vitamin D_3.[22] A significant amount (i.e. 3 per cent) of ^{3}H-vitamin D_3 is also detectable in the urine during the 48- to 72-hour period following an intravenous dosage.[22]

DIETARY IMPLICATIONS

Because most foodstuffs are fortified with vitamin D, the daily vitamin requirement (*i.e.* 400 IU) can be achieved without vitamin supplementation.[23] However, rickets can occur in breast-fed infants and those fed unfortified milk,[24] in which case a vitamin D supplement is recommended (*e.g.* 400 IU daily). It is currently suggested that prophylactic doses of vitamin D in excess of 1,000 IU daily are inadvisable.[25] However, Fomon and associates have shown that moderate overdoses of vitamin D (*i.e.* 1,380 to 2,370 IU daily), common in a substantial number of children in the United States, had no detrimental effect on growth.[26] A high frequency of a mild form of idiopathic hypercalcemia in Great Britain has been associated with a vitamin intake of 4,000 IU daily, due mainly to fortified infant foods.[27] Of course, an excessive intake of vitamin D (*i.e.* 50,000 to 100,000 IU daily) is potentially dangerous to normal children[38] and adults[29] and should be avoided.

There should also be an awareness that improper dietary intakes of calcium and/or phosphorus can be manifest by improper growth and bone diseases. Infants require 400 to 600 mg of calcium daily, children (1 to 10 years) and adults (over 18 years) require 800 mg daily, while growing children (10 to 18 years) and women during pregnancy need 1300 mg daily.[24] Phosphorus should be consumed at a level equivalent to calcium with the dietary ratio of the two ions approximating 1:1. A high phosphorus diet as afforded by cow's milk may prompt the occurrence of hypocalcemic tetany during early infancy.[30] The high phosphate intake in the United States afforded through soft drinks and food preservatives is also of interest concerning possible long-term effects in children and adults alike. High phosphate diets effectively decrease the absorption of calcium by the formation of an insoluble calcium complex. Phytate in bread and certain cereals forms insoluble calcium phytate which also interferes with intestinal calcium absorption.[31]

One resultant effect of low blood calcium and phosphorus is the softening and deformity of the maxillary bones. Mellanby and Mellanby reported that in London between 1945 and 1947 children (*i.e.* up to 5 years) who had increased availability of calcium and vitamin D possessed markedly improved dental status.[32]

METABOLITES OF VITAMIN D

Column chromatography of chloroform tissue extracts from rats and chicks, injected with ^{3}H-vitamin D_3, results in the separation of several vitamin D metabolites. A sulfated vitamin D^{33} and a long-chain fatty acid ester of the vitamin[34] have been identified. Recently, interest has developed concerning polar metabolites which possess additional hydroxy groupings. The major circulating form of the vitamin *in vivo* has been identified as 25-hydroxycholecalciferol (25-HCC) by Blunt and associates.[35] This polar compound appears to be hydroxylated further wherein 21,25-dihydroxycholecalciferol (21,25-DHCC)[36] and 25,26-dihydroxycholecalciferol (25,26-DHCC)[37] have been isolated from hog plasma. In addition Holick and co-workers[38,39] have succeeded in identifying 1,25-dihydroxycholecalciferol (1,25-DHCC) from the intestine of chickens. This metabolite is present in intestine at a concentration of only 0.5 to 1 ng/gm tissue and is extremely active in stimulating intestinal calcium transport.

The biological action of the 25-hydroxy derivatives can be summarized with respect to an equivalent dose of vitamin D_3 as follows:

25-HCC demonstrates faster action in stimulation of calcium transport, 40 per cent greater antirachitic activity and greater activity in mobilization of bone mineral.

21,25-DHCC is only 50 per cent as active in the cure of rickets and enhancement of intestinal calcium transport while it is more active in the mobilization of bone mineral.

25,26-DHCC is about 50 per cent as active in the stimulation of intestinal calcium transport but shows little antirachitic or bone mineral mobilization activity.

1,25-DHCC is the most potent and quickest acting metabolite with regard to enhancement of intestinal calcium transport. An effect on calcium absorption is evident 3 hours following a 5-IU dose to rachitic chicks. The metabolite is probably more potent and may be quicker acting with regard to bone mobilization, however, to date it has elicited only normal antirachitic activity.

VITAMIN D AND CALCIUM HOMEOSTASIS

Parathyroid hormone (PTH, from chief cells of parathyroid), thyrocalcitonin (TCT, from c cells of thyroid) and vitamin D work in concert to maintain plasma calcium concentration at the population mean of 10 mg/100 ml. Current results suggest an inverse control mechanism between plasma calcium and PTH release.[40] PTH appears to effect its hypercalcemic action through bone mineral mobilization,[41] phosphate diuresis[42] and possibly calcium absorption.[43] The action of PTH on bone resorption and calcium absorption is vitamin D dependent, while its action on phosphate diuresis is not.[42,43]

The major site of action for TCT appears to be bone.[44,45] Neither the kidney[46] nor the gastrointestinal tract[44] is necessary for demonstration of TCT's hypocalcemic effect. TCT is secreted in response to hypercalcemia and functions in controlling plasma calcium concentration when it rises above normal. The action of TCT is independent of the PTH system, as illustrated by its activity in parathyroidectomized, intact and vitamin D-deficient rats.[47]

Dihydrotachysterol,[48] vitamin D and especially 25-HCC can effectively mobilize bone, in the apparent absence of PTH,[49,50] when given in pharmacological quantities. Such is evident from the fact that hypoparathyroid patients can be adequately managed with high doses of vitamin D (25,000 to 200,000 IU daily) as the only treatment.[50]

Vitamin D is also required for adaptation to low calcium intakes. The adaptive response results in increased efficiency of calcium absorption beyond that observed for a normal calcium diet.[51] Calcium-binding protein (CaBP) activity also increases in animals fed a low-calcium diet.[52a] Thyroparathyroidectomy does not inhibit the adaptive phe-

nomenon.[51,52b] It has been presumed, since the early work of Nicolaysen,[53] that the adaptive mechanism responds to the state of mineralization of the skeleton. However, studies now in progress in the authors' laboratory indicate that dietary calcium in some manner affects the metabolism of vitamin D, which in turn could affect calcium absorption (private communication).

CALCIUM TRANSPORT

Vitamin D has been implicated in calcium absorption since the pioneering work of Nicolaysen.[54] It should be noted that the intestinal calcium absorption mechanism is one of active transport in which cellular energy is required to transfer calcium against an electrochemical potential gradient.[55,56] Sodium ions are required for the expulsion of calcium into the serosal fluid[57] but not in the calcium uptake process. There is still some disagreement as to whether vitamin D is involved in the active portion of the transport process.[58,59]

Regardless of the mechanism, it is now apparent that a vitamin D metabolite (e.g. 1,25-DHCC) affects that portion of the process which functions in the intestinal translocation of calcium. From more recent studies it is apparent that vitamin D is metabolized to 25-HCC in the liver[20] which is further hydroxylated to 1,25-DHCC in the kidney.[60] The 1,25-DHCC is sequestered by the intestine where it then effects assembly of the cellular calcium transport system. A vitamin D-dependent calcium-binding protein has been identified from both chick[61] and rat[62] intestine and could be a constituent of the transport system. The action of vitamin D in the intestine is blocked by protein synthesis inhibitors[63] and dietary strontium.[64] However, recent results from the rat suggest that 1,25-DHCC can act in the intestine in the presence of actinomycin D.[65]

In the deficient state, a major barrier to calcium translocation across the epithelial cell is presented by the brush border surface.[55] A vitamin D-dependent calcium ATPase has been isolated from rat and chick brush border preparations[66] and could work synergistically with the calcium-binding protein to enhance the movement of calcium across the mucosal barrier. Work with filipin[67] also suggests an effect of vitamin D on the apical border of the columnar epithelial cell.

VITAMIN D DEFICIENCY AND DISEASE STATES

Numerous biochemical and physiological imbalances occur in the deficient state, which if not corrected result in rickets in growing children and osteomalacia in adults. Characteristic biochemical changes include low plasma calcium (mainly in children) and inorganic phosphorus with a concomitant high plasma alkaline phosphatase. Early in deficiency a defect in calcium absorption occurs. This often leads to secondary hyperparathyroidism in which PTH is secreted in response to a low plasma calcium concentration. Rickets occurs when the newly synthesized organic matrix fails to mineralize, resulting in soft bones. Most striking is the failure of endochondral calcification, resulting in widening of the epiphyseal plate and the build up of osteoid tissue.

Vitamin D affects citrate metabolism as evidenced by the serum citrate from 10 rachitic infants which was 1.5 mg/100 ml compared to 2.5 mg/100 ml in normal infants.[68] Vitamin D treatment (*i.e.* 600,000 IU) resulted in elevation of the serum citrate; however, it is now clear that the citrate response is a consequence of, rather than a participant in, the vitamin-induced changes in mineral metabolism.[69]

Diagnosis of rickets is usually made from the characteristic bony deformities seen on radiographs. The non-calcified epiphyseal plate becomes more apparent and there are broadening and irregularity in the adjacent regions of the epiphysis and metaphysis.

Although D-deficient rickets is now rare in the western world, several disorders still exist in which there is an apparent lack of the vitamin's action within the calcium homeostatic system. It is now clear that vitamin D is converted to active metabolites in specific organs[55] and that these metabolites may act as the signal to the target tissue, resulting in a specific physiological action. Isolation of several metabolites and the realization that some disease states may stem from an inability to synthesize these metabolites have generated new enthusiasm for the treatment of vitamin D-related diseases.

REFRACTORY OR VITAMIN D-RESISTANT RICKETS (FAMILIAL HYPOPHOSPHATEMIA)

This disease is usually manifest in early childhood[70] and is characterized by hypophosphatemia. The syndrome often appears due to a single dominant gene. Although the exact defect which causes the disease is not known, the most characteristic dysfunction is a renal wasting of phosphate. In addition, intestinal calcium absorption is below normal. Abnormal vitamin D metabolism has been reported in this disease,[71] however, it is certainly not merely a failure of 25-hydroxylation since physiologic amounts of 25-HCC fail to cure the disease. It is of interest that the disease does not apparently result from secondary hyperparathyroidism wherein phosphate infusion will cause an increase in intestinal calcium absorption in affected patients.[72] It is likely that the defect involves renal handling of phosphate which may or may not be related to abnormal vitamin D metabolism.

Treatment with massive doses of vitamin D (*e.g.* 50,000 to 100,000 IU daily) gives quite variable results.[73] Some investigators have reported better success by using lower amounts of vitamin D (*e.g.* 15,000 to 50,000 IU daily) in conjunction with oral phosphate supplements.[74]

Recently 25-HCC has been used in the treatment of vitamin D-refractory rickets. The dosages required are much less than vitamin D_3. A response can be obtained with as little as 10,000 IU daily in some patients, while others have not responded to doses of 25,000 IU daily.[75a,b] The 25-HCC is therefore more effective as a therapeutic drug and is much safer to use because it is more rapidly eliminated than vitamin D_3.

HYPOPARATHYROIDISM

Hypoparathyroidism usually occurs from the injury or accidental removal of the glands during surgical operations. Idiopathic hypo-parathyroidism is uncommon. This rare disease frequently persists with major convulsive seizures in addition to tetanic spasms. Such patients have often had years of anticonvulsant therapy before the underlying pathologic condition is detected. In this context it is interesting that the long-term use of anticonvulsant drugs apparently accelerates the metabolic breakdown of vitamin D.[76,77]

Hypoparathyroidism is usually treated with high doses of dihydrotachysterol or vitamin D_2. Dihydrotachysterol is reported to be the more active compound on a weight basis.[77] Occasionally hypoparathyroid patients develop a resistance to treatment with vitamin D and dihydrotachysterol, necessitating the search for derivatives which may be more active. To date 25-HCC[35] and 25-hydroxy-dihydrotachysterol[78,79] have been synthesized and found to be more active than the parent compound in mobilization of bone mineral.

It has recently been suggested that patients with renal failure and resistant rickets show abnormalities in vitamin D metabolism.[71] It is interesting, therefore, that 25-HCC is more effective in the treatment of both D-resistant and uncomplicated hypoparathyroidism[80] in which patients respond to a dose of 2,000 to 25,000 IU daily. However, one patient with moderate renal failure did not respond to 25-HCC treatment. It is possible that 25-HCC requires further metabolism and that one of the resultant metabolites (*e.g.* 1,25-DHCC, synthesized in the kidney) will then act beyond a metabolic block present in vitamin D-resistant hypoparathyroid patients.

PSEUDO VITAMIN D DEFICIENCY

Prader and his associates have described a D-resistant rickets in children which is completely curable with doses of vitamin D ranging from 50,000 to 100,000 IU daily.[81] A lower level of 25-HCC (*i.e.* 6,000 to 10,000 IU/day) effects a similar cure.[75b] The pseudo deficiency differs from familial hypophosphatemia in that the latter does not respond completely to vitamin D. Several children suffering from this disease have responded to

6,000 to 24,000 IU 25-HCC daily.[75b] Again this disease is not a simple block in 25-hydroxylation of vitamin D, although 25-HCC is a more satisfactory therapeutic agent.

AZOTEMIC CHRONIC RENAL FAILURE

Patients suffering from chronic renal failure often present abnormally low intestinal calcium absorption, low plasma calcium, secondary hyperparathyroidism and an osteodystrophy.[82,83] Such patients have features of both osteitis fibrosa cystica and/or osteomalacia. They are resistant to vitamin D and show abnormal vitamin D metabolism.[84] These patients respond satisfactorily to 10,000 IU/day of 25-HCC as compared to much larger doses of vitamin D.[85] Recently it has been shown that renal tissue is responsible for the further metabolism of 25-HCC to 1,25-DHCC,[55] the probable metabolically active form of vitamin D in the intestine. It is attractive to consider that, in chronic renal disease, 1,25-DHCC is not made in sufficient amounts and thus a "vitamin D"-deficient intestine results. The resulting hypocalcemia brings about secondary hyperparathyroidism and osteodystrophy. The 1,25-DHCC satisfactorily restores calcium absorption in nephrectomized rats to normal (I. Boyle, L. Miravet, and H. F. DeLuca, unpublished results). Therefore, 1,25-DHCC or a closely related compound should be of obvious benefit in this disease.

Other bone diseases may also be of interest in regard to vitamin D metabolism. The vitamin D resistance of such diseases as hepatic rickets and Fanconi syndrome makes the investigation into the use of vitamin D metabolites for the treatment of such illnesses an exciting area of clinical investigation.

HYPERVITAMINOSIS D (VITAMIN D TOXICITY)

Care should be taken when using large doses of vitamin D to detect any increase in serum calcium which could be indicative of hypercalcemia. Irreversible renal damage is

known to result from prolonged hypercalcemia. However, the detected increase in
serum calcium need not exceed the often
quoted physiological limit of 11 mg/100 ml in
order to prompt renal damage.[72]

Treatment in mild cases consists of withdrawing vitamin D until serum calcium falls,
which necessitates the readministration of
vitamin D, usually at a reduced level. More
severe cases may require the use of glucocorticoids.[86] Calcitonin may also be occasionally used in the treatment of hypervitaminosis D[87] when it becomes available
for clinical use.

In summary, the mode of action for vitamin D is becoming increasingly clear due to
the recent discovery of several metabolites
which differ from the parent vitamin by
containing specific additional hydroxyl functions. Vitamin D is first hydroxylated in the
liver to 25-HCC, which represents the major
circulating form of the vitamin in blood.
Further hydroxylation of 25-HCC to 1,25-
DHCC occurs in the kidney. It is the latter
compound which acts directly on the intestine
to enhance intestinal calcium absorption.
To date, both 25-HCC and 1,25-DHCC
promote bone mineral mobilization.

The realization that vitamin D serves only
as a precursor for the synthesis of active
metabolites suggests that some vitamin D-related diseases may involve a blockage in the
production of the active form(s) of the vitamin. Although 25-HCC is more active than
vitamin D in several disease states, a complete
cure is not observed. Possibly, correction of
such disease may require a further metabolite
of 25-HCC (*e.g.* 1,25-DHCC). Clinical testing of 1,25-DHCC is about to begin and
should provide valuable information concerning possible metabolic blocks.

BIBLIOGRAPHY

1. Griffenhagen: Bull. Natl. Inst. Nutr., *2*, No. 9, 1952.
2. Bennett: *Treatise on the Oleum Jecoris Aselli or Cod-Liver Oil*, Edinburgh, 1848.
3. Palm: The Practitioner, *45*, 270, 1890.
4. Mellanby: J. Physiol., *52*, Liii, 1919.
5. McCollum, Simonds, Becker and Shipley: J. Biol. Chem., *53*, 293, 1922.
6. ———: Bull. Johns Hopkins Hosp., *33*, 229, 1922.
7. Steenbock and Black: J. Biol. Chem., *61*, 405, 1924.
8. Steenbock: Science, *60*, 224, 1924.
9. Askew, Bourdillon, Bruce, Jenkins and Webster: Proc. Roy. Soc., *B107*, 76, 1931.
10. Windaus, Schenck, and Von Werder: Hoppe-Seyler's Z. Physiol. Chem., *241*, 100, 1936.
11. Bernstein, Oleson, Ritter and Sax: J. Am. Chem. Soc., *71*, 2576, 1949.
12. Bernstein and Sax: J. Org. Chem., *16*, 685, 1951.
13. Parfitt: Aust. Ann. Med., *16*, 114, 1967.
14. Panalaks: Internat. J. Vit. Res., *39*, 426, 1969.
15. *U.S. Pharmacopoeia*, 15th revision, U.S.P. XV, p. 889, Easton, Pa., Mack Publishing Co., 1955.
16. Association of Official Analytical Chemists, Horwitz, ed. Box 540, Benjamin Franklin Station, Washington, D.C.
17. Thompson, Lewis and Booth: J. Clin. Invest., *45*, 94, 1966.
18. Schachter, Finkelstein, and Kowarski: J. Clin. Invest., *43*, 787, 1964.
19. Blomstrand and Forsgren: Acta Chem. Scand., *21*, 1662, 1967.
20. Ponchon and DeLuca: J. Clin. Invest., *48*, 1273, 1969.
21. Rikkers and DeLuca: Am. J. Physiol., *213*, 380, 1967.
22. Avioli, Williams, Lund and DeLuca: J. Clin. Invest., *46*, 1907, 1967.
23. National Research Council, Food and Nutrition Board, *Recommended Dietary Allowances*, Washington, D.C., revised 1968.
24. National Research Council, Food and Nutrition Board, *Maternal Nutrition and Child Health*, Bull. 123, Washington D.C., 1950 (reprinted 1957).
25. Fraser and Salter: Ped. Clin. N. A., p. 417, 1958.
26. Fomon, Younozai and Thomas: J. Nutr., *89*, 345, 1966.
27. Fellers and Schwartz: New Eng. J. Med., *259*, 1050, 1958.
28. Anning, Dawson, Dolby and Ingram: Quart. J. Med., *17*, 203, 1948.
29. Hess and Lewis: J.A.M.A., *91*, 783, 1928.
30. Gardner: Pediatrics, *9*, 534, 1952.
31. Bruce and Callow: Biochem. J., *28*, 517, 1934.
32. Mellanby and Mellanby: Brit. Med. J., *2*, 409, 1948.
33. Higaki, Takahashi, Suzuki and Sahashi: J. Vitaminol., *11*, 261, 1956.
34. Lund, DeLuca, and Horsting: Arch. Biochem. Biophys., *120*, 513, 1967.
35. Blunt, DeLuca, and Schnoes: Biochemistry, *7*, 3317, 1968.
36. Suda, DeLuca, Schnoes, Ponchon, Tanaka and Holick: Biochemistry, *9*, 2917, 1970.
37. Suda, DeLuca, Schnoes, Tanaka and Holick: Biochemistry, *9*, 4776, 1970.
38. Holick, DeLuca and Schnoes: Proc. Nat. Acad. Sci. USA, *68*, 803, 1971.
39. Holick, Schnoes, DeLuca, Suda and Cousins: Biochemistry, *10*, 2799, 1971.
40. Sherwood, Mayer, Ramberg, Kronfield, Aurbach and Potts: Endocrinology, *83*, 1043, 1968.

41. Raisz: J. Clin. Invest., *44*, 103, 1965.
42. Rasmussen, DeLuca, Arnaud, Hawker and Von Stedingk: J. Clin. Invest., *42*, 1940, 1963.
43. Lifshitz, Harrison and Harrison: Endocrinology, *84*, 912, 1969.
44. Wase, Peterson, Rickes and Solewski: Endocrinology, *79*, 687, 1966.
45. Aliapoulios, Goldhaber and Munson: Science, *151*, 330, 1966.
46. Hirsch, Voelkel, and Munson: Science, *146*, 412, 1964.
47. Morii and DeLuca: Am. J. Physiol., *213*, 358, 1967.
48. Harrison, Harrison and Lifshitz: In Talmage and Belanger (eds.), Proceedings of the Third Parathyroid Conference, Montreal, Excerpta Medica Foundation, Amsterdam, p. 455, 1968.
49. Raisz: Arch. Intern. Med., *126*, 887 1970.
50. Krane, J.A.M.A., *78*, 472, 1961.
51. Kimberg, Schachter, and Schenker: Am. J. Physiol., *200*, 1256, 1961.
52a. Wasserman and Taylor: J. Biol. Chem., *243*, 3987, 1968.
52b. Bronner and Maddaiah: Discussion In: *Symposium on Membrane Proteins*, Boston, Little, Brown and Co., p. 134–136, 1969.
53. Nicolaysen: Acta Physiol. Scand., *5*, 200, 1943.
54. ———: Biochem. J., *31*, 323, 1937.
55. Martin and DeLuca: Arch. Biochem. Biophys., *134*, 139, 1969.
56. Schachter, Kowarski, Finkelstein and Ma: Am. J. Physiol., *211*, 1131, 1966.
57. Martin and DeLuca: Am. J. Physiol., *216*, 1351, 1969.
58. Harrison and Harrison: Am. J. Physiol., *208*, 370, 1965.
59. Wasserman, Taylor and Kallfelz: Am. J. Physiol., *211*, 419, 1966.
60. Fraser and Kodicek: Nature, *228*, 765, 1971.
61. Wasserman, Corradino and Taylor: J. Biol. Chem., *243*, 3978, 1968.
62. Drescher and DeLuca: Biochemistry, *10*, 2302, 1971.
63. Zull, Czarnowska-Misztal and DeLuca: Proc. Natl. Acad. Sci. USA, *55*, 177, 1966.
64. Corradino and Wasserman: Proc. Soc. Exptl. Biol. Med., *133*, 960, 1970.
65. Tanaka, DeLuca, Omdahl and Holick: Proc. Natl. Acad. Sci. USA, *68*, 1286, 1971.
66. Melancon and DeLuca: Biochemistry, *9*, 1658, 1970.
67. Adams, Wong and Norman: J. Biol. Chem., *245*, 4432, 1970.
68. Harrison and Harrison: Yale J. Biol. Med., *24*, 273, 1952.
69. ———: Am. J. Physiol., *199*, 265, 1960.
70. Fanconi and Girardet: Helvet. Paediat. Acta, *7*, 14, 1952.
71. Avioli, Williams, Lund and DeLuca: J. Clin. Invest., *46*, 1907, 1967.
72. Yendt, DeLuca, Garcia and Cohanim: In: DeLuca and Suttie (eds), *The Fat Soluble Vitamins*, Madison, University of Wisconsin Press, p. 125, 1969.
73. Harrison: J. Pediat. *64*, 618, 1964.
74. Wilson, York, Jaworski and Yendt: Medicine, *44*, 99, 1965.
75a. Yendt: personal communication.
75b. Balsan and Garabedian: J. Clin. Invest., *51*, 749, 1972.
76. Rickens and Rowe: British Med. J., *4*, 73, 1970.
77. Harrison, Lifshitz and Blizzard: New Eng. J. Med., *276*, 894, 1967.
78. Hallick and DeLuca: J. Biol. Chem., *246*, 5733, 1971.
79. Suda, Hallick, DeLuca and Schnoes: Biochemistry, *9*, 1651, 1970.
80. Pak, DeLuca, Chavez de los Rios, Suda, Ruskin and Delea: Arch. Int. Med., *126*, 239, 1970.
81. Prader, Illig and Heierli: Helv. Paediat. Acta, *16*, 452, 1961.
82. Stanbury and Lumb: Medicine, *41*, 1, 1962.
83. Kimberg, Baerg and Gershon: Arch. Int. Med., *126*, 891, 1970.
84. Avioli, Birge, Lee and Slatopolsky: J. Clin. Invest., *47*, 2239, 1968.
85. DeLuca and Avioli: Arch. Intern. Med., *126*, 896, 1970.
86. Connor, Hopkins, Thomas, Carey and Howard: J. Clin. Endocrinol., *16*, 945, 1956.
87. Milhaud: In Talmage and Belanger (eds.), *Parathyroid Hormone and Thyrocalcitonin (Calcitonin)*, Proceedings of the Third Parathyroid Conference, New York, Excerpta Medica Foundation, p. 86, 1968.

Chapter

5

Section C   Vitamin K

Robert. E. Olson

INTRODUCTION

While studying cholesterol biosynthesis in chicks fed a fat-extracted diet, Dam in 1929[1] observed an unexpected hemorrhagic disease. He soon demonstrated that the hemorrhagic disease was due to a deficiency of a previously unrecognized fat-soluble substance in the diet. This factor was not identical with any known lipid or the then known fat-soluble vitamins A, D, and E, and was found to be broadly distributed in the plant kingdom, particularly in green leafy vegetables. Dam christened the new substance "vitamin K" for *Koagulation*

vitamin. McFarland *et al.* in 1931[2] confirmed Dam's finding and reported that fishmeal was a source of the new vitamin K.

Efforts were then initiated to attempt to isolate the new factor from both alfalfa and fishmeal, the vitamin K content of which was greatly increased by intentional putrefaction.[3] In 1939, Doisy and his colleagues[4] and Dam and his colleagues[5] announced the isolation of vitamin K from alfalfa. In addition, Doisy's group reported the isolation of a related but not identical vitamin K from putrefied fishmeal.[6] They named these compounds "vitamins K_1 and K_2."

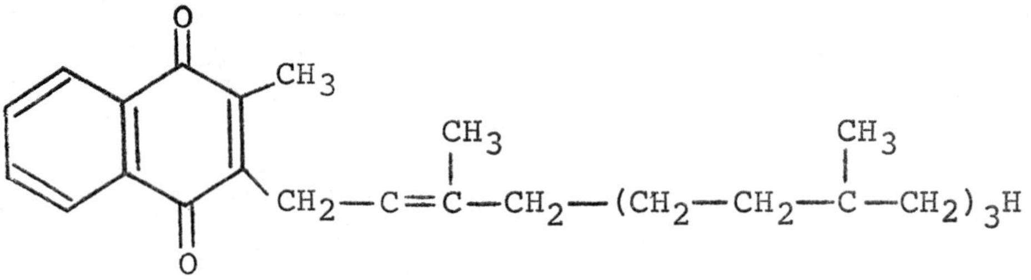

Phylloquinone (Vitamin K_1)

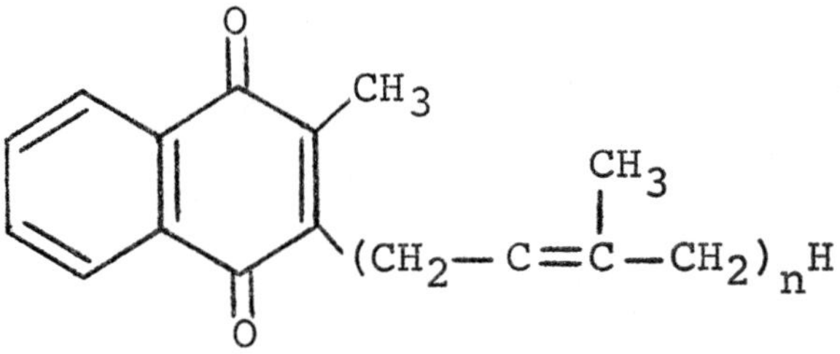

Menaquinone-n (MK-n, Vitamins K_2)

Fig. 5C-1

166

CHEMISTRY OF THE K VITAMINS

Vitamin K_1, now known as phylloquinone, was identified by Doisy's group[7] as 2-methyl-3-phytyl-1,4-naphthoquinone; shown in Figure 5C–1. It is the only homologue of vitamin K synthesized by plants. Vitamin K_2 isolated from fishmeal was originally believed to be 2-methyl-3-difarnesyl-1,4-naphthoquinone,[8] but has since been shown to have 7 isoprene units in the side chain instead of 6, and is now called menaquinone-7.[9] Traces of MK-6 were also found. The menaquinone family of vitamin K_2 homologues is a large series of vitamins containing unsaturated side chains, which differ in the number of isoprenyl units. Menaquinone-4 is synthesized in animals and birds from menadione (2-methyl-1,4-naphthoquinone),[10] formerly known as vitamin K_3, by alkylation with digeranyl-pyrophosphate. The enzyme has been partially purified and characterized from chick and rat liver microsomes.[11] The other menaquinones are products of bacterial biosynthesis and range from menaquinone-6 to menaquinone-13.[12,13] Partially saturated menaquinones, menaquinone-9-H[14] and menaquinone-8-H,[15] are known.

ESTIMATION OF VITAMIN K

Except for vitamin K-rich foods, vitamin K is present in animal and plant tissues in concentrations less than 1 μg/gm of fresh weight. Such a low concentration makes chemical determinations difficult, particularly since all the vitamin K homologues are labile to alkali and light. Extraction of desiccated tissue with neutral solvents, followed by column and thin-layer chromatography, has resulted in the isolation of a variety of vitamin K homologues from various tissues.[16,17] When purified in sufficient quantity, the vitamin Ks can be identified by a distinctive absorption spectrum: the molecular extinction coefficient at 248 mμ being 19,000.

The most commonly used technique for measuring the vitamin K content of foods is the chick bioassay, which is sensitive to 0.1 μg phylloquinone/gm of diet. Chicks made deficient in vitamin K, by feeding a vitamin K-free diet for 10 days, are then fed a supplement containing the assay food. The pro-thrombin level of the blood is then compared with a standard curve resulting from the feeding of known amounts of phylloquinone.[18,19]

THE VITAMIN K CONTENT OF FOODS

The vitamin K content of common foods as determined by bioassay in chicks is presented in Table 5C–1. In general, green leafy vegetables are high, fruits and cereals are low, and meats and dairy products intermediate. These bioassays were done on an "as is" basis, without extraction, which, in the instances of green vegetables, gave less than the actual content of vitamin K_1. In fact, the intestinal absorption of vitamin K from plant sources ranges from 30 to 70 per cent of the actual content determined by extraction. It appears that tobacco is one of the richest sources of phylloquinone known. It contains about 5 mg per 100 gm, a small percentage of which is volatilized in smoking and absorbed through the mucous membranes of the nasopharynx and bronchi.[20]

ABSORPTION, DISTRIBUTION, AND METABOLISM OF VITAMIN K

The absorption of phylloquinone and the menaquinones requires bile and pancreatic juice for maximum effectiveness.[21] These alkylated lipid-soluble homologues are incorporated into chylomicrons and appear in the lymph.[22] Efficiency of absorption has been measured from 10 to 70 per cent, depending upon the vehicle in which the vitamin is administered and the extent of the entero-hepatic circulation generally characteristic of isoprenoid lipids. When isotopically labeled phylloquinone was administered by mouth in doses ranging from the physiological to the pharmacological to animals[23] and man,[24] the vitamin appeared in the plasma within 20 minutes and peaked in the plasma at 2 hours. It then declined exponentially to low values over a period of 48 to 72 hours. During this period, it appeared to be transferred from the chylomicrons to the β-lipoproteins. Between 8 and 30 per cent of the administered radioactivity was recovered in the urine

Table 5C-1.   Average Vitamin K Content of Some Ordinary Foods*

Food	Vitamin K μg/100 gm	Food	Vitamin K μg/100 gm
Milk & Milk Products		*Vegetables*	
Milk (Cows)	3	Asparagus	57
Cheese	35	Beans, Green	14
Butter	30	Broccoli	200
		Cabbage	125
		Lettuce	129
Eggs		Peas, Green	19
		Spinach	89
Hens (Whole)	11	Turnip Greens	650
		Potato	3
		Pumpkin	2
Meat & Meat Products		Tomato	5
		Watercress	57
Ground Beef	7		
Beef Liver	92		
Ham	15	*Fruits*	
Pork Tenderloin	11		
Chicken Liver	7	Applesauce	2
Pork Liver	25	Banana	2
Bacon	46	Orange	1
		Peach	8
		Raisins	6
Fats		Strawberries	—
Corn Oil	10		
Safflower Oil	—	*Beverages*	
		Coffee	38
Cereals & Grain Products		Cola	2
		Tea, Green	712
Rice	—	Tea, Black	—
Maize	5		
Whole Wheat	17		
Wheat Flour	4		
Bread	4		
Oats	20		

* Data taken from the studies of Dam and Glavind,[18] Richardson[91] and Doisy.[20]

over a 3-day period in both animals and man, whereas total fecal radioactivity accounted for 45 to 60 per cent of the administered dose over a 5-day period. About one third of this was unchanged vitamin K_1. The administration of non-absorbable lipids, such as mineral oil or squalene, greatly reduced the absorption of vitamin K in animals.[25]

As much as 50 per cent of a parenterally administered dose of vitamin K_1 may appear in the liver within 1 hour. After oral administration, the liver may contain as much as 20 per cent of the administered dose

in 2 hours, which then declines to low values after 24 hours. The relative concentration of vitamin K in kidney, heart, skin, and muscle increased to maximum values over a 24-hour period, and then declined. The principal sites of uptake, after liver, were skin and muscle. Fractionation of liver tissue, after the administration of phylloquinone-^{3}H to rats, showed the following relative distribution of radioactivity: nuclei, 13 per cent; mitochondria, 9 per cent; microsomes, 63 per cent and cytosol, 14 per cent.[26] In omnivorous animals, like man, both phylloquinone

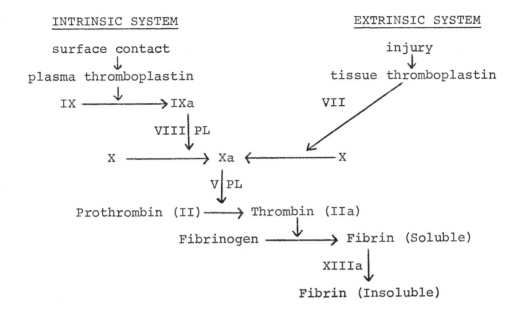

Fig. 5C-2. Factors II, prothrombin; VII, proconvertin; IX, Christmas factor; and X, Stuart-Prower factor are vitamin K-dependent and occupy the core of the clotting scheme. Factor V is acceleration globulin; factor VIII is antihemophilic globulin; factor XIII is fibrin-stabilizing factor, a transpeptidase; PL is phospholipid; factor a is active enzyme.

and the higher molecular weight menaquinones (MK-7 to MK-13) of bacterial origin, and most likely derived from intestinal flora, are found in the liver.[27,28]

Wiss et al.[29] observed that the principal excretory form of vitamin K in rat urine was a metabolite resembling the lactone of vitamin E first described by Simon, Gross and Milhorat.[30] It was identified as a chain-shortened and oxidized derivative of vitamin K, which forms a gamma-lactone and is probably excreted as a glucuronide. Vitamin K oxide has also been identified as a metabolite of vitamin K in rats.[31]

When menadione (2-methyl-1,4-naphthoquinone) is administered to animals or man, only a small percentage (0.05 to 1.0 per cent) is converted to an active vitamin, menaquinone-4.[32-34] The principal metabolites of menadione are the sulfate and glucuronide of dihydromenadione.[35] Menadione also reacts with free sulfhydryl groups in proteins to form a thioether linkage, first described by Fieser,[36] which may account for some of its reported toxicity.[37]

PHYSIOLOGICAL FUNCTION OF VITAMIN K

Shortly after the discovery of vitamin K, Dam et al.[38] demonstrated that the anticoagulant effect of vitamin K deficiency in the chick was due to a reduction in the content of plasma prothrombin. Subsequently, it was learned that three other coagulation proteins, factor VII,[39] factor IX[40] and factor X,[41] were also regulated by vitamin K. An abbreviated clotting scheme depicting the proteolytic cascade hypothesis proposed by Biggs and McFarlane[42] and by Davie and Ratnoff,[43] and showing the role of the vitamin K-dependent factors, is shown in Figure 5C-2.

The four vitamin K-dependent coagulation factors are distributed in the extrinsic system, which is activated by injury, the intrinsic system, which is activated by platelets, and the final common pathway leading to the conversion of fibrinogen to fibrin. In deficient animals or man, the administration of vitamin K brings about a prompt response and return toward normal of depressed coagulation factors in 4 to 6 hours. In the absence of the liver, this response does not occur.[44] Various ideas about the mode of action of vitamin K at the molecular level have been proposed, including the idea that vitamin K might be a part of the prothrombin molecule, that vitamin K might indirectly effect protein synthesis by depressing ATP synthesis and electron transport[45] or that vitamin K might function as a coenzyme for the enzyme "involved in the synthesis of prothrombin."[46]

Real insight into the mode of action of vitamin K in stimulating the synthesis of these factors by the liver was not available until general advances were made in the understanding of the molecular biology of protein synthesis.[47] In 1961, Jacob and Monod[48] proposed a scheme for the induction of protein synthesis in bacteria which postulated the existence of regulatory genes whose products were repressor proteins capable of interacting with DNA and regulating the expression of genetic information. The possibility that vitamin K could act as an effector in the Jacob and Monod model was explored first by Olson,[49] who indeed found that actinomycin D, administered 4 hours prior to vitamin K, could block the action of the vitamin in stimulating the appearance of prothrombin in the blood of vitamin K-deficient chicks over a 6-hour period. Subsequently, Olson found[50] that the degree of inhibition of the action of vitamin K by actinomycin D varied with the time of administration of the antibiotic and that puromycin was a more effective blocker for vitamin K-induced prothrombin synthesis than actinomycin D in vitamin K-deficient chicks.[51] Olson proposed that regulatory control by vitamin K was most likely exercised at the level of translation, a view also proposed independently by B. C. Johnson and his group.[52,53] The demonstration by Barnhart and Anderson[54] that liver cells of dogs treated with a vitamin K antagonist, Dicumarol, were devoid of prothrombin by the immunofluorescent antibody technique, and that the administration of vitamin K gave a prompt appearance of immunofluorescence in hepatocytes speaks for the primary role of vitamin K in stimulating the synthesis of prothrombin. Olson and his colleagues[55] demonstrated that vitamin K stimulated the synthesis of radioactive prothrombin by the isolated perfused liver in the presence of radioactive leucine.

Many lines of study in the intact animals, isolated perfused liver, and isolated microsomes, however,[53,56,57] have shown that there is no change in general protein synthesis in vitamin K deficiency or in coumarin drug-induced anticoagulant states in vivo. The action of vitamin K appears thus to be confined to the control of the synthesis of vitamin K-dependent proteins only. Johnston and Olson,[58,59] furthermore, were able to identify both radioactive prothrombin and serum albumin in sonicates of light hepatic microsomes after incubation with radioactive L-leucine-1-^{14}C, using specific antibody to precipitate the newly synthesized proteins. The microsomes from vitamin K-deficient rats, vitamin K-deficient rats treated with vitamin K and normal rats treated with the anticoagulant warfarin were studied for their capacity to synthesize prothrombin in vitro. Both vitamin K-deficient and coumarin-antagonized rats demonstrated negligible synthesis of prothrombin, although their total protein and albumin synthesis were within normal limits. The microsomes of vitamin K-deficient rats given vitamin K showed much better incorporation of L-leucine-U-^{14}C into prothrombin than did normal rats.

These data strongly suggest that vitamin K regulates the synthesis of vitamin K-dependent coagulation proteins at the ribosomal level.[60,61] Conflicting effects of inhibitors of protein synthesis upon the action of vitamin K in whole animals have led to some unnecessary controversy.[62-64]

COUMARIN ANTICOAGULANT DRUGS

A hemorrhagic disease in cattle which had consumed spoiled clover was described by Schofield[65] in 1922 and attributed to a depressed prothrombin level in 1931.[66] In 1941, Link and his associates[67] demonstrated that the active agent in spoiled clover was

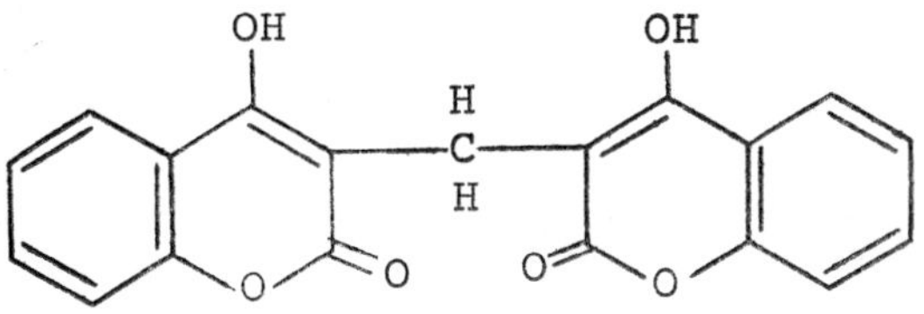

DICUMAROL

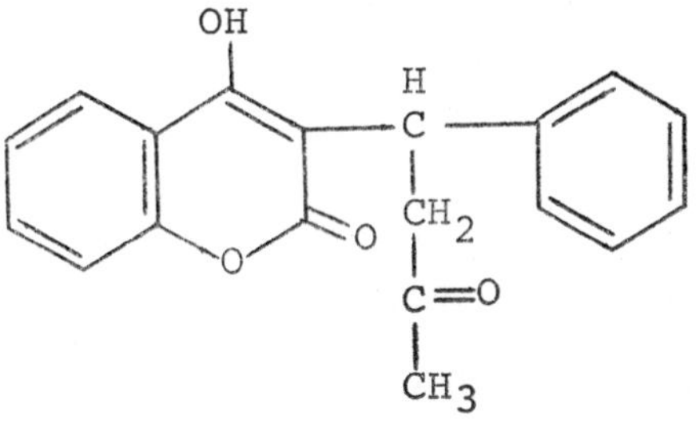

WARFARIN

Fig. 5C-3.

bishydroxycoumarin (Dicumarol). A variety of related compounds, either derivatives of 4-hydroxy-coumarin or phenindandione, have been synthesized and tested for anticoagulant activity in animals and man. One of the more popular ones in the U.S. is warfarin (3-(α-acetonylbenzyl)-4-hydroxycoumarin), which is more soluble than Dicumarol. Their structures are shown in Figure 5C-3.

The oral anticoagulant agents regulate the biosynthesis of prothrombin (factor II) and factors VII, IX and X in the liver. They also induce hypoprothrombinemia at the same rate when given in saturating doses, even though the half-life of various drugs varies from hours to days. As soon as there is an effective concentration of the drug, prothrombin biosynthesis by liver is shut off and the factors then decay in plasma at their specific half-lives.[68] Hydroxylated products of these drugs, generated by the enzymes in the liver microsomes, are inactive.

There is presently a controversy on the mode of antagonism of the coumarin drugs and vitamin K. Some believe that the interaction is competitive at some common site on a regulatory protein or enzyme involved in prothrombin synthesis[46,69] and others feel that the kinetics are not competitive[68,70,71] and are probably allosteric.[72]

The likelihood that vitamin K and the coumarin anticoagulant drugs combine allosterically with a single regulatory protein concerned with prothrombin synthesis is consistent with the discovery of O'Reilly et al.[73] of a kindred of genetically determined resistance to the anticoagulant action of coumarin drugs. The genetic defect may be a reduced affinity of the regulatory protein for coumarin drugs. Responsiveness to vitamin K in these patients was normal. A related group of coumarin-resistant rats[69,74,75] appears to have a high resistance to coumarin drugs and a slightly increased vitamin K requirement, suggesting that the mutant protein in the rat may have altered sites for both coumarin and vitamin K.

When overdosage with coumarin drugs occurs in patients who are anticoagulated to prevent thrombosis (coronary artery disease, pulmonary embolic disease), the intravenous administration of pharmacologic doses of vitamin K_1 in the milligram range reinitiates prothrombin synthesis within minutes, gives protective levels of prothrombin within hours and normal values in 24 hours. Water-soluble derivatives of menadione (e.g. Synkavite) are largely ineffective against the coumarin anticoagulant drugs because, as previously mentioned, the rate of conversion to menaquinone-4 is so slow that pharmacologically effective levels of the alkylated vitamin are not attained.[76,77]

VITAMIN K DEFICIENCY

Primary vitamin K deficiency is uncommon in man. This is due to the widespread distribution of vitamin K in plant and animal tissues and to the microbiologic flora of the normal gut, which synthesize the menaquinones in amounts that may supply the bulk of the requirement for vitamin K.

Newborn infants represent a special case of vitamin K nutrition because (1) the placenta is a relatively poor organ for the transmission of lipids and (2) the gut is sterile during the first few days. In normal infants, the plasma prothrombin concentration may decrease to as low as 20 per cent in the second and third days of life, and then gradually climb to normal adult values over a period of weeks. If values fall below 10 per cent, hemorrhagic disease of the newborn may occur.[78] Both water-soluble and lipid-soluble forms of vitamin K are effective in restoring prothrombin levels and controlling hemorrhage in these infants.[79,80] The advisability of giving vitamin K routinely to expectant mothers is controversial.[81,82]

Healthy adult subjects fed low vitamin K diets (less than 20 μg per day) for periods of several weeks show minimal signs of vitamin K deficiency, i.e., plasma prothrombin values of 60 to 90 per cent, unless they are also given bowel-sterilizing antibiotics, such as neomycin.[20,83,84] In one study, intravenous nutrition of apoplectic patients plus neomycin was required to lower the vitamin K-dependent clotting factors to below 20 per cent of normal[84] in 4 weeks. The intravenous administration of vitamin K in various doses, from 0.03 to 1.5 μg/kg, to these patients caused a proportional rise in the concentration of these depressed values to normal.

Udall[83] showed that large amounts of vitamin K (of the order of 500 mg/day) instilled into the cecum did not elevate depressed coagulation factors in anticoagulated patients, whereas the same dose given orally gave a prompt response. It appears that the microorganisms synthesizing vitamin K in the gut must reside in the ileum, where absorption of vitamin K is possible. In unusual cases, self-imposed dietary restriction has been observed to induce hypoprothrombinemia with hemorrhage responsive to oral vitamin K.[85,86]

Any disorder that hinders the delivery of bile to the small bowel, such as obstructive jaundice or bile fistula, reduces the absorption of vitamin K from the bowel, and causes a reduction in plasma concentration of the vitamin K-dependent factors that can be prevented or relieved by the administration of parenteral vitamin K, or oral vitamin K plus bile salts. Malabsorption syndromes associated with sprue, pellagra, bowel shunts, regional ileitis, and ulcerative colitis also cause a secondary vitamin K deficiency.[87]

In chronic liver disease, hypoprothrombinemia with bleeding may occur because of lack of functional hepatic ribosomes to respond to vitamin K.

NUTRITIONAL REQUIREMENTS FOR VITAMIN K

The vitamin K requirement of mammals is met by a combination of dietary intake and microbiological biosynthesis in the gut. Furthermore, there are, no doubt, genetic factors which influence the vitamin K requirement in both animals and man. In conventional rats, the vitamin K requirement is about 10 μg/kg/day, whereas in germ-free rats, the requirement is more than doubled to about 25 μg/kg/day.[88]

In human subjects, the vitamin K homologues stored in the liver suggest that about 40 to 50 per cent of the daily requirement is derived from plant sources, i.e. vitamin K_1, and the remainder from microbiological biosynthesis. Rietz, Gloor and Wiss[28] reported that 50 per cent of the vitamin K of human liver was vitamin K_1 and the remainder a mixture of MK-7, MK-8, MK-9, MK-10, and MK-11.

If one assumes that the intravenous dose of vitamin K required to raise depressed vitamin K to normal for 1 day is 1 μg/kg,[84] and that 50 per cent of the vitamin K appearing in the lumen of the gut each day is absorbed, the total daily requirement for the vitamin would be 2 μg/kg per day. If, on the other hand, one assumes that 50 per cent of the requirement is derived from intestinal microorganisms, then the dietary requirement would be reduced again to 1 μg/kg per day. With the information at hand, this is a rough estimate, particularly since there is controversy on the relative activity of phylloquinone and the menaquinones in stimulating prothrombin synthesis.[89,90] From the dietary information presented in Table 5C-1, one can calculate that a "normal mixed diet" in the U.S. will contain from 300 to 500 μg of vitamin K per day, an amount more than adequate to supply the dietary requirement for vitamin K.

BIBLIOGRAPHY

1. Dam: Biochem. Zeit., *215*, 475, 1929.
2. McFarland, Graham and Richardson: Biochem. J., *25*, 358, 1931.
3. Almquist and Stokstad: J. Nutr., *12*, 329, 1936.
4. Binkley, MacCorquodale, Thayer and Doisy: J. Biol. Chem., *130*, 219, 1939.
5. Dam, Geiger, Glavind, Karrer, Karrer, Rothchild and Salomon: Helv. Chim. Acta, *22*, 310, 1939.
6. McKee, Binkley, Thayer, MacCorquodale, and Doisy: J. Biol. Chem., *131*, 327, 1939.
7. Binkley, Cheney, Holcomb, McKee, Thayer, MacCorquodale and Doisy: J. Am. Chem. Soc., *61*, 2558, 1939.
8. Binkley, McKee, Thayer and Doisy: J. Biol. Chem., *133*, 721, 1940.
9. Isler, Rüegg, Chopard-dit-Jean, Winterstein and Wiss: Helv. Chim. Acta, *41*, 786, 1958.
10. Martius and Esser: Biochem. Zeit., *331*, 1, 1958.
11. Dialameh, Yekundi and Olson: Biochim. Biophys. Acta, *223*, 332, 1970.
12. Matschiner, Taggart and Amelotti: Biochemistry, *6*, 1243, 1967.
13. Pennock: Vitamins and Hormones, *24*, 307, 1966.
14. Gale, Arison, Trenner, Page and Folkers: Biochemistry, *2*, 200, 1963.
15. Scholes and King: Biochem. J., *97*, 766, 1965.
16. Martius: Amer. J. Clin. Nutr., *9*, Part 2, 97, 1961.
17. Matschiner and Taggart: Anal. Biochem., *18*, 88, 1967.
18. Dam and Glavind: Biochem. J., *32*, 485, 1938.
19. Matschiner and Doisy: J. Nutr., *90*, 97, 1966.
20. Doisy: Unpublished work.
21. Mann, Mann and Bollman: Amer. J. Physiol., *158*, 311, 1949.
22. Blomstrand and Forsgren: Internat. J. Vit. Res., *38*, 45, 1968.
23. Wiss and Gloor: Vitamins and Hormones, *24*, 575, 1966.
24. Shearer, Barkhan and Webster: Brit. J. Haematol., *18*, 297, 1970.
25. Matschiner, Hsia and Doisy: J. Nutr., *91*, 299, 1967.
26. Bell and Matschiner: Biochim. Biophys. Acta, *184*, 597, 1969.
27. Matschiner and Amelotti: J. Lipid Res., *9*, 176, 1968.
28. Rietz, Gloor and Wiss: Internat. J. Vit. Res., *40*, 351, 1970.
29. Wiss and Gloor: Vitamins and Hormones, *24*, 575, 1966.
30. Simon, Gross and Milhorat: J. Biol. Chem., *221*, 797, 1956.
31. Matschiner, Bell, Amelotti and Knauer: Biochem. Biophys. Acta, *201*, 309, 1970.
32. Billeter, Bolliger and Martius: Biochem. Zeit., *340*, 290 1964.
33. Taggart and Matschiner: Biochemistry, *8*, 1141, 1969.
34. Dialameh, Taggart, Matschiner and Olson: Internat. J. Vit. Nutr. Res., *41*, 391, 1971.
35. Losito, Owen and Flock: Biochemistry, *6*, 62, 1967.
36. Fieser and Turner: J. Amer. Chem. Soc., *69*, 2335, 1947.
37. Mezick and Cornwell: Biochim. Biophys. Acta, *219*, 361, 1970.
38. Dam, Schønheyder and Tage-Hansen: Biochem. J., *30*, 1075, 1936.
39. Owen: Bull. Amer. Coll. Surg., *32*, 256, 1947.
40. Naeye: Proc. Soc. Expt. Biol. Med., *97*, 101, 1956.
41. Hougie, Barrow and Graham: J. Clin. Invest., *36*, 485, 1957.
42. Biggs and McFarlane: *Human Blood Coagulation and Its Disorders*, 3rd Ed., Philadelphia, F. A. Davis Co., 1962.
43. Davie and Ratnoff: Science, *145*, 1310, 1964.
44. Andrus, Lord and Moore: Surgery, *6*, 899, 1939.
45. Martius and Nitz-Litzow: Biochim. Biophys. Acta, *13*, 152, 1954.
46. Quick and Collentine: J. Lab. Clin. Med., *36*, 976, 1950.
47. Crick: Cold Spring Harbor Symposium, Quant. Biol., *31*, 3, 1966.
48. Jacob and Monod: J. Mol. Biol., *3*, 318, 1961.
49. Olson: Science, *145*, 926, 1964.
50. Olson: Canad. J. Biochem., *43*, 1565, 1965.
51. Olson: Adv. Enzym. Reg., *4*, 181, 1966.
52. Johnson, Hill, Alden and Ranhotra: Life Sci., *5*, 385, 1966.
53. Hill, Gaetani, Paolucci, Rama Rao, Alden, Ranhotra, Shah, Shah and Johnson: J. Biol. Chem., *243*, 3930, 1968.
54. Barnhart and Anderson: Biochem. Pharmacol., *9*, 23, 1962.
55. Li, Kipfer and Olson: Arch. Biochem. Biophys., *137*, 494, 1970.
56. Berry, Philipps and Olson: Biochem. Pharmacol., *20*, 853, 1971.
57. Olson, Kipfer and Li: Adv. Enzym. Reg., *7*, 83, 1969.
58. Johnston and Olson: J. Biol. Chem., *247*, 3994, 1972.
59. Johnston and Olson: J. Biol. Chem., *247*, 4001, 1972.
60. Olson: *The Fat-Soluble Vitamins*, 1st Ed., Madison, Wisconsin, The University of Wisconsin Press, p. 463, 1970.
61. Olson: Nutr. Rev., *28*, 171, 1970.
62. Suttie: Arch. Biochem. Biophys., *141*, 571, 1970.
63. Johnson, Martinovic and Johnson: Biochem. Biophys. Res. Commun., *43*, 1040, 1971.
64. Babior: Biochim. Biophys. Acta, *123*, 606, 1966.
65. Schofield: Canad. Vet. Rec., *3*, 74, 1922.
66. Roderick: Am. J. Physiol., *96*, 413, 1931.
67. Campbell, Smith, Roberts and Link: J. Biol. Chem., *138*, 1, 1941.
68. O'Reilly and Aggeler: Pharmacol. Rev., *22*, 35, 1970.
69. Hermodson, Suttie and Link: Amer. J. Physiol., *217*, 1316, 1969.

70. Babson, Malament, Mangun and Phillips: Clin. Chem., *2*, 243, 1956.
71. Woolley: Physiol. Rev., *27*, 308, 1947.
72. Olson, Philipps and Wang: Adv. Enzym. Reg., *6*, 213, 1968.
73. O'Reilly, Aggeler, Hoag, Leong and Kropatkin: New Eng. J. Med., *271*, 809, 1964.
74. Greaves and Ayres: Nature, *215*, 877, 1967.
75. Pool, O'Reilly, Schneiderman and Alexander: Amer. J. Physiol., *215*, 627, 1968.
76. Douglas and Brown: Brit. Med. J., *1*, 412, 1952.
77. Dam: Vitamins and Hormones, *24*, 295, 1966.
78. Brinkhous, Smith and Warner: Amer. J. Med. Sci., *193*, 475, 1937.
79. Dam, Tage-Hansen and Plum: Lancet, *237*, 1157. 1939.
80. Brinkhous: Medicine, *19*, 329, 1940.

81. Potter: Amer. J. Obst. Gynec., *50*, 235, 1945.
82. Webster and Fitzgerald: Surg. Clin. North America, *23*, 85, 1943.
83. Udall: J.A.M.A., *194*, 107, 1965.
84. Frick, Riedler and Brogli: J. Applied Physiol., *23*, 387, 1967.
85. Kark and Lozner: Lancet, *2*, 1162, 1939.
86. Aggeler, Lucia and Fishbon: Amer. J. Dig. Dis., *9*, 227, 1942.
87. Clark, Dixon, Butt and Snell: Mayo Clin. Proc., *14*, 407, 1939.
88. Gustafsson, Daft, McDaniel, Smith and Fitzgerald: J. Nutr., *78*, 461, 1962.
89. Matschiner and Taggart: J. Nutr., *94*, 57, 1968.
90. Isler and Wiss: Vitamins and Hormones, *17*, 53, 1959.
91. Richardson, Wilkes and Ritchey: J. Nutr., *73*, 363, 1961.

Chapter

5

Section D   Vitamin E

M. K. HORWITT

INTRODUCTION

In 1922, Evans and Bishop[1] noted that a fat-soluble factor prevented fetal resorption in animals that had been fed a rancid lard diet. This was confirmed by Mattill *et al.*[2] and designated as vitamin E by Sure[3] in 1924. The term "tocopherol" was proposed by Evans from the Greek word "*tocos*" meaning childbirth or offspring, the Greek noun "*phero*," to bring forth, and "*ol*" for alcohol. The usefulness of the study of fetal resorption as an assay method overwhelmed the significance of the early study of Olcott and Emerson[4] on the antioxidant properties of tocopherol which was amply supported by Moore,[4a] Dam,[5] Filer *et al.*,[6] and others.[7–9] In more recent times, the function of α-tocopherol as an antioxidant of the poly-unsaturated fatty acids in the tissues has been supported by Tappel,[10] Horwitt,[11] Draper,[12] and Witting.[13] That it can also protect coenzyme Q has been claimed by Folkers.[14] Since coenzyme Q is involved in the transfer of electrons, additional studies on this relationship to vitamin E may serve to resolve a current controversy—whether α-tocopherol is an integral part of an enzyme system[15,16] or whether it protects the integrity of the lipid component of enzyme systems or of the cellular structures that produce or support the enzymes. The possibility that vitamin E is both a biological antioxidant and a component of some enzyme systems cannot be precluded.

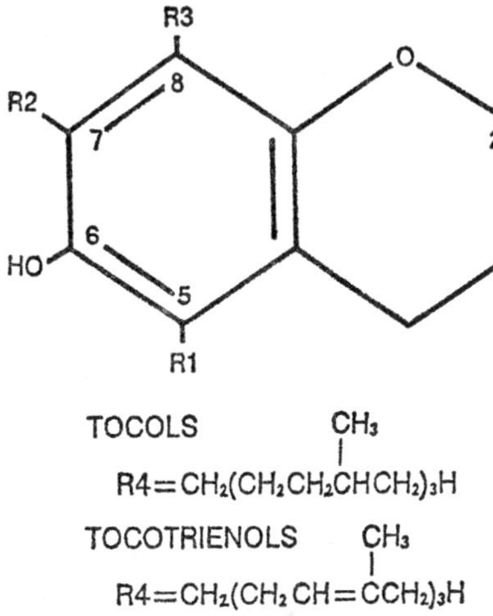

CHEMISTRY

Pure vitamin E was first isolated by Evans and the Emersons[17] from the unsaponifiable fraction of wheat germ oil in 1936. Its chemical structure[18] and synthesis[19] were reported in 1938. Although α-tocopherol is the active compound most often designated as vitamin E, there are seven other naturally occurring tocopherols. These are designated[20] by the number and position of the methyl groups on either the tocol or tocotrienol complex (Fig. 5D–1) as shown in Table 5D–1. The alpha, beta, zeta and gamma tocopherols have approximately 135, 50, 30, and 10 per cent relative biological activity,[21] respectively. Not as much is known about the others but their relative biological activities are quite low, ranging from 5 for epsilon tocopherol to 1 for delta tocopherol.

TOCOLS

$$R4 = CH_2(CH_2CH_2\overset{\displaystyle CH_3}{\overset{|}{C}HCH_2})_3H$$

TOCOTRIENOLS

$$R4 = CH_2(CH_2CH = \overset{\displaystyle CH_3}{\overset{|}{C}}CH_2)_3H$$

Fig. 5D-1. Structural formulae of vitamin E compounds.

Table 5D-1. Naturally Occurring
Tocopherols

Tocol	Tocotrienol	Methyl Positions
α-(alpha)	ζ-(zeta)	5, 7, 8
β-(beta)	ε-(epsilon)	5, 8
γ-(gamma)	η-(eta)	7, 8
δ-(delta)	8-methyl-tocotrienol	8

The most important sources of the tocopherols are the various vegetable oils.
Usually, the amount of α-tocopherol present
is related to the percentage of linoleic acid in
the triglyceride.[8] Thus, safflower oil which is
about 80 per cent linoleate has one of the
highest contents of α-tocopherol. An exception to this rule is corn oil which, although
containing about 50 per cent linoleic acid,
has about 90 per cent of the total tocopherol
in the gamma tocopherol form. The amounts
of total tocopherol present in commercial oils
vary greatly with the refining process used.

Differences in activity between the tocopherols are probably a function of the ability
of cellular components to distinguish between
the compounds and to remove them at different rates. There seems to be no significant
difference in the rate at which the individual
tocopherols are absorbed from the intestine.
Tocopherol acetate, which has no antioxidant
activity before the acetate is removed by cellular esterases, is partially hydrolyzed in the
intestine and partially absorbed as the intact
ester.[22] Maximum liver storage also occurs
sooner with the free tocopherol than with the
acetate derivatives. However, there may be
some theoretical advantage to the slower
utilization of the acetates. Not only are they
less likely to be oxidized before absorption,
but it has been demonstrated in rats and in
chicks fed tocopherol-deficient diets containing different levels of polyunsaturated fatty
acids that dividing a tocopherol supplement
into smaller more frequent doses protects
better than giving the same total amount
once a week.

Various metabolites of α-tocopherol have
been investigated for biologic activity: among
these are α-tocopherylquinone, the hydro-

quinone and tocopheronolactone. Both the
quinone and hydroquinone derivatives are
active in restoring the fertility of rats on E-
deficient diets[22,23] and can prevent or cure
nutritional muscular dystrophy induced by
vitamin E deficiency in the rat and rabbit.[24]
Tocopheronolactone has no effect on the fertility of deficient rats as measured by the ges-
tation-resorption test. Like the former derivatives however, it maintains tissue levels
of coenzyme Q.[25]

Knowledge of the chemistry of α-tocopherol
and its oxidation products is still far from
complete. Similarly, the metabolic fate of
tocopherol in man is largely unknown, although two conjugated urinary metabolites
have been described following the ingestion
of large quantities of vitamin E.[26] These
may represent final degradation products or
intermediates in the formation of other
metabolites. However, the possibility exists
that some of the presumed metabolites
described recently may be formed in vitro,
post mortem or during isolation.[27]

UNITS OF MEASUREMENT

One mg of dl-α-tocopherol has been designated as having 1 International Unit. On
the basis of relative biological activity, which
in the past has been a function of efficacy in
the prevention of fetal resorption in rats,
dl-α-tocopherol, d-α-tocopherol acetate and
d-α-tocopherol have been assigned International Units of 1.1, 1.36 and 1.49, respectively. An approximate confirmation of this
relationship between d- and dl-α-tocopherol
acetate was obtained during resupplementa-
tion of adult men whose stores of α-tocopherol
had been depleted[28] under controlled experimental conditions.

EFFECTS OF DEFICIENCY ON PHYSIOLOGICAL FUNCTION

Experimental deprivation of vitamin E in
animals is followed by a more baffling array
of diverse physiological abnormalities than
has been encountered with any other vitamin.
For the sake of discussion, although all the
syndromes have proven to be related, at least
in part, to the levels of polyunsaturated fats

in the diet and the tissues affected, the pathological changes studied in mammals may be divided into effects upon the reproductive system, the musculature, the nervous system, and the vascular system, respectively. These changes have been described in detail by Mason.[29]

Reproductive System

The seminiferous epithelium of vitamin E-deficient male rats shows no injury until active spermatogenesis begins during the third month of life when there is a relatively rapid degeneration of the epithelium. To prevent these changes, tocopherol must be given about 2 weeks prior to the appearance of histological injury. The degeneration is characterized by the following sequence of events: (1) inhibition of spermatogenesis with abnormal swelling and fusion of mature sperm, (2) marked diminution of sperm and nuclear chromolysis in spermatids and secondary spermatocytes, (3) sloughing of germ cells, and fusion of many into large multinucleate cells, (4) nuclear fragmentation and hydropic degeneration of remaining germ cells, (5) eventually the shrunken tubules are lined by a vacuolated, fibrous Sertoli syncytium. The testes are grossly atrophied, brownish, flabby and watery when cut. The rabbit, dog, and monkey show testes damage resembling the early phases of injury in the rat but the mouse is remarkably resistant taking many more months before marked atrophy of the germinal epithelium takes place.

In the female rat, all reproductive events are apparently normal up to the time of implantation which occurs at about the 7th day after insemination. Impaired vascular relationships between fetal and maternal components of the placenta appear to be responsible for asphyxia, starvation and death of the fetus. Fetal resorption can be prevented if sufficient tocopherol is given during the first week of pregnancy. In rats given doses that are less than adequate, death may be delayed but pronounced changes may show up in the vascular system prior to death. Changes in the ovaries of young rats have not been demonstrated; the pathologic condition noted seems to be due to uterine dysfunction.

Similar intrauterine effects of vitamin E deficiency have been noted in the mouse, hamster and guinea pig. There is no good evidence to relate malfunction of the reproduction process in man with an increased need for vitamin E.

Muscular System

The term "nutritional muscular dystrophy" refers to a form of myopathy which is noted in animals on vitamin E-deficient diets and should not be confused with human "muscular dystrophy." Although it may be proper to consider that nutritional muscular dystrophy can be produced in man,[30] under specially defined conditions, the distinction between the disorder that can be produced by nutritional means and the hereditary disease termed human "muscular dystrophy" should be emphasized.

In animals, it is possible to produce a form of muscle paralysis, usually preceded by a pronounced creatinuria,[31] by decreasing the ratio of tocopherol to polyunsaturated fats fed or by inhibiting the optimum utilization of tocopherol by feeding diets which are deficient in either selenium and/or sulfur amino acids.[32] Grossly, the skeletal muscle may be pale, ischemic, and gritty owing to calcium deposition. Microscopically there may be edema, leukocyte infiltration and segmental fragmentation of the muscle fibers. The amount of such changes may depend on the severity of the disorder which is a function of the degree of deficiency, the level of polyunsaturated lipids in the tissues, time of onset and of many related stresses and other nutritional imbalances which can alter the picture.

Herbivorous animals appear to be particularly susceptible to such nutritional myopathies but it is not certain how much of this increased susceptibility may be related to the higher levels of polyunsaturated fat in the usual diets of these animals.[33] The cardiac muscles of herbivorous animals (rabbit, sheep and cattle) are particularly sensitive to low tocopherol regimens;[34] sudden death through myocardial failure may appear before the development of the acid-fast pigment that is characteristic of deficiency in other animals.

The accumulations of the acid-fast pigments have been studied most intensively in the smooth muscle of rats. The changes in the uterus constitute a prototype for those observed elsewhere.

Pigment granules, which give the uterus a chestnut brown fluorescent color, appear first at the pole of the nucleus and gradually push the myofibrillae peripherally, eventually distorting the muscle cells. A similar pigment referred to as lipofuscin or ceroid pigment has been found in the smooth muscle of the stomach, intestine, bronchial wall and bladder of children dying with cystic fibrosis of the pancreas,[35] especially if they were over 2 years of age. They have also been described in adults with chronic pancreatitis.[36] It is noteworthy that the children with cystic fibrosis of the pancreas showed an excessive creatinuria which could be diminished by administering α-tocopherol.[37] In addition, one adult male patient with pronounced muscular weakness and high creatinuria showed marked improvement after tocopherol therapy. A thorough study of the latter patient,[30] in which remission and exacerbation of the symptoms could be controlled by providing or withholding tocopherol, indicated that the basic difficulty might be secondary to the malabsorption of lipids due to a deficiency of pancreatic lipase.

Nervous System

Although extensive lesions in the vestibular nuclei and pyramidal tracts as well as changes in the motor horn cells of the spinal tract of animals[38] have been reported in experimental animals, interpretations as to whether these are the causes or effects of muscular degeneration have been controversial. Pigment accumulation in vitamin E-deficient rats has been confirmed in the anterior horn cells, glial cells and macrophages; however, only occasional sclerotic motor cells in the spinal cord have been noted in more recent work.[39] In another study the claim is made that the metabolic derangements may affect the muscles and nervous system independently.[40]

Nutritional encephalomalacia in the chick is apparently also a function of the relative ratio of tocopherol to polyunsaturated fats in the diet.[41] It is characterized by motor incoordination, ataxia, head retraction followed by prostration and death. Two cases of human cerebellar encephalomalacia[42] related to tocopherol deficiency have been reported, but in only one of these was there a satisfactory dietary history. In that one,[43] an infant had been given, intravenously, a lipid preparation which provided a high proportion of linoleic acid without compensatory high levels of tocopherol. Necropsy did not reveal abnormalities in the cerebral hemispheres, but the cerebellum was the site of widespread hemorrhages, proliferation of capillaries and absence of Purkinje cells. The histopathology could be differentiated from that found in Wernicke's encephalitis.

Vascular System

Hemorrhage is a common manifestation in vitamin E deficiency. Those in the brain have already been noted. The syndrome called exudative diathesis in chicks is usually manifested by the appearance of large patches of subcutaneous edema on the breast and abdomen. There is increased permeability of the capillaries with interfascial accumulations of a fluid colored greenish by decomposed hemoglobin.

The decreased ability of the erythrocyte to withstand peroxidative deterioration by hydrogen peroxide, when the level of tocopherol in the blood is low, has become the basis for the so-called peroxide hemolysis test.[44] The erythrocytes of premature and newborn infants are particularly susceptible to peroxide hemolysis. It may be generalized that when the plasma tocopherol level is below 0.5 mg/100 ml such hemolysis tests are positive.

An evaluation of the peroxide hemolysis test in adult men was made in a study sponsored by the Food and Nutrition Board of the National Research Council in which the diet was limited to approximately 3 mg of α-tocopherol per day for over 6 years.[45] The erythrocytes of the men on this diet showed a gradual increase in peroxide hemolysis which was almost maximal within 2 years in most of the subjects. When the fat in the diet, which had been "stripped" lard, was changed to

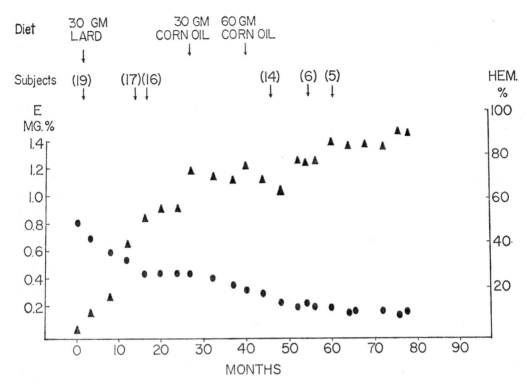

Fig. 5D-2. Decrease in average plasma total tocopherols (●) and increase of peroxide hemolysis test results (▲) with time and with progressive increase in dietary content of polyunsaturated fatty acids. Figures in parentheses indicate number of adult male subjects remaining on controlled depletion regimen at times indicated. (This figure is an extension of one previously reported[28]).

"stripped" corn oil, in order to increase the amounts of polyunsaturated fat consumed, there was a further increase in the degree of peroxide hemolysis along with a decrease in levels of tocopherol in the plasma, although there was appreciably more tocopherol remaining in the stripped corn oil than in the stripped lard.[28] Figure 5D-2 gives the trend of the average data obtained in the depleted subjects and further shows that when the stripped corn oil intake was doubled from 30 to 60 gm per day there was a further decrease in the plasma tocopherol levels.

After over 6 years on the diet, when the plasma tocopherol had reached a plateau approximating 0.2 mg of tocopherol per 100 ml of plasma, there was a small but significant decrease in erythrocyte survival time[46] as measured by ⁵¹Cr erythrocyte-life techniques. It should be emphasized that these subjects were not anemic, possibly because special controls were built into the experiment to supply protein, ascorbic acid and iron in amounts considered adequate to forestall anemia. Nevertheless, when they were supplemented with 300 mg d-α-tocopherol acetate per day, 4 out of 5 depleted subjects showed a small but significant increase in reticulocytes, which was not obtained in any patients in the control groups who were similarly supplemented.[47] These small changes in reticulocyte response would not have been convincing but for the studies of Dinning[48] and of Fitch[49] who obtained marked erythropoietic responses when α-tocopherol was administered to vitamin E-deficient monkeys. The beneficial effect of α-tocopherol administration on red cell survival in patients with proven malabsorption and low serum tocopherols has recently been confirmed by Leonard and Losowsky.[50]

A direct relationship between erythrocyte

stability *in vivo* and the *in vitro* peroxide hemolysis test cannot be made since the sensitivity of the erythrocyte to dilute peroxide is far greater than to anything that it normally encounters. It has been shown in man[51] and more recently confirmed and elaborated by Bieri and Poukka[52] in studies of rat erythrocytes that the peroxide hemolysis test is primarily related to the level of tocopherols in the plasma and only secondarily a function of the level of polyunsaturated fatty acids in the erythrocyte. The phospholipids in the erythrocyte membrane are peroxidized[53] at a rate related to the amount of tocopherols present.

Currently, there is a debate on whether vitamin E has a hemopoietic effect in children with protein-calorie malnutrition. Since children with protein-calorie malnutrition usually have low levels of lipoproteins in their blood and the serum tocopherol levels are related to the level of blood lipids, it is possible that many such children with low levels of serum tocopherol had adequate levels of vitamin E in their tissues. Thus, different workers may have been treating patients who were not equivalent in their states of vitamin E deficiency. The direct relationship between total blood lipid levels and serum tocopherol levels, which are now being studied,[54] may make it necessary to report levels of serum tocopherols as a function of the level of blood lipids rather than as mg per 100 ml as has been done in the past.

MODE OF ACTION

The disagreement among investigators with respect to the function of vitamin E has not been resolved despite many years of work in this field. There is relative harmony regarding the following:

(1) When polyunsaturated fatty acids (PUFA) intake is only sufficient to supply the minimal needs for health, relatively little vitamin E seems to be required. Increasing the levels of the more unsaturated lipids in the diet, which, in turn, increases the levels of PUFA in the various tissues at different rates, increases the requirement for vitamin E. This is true for chicks,[41] rats,[31] cattle,[55] and man.[11] It is noteworthy that tissues, like the

testes, which accumulate the more unsaturated fatty acids to a higher degree are among the first to break down during vitamin E deficiency.[56]

(2) The amount of lipofuscin pigment found in the tissues is a function of time, increased ingestion of PUFA and decreased ingestion of vitamin E.[57,58]

(3) The substitution of other lipid antioxidants for α-tocopherol can prevent or diminish the incidence of vitamin E deficiency in animals fed diets containing no detectable amount of tocopherols.[59] The efficacy of such antioxidants is limited by their different absorbabilities, transport and the fact that they are foreign to the body.

The opponents of the antioxidant theory contend that so vital a compound as vitamin E must be a component of an enzyme or transport system in an action unrelated to its antioxidant function. In consequence, since a vitamin E-deficient animal presents a staggering list of apparently unrelated histopathological sequelae, many deficient enzyme systems have been reported to be present in vitamin E deficiency. Arguments that the breakdown by peroxidation or free radical reactions of membrane phospholipids, coenzyme Q, vitamin A and other compounds could cause such enzyme dysfunctions are not considered conclusive. And arguments that other antioxidants can prevent pathology are countered with the belief that only minute amounts of tocopherol are needed when other antioxidants are present.

It is hoped that future research will prove that both the "antioxidant" and "enzyme" proponents for vitamin E function will prove to be correct.

DISTRIBUTION, FOOD SOURCES AND STORAGE

The vegetable and seed oils are the largest contributors of the tocopherols to the diet. It is interesting that in nature there is a rough proportionality between the level of the tocopherols in a seed oil and the concentration of linoleic acid in the oil,[8] as though the antioxidant were placed there to protect the PUFA from autooxidation. Unfortunately, the different tocopherols are not uniformly distributed so that the amounts of α-tocopherol available to the consumer may not always be optimal. Thus, in corn oil, which has approximately 50 per cent linoleic acid, there are 100 mg of total tocopherol per 100 gm, of which only about 10 per cent is α-tocopherol. In cottonseed oil, approximately 60 per cent of the total tocopherols is α-tocopherol; in safflower oil, approximately 90 per cent of the total is α-tocopherol.

Animal products are relatively poor sources of α-tocopherol but variations are quite large, depending upon the source of fat in the animal's diet.

The losses of natural concentrations of α-tocopherol[60] during cooking procedures and commercial processes are quite substantial. In the preparation of wheat flour, in addition to the large losses incurred during the separation of the bran and the sperm, the flours may lose nearly all of the remaining tocopherol if chlorine dioxide is used in the bleaching process.[61] Much tocopherol is removed from oils by purification processes before they reach the market; in fact, the by-products of such processes serve as important sources for the production of tocopherol concentrates sold for human and animal supplementation. The depot fats and the liver may be the chief repositories of tocopherol and serve as convenient indices of previous intake in animal studies. The pituitary and the adrenals become very rich in tocopherol[62] soon after tocopherol is fed. However, these observations become less spectacular if the level of tocopherol is expressed in terms of mg tocopherol per gm of fat, after which the relative levels in blood and in the tissues with the more unsaturated lipids, the adrenals, pituitary and testes, become quite similar. Thus, the ratio of approximately 1 mg tocopherols per gm lipid, a ratio which is in the same range noted in vegetable oils, is found in some animal tissue fats.

The amounts of α-tocopherol found in the ordinary components of human diets differ much more than is usually appreciated, depending upon source, preparation and age of the food. Dicks[63] has surveyed the literature to show that the tocopherol content of most foods may vary severalfold. Accordingly, the data given in Table 5D–2, which

Table 5D-2. Fat and d-α-Tocopherol in Various Food Groups Available for Consumption in the United States in 1960

	Fat (gm/day)	d-α-Tocopherol Content (mg/100 gm fat)	d-α-Tocopherol Amount (mg/day)
Visible fats			
Butter	7.19	1.6	0.115
Lard	9.55	2.3	0.220
Margarine	9.42	10.2	0.961
Shortening	15.62	10.0	1.562
Other fats and oils	14.14	50.0	7.063
Total	55.92	..	9.921
Other food fats			
Dairy products	23.31	1.6	0.378
Eggs	5.33	10.7	0.572
Meats, etc.	52.08	1.7	0.893
Beans, peas, nuts, etc.	5.33	9.3	0.496
Fruits and vegetables	1.74	91.7	1.597
Grain products	2.23	48.9	1.092
Total	90.02	..	5.028
Totals	145.94	..	14.949

(Harris and Embree: Am. J. Clin. Nutrition, 13, 385, 1963.)

show an average consumption of 15 mg of α-tocopherol per day, should be interpreted as only an approximation of average consumption in the U.S.

NUTRITIONAL REQUIREMENTS

The average intake of α-tocopherol by adults is 15 mg per day but the range of intake must be considered to be quite large, since individuals fed high protein-low plant fat diets would consume less than 10 mg per day, whereas those fed diets high in polyunsaturated oils could be ingesting over 60 mg per day. Since, in both cases, the amount of tocopherol consumed most likely is close to the requirement, the question of what to recommend as a universal requirement is not easy to resolve. Harris and Embree,[64] using the Elgin studies[28] as a basis, suggested that the E:PUFA ratio should be 0.6. Thus, a man consuming 60 gm of PUFA, which is 50 per cent polyunsaturated, would require 21.6 mg of α-tocopherol or 32 IU. Extrapolation of studies of various animals of different sizes tends to confirm the estimate of 30 IU for a 70-kg man.[65] A similar calculation for infants gives 3 to 6 IU of vitamin E, which is in good agreement with the range suggested by clinical studies[66] and is readily supplied by their normal diets.

Some certification of the tocopherol requirement when the diet contained approximately 38 gm of linoleic acid a day is supplied by data from the Elgin studies, in which adult male patients were maintained on 3 mg of α-tocopherol for over 6 years (Fig. 5D-2). Control subjects on the same diet, who were supplemented with 15 mg of α-tocopherol acetate (a total of approximately 24 IU per day), showed no signs of vitamin E deficiency but they also had no reserves, since examination of their erythrocytes showed a rapid increase in "peroxide hemolysis" soon after the supplement was removed.[28] Supplementation of nine depleted subjects at 54 months with various levels of vitamin E, as shown in Table 5D-3, indicated that the addition of 20 IU to the 4.5 IU in the diet was not sufficient to maintain blood levels even after 138 days of supplementation.

It should be understood that an adult does not require 30 IU per day unless he is consuming the equivalent of 60 gm of an unsaturated oil per day. And, if he is, he is probably obtaining the required amounts of tocopherols from the oil being consumed. The need for a stated requirement is not so much for normal individuals fed normal diets as for those who have absorptive difficulties or who for various reasons are consuming oxidized fats or large amounts of fish oils. Fish oils have a high peroxidative

Table 5D-3. Effect of Tocopherol Supplements on Subjects Who Had Been on Basal Diet for 54 Months*

Subject	Tocopherol Supplement	Period of Supplement (days)	Plasma Tocopherol (mg %)	Peroxide Hemolysis (%)
B 3	None	0	0.12	83
		3	0.24	80
		6	0.20	85
		13	0.26	86
		21	0.25	86
		50	0.20	76
		138	0.16	90
BS 10	7.5 mg/day d-α-tocopherol acetate	0	0.18	86
		3	0.34	82
		6	0.37	80
		13	0.45	82
		21	0.42	90
		50	0.52	85
		138	0.56	91
BS 14	10 mg/day dl-α-tocopherol acetate	0	0.22	67
		3	0.29	70
		6	0.40	78
		13	0.34	78
		21	0.28	80
		50	0.30	52
		138	0.29	79

Table 5D-3. Effect of Tocopherol Supplements on Subjects Who Had Been
on Basal Diet for 54 Months* (Continued)

Subject	Tocopherol Supplement	Period of Supplement (days)	Plasma Tocopherol (mg %)	Peroxide Hemolysis (%)
BS 13	15 mg/day d-α-tocopherol acetate	0	0.46	75
		3	0.66	35
		6	0.80	40
		13	0.64	32
		21	0.70	10
		50	0.71	10
		138	0.72	34
BS 6	20 mg/day dl-α-tocopherol acetate	0	0.18	85
		3	0.38	79
		6	0.37	70
		13	0.45	22
		21	0.41	40
		50	0.53	20
		138	0.57	25
BS 7	60 mg/day d-α-tocopherol acetate	0	0.30	73
		3	1.13	0
		6	1.16	0
		13	1.22	0
		21	1.16	2
		50	1.24	2
		138	1.29	1
BS 11	80 mg/day dl-α-tocopherol acetate	0	0.29	85
		3	0.60	0
		6	0.56	12
		13	0.70	2
		21	0.68	4
		50	0.74	2
		138	0.89	3
BS 8	240 mg/day d-α-tocopherol acetate	0	0.30	85
		3	1.38	0
		6	1.49	0
		13	1.47	2
		21	1.24	1
		50	1.18	1
		138	1.27	3
BS 12	320 mg/day d-α-tocopherol acetate	0	0.31	87
		3	1.14	1
		6	1.25	1
		13	1.34	1
		21	0.95	2
		50	0.99	2
		138	1.05	2

* Experimental diet furnished 2 to 4 mg of tocopherol per day, and contained varying amounts of linoleic acid as described in text. Supplement withdrawn for 44 hours before obtaining blood to allow time for plasma clearance of recently ingested tocopherol.
(Horwitt,[28] courtesy of Am. J. Clin. Nutrition)

potential[47] and relatively low levels of to-copherols. In other words, the need for sup-plementation of normal diets which happen to have low levels of PUFA and correspond-ing low levels of vitamin E is not indicated in normal individuals on the basis of current evidence.

DEFICIENCY IN MAN

Although mammals on prescribed diets that are deficient in vitamin E can show a bewildering spectrum of pathological symp-toms, there is no good evidence to indicate that the healthy man is susceptible to vitamin E deficiency when he consumes and absorbs the constituents of the average U.S. diets. What happens when his absorption of lipids is deficient is another matter, as has been noted in the above section on effects of de-ficiency on physiological function. As early as 1908, a peculiar lesion of muscle was re-ported in a patient with sprue.[67] In children with cystic fibrosis of the pancreas, who have steatorrhea, many had excessive creatinuria while fed a low-creatine diet,[68–70] which was decreased after supplementation with vitamin E. More recently, a study of adult patients with proven malabsorption was reported in which impaired red cell survival was demon-strated.[50]

A syndrome consisting of edema, skin lesions, an elevated platelet count and mor-phological changes in erythrocytes has been described in premature infants receiving for-mula mixtures that contained relatively high levels of PUFA.[71] The abnormalities dis-appeared rapidly after the administration of vitamin E and were not observed in infants fed identical diets supplemented with vitamin E.

Although the requirement for vitamin E for what is considered normal health is relatively non-controversial, the possible need for antioxidants to promote improved func-tion and decreased rate of aging is another matter.[72] The hypothesis supporting the belief that aging is, at least in part, a progres-sive accumulation of cellular deteriorations that come from free-radical damage, either from cosmic rays, pollution, or peroxidative sequelae, has found many proponents. The

story of free radical pathologic condition and the possibility that antioxidants can in-hibit such a condition has been reviewed by Pryor.[73] The most that can be said for this theory is that it is attractive, that the clues of prolonged survival of small animals given antioxidants are most interesting, but con-crete evidence to support it has not yet been published. There is the possibility that the accumulated effects of small changes over a 60-year period cannot be demonstrated in the cells of small animals with relatively short life spans.

So much α-tocopherol acetate has been ingested by so many that one may conclude, in the absence of any apparent physiological signs, that this is one of the least toxic of all the vitamins. It has been consumed by many at levels of more than a gram per day for many months, despite the fact that the bene-fits claimed remain to be proved.

BIBLIOGRAPHY

1. Evans and Bishop: Science, 56, 650, 1922.
2. Mattill, Carman and Clayton: J. Biol. Chem., 61, 729, 1924.
3. Sure: J. Biol. Chem., 58, 693, 1924.
4. Olcott and Emerson: J. Am. Chem. Soc., 59, 1008, 1937.
4a. Moore: Biochem. J., 34, 1321, 1940.
5. Dam: Pharmacol. Rev., 9, 1, 1957.
6. Filer Rumery and Mason: Trans. First Conf. on Biological Antioxidants, New York, Josiah Macy Foundation, 1946, pp. 67–77.
7. Hickman: Record of Chem. Prog., 9, 104, 1948.
8. Hove and Harris: J. Am. Oil Chem. Soc., 28, 405, 1951.
9. Hove: Am. J. Clin. Nutr., 3, 328, 1955.
10. Tappel: Vitamins and Hormones, 20, 493, 1962.
11. Horwitt: Borden's Rev. of Nutr. Res., 22, 1, 1961.
12. Draper: In Int. Encyclopedia of Food and Nutrition, Vol. 9, "Fat-Soluble Vitamins," Ed. by Morton, New York, Pergamon Press, 1970, p. 333.
13. Witting: Lipids, 2, 109, 1967.
14. Folkers: Int. J. Vitamin Res., 39, 334, 1969.
15. Boguth: Vitamins and Hormones, 27, 1, 1969.
16. Green and Bunyan: Nutrition Abs. and Rev., 39, 321, 1969.
17. Evans, Emerson and Emerson: J. Biol. Chem., 113, 319, 1936.
18. Fernholz: J. Am. Chem. Soc., 60, 700, 1938.
19. Karrer, Fritzsche, Ringier, and Salomon: Helv. Chim. Acta, 21, 520, 1938.
20. Pennock, Hemming, and Kerr: Biochem. Bio-phys. Res. Commun., 17, 542, 1964.
21. Century and Horwitt: Fed. Proc., 24, 906, 1965.

22. Wiss, Bunnell, and Gloor: Vitamins and Hormones, *20*, 441, 1962.
23. Green, Edwin, Diplock and Bunyan: Biochim. Biophys. Acta, *49*, 417, 1961.
24. MacKensie and MacKensie: J. Nutrition, *72*, 322, 1960.
25. Green, Diplock, Bunyan, Edwin, and McHale: Nature, *189*, 747, 1961.
26. Simon, Eisengart, Sundhein, and Milhorat: J. Biol. Chem., *221*, 807, 1956.
27. Plack and Bieri: Biochim. Biophys. Acta, *84*, 729, 1963.
28. Horwitt: Am. J. Clin. Nutrition, *8*, 451, 1960.
29. Mason: In *The Vitamins*, Ed. by Sebrell and Harris, New York, Academic Press, Vol. 3, pp. 514–538.
30. Vester and Williams: Clin. Res., *11*, 180, 1963.
31. Witting and Horwitt: J. Nutrition, *82*, 19, 1964.
32. Witting and Horwitt: J. Nutrition, *84*, 351, 1964.
33. Blaxter: Vitamins and Hormones, *20*, 633, 1962.
34. Swahn and Thafvelin: Vitamins and Hormones, *20*, 645, 1962.
35. Kerner and Goldbloom: J. Dis. Child., *99*, 597, 1960.
36. Braunstein: Gastroenterology, *40*, 224, 1961.
37. Nitowsky, Hsu and Gordon: Vitamins and Hormones, *20*, 559, 1962.
38. Einarson: J. Neurol. Neurosurg. Psychiat., *16*, 98, 1953.
39. Mason: In *Pharmacology and Disease*, Edited by Bourne, New York, Academic Press, 1960, p. 171.
40. West: In *Muscular Dystrophy in Man and Animals*, Ed. by Bourne and Golarz, New York, Hafner Publishing Co., 1963, p. 367.
41. Century, Horwitt and Bailey: Arch. Gen. Psychiat., *1*, 420, 1959.
42. Bailey: Am. J. Clin. Nutrition, *12*, 275, 1963.
43. Horwitt and Bailey: Arch. Neurol., *1*, 312, 1959.
44. György, Cogan and Rose: Proc. Soc. Exptl. Biol. Med., *81*, 536, 1952.
45. Horwitt, Harvey, Duncan, and Wilson: Am. J. Clin. Nutrition, *4*, 408, 1956.
46. Horwitt, Century and Zeman: Am. J. Clin. Nutrition, *12*, 99, 1963.

47. Horwitt: Vitamins and Hormones, *20*, 541, 1962.
48. Dinning: Nutrition Rev., *21*, 289, 1963.
49. Fitch: Vitamins and Hormones, *26*, 501, 1968.
50. Leonard and Losowsky: Am. J. Clin. Nutrition, *24*, 388, 1971.
51. Horwitt, Harvey and Harmon: Vitamins and Hormones, *26*, 487, 1968.
52. Bieri and Poukka: J. Nutrition, *100*, 557, 1970.
53. Heikkila, Mezick and Cornwell: Physiol. Chem. and Physics, *3*, 93, 1971.
54. Horwitt, Harvey and Searcey: Fed. Proc., *30*, 640, 1971 (Abstract).
55. Blaxter: In "Vitamin E," Atti del terzo Congresso Internationale Venezia, Edizioni Valdonega Verona, 1956, p. 622.
56. Witting, Likhite and Horwitt: Lipids, *2*, 103, 1967.
57. Sulkin and Srivanij: J. Geront., *15*, 2, 1960.
58. Witting, Theron and Horwitt: Lipids, *2*, 97, 1967.
59. Draper, Bergan, Chiu, Csallany, and Boaro: J. Nutrition, *84*, 395, 1964.
60. Harris: Vitamins and Hormones, *20*, 603, 1962.
61. Moore: Brit. Med. Bull., *12*, 44, 1956.
62. Quaife, Swanson, Dju and Harris: Ann. N.Y. Acad. Sci., *52*, 300, 1949.
63. Dicks: Vitamin E Content of Foods and Feeds for Human and Animal Consumption, Agric. Exp. Station Bull., 435, Univ. of Wyoming, Laramie, 1965.
64. Harris and Embree: Am. J. Clin. Nutrition, *13*, 385, 1963.
65. Harris: Ann. N.Y. Acad. Sci., *52*, 240, 1949.
66. MacKensie: Pediat., *13*, 346, 1954.
67. Bramwell and Muir: Quart. J. Med., *1*, 1, 1907–8.
68. Gordon, Nitowsky and Cornblath: Am. J. Dis. Child., *90*, 669, 1955.
69. Nitowsky, Cornblath and Gordon: Am. J. Dis. Child., *92*, 164, 1956.
70. Nitowsky, Tildon, Levin, and Gordon: Am. J. Clin. Nutrition, *10*, 368, 1962.
71. Hassan, Hashim, Van Itallie, and Sebrell: Am. J. Clin. Nutrition, *19*, 147, 1966.
72. Tappel: Geriatrics, *23*, 97, 1968.
73. Pryor: Chem. Eng. News, pp. 34–51, June 7, 1971.

Chapter

5

Section E Thiamin

ROBERT A. NEAL

AND

HOWERDE E. SAUBERLICH

HISTORY

Recognition of vitamin B_1 activity dates back to 1890 when the Dutch physician Eijkman observed that chickens fed a diet which consisted mainly of polished rice developed polyneuritic symptoms similar to those common to beriberi patients. Additional studies showed that the paralysis resulting from feeding polished rice could be cured by adding rice polishings to the diet. As a result of these studies Eikjman suggested the toxic principle was contained in polished rice but could be neutralized by some protective factor in rice polishings.

Takaki of Japan was the first to advance an explanation that beriberi was actually a nutritional deficiency. Starting in 1884, he began experiments in which he modified the diet fed sailors aboard ships of the Japanese Navy in an attempt to decrease the disastrous incidence of beriberi. The major modification was the inclusion of dry milk and additional meat in the diet. The modified diet resulted in a dramatic decrease in the incidence of beriberi.[1] He concluded from these experiments that beriberi was caused by a lack of nitrogenous food components in association with excessive intake of non-nitrogenous food.

The correct explanation for the etiology of beriberi was proposed in 1901 by Grijns.[2] Grijns found that in addition to rice polishings, *Katjang hidioe*, a green bean and meat could also prevent beriberi in fowl fed a diet consisting mainly of starch. As a result of these studies he postulated that natural foodstuffs contained an unknown factor, absent in polished rice, which prevented the development of polyneuritis.

Funk[3] reported the isolation of a substance from rice polishings which cured beriberi, and named it Vitamine. However, the active product he isolated still contained little of the active principle.

Jansen and Donath,[4] employing adsorption onto fuller's earth, were able to isolate crystalline material which cured polyneuritis in rice birds. The trivial name Aneurine was suggested by Jansen. This name was commonly used throughout Europe for a considerable time. However, this nomenclature was not accepted in the United States because of its therapeutic implications. The name Aneurine was eventually replaced by thiamin (thiamine).

In 1934 R. R. Williams and his colleagues,[5] using an improved process, isolated sufficient quantity of the vitamin to make structure elucidation possible.

STRUCTURE, CHEMICAL SYNTHESIS, CHEMICAL AND PHYSICAL PROPERTIES

Work by R. R. Williams and his colleagues made it clear that thiamin was composed of a pyrimidine and a thiazole moiety and in 1936 established its structure as 3-(2'-methyl-4'-amino-5'-pyrimidylmethyl)-5-(2-hydroxyethyl)-4-methylthiazole.[6]

Thiamin

Thiamin has been synthesized by the formation of the pyrimidine and thiazole moieties separately followed by a coupling of the two moieties or by synthesizing the pyrimidine with a suitable side chain which can be reacted with a second compound to form the thiazole ring.

Williams and Cline[7] used the first method in their original synthesis of thiamin. The 4-hydroxy pyrimidine was synthesized in a reaction between acetamidine and the sodio derivative of ethyl-2-ethoxy-1-formylpropionate. The 4-hydroxy pyrimidine was converted in a series of steps to 2-methyl-4-amino-5-bromomethylpyrimidine. The thiazole moiety was synthesized by reacting 3-acetyl-3-chloropropanol with thioformamide. The coupling of the two moieties gave thiamin bromide hydrobromide.

An example of the second type of synthesis is that of Todd and Bergel.[8] These workers condensed ethyl-1-ethoxy-methylene-1-cyanoacetate with acetamidine to form 5-cyano-4-hydroxy-2-methylpyrimidine. This compound was converted in a series of steps to 2-methyl-4-amino-5-aminomethylpyrimidine. Reaction of this latter compound with potassium dithioformate yielded 2-methyl-4-amino-5-thioformamidomethylpyrimidine. Condensation of this compound with 3-acetyl-3-chloropropanol yielded thiamin.

One gram of thiamin chloride hydrochloride can dissolve in 1 ml of water. It is soluble to about 1 per cent in ethanol but rather insoluble in other common organic solvents. The hemihydrate of thiamin melts at 248 to 250° C. Thiamin has a characteristic odor very much like that of yeast.

The vitamin exhibits absorption bands in the ultraviolet region of the spectrum. At pH 7 in aqueous solution the absorption maxima are at 235 and 267 nm corresponding to the pyrimidine and thiazole moieties respectively. At pH 1 there is one maximum

at 247 and a shoulder at 260 nm again corresponding to the pyrimidine and thiazole moieties respectively.

Thiamin is destroyed at elevated temperature unless the pH is below 5. At pH values above 7 thiamin rapidly loses its biological activity. In alkaline solution under oxidizing conditions (*e.g.* potassium ferricyanide) thiamin is oxidized to the fluorescent compound thiochrome, a reaction widely used for the detection and quantitation of thiamin.

Thiochrome

Sulfite ion at room temperature attacks the methylene bridge between the two ring systems of thiamin to yield the separate pyrimidine and thiazole moiety.[6] The products of this reaction are 2-methyl-4-amino-5-pyrimidylmethylsulfonic acid and 5-(2-hydroxyethyl)-4-methylthiazole.

BIOLOGICAL FUNCTIONS OF THIAMIN

Thiamin in the form of pyrophosphate participates as a coenzyme in the oxidative decarboxylation of alpha ketoacids to aldehydes. The most important substrates for this type of reaction are pyruvate which is metabolized to acetyl coenzyme A and alpha ketoglutarate which is metabolized to succinyl coenzyme A. Both these reactions require the participation of lipoic acid, NAD, and coenzyme A. The mechanism of these reactions involves first the formation of an "active aldehyde" intermediate between the substrate (pyruvate or alpha ketoglutarate) and enzyme-bound thiamin pyrophosphate. The intermediate in the decarboxylation of pyruvate is 2-(1-hydroxyethyl)-thiamin pyrophosphate. In the decarboxylation of alpha ketoglutarate the intermediate is 2-(1-hydroxy-3-carboxypropyl)-thiamin pyrophosphate.

The next step is the transfer of the two-carbon fragment in the case of pyruvate and the four-carbon fragment in the case of alpha ketoglutarate to lipoic acid. This transfer may take place either by an electrophilic attack by oxidized lipoic acid on the number one carbon of the fragment displacing thiamin pyrophosphate or by a preliminary oxidation of the "active aldehyde" intermediate to yield an acyl thiamin pyrophosphate followed by nucleophilic attack of reduced lipoic acid to displace thiamin pyrophosphate. There is some evidence to indicate the latter route may be the correct one.

The final step in the oxidative decarboxylation of pyruvate and alpha ketoglutarate is the transfer of acetate and succinate respectively from lipoic acid to coenzyme A. The oxidative decarboxylation reactions of pyruvate and alpha ketoglutarate are important from the standpoint of energy production in plants and in animal organisms.

An additional important thiamin pyrophosphate requiring enzyme in plants and animals is transketolase. The enzyme catalyzes the reaction

xylulose-5-phosphate + ribose-5-phosphate ⟶ sedoheptulose-7-phosphate + glyceraldehyde-3-phosphate.

In this reaction xylulose-5-phosphate is cleaved between carbons 2 and 3 to form a 2-(1,2-dihydroxyethyl)-thiamin pyrophosphate intermediate and glyceraldehyde-3-phosphate. The 1,2-dihydroxyethyl group is then transferred from thiamin to the number one carbon of ribose-5-phosphate to yield sedoheptulose-7-phosphate. This reaction is important in the phosphogluconate pathway, a reaction sequence which carries out the interconversion of three-, four-, five-, six-, and seven-carbon sugars. This pathway is also an important source of reduced NADP.

Other enzyme-catalyzed reactions requiring thiamin as a coenzyme are the nonoxidative decarboxylation of alpha keto acids and the phosphoketolase reaction, both of which are important only in microorganisms. The latter reaction involves the cleavage of a ketopentose phosphate to triose phosphate and acetyl phosphate.

METHODS OF ASSAY

There are various methods for assay for thiamin in biological materials. These include animal assays as well as chemical and microbiological assays.

The thiochrome procedure[9] is the most widely used chemical method for assay of thiamin in biological materials. This method depends on the alkaline oxidation of thiamin to thiochrome. Thiochrome exhibits an intense blue fluorescence and can be measured fluorimetrically. In this procedure thiamin is isolated from biological materials by passing a solution containing the vitamin over a column of the synthetic zeolite Decalso. The thiamin absorbed to the Decalso is eluted and oxidized to thiochrome using an alkaline solution of ferricyanide. The thiochrome is extracted into isobutanol and quantitated by measuring the fluorescence of the isobutanol solution. Since thiamin pyrophosphate forms a thiochrome derivative poorly soluble in isobutanol, the thiochrome procedure can be used to distinguish between free thiamin and its pyrophosphate forms by assaying an extract before and after incubation with a phosphatase enzyme.

Other chemical tests for thiamin are the formaldehyde-diazotized sulphanilic acid method,[10] the diazotized p-aminoacetophenone method,[11,12] and the bromothymol blue method.[13]

The microbiological method which is most widely used currently is assay with *Lactobacillus viridescens*.[14] This organism requires the intact thiamin molecule for growth; neither the thiazole nor pyrimidine moieties nor their phosphorylated forms are active. Thiamin monophosphate and diphosphate are as active as thiamin while the hydroxyethyl derivative of thiamin is only 80 per cent as active.

Other useful but less widely used microorganisms for thiamin assay include *Phycomyces blakesleeanus*,[15] *Kloeckera brevis*,[16] *Lactobacillus fermenti*,[17] and *Ochromonas danica*.[18]

With the development of chemical and microbiological assays for thiamin, the applicability of animal assays decreased. Animal assays are still useful, however, for determining the availability of thiamin in a food source or a new form or preparation of the vitamin. The response may be measured in various animals including pigeons and chicks, but the rat is the animal of choice. The rat assay measures the curative effect of the food source or new preparation containing thiamin on rats which have been made thiamin deficient. The response is compared to the curative effect of pure synthetic thiamin hydrochloride. The response more commonly measured is growth, although the length of cure of bradycardia or of polyneuritis is sometimes used.

Numerous methods have been used to assess the state of thiamin nutrition in man.[32] The most important of these are the measurement of the activity of erythrocyte transketolase, a thiamin pyrophosphate-requiring enzyme, the measurement of blood or urinary levels of thiamin using various chemical and microbiological techniques, and measurement of blood levels of pyruvate and alpha ketoglutarate. The best methods currently in use appear to be the erythrocyte transketolase method of Brin[19] as modified by others,[20-22] and the measurement of thiamin in urine using the modified thiochrome procedure of Hennessy and Cerecedo.[9]

DEFICIENCY IN EXPERIMENTAL ANIMALS AND MAN

One of the first recorded signs of thiamin deficiency in experimental animals was the characteristic head retraction in the pigeon.[23] Thiamin-deficient pigeons also show ataxia and leg weakness, cardiac failure with tachycardia, abnormalities of the electrocardiogram and necrosis of the heart muscle. Chicks respond to thiamin deficiency in a way very similar to pigeons.

The major symptoms of thiamin deficiency in rats are loss of appetite (anorexia), weight loss, convulsions, slowing of the heart rate (bradycardia), and lowering of the body temperature. Loss of muscular tone and lesions of the nervous system may also develop. The urine of deficient rats contains a higher pyruvate:lactate ratio than that of normal animals. Thiamin-deficient rats also exhibit a reduced erythrocyte transketolase activity. The administration of thiamin to rats brings about a remarkable reversal of the deficiency in 24 hours.

The classical pathological condition arising from thiamin deficiency in man is called beriberi. The symptoms and treatment of beriberi will be discussed in detail in the chapter entitled "Clinical Manifestations of Certain Vitamin Deficiencies."

NUTRITIONAL REQUIREMENT

The requirements for thiamin in human nutrition are usually based on caloric intake. Various investigators have indicated the daily adult requirement for thiamin is from 0.23 to 0.5 mg per 1000 calories.[21,24-26]

The Food and Nutrition Board recommends 0.5 mg of thiamin for each 1,000 calories in the diet. Therefore the recommended average intake of thiamin for men is 1.2 to 1.4 mg and 1 mg for women. In women during pregnancy the recommended intake is increased to 1.2 mg and during lactation to 1.5 mg.

The recommended daily intakes for children are: infants 0 to 2 mo., 0.2 mg; infants 2 to 6 mo., 0.4 mg; 6 mo. to 1 yr., 0.5 mg; 1 to 3 yr., 0.6 mg; 3 to 4 yr., 0.7 mg; 4 to 6 yr., 0.8 mg; 6 to 8 yr., 1.0 mg; 8 to 10 yr., 1.1 mg; boys 10 to 12 yr., 1.3 mg; boys 12 to 14 yr., 1.4 mg; boys 14 to 18, 1.5 mg; girls 10 to 12 yr., 1.1 mg; and girls 12 to 18 yr., 1.2 mg.

Good sources of thiamin are pork, beef, organ meats, wheat or other whole or enriched grains, and fresh vegetables, especially peas and beans (see Table 5I-1).

TOXICITY

Thiamin produces a variety of pharmacological effects when administered in large amounts. However, these effects are seen only in doses which are thousands of times larger than those required for optimum nutrition.

Death after intravenous injection of thiamin in animals is due to depression of the respiratory center.[27] The lethal dose of thiamin administered by intravenous injection is 125 mg per kg in mice; 250 mg per kg in rats; 300 mg per kg in rabbits; and 350 mg per kg in dogs.[28] The ratios of the lethal doses on intravenous injection to those on subcutaneous and oral administration were found to be 1:6:40. In monkeys, intravenous administration of 200 mg per kg failed to elicit any symptoms[28] and only 600 mg per kg caused any toxic effects.

Rats have been maintained for three generations on a daily intake of 0.08 to 1.0 mg of thiamin without harmful effects.[6] These are doses up to 100 times the daily requirement for the vitamin.

No toxic effects of thiamin administered by mouth have been reported in man. Generally toxic effects have not been reported on subcutaneous, intramuscular, intraspinal, or intravenous injection of doses 1 to 200 times larger than the daily maintenance doses. In rare cases, however, thiamin has caused reactions resembling anaphylactic shock in man. The majority of these cases are in patients who had previously received large doses of thiamin by injection. Thus, they apparently developed a hypersensitivity to thiamin.

THIAMIN METABOLISM

Over two dozen metabolites of thiamin have been noted to occur in the urine of rats[29,30] and of men[31-33] given the vitamin labeled in either the pyrimidine or thiazole moieties. Only six of these have so far been identified. These are 2-methyl-4-amino-5-pyrimidine carboxylic acid,[31] 4-methylthiazole-5-acetic acid,[33,34,35] 2-methyl-4-amino-5-hydroxymethylpyrimidine,[36] 5-(2-hydroxyethyl)-4-methylthiazole,[37] [3-(2'-methyl-4'-amino-5'-pyrimidylmethyl)-4-methylthiazole-5 acetic acid] (thiamin acetic acid),[37] and 2-methyl-4-amino-5-formylaminomethylpyrimidine.[37]

BIBLIOGRAPHY

1. Takaki: Lancet, 2, 189, 1887.
2. Grijns: Research on Vitamins 1900–1911, J. Noorduyn, Gorinchem. pp. 37, 38, 1935.
3. Funk: J. State Med., 20, 341, 1912.
4. Jansen and Donath: Koninkl. Ned. Akad. Wetenschap., Proc. 29, 1390, 1926.
5. Williams, Waterman and Keresztesy: J. Am. Chem. Soc., 56, 1187, 1934.
6. Williams and Spies: Vitamin B1. New York, The Macmillan Co., 1938.
7. Williams and Cline: J. Am. Chem. Soc., 58, 1504, 1936.
8. Todd and Bergel: J. Chem. Soc., 364, 1937.
9. Hennessy and Cerecedo: J. Am. Chem. Soc., 61, 179, 1939.
10. Kinnersley and Peters: Biochem. J. 32, 1516, 1938.
11. Prebluda and McCollum: J. Biol. Chem., 127, 495, 1939.
12. Melnick and Field: J. Biol. Chem., 130, 97, 1939.
13. Gupta and Cadwallader: J. Pharmaceut. Sci., 57, 112, 1968.
14. Deibel, Evans and Niven: J. Bac. 74, 818, 1957.
15. Schopfer and Jung: Compt. Rend. 5th Congr. Intern. Tech. Chem. Ind. Agr. Scheveningen, 1, 22, 1937.
16. Hoff-Jorgensen and Hansen: Acta Chem. Scand., 9, 552, 1955.
17. Sarett and Cheldelin: J. Biol. Chem., 155, 153, 1944.
18. Baker, Pasher, Frank, Hutner, Aaronson and Sobotka: Clin. Chem., 5, 13, 1959.
19. Brin: Ann. N.Y. Acad. Sci., 98, 528, 1962.
20. Warnock: J. Nutrition, 100, 1057, 1970.
21. Ziporin, Nunes, Powell, Waring and Sauberlich: J. Nutrition 85, 297, 1965.
22. Stevens, Sauberlich and Long: In Automation in Analytical Chemistry, New York, Mediad Incorporated, 1968.
23. Suzuki, Shamimura and Okade: Biochem. Z., 43, 89, 1912.
24. National Acad. Sci.—Natl. Res. Council, Publ. 1964, Washington, D.C., 1968.
25. Ziporin, Nunes, Powell, Waring and Sauberlich: J. Nutrition, 85, 287, 1965.
26. Sauberlich, Herman and Stevens: Am. J. Clin. Nutrition, 23, 671, 1970.
27. Haley: Proc. Soc. Exptl. Biol. Med., 68, 153, 1948.
28. Mouriquand and Coisnard: Presse Med., 53, 369, 1945.
29. Neal and Pearson: J. Nutrition, 83, 343, 1964.
30. Balaghi and Pearson: J. Nutrition, 89, 265, 1966.
31. Neal and Pearson: J. Nutrition, 83, 351, 1964.
32. Sauberlich: Am. J. Clin. Nutrition, 20, 528, 1967.
33. Ariaey-Nejad, Balaghi, Baker and Sauberlich: Am. J. Clin. Nutrition, 23, 764, 1970.
34. Ariaey-Nejad and Pearson: J. Nutrition, 96, 445, 1968.
35. Suzuoki, Tominaga, Matsuo, Sumi and Miyakawa: J. Nutrition, 96, 433, 1968.
36. White, Amos and Neal: J. Nutrition, 100, 1053, 1970.
37. Amos and Neal: J. Biol. Chem., 245, 5643, 1970.

Chapter

5

Section F Riboflavin

M. K. Horwitt

INTRODUCTION

The food fraction termed "water-soluble B" reported by McCollum and Kennedy[1] in 1916 with the suggestion that it might be identical with the antiberiberi substance was first shown to be dual in nature in 1920 by Emmett and Luros.[2] This was further studied by Smith and Hendrick[3] who, in 1926, divided the complex into a beriberi preventative material which was destroyed by heat and an antipellagric substance which was more heat stable. About the same time Goldberger and Lillie[4] were making their classical demonstrations that pellagra could be cured by dietary means and the term "vitamin B_1" began to represent the water-soluble, heat-labile, antineuritic fraction, and vitamin B_2 or G, the heat-stable antipellagric fraction. Soon after Warburg and Christian[5] discovered the first flavoprotein in 1932, the close correlation between the vitamins and biological oxidations was recognized from the combined observations of Ellinger and Koschara,[6] Booher,[7] and Kuhn *et al.*[8] and riboflavin deficiency was proved responsible for some of the pathology formerly associated with pellagra.

ISOLATION AND CHEMICAL NATURE

Although the water-soluble, yellow-green fluorescent compound in whey was known to chemists in the 19th century,[9] it was not isolated from milk and shown to be a part of the B-complex until 1933 by Kuhn, György and Wagner-Jauregg.[8] In the meantime Warburg and Christian[5] while studying yellow-fluorescent tissue extracts as parts of various enzyme systems in tissues had reported sufficient revealing chemical data to uncover the close relationship of their yellow enzyme to the vitamin-like yellow fluorescent compound in milk. The identification of the colored component of the "yellow oxidation enzyme" with the vitamin made the recognition of riboflavin as the prosthetic group of the active flavoprotein enzymes possible. At about the same time Booher[7] confirmed the fact that the growth promoting property of whey was associated with its water-soluble yellow fluorescent pigment.

The synthesis of riboflavin was accomplished by Kuhn[10] and Karrer[11] and associates in 1935 who showed that the compound was 6,7-dimethyl-9-(dl′-ribityl)isoalloxazine.

Riboflavin
6,7-dimethyl-9-(dl′-ribityl)isoalloxazine

The methods of isolation varied somewhat with the source of the material but nearly all the early workers used adsorption on fuller's earth for slightly acid extracts. The resulting adsorbate was extracted with pyridine solutions or dilute ammonia, and the eluate, after concentration, was precipitated with a heavy metal to form a salt of flavine. Until it was recognized that all were dealing with the same substance, the pigments were given specific names like ovoflavin, lactoflavin, hepatoflavin, and uroflavin.

Riboflavin crystallizes in yellowish brown needles. Solubility is relatively slight, being only 12 mg per 100 ml at 27.5° C. Riboflavin-5-phosphate, the "flavin mononuceotide," is much more soluble. Both riboflavin and its phosphate are decomposed by exposure to light and in strongly alkaline solutions. The typical fluorescence of riboflavin is dependent upon the presence of a free 3-imino group, and neither 3-substituted riboflavin nor the enzyme systems will fluoresce.

The Estimation of Riboflavin. Although the growth of rats[12] and chicks[13] may occasionally be used to assay riboflavin in mixed diets, the biological method of assay has been generally superseded by the microbiological method of Snell and Strong.[14] This measures the lactic acid production of a lactic acid-producing organism which is dependent upon the presence of riboflavin in the medium.

The chemical assay of riboflavin relies upon the fact that the fluorescence of riboflavin is proportional to its concentration under controlled conditions of salt concentration, pH and temperature. Interfering substances may be removed by potassium permanganate,[15] or by adsorption on Florisil.[16]

The present U.S.P. Reference Standard is a recrystallized sample of riboflavin obtainable from the U.S.P. Reference Standard Committee. Comparisons of purified riboflavin with biological units have shown that one Bourguin-Sherman rat growth unit,[17] which upon daily addition will produce an average gain of 3 gm per rat per week, is equal to about 2.5 mcg of riboflavin. Von Euler[18] proposed a unit of 5 mcg of riboflavin, an amount which produced an increase in weight of 0.8 to 1.0 gm per day in young rats. A Cornell unit[19] is defined as the growth effect on chicks equivalent to that produced by 1 mcg of riboflavin.

The need for biological standards of activity continues to exist especially in the study of derivatives of riboflavin. For example, in the assay of a water-soluble derivative prepared by Stone,[20] fluorometric assay yielded a value of 57.2 per cent riboflavin, a microbiological assay by U.S.P. XIII revision method gave a value of 33 per cent riboflavin, whereas the biological assay by rat growth method showed that the riboflavin potency was negligible.

DEFICIENCY IN EXPERIMENTAL ANIMALS

The effects of riboflavin deficiency in rats, dogs, foxes, pigs, young ruminants, other mammals and birds have been reviewed by Horwitt.[21] The primary effect of riboflavin restriction is the cessation of growth. When less than the minimum requirement is provided rats show severe ophthalmia and a bilateral, symmetrical alopecia which almost completely denudes the head, neck and trunk. An eczematous condition of the skin especially affects the nostrils and eyes. The eyelids become denuded of hair and may be stuck together with a serous exudate. Conjunctivitis, blepharitis, corneal opacities and vascularization of the cornea are common manifestations of rat ariboflavinosis.

The importance of riboflavin in the reproductive cycle is often overlooked. Its absence from the diet of rats may produce anestrus and the damage is irreparable[22] if riboflavin is not restored in 10 weeks. Riboflavin-deficient female rats gave birth to litters with congenital malformations.[23]

The deficiency of riboflavin in dogs was evaluated by Sebrell[24,25] who noted a characteristic fatty liver followed by collapse, coma and death in about 3 months. Patek et al.[26] characterized riboflavin deficiency in the pig as a syndrome which included retarded growth, corneal opacities, dermatitis, changes in the hair and hoofs and terminal collapse associated with hypoglycemia. Mitchell et al.[27] considered the absolute and relative neutrophilic granulocyte concentrations in the blood as the most sensitive indices of riboflavin deficiency in the pig. Rhesus monkeys[28] develop a freckled type of dermatitis on the face, hands, legs and groin. Foy and Kondi[29] have studied ariboflavinosis in the baboon which, after 10 weeks, developed swollen and edematous bleeding gums, and ulcerated seborrheic keratitis of the face, nose, eyebrows, armpits and scrotum.

BIOCHEMICAL AND PHYSIOLOGICAL FUNCTIONS OF RIBOFLAVIN

Knowledge of the close relationship between the vitamins and biological oxidations may be said to date from 1932, the year in which the first flavoprotein was discovered. This compound, often referred to as the "old yellow enzyme," was soon separated into a protein and a yellow prosthetic group.[5] Stern and Holiday[30] found that the prosthetic group of Warburg's yellow enzyme was a derivative of alloxazine. This fact, when combined with the observations of correlations between vitamin B_2 requirements and concentration of the yellow-green fluorescence, was soon corroborated by the synthesis of riboflavin. Theorell's[31] demonstration that Warburg's enzyme contained one molecule of phosphate and the proof of constitution of riboflavin-5'-phosphate were the concluding steps in the first separation, identification and synthesis of the prosthetic group of an enzyme.

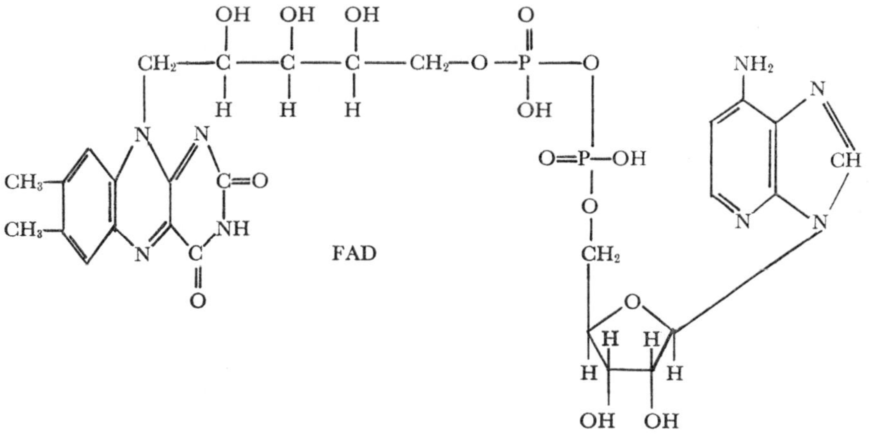

Riboflavin is a constituent of two coenzymes, riboflavin-5'-phosphate, erroneously called flavin mononucleotide (FMN) since ribitol is an alcohol, and flavin adenine dinucleotide (FAD). The formulas are as follows:

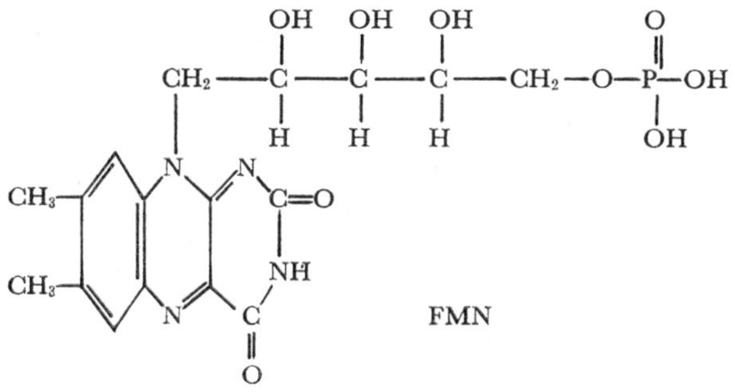

The riboflavin coenzymes are essential parts of a number of oxidative enzyme systems involved in electron transport. These include the amino acid oxidases, xanthine oxidase, the succinic dehydrogenase complex, glutathione reductase and many others. Some of the relationships of deficiencies in such enzyme systems to endocrine imbalances have been reviewed by Rivlin.[31a]

It is axiomatic that cellular growth cannot

evolve in the absence of riboflavin. During periods of riboflavin deficiency, negligible amounts of riboflavin are excreted in the urine and one might surmise that the body is capable of utilizing much of the riboflavin released by its own catabolic processes. However, the day-by-day needs of this vitamin for tissue turnover in the adult appear to be greater than 0.5 mg per day, and the decomposition products of riboflavin must be excreted in forms not recognized at present.

It is reasonable that any local trauma to the skin must be repaired by new growth.[32] Such trauma might range from erosions at the angles of the mouth, an area that is constantly flexed, to surgical intervention. The lesions formed are repaired by local growth only to the extent that riboflavin and protein are available. In the absence of riboflavin, minor injuries become aggravated, and the so-called specific manifestations of ariboflavinosis become apparent.

CLINICAL ASPECTS OF RIBOFLAVIN DEFICIENCY

The first description of the clinical findings, which have subsequently become known as ariboflavinosis, was published by Stannus in 1912,[33] 20 years before riboflavin itself was discovered. His findings were confirmed and augmented by Bahr[34] in Ceylon, Scott[35] in Jamaica, Moore[36] in West Africa, Landor and Pallister[37] in Singapore, Aykroyd and Krishnan[38] in South India, and Goldberger and Wheeler[39] and Tanner[40] in the United States. It was generally recognized that the lesions were on the basis of some dietary deficiency and that they could be cured by administration of vitamin B complex.

Lesions of the eye, in particular corneal vascularization, were described in the rat by Bessey and Wolbach[41] and by Spies,[42] Sydenstriker[43] and Kruse[44] in the human being. Extensive corneal vascularization among members of the Royal Canadian Air Force which seemed to respond to riboflavin administration was observed by Tisdall, McCreary and Pearce.[45]

The concept of riboflavin deficiency in man as a syndrome characterized by angular stomatitis, glossitis, seborrheic dermatitis about the nose and scrotum, and vascularization of the cornea has been generally accepted since the publication of the findings of Sebrell and Butler.[46] This was confirmed and extended by the controlled experiment of Horwitt, Hills et al.[32] In the latter study,[32,47] although scrotal dermatitis was observed frequently, no evidence of circumcorneal injection or unusual vascularization of the cornea was observed. The tendency of small vascular twigs in the margins of the cornea to disappear and reappear months later was frequently noted, but no proliferation of the vessels of the limbic plexus was seen. Also, no other ocular abnormalities were noted except for a tendency on the part of three subjects in the deficient group whose flicker fusion thresholds were increased. None of the subjects had any evidence of glossitis. There was nothing to suggest "magenta" tongue, "red" tongue or loss of the normal papillae. Studies of the capillary bed mentioned earlier failed to reveal any evidence of a "capillary dyskinesia," suggested by Stannus[48] to be the fundamental pathologic change of hyporiboflavinosis. None of the results of these tests in themselves is entirely satisfactory, but taken as a group they are suggestive that no significant changes took place in the general capillary bed. There were no neurologic abnormalities, and no change of attitude, activity or appetite, such as appears in thiamine deficiency, was noted. Biochemically there was a sharp contrast between the behavior of these subjects and that of those exposed to deficiency of thiamin as previously reported,[49,50] in that the "double metabolic load" of glucose plus exercise failed to reveal any abnormality of the levels of lactic and pyruvic acids in the blood. This was surprising because of the intimate role played by both these vitamins in the enzyme systems involved in the metabolism of carbohydrate.

RIBOFLAVIN REQUIREMENTS OF MAN

Evidence of ariboflavinosis has not been confirmed on experimental diets which provided 0.8 to 0.9 mg per day[49,51] for over 2 years. Interpretation of the results of urinary excretions at different levels of riboflavin intake[52] has indicated that a tissue reserve of riboflavin may not be maintained in adult men at levels of intake below 1.2 mg per day. When intake was restricted to levels between 0.55 and 1.1 mg per day, less than 10 per cent of the ingested riboflavin was excreted in the urine. At levels of 1.3 mg per day or higher, over 20 per cent was excreted. Similar results have been obtained in female adults.[53,54]

The requirement for riboflavin does not appear to be related to calorie requirement or to muscular activity. However, the urinary excretion is markedly affected by alterations in nitrogen balance.[55-57] Less is excreted in the urine, on a given intake, when tissue growth is rapid, as during convalescence after severe trauma,[58] during lactation,[59] or after administration of testosterone propionate;[60] more is excreted after severe burns or surgical procedures where protein losses indicate cellular decomposition.[61] As a consequence of these observations, and the knowledge that in animal growth studies the amounts of riboflavin and protein in the diet are proportionately limiting, this reviewer has suggested that the daily mg riboflavin allowances be computed from the daily grams of protein allowances, because protein utilized has been related to changes in the lean body mass[62] by those responsible for estimating protein requirements. This correlates similar conditions which increase the need for riboflavin and protein simultaneously, such as growth, pregnancy, lactation, and wound healing. One advantage of relating the riboflavin and protein allowances is in facilitating a simple calculation of the needs of individuals who are growing faster than the average, or for those who, for a time, need more protein and riboflavin for tissue repair as a consequence of surgery, burns or other trauma.

In recent years there has been a tendency to relate riboflavin requirements to metabolic body size. Thus the Food and Nutrition Board has recommended that the allowance be calculated as a function of kg of body weight to the 0.75 power. The assumption is made that infants require 0.1, children 0.08, and adults 0.07 $mg/kg^{0.75}$. In effect, this relates somewhat the riboflavin requirement to the protein requirement and curbs recommendations that would make it necessary to drink large amounts of milk when expending large amounts of energy. Included in current Recommended Dietary Allowances is an increased riboflavin intake of 0.3 mg/day during pregnancy and 0.5 mg/day during lactation. On this basis, infants need 0.4 to 0.6 mg, children 0.6 to 1.2 mg, adults 1.3 to 1.7 mg and pregnant and lactating women 1.8 and 2.0 mg/day, respectively.

SOURCES OF RIBOFLAVIN

It is not difficult to conceive a riboflavin-deficient diet if dairy foods and other animal protein sources are omitted.[63] Conversely, a mixed diet that contains a pint of milk and the usual portions of meat products is not likely to be deficient in riboflavin. Fortunately, the relative heat stability of riboflavin in the absence of light favors its preservation in ordinary cooking procedures.[64] The major losses which may occur are probably attributable to the extraction of the vitamin by the water used in cooking or blanching.[65-67] Loss due to exposure to light during cooking[68] may be important.

The relative insolubility of riboflavin makes it logical to give divided doses during therapeutic administration of the vitamin. However, a daily oral administration of 6 mg appears to be assimilated as satisfactorily as three 2-mg doses at 4-hour intervals.[52] Where more rapid saturation is desired, a single dose of 25 mg of the sodium salt of riboflavin phosphate may be administered[69] intramuscularly. The intramuscular administration is preferred, since the intravenous injection of 50 mg in 1 minute produced evidence of a slight decrease in pulse rate in all of 5 adult subjects tested.

TOXICITY

The low solubility of riboflavin may be responsible for its low toxicity. The oral administration of 10 gm per kg to rats and 2 gm per kg to dogs produced no ill effects.[70] Mice receiving 340 mg per kg intraperitoneally, which is 5,000 times the therapeutic dose, or an equivalent of 20 gm per day for a man, showed no apparent effect. The rat

LD_{50} following intraperitoneal administration was 560 mg per kg.[70]

BIBLIOGRAPHY

1. McCollum and Kennedy: J. Biol. Chem., *24*, 491, 1916.
2. Emmett and Luros: J. Biol. Chem., *43*, 265, 1920.
3. Smith and Hendrick: Pub. Health Rep., *41*, 201, 1926.
4. Goldberger and Lillie: Pub. Health Rep., *41*, 1025, 1926.
5. Warburg and Christian: Biochem. Z., *266*, 377, 1933.
6. Ellinger and Koschara: Ber., *66*, 315, 808, 1933.
7. Booher: J. Biol. Chem., *102*, 39, 1933.
8. Kuhn, György and Wagner-Jauregg: Ber., *66*, 317, 576, 1034, 1933.
9. Blyth: J. Chem. Soc., *35*, 530, 1879.
10. Kuhn, Reinemund, Weygand, and Strobele: Ber., *68*, 1765, 1935.
11. Karrer, Salomon, Schopp, and Benz: Helv. Chem. Acta, *18*, 1143, 1935.
12. von Euler and Malmberg: Z. physiol. Chem., *250*, 158, 1937.
13. Jukes: J. Nutrition, *14*, 223, 1937.
14. Snell and Strong: Ind. Eng. Chem., Anal. Ed., *11*, 346, 1939.
15. van Eekelen and Emmerie: Acta Brevia Neerland, *5*, 77, 1935.
16. Andrews: Cereal Chem., *21*, 398, 1944.
17. Bourguin and Sherman: J. Am. Chem. Soc., *53*, 3501, 1931.
18. von Euler: Institut international di Chimie Solvay, Sixieme Conseil de Chimie, rapport et discussions Sur Les Vitamines et les Hormones, p. 198, Paris, 1938.
19. Norris, Wilgus, Ringrose, Heiman and Heuser: Cornell Univ. Agr. Exptl. Sta. Bull., *660*, 3, 1936.
20. Stone: Science, *111*, 283, 1950.
21. Horwitt: *The Vitamins*, Vol. 3, edited by Sebrell and Harris, New York, Academic Press, 1954, p. 380.
22. Coward, Morgan, and Waller: J. Physiol., *100*, 423, 1942.
23. Warkany: Vitamins and Hormones, *3*, 73, 1945.
24. Sebrell: Nat. Inst. Health Bull., *162*, Part 3, 23, 1933.
25. Sebrell and Onstatt: Public Health Rep., *53*, 83, 1938.
26. Patek, Post and Victor: Am. J. Physiol., *133*, 47, 1941.
27. Mitchell, Johnson, Hamilton and Haines: J. Nutrition, *41*, 317, 1950.
28. Cooperman, Waisman, McCall and Elvehjem: J. Nutrition, *30*, 45, 1945.
29. Foy and Kondi: Vitamins and Hormones, *26*, 653, 1968.
30. Stern and Holiday: Ber., *67*, 1104, 1442, 1934.
31. Theorell: Biochem. Z., *272*, 155, 1934.
31a. Rivlin: New Eng. J. Med., *283*, 463 1970.
32. Horwitt, Hills, Liebert and Steinberg: J. Nutrition, *39*, 357, 1949.
33. Stannus: Tr. Roy. Soc. Trop. Med. & Hyg., *5*, 112, 1912.
34. Bahr: *Researches on Sprue in Ceylon*, 1912–1914, London, Cambridge University Press, 1915.
35. Scott: Ann. Trop. Med., *12*, 109, 1918.
36. Moore: West African M. J., *4*, 46, 1930; J. Trop. Med., *42*, 109, 1939.
37. Landor and Pallister: Tr. Roy. Soc. Trop. Med. & Hyg., *19*, 121, 1935.
38. Aykroyd and Krishnan: Indian J. M. Research, *24*, 411, 1936.
39. Goldberger and Wheeler: Hygienic Laboratory Bulletin, No. 120, U.S. Treasury Dept. Public Health Service, 1920, p. 116.
40. Goldberger and Tanner: Pub. Health Rep., *40*, 54, 1925.
41. Bessey and Wolbach: J. Exper. Med., *69*, 1, 1939.
42. Spies, Vilter and Ashe: J.A.M.A., *113*, 931, 1939; Spies, Bean, and Ashe: Ann. Int. Med., *12*, 1830, 1939.
43. Sydenstricker, Geeslin, Templeton and Weaver: J.A.M.A., *113*, 1697, 1939.
44. Kruse, Sydenstricker, Sebrell and Cleckley: Pub. Health Rep., *55*, 157, 1940.
45. Tisdall, McCreary, and Pearce: Canad. M.A.J., *49*, 5, 1943.
46. Sebrell and Butler: Pub. Health Rep., *53*, 2282, 1938.
47. Hills, Liebert, Steinberg, and Horwitt: Arch. Int. Med., *87*, 682, 1951.
48. Stannus: Brit. M. J., *2*, 103, 1944.
49. Horwitt, Liebert, Kreisler and Wittman: National Research Council Bull., *116*, Washington, D.C., 1948.
50. Horwitt and Kreisler: J. Nutrition, *37*, 411, 1949.
51. Williams, Mason, Cusick and Wilder: J. Nutrition, *25*, 361, 1943.
52. Horwitt, Harvey, Hills and Liebert: J. Nutrition, *41*, 247, 1950.
53. Davis, Oldham and Roberts: J. Nutrition, *32*, 143, 1946.
54. Brewer, Porter, Ingalls and Ohlson: J. Nutrition, *32*, 583, 1946.
55. Sarett and Perlzweig: J. Nutrition, *25*, 173, 1943.
56. Sarett, Klein and Perlzweig: J. Nutrition, *24*, 295, 1942.
57. Pollack and Bookman: J. Lab. & Clin. Med., *38*, 561, 1951.
58. Andrea, Schenker and Browne: Federation Proc., *5*, 3, 1946.
59. Roderick, Coryell, Williams and Macy: J. Nutrition, *32*, 267, 1946.
60. Beher and Gaebler: J. Nutrition, *41*, 447, 1950.
61. Pollack and Halpern: *Therapeutic Nutrition*, National Research Council, 1951.
62. Horwitt: Am. J. Clin. Nutrition, *18*, 458, 1966.
63. Horwitt, Sampson, Hills and Steinberg: J. Am. Dietet. Assoc., *25*, 591, 1949.
64. Levine and Remington: J. Nutrition, *13*, 525, 1937.

65. Mayfield and Hedrick: J. Am. Dietet. Assoc., 25, 1024, 1949.
66. Wagner, Strong and Elvehjem: Ind. Eng. Chem., 39, 985, 1947.
67. Krehl and Winters: J. Am. Dietet. Assoc., 26, 966, 1950.
68. Cheldelin, Woods, and Williams: J. Nutrition, 26, 477, 1943.
69. Horwitt and Wilson: Unpublished.
70. Unna and Greslin: J. Pharm. Exptl. Therap., 76, 75, 1942.
71. Kuhn and Boulanger: Z. Physiol. Chem., 241, 233, 1936.
72. Kuhn: Klin. Wochschr., 77, 222, 1938.
73. Demole: Z. Vitaminforsch., 7, 138, 1938.

Chapter

5

Section G   Niacin

M. K. HORWITT

Pellagra first appeared in Europe about 1720, which coincided with the introduction of corn (maize) planting. The first recorded description of symptoms of pellagra as an individual disease was by Casal, a Spanish physician, in 1735. The term "pellagra," or rough skin, which had been used by the peasantry in Italy to describe the symptoms, was not published until 1771 by Frapolli. Despite its antiquity, the recognition that this was a dietary deficiency disease did not evolve until after Goldberger's classical studies which began in 1913, when the U.S. Public Health Service undertook an investigation of an epidemic in the South where about 200,000 cases a year were being recorded. As early as 1913, Sandwith had suggested that pellagra was due to a deficiency of tryptophan in maize.[1] Wilson,[2] working in Egypt, had claimed, in 1920, that pellagra was due to the poor biological value of the protein in corn, a point with which Goldberger[3] concurred. In fact, Tanner, an associate of Goldberger (quoted by Sebrell[4]), in a letter written in 1921 describes the rapid cure of a pellagrous patient by the administration of tryptophan. However, the discovery that a yeast extract devoid of amino nitrogen was effective in curing pellagra delayed the recognition of the significance of these observations. It was not until 1937, when Elvehjem et al.[5] demonstrated that nicotinic acid could cure the animal analogs of pellagra, that the direct correlation between human pellagra and nicotinic acid became apparent.[6-10] Almost 8 years more were to pass before the biological transformation of tryptophan to niacin was fully appreciated.[11] Even today one finds tables in textbooks in use that report the niacin content of foods without reference to the tryptophan content.

DISCOVERY AND CHEMICAL NATURE

Although nicotinic acid was prepared as a pure chemical substance in 1867[12] and isolated from rice polishings by Funk in 1911,[13] its recognition as a vitamin was not fully established until 1937 when Elvehjem,

Nicotinic acid (Niacin)
pyridine-3-carboxylic acid

Nicotinamide (Nicotinic Acid Amide; Niacinamide)
pyridine-3-carboxylic acid amide

Madden, Strong and Woolley[5] showed that the deficiency disease, black tongue in dogs, was cured by this substance. The recognition that nicotinic acid (niacin) was the human antipellagric vitamin was soon confirmed by numerous investigators.

Niacin is β-pyridine carboxylic acid. This is easily converted to the physiologically active nicotinic acid amide (niacinamide). Niacin is a nonhygroscopic, stable, white, crystalline solid which sublimes without decomposition at about 230° C. It is soluble in water (1 gm to 60 ml at 25° C) and in alcohol (1 gm in 80 ml at 25° C) and insoluble in ether. Niacinamide is much more soluble in water (1 gm in 1 ml) and in alcohol (1 gm in 1.5 ml) and is also soluble in ether.

THE ESTIMATION OF NICOTINIC ACID

Although animals have never been completely satisfactory subjects for the assay of the pellagra-preventive factor, dogs have been used to produce uncomplicated niacin deficiency.[14,15] The chemical technique most often used depends upon the König reaction[16] in which the pyridine compound reacts with cyanogen bromide and an organic base to form a yellow color.[17,18] In recent years the microbiological methods as illustrated by that of Snell and Wright[19] have been more popular. This depends upon the amount of lactic acid produced by *L. arabinosus* on a synthetic medium containing all known growth factors except niacin.

THE BIOLOGICAL FUNCTION OF NICOTINIC ACID

The physiologic significance of nicotinic acid was understood in 1935 by Warburg and Christian[20] before its importance in nutrition was recognized. Their isolation of coenzyme II, a compound of adenine, nicotinamide, two molecules of ribose and three molecules of phosphoric acid, was followed by the recognition that this coenzyme, triphosphopyridine nucleotide (TPN) was a specific codehydrogenase for a series of dehydrogenases which included, among other enzymes, those involved in changing glucose-6-monophosphate to phosphogluconic acid, and citric acid to α-ketoglutaric acid. Coenzyme I (cozymase) or diphosphopyridine nucleotide (DPN) is similar in general action and in structure except that it contains two molecules of phosphoric acid. It is a specific codehydrogenase for enzymes responsible for converting lactic acid to pyruvic acid, alcohol to acetaldehyde, β-hydroxybutyric to acetaldehyde, and for many other reactions. The modern terminology for DPN and TPN is NAD and NADP which are the currently accepted abbreviations for nicotinamide adenine dinucleotide and nicotinamide adenine dinucleotide phosphate, respectively.

NAD and NADP serve as parts of the intracellular respiratory mechanism of all cells. They assist in the stepwise transfer of hydrogen from a product of glycolysis to flavin mononucleotide which in turn, with the help of specific enzymes, transfers this hydrogen to the cytochromes which in turn transfer the hydrogen to oxygen to form water. NAD and NADP can accept electrons from many biological substrates. Reduced NAD (NADH) usually donates its hydrogens to flavin adenine dinucleotide (FAD) in the cell respiratory chain responsible for energy release. NADPH gives up its hydrogens most often to cellular biosynthetic processes like the synthesis of fatty acids.

CLINICAL ASPECTS OF NICOTINIC ACID DEFICIENCY

Although the disease, pellagra, has been endemic in corn-eating areas of the world for over 200 years, it was not until about 1908 that the diagnostic symptoms of pellagra were clearly recognized.[21] Usually, the early symptoms are weakness, lassitude, anorexia, and indigestion. These are followed by the classic "three D's," dermatitis, diarrhea and dementia.

The dermatitis has a characteristic appearance on those parts of the body exposed to sunlight, heat, or mild trauma. The lesions are distributed on the face, neck, and surfaces of the hands, feet, elbows and other parts of the body which may be subject to mechanical irritations or to contact with body secretions. Usually the lesions of pellagra are bilaterally symmetrical. In a study by Goldsmith et al.[22] of experimentally produced pellagra, the importance of oral lesions as diagnostic signs was confirmed.

Although diarrhea is a prominent feature in the pellagric patient, it may not develop in all cases.[23] The diarrhea may be severe and may be accompanied by vomiting and a dysphagia, a mouth inflammation which may be so painful that the patient refuses food, and becomes emaciated.

The mental symptoms develop in untreated cases.[24] Irritability, headaches, sleeplessness, loss of memory or other signs of emotional instability often accompany the early signs of pellagra. In advanced cases, a toxic confusional psychosis with symptoms of acute delirium and catatonia has been observed.

Lesions of the nervous system are nonspecific. Scattered degeneration of the axis cylinders of the pyramidal cells of the cortex and a myelin degeneration of fibers of the spinal column have been found.[25] Peripheral lesions are uncommon.

Recognition of the deficiency of dietary intake of nicotinic acid, or tryptophan-containing proteins, can be obtained by analyzing the urine for its N^1-methylnicotinamide content. Whereas the normal daily excretion is usually over 3 mg, subjects on a restricted diet providing 4.7 mg of niacin and 190 mg of tryptophan for 60 days had excretions of approximately 0.5 mg per day.[22] Slightly higher excretions of N^1-methylnicotinamide were obtained in another study in which a diet providing 5.8 mg niacin and 265 mg of tryptophan daily was fed for more than a year.[26] The latter study also showed that the pyridone of N^1-methylnicotinamide was not excreted unless the excretion of N^1-methylnicotinamide approached satisfactory levels. In effect, if the pyridone is found in the urine at minimal levels one should expect the diet to be adequate in niacin-tryptophan.

NICOTINIC ACID REQUIREMENTS OF MAN

Dietary levels of less than 7.5 mg a day have been associated with the production of pellagra[22,27,28] but it is not correct to speak about nicotinic acid needs without considering the amount of tryptophan in the diet. Not only can tryptophan alone heal the lesions of pellagra[29-31] but it may be more nearly correct to think of pellagra as a tryptophan deficiency, since corn products are relatively more deficient in tryptophan than in nicotinic acid.[32,33]

The term "niacin-equivalent"[32] was introduced to facilitate the calculation of the combined effects of nicotinic acid and tryptophan in the diet. The amount of tryptophan chosen to be equivalent to 1 mg of nicotinic acid was 60 mg. This ratio is a compromise based upon studies of the amounts of tryptophan converted to N^1-methylnicotinamide and its metabolites in human subjects.[26,34] Obviously, such a relationship cannot be expected to be inflexibile under all conditions of genetic, physiologic, and dietary variations, but the fact that some protein foods, practically devoid of nicotinic acid, can supply all the niacin-equivalents necessary for optimal health makes it practical to have some estimation of the amounts of tryptophan in the diet in order to evaluate nicotinic acid requirements. This is illustrated in Table 5G–1.

It should be emphasized that although most studies[35-38] have confirmed that an average of 60 mg of tryptophan is converted to 1 mg of niacin, this equivalence will vary from individual to individual. Of special interest are data[39] from women in the third trimester of pregnancy who can convert tryptophan to niacin metabolites 3 times as efficiently as non-pregnant females. It would appear from

Table 5G-1. Niacin-Equivalents of Representative Foods[26]

Food	Niacin mg/1000 calories	Trypto-phan mg/1000 calories	Niacin-Equivalent per 1000 calories
Cow's milk	1.21	673	12.4
Human milk	2.46	443	9.84
Beef, round	24.7	1280	46.0
Whole eggs	0.60	1150	10.8
Salt pork	1.15	61	2.17
Wheat flour	2.48	297	7.43
Corn grits	1.83	70	3.00
Corn	4.97	106	6.74

interpretation of studies on the effect of tryptophan load tests during pregnancy or after ingestion of contraceptive steroids or steroid hormones that the estrogens cause stimulation of tryptophan oxygenase which is apparently the rate-limiting enzyme in the tryptophan-nicotinic acid ribonucleotide pathway.[40,41]

An interesting point that comes out of studies of human requirements is the calculation that the requirement for niacin-equivalents is dependent upon the total caloric intake either as a function of metabolism plus work or of body size. Accordingly, it may be necessary to think of niacin-tryptophan requirements, as one does for thiamine requirements, as being related to calories consumed. An illustration of this may be had from comparing the experimental pellagra-producing diet used by Goldberger[27] with those used by Goldsmith et al.,[22] and in the Elgin studies.[26] The Goldberger diet provided 6.7 mg nicotinamide and 330 mg tryptophan in 3000 calories, or 4.1 niacin-equivalents per 1000 calories, whereas diets in the other studies, which provided 5.2 mg of nicotinamide plus 235 mg tryptophan in 2000 calories or 4.4 niacin-equivalents per 1000 calories, did not produce pellagra. In the Tulane studies,[22] diets which provided less than 4.4 niacin-equivalents per 1000 calories at levels of intake of 2000 calories did produce pellagra.

To put the figure of 4.4 mg of niacin-equivalent per 1000 calories in proper perspective, it should be compared with levels of intake of thiamine and riboflavin below which pathologic symptoms appear. This would be about 0.18 mg of thiamine per 1000 calories and about 0.6 mg of riboflavin per day.

THERAPY

Since the ingestion of large, therapeutic amounts of nicotinic acid usually produces a flushing reaction, niacin prescribed for correction of nutritional deficiency is more often administered as the nicotinamide (niacinamide). The amounts of nicotinamide generally recommended for therapeutic purposes are about 10 times the daily minimum requirement (assuming adequacy of protein) and

range from 50 to 250 mg per day. Recommended allowances as defined by the Food and Nutrition Board range from 5 to 8 niacin-equivalents for infants to 20 niacin-equivalents for lactating females. Since 75 gm of good protein will supply about 15 mg niacin-equivalents from its tryptophan content and practically all mixed diets with adequate calories will add more than 5 mg of niacin, this allowance of 20 mg niacin-equivalents is easy to achieve.

Large doses of nicotinic acid, from 3 to 6 gm per day, reduce the levels of cholesterol, beta-lipoproteins and triglycerides in the blood.[42,43] Nicotinamide is ineffective. The flushing reaction and itching resulting from oral ingestion of nicotinic acid disappear after about 3 days of therapy, but prolonged use has raised some problems of gastrointestinal irritation and possible liver damage.[44]

BIBLIOGRAPHY

1. Sandwith: Trans. Soc. Trop. Med. and Hyg., 6, 143, 1913.
2. Wilson: J. Hyg., 20, 1, 1921.
3. Goldberger: J.A.M.A., 78, 1676, 1922.
4. Sebrell: J. Nutr., 55, 3, 1955.
5. Elvehjem, Madden, Strong and Woolley: J. Am. Chem. Soc., 59, 1767, 1937; J. Biol. Chem., 123, 137, 1938.
6. Fouts, Helmer, Lepkovsky, and Jukes: Proc. Soc. Exper. Biol. & Med., 37, 405, 1937.
7. Smith, Ruffin and Smith: J.A.M.A., 109, 2054, 1937.
8. Spies, Cooper and Blankenhorn: J.A.M.A., 110, 622, 1938.
9. Spies, Bean and Stone: J.A.M.A., 111, 584, 1938.
10. Schmidt and Sydenstricker: J.A.M.A., 110, 2065, 1938; Sydenstricker: Arch Int. Med., 67, 746, 1941; Sydenstricker and Cleckley: Am. J. Psychiat., 98, 83, 1941.
11. Krehl, Sarma, Teply and Elvehjem: J. Nutrition, 31, 85, 1946.
12. Huber: Liebeg's Ann. Chem., 141, 271, 1867.
13. Funk: J. Physiol. 43, 395, 1911; J.A.M.A., 109, 2086, 1937.
14. Waisman, Mickelsen, McKibbin and Elvehjem: J. Nutrition, 19, 483, 1940; McKibbin, Waisman, Mickelsen and Elvehjem: Wisconsin Agric. Exp. Sta. Bull. No. 446.
15. Schaefer, McKibbin and Elvehjem: J. Biol. Chem., 144, 679, 1942.
16. König: J. prakt. Chem., 69, 105, 1904, 70, 19, 1904.
17. Swaminathan: Nature, 141, 830, 1938.
18. Bandier and Hald: Biochem. J., 33, 264, 1939.
19. Snell and Wright: J. Biol. Chem., 139, 675, 1941.

20. Warburg and Christian: Biochem. Z., *275*, 464, 1935.
21. Elvehjem: Physiol. Rev., *20*, 249, 1940.
22. Goldsmith, Sarett, Register, and Gibbons: J. Clin. Invest., *31*, 533, 1952.
23. Bicknell and Prescott: *Vitamins in Medicine*, 3rd Ed., New York, Grune & Stratton, 1953.
24. Frostig and Spies: Am. J. Med. Sci., *199*, 268, 1940.
25. Youmans: *Nutritional Deficiencies*, Philadelphia, J. B. Lippincott Co., 1943.
26. Horwitt, Harvey, Rothwell, Cutler and Haffron: J. Nutrition, *60*, Supplement 1, 1956.
27. Goldberger and Wheeler: Arch. Int. Med., *25*, 451, 1920.
28. Frazier and Friedeman: Quart. Bull. Northwestern Med. School, *20*, 24, 1946.
29. Bean, Franklin and Daum: J. Lab. & Clin. Med., *38*, 167, 1951.
30. Sarett: J. Biol. Chem., *193*, 627, 1951.
31. Vilter, Mueller and Bean: J. Lab. & Clin. Med., *34*, 409, 1949.
32. Horwitt: Am. J. Clin. Nutrition, *3*, 244, 1955.
33. ———: J. Amer. Dietet. Assoc., *34*, 914, 1958.
34. Goldsmith: Am. J. Clin. Nutrition, *6*, 479, 1958.
35. Goldsmith, Miller and Unglaub: J. Nutr., *73*, 172, 1961.
36. Moyer, Goldsmith, Miller and Miller: J. Nutr., *79*, 423, 1963.
37. deLange and Joubert: Am. J. Clin. Nutr. *15*, 169, 1964.
38. Vivian: J. Nutr. *82*, 395, 1964.
39. Wertz, Lojkin, Bouchard and Derby: J. Nutr., *64*, 339, 1958.
40. Rose and Braidman: Am. J. Clin. Nutr., *24*, 673, 1971.
41. Brin: Am. J. Clin. Nutr., *24*, 704, 1971.
42. Miller, Hamilton and Goldsmith: Am. J. Clin. Nutr., *8*, 480, 1960.
43. Shawver, Scarborough and Tarnowski: Am. J. Psychiat., *117*, 741, 1961.
44. Christensen, Achor, Berge and Mason: Dis. Chest, *46*, 411, 1964.

Chapter

5

Section H Pantothenic Acid

HOWERDE E. SAUBERLICH

INTRODUCTION

Pantothenic acid was recognized in 1933[1] as a growth factor for yeast. Following its isolation[2,3] and synthesis,[4] it was recognized that the vitamin could prevent or cure chick dermatitis.[5,6] Subsequently it was recognized as an essential nutrient for the rat, mouse, monkey, pig, dog, fox, turkey, fish, hamster, and other species. It is widely distributed in nature and has been found in all forms of living things. Liver, meat, cereal, milk, egg yolk, fresh vegetables, and many other foods are good sources (Table 5I–1).[7]

CHEMISTRY AND BIOCHEMICAL FUNCTIONS OF PANTOTHENIC ACID

Pantothenic acid has a molecular weight of 219 and consists of α, γ-dihydroxy β, β' di-methyl butyric acid and β-alanine joined by a peptide linkage. Since the vitamin itself is a pale yellow viscous oil, it is commonly available as a synthetic, white crystalline calcium salt. The vitamin is stable in neutral solution but is readily destroyed by heat at either alkaline or acid pH.

Pantothenic acid is converted via pan-

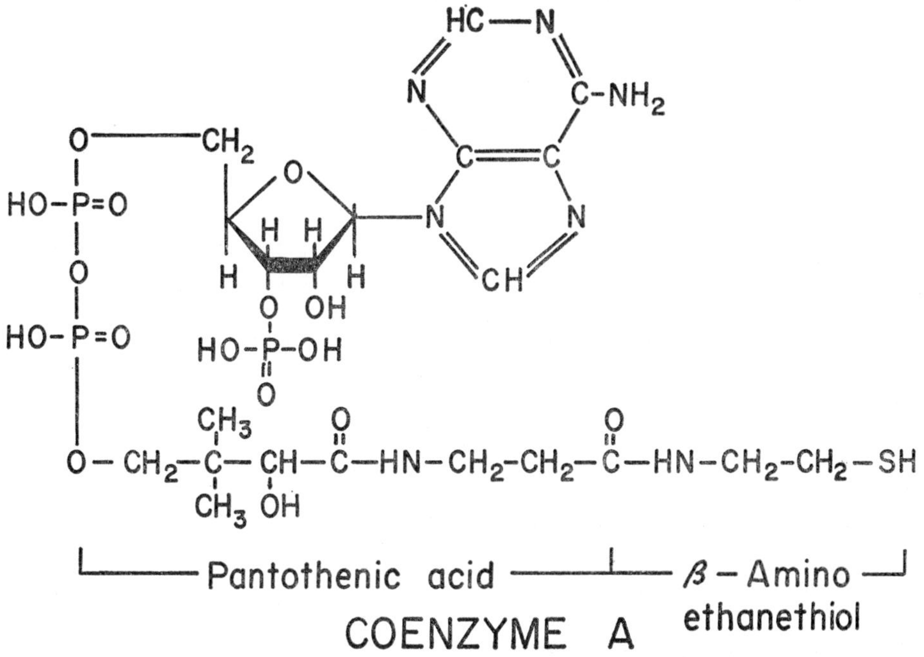

Fig. 5H-1

tetheine to coenzyme A which is an important catalyst of biological acetylation reactions,[8–11] or in a broader sense in acyl transfers. Coenzyme A contains β-mercaptoethylamine whose terminal sulfhydryl group is the reactive site of the molecule in biological reactions.[12,13] All known acyl derivatives of coenzyme A are thiol esters. These acyl derivatives of coenzyme A may participate in a number of metabolic reactions. Thus coenzyme A is involved in condensation and addition reactions, acyl group interchanges, and nucleophilic attack. In this manner, coenzyme A is enzymatically involved in the (a) acetylation of choline and certain aromatic amines such as sulfonamides; (b) oxidation of fatty acids, pyruvate, α-ketoglutarate and acetaldehyde; and (c) synthesis of fatty acids, cholesterol, sphingosine, citrate, acetoacetate, porphyrin and sterols. Thus coenzyme A may serve not only as an acetyl acceptor or acetyl donor but also as an acceptor or donor of acyl groups.[14–17]

Pyruvate and α-ketoglutarate are converted to acetyl coenzyme A and to succinyl coenzyme A, respectively, through the participation of thiamin pyrophosphate, niacin adenine dinucleotide (NAD) and lipoic acid. Additional roles of coenzyme A in carbohydrate metabolism have been noted.[18–20] Acetoacetyl coenzyme A may conjugate in the liver with acetyl coenzyme A to form β-hydroxy-β-methylglutaryl coenzyme A, an important precursor of cholesterol and other sterols. Coenzyme A participates in the biosynthesis of sphingosine and ceramide.[21] Histones of liver nuclei are acetylated by coenzyme A.[22]

Fatty acids are converted into an active state for oxidation in the mitochondria by the formation of fatty acyl-coenzyme A esters by the catalyzed reactions of enzymes such as thiophorases, acetate thiokinase, medium- and long-chain fatty acid thiokinases and a guanine triphosphate-specific acid thiokinase.[23,24] Enzymatic β-oxidation of the straight-chain fatty acids with even number carbon atoms results in the production of acetyl coenzyme A. Quantities of propionyl coenzyme A and methylmalonyl coenzyme A result from the oxidation of odd carbon or branched-chain fatty acids and unsaturated fatty acids.[25] Propionyl coenzyme A is converted by the biotin requiring propionyl carboxylase enzyme into methylmalonyl coenzyme A. The vitamin B_{12} containing methylmalonyl mutase enzyme converts methylmalonyl coenzyme A into succinyl coenzyme A which may then enter the tricarboxylic acid cycle.[26]

The de novo synthesis of long-chain fatty acids proceeds mainly through malonyl coenzyme A as an intermediate.[27–30] Malonyl coenzyme A is formed by carboxylation of acetyl coenzyme A through the action of acetyl coenzyme A carboxylase. This enzyme appears to play an important role in the control of fatty acid synthesis.[28] Through the involvement of a cytoplasmic multienzyme complex, acetyl coenzyme A and malonyl coenzyme A are converted to palmityl coenzyme A and stearyl coenzyme A.[31] Further elongation may occur in the mitochondria with the participation of acetyl coenzyme A or in the microsomes with the participation of malonyl coenzyme A.[32] The metabolism of medium-chain fatty acids likewise involves coenzyme A.[17,33,34]

Fatty acid biosynthesis in the cytoplasm and mitochondria involves an additional role of pantothenic acid in the form of the cofactor, 4′-phosphopantetheine. This factor is bound to a protein commonly referred to as the acyl carrier protein (ACP).[36] This protein, with 4′-phosphopantetheine, ap-

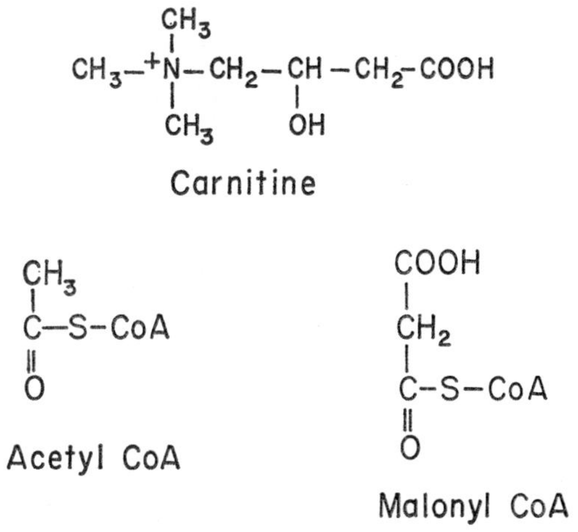

$$CH_3-{}^+N-CH_2-CH-CH_2-COOH$$

with CH_3 groups on N and OH on the carbon

Carnitine

$$CH_3-C(=O)-S-CoA$$

Acetyl CoA

$$COOH-CH_2-C(=O)-S-CoA$$

Malonyl CoA

Fig. 5H-2

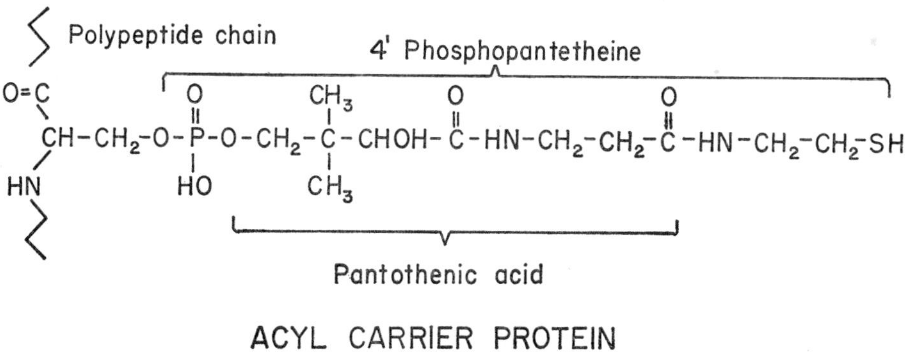

ACYL CARRIER PROTEIN

Fig. 5H-3

pears to be involved in all fatty acid synthesizing systems.[30,37-39] The acyl intermediates formed during fatty acid synthesis are esterified to the sulfhydryl group of the 4'-phosphopantetheine linked to the acyl carrier protein. Phosphopantetheine is a cofactor bound to the guanosine triphosphate-dependent acyl coenzyme A synthetase.[40] Thus, 4'-phosphopantetheine serves in a capacity during fatty acid synthesis analogous to that of coenzyme A during fatty acid oxidation. The fatty acids formed may be converted to triglycerides via the participation of their fatty acyl coenzyme A esters.[41] Coenzyme A also participates in the biosynthesis of ceramides.

Carnitine reacts with fatty acyl coenzyme A esters to form fatty acyl carnitine esters. The acylated carnitines are capable of crossing the mitochondrial membrane which is impermeable to acyl coenzyme A.[27,42-44] Following passage into the mitochondria, the fatty acyl group is transferred from carnitine to coenzyme A again to form fatty acyl coenzyme A. Coenzyme A is synthesized within the cells as blood coenzyme A fails to permeate liver cells.[45]

METHODS OF ASSAY

Pantothenic acid may be measured with the use of chemical methods, microbiological procedures and the chick curative bioassay. Although the chick and rat prophylactic and curative bioassays were commonly used in early studies on pantothenic acid, they have been replaced by microbiological procedures for assaying natural products.[46] Pantothenic acid, pantetheine and coenzyme A are equally active in the animal bioassays. The microbiological assays use either *Saccharomyces carlsbergenis*, *Lactobacillus casei* or *L. plantarum* (*L. arabinosus*) as the test organism.[47-49] More recently, some investigators have employed the protozoan *Tetrahymena pyriformis*[50] for measuring pantothenic acid levels in natural products and biological fluids. The majority of the pantothenic acid in foods and biological materials exists as coenzyme A and other bound forms. Microbiological assays for total pantothenic acid content require enzymatic hydrolysis of the samples to provide free pantothenic acid. Pantethine and pantetheine have been estimated in samples with the use of *L. helveticus*.[47,51] Pharmaceutical preparations of pantothenic acid can be readily assayed with the use of *L. plantarum*.[52] Pantothenyl alcohol (panthenol), a compound with equivalent pantothenic acid activity for animals and man,[53] can be measured in pharmaceutical products with the use of *Leuconostoc mesenteroides*.[47,54] Chemical procedures, including gas chromatography[108] are also available for determining pantothenic acid and pantothenyl alcohol in dry or liquid multivitamin preparations.[47,55-57] Pantoic acid, a metabolite and constituent of pantothenic acid, can be estimated with the use of an *Escherichia coli* mutant.[58] Procedures for measuring coenzyme A have also been described.[59,60]

DEFICIENCIES IN EXPERIMENTAL ANIMALS

Although the effects of a pantothenic acid deficiency vary greatly from species to species certain common denominators exist, particularly that of growth failure.[61] In addition, a deficiency of the vitamin in the rat results in dermatitis, achromotrichia (graying), adrenal necrosis and hemorrhage, "spectacled eyes" (hair loss about the eyes), spastic gait, anemia, leukopenia, impaired antibody production, gonadal atrophy, infertility and duodenal ulcer. Congenital malformations may occur in offspring of pantothenic-deficient rats.[62,63] Increased levels of fat in the diet did not increase the requirement for pantothenic acid in the rat based upon body weight changes, adrenal weights or onset and incidence of graying of the hair. Pantothenic acid-deficient rats did, however, have lower liver conenzyme A values when fed a high fat diet.[64] A pantothenic acid deficiency in the mouse resembles that in the rat. The mouse, however, does not develop hemorrhagic and necrotic adrenals but exhibits a partial paralysis of the hind legs with nerve tissue degeneration.

Dogs develop hair changes, decreased appetite, irritability, fatty livers, gastrointestinal tract disturbances, hypoglycemia, convulsions, coma and death. Similar observations have been reported for the monkey. Swine develop dermatitis, spastic gait ("goose-stepping"), hair loss, excessive nasal secretions, diarrhea, ulcerative colitis, degenerative lesions of the spinal cord and peripheral nerves and alterations in sodium, potassium, and glucose absorption.[65] The coenzyme A activity of cells from colonic mucosa was markedly reduced in pantothenic acid-deficient swine.[65] These observations suggest a relationship between coenzyme A content of colonic tissue and diarrhea and ulcerative colitis.

A pantothenic acid deficiency in the chick results in the classical dermatitis in the corners of the mouth and of the toes and upper surface of the foot. Other signs of a deficiency include poor feathering, spinal cord degeneration, incoordination, paralysis, involution of the thymus, fatty degeneration of the liver and death.[66] Symptoms of a pantothenic acid deficiency in turkeys resemble closely those in chickens.[67] In addition, ducks deficient in pantothenic acid develop anemia and show an impaired ability to develop antibodies when stimulated with bacterial, viral or erythrocyte antigens.[68,69] A pantothenic acid deficiency can be induced in other species, including the guinea pig and cat.[70]

DEFICIENCIES IN MAN

Pantothenic acid is of such widespread distribution in foods that an occurrence of a deficiency in the vitamin is probably exceedingly rare. In malnutrition, however, multiple deficiencies frequently exist and a deficiency in pantothenic acid may not be recognized as part of the condition. Means of detecting and evaluating a pantothenic acid deficiency are limited. In studies in which attempts were made to control dietary intakes of pantothenic acid, results indicate that the urinary excretion of the vitamin by man is related to its dietary intake.[71,72] Urinary excretions of less than 1.0 mg per day are considered abnormally low for the human adult. Both serum and erythrocytes contain relatively high levels of pantothenic acid but whether changes in these levels can indicate a pantothenic acid deficiency is uncertain.[50,73,74] The measurement of changes in the blood and urine levels of the vitamin after test loads of 10 to 50 mg of the vitamin is not very useful in the diagnosis of pantothenic acid deficiency.[75,76] Patients with chronic malnutrition tend to have lower levels of pantothenic acid in blood and urine.[77,78] Poorly nourished alcoholic patients have been observed to have low serum levels of pantothenic acid.[79] The elevated serum copper levels noted in pellagrins were lowered significantly by injections of pantothenic acid.[80] The vitamin has been reported to afford relief in nutritional neuropathy and Korsakoff's psychosis.[81] Pantothenic acid treatment improved the burning or electric foot syndrome (nutritional melalgia),[82,83] which was noted in prisoners of the Japanese during World War II.[84–86] Subjects with this syndrome have been reported to have a reduced ability to acetylate para-aminobenzoic acid.[87] Pantothenic acid has been reported to improve the ability of well-nourished subjects to withstand stress.[88,89]

The most well-defined signs and symptoms of a pantothenic acid deficiency have been those observed in human volunteers maintained on a diet deficient in pantothenic acid and on a pantothenic acid antagonist, omega methyl pantothenic acid.[90-94] Subjects on the pantothenic-deficient diet developed vomiting, malaise, abdominal distress and burning cramps. Later during the deficiency, tenderness in the heels, fatigue and insomnia occurred. Subjects who received both omega methyl pantothenic acid and the deficient diet developed similar symptoms somewhat earlier. The subjects were observed to have pain and soreness in the abdomen, nausea, some personality changes, insomnia, weakness and cramps in the legs, and paresthesia in the hands and feet. There was an impaired eosinopenic response to ACTH and an elevated sedimentation rate. Adrenocortical function appeared to remain normal. Antibody production against tetanus was impaired by the pantothenic acid deficiency. The combination of pantothenic acid and pyridoxine deficiencies exaggerated the impaired antigenic response when bacterial antigens were used, but not when polio virus was employed. Administration of large doses of pantothenic acid reversed most of the signs and symptoms and laboratory changes ascribed to the pantothenic acid deficiency.

NUTRITIONAL REQUIREMENT

The usual diet of a human adult provides approximately 10 to 15 mg of pantothenic acid daily, with a range of 9 to 20 mg.[95] Diets adequate for children of 7 to 9 years of age provide about 4 to 5 mg of pantothenic acid.[72] The Food and Nutrition Board has not established a recommended dietary allowance for pantothenic acid but states that a daily intake of 5 to 10 mg is probably adequate for children and adults.[96] Pantothenic acid is unstable to heat with losses ranging from 15 to 30 per cent in heat-dried and in canned and in cooked meats.[97]

8

THERAPEUTIC USE, TOXICITY, AND METABOLISM

Although pantothenic acid has been reported as an anti-gray hair factor in man and to relieve postoperative paralytic ileus and to provide benefit in cases of burn and skin lesions, these effects have not been corroborated.[89,98-102] At present, no clearly defined therapeutic use of pantothenic acid exists, although the vitamin is commonly present in multi-vitamin preparations and in products employed in intravenous and oral alimentation. Synthetic calcium pantothenate is usually employed for these purposes, although the sodium salt is used in aqueous dispersions where the calcium ion must be avoided. Only the D (+) enantiomorph has biological activity. Pantothenyl alcohol may also be used in the preparation of injectable and other liquid pharmaceutical preparations.

Pantothenic acid has been administered to human subjects in the amounts of 10 to 20 gm as the calcium salt. The only evidence of toxicity from these high intakes was an occasional diarrhea.[103,104]

The metabolism of pantothenic acid has not been studied in depth in man. Although the germ-free rat has been reported not to metabolize and break down pantothenic acid[105] limited information suggests that man does metabolize daily a quantity of the vitamin.[89] Antagonists of pantothenic acid have been reported to possess antimalarial properties.[106,107]

BIBLIOGRAPHY

1. Williams, Lyman, Goodyear, Truesdail and Holaday: J. Am. Chem. Soc., 55, 2912, 1933.
2. Williams: Science, 89, 486, 1939.
3. Williams, Weinstock, Rohrmann, Truesdail, Mitchell and Meyer: J. Am. Chem. Soc., 61, 454, 1939.
4. Williams and Major: Science, 91, 246, 1940.
5. Jukes: J. Am. Chem. Soc., 61, 975, 1939.
6. Woolley, Waisman and Elvehjem: J. Am. Chem. Soc., 61, 977, 1939.
7. Orr: Pantothenic Acid, Vitamin B6 and Vitamin B12 in Foods. Home Economics Research Report No. 36, U. S. Dept. of Agric., 1969.
8. Lipmann, Kaplan, Novelli, Tuttle and Guirard: J. Biol. Chem., 167, 869, 1947.
9. Baddiley: Adv. Enzymol., 16, 1, 1955.

10. Lipmann: Bacteriological Revs., *17*, 1, 1953.
11. Jaenicke and Lynen: In *The Enzymes*, Boyer, Lardy and Myrbäck, Editors, New York, Academic Press, 1960, Vol. 3, p. 3.
12. Stern and Ochoa: J. Biol. Chem., *179*, 491, 1949.
13. Lynen, Reichert and Rueff: Ann. Chem., Justus Liebigs, *574*, 1, 1951.
14. Clayton: Quart. Rev., *19*, 168, 1965.
15. Frantz and Shroepfer: Ann. Rev. Biochem., *36*, 691, 1967.
16. Lennarz: Ann. Rev. Biochem., *39*, 359, 1970.
17. Shapiro: Ann. Rev. Biochem., *36*, 247, 1967.
18. Cooper and Bendict: Biochemistry (Wash.), *7*, 3032, 1968.
19. Nakashima, Pontremoli and Horecker: Proc. Nat. Acad. Sci., U.S.A., *64*, 947, 1969.
20. Weber, Lea and Stamm: Lipids, *4*, 388, 1969.
21. Morell: J. Biol. Chem., *245*, 342, 1970.
22. Gallwitz and Sekeris: Hoppe Seylers Z. Physiol. Chem., *350*, 150, 1969.
23. Galigzna, Rossi, Sartorelli and Gibson: J. Biol. Chem., *242*, 2111, 1967.
24. Greville and Tubbs: *Essays in Biochemistry*, New York, Academic Press, 1968, Vol. IV.
25. Dupont and Mathias: Lipids, *4*, 478, 1969.
26. Hogenkamp: Ann. Rev. Biochem., *37*, 225, 1968.
27. Stumpf: Ann Rev. Biochem., *38*, 159, 1969.
28. Numa, Nakanishi, Hashimoto, Iritani, and Akazaki: Vitamins and Hormones, *28*, 213, 1970.
29. Vagelos: Ann. Rev. Biochem., *33*, 139, 1964.
30. Schweizer, Willecke, Winnewisser and Lynen: Vitamins and Hormones, *28*, 329, 1970.
31. Hansen and Hanser: Acta Chem. Scand., *23*, 2180, 1969.
32. Seubert, Lamberts and Kramer: Biochim. Biophys. Acta, *164*, 498, 1968.
33. Bar-Tana and Rose: Biochem. J., *109*, 283, 1968.
34. Bar-Tana, Rose and Shapiro: Biochem. J., *109*, 269, 1968.
35. Mooney and Barron: Biochemistry (Wash.), *9*, 2138, 1970.
36. Majerus and Vagelos: Adv. Lipid Res., *5*, 2, 1967.
37. Pugh and Wakil: J. Biol. Chem., *240*, 4727, 1965.
38. Larrabee, McDaniel, Bakerman, and Vagelos: Proc. Nat. Acad. Sci. U.S., *54*, 267, 1965.
39. Vanaman, Wakil and Hill: J. Biol. Chem., *243*, 6420, 1968.
40. Rossi, Alexandre and Galzigna: J. Biol. Chem., *245*, 3110, 1970.
41. Dagley and Nicholson: *An Introduction to Metabolic Pathways*, New York, John Wiley and Sons, Inc., 1970.
42. Fritz and Yue: J. Lipid Res., *4*, 279, 1963.
43. Rossi, Alexandre and Sartorelli: Eur. J. Biochem., *4*, 31, 1968.
44. Thomitzek: Ergebn. Physiol., *62*, 68, 1970.
45. Domschke, Liersch and Decker: Hoppe Seylers Z. Physiol. Chem., *352*, 85, 1971.
46. Bliss, Bird and Thompson: *The Vitamins*, 2nd Ed., György and Pearson, Editors, New York, Academic Press, 1967, Vol. VII, p. 237.
47. Bird and Thompson: *The Vitamins*, 2nd Ed., György and Pearson, Editors, New York, Academic Press, 1967, Vol. VII, p. 209.
48. Atkin, Williams, Schultz and Frey: Ind. Eng. Chem., Anal. Ed., *16*, 67, 1944.
49. Clarke: Anal. Chem., *29*, 135, 1957.
50. Baker and Frank: *Clinical Vitaminology*, New York, Interscience Publishers, 1968.
51. Snell and Wittle: In, *Methods in Enzymology*, Colowick and Kaplan, Editors, New York, Academic Press, 1957, Vol. III, p. 918.
52. *U. S. Pharmacopeia*, Revision XVI, p. 871, Mack Publ., Easton, Pa., 1960.
53. Abiko, Tomikawa and Shimizu: J. Vitamin (Kyoto), *15*, 59, 1969.
54. Bird and McCready: Anal. Chem., *30*, 2045, 1958.
55. Panier and Close: J. Pharm. Sci., *53*, 108, 1964.
56. Zappala and Simpson: J. Pharm. Sci., *50*, 845, 1961.
57. Sheppard and Prosser: In, *Methods in Enzymology*, McCormick and Wright, Editors, New York, Academic Press, 1970, Vol. XVIII, Part A, p. 311.
58. Rogers and Campbell: Anal. Chem., *32*, 1662, 1960.
59. Allred: Anal. Biochem., *29*, 293, 1969.
60. Abiko: In, *Methods in Enzymology*, McCormick and Wright, Editors, New York, Academic Press, 1970, Vol. XVIII, Part A, p. 314.
61. Follis: In, *Deficiency Disease*, Springfield, Charles C Thomas, 1958, p. 223.
62. Jennings: In, *Vitamins in Endocrine Metabolism*, Springfield, Charles C Thomas, 1970.
63. Nelson, Wright, Baird and Evans: J. Nutrition, *62*, 395, 1957.
64. Williams, Chu, McIntosh and Hincenbergs: J. Nutrition, *94*, 377, 1968.
65. Nelson: Am. J. Clin. Nutrition, *21*, 495, 1968.
66. Milligan and Briggs: Poultry Sci., *28*, 202, 1949.
67. Kratzer and Williams: Poultry Sci., *27*, 518, 1948.
68. Schulman and Rickert: J. Biol. Chem., *226*, 181, 1957.
69. Axelrod and Hopper: J. Nutrition, *72*, 325, 1960.
70. Gershoff and Gottlieb: J. Nutrition, *82*, 135, 1964.
71. Fox and Linkwiler: J. Nutrition, *75*, 451, 1961.
72. Pace, Stier, Taylor and Goodman: J. Nutrition, *74*, 345, 1961.
73. Stanbery, Snell and Spies: J. Biol. Chem., *135*, 353, 1940.
74. Pelezar and Porter: Proc. Soc. Exp. Biol. and Med., *47*, 3, 1941.
75. Spies, Stanbery, Williams, Jukes and Babcock: J.A.M.A., *115*, 523, 1940.
76. Krahnke and Gordon: J.A.M.A., *116*, 2431, 1941.

77. Makila: Int. Z. Vitaminforsch., *40*, 81, 1970.
78. Kerrey, Crispin and Fox: Am. J. Clin. Nutr., *21*, 1274, 1968.
79. Leevy, Baker, ten Houe, Frank and Cherrick: Am. J. Clin. Nutr., *16*, 339, 1965.
80. Findlay and Venter: J. Invest. Dermatol., *31*, 11, 1958.
81. Gordon: Pantothenic Acid in Human Nutrition, University of Chicago Symposium on Biol. Action Vitamins, pp. 136–143, 1942.
82. Harrison: Lancet, *1*, 961, 1946.
83. Cruickshank: Lancet, *2*, 369, 1946.
84. Gopalan: Indian M. Gaz., *81*, 23, 1946.
85. Glusman: Am. J. Med., *3*, 211, 1947.
86. Denny-Brown: Medicine, *26*, 41, 1947.
87. Sarma, Menon and Venkatachalam: Current Science, *18*, 367, 1949.
88. Ralli: Nutrition Symposium Series, *5*, 78, 1952.
89. Ralli: In, *The Vitamins*, Sebrell and Harris, Editors, New York, Academic Press, 1954, Vol. II, pp. 669.
90. Hodges, Bean, Ohlson and Bleiler: Am. J. Clin. Nutrition, *11*, 85, 1962.
91. Hodges, Bean, Ohlson and Bleiler: Am. J. Clin. Nutrition, *11*, 187, 1962.
92. Bean and Hodges: Proc. Soc. Exp. Biol. and Med., *86*, 693, 1954.
93. Hodges, Ohlson and Bean: J. Clin. Invest., *37*, 1642, 1958.
94. Hodges, Bean, Ohlson and Bleiler: J. Clin. Invest., *39*, 1421, 1959.
95. Mangay Chung, Pearson, Darby, Miller and Goldsmith: Am. J. Clin. Nutrition, *9*, 573, 1961.
96. Recommended Dietary Allowances. Natl. Acad. Sci.—Natl. Res. Council, Publ. 1964, Washington, D.C., 1968.
97. Anon.: Nutrition Reviews, *20*, 257, 1962.
98. Goldman: J. Invest. Dermatol., *11*, 95, 1948.
98a.Scichounoff and Naz: Schweiz. med. Wochschr., *75*, 767, 1945.
99. Combs and Zuckerman: J. Invest. Dermatol., *16*, 379, 1951.
100. Frost: Physiol. Rev., *28*, 368, 1948.
101. Jacques: Lancet, *2*, 861, 1951.
102. Watne, Mendoza, Rosen, Nadler and Case: J.A.M.A., *181*, 827, 1962.
103. Gershberg, Rubin and Ralli: J. Nutrition, *39*, 107, 1949.
104. Gershberg and Kuhl: J. Clin. Invest., *29*, 1625, 1950.
105. Anon.: Nutrition Reviews, *14*, 116, 1956.
106. Elslager, Hutt and Werbel: J. Med. Chem., *11*, 1071, 1968.
107. Razdan, Reinsel and Zitko: J. Med. Chem., *13*, 546, 1970.
108. Prosser and Sheppard: J. Pharm. Sci., *58*, 718, 1969.

Chapter

5

Section I   Vitamin B-6

HOWERDE E. SAUBERLICH

AND

JOHN E. CANHAM

INTRODUCTION

In 1934, a factor was recognized that prevented skin lesions in the rat ("rat acrodynia") with the name "vitamin B-6" proposed by György for this factor.[1-3] The crystalline compound was isolated and reported on by three groups of investigators in 1938.[4-6] Subsequently, the vitamin was characterized[7-9] and synthesized.[10] Following the knowledge of the structure of the molecule, the term "pyridoxine" came into use for the synthesized vitamin. Bacterial studies later revealed the existence of two other natural forms of the vitamin—pyridoxal and pyridoxamine.[11,12] Since the three forms are essentially equally effective in animal nutrition, the group of compounds is referred to collectively as vitamin B-6. The vitamin is essential for man, rat, mouse, chick, pig, dog, turkey and other species, including many microorganisms. Once the rumen has developed, cattle and sheep and other ruminants do not require a dietary source of vitamin B-6. Horses similarly synthesize the vitamin in the cecum. Vitamin B-6 occurs widespread in foods, with meats, cereals, lentils, nuts, and some fruits and vegetables rich sources (Table 5I-1). The vitamin occurs in animal products largely in its pyridoxal and pyridoxamine forms while pyridoxine is the more prevalent form in most products of vegetable origin.[11,13,14] Several comprehensive reviews on vitamin B-6 are available.[15-21]

CHEMISTRY AND BIOCHEMICAL FUNCTIONS OF VITAMIN B-6

Pyridoxine hydrochloride, the commonly available synthetic form, has a molecular weight of 205.6 and occurs as white platelets readily soluble in water. Pyridoxine is quite stable in acid solutions, but rapid destruction by light occurs in neutral and alkaline solutions. Pyridoxal and pyridoxamine are also available but less used. The coenzyme activities of vitamin B-6 were recognized with the discovery and identification of pyridoxal-5-phosphate.[22-25] The phosphorylated form of pyridoxamine was subsequently shown to occur naturally.[26] Additional information on the early history of vitamin B-6 may be found in reviews.[27-30]

Pyridoxal-5-phosphate represents the coenzyme form of vitamin B-6, although pyridoxamine can also activate a number of vitamin B-6-dependent enzymes.[28-34] Pyridoxine, pyridoxamine and pyridoxal are converted through enzymatic pathways to the coenzyme form.[16,20,28,35,36] A number of compounds structurally related to pyridoxine have been synthesized with some possessing vitamin B-6 activity.[16,20,28,37] Other analogs possess antivitamin B-6 action.[15,16,19,20] 4-Deoxypyridoxine, for example, has been used to induce vitamin B-6-deficiency symptoms in animals and man.[16,19,37-43] Other antagonists function as binding agents to inactivate vitamin B-6. Included in this group are isoniazid (INH), penicillamine, semicarbazide and cycloserine.[15,16,19]

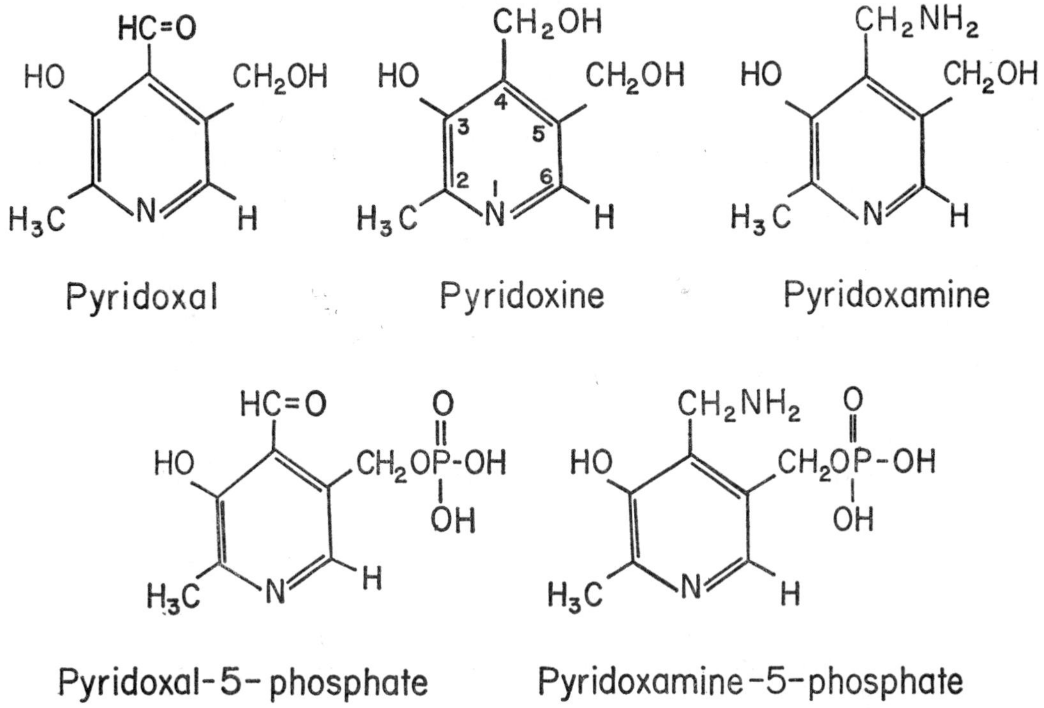

Pyridoxal   Pyridoxine   Pyridoxamine

Pyridoxal-5-phosphate   Pyridoxamine-5-phosphate

Fig. 5I-1

Vitamin B-6, in the coenzyme form, is concerned with a vast number and variety of enzyme systems almost entirely associated with nitrogen metabolism. Well over sixty pyridoxal phosphate-dependent enzymes are known.

Some of the reactions catalyzed by these enzymes involving amino acids include trans-

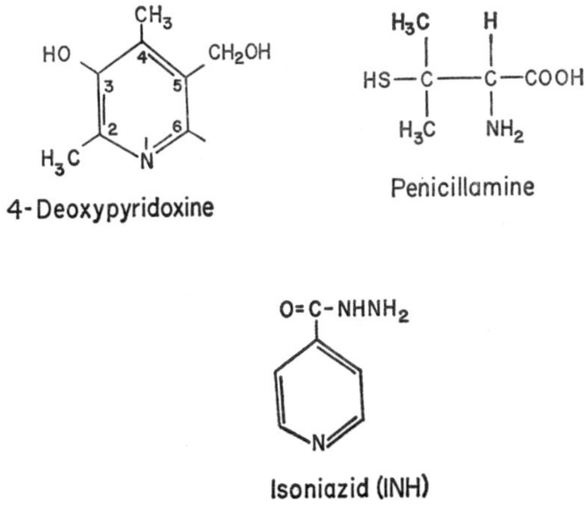

4-Deoxypyridoxine

Penicillamine

Isoniazid (INH)

Fig. 5I-2

amination, racemization, decarboxylation, cleavage, synthesis, dehydration, and desulfhydration. The transaminases represent a major group of the pyridoxal phosphate-catalyzed enzymes. The α-amino group of amino acids such as alanine, arginine, asparagine, aspartic acid, cysteine, isoleucine, lysine, phenylalanine, tryptophan, tyrosine and valine is removed by transamination. Usually α-ketoglutarate serves as the final acceptor of the amino groups for channeling into reactions whereby the nitrogenous end products such as urea are formed. Following deamination, the carbon skeletons of the amino acids undergo oxidative degradation to compounds that are metabolized in the tricarboxylic acid cycle. Pyridoxal phosphate functions in transaminases in a Schiff base (ketimine) mechanism.[15-19,45,46] Glutamic-oxaloacetic acid transaminase (GOT) and glutamic-pyruvic acid transaminase (GPT) and other transaminases are located almost entirely within the cell. Elevated levels of serum transaminase activity are commonly employed as a diagnostic aid for following

Table 5I-1. Vitamin Content of Selected Foods
(per 100 gm of edible portion)

Food Item	Pantothenic acid[1] (mg)	Vitamin B-6[1] (µg)	Thiamin[2] (µg)
Meats			
Beef (raw)			
Liver	7.700	840	250
Round	0.470	330	90
Kidney	3.850	430	360
Heart	2.500	250	530
Pork (raw)			
Ham (cured), lean	0.525	320	890
Loin	0.600	350	980
Liver	6.400	650	300
Veal (raw)			
Loin	0.900	340	140
Frankfurters (all-meat)	0.430	140	160
Lamb (raw)			
Leg	0.550	275	180
Fish			
Ocean perch fillet (raw)	0.360	230	100
Halibut, fresh (raw)	0.275	430	70
Tuna, canned	0.320	425	50
Salmon, canned	0.550	300	30
Chicken (raw)			
Dark	1.000	325	80
Light	0.800	683	50
Eggs (raw)			
Whites	0.200	2	Trace
Yolk	4.400	300	220
Whole	1.600	110	110
Cheese			
Cheddar	0.500	80	30
Cottage	0.220	40	30
Milk			
Cow			
Whole	0.340	40	30
Skim	0.370	42	40
Evaporated	0.640	50	40
Condensed	0.680	60	80
Dry, whole	2.400	270	290
Dry, skim	3.600	380	350
Human	0.220	10	10
Cereals and Grain Products			
Bread, white	0.430	40	250
Bread, whole wheat	0.760	180	260
Oatmeal, dry	1.500	140	600
Corn grits, dry (enriched)	——	147	440
Cornmeal (enriched)	0.580	250	440
Corn flakes (cereal)	0.185	65	430
Rice, dry, regular (enriched)	0.550	170	440
Rice, pre-cooked (enriched)	0.285	34	440
Shredded wheat (cereal)	0.706	244	220
Flour, all-purpose (enriched)	0.465	60	440

Table 5I-1. Vitamin Content of Selected Foods (Continued)

Food Item	Pantothenic acid[1] (mg)	Vitamin B-6[1] (μg)	Thiamin[2] (μg)
Cereals and Grain Products (Cont.)			
Soybean flour (defatted)	2.220	724	1090
Macaroni, dry (enriched)	——	64	880
Noodles, egg, dry (enriched)	——	88	880
Fruits and Vegetables			
Apples (raw)	0.100	30	30
Bananas (raw)	0.260	510	50
Apricots (canned)	0.092	54	20
Avocados (raw)	1.070	420	110
Blueberries (canned)	0.068	39	10
Cherries, sour (canned)	0.105	44	30
Grapefruit (raw)	0.283	34	40
Grapes (raw)	0.075	80	50
Oranges (raw)	0.250	60	100
Plums (canned)	0.072	27	20
Peaches (canned)	0.050	19	100
Pears (canned)	0.022	14	100
Pineapple (canned)	0.100	74	80
Strawberries (raw)	0.340	55	30
Cantaloupe (raw)	0.250	86	40
Cranberries (raw)	0.219	35	30
Cabbage (raw)	0.205	160	50
Cauliflower (raw)	1.000	210	110
Lettuce (raw)	0.200	55	60
Peas, green (raw)	0.750	160	350
Potatoes, white (raw)	0.380	250	100
Potatoes, sweet (raw)	0.820	218	100
Squash, summer (raw)	0.360	82	50
Turnip greens (frozen)	0.140	100	60
Beans, green snap (fresh)	0.190	80	80
Navy beans (dried)	0.725	560	650
Corn, yellow (canned)	0.220	200	30
Spinach, leaf (frozen)	0.150	150	100
Tomatoes, ripe (raw)	0.330	100	60
Nuts			
Almonds (dry)	0.470	100	240
Peanuts (roasted)	2.100	400	320
Pecans	1.707	183	860
Walnuts (English)	0.900	730	330
Dried Fruits			
Dates	0.780	153	90
Figs	0.435	175	100
Peaches	——	100	100
Prunes	0.460	240	90
Raisins (seedless)	0.045	240	110
Beverages, alcoholic			
Beer	0.080	60	Trace
Wine	0.030	40	Trace

[1]From Home Economic Research Report No. 36, August 1969, U.S. Department of Agriculture.
[2]From Agriculture Handbook No. 8, December 1963, U.S. Department of Agriculture.

cellular involvement in certain disease processes.[51]

The pyridoxal phosphate-dependent decarboxylases are of considerable importance in mammalian tissues.[15–19,45,46] Thus, aromatic L-amino acid decarboxylase reacts on tyrosine, histidine, dopa and tryptophan to form their respective amines. Serotonin is produced by the action of this enzyme on 5-hydroxytryptophan.[47] Glutamic acid decarboxylase catalyzes the formation of γ-aminobutyric acid from glutamic acid in the central nervous system.[48] Cysteine sulfinic acid decarboxylase converts cysteine to taurine. Tryptophan metabolism, including its conversion to nicotinic acid, requires a number of pyridoxal phosphate-catalyzed reactions.[15,16,49,50] Consequently, when a deficiency in vitamin B-6 occurs, tryptophan metabolism is altered giving rise to excessive urinary excretion of xanthurenic acid, kynurenine, 3-hydroxykynurenine and quinolic acid, while the excretion of nicotinic acid and N^1-methylnicotinamide may be reduced.[51–61,167]

The vitamin is also required in the conversion of cysteine to pyruvic acid[62] and oxalate to glycine,[63] and in the synthesis of δ-aminolevulinic acid,[16,64–66] an intermediate in the formation of porphyrin. Pyridoxal phosphate is a cofactor for a number of dehydratases, racemases, transferases, hydroxylases, synthetases and other classes of enzymes.[16–18] Unique of the enzymes requiring pyridoxal phosphate is phosphorylase,[18,67,68] the enzyme that catalyzes the breakdown of glycogen to form glucose-1-phosphate. The coenzyme plays an important conformational or structural role in this enzyme, but whether it also plays an essential catalytic role is unclear. Although vitamin B-6 has been implicated in lipid metabolism, the role appears to be mediated through secondary effects.[16,69–72] Additional information on the biochemical roles of vitamin B-6 is available in the cited reviews.[15–20,46,73,74]

METHODS OF ASSAY

Microbiological assay, chemical methods and animal bioassay procedures are available to measure vitamin B-6. The animal bioassays, using either the rat or chick,[75,76] are time-consuming, expensive and variable and therefore have been generally replaced by microbiological and chemical methods. *Saccharomyces carlsbergensis* is the test organism commonly used in the microbiological method since pyridoxine, pyridoxal and pyridoxamine are equally active on a molar basis for this organism.[21,77] The individual forms may be determined by a differential assay employing *Lactobacillus casei* to measure pyridoxal, *Streptococcus faecalis* to measure combined pyridoxal and pyridoxamine, and *S. carlsbergensis* to measure total vitamin B-6 content.[20,21,78–80] A more recent procedure involves the chromatographic separation of the three forms of vitamin B-6 followed by assay of the eluates with *S. carlsbergensis*.[20,21,81–85] The protozoan *Tetrahymena pyriformis* has also been used to measure vitamin B-6 in biological materials.[108,109] Since the majority of the forms of vitamin B-6 occur in natural substances in phosphorylated and bound forms, extraction and hydrolytic procedures are required prior to assay.[21,86] Fluorometric and enzymatic procedures have been described for measuring pyridoxal and pyridoxal phosphate in biological material.[20,21,87–89,169–171] Thin-layer chromatography and gas-liquid chromatography methods appear promising for application to pharmaceutical preparations.[20,90–92] The major metabolite of vitamin B-6 is 4-pyridoxic acid for which fluorometric procedures are available.[21,93,94] Measurement of this metabolite has been useful in clinical and research studies on vitamin B-6 nutrition and metabolism.[60]

DEFICIENCIES IN EXPERIMENTAL ANIMALS

Dermatitis (acrodynia) is the characteristic sign of a vitamin B-6 deficiency in the rat. The lesions occur on the paws, ears, nose, chin, submental region, and upper thorax.[16,96–97] The acrodynia resembles the dermatological effects of an essential fatty acid deficiency, but the nature of the relationship is not clear.[69,96,99] A high fat diet will delay the appearance of pyridoxine-deficiency dermatitis[100] and pyridoxine has a similar effect on the dermatitis of essential fatty acid deficiency.[101] A pyridoxine deficiency in the rat also induces poor growth, muscular weakness, fatty livers, convulsive seizures,[102] anemia,[103] reproductive impairment,[104] edema, nerve degeneration, enlarged adrenal glands, increased excretion of xanthurenic acid, urea and oxalate, decreased transaminase activities, reduced synthesis of ribosomal and messenger ribonucleic acid and deoxyribonucleic acid,[105,106] impaired immune responses and numerous other alterations in biochemical processes.[16] Lesions noted in the pyridoxine-deficient mouse resemble those in the rat.[107] As with the rat, high protein intakes induce more readily the characteristic skin lesions and death in animals fed a vitamin B-6-deficient diet.

Similar alterations have been noted in vitamin B-6-deficient chicks, hamsters, dogs, monkeys, swine, calves, turkeys and rabbits. The most commonly observed effects of a deficiency in these species have been microcytic hypochromic anemia, degeneration of nervous tissues and convulsions.[16,98]

DEFICIENCY IN MAN

The first evidence of the essentiality of vitamin B-6 for the human was reported in 1939.[110] Patients on poor diets were observed to have an ill-defined syndrome characterized by weakness, irritability and nervousness, insomnia and difficulty in walking. Although the symptoms did not respond to treatment with other members of the B-complex, relief was obtained within 24 hours when pyridoxine was administered. Shortly thereafter pyridoxine was reported to be effective in healing cheilosis which did not respond to riboflavin.[111] Convincing evidence of the essentiality of vitamin B-6 in human nutrition was the reports on the widespread occurrence of convulsive seizures and nervous irritability in infants fed an autoclaved commercial liquid milk formula low in vitamin B-6.[112–116] Approximately 300 cases with overt symptoms responsive to pyridoxine therapy were noted.[116] The clinical improvement was corroborated by return of the abnormal electroencephalographic patterns to normal.[15,115]

More clearly defined symptoms of a vitamin B-6 deficiency in man have been obtained with the use of experimental subjects placed on diets low in the vitamin and with the administration of certain anti-vitamin B-6 compounds.[15,16,19,60,61] The earliest such study was conducted in 1948 by administering a purified diet deficient in vitamin B-6 to an adult for 55 days.[117] No clear-cut symptoms of a pyridoxine deficiency appeared though mental depression was noted. Derangement of tryptophan metabolism, manifested by the excretion of xanthurenic acid, was observed within 3 weeks in adult human subjects maintained on a vitamin B-6-deficient diet.[118] In subsequent years, the tryptophan load test has commonly been used in vitamin B-6-deficiency and -requirement studies.[15,16,19,60,61]

Convincing deficiency symptoms were produced in two infants placed on a vitamin B-6-deficient diet.[55] The infants ceased to gain weight after several months. Pyridoxic acid disappeared from the urine and urinary pyridoxine was reduced to very low values. The ability to convert tryptophan to nicotinic acid was lost. Convulsions occurred in one and hypochromic anemia in the other. The administration of pyridoxine readily corrected these abnormalities, except for the ability to convert tryptophan to nicotinic acid which was slower to respond.

Vitamin B-6 deficiency has been induced in 50 human adults with the associated use of the pyridoxine antagonist, 4-deoxypyridoxine.[38,39] Seborrhea-like lesions appeared about the eyes, in the nasolabial folds and around the mouth. These lesions spread to involve the face, forehead, eyebrows and the skin behind the ears. The scrotal and perineal regions were involved occasionally. Intertrigo developed under the breasts and in other moist areas. Hyperpigmented scaly pellagra-like dermatitis also developed occasionally in the collar region and on the forearms, elbows and thighs. Cheilosis, glossitis and stomatitis occurred which were morphologically indistinguishable from the oral lesions of nicotinic acid and riboflavin deficiency. Three patients developed peripheral neuropathy of a sensory type; motor function was impaired later. Weight loss was noted in all subjects, with apathy, somnolence and increased irritability occurring in some. Although there was a strong tendency to develop infections, particularly of the genitourinary tract, production of antibodies to typhoid and erythrocyte antigens was not measurably impaired.[119]

Another group of investigators similarly induced a B-6 deficiency in human subjects with the use of a deficient diet and deoxypyridoxine.[43] In this study there was a very slight impairment of the formation of antibodies against tetanus and typhoid in the deficient subjects. The majority of the subjects, including all those who developed clinical signs of deficiency, excreted large amounts of xanthurenic acid in the urine after a test dose of tryptophan, but their ability to convert tryptophan to N^1-methylnicotinamide was not impaired. In a companion study, subjects were given a diet deficient in pantothenic acid and pyridoxine and supplemented with deoxypyridoxine and omega methylpantothenic acid.[120] These subjects became ill and were completely unable to respond to tetanus and to typhoid "O" antigen.

In more recent years, vitamin B-6 deficiency has been induced in human volunteer subjects without the use of pyridoxine antagonists.[15,16,19,53,54,56,60,61,121—127] Subjects on a vitamin B-6-deficient diet have been observed to develop personality changes manifested by irritability, depression, and loss of the sense of responsibility.[61] The subjects also developed filiform hypertrophy of the lingual papilla, aphthous stomatitis, nasolabial seborrhea and an acneiform papular rash of the forehead. Abnormal electroencephalograms were observed. Tryptophan metabolism was altered, with high urinary excretions of xanthurenic acid occurring after tryptophan loading. Pyridoxine repletion corrected all of the abnormalities noted. Vitamin B-6 in natural foods was as available as crystalline pyridoxine.[15,16] Although there appears to be no apparent effect of increased caloric utilization on vitamin B-6 requirements,[61] high intakes of protein hastened the onset of a vitamin B-6

deficiency.[15,19,61,121,123,124]   A tryptophan load induces in the vitamin B-6-deficient subject not only marked urinary excretions of xanthurenic acid, but also of kynurenine, hydroxykynurenine, kynurenic acid, acetylkynurenine, and quinolinic acid.[53,56,121,123] Plasma and blood levels of vitamin B-6 and urinary excretions of vitamin B-6 and 4-pyridoxic acid fall with decreased intakes of the vitamin.[19,121,124,126,133,147,148]   Cysteine metabolism appeared to be only slightly altered with pyridoxine deficiency.[60,125] Glutamic-oxaloacetate transaminase (GOT) and glutamic-pyruvate transaminase (GPT) activities in blood and its components are lowered in vitamin B-6 deficiency.[15,19,60,61,122,126—132,147] Changes in plasma and urinary levels of free amino acids may occur in pyridoxine deficiency.[19,127,134]   Certain metabolic defects appear to respond to increased intakes of pyridoxine.[146] Several infants with convulsive seizures dating from shortly after birth have been found to respond to 2 mg of pyridoxine daily.[135—137] A number of patients with pyridoxine-responsive anemia, classified as sideroblastic anemia, have been reported.[15,16,19,138—144] In these individuals the production of hemoglobin and erythrocytes is dependent upon the administration of 2.5 mg or more of vitamin B-6 daily. Iron, folic acid and vitamin B-12 are without effect. Other types of vitamin B-6-dependency syndromes have been reported.[146] Oxaluria may occur in persons receiving deoxypyridoxine or isoniazid.[45,145,160]   Evidence of vitamin B-6 deficiency occurring in chronic alcoholic patients has been reported.[149,172]

A metabolic interrelationship between steroid hormones and vitamin B-6 has been observed.[16] Women taking steroid hormones for contraceptive purposes have been observed to excrete grossly increased amounts of tryptophan metabolites following a tryptophan load.[19,61,150—155,167,173,174] Vitamin B-6 supplementation corrects this abnormality. At present, the effects of estrogens on tryptophan and vitamin B-6 metabolism have no satisfactory molecular explanation.[19] Pregnant women may excrete abnormal amounts of kynurenine, xanthurenic acid and 3-hydroxykynurenine which may be decreased with pyridoxine supplements.[15,16,156,157,167]

Supplements of vitamin B-6 failed to change complications of pregnancy.[158] Evidence has been reported indicating the vitamin B-6 requirement is increased in patients with hyperthyroidism.[159]

NUTRITIONAL REQUIREMENT

The Food and Nutrition Board[161] has established a recommended daily dietary allowance of 2.0 mg of vitamin B-6 for adult men and women. During pregnancy and lactation, an allowance of 2.5 mg per day is recommended. For younger age groups, lesser amounts have been suggested as being adequate. Vitamin B-6 requirements for the adult have been reasonably well established from controlled depletion and repletion experimental human investigations.[15,16,19,60,61,121-126] These studies have demonstrated an influence of protein intake on the requirement for vitamin B-6.[16] Adult males ingesting 100 gm of protein daily appeared to have a daily vitamin B-6 requirement of 1.75 to 2.0 mg, while persons on a low protein intake had a requirement of 1.25 to 1.5 mg per day. An intake of 1.5 mg of vitamin B-6 has been suggested as adequate for young women. Information as to the actual pyridoxine requirement of infants and children is exceedingly limited.[15,16,161] A daily allowance of 0.4 mg of vitamin B-6 for artificially fed infants has been considered to amply provide for their needs. The average diet in the U.S.A. provides the amounts of vitamin B-6 recommended, though certain poor or restricted diets do not.[95] Although meats serve as a good source of vitamin B-6, a considerable loss of the vitamin occurs during cooking.[14,168]

THERAPEUTIC USE, TOXICITY, AND METABOLISM

Pyridoxine hydrochloride is frequently present in multi-vitamin preparations. The compound is used as an adjunct in prophylaxis and treatment of multiple vitamin B-complex deficiencies and is included in preparations designed for intravenous and oral alimentation. It has also been used in the treatment of dermatoses, neuromuscular and neurological diseases. Oral doses of 1 to 150 mg per day have been used. Similar levels have been used in treating pyridoxine-responsive anemias. Pyridoxine supplements are commonly employed as a precautionary measure when isoniazid is used in the treatment of tuberculosis.[162] Where other drugs possessing anti-vitamin B-6 properties are used for extended periods, such as penicillamine in the treatment of Wilson's disease and other conditions, pyridoxine supplements are recommended.[19,163] Pyridoxine has been used for a number of years by obstetricians for the control of nausea and vomiting of pregnancy. The effectiveness of this treatment has not been proved by carefully controlled studies. Pyridoxine has been employed in the treatment of hyperoxaluria and recurring oxalate kidney stones,[175,176] chorea,[177] isoniazid toxicty[178] and levodopa-induced dystonia.[179-181] Excess pyridoxine, however, can reduce the clinical benefits of levodopa therapy in Parkinson's disease.[182,183] Pyridoxal-5-phosphate (as the calcium salt) has also been used for prophylaxis and treatment of vitamin B-6 deficiency. Pyridoxamine dihydrochloride possesses hypnotic properties.

The toxicity of pyridoxine is extremely low. Doses up to 1 gm per kg of body weight were tolerated without ill effects by dogs, rats and rabbits. The pharmacodynamic effects are few and none has been observed in man. The toxicity of pyridoxamine and pyridoxal is also very low, although pyridoxal was about twice as toxic as pyridoxine or pyridoxamine for animals.[16,164]

Vitamin B-6 is extensively metabolized by man. The major metabolite is 4-pyridoxic acid which accounts for 20 to 40 per cent of the vitamin metabolized daily.[124,165,166] Isotopic studies indicate the presence in the urine of a number of unknown metabolites derived from pyridoxine. Small amounts of pyridoxal, pyridoxamine and pyridoxine and their phosphorylated analogs are present in the urine.[124,165]

BIBLIOGRAPHY

1. György: Nature, 133, 498, 1934.
2. Birch, György and Harris: Biochem. J., 29, 2830, 1935.
3. Birch and György: Biochem. J., 30, 304, 1936.

4. Lepkovsky: Science, *87*, 169, 1938.
5. Keresztesy and Stevens: Proc. Soc. Expt. Biol. and Med., *38*, 64, 1938.
6. György: J. Am. Chem. Soc., *60*, 983, 1938.
7. Stiller, Keresztesy and Stevens: J. Am. Chem. Soc., *61*, 1237, 1939.
8. Kuhn, Wendt and Westphal: Chem. Ber., *72B*, 310, 1939.
9. Harris, Stiller and Folkers: J. Am. Chem. Soc., *61*, 1242, 1939.
10. Harris and Folkers: Science, *89*, 347, 1939.
11. Snell: J. Biol. Chem., *157*, 491, 1945.
12. Snell, Guirard and Williams: J. Biol. Chem., *143*, 519, 1942.
13. Rabinowitz and Snell: J. Biol. Chem., *176*, 1157, 1948.
14. Orr: Pantothenic Acid, Vitamin B-6 and Vitamin B-12 in Foods. Home Economics Research Report No. 36, U.S. Dept. of Agric., 1969.
15. Harris, Wool and Loraine, Editors: *Vitamins and Hormones*, Vol. 22, New York, Academic Press, Inc., 1964.
16. Sebrell and Harris, Editors: *The Vitamins*, New York, Academic Press, 1968, Vol. II, pp. 2–117.
17. Snell and DiMari: In *The Enzymes*, Boyer, Editor, New York, Academic Press, 1970, Vol. II (3rd Edition), p. 335.
18. Harris, Muson and Diczfalusy, Editors: *Vitamins and Hormones*, Vol. 28, New York, Academic Press, Inc., 1970, p. 265.
19. Kelsall, Editor: Ann. N.Y. Acad. Sci., *166*, 1–364, 1969.
20. McCormick and Wright, Editors: *Methods in Enzymology*, New York, Academic Press, 1970, Vol. XVIII, Part A, p. 431.
21. Sauberlich: In *The Vitamins*, György and Pearson, Editors, New York, Academic Press, 1967, Vol. VII, p. 169.
22. Gunsalus, Bellamy and Umbreit: J. Biol. Chem., *155*, 685, 1944.
23. Heyl, Luz, Harris and Folkers: J. Am. Chem. Soc., *73*, 3430, 1951.
24. Baddiley and Mathias: J. Chem. Soc., 2583, 1952.
25. Schlenk and Snell: J. Biol. Chem., *157*, 425, 1945.
26. Rabinowitz and Snell: J. Biol. Chem., *169*, 643, 1947.
27. Robinson: *The Vitamin B Complex*, New York, John Wiley and Sons, Inc., 1951.
28. Snell: Vitamins and Hormones, *16*, 77, 1958.
29. Meister: In *The Enzymes*, Boyer, Lardy and Myrbäck, Editors, New York, Academic Press, 1962, Vol. 6, p. 193.
30. Braunstein: In *The Enzymes*, Boyer, Lardy and Myrbäck, Editors, New York, Academic Press, 1960, Vol. 2, Part A, p. 113.
31. Meister: Adv. Enzymol., *16*, 185, 1955.
32. Velick and Vavra: In *The Enzymes*, Boyer, Lardy and Myrbäck, Editors, New York, Academic Press, 1962, Vol. 6, p. 219.
33. Ellis and Davies: Biochem. J., *78*, 615, 1961.
34. Davies and Ellis: Biochem. J., *78*, 623, 1961.

35. Brown and Reynolds: Ann. Rev. Biochem., *32*, 447, 1963.
36. Wada and Snell: J. Biol. Chem., *236*, 2089, 1961.
37. Snell: In *Comprehensive Biochemistry*, Florkin and Stotz, Editors, Amsterdam, Elsevier Publishing Co., 1963, Vol. II.
38. Mueller and Vilter: J. Clin. Invest., *29*, 193, 1950.
39. Vilter, Mueller, Glazer, Jarrold, Abraham, Thompson, and Hawkins: J. Lab. Clin. Med., *42*, 335, 1953.
40. Glazer, Mueller, Thompson, Hawkins and Vilter: Arch. Biochem. Biophys., *33*, 243, 1951.
41. Will, Repasky, Mueller and Glazer: Am. J. Clin. Nutr., *9*, 245, 1961.
42. Muller and Iacono: Am. J. Clin. Nutr., *12*, 358, 1963.
43. Hodges, Bean, Ohlson and Bleiler: Am. J. Clin. Nutr., *11*, 180, 1962.
44. Faber, Feitler, Bleiler, Ohlson and Hodges: Am. J. Clin. Nutr., *12*, 406, 1963.
45. Guirard and Snell: In *Comprehensive Biochemistry*, Florkin and Stotz, Editors, Amsterdam, Elsevier Publishing Co., 1964, Vol. 15.
46. Yamada, Katunuma and Wada, Editors, *Symposium on Pyridoxal Enzymes*, Tokyo, Maruzen, 1968.
47. Weissbach, Bogdanski, Redfield and Udenfriend: J. Biol. Chem., *227*, 617, 1957.
48. Kellam and Bain: J. Pharm. Exp. Therap., *119*, 225, 1956.
49. Henderson, Gholson and Dalgliesh: In *Comprehensive Biochemistry*, Florkin and Stotz, Editors, Amsterdam, Elsevier Publishing Co., 1962, Vol. 4, Part B, p. 288.
50. Coursin: Am. J. Clin. Nutr., *14*, 56, 1964.
51. Searcy: *Diagnostic Biochemistry*, New York, McGraw-Hill Book Co., 1969, p. 510.
52. Price, Brown and Larson: J. Clin. Invest., *36*, 1600, 1957.
53. Yess, Price, Brown, Swan and Linkswiler: J. Nutrition, *84*, 229, 1964.
54. Brown, Yess, Price, Linkswiler, Swan and Hankes: J. Nutrition, *87*, 419, 1965.
55. Snyderman, Holt, Carretero and Jacobs: Am. J. Clin. Nutr., *1*, 200, 1953.
56. Kelsay, Miller and Linkswiler: J. Nutrition, *94*, 27, 1968.
57. Fouts and Lepkovsky: Proc. Soc. Expt. Biol. Med., *50*, 221, 1942.
58. Greenberg, Bohr, McGrath and Rinehart: Arch. Biochem., *21*, 237, 1945.
59. Lepkovsky and Nielson: J. Biol. Chem., *144*, 135, 1942.
60. Linkswiler: Am. J. Clin. Nutrition, *20*, 547, 1967.
61. Sauberlich, Canham, Baker, Raica and Herman: J. Scientific and Ind. Res., *29*, No. 8, p. S28, 1970.
62. Binkley, Christensen and Jensen: J. Biol. Chem., *194*, 109, 1952.
63. Pasquarillo and Tenconi: Acta Vitaminol., *15*, 163, 1961.

64. Schulman and Richert: J. Biol. Chem., *226*, 181, 1957.
65. Richert and Schulman: Am. J. Clin. Nutrition, *7*, 416, 1959.
66. Burnham and Lascilles: Biochem. J., *87*, 462, 1963.
67. Illingworth, Jansz, Brown and Cori: Proc. Natl. Acad. Sci., U.S., *44*, 1180, 1958.
68. Brown and Cori: In *The Enzymes*, Boyer, Lardy and Myrbäck, Editors, New York, Academic Press, 1961, Vol. 5, Part B, p. 207.
69. Witten and Holman: Arch. Biochem. Biophys., *41*, 266, 1952.
70. Swell, Law, Schools and Treadwell: J. Nutrition, *74*, 148, 1961.
71. Rosen and Nichol: Vitamins and Hormones, *21*, 135, 1963.
72. Goswami and Coniglio: J. Nutrition, *89*, 210, 1966.
73. Dagley and Nicholson: *An Introduction to Metabolic Pathways*, New York, John Wiley and Sons, Inc., 1970.
74. Fasella: Ann. Rev. Biochem., *36*, 185, 1967.
75. Bliss and György: In *The Vitamins*, György and Pearson, Editors, New York, Academic Press, 1967, Vol. VII, p. 205.
76. Sarma, Snell and Elvehjem: J. Biol. Chem., *165*, 55, 1946.
77. Atkin, Schultz, Williams and Frey: Ind. Eng. Chem., Anal. Ed., *15*, 141, 1943.
78. Rabinowitz and Snell: J. Biol. Chem., *176*, 1157, 1948.
79. Gregory: J. Dairy Res. (London), *26*, 203, 1959.
80. Gregory and Mabbitt: J. Dairy Res. (London), *28*, 293, 1961.
81. MacArthur and Lehmann: Assoc. Off. Agr. Chem. J., *42*, 619, 1959.
82. Polansky and Murphy: Am. Diet. Assoc. J., *48*, 109, 1966.
83. Toepfer and Lehmann: Assoc. Off. Agr. Chem. J., *44*, 426, 1961.
83a. Thiele and Brin: J. Nutrition, *90*, 347, 1966.
84. Toepfer, MacArthur and Lehmann: Assoc. Off. Agr. Chem. J., *43*, 57, 1960.
85. Toepfer, Polansky, Richardson and Wilkes: J. Agr. Food Chem., *11*, 523, 1963.
86. Woodring and Storvick: Assoc. Off. Agr. Chem. J., *43*, 63, 1960.
87. Storvick, Benson, Edwards and Woodring: Meth. Biochem. Anal., *12*, 183, 1964.
88. Donald and Ferguson: Anal. Biochem., *7*, 335, 1964.
89. Boxer, Pruss and Goodhart: J. Nutrition, *63*, 623, 1957.
90. Ahrens and Karytnyk: Anal. Biochem., *30*, 413, 1969.
91. Prosser, Sheppard and Libby: Assoc. Off. Anal. Chem. J., *50*, 1348, 1967.
92. Korytnyk, Fricke and Paul: Anal. Biochem., *17*, 66, 1966.
93. Reddy, Reynolds and Price: J. Biol. Chem., *233*, 691, 1958.
94. Woodring, Fisher and Storvick: Clin. Chem., *10*, 479, 1964.
95. Mangay Chung, Pearson, Darby, Miller and Goldsmith: Am. J. Clin. Nutrition, *9*, 573, 1961.
96. Sullivan and Nicholls: J. Invest. Dermat., *3*, 317, 1940.
97. Antopol and Unna: Arch. Path., *33*, 241, 1942.
98. Follis: *Deficiency Disease*, Springfield, Charles C Thomas, 1958, p. 235.
99. Carter and Phizackerley: Biochem. J., *49*, 227, 1951.
100. Birch: J. Biol. Chem., *124*, 775, 1938.
101. Schneider, Steenback and Platz: J. Biol. Chem., *132*, 539, 1940.
102. Chick, Sadr and Worden: Biochem. J., *34*, 595, 1940.
103. Batchen, Cheesman, Copping and Trusler: Brit. J. Nutrition, *9*, 49, 1955.
104. Nelson and Evans: J. Nutrition, *43*, 281, 1951.
105. Montjar, Axelrod and Trakatellis: J. Nutrition, *85*, 45, 1965.
106. Trakatellis and Axelrod: Biochem. J., *95*, 344, 1965.
107. Boutwell, Rusch and Chiang: Proc. Soc. Expt. Biol. Med., *77*, 860, 1951.
108. Baker, Frank, Ning, Gellene, Hutner and Leevy: Am. J. Clin. Nutrition, *18*, 123, 1966.
109. Baker and Frank: *Clinical Vitaminology*, New York, Interscience Publishers, 1968.
110. Spies, Bean and Ashe: J.A.M.A., *112*, 2414, 1939.
111. Smith and Martin: Proc. Soc. Exp. Biol. Med., *43*, 660, 1940.
112. Vitamin B-6 in Human Nutrition: M. and R. Conference, Chicago, Nov. 19, 1953.
113. Coursin: Vit. and Hormones, *22*, 756, 1964.
114. Malony and Parmelee: J.A.M.A., *154*, 405, 1954.
115. Coursin: J.A.M.A., *154*, 406, 1954.
116. Hawkins: Science, *121*, 880, 1955.
117. Hawkins and Barsky: Science, *108*, 284, 1948.
118. Greenberg, Bohr, McGrath and Rinehart: Arch. Biochem., *21*, 237, 1949.
119. Wayne, Will, Friedman, Becker and Vilter: Arch. Int. Med., *101*, 143, 1958.
120. Hodges, Bean, Ohlson and Bleiler: Am. J. Clin. Nutrition, *11*, 187, 1962.
121. Baker, Canham, Nunes, Sauberlich and McDowell: Am. J. Clin. Nutrition, *15*, 59, 1964.
122. Canham, Baker, Raica and Sauberlich: Proc. Seventh Int. Cong. of Nutrition, *5*, 558, 1966.
123. Miller and Linkswiler: J. Nutrition, *93*, 53, 1967.
124. Kelsay, Bysal and Linkswiler: J. Nutrition, *94*, 490, 1968.
125. Swan, Wentworth and Linkswiler: J. Nutrition, *84*, 220, 1964.
126. Baysal, Johnson and Linkswiler: J. Nutrition, *89*, 19, 1966.
127. Aly, Donald, and Simpson: Am. J. Clin. Nutrition, *24*, 297, 1971.
128. Raica and Sauberlich: Am. J. Clin. Nutrition, *15*, 67, 1964.

129. Jacobs, Cavill and Hughes: Am. J. Clin. Nutrition, *21*, 502, 1968.
130. Woodring and Storvick: Am. J. Clin. Nutrition, *23*, 1385, 1970.
131. Cinnamon and Beaton: Am. J. Clin. Nutrition, *23*, 696, 1970.
132. Cheney, Sabry and Beaton: Am. J. Clin. Nutrition, *16*, 337, 1965.
133. Baker and Frank: World Rev. Nutr. and Dietetics, *9*, 124, 1968.
134. Harding, Sauberlich and Canham: In *Automation in Analytical Chemistry*—Technicon Symposia, Skeggs, Editor, New York, Mediad Inc., 1965, p. 643.
135. Hunt, Stokes, McCrory and Stroud: Pediatrics, *13*, 140, 1954.
136. Bessey, Adam and Hansen: Pediatrics, *20*, 33, 1957.
137. Waldinger and Berg: Pediatrics, *32*, 161, 1963.
138. Harris, Whittington, Wesiman and Horrigan: Proc. Soc. Expt. Biol. Med., *91*, 427, 1956.
139. Bickers, Brown and Sprague: Blood, *19*, 304, 1962.
140. Hines and Harris: Am. J. Clin. Nutrition, *14*, 137, 1964.
141. Horrigan and Harris: Vitamins and Hormones, *22*, 722, 1964.
142. Nordio and Massino: Ann. Paediat., *207*, 160, 1966.
143. Weintraub, Conrad and Crosby: New Eng. J. Med., *275*, 169, 1966.
144. Wohllebe and Paul: Folia Haematol., *86*, 445, 1966.
145. Johnston and Donald: Am. J. Clin. Nutrition, *12*, 413, 1963.
146. Frimpter, Andelman and George: Am. J. Clin. Nutrition, *22*, 794, 1969.
147. Gailani, Holland, Nussbaum and Olson: Cancer, *21*, 975, 1968.
148. Ziegler, Reinken and Berger: Int. Z. Vit. Forschung, *39*, 192, 1969.
149. Walsh, Howorth and Marks: Am. J. Clin. Nutrition, *19*, 379, 1966.
150. Rose: Clin. Sci., *31*, 265, 1966.
151. Rose: Nature (London), *210*, 196, 1966.
152. Price, Brown and Thornton: Am. J. Clin. Nutrition, *18*, 312, 1966.
153. Price, Brown and Yess: *Advances in Metabolic Disorders,*, 2, 159, 1965.
154. Wolf, Price, Brown and Kawamura: *Eighth Int. Cong. of Nutrition*, Prague, 1969, Abstracts, W-16.
155. Brown, Thornton and Price: J. Clin. Invest., *40*, 617, 1961.
156. Wachstein, Moore and Graffeo: Proc. Soc. Expt. Biol. Med., *96*, 326, 1957.
157. Friedman, Becker, Thompson and Vilter: J. Lab. and Clin. Med., *46*, 817, 1955.
158. Hillman, Cabaud, Nilsson, Arpin and Tufano: Am. J. Clin. Nutrition, *12*, 427, 1963.
159. Wohl, Levy, Szutka and Maldia: Proc. Soc. Expt. Biol. Med., *105*, 523, 1960.
160. McCoy, Anast and Naylor: J. Ped., *65*, 208, 1965.
161. Recommended Dietary Allowances. Natl. Acad. Sci.—Natl. Res. Council, Publ. 1964, Washington, D.C., 1968.
162. McKusick and Hsu: Arthritis and Rheum., *4*, 426, 1961.
163. Jaffe, Altman and Merryman: Clin. Invest., *43*, 1869, 1964.
164. Kraft, Fiebig and Hotovy: Arzneimittel Forsch., *11*, 922, 1961.
165. Tillotson, Sauberlich, Baker, and Canham: Proc. Seventh International Congress of Nutr., *5*, 554, 1966.
166. Johansson, Lindstedt, Register, and Wadström: Am. J. Clin. Nutrition, *18*, 185, 1966.
167. Brown: Am. J. Clin. Nutr., *24*, 653, 1971.
168. Schroeder: Am. J. Clin. Nutr., *24*, 562, 1971.
169. Chabner and Livingston: Anal. Biochem., *34*, 413, 1970.
170. Takanashi, Matsunaga and Tamura: J. Vitamin (Kyoto), *16*, 132, 1970.
171. Evangelopoulos, Karni-Katsadimas and Kalogerakos: Enzymologia, *40*, 37, 1971.
172. French: New Eng. J. Med., *283*, 1173, 1970.
173. Baumblatt and Winston: Lancet, *1*, 832, 1970.
174. Luhby, Davis and Murphy: Lancet, *2*, 1083, 1970.
175. Gibbs and Watts: Clin. Sci., *38*, 277, 1970.
176. Gershoff and Prien: Am. J. Clin. Nutrition, *20*, 393, 1967.
177. Paulson: Am. J. Psychiatry, *127*, 1091, 1971.
178. Katz and Jobin: Amer. Rev. Resp. Dis., *101*, 991, 1970.
179. Jameson: J.A.M.A., *211*, 1700, 1970.
180. Friedman: J.A.M.A., *214*, 1563, 1970.
181. Golden, Mortati and Schroeter: J.A.M.A., *213*, 628, 1970.
182. Du Voison, Yahr and Cote: Trans. Amer. Neurol. Assoc., *94*, 81, 1969.
183. Cogzias: J.A.M.A., *210*. 1255, 1969.

Chapter

5

Section J Folic Acid and Vitamin B$_{12}$*

VICTOR HERBERT, M.D.

HISTORY[1,2,3]

In 1822, Combe[4] reported to the Royal Medical and Surgical Society of Edinburgh on the "history of a case of anemia" which he surmised was due to "some disorder of the digestive and assimilative organs." Thus was launched the study of pernicious anemia in particular and megaloblastic anemia in general, after re-stimulation by Addison's description, in 1849 and 1855,[5] of what his contemporaries evidently recognized as pernicious anemia, even though he did not mention glossitis, jaundice, or nerve damage. He did mention "the disease having uniformly occurred in fat people," which would imply deficiency of vitamin B$_{12}$ rather than of folate, since deficiency of the latter tends to be associated with wasting. Barclay,[6] in 1851, had reported death from an anemia which was probably megaloblastic anemia due to folate deficiency, resulting from several pregnancies superimposed on a bad diet.

The nutritional basis of pernicious anemia was suspected by Flint[7] in 1860, when he stated that "in these cases there exists degenerative disease of the glandular tubuli of the stomach." Another two-thirds of a century had passed when the classic work of Castle[8] and his associates demonstrated that normal human gastric juice contains an "intrinsic factor" that combines with an "extrinsic factor" contained in animal pro-

tein to result in absorption of the "anti-pernicious anemia principle." When vitamin B$_{12}$ was isolated in 1948 almost simultaneously in the United States[9] and England,[10] Berk and his associates[11] showed that this vitamin was both "extrinsic factor" and "anti-pernicious anemia principle."

In the 1930's, Wills and her associates[12] described a macrocytic anemia in Hindu women in Bombay, usually associated with pregnancy, that responded to therapy with a commercial preparation of autolyzed yeast called Marmite. By feeding the same type of diet ingested by their patients to monkeys, they produced in them a similar macrocytic anemia, which responded to a "Wills factor" present in crude but not purified liver extracts. We now know that the more purified extract consisted of a fairly pure solution of vitamin B$_{12}$, and that the "Wills factor" removed from the crude liver extract in the process of purification is folic acid. This gradually became clear after the purification of pteroylglutamic acid in 1943 by Stokstad,[13] its crystallization from liver in the same year by Pfiffner and associates,[14] its synthesis and structural identification by Angier and his co-workers,[15] and the 1948 isolation of crystalline vitamin B$_{12}$. The rapid isolation of vitamin B$_{12}$ by the American workers was greatly aided by a microbiologic assay based on Shorb's[16] discovery that "LLD factor," a growth factor required by *Lactobacillus lactis Dorner*, was not only the "animal protein factor" necessary for proper growth and function in animals fed an all-vegetable diet, but was also present in liver

* Supported in part by U.S.P.H.S. Grants #AM 15163 and 15164, by Career Scientist Award #I–683 of the Health Research Council of the City of New York, and by a Veterans Administration Medical Investigatorship.

extracts in amounts that closely paralleled their potency in the treatment of pernicious anemia.

Folic acid proved to be not only the "Wills factor," but also the vitamin M contained in dried brewer's yeast which corrected the deficiency anemia, leukopenia, diarrhea, and gingivitis of monkeys studied by Day and associates.[17] It also proved to be the vitamin B_c, contained in yeast, that corrected the deficiency syndrome in chicks characterized by anemia and growth failure. Furthermore, folic acid proved to be the norite eluate factor (i.e., it could be adsorbed on and eluted from charcoal) of liver, described by Snell and Peterson[18] as essential to the growth of *Lactobacillus casei* (and therefore also called the "*L. casei* factor"). The term "folic acid" was coined by Mitchell and co-workers[19] because they found this material in a leafy vegetable (spinach) At that time, it was not recognized that vitamin B_{12}, and not folic acid, was the active ingredient in the oral liver therapy which Minot and Murphy[20] reported in 1926 as successful in treating pernicious anemia (for which work they received the Nobel Prize in Medicine in 1934).

CHEMISTRY[3,21,22]

Neither vitamin B_{12} (cyanocobalamin) nor folic acid (pteroylglutamic acid) is present as such in significant quantity in either the human body or the various foods from which these agents were isolated. In the body and in foods, they are present in various reduced metabolically active coenzyme forms, often conjugated (in the case of B_{12} to peptide and in the case of folate to one or more glutamates) in peptide linkage. During the extraction procedure these labile active forms are either oxidatively destroyed (particularly folates), or oxidized and converted to cyanocobalamin or pteroylglutamic acid, which are the stable forms of the respective vitamins.

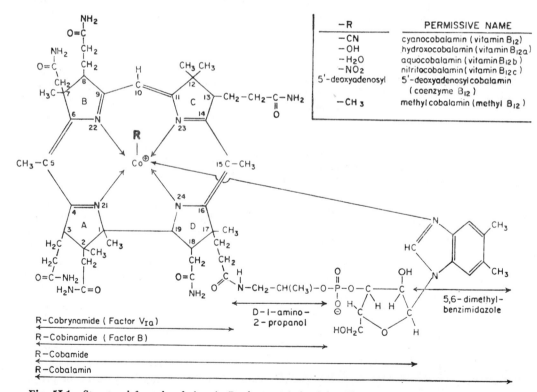

−R	PERMISSIVE NAME
−CN	cyanocobalamin (vitamin B_{12})
−OH	hydroxocobalamin (vitamin B_{12a})
−H_2O	aquocobalamin (vitamin B_{12b})
−NO_2	nitritocobalamin (vitamin B_{12c})
5'−deoxyadenosyl	5'−deoxyadenosylcobalamin (coenzyme B_{12})
−CH_3	methylcobalamin (methyl B_{12})

R−Cobrynamide (Factor V_{Ia})

R−Cobinamide (Factor B)

R−Cobamide

R−Cobalamin

Fig. 5J-1. Structural formula of vitamin B_{12} (cyanocobalamin). The numbering system for the corrin nucleus is made to correspond to that of the porphin nucleus by omitting the number 20. (Modified from Brown and Reynolds: Biogenesis of Water-Soluble Vitamins. *Annual Review of Biochemistry, 32,* 419–462, 1963.)

These stable forms are partially oxidized and not known to be metabolically active; it is not until they are reduced by metabolic systems present within gut and other tissue cells that they become metabolically active.

Vitamin B_{12}.[3,21,23—25] Figure 5J–1 shows the structural formula of vitamin B_{12} (cyanocobalamin); delineation of this structure, using x-ray crystallography, by Hodgkin and her co-workers was partly responsible for her winning the 1964 Nobel Prize in Chemistry. The chemistry of the vitamin has been reviewed by Smith.[21] The two major portions of the molecule are the corrin nucleus (a planar group), and a "nucleotide" lying in a plane nearly at right angles to the corrin nucleus and linked to it by D-1-amino-2-propanol. The "nucelotide" (5,6-dimethyl-benzimidazole) is attached to ribose by an alpha-glycoside linkage. A second bond between the two major parts of the molecule is the coordinate linkage of the cobalt atom to one of the nitrogen atoms of the "nucleotide."

In cyanocobalamin, the anionic (–R) group in coordinate linkage with the cobalt is cyanide. Fortuitously, the original isolation of B_{12} from liver yielded a stable product, cyanocobalamin, because the unstable linkage of the 5'-deoxyadenosyl anionic group to the rest of the molecule in coenzyme B_{12} (the form naturally present in liver) was ruptured and replaced by cyanide which leached from the charcoal columns used in the isolation procedure.

Cyanocobalamin crystals are dark red, the substance absorbs water, and the product official in the USP contains 12 per cent absorbed moisture. The activity is destroyed by heavy metals and strong oxidizing or reducing agents, but not by autoclaving for short periods at 121° C. It is soluble 1:80 in water, and stable in solution. Aqueous solutions are neutral; maximal stability is at pH 4.5 to 5.

Coenzyme B_{12} (5'-deoxyadenosylcobalamin) and methyl-cobalamin (methyl-B_{12}) are the two vitamin B_{12} coenzymes known to be metabolically active in man, and constitute the dominant forms of B_{12} in mammalian tissues. Both are unstable in light, and undergo photolysis with formation of aquocobala-min, or, in the presence of potassium cyanide, cyanocobalamin. Under the rules of the International Union of Pure and Applied Chemistry (IUPAC) Commission on Biochemical Nomenclature,[26] cyanocobalamin is a permissive (semi-systematic) name for vitamin B_{12}, and the term "vitamin B_{12}" without qualification means cyanocobalamin exclusively. However, the term is also entrenched in the literature as a generic term for all the cobalamins active in man. The permissive term "cobalamin" (or B_{12}) is used to describe the vitamin B_{12} molecule minus the cyanide group, and is prefixed by the designation of the anionic R group (see Figure 5J–1) attached to the cobalt. The terms "coenzyme B_{12}" and "vitamin B_{12} coenzyme" are not interchangeable; the former means 5'-deoxyadenosylcobalamin exclusively, and the latter applies to any coenzyme form of B_{12}.

Figure 5J–1 delineates some of the family of natural and semi-synthetic cobalamins; others include di-cyanocobalamin, thio cyanatocobalamin, chlorocobalamin, and sulfitocobalamin. The alphabetical congeners of vitamin B_{12} (B_{12a}, B_{12b}, B_{12c}) listed in Figure 5J–1 are believed equipotent in treatment of vitamin B_{12} deficiency (unless that deficiency is due to a congenital or acquired defect in enzymes involved in converting one B_{12} form to another). However, minimal dose therapy suggests[27] that coenzyme B_{12} is more potent therapeutically than cyanocobalamin; therapy with doses greater than minimal is always

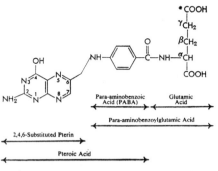

*Site of attachment of extra glutamate residue(s) of pteroyl di-, tri-, or hepta-glutamate.

Folic Acid (Pteroylmonoglutamic Acid)

Fig. 5J-2. The structural formula of folic acid (pteroylglutamic acid). (From Herbert: In *The Pharmacological Basis of Therapeutics*, 4th ed. Goodman and Gilman, Editors. New York, The Macmillan Company, 1970.)

used clinically, and all forms of B_{12} appear equipotent when used in greater than minimal doses.

Folic Acid.[3,22,28] Figure 5J–2 presents the structural formula of folic acid (pteroyl-glutamic acid), and Figure 5J–3 presents the major coenzymatically active forms of the vitamin. The major portions of the molecule are the pteridine moiety linked by a methylene bridge to para-aminobenzoic acid, which itself is joined in peptide-like linkage to glutamic acid.

Crystalline folic acid is yellow. The free acid is almost insoluble in cold water, but the disodium salt is more soluble (about 1.5 gm%). Injectable solutions are prepared by dissolving folic acid in isotonic sodium bicarbonate solution, or by using the disodium salt. Folic acid is destroyed at pH below 4, but is relatively stable above pH 5, with no destruction in 1 hour at 100° C.

The molecule usually splits into pteridine and para-aminobenzoyl glutamate.

The rules of the International Union of Pure and Applied Chemistry[26] are that pteroylglutamic acid may be designated generically as folic acid, and that the pure substance hitherto known as folic acid, folacine, or vitamin B_c shall be named "pteroylglutamic acid." However, the term "folic acid" is entrenched in the literature not only generically but also as a synonym for pteroylglutamic acid. Therefore, when the context does not make the meaning clear, it is preferable to use the term "folate" for the generic meaning (as done by WHO Scientific Group, 1968[29] and FAO/WHO Expert Group, 1970).[30]

5-Formyl-tetrahydrofolic acid is also known as folinic acid, and as citrovorum factor.

Pteroylglutamic acid is not normally found in foods or in the human body in

	R	OXIDATION STATE
N^5 formyl THFA	—CHO	formate
N^{10} formyl THFA	—CHO	formate
N^5 formimino THFA	—CH=NH	formate
$N^{5,10}$ methenyl THFA	>CH	formate
$N^{5,10}$ methylene THFA	>CH_2	formaldehyde
N^5 methyl THFA	—CH_3	methanol

*Broken lines indicate the N^5 and/or N^{10} site of attachment of various 1-carbon units for which THFA acts as a carrier.

5,6,7,8-Tetrahydrofolic Acid (THFA)(FH₄)(R=—H)

Fig. 5J-3. Structures and nomenclature in the folate field. The table above the formula lists some of the possible 1-carbon adducts formed with THFA. (From Herbert: In *The Pharmacological Basis of Therapeutics*, 4th ed. Goodman and Gilman, Editors. New York, The Macmillan Co., 1970.)

significant concentrations. The forms which are found in such sources are indicated in Figure 5J–3; they are THFA and various 1-carbon adducts formed with THFA, which is produced from pteroylglutamic acid by action of the enzyme dihydrofolate reductase splitting the double bond between the 5,6 and between the 7,8 position, adding a hydrogen at each of these four positions. In addition to being reduced folates, the naturally occurring forms are usually conjugated in peptide-like linkage through their gamma-carboxyl groups (see Fig. 5J–2) to one or more glutamic acid residues; in such folyl peptides, each glutamic acid residue is linked through its amino group to the gamma-carboxyl of the preceding residue.

UNITS OF MEASUREMENT AND METHODS OF ASSAY

Vitamin B_{12}.[3,21,31] Human serum levels of vitamin B_{12} are measured in picograms (pg; 10^{-12} grams; $\mu\mu g$; micromicrograms) per ml of serum; normal values range from 200 to 900 pg/ml; values below 80 pg/ml represent unequivocal B_{12} deficiency according to the WHO Scientific Group on Nutritional Anemias.[29] This tiny quantity of vitamin B_{12} activity may only be measured microbiologically or by radioassay. Many microorganisms require vitamin B_{12} in order to grow, and therefore, there are many microbiologic assays for vitamin B_{12}. Radioassay for vitamin B_{12} has the advantage over microbiologic assay in that false low results do not occur if serum contains antibiotic or other substances which inhibit growth of microorganisms, whereas the microbiologic assays do yield false low results in such circumstances. Radioassay for vitamin B_{12} was first described in 1958;[32] the most widely used such assay applies coated charcoal[33,34] to separate free from bound vitamin B_{12}.

Larger quantities of vitamin B_{12} may be assayed colorimetrically, spectroscopically, fluorometrically, or chemically.

The U.S.P. assay for vitamin B_{12} is spectrophotometric. Although liver extract for injection was deleted from the U.S.P. in 1960, such products are still being used, assayed by a microbiological method for their vitamin B_{12} content. Such preparations are still in the National Formulary; for clinical purposes the injectable unit is approximately the equivalent of 1.33 micrograms of vitamin B_{12}. It should be noted that preparations of liver extract contain hematopoietic materials other than vitamin B_{12} (*e.g.*, folic acid, folinic acid); they constitute shotgun therapy, like many other multi-ingredient therapies.

Folic Acid.[3,35] Normal human serum contains 7 to 16 nanograms (ng; 10^{-9} grams; $m\mu g$; millimicrograms) of folic acid activity per ml of serum. These tiny quantities could only be measured microbiologically, as originally described in 1959,[36–40] until 1970, when a radioisotopic assay was described.[41] Since the dominant form of folate in human serum is 5-methyltetrahydrofolate, on which only *Lactobacillus casei* but no other microorganism grows well, the only microbiologic assay which adequately measures serum folate in man uses *L. casei*. Since serum folate is labile, false low values for serum folate activity occur if the serum has not been protected against oxidative destruction prior to assay. Such protection is brought about by storing the serum frozen, storing it in the presence of a reducing agent such as ascorbate, or both.

Larger quantities of folate activity than those normally present in human serum may be measured chemically, fluorometrically, by paper and thin-layer chromatography, enzymatically, or by animal assay.[35]

THE CAUSES OF NUTRITIONAL DEFICIENCY OF VITAMIN B_{12} AND FOLIC ACID

In the final analysis, nutritional deficiency means there is inadequate usage of a nutrient, in one or more intracellular systems, to sustain normal biochemical functions. Such inadequate usage falls in one or more of five basic categories, *viz.*:

1. Inadequate ingestion;
2. Inadequate absorption;
3. Inadequate utilization;
4. Increased requirement;
5. Increased excretion.

Any one or combination of these three inadequacies and two excesses may result in

Table 5J-1.   Etiologic Classification of Vitamin B_{12} and Folate Deficiency in Man*

I. Vitamin B_{12} Deficiency (normal B_{12} body stores last 3–6 years after cessation of B_{12} absorption)
  A. *Indequate Ingestion*
    1. *Poor diet* (lacking animal protein and microorganisms, the sole B_{12} sources)
      a. Vegans
      b. Chronic alcoholism (folate deficiency more common)
      c. Poverty, religious tenets, ignorance, dietary faddism
  B. *Inadequate Absorption*
    1. *Inadequate or absent secretion of gastric intrinsic factor*
      a. Failure of the stomach to adequately secrete intrinsic factor
        1. Addisonian pernicious anemia
          a. Hereditary failure of intrinsic factor secretion
          b. Hereditary degenerative gastric atrophy
          c. Gastric atrophy as the end result of superficial inflammatory gastritis; superficial gastritis with atrophy
          d. Autoimmunity producing gastric atrophy?
        2. Lesions which destroy the gastric mucosa (ingested corrosives, linitis plastica, etc.)
        3. Endocrine disorders (hypothyroidism, polyendocrinopathy, etc.)
      b. Gastrectomy
        1. Total
        2. Subtotal
          a. Proximal
          b. Distal
      c. Intrinsic factor inhibitor in gastric secretion
        1. Antibody to intrinsic factor (in saliva or gastric juice)
          a. Blocking antibody
          b. Binding antibody
    2. *Small intestine disorder* (affecting ileum, which is the main site of B_{12} absorption)
      a. Gluten-induced enteropathy (childhood celiac disease; adult celiac disease) (idiopathic steatorrhea, non-tropical sprue)
      b. Tropical sprue
      c. Regional ileitis
      d. Strictures or anastomoses of the small bowel
      e. Intestinal resection
      f. Malignancies and granulomatous lesions involving the small intestine
      g. Other conditions characterized by chronically disturbed intestinal function
      h. Drugs
        1. Para-aminosalicylic acid (PAS)
        2. Colchicine
        3. Neomycin
        4. Ethanol
        5. Oral contraceptive agents?
      i. Specific malabsorption for vitamin B_{12}
        1. Due to long-term ingestion of calcium-chelating agents
        2. Due to inadequately alkaline pH in ileum
        3. Unknown causes (absence of intestinal receptors for B_{12}-intrinsic factor complex? absence of "releasing factor"?)
          a. Congenital (Imerslund-Grasbeck syndrome)
          b. Acquired (form fruste of sprue)
        4. Inadequate pancreatic exocrine secretion
    3. *Competition for vitamin B_{12} by intestinal parasites or bacteria*
      a. Fish tapeworm (Diphyllobothrium latum)
      b. Bacteria: The blind loop syndrome (B_{12}-greedy bacteria)
  C. *Inadequate Utilization*
    1. Vitamin B_{12} antagonists
      a. Substituted B_{12} amides and anilides
      b. Cobaloximes

Table 5J-1.   Etiologic Classification of Vitamin B_{12} and Folate Deficiency in Man (Continued)

    2. Protein malnutrition?
    3. Malignancy?
    4. Liver disease?
    5. Renal disease?
    6. Thiocyanate intoxication?
    7. Congenital or acquired enzyme deficiency or deletion
      a. Methylmalonyl-CoA mutase
      b. Methyltetrahydrofolate-homocysteine methyltransferase
      c. B_{12a} reductase
      d. $B_{12\gamma}$ reductase
      e. Deoxyadenosyltransferase
      f. Other enzyme reduction or deletion
    8. Abnormal B_{12}-binding protein in serum, irreversibly binding B_{12} and making it unavailable to tissues
      a. Abnormal α (myeloproliferative disorders)
      b. Abnormal β (liver disease)
    9. Inadequate serum B_{12}-binding protein
      a. α
      b. β
  D. *Increased Requirement*
    1. Hyperthyroidism
    2. Increased hematopoiesis?
    3. Infancy?
    4. Parasitization
      a. By fetus
      b. By malignant tissue?
  E. *Increased Excretion*
    1. Inadequate B_{12}-binding protein in serum?
    2. Liver disease (inadequate retention of B_{12})
    3. Renal disease?
II. Folic Acid Deficiency (normal folate body stores will last only 3–6 months after cessation of folate ingestion)
  A. *Inadequate Ingestion*
    1. *Poor diet* (lacking unprocessed fresh, uncooked or slightly-cooked food) (folates are heat-labile)
      a. Nutritional megaloblastic anemia
        1. Tropical
        2. Nontropical
        3. Scurvy (diets poor in vitamin C are also poor in folate)
      b. Chronic alcoholism with or without cirrhosis
  B. *Inadequate Absorption* (affecting upper $\frac{1}{3}$ of small intestine which is the main site of folate absorption)
    1. *Malabsorption syndromes*
      a. Gluten-induced enteroptahy (childhood and adult celiac disease) (idiopathic steatorrhea, nontropical sprue)
      b. Any chronic functional or structural disorder involving the upper small intestine
        1. Tropical sprue
      c. Drugs
        1. Diphenylhydantoin (Dilantin)
        2. Primidone
        3. Barbiturates
        4. Oral contraceptive agents (?)
        5. Cycloserine
        6. Ethanol
    2. *Specific malabsorption for folate*
      a. Congenital
      b. Acquired

Table 5J-1. Etiologic Classification of Vitamin B₁₂ and Folate Deficiency in Man (Continued)

    3. *Blind loop syndrome* (folate-greedy bacteria)
C. *Inadequate Utilization* (metabolic block)
    1. Folic acid antagonists (dihydrofolate reductase inhibitors)

a. 4-amino-4-deoxyfolates (*i.e.* methotrexate)	(Chemotherapy, immunosuppression, psoriasis)
b. 2,4-diaminopyrimidine (*i.e.* pyrimethamine)	(Malaria, toxoplasmosis)
c. Triamterene	(Diuretic)
d. Diamidine compounds (*i.e.* pentamidine isethionate)	(Pneumocystis carinii, protozoacidal)
e. Trimethoprim	(Antibacterial)

    2. Anticonvulsants?
    3. Enzyme deficiency
        a. Congenital
            1. Formiminotransferase
            2. Dihydrofolate reductase
            3. Methyltetrahydrofolate transmethylase
            4. Other enzymes
        b. Acquired
            1. Liver disease
                a. Formiminotransferase
                b. Other enzymes
    4. Vitamin B₁₂ deficiency
    5. Alcohol
    6. Ascorbic acid deficiency?
    7. Dietary amino acid excess (glycine, methionine)
D. *Increased Requirement*
    1. Parasitization
        a. By fetus (especially in multiple and twin pregnancies)
        b. By malignant tissue (especially lymphoproliferative disorders; myeloproliferative disorders to a lesser extent; extensive carcinomatosis, etc.)
    2. Infancy
    3. Increased hematopoiesis (hemolytic anemias; chronic blood loss [including scurvy])
    4. Increased metabolic activity (*e.g.*, hyperthyroidism)
E. *Increased Excretion*
    1. Vitamin B₁₂ deficiency? (? of obligatory excretion of folate in urine and bile) (due partly to inability to incorporate folate in cells)
    2. Liver disease?

* Compiled mainly from information in "Symposium on Vitamin B₁₂ and Folate" (Herbert, V., guest editor), Am. J. Med. *48*:539–670, 1970, and from Herbert, V. "Megaloblastic Anemias—Mechanisms & Management," Disease-a-Month, Year Book Medical Publishers, Chicago, August, 1965.

nutritional deficiency. Table 5J–1 presents the currently known possible etiologic factors in each of these five categories which may produce nutritional deficiency of vitamin B₁₂ or folic acid. The ensuing sections will discuss in more detail mechanisms of inadequate absorption and utilization of these two vitamins.

Absorption of Vitamin B₁₂.[3,23,42–46] There are two separate and distinct mechanisms for the absorption of vitamin B₁₂. The *physiologic* mechanism, whose derangement accounts for much human vitamin B₁₂ deficiency, is capable of handling a maximum of 1.5 to 3 micrograms of free vitamin B₁₂ at any one time. This mechanism operates as follows: (1) ingested vitamin B₁₂ is freed from its polypeptide linkages to food by gastric acid and gastric and intestinal enzymes; (2) the free vitamin B₁₂ attaches to the gastric intrinsic factor of Castle (a glycoprotein of molecular weight in the range of 50,000, produced by normal gastric parietal cells, which dimerizes on combination with vitamin B_{12} so that a complex is formed consisting of two molecules of intrinsic factor and two molecules of vitamin B_{12}); (3) the vitamin B_{12}-intrinsic factor complex is carried down to the ileum, where it is plastered onto the brush border of the ileal mucosal cells in the presence of ionic calcium and a pH above 6; (4) via a currently-uncertain mechanism, the vitamin B_{12} is released from its complex with intrinsic factor probably at but possibly within the ileal enterocyte (epithelial cell); (5) the vitamin then finds its way across the enterocyte into the portal venous blood, at which point it is attached to serum vitamin B_{12}-binding glycoprotein (see Fig. 5J–4).

The other, or *pharmacologic*, mechanism of vitamin B_{12} absorption appears to be diffusion. It accounts for the absorption along the entire length of the small intestine of approximately 1 per cent of *any* quantity of *free* vitamin B_{12} in the small bowel. This is the mechanism which makes possible oral (rather than parenteral) therapy of vitamin B_{12} deficiency due to vitamin B_{12} malabsorption. However, such therapy is less reliable than parenteral therapy.[3]

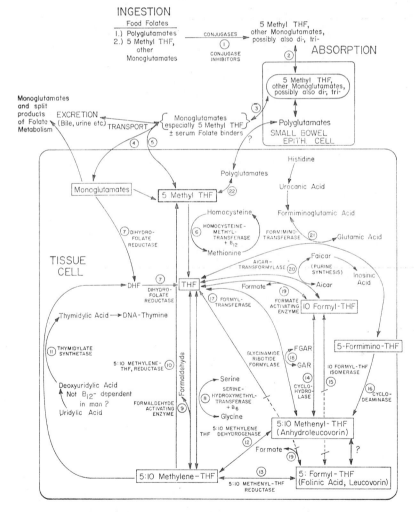

Fig. 5J-4A. Flow chart of folate metabolism in man. Circled numbers identify individual steps in folate metabolism. THF = tetrahydrofolate; DHF = dihydrofolate. (From V. Herbert and G. Tisman, in *Biology of Brain Dysfunction* [G. E. Gaull, editor]. Plenum Press, N.Y., 1972.)

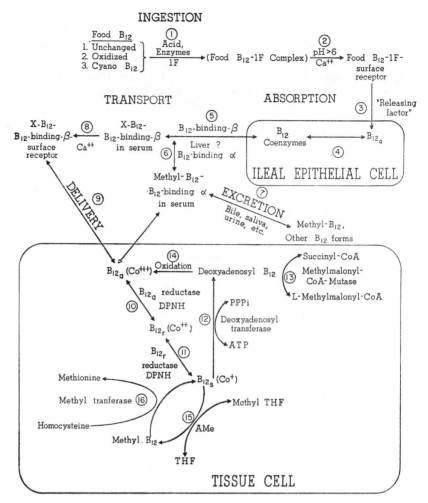

Fig. 5J-4B. Cobalamin (B_{12}) metabolism in man. (Herbert in Arstein and Wrighton, courtesy of J. & A. Churchill.)

Absorption of Folic Acid.[3,43,47–51] Current evidence suggests that food folate is absorbed primarily from the proximal third of the small intestine, although it is capable of being absorbed from the entire length of the small bowel. Folate in food is present primarily in polyglutamate form. Prior to the absorption of the vitamin, the "excess" glutamates are split off the side chain of the vitamin molecule by conjugases. The amount of food folate which can be absorbed is limited both by the efficiency of the deconjugating mechanism and by the presence of conjugase inhibitors in some foods, such as yeast.

Though it is not yet established with certainty, it is probable that for folate, as for vitamin B_{12}, there are two separate and distinct absorption mechanisms. The active mechanism requires energy and is accelerated by the presence of glucose. The passive mechanism is probably diffusion, and accounts for absorption of a small but relatively unchanging percentage of any quantity of free (*i.e.*, unconjugated) folate in the small intestine.

Vitamin B_{12} Transport, Distribution, Storage, Fate, and Excretion (see Fig. 5J-4).[3,23,44,52,53] When absorbed into the blood stream, vitamin B_{12} appears to be instantly and tightly bound to glycoproteins, mainly two which move electrophoretically as alpha- and beta-globulin. Vitamin B_{12}-binding beta-globulin ("transcobalamin II") appears to be primarily a transport and delivery protein for vitamin B_{12}. Vitamin B_{12}-binding alpha-globulin ("transcobalamin I") appears to be primarily a storage protein for vitamin B_{12}, with a possible minor delivery function. The molecular weight of the B_{12}-binding beta-globulin is in the range of 35,000, and that of the B_{12}-binding alpha-globulin is in the range of 60,000. A significant portion of the B_{12}-binding alpha-globulin is made by granulocytes;[44,53,55] these cells may also make some of the B_{12}-binding beta-globulin.[56] There is some speculation that the B_{12}-binding alpha is a dimer of the B_{12}-binding beta-globulin. A third vitamin B_{12}-binding protein is present in serum, normally in smaller quantity and with different electrophoretic mobility from the other two.[52,53]

Serum B_{12}-binding protein delivers the vitamin to liver,[32] bone marrow cells, reticulocytes,[57] and possibly other tissues as well, via a mechanism closely similar to that by which intrinsic factor delivers the vitamin to ileal mucosal cells. Bone marrow cells and reticulocytes contain on their surfaces "receptor sites" for the complex of vitamin B_{12}-binding beta-globulin and vitamin B_{12}; these sites will only take up the complex in the presence of ionic calcium and a pH greater than 6.[57] Thus, delivery of B_{12} to both the gut enterocyte and the immature blood erythrocyte require: (1) a transport glycoprotein, (2) pH above 6, (3) ionic calcium, and (4) a receptor site for the glycoprotein-vitamin B_{12} complex on the surface of the cell. However, gastric intrinsic factor and B_{12}-binding beta-globulin are not the same glycoprotein, since neither will substitute functionally for the other, and they are immunologically distinct and have different molecular weights.

The vitamin B_{12} picked up from the ileum by serum vitamin B_{12}-binding beta-globulin is so rapidly delivered to tissues that, when one draws a sample of human blood, one normally finds little B_{12} attached to beta-globulin.

Characteristically, human serum has a total vitamin B_{12}-binding capacity in the range of 1800 picograms (pg, $\mu\mu g$) per ml, of which approximately one-third to one-fifth is saturated with vitamin B_{12}.[53] This third-to-fifth is all alpha-globulin. Of the two-thirds to four-fifths of the total serum vitamin B_{12}-binding capacity which is unsaturated (i.e., the "UBBC" or "unsaturated B_{12}-binding capacity"), approximately 80 per cent is beta- and 20 per cent is alpha-globulin vitamin B_{12}-binding protein. TBBC (total B_{12}-binding capacity), UBBC, and serum vitamin B_{12} level all tend to be elevated in any situation in which the total body neutrophil pool is increased (as in myeloproliferative disorders), in which conditions the dominant elevation is in B_{12}-binding alpha-globulin. (These parameters also tend to be elevated in acute and chronic liver disease, which throws into the blood stream an abnormal B_{12}-binding beta-globulin.) The dominant B_{12}-binding alpha-globulin in myeloproliferative disorders does not deliver its load of vitamin to tissues, as illustrated by the fact that a patient with chronic myelogenous leukemia and pernicious anemia may have a normal serum vitamin B_{12} level and yet have tissues severely depleted of the vitamin, to the point where biochemical deficiency is severe.[58]

"Normal" stores of vitamin B_{12} range between 1 and 10 mg,[29,30,59] with the liver containing 50 to 90 per cent of the total stored vitamin (averaging 1 μg B_{12}/gm of liver). Average stores range between 2 and 5 mg. There is no evidence for significant catabolism of vitamin B_{12} by man, and it is probable that loss occurs only by excretion, mainly in the bile. The whole body turnover of vitamin B_{12} is between 0.1 and 0.2 per cent daily, regardless of whether body stores are normal or reduced. Coenzyme B_{12} appears to be the main storage form, and methyl-B_{12} appears to be the main serum transport form.[23]

There is normally an enterohepatic circulation of vitamin B_{12} which may account for from approximately 0.6 to approximately 6 μg of the vitamin excreted daily in the bile and reabsorbed in the ileum.[3,60-62] This almost total conservation of vitamin B_{12} explains why pure vegetarians, who eat almost no vitamin B_{12}, take decades to develop deficiency of the vitamin. It is only when the reabsorption phase of the enterohepatic circulation of the vitamin is damaged, by damage to the stomach or the ileum, that vitamin B_{12} deficiency disease develops more rapidly (*i.e.*, in 3 to 6 years).

Folate Transport, Distribution, Storage, Fate and Excretion.[3,52] Folate, like vitamin B_{12}, is probably transported in the blood serum bound to a protein, although this bond is much weaker[63] than that between vitamin B_{12} and its serum transport protein (Fig. 5J–4A).

Folate is delivered to bone marrow cells and reticulocytes[64] (and probably other tissue cells, as well) in both an energy-dependent active manner and, to a considerably lesser extent, probably also by passive diffusion. Methyl-folate (N^5-methyl-tetrahydrofolate) appears to be the main form of the vitamin in serum, liver and other tissues;[65] it also appears to be preferentially taken up by bone marrow cells and reticulocytes as compared to the oxidized, stable, medicinal form of folic acid (pteroylglutamic acid). It has not yet been determined whether reduced folate is preferentially absorbed by the intestine as compared to oxidized folate.

Normal total body folate stores are in the range of 5 to 10 mg, of which approximately half is in the liver.[29,30] As is true for B_{12}, there is also an enterohepatic circulation of folate. Approximately 0.1 mg of folate is normally excreted in the bile daily.[3]

NUTRITIONAL REQUIREMENTS AND NATURAL SOURCES

The term "minimal daily requirement" (MDR), as used in this chapter, means the minimal daily requirement *from exogenous sources* required to sustain normality, with normality defined as the absence of any biochemical hypofunction which is correctable by addition of greater quantities of the vitamin. By this definition, the minimal daily requirement for vitamin B_{12} of a normal subject would be only 0.1 microgram, since this quantity will sustain normality in a normal subject.[67,68] The minimal daily requirement for vitamin B_{12} of a patient with gastric or ileal structural or functional damage would

be greater, since such damage not only eliminates the normal absorption of vitamin B_{12} from exogenous (food) sources, but also eliminates the normal daily reabsorption from the ileum of almost all the vitamin B_{12} normally excreted each day in bile.

The minimal daily requirement can be reduced to a formula[66] applicable generally to essential (*i.e.*, required from exogenous sources) nutrient deficiency, as follows:

$$(1) \quad \text{MDR (units/day)} = \frac{\text{UBS (units)}}{\text{D (days)}}$$

where:

MDR = Minimal daily requirement of nutrient from exogenous sources.
UBS = Utilizable body stores of nutrient.
  D = Number of days required to develop tissue deficiency after cessation of absorption from exogenous sources of nutrient (with appropriate correction for *incomplete* cessation of absorption).

The above formula may also be written as:

$$(2) \qquad D = \frac{\text{UBS}}{\text{MDR}}$$

or

$$(3) \qquad \text{UBS} = D \times \text{MDR}$$

As suggested above, one can predict the time it would take any given nutrient deficiency to develop in any given person after reduction or cessation of absorption of the nutrient if one knows (or can reasonably estimate) the MDR for the nutrient and the utilizable body stores thereof.

Vitamin B_{12}. *Nutritional Requirements.*[3,27,29,30,67,68] Vitamin B_{12} requirements have been estimated from three different types of study:[30] (1) those designed to determine the minimal amount needed to prevent or cure megaloblastic anemia resulting from vitamin B_{12} deficiency, (2) those correlating the relationship between the levels of vitamin B_{12} in serum and in liver in deficient and healthy subjects, and (3) those correlating body stores and turnover rates of vitamin B_{12}.

The results of such studies[30] demonstrated

that: (1) the minimal quantity of vitamin B_{12} which would produce hematologic response in patients with uncomplicated vitamin B_{12} deficiency was in the range of 0.1 microgram daily, and 0.5 to 1 microgram of the vitamin daily produces maximum hematological responses, with similar amounts maintaining a normal picture; (2) patients with moderate vitamin B_{12} deficiency resulting from B_{12} malabsorption had an average liver vitamin B_{12} content of 0.16 μg per gm wet weight of liver, associated with serum vitamin B_{12} levels ranging from 80 to 130 pg per ml, and an average total body B_{12} of approximately 250 μg. (a second group of individuals who were also suffering from vitamin B_{12} malabsorption, but who had not yet developed morphological evidence of blood damage due to vitamin B_{12} deficiency, all had serum levels between 130 and 200 pg per ml, associated with approximately 0.28 μg of vitamin B_{12} per gm wet weight of liver and an average total body vitamin B_{12} content of approximately 525 μg); (3) the daily whole body turnover of vitamin B_{12} measured with tracer doses of radioactive vitamin indicates a radioactivity turnover of between 0.1 and 0.2 per cent daily, regardless of whether the body vitamin B_{12} stores are normal or reduced.

Loss of 0.1 to 0.2 per cent of radioactive vitamin B_{12} daily means less than that quantity of vitamin is lost from the body stores daily, since the radioactive B_{12} excreted in the bile mixes with nonradioactive B_{12} in the diet, and some of the radioactive B_{12} that would otherwise be reabsorbed in the ileum is replaced by absorbed nonradioactive vitamin. The net result is a gradual reduction in the radioactivity of the body vitamin B_{12} stores, but a much lesser reduction in the actual vitamin B_{12} content of those stores.

The Food and Nutrition Board of the National Research Council (NRC) states[67] that, "if absorption is normal, a dietary intake of 5 micrograms per day of vitamin B_{12} is required to insure the replacement of normal losses." That is their "recommended daily allowance (RDA) for adults." On the other hand, the Joint FAO/WHO Expert Group[30] recommends a daily intake of 2 μg of vitamin B_{12} for the normal adult. The recommendation of the NRC group is based almost entirely on studies of the body turnover of radioactive vitamin B_{12}, studies that seem to have no relation to minimal daily requirement, since such turnover tends to be a fixed percentage of body stores regardless of the size of body stores. On the other hand, the 2 μg daily intake recommended for adults by the FAO/WHO group is based not only on the same radioactivity turnover studies on which the NRC relied almost exclusively, but also on studies of minimal amounts needed to prevent or cure megaloblastic anemia resulting from vitamin B_{12} deficiency, and on studies of the relationship between the levels of vitamin B_{12} in serum and in liver in deficient and healthy subjects. Therefore, the recommended daily allowance (RDA) of 5 μg of vitamin B_{12} for adults by the NRC group carries a considerable margin above normal physiological requirements and bears no direct relationship to minimal daily requirement, whereas the recommended daily intake of 2 μg of vitamin B_{12} of the Joint FAO/WHO Expert Group, while also carrying a substantial margin above normal physiological requirements (i.e., above the MDR), does bear a direct relationship to the normal adult minimal daily requirement (MDR).

Vitamin B_{12} deficiency does not occur in breast-fed infants unless their mothers are deficient in the vitamin. Infants showing such deficiency respond hematologically to 0.1 μg of vitamin B_{12} orally. In the economically advanced countries, breast milk supplies 0.3 μg of vitamin B_{12} daily, which is clearly adequate as manifested by lack of evidence of any deficiency in the infant. Available evidence suggests that the milk from mothers whose serum contains vitamin B_{12} concentrations close to the lower limit of normality (i.e., 200 pg/ml) is also adequate. The Joint FAO/WHO Expert Group therefore recommends 0.3 μg of vitamin B_{12} daily as the intake for infants on artificial feeding.[30]

Vitamin B_{12} deficiency does not occur in normal children on adequate calorie and animal protein intakes. Therefore, the Joint FAO/WHO Expert Group calculated desirable intakes of vitamin B_{12} for different ages in relation to the calorie intakes recommended for the respective age groups: 0.9 μg daily for children age 1 to 3 years, 1.5 for children age 4 to 9 years, 2 μg for children age 10 years and over, and 2 μg daily for adults.[30]

Pregnancy produces an increased requirement for vitamin B_{12} due to the fetal drain on maternal stores. The fetus removes approximately 0.2 μg of vitamin B_{12} daily from the maternal stores in the latter half of pregnancy; the total recommended daily intake of vitamin B_{12} in pregnancy is 3 μg.[30]

Total recommended intake during lactation is 2.5 μg per day, based on the recommended daily intake of 2 for the normal adult plus an additional 0.5 μg to accommodate the approximately 0.3 μg lost in the milk of nursing mothers.[30]

Eight per cent of the vitamin B_{12} in the liver is lost by boiling at 100° C for 5 minutes, while boiling muscle meat at 170° C for 45 minutes results in a loss of 30 per cent of the vitamin from the meat. Milk pasteurized for 2 to 3 seconds loses 7 per cent of its available vitamin B_{12}; when boiled for 2 to 5 minutes, it loses 30 per cent; sterilization in a bottle for 13 minutes at 119 to 120° C causes a loss of 77 per cent; rapid sterilization (3 to 4 seconds) with superheated steam at 143° C destroys only about 10 per cent of the vitamin.[30]

Natural Sources.[2,3,21,23,24,25,29,30,67,69] The sole source of vitamin B_{12} in nature is synthesis by microorganisms. The vitamin is absent from plants except when they are contaminated by microorganisms (for example, the root nodules of certain legumes contain microorganisms which make vitamin B_{12}; ingestion of these root nodules with their contained microorganisms may well provide the only dietary source of vitamin B_{12} for strict vegetarians, except for the vitamin B_{12} contained in ingested fecal matter on unwashed foods). Fruits and vegetables and grains and grain products are usually devoid of vitamin B_{12}. The usual dietary sources are meat and meat products (including shellfish, fish, and poultry), and, to a lesser extent, milk and milk products.

Rich sources of vitamin B_{12} (greater than 10 μg per 100 gm of wet weight) are organ meats such as lamb and beef liver, kidney and heart, and bivalves (clams, oysters) which siphon large quantities of vitamin B_{12}-synthesizing microorganisms from the sea. Moderately high amounts (3 to 10 μg per 100 gm of net weight) are present in non-fat dry milk, some seafood (crabs, rock fish, salmon, sardines), and egg yolk. Moderate amounts (1 to 3 μg per 100 gm wet weight) are found in muscle meats, some seafood (lobster, scallops, flounder, haddock, swordfish, tuna), and fermenting cheeses (Camembert, Limburger). There is less than 1 μg per 100 gm of wet weight in fluid milk products and in cream, Cheddar, and cottage cheese.

The vitamin B_{12} molecule is almost indestructible, unless heated in alkali at temperatures in excess of 100° C; the molecule splits at 250° C. Thus, hamburgers cooked on a hot griddle may lose some of their B_{12} from the surface flat against the hot griddle, but the vitamin B_{12} deep within the patty is preserved.

The enzymatically active forms of vitamin B_{12} (coenzyme B_{12} and methylcobalamin) are dominant forms in foodstuffs, in which they are generally attached to polypeptides. Cyanocobalamin *per se* is probably not present to a significant extent in any natural source. This stable form of vitamin B_{12} results from the action of cyanide on natural vitamin B_{12} coenzymes; thiocyanate ingestion and absorption of tobacco smoke (which contains cyanide) may convert a small amount of enzymatically active cobalamins in blood and tissues to cyanocobalamin.

Folic Acid. *Nutritional Requirements.*[3,29,30,65,67,68,70,71] The minimal daily requirement (MDR) for folate is in the range of 50 μg for adults. The FAO/WHO Expert Group recommends[30] a daily dietary intake (allowing for less than 100 per cent absorption) of 200 μg of "free" folate (defined as folate available to the microorganism *L. casei* without conjugase treatment) for adults, 50 μg for infants, 100 μg for children, 400 μg during pregnancy, and 300 μg during lactation. Since the daily folate requirement is hinged to the daily metabolic and cell turnover rates, it is increased by anything which increases metabolic rate (such as infection and hyperthyroidism), and anything which increases

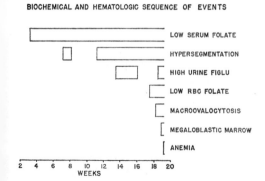

DIETARY FOLIC ACID DEPRIVATION IN MAN:
BIOCHEMICAL AND HEMATOLOGIC SEQUENCE OF EVENTS

LOW SERUM FOLATE

HYPERSEGMENTATION

HIGH URINE FIGLU

LOW RBC FOLATE

MACROOVALOCYTOSIS

MEGALOBLASTIC MARROW

ANEMIA

Fig. 5J-5. Biochemical and hematologic sequence of events in developing dietary folate deficiency in man. (Herbert: Trans. Assoc. Am. Phys. 75:307–320, 1962.)

cell turnover (such as hemolytic anemia and rapid tissue growth in the fetus and malignant tumors). Folate consumption by individual cells is proportional to their rate of 1-carbon-unit transfer. Alcohol interferes with folate utilization, and thereby increases folate requirement.[72]

The sequence of events in developing folate deficiency in man is depicted in Figure 5J-5.

Natural Sources of Folate.[3,22,30,67,73–76] Unlike vitamin B_{12}, which is present only in animal protein, folates are ubiquitous in nature, being present in nearly all natural foods. Unlike vitamin B_{12}, folate is highly susceptible to oxidative destruction; 50 to 95 per cent of the folate content of foods may be destroyed by protracted cooking or other processing, such as canning, and all folate is lost from refined foods such as hard liquor and hard candies. Foods with the highest folate content per unit of dry weight include yeast, liver and other organ meats, fresh green vegetables, and some fresh fruits.

The naturally occurring folates are active metabolic forms, usually in polyglutamate linkage (with pteroylheptaglutamates dominant in yeast). Conjugases present in vegetable and mammalian tissues (including human intestine) liberate pteroyldiglutamates and pteroylmonoglutamates from the conjugates, thereby making the folate available for absorption. About 90 per cent of mono-

glutamate, but only about half of heptaglutamate, is absorbed by man.[47–50]

The pharmaceutical product pteroylglutamic acid (PGA), like the pharmaceutical product cyanocobalamin, is not usually found as such in natural sources. Its isolation from natural sources, like the isolation of cyanocobalamin, was the result of oxidation and deconjugation of the naturally occurring conjugated forms to a stable form.

METABOLIC FUNCTIONS

Interrelations of Vitamin B_{12} and Folic Acid.[2,3,23,52,76,77] *DNA Synthesis.* As illustrated in Figure 5J-6, both vitamin B_{12} and folic acid are required for synthesis of thymidylate, and therefore of DNA. A vitamin B_{12}-containing enzyme removes a methyl group from methyl folate and delivers it to homocysteine, thereby converting homocysteine to methionine (methyl-homocysteine) and regenerating THFA,[78] from which the 5,10-methylene THFA involved in thymidylate synthesis is made. Since methyl folate is the dominant form of folate in human serum and liver, and probably also in other body storage depots for folate, and since methyl folate may only return to the body's folate pool via a vitamin B_{12}-dependent step, when a patient suffers from vitamin B_{12} deficiency much of his folate is "trapped" as methyl folate, and thus is metabolically useless. This "folate trap" hypothesis[52,76,79] may provide much of the explanation of why the hematologic damage of vitamin B_{12} deficiency is not clinically distinguishable from that of folate deficiency. In both instances, the hematologic damage results from lack of adequate 5,10-methylene THFA, which delivers its methyl group to deoxyuridylate to convert that substance to thymidylate, and thus makes DNA during the S phase. In either deficiency lack of adequate DNA synthesis causes many hematopoietic cells to die in the bone marrow, very possibly without ever completing the S phase of cell replication (*i.e.*, a form of "ineffective erythropoiesis").

Megaloblastosis (the presence of giant germ cells) is the end product of deranged DNA synthesis of any cause. It is most easily

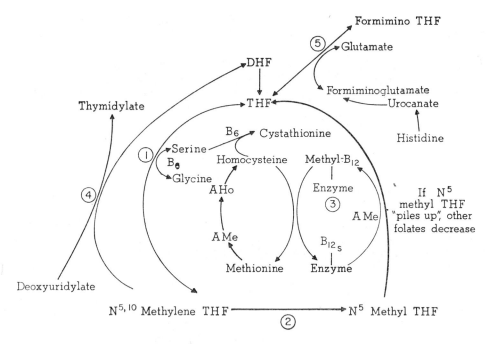

Fig. 5J-6. Interrelationships of vitamin B_{12}, B_6 and folate. (Herbert in Arstein and Wrighton, courtesy of J. & A. Churchill.)

understood as an arrest in the S (synthesis) phase of cell replication, usually due to inadequate availability of vitamin B_{12} or folate, with most replicating cells in the body, instead of being in a resting phase, being in process of attempting (with poor success) to double their DNA in order to divide. This is most striking in bone marrow cells, with the "ineffective hematopoiesis" resulting in peripheral blood pancytopenia (anemia, leukopenia, and thrombopenia). However, megaloblastosis is also present in all other duplicating cells of the body,[3,83] and may be strikingly noted in the epithelial cells of the entire alimentary tract, producing glossitis and variable degrees of megaloblastosis along the entire alimentary tract epithelium. It is not yet clear why gut changes associated with vitamin B_{12} deficiency are more often associated with constipation, whereas those associated with folate deficiency are more commonly associated with diarrhea; these differences may be related to phenomena other than the nutrient deficiency *per se.*

Since growth is dependent on cell replication, and cell replication is dependent on DNA synthesis, both vitamin B_{12} and folic acid are required for growth.

Packaging Folate in Cells. Another important interrelationship of these two vitamins appears to be an involvement of B_{12} in the packaging of folate into cells.[80-82] When the supply of vitamin B_{12} is not adequate, folic acid does not appear to be incorporated into red cells in adequate quantity. Furthermore, when the vitamin B_{12} stores of sheep have fallen to about 10 per cent of normal levels, the liver folate stores suddenly appear to "wash away."

Inadequate myelin synthesis with resultant neurologic damage results from vitamin B_{12} deficiency, but not from folate deficiency.[3,83] The biochemical basis for this defective myelin synthesis is unknown. Since myelin is lipoprotein, vitamin B_{12} must have some as yet undetermined role in synthesis of either the lipid or the protein component of myelin. It has been proposed that the neurologic damage relates to the B_{12} requirement for the propionate-methylmalonate conversion, but this is probably not so because infants born lacking the apoenzyme for this conversion do not have damaged myelin, and the abnormalities reported in fatty acids in myelin of vitamin B_{12}-deficient subjects[84] may well relate to plasmalogen[85] rather than to B_{12} deficiency. The nervous system damage due to vitamin B_{12} deficiency involves,[83] in addition to myelinated peripheral nerves, the myelinated posterior and lateral cords of the spinal column, and therefore nervous system damage due to vitamin B_{12} deficiency has been variously termed "subacute combined degeneration," "combined system disease," "postero-lateral sclerosis," and "funicular degeneration." However, the disease usually starts insidiously and not subacutely, combined lesions are often absent, and lesions of the peripheral nerves occur more frequently and earlier than lesions of the central nervous system. For these reasons, the nervous system changes are more accurately described by direct reference to the actual involvement (i.e., peripheral nerve or spinal cord or cerebral damage due to vitamin B_{12} deficiency).

The various neurologic symptoms and signs resulting from the inadequate myelin synthesis due to vitamin B_{12} deficiency include paresthesia, especially numbness and tingling in the hands and feet, diminution of vibration sense and/or position sense (usually but not always occurring first in the ankles and feet), unsteadiness, poor muscular coordination with ataxia, moodiness, mental slowness, poor memory, confusion, agitation, depression, and central scotomata (sometimes with dim vision due to optic atrophy or tobacco amblyopia); delusions, hallucinations, and even overt psychosis (usually with paranoid ideas) may occur. The wide variety of sensory and motor changes tend to be symmetrical, especially if present for a period of weeks or months.

It has been our observation that economically advantaged people with vitamin B_{12} deficiency tend to have relatively severe neurologic damage and relatively mild hematologic damage, whereas poor people with vitamin B_{12} deficiency tend to have relatively equal severity of neurologic and hematologic damage. We believe that a major explanation for the variable degree of hematologic damage with a fixed amount of neurologic damage in vitamin B_{12} deficiency is the quantity of folate in the diet. Well-to-do people tend to eat better diets, richer in high-folate-containing foods such as fresh fruits and fresh vegetables, as well as fresh meats. The folate retards development of hematologic damage, while allowing neurologic damage to progress.

Folate deficiency does not damage myelin, but it is associated with a high frequency of irritability, forgetfulness, and, often, hostility and paranoid behavior. These phenomena often strikingly improve within 24 hours of the start of therapy with folic acid.

Cerebration may improve rapidly when vitamin B_{12} deficiency is appropriately treated, but the neurological damage resulting from inadequate myelin synthesis heals most slowly. Since the nerve damage is related to deterioration of the axon underneath the deteriorated myelin, healing is related to the speed of regeneration of damaged axons, this regeneration creeps peripherally from the nerve head at the rate of 0.1 mm per day.

B_{12} in Fat and Carbohydrate Metabolism.[3,21,23,25,28,86] Since coenzyme B_{12} is required for the hydrogen transfer and isomerization whereby methylmalonate is converted to succinate,[23,25] B_{12} is involved in both fat and carbohydrate metabolism. As indicated above, although it is an attractive speculation that one reason for the neurologic damage of patients with vitamin B_{12} deficiency is inability to make the lipid portion of the lipoprotein myelin sheath (due to inadequate propionic acid utilization related to inadequate interconversion of methylmalonate and succinate), there is not yet evidence to tie this to the neurologic damage of vitamin B_{12} deficiency in man.

B_{12} in Protein and Fat Metabolism.[21,23,25,28] Vitamin B_{12} is involved in protein synthesis through its role in the synthesis of the amino acid methionine, and possibly in other ways as well. Since methionine is involved in making available more of the lipotropic substances, choline and betaine, this is another point where cobalamin may play a role in lipid metabolism.

B_{12} as a Reducing Agent.[3,21,87] Vitamin B_{12} appears concerned in maintenance of sulfhydryl groups in the reduced form necessary for function of many SH-activated enzyme systems. Vitamin B_{12} deficiency is characterized by a decrease in reduced glutathione (which is changed from GSH to GSSG) of erythrocytes and liver. This is correctable by administration of vitamin B_{12}. *In vitro*, vitamin B_{12} derivatives catalyze the non-enzymatic oxidation of sulfhydryl derivatives.

Folates in One-carbon-unit Transfers.[3,22,28,70] Folate coenzymes are concerned with mammalian metabolic systems involving transfer of a one-carbon unit. These reactions include

(see Fig. 5J–7): (1) *de novo* purine synthesis (formylation of glycinamide ribonucleotide [GAR] and 5-amino-4-imidazole carboxamide ribonucleotide [AICAR]); (2) pyrimidine nucleotide biosynthesis (methylation of deoxyuridylic acid to thymidylic acid); (3) three amino acid conversions: (*a*) the interconversion of serine and glycine (which also requires vitamin B_6); (*b*) catabolism of histidine to glutamic acid; (*c*) conversion of homocysteine to methionine (which also requires vitamin B_6); (4) generation of formate

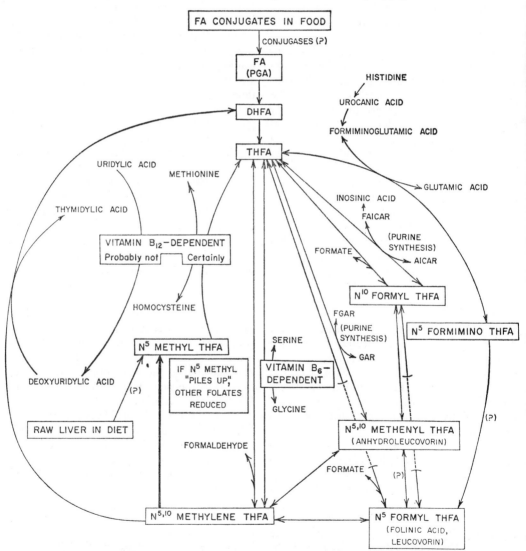

Fig. 5J-7.   Functions and interrelations of the various folate coenzymes. (Herbert in Goodman and Gilman, courtesy of The Macmillan Co.)

into the formate pool (and utilization of formate).

Role of Ascorbic Acid. It is possible that ascorbate *in vivo* may aid in the protection against oxidative destruction of reduced folates in the body. There is no evidence that ascorbate plays any role in the reduction of pteroylglutamic acid to tetrahydrofolic acid, a reaction mediated by folate reductases; the original such evidence proved to be protection by ascorbate of the end product against oxidative destruction.

THERAPY[3]

The only established therapeutic use of vitamin B_{12} or folic acid is in treating deficiency of the respective vitamin. Claims made for nutritional value of either of these vitamins in clinical situations in which de-

---

Table 5J-2.   Clinical Picture of the Megaloblastic Anemias

---

1. *Symptoms*
   Weakness, tiredness
   Dyspnea
   Sore tongue
   Paresthesia (B_{12} deficiency only)
   Diarrhea (especially folate deficiency)
   Constipation (especially B_{12} deficiency)
   Irritability and forgetfulness (especially folate deficiency)
   Anorexia
   Syncope
   Headache
   Palpitation
2. *Signs*
   Anemia, leukopenia, thrombocytopenia, with macroovalocytes (normal MVC $= 87 \pm 5$ cu. μ) and "hypersegmented polys" (normal "Arneth count"; 2 lobes $= 20$–40%; 3 lobes $= 40$–50%; 4 lobes $= 15$–25%; 5 lobes $= 0$–5%; 6 lobes $= 0$–0.1%; more than 6 lobes $= 0$) (normal "lobe average" $= 3.17 \pm 0.25$) (Rule of Fives! When 100 neutrophils counted, the presence of five or more with five or more lobes means hypersegmentation.)
   Morphologic "red herrings": congenital hypersegmentation (approx. 1% of population) : hypersegmentation with renal disease; twinning deformities; macrocytes of pyruvate kinase deficiency, aplastic anemia, reticulocytosis
   Fever
   Icterus
   Glossitis
     Acute
     Chronic atrophic
   Neurologic damage (only B_{12} deficiency damages myelin)
     Vibration sense diminished
     Position sense diminished; ataxia
     Impaired mentation, paranoid ideation.
   Malabsorption
   Achylia gastrica (primary with B_{12} deficiency; secondary with folate deficiency)
   Splenomegaly (in approximately $\frac{1}{3}$ of cases, if looked for radiologically)
   Weight loss (especially folate deficiency)
   Pigmentation
   Postural hypotension (especially B_{12} deficiency)
   Low serum vitamin B_{12} or folate level
   Elevated serum lactic dehydrogenase (LDH)
   Elevated urine formiminoglutamate
   Methylmalonic aciduria (B_{12} deficiency only)
   High serum iron, increased saturation of iron-binding capacity of serum, increased bone marrow iron stores

---

ficiency of the vitamin does not exist are without foundation in fact.

When the deficiency is of vitamin B_{12}, only this vitamin should be used for therapy; conversely, when the deficiency is of folate, only that vitamin should be used for therapy. The use of folic acid in the treatment of a patient whose deficiency is of vitamin B_{12} will often produce hematologic improvement of a temporary nature, but will allow the neurologic damage of the underlying vitamin B_{12} deficiency to progress, often to an irreversible state.

Signs and Symptoms of Deficiency of Vitamin B_{12} or Folate in Man.[1-3,83,88,90,93] These are listed in Table 5J–2.

Therapy of the Critically Ill Patient. It is rarely necessary to institute immediate therapy prior to determining the cause of megaloblastic anemia. Major indications for emergency therapy include severe thrombocytopenia (platelet count less than 50,000/mm^3) associated with bleeding, severe leukopenia (white cell count less than 3,000/mm^3) associated with infection, infection itself, coma, severe disorientation, marked neurologic damage, severe hepatic disease, uremia, or other debilitating illness complicating the anemia. The anemia itself is not a problem since the dyspnea and occasional angina which may accompany a hematocrit of less than 15 volumes per cent are relieved by a transfusion of 1 to 2 units of packed erythrocytes. Transfusion is unwarranted in the absence of symptoms of anemia. When venous pressure is elevated, transfusion of packed erythrocytes should be accompanied by withdrawal of equivalent or slightly smaller quantities of whole blood. This will reduce rather than raise the venous pressure; transfusion of whole blood without withdrawal of blood has been responsible for acute rises in venous pressure with resultant irreversible congestive failure in elderly patients with megaloblastic anemia and unrecognized elevated venous pressure. Ideally, venous pressure should be determined prior to transfusion, and monitored during both the transfusion of packed cells and the simultaneous withdrawal of whole blood. This may easily be done by use of a three-way stopcock, injecting the packed cells in units

of 50 ml, followed by determination of venous pressure change and withdrawal of 30 to 50 ml of whole blood, prior to repeating the whole procedure with injection of another 50 ml of erythrocytes.

When, for one or more of the reasons discussed above, immediate vitamin therapy is necessary before etiological diagnosis, 100 μg of cyanocobalamin and 15 mg of folic acid are given intramuscularly, followed by 5 mg of folic acid by mouth and 100 μg of vitamin B_{12} intramuscularly daily, for a week. Such treatment will produce excellent hematologic response except in cases in which hematopoiesis is suppressed by infection, uremia, chloramphenicol administration, or some other factor.

Vitamin B_{12} Therapy.[3] Vitamin B_{12} deficiency in man is nearly always due to inadequate ingestion and/or inadequate absorption, and therapy is guided by adequate etiologic diagnosis (Table 5J–1).

Inadequate ingestion of vitamin B_{12} is corrected by adding to the daily diet any food containing vitamin B_{12} (*i.e.*, meat or meat product, including fish, shellfish, or poultry). If the patient, because of poverty, cannot afford meat or meat products, or, for religious or other reasons, is a strict vegetarian, adequate treatment consists of 1 μg of vitamin B_{12} orally daily supplied as liquid or tablet.

When the vitamin B_{12} deficiency is due to inadequate absorption, 1 μg of vitamin B_{12} parenterally (subcutaneously or intramuscularly) daily constitutes adequate therapy. A single injection of 100 μg or more of vitamin B_{12} will produce a complete therapeutic remission in any patient whose vitamin B_{12} deficiency is not complicated by unrelated systemic disease or other factors. The remission is sustained for life by monthly injections of 100 μg of vitamin B_{12}. It is important to point out to the patient who has permanent gastric or ileal damage that he must receive monthly injections of vitamin B_{12} for life.

For simultaneous differential diagnosis and therapy, patients should be treated with an injection of 1 μg of vitamin B_{12} daily for 10 days, after a control period of a few days to establish the constancy of the reticulocyte level, elimination of dietary sources of vitamin B_{12} and folic acid (by provision of a diet con-

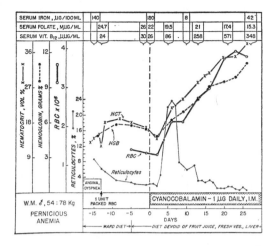

Fig. 5J-8. Response of a patient with uncomplicated vitamin B_{12} deficiency to therapy with 1 μg daily of parenteral vitamin B_{12}. (Herbert: New Eng. J. Med. *268*, 201, 1963.)

sisting exclusively of well-cooked finely particulate grains or vegetables [such as rice and beans] and beverages devoid of vitamin B_{12} and folate such as tea, coffee, and soft drinks). Such a therapeutic trial is illustrated in Figure 5J-8, from reference 88. Not shown in the figure is the leukopenia or thrombopenia often seen in untreated megaloblastic anemia; granulocytes and platelets return to normal levels within 1 week after the start of therapy, at approximately the time reticulocytes reach their peak level.

Initial therapy with doses of vitamin B_{12} greater than 1 μg daily is desirable when the vitamin B_{12} deficiency is complicated with other debilitating illness such as infection, hepatic disease, uremia, coma, severe disorientation, or marked neurologic damage. In such cases, 30 μg or more of vitamin B_{12} is given daily parenterally for 5 to 10 days. Daily parenteral doses larger than 30 μg have no proven therapeutic advantage, and much of the excess is rapidly excreted in the urine.

Hydroxocobalamin and other depot preparations of vitamin B_{12} may be retained longer at the site of injection and in serum, but this possible slight therapeutic advantage over cyanocobalamin does not warrant their greater cost; they also may have undesirable side effects. More detailed discussion of vitamin B_{12} preparations, routes of administration, dosage, and therapeutic responses may be found in *The Pharmacological Basis of Therapeutics*.[3]

Folic Acid Therapy.[3] For combined differential diagnosis and therapy, the patient is treated with 100 μg of folic acid orally daily (if the suspected diagnosis is dietary inadequacy), or parenterally (if the suspected diagnosis is folate malabsorption). This dosage will produce a maximal hematologic response in patients with folate deficiency, but will not produce hematologic response in patients with vitamin B_{12} deficiency. Therapeutic trial with a parenteral dose of 50 μg of pteroylglutamic acid daily in a patient with folate deficiency is shown in Figure 5J–9, from reference 88. Note in the figure that ascorbic acid *per se* has no hematopoietic effect in folate deficiency. The expected sharp fall in plasma iron level does not occur when ascorbate therapy is used, because vitamin C produces a rise in serum iron which cancels out the early fall that otherwise develops when folate deficiency is treated with folate (or vitamin B_{12} deficiency is treated with vitamin B_{12}).[89] As in treated vitamin B_{12} deficiency, treatment of folate deficiency returns sub-

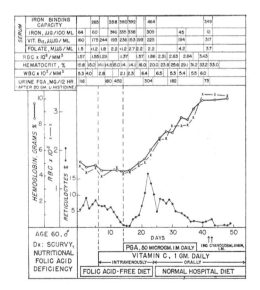

Fig. 5J-9. Hematologic response to parenteral administration of 50 μg of folic (pteroylglutamic) acid daily, in a patient with nutritional folate deficiency and treated scurvy. (Herbert: New Eng. J. Med. *268*, 201, 1963.)

normal leukocyte and platelet levels to normal within a week after the start of therapy, at approximately the time of the reticulocyte peak.

Therapy with doses of folic acid larger than 0.1 mg daily is desirable when the folate deficiency state is complicated by conditions which may suppress hematopoiesis (such as unrelated systemic disease), conditions that increase folate requirement (pregnancy, hypermetabolic states, alcoholism, hemolytic anemia), and conditions that reduce folate absorption. Therapy should then be with 0.5 to 1 mg daily. There is no evidence that doses greater than 1 mg daily have any greater efficacy; additionally, loss of folate in the urine becomes roughly logarithmic as the amount administered exceeds 1 mg.

Maintenance therapy is normally 0.1 mg of folic acid daily for 1 to 4 months, and then should be stopped only if the diet contains at least one fresh fruit or fresh vegetable daily. If the daily folate requirement is increased due to an increased metabolic or cell-turnover rate the maintenance dose should be 0.2 to 0.5 mg daily.

Ideal nutritional therapy for dietary folate deficiency is the ingestion of one fresh fruit or one fresh vegetable daily; such a diet would probably wipe nutritional folate deficiency from the face of the earth.[90] As it is, nutritional folate deficiency probably encompasses approximately a third of all the pregnant women in the world.[30]

TOXICITY[3]

It is hard to accept that either vitamin B_{12} or folic acid, being necessary for life, could, in quantities close to minimal daily requirements, be toxic in man. In fact, these substances are non-toxic in man not only in small doses but also in doses which exceed the minimal daily adult human requirement by ten thousand-fold for vitamin B_{12} and one thousand fold for folic acid. Being water-soluble, excesses of these vitamins tend to be excreted in the urine rather than, like the fat-soluble vitamins, being stored in tissues. Vitamin B_{12} and folic acid both appear to require binding to polypeptides as a pre-condition of storage; excesses above the limited

serum- and tissue-available-binding capacity tend to be excreted rather than retained.

A rare allergic reaction has been reported, possibly due to impurities in a rare preparation of crystalline cyanocobalamin.[23] Hydroxocobalamin injections and injections of various depot preparations of cyanocobalamin have been associated with the appearance of antibody to plasma vitamin B_{12}-binding protein;[91] while the significance of this antibody is not yet clear, such preparations offer no clear advantage over cyanocobalamin to warrant their use, especially in view of their greater cost and the pain on injection of some of the depot preparations.

One questionable instance of an allergic reaction to folic acid has been reported in man.[2] Daily doses of up to 15 mg in man are without toxic effects; this daily dose is well below that which could lead to precipitation of crystalline folic acid in the kidneys (precipitation produces renal toxicity in rats given massive doses of folic acid). Folic acid has been reported to partially reverse the anti-epileptic effects of pheno barbital, diphenylhydantoin, and primidine, and thereby increase seizure frequency in patients getting anti-convulsant therapy.[92]

Note: The prior edition of this text contains excellent well-referenced chapters by R. W. Vilter on the subjects of vitamin B_{12} and folic acid.

BIBLIOGRAPHY

1. Castle: Trans. Am. Clin. Climatological Ass., *73*, 53, 1961.
2. Chanarin: *The Megaloblastic Anemias*, Philadelphia, F. A. Davis, 1969.
3. Herbert: *Drugs Effective in Megaloblastic Anemias: Vitamin B_{12} and Folic Acid* in *The Pharmacological Basis of Therapeutics*, 4th ed. (ed. by L. S. Goodman & A. Gilman), New York, The Macmillan Co., 1414, 1970.
4. Combe: Trans. Roy. med Chir. Soc. Edinburgh, *1*, 194, 1822.
5. Addison: *On the Constitutional and Local Effects of Disease of the Suprarenal Capsules*. London, S. Highley, 1855.
6. Barclay, 1851. Quoted by Castle, ref. 1.
7. Flint: Am. med. Times, *1*, 181, 1860.
8. Castle: Am. J. med. Sci., *178*, 748, 1929.
9. Rickes, Brink, Koniuszy, Wood and Folkers: Science, *107*, 396, 1948.
10. Smith and Parker: Biochem. J., *43*, viii, 1948.

11. Berk, Castle, Welch, Heinie, Anker and Epstein: New Eng. J. Med., *239*, 911, 1948.
12. Wills, Clutterbuck, and Evans: Biochem. J., *31*, 2136, 1937.
13. Stokstad: J. Biol. Chem., *149*, 573, 1943.
14. Pfiffner, Binkley, Bloom, Brown, Bird, and Emmett: Science, *97*, 404, 1943.
15. Angier, Boothe, Hutchings, Mowat, Semb, Stokstad, Subba Row, Walter, Cosulich, Farrenbach, Hultquist, Kuh, Northey, Seeger, Sickels, and Smith: J. Am. Chem. Soc., *103*, 667, 1946.
16. Shorb: Science, *107*, 397, 1948.
17. Day, Mims, Totter, Stokstad, Hutchings and Sloane: J. Biol. Chem., *157*, 423, 1945.
18. Snell and Peterson: J. Bact., *39*, 273, 1940.
19. Mitchell, Snell and Williams: J. Am. Chem. Soc., *63*, 2284, 1941.
20. Minot and Murphy: J.A.M.A., *87*, 470, 1926.
21. Smith: *Vitamin B12*, 3rd edition, London, Methuen & Co.; New York, John Wiley & Sons, Inc., 1965.
22. Blakley: *The Biochemistry of Folic Acid and Related Pteridines*. New York, John Wiley & Sons, Inc., 1969.
23. Symposium: *The Cobalamins* (ed. by H. Arnstein and R. Wrighton), London, J. & A. Churchill, 1971.
24. Symposium (2nd European): *Vitamin B12 and Intrinsic Factor.* (ed. by H. C. Heinrich), Stuttgart, Ferdinand Enke Verlag, 1962.
25. Symposium: *Vitamin B12 Coenzymes.* (ed. by D. Perlman) Ann. N.Y. Acad. Sci., *112*, 547, 1964.
26. IUPAC-IUB Commission on Biochemical Nomenclature: Nomenclature of vitamins, coenzymes and related compounds. Tentative rules. J. Biol. Chem., *241*, 2991, 1966.
27. Sullivan and Herbert: New Eng. J. Med., *272*, 340, 1965.
28. Huennekens: *Folate and B12 Coenzymes in Biological Oxidations* (ed. by T. P. Singer), New York, Interscience, 439, 1968.
29. WHO Scientific Group: *Nutritional Anemias:* Wld Hlth. Org. Techn. Rep. Ser., #405, 1968.
30. FAO-WHO Expert Group: *Requirements of ascorbic acid, vitamin D, vitamin B12, folate, and iron.* WHO Techn. Rep. Ser., #452, 1970.
31. Skeggs: *Vitamin B12 in The Vitamins: Chemistry, Physiology, Pathology, Methods*, 2nd ed., Vol. VII (ed. by P. Gyorgy and W. Pearson), New York, Academic Press, 277, 1967.
32. Herbert: Am. J. Clin. Nutr., *7*, 433, 1959.
33. Lau, Gottlieb, Wasserman, and Herbert: Blood, *26*, 202, 1965.
34. Herbert: *B12 and Folate Analysis with Radionuclides* in *Hematopoietic and Gastrointestinal Investigations with Radionuclides* (ed. by A. Gilson & W. Smoak), Springfield, Charles C Thomas, 1972.
35. Herbert and Bertino: *Folic Acid in The Vitamins: Chemistry, Physiology, Pathology, Methods*, 2nd ed., Vol. VII (ed. by P. Gyorgy and W. Pearson), New York, Academic Press, 243, 1967.
36. Herbert, Wasserman, Frank, Pasher and Baker: Fed. Proc., *18*, 246, 1959.
37. Baker, Herbert, Frank, Pasher, Hutner, Wasserman and Sobotka: Clin. Chem., *5*, 275, 1959.
38. Herbert, Baker, Frank, Pasher, Sobotka and Wasserman: Blood, *15*, 228, 1960.
39. Herbert: J. Clin. Invest., *40*, 81, 1961.
40. Herbert: J. Clin. Path., *19*, 12, 1966.
41. Waxman, Schreiber and Herbert: Blood, *36*, 858, 1970; *38*, 219, 1971; Rothenberg, da Costa and Rosenberg: New Eng. J. Med., *286*, 1335, 1972.
42. Glass: Physiol. Rev., *43*, 529, 1963.
43. Herbert: Gastroenterology, *54*, 110, 1968.
44. Grasbeck: *Intrinsic Factor and the Other Vitamin B12 Transport Proteins* in *Progress in Hematology, VI* (ed. by E. B. Brown & C. V. Moore), New York, Grune & Stratton, Inc., 233, 1969.
45. Carmel, Rosenberg, Lau, Streiff and Herbert: Gastroenterology, *56*, 548, 1969.
46. Corcino, Waxman and Herbert: Am. J. Med., *48*, 562, 1970; Chanarin: J. Clin. Path., *24*, Suppl. (Roy. Coll. Path.) 5, 60, 1971.
47. Bernstein, Gutstein, Weiner, and Efron: Am. J. Med., *48*, 570, 1970.
48. Butterworth, Baugh and Krumdieck: J. Clin. Invest., *48*, 1131, 1969.
49. Butterworth: Am. J. Clin. Nutr., *21*, 1121, 1968.
50. Rosenberg and Godwin: Gastroenterology, *60*, 445, 1971; Hoffbrand: J. Clin. Path., *24*, Suppl. (Roy. Coll. Path.), *5*, 66, 1971.
51. Gerson, Cohen, Hepner, Brown, Herbert and Janowitz: Clin. Res., *17*, 593, 1969; Gastroenterology, *51*, 624, 1971.
52. Hall: Ann. Int. Med., *75*, 297, 1971.
53. Herbert: Blood, *32*, 305, 1968; Carmel and Herbert: Blood, *40*, in press, 1972.
54. Hall and Finkler: *Isolation and evaluation of the various vitamin B12 binding proteins in human plasma* in *Vitamins and Coenzymes* (ed. by D. M. McCormick and L. D. Wright), New York, Academic Press, 1970.
55. Corcino, Krauss, Waxman and Herbert: J. Clin. Invest., *49*, 2250, 1970.
56. Chikkappa, Corcino, Greenberg and Herbert: Blood, *37*, 124, 1971.
57. Retief, Gottlieb, and Herbert: J. Clin. Invest., *45*, 1907, 1966.
58. Corcino, Zalusky, Greenberg and Herbert: Brit. J. Haemat., *20*, 511, 1971.
59. Rappazzo, Salmi and Hall: Brit. J. Haemat., *18*, 427, 1970.
60. Okuda, Grasbeck and Chow: J. Lab. Clin. Med., *51*, 17, 1958.
61. Grasbeck, Nyberg and Reizenstein: Proc. Soc. Exp. Biol. & Med., *97*, 780, 1958.
62. Heinrich; Seminars Hemat., *1*, 199, 1964.
63. Metz, Zalusky and Herbert: Am. J. Clin. Nutr., *21*, 289, 1968.
64. Corcino, Waxman and Herbert: Brit. J. Haemat., *20*, 503, 1971.
65. Herbert: *Folic acid deficiency in man* in *Vitamins and Hormones*, Vol. 26, New York, Academic Press, 525, 1968.
66. Herbert: New Eng. J. Med., *284*, 976, 1971.

67. Food and Nutrition Board, National Research Council: *Recommended Dietary Allowances*, 7th Ed., National Academy of Sciences, Washington, D.C., 1968.
68. Herbert: Am. J. Clin. Nutr., *21*, 743, 1968.
69. Lichtenstein, Beloian and Murphy: *Vitamin B₁₂: Microbiological Assay Methods and Distribution in Selected Foods.* Home Economics Research Report #13, U. S. Dept. of Agriculture, Washington, D. C., 1961.
70. Sullivan: *Folates in human nutrition* in *Newer Methods of Nutritional Biochemistry*, Vol. 3 (ed. by A. A. Albanese), New York, Academic Press, 365, 1967.
71. Streiff: Sem. Hemat., *7*, 23, 1970.
72. Sullivan and Herbert: J. Clin. Invest., *43*, 2048, 1964.
73. Butterworth: Brit. J. Haemat., *14*, 339, 1968.
74. Herbert: Am. J. Clin. Nutr., *12*, 17, 1963.
75. Hurdle, Barton and Searles: Am. J. Clin. Nutr., *21*, 1202, 1968.
76. Herbert and Zalusky: J. Clin. Invest., *41*, 1263, 1962.
77. Metz, Kelly, Swett, Waxman and Herbert: Brit. J. Haemat., *14*, 575, 1968.
78. Weissbach and Taylor: Vitamins and Hormones, *28*, 415, 1970.
79. Noronha and Silverman: *On folic acid, vitamin B₁₂, methionine and formiminoglutamic acid metabolism* in *Vitamin B₁₂ and Intrinsic Factor, 2nd European Symposium.* Stuttgart, Enke, 728, 1962.
80. Herbert: Proc. Roy. Soc. Med., *57*, 377, 1964.
81. Cooper and Lowenstein: Blood, *24*, 502, 1964.
82. Herbert: *Recent developments in cobalamin metabolism* in *Symposium: The Cobalamins* (ed. by H. R. V. Arnstein and R. J. Wrighton), London, J. & A. Churchill, 1971.
83. Herbert, V.: *The Megaloblastic Anemias*, New York, Grune & Stratton, 1959.
84. Frenkel: J. Clin. Invest., *50*, 33a, 1971.
85. Marcus, Ullman, Safier and Ballard: J. Clin. Invest., *41*, 2198, 1962.
86. Weissbach and Taylor: Vitamins and Hormones, *28*, 395, 1968.
87. Ellenbogen: *Vitamin B₁₂ and intrinsic factor* in *Newer Methods of Nutritional Biochemistry*, Vol. 1 (ed. by A. A. Albanese), New York, Academic Press, 1963.
88. Herbert: New Eng. J. Med., *268*, 201 and 368, 1963.
89. Zalusky and Herbert: New Eng. J. Med., *265*, 1033, 1961.
90. Herbert: Sem. Hemat., *7*, 2, 1970.
91. Hom, Olesen, and Schwartz: Scand. J. Haemat., *5*, 107, 1068.
92. Reynolds: Brain, *91*, 197, 1968; Herbert and Tisman: in *Biology of Brain Dysfunction* (G. B. Gaul, Ed.), New York, Plenum Press, 1972.
93. Herbert: *Megaloblastic anemias—mechanisms and management* in *Disease-a-Month*, Chicago, Year Book Medical Publishers, 1965.

Chapter

5

Section K Ascorbic Acid

Robert E. Hodges

and

Eugene M. Baker

HISTORY

Although ascorbic acid itself was not identified until about 40 years ago, the disease which results from lack of it in the diet of man was recognized and feared in ancient times. It was described by ancient Egyptians in the Papyrus Ebers about 1550 B.C.[1] and the writings of the ancient Greeks and Romans refer to a plague that was almost certainly scurvy.[2] Scurvy shaped the course of history because many military campaigns came to a spontaneous end when army or navy rations contained inadequate amounts of vitamin C.[3] Vivid accounts of scurvy appear in the writings of explorers who lived in the 16th, 17th, and 18th centuries A.D.[4,5]

Although the authors of most textbooks give original credit to the Scottish naval surgeon James Lind, who performed a controlled study onboard the Salisbury at sea and demonstrated that lemons and oranges were the best treatment for scurvy, he actually was only repeating the work of others.[6,7] It is entirely likely that many cures for scurvy were found, then forgotten, then rediscovered by a succession of explorers and scientists, only a few of whom recorded their observations for posterity. In 1536, Jacques Cartier, then in Newfoundland, was gravely concerned because most of his crew were ill with scurvy.[8] He was advised by the Indians to give an extract of the arborvitae tree (a white cedar).* This promptly cured the survivors

* Other sources refer to Ameda or Hanneda (thought to be a sassafras) tree.

of scurvy. We know that in 1593 Sir Richard Hawkins described the use of oranges and lemons in the treatment of scurvy among British sailors.[5] We also know that, in Sweden, Urban Hiaerne recommended cloudberries for the treatment of scurvy about 1665.[9]

A fascinating although disjointed collection of various forms of treatment of scurvy appears in the first edition of the Encyclopedia Britannica—1771.[5] This is so poorly documented it is impossible to tell which forms of treatment antedated others. Many of the recommended therapies seem to be without value yet the majority of them undoubtedly helped, for these foods or potions contained varying quantities of ascorbic acid. A few of these forms of therapy included "plenty of fresh greens or vegetables ... particularly sallads of garden cresses." In referring to James Lind's treatise, the encyclopedia reported "the oranges and lemons had the best effect" and ... "next to the oranges, the cyder had the best effect" ... and later— "but as oranges and lemons are apt to spoil, let the juice of these fruits be well-cleared from the pulp, and depurated by standing some time; after which it may be poured off from the gross sediment. Let it then be poured into any clean open vessel of china or stoneware ... that it may evaporate more readily. Put this into a pan of water over a clear fire; let the water come almost to a boil, and continue nearly in that state with the bowl full of juice in the middle of it, till the

245

juice is found of the consistence of a thick syrup when cold. When it is cold it is to be corked up in a bottle for use. Two dozen of good oranges weighing five pounds, when evaporated . . . will be equal to less than three ounces . . . and the virtues of this extract, thus made, . . . will serve one man at sea several years. . . ."

The Encyclopedia Britannica goes on to say "it will likewise be of great use to seamen to have gooseberries . . . preserved in bottles . . . also small onions pickled in vinegar; cabbage, french beans, etc. may be preserved by putting them in clean dry stone jars, with a layer of salt on the bottom then a thin layer of the vegetable covered with salt, and so alternately till the jar is full." Also, ". . . this is the manner in which they preserve that never-failing remedy, Greenland scurvy-grass.

"Poor people that winter in Greenland . . . preserved themselves from the scurvy by spruce-beer which is their common drink." "Likewise, the simple decoction of fir tops has done wonders. The shrub black spruce of America makes this most wholesome drink. . . ." "A simple decoction of the tops, cones, leaves, or even of the green bark or wood of these is an excellent antiscorbutic, but perhaps it is much more so when fermented. By carrying a few bags of spruce to sea this wholesome drink can be made at any time. . . ." Patients with scurvy were treated . . . "with raisins or currants . . . but more particularly pickled cabbage and small onions boiled. Most of their food ought to be well-acidulated with orange or lemon juice . . . and salads of all kinds are beneficial, but more particularly dandelion, sorrell, endive, lettuce, sumitory, and purslane; to which may be added scurvy grass, cresses, and the like." "Summer fruits are all good, as oranges, lemons, citrons, apples, etc. In the winter-time, genuine spruce beer, with lemons and orange juice is proper; or antiscorbutic ale made of an infusion of wormwood, horse-radish, mustard-seed, and the like.

"Van Swieten says, he has often seen whole families cured of the scurvy in Holland, by the use of a cask of ale in which were put heads of red cabbage cut small, twelve handfuls of scurvy grass, and a pound of fresh horse-radish, freshly infused."

With this background of information and some misinformation, the British admiralty undoubtedly was sorely vexed when their admiral, George A. Anson, undertook a voyage around the world in the ship Centurion between 1740 and 1744.[3] He started with 6 ships and 1,955 men, yet only the flagship returned. One thousand fifty-one died, chiefly of scurvy. These losses inspired James Lind (or perhaps he was ordered) to seek the cure of scurvy. No doubt he was aware of at least some of the aforementioned forms of treatment when, on the ship Salisbury, he performed his classical experiment on the 20th of May, 1747.[7] He did not publish his treatise until 7 years later, and it was not until 1795 (48 years after Lind's experiment) that the Admiralty prescribed lemon juice for all British sailors (hence the nickname limey). But Lind's studies did have a prompt and profound effect upon a close friend, the enthusiastic Captain James Cook.[10,11] Cook was not content with only the recommendations of James Lind for he also insisted upon unprecedented cleanliness and hygienic measures aboard ship. He sent men ashore at every opportunity to gather all manner of greens, even grasses, which were prepared, served, and eaten. He employed the ingenious technique of insisting that his officers eat this food in front of the men, whereupon they deemed it more than suitable and ate their share. By these methods Captain Cook was the first to demonstrate that prolonged ocean voyages did not necessarily result in scurvy among the crew. His first voyage from 1768 to 1771 and his second from 1772 to 1775 conclusively demonstrated that scurvy could be prevented. His third and final voyage began in 1776 and unfortunately 3 years later he was killed by natives in Hawaii.

Yet the efforts of many early explorers and later of James Lind and Captain James Cook were insufficient to impress upon the civilized world the lesson they sought to teach. Indeed, as recently as 1912, when Captain Robert Falcon Scott explored the South pole, he and his team met with tragic death as a result of scurvy.[12] And, in the mid-nineteenth century during the American Civil War,[13] scurvy was rampant among the troops of both the North and the South. Only in the past half-century has scurvy become an uncommon disease.

CHEMISTRY

Between 1910 and 1920, Zilva and his co-workers worked at the isolation and synthesis of vitamin C. They also demonstrated that this substance was necessary for normal development of teeth in susceptible species of animals.[14]

The actual isolation of ascorbic acid was accomplished independently in 1928 by two different teams of investigators: one, headed by Szent-Györgyi, isolated "hexuronic acid" from orange juice, cabbage juice, and adrenal glands;[15] and the other, headed by King, not only isolated vitamin C from lemon juice but demonstrated that the hexuronic acid described by Szent-Györgyi was identical to vitamin C.[16] It was only a short step from this discovery to the synthesis of ascorbic acid by two men; Haworth,[17] who determined its structure, and Reichstein,[18] who finally synthesized it.

By this time an astonishing fact had become apparent; only a few species of animals must consume ascorbic acid in their diet, whereas most other species synthesize their own.[19] Herein lies one of the great genetic mysteries which still is only partially solved.[20]

Chemically, L-ascorbic acid, or vitamin C, is a rather simple compound with the empiric formula, $C_6H_8O_6$. It has a molecular weight of 176, is very soluble in water, less so in ethyl alcohol, and quite insoluble in most lipid solvents. L-Ascorbic acid has been considered to be the active form of vitamin C but recent work has focused attention on ascorbate 3 sulfate* as a metabolically active derivative.[21–24] Dehydro-L-ascorbic acid is a potent antiscorbutic agent, but other analogs have weaker antiscorbutic activity. The D isomer of arabo-ascorbic acid is of questionable value in curing scurvy. Vitamin C is easily destroyed by oxidation, but its perishability in foods has been somewhat exag-

* Some consider this to be ascorbate 2 sulfate.

gerated. Heat, exposure to air and an alkaline medium hasten oxidation, especially when the food is in contact with copper, iron, or various oxidative enzymes. Fortunately, many foods which contain ascorbic acid also contain factors such as other organic acids and antioxidants which help to protect and preserve the vitamin C contained therein. Prolonged cooking, especially if the cooking water is discarded, results in heavy losses of vitamin C.

Ascorbic acid is widely distributed throughout the foods of the world but is found chiefly in plant products, especially rapidly growing vegetables and fruits, whereas grains and cereals contain almost none. A convenient way to remember the best sources of vitamin C is to divide them into three categories; excellent, good, and fair. The "excellent" category includes foods containing more than 100 mg/100 gm. This includes broccoli greens, brussels sprouts, collards, black currants, guava, horseradish, kale, turnip greens, parsley and sweet peppers. The second or "good" category of foods, containing 50 to 99 mg/100 gm, includes cabbage, cauliflower, chives, kohlrabi, orange pulp, lemon pulp, mustard greens, beet greens, papaya, spinach, strawberries, and watercress. The third or "fair" category of foods, with 30 to 49 mg/100 gm, includes asparagus, lima beans, swiss chard, gooseberries, currants, grapefruit, limes, loganberries, melons (cantaloupe), okra, tangerines, potatoes, and turnips. Note that potatoes and cabbage, which may be consumed in large quantities by low-economic groups, can provide rather large intakes of ascorbic acid.

Ascorbic acid may function in hydrogen ion transfer systems and aid in regulation of intracellular oxidation-reduction potentials. It is a powerful water-soluble antioxidant itself and probably helps to protect other antioxidants, even the lipid-soluble vitamin E, the polyunsaturated fatty acids, and vitamin A. It also aids in the conversion of folic acid to folinic acid and it facilitates gastrointestinal absorption of iron under certain circumstances. Ascorbic acid may also play a role in the detoxification of certain poisonous compounds by virtue of its co-factorial role in hydroxylation reactions.

UNITS OF MEASUREMENT

Unlike many other vitamins, ascorbic acid has always been measured in milligrams rather than arbitrary international units. Quantitative estimation of L-ascorbic acid is generally accomplished by taking advantage of its reducing properties. An example of this is the 2,6,dichlorophenolindophenol method of Bessey.[25] This technique is, however, time consuming and measures principally reduced L-ascorbic acid, whereas the popular 2,4,dinitrophenylhydrazine method measures "total" ascorbic acid.[26]

Many investigators have employed a variety of chemical techniques for ascertaining the state of ascorbic acid nutrition of animals or of man. The simplest of these is measurement of the vitamin C content of serum or plasma. Another method employs whole blood, whereas still another measures the ascorbic acid content of the buffy coat of centrifuged blood.[27] This layer is composed chiefly of leukocytes and platelets. A variety of values can be obtained from the literature. Table 5K–1 gives a composite approximation of values suggested by a number of investigators. It should be emphasized that neither serum nor whole blood nor buffy coat concentrations of ascorbic acid can provide a valid estimate of nutritional stores. These can only be measured by isotopic techniques, which are not suitable for routine clinical use. For purposes of comparison, however, a fourth column has been included to show body pool size as determined by these isotopic methods.

Throughout the years physicians have attempted to ascertain the ascorbic acid status of patients through a variety of "load tests." These are based upon the principle of "tissue saturation," a term which actually implied a finite body pool that can be saturated by giving enough ascorbic acid. The methods employed generally consisted of administering, either orally or parenterally, one or several doses of ascorbic acid and collecting, at intervals, samples of blood or urine or both. By measuring the rate of increase in the concentration of ascorbic acid in these biologic fluids, one could then estimate the degree of deficiency.

The most precise and specific technique employs L-ascorbic acid radioactively labeled with either ^{14}C or ^3H. A sufficient period of time for equilibration must be allowed after administering the labeling dose in order to permit complete mixing. By determining the specific radioactivity of L-ascorbic acid in plasma or blood, one can estimate the body pool size quite accurately. Since excretion of radioactive materials occurs largely in the urine, with almost negligible amounts being lost in feces, sweat, and expired CO_2,[28] the daily rate of excretion of radioactivity in the urine gives an estimate of the rate of catabolism of ascorbic acid. Metabolic studies of guinea pigs labeled with radioactive L-ascorbic acid disclosed that the distribution of this nutrient is highest in the adrenals and occurs in decreasing concentrations in the spleen, small intestine, bone marrow, stomach, liver, kidneys, and muscle.[29] Other investigators have reported high concentrations in the eyes, the pituitary gland, and the brain.[30]

Table 5K-1. L-Ascorbic Acid Nutritional Status of Man

	Serum or Plasma Concentration mg/100 ml	Whole Blood Concentration mg/100 ml	Buffy Coat Concentration μg/10⁸ cells	Body Pool Size mg
Well nourished*	>0.60	>1.0	>16	1500
Adequate*	0.40–0.59	0.60–0.99	11–15	600–1499
Low	0.10–0.39	0.30–0.59	2–10	300–599
Deficient	<0.10	<0.30	<2	0–299

* These represent approximate ranges, not absolute values. This table is offered only as a guide to interpret current publications.

DEFICIENCY IN EXPERIMENTAL ANIMALS

Most species of animals can synthesize ascorbic acid from glucose. The few exceptions include man and other primates, guinea pigs, the red vented bulbul, the fruit-eating bat, and at least two kinds of fish, the rainbow trout and the Coho salmon.[31] These species all must have ascorbic acid in their diets in order to avoid a deficiency syndrome known as scurvy. This disease may be fatal within a relatively short period of time, especially in young rapidly growing animals. Its major manifestations result from interference with the metabolism of mesenchymal tissues and apparent interference with blood clotting mechanisms. In the young, bone formation is impaired, dentition is disrupted, and synthesis of collagen is halted.[32,33] Biochemical studies have demonstrated defects in the metabolism of tyrosine,[34,35] in the formation of glycoproteins[36,37] and in the process of hydroxylation of proline, which is needed for formation of fibrous tissue.[38-40] In adult animals and in man, scurvy may result in a form of arthritis accompanied by effusions in the joints.[41,42] Wound healing has been reported to be seriously impaired in both animals and man, presumably as a result of impairment of collagen synthesis.[38,43] In both the British Medical Research Council Study[44] and the Iowa City Studies[45,46] of scurvy, however, impairment of wound healing could not be demonstrated. In other instances of both experimental and spontaneous scurvy, however, there has been unequivocal impairment of wound healing[47,48] and faulty healing of bony fractures.

The hemorrhagic manifestations of scurvy[49] include subperiosteal bleeding, petechial hemorrhages, ecchymoses, bleeding into joints, into the peritoneal cavity, and into the pericardial sac. Massive hemorrhage into the adrenals has been described in scorbutic guinea pigs and presumably may be a major cause of death.

The explanation for the hemorrhagic phenomena of scurvy is no longer self-evident. For many years, the theory of Wolbach and Howe[32] that lack of intercellular cement permitted disruption of the endothelial membrane and resulted in capillary hemorrhages was a very attractive explanation. This was particularly so in view of the many negative results of attempts to detect impairment of any of the blood clotting factors in either animal or human scurvy. Recent electron microscope studies, however, of tissues taken from patients with scurvy at a time when they had abundant evidence of hemorrhagic phenomena failed to demonstrate any capillary disruption or loss of the hypothetical intercellular cement.[45] Perhaps another explanation will be found for the hemorrhagic manifestations of scurvy.

Infectious diseases have consistently been much more common among people with scurvy.[50] Animal experiments have supported these observations.[51] Despite this, however, both the leukocyte count[45] and the immune response to antigenic challenge remain normal in scorbutic animals[52] and man.[46] Perhaps disruption of epithelial surfaces and impairment of mucus secretions play a role.

The finding of a high concentration of ascorbic acid in the adrenal cortex suggests that deficiency of vitamin C might result in impairment of adrenal cortical function.[53] This, however, has not been the case in a number of carefully controlled studies. In fact, it appears that adrenal cortical activity is increased in experimental scurvy.[54,55]

A series of studies has demonstrated impairment of vascular responses in scorbutic animals and faulty metabolism of sympathetic amines.[56-58] A recent report of experimental scurvy in man also described impairment of vascular reactivity, but the mechanism was not apparent.[59] Nonetheless, the occurrence of this phenomenon could explain sudden death in scurvy.

BIOCHEMISTRY AND PHYSIOLOGY

Although the exact mechanisms of action of ascorbic acid remain to be determined, certain functions have been clearly identified. L-Ascorbic acid is a coenzyme or a co-factor in some situations where the rate of reaction is important. For example, in hydroxylation reactions, where either copper or iron must remain in a reduced state for the function of an enzyme, ascorbic acid has proven to be critical.[60,61] It has been reported to be necessary for the metabolism of several amino acids; for example, hydroxylation of proline in the synthesis of collagen,[62] and hydroxylation of tryptophan to 5-hydroxytryptophan.[63] Metabolism of 3,4-dihydroxyphenylethylamine to norepinephrine,[64,65] which presumably might account for some of the aberrations of vascular reactivity and some of the mental and psychological changes that accompany scurvy,[66] was once thought to be ascorbate-dependent but this seems doubtful. Ascorbic acid is, however, necessary for conversion of hydroxyphenylpyruvate to homogentisic acid in the formation of tyrosine.[67,68]

Metabolically, ascorbic acid behaves somewhat like glucose to which it is chemically related. It is readily absorbed from the gastrointestinal tract* and is conserved by a tubular re-absorptive enzyme in the renal tubules. A large amount of ascorbic acid given orally or parenterally will not result in sustained high concentrations in the blood. The renal threshold of the kidneys prevents hyperascorbemia by means of a tubular maximum (TM) which "turns off" the re-absorptive mechanism and allows rapid urinary excretion of the substance. The practical consequence of this is that even massive intakes of ascorbic acid fail to maintain the plasma level much above 1.5 to 2.0 mg/100 ml. At concentrations above 1.4 mg/100 ml the clearance rises rapidly.[69,70] Probably this is fortunate, because ascorbic acid is a highly reactive substance.

Ascorbic acid deficiency sometimes is accompanied by anemia. Much controversy surrounds the question of whether ascorbic acid is necessary for utilization of folic acid[71] and vitamin B_{12}.[72,73] In any event anemic scorbutic patients often respond rapidly to ascorbic acid alone.[74-77]

Protein metabolism may be altered in scurvy. In both animals[78] and man,[28] deficiency of ascorbic acid leads to changes in serum protein fractions (lowering of serum albumin with an accompanying rise of one or another of the globulin fractions) and to an excessive rate of urinary loss of nitrogen.[46]

* Very large amounts are only partially absorbed

Cholesterol metabolism may in some way be related to ascorbic acid.[79] For many years Russian physicians have recommended a high intake of ascorbic acid as a means of avoiding hypercholesterolemia in the hope of preventing atherosclerosis.[80] Although most American investigators have failed to confirm these observations, it is of interest that Fox and Dangerfield in South Africa[81] and Hodges et al. in the United States[46] observed a significant rise in serum cholesterol of scorbutic subjects given repleting doses of vitamin C. These changes occurred without any other modification of the diet. Recent preliminary reports by Mumma et al.[21,24] suggest that ascorbate 3 sulfate can mobilize tissue stores of cholesterol. At the present time there does not seem to be sufficient evidence to support the claims that ascorbic acid can prevent atherosclerosis but enough interest has been generated to warrant further investigation.

The demonstration of ascorbate 3 sulfate in human urine, as well as in guinea pig, rat, and trout urine suggests that this compound is a fairly ubiquitous metabolite of ascorbic acid. Thus the biological role of ascorbate sulfate is of some interest. It could act as a sulfate donor, as has been suggested by Chu and Slaunwhite[82] and Mumma. It could have a function in transport across cellular membranes, inasmuch as ascorbate 3 sulfate is a di-negative ion at physiological pH concentrations and appears to interact strongly with metal ions. It could also be part of the ascorbate pool in man and animals. Ascorbate sulfate might play a part in the transfer of ascorbate across the blood-brain barrier thus affecting the concentration of ascorbate in brain tissue. Hammarström and others have demonstrated that *free* ascorbate does not rapidly cross this barrier.[83] Blaschke and Hertting[84] have recently demonstrated two metal-ascorbates in the rat. Earlier Kiss and Neukom[85] suggested that a metal-ascorbate was the ascorbigen of cabbage. In addition, a variety of 2- and 3-ascorbate derivates have been prepared by chemical means. The presence of a number of as yet unidentified 6-carbon metabolites in human and guinea pig urine indicates the complexities of "essential ascorbate" metabolism.

NUTRITIONAL REQUIREMENTS VS RECOMMENDED ALLOWANCES

Perhaps because ascorbic acid is an essential nutrient for only a few species of animals, scientists have long regarded it as a special substance, somewhat apart from the other vitamins or accessory food factors. In any event, the recommended level of intake for ascorbic acid has varied greatly from time to time and from country to country. According to the Recommended Dietary Allowances of the National Research Council in 1968,[86] the allowance of ascorbic acid for an adult man varies from 30 mg daily in the United Kingdom to 75 mg in West Germany. In the United States, the recommended level of intake which once was 150 mg daily, now is 60 mg.*

This brings us to the important difference between *requirements* and *allowances*. The former is *that amount which must be consumed daily to avoid deficiency*. The latter is *a generous surplus to compensate for fluctuations in the nutrient content of foods, perishability of a given essential nutrient, and individual variations.* The British Medical Research Council study clearly indicated that 10 mg of ascorbic acid daily (perhaps somewhat less) could prevent or cure scurvy in adult man. These observations were fully confirmed in two separate studies in Iowa City a quarter of a century later.

But no one pretends that mere avoidance of deficiency diseases represents optimal nutrition for man. Indeed, for many years authorities have stressed "tissue saturation" when referring to ascorbic acid and have endeavored to ascertain that daily dose of vitamin C which would maintain *full saturation.* For herein lay the magic key to unlock the portals to "superior health, great stamina, resistance to infection, superior mental prowess, enhanced fertility, ability to inactivate toxins, and resistance to malignant disease." Truly, vitamin C must be a wondrous drug. Note that we are no longer talking about an accessory food factor needed in trace amounts, but a *protective drug* that allegedly can be taken in large "health-giving" quantities; "the more the better."

* The new RDAs are not yet published, but may be reduced.

To return to reality, we note that the joint FAO/WHO Expert Group recommended an adult daily allowance of 30 mg; the same amount recommended by the Committee on Medical Aspects of Food Policy for the United Kingdom.

In support of a similar allowance, we have drawn a mathematical model of the rate of catabolism and the body pool size of ascorbic acid in man. This is based on studies of nine men labeled with ^{14}C ascorbic acid and fed a scorbutogenic diet until they had scurvy (Fig. 5K–1). In this model, the saturated body pool approximates 1500 mg and the rate of catabolism of ascorbic acid is about 3 per cent of the existing body pool per day. At the start, the rate of catabolism would be 45 mg daily so an intake of this amount should maintain the pool at or near its maximum. At an intake of 30 mg daily, a body pool size of about 1,000 mg would be maintained. At 10 mg daily the pool would be only 333 mg. It is noteworthy that the subjects began to manifest scurvy when their body pool fell below 300 mg.[28]

Thus one might justify a recommendation of any level of intake of ascorbic acid between 10 and 50 mg daily.[87] We doubt whether there is any important difference between 30 and 50 mg. Certainly the people of the United States do not seem to be any healthier than the people of the United Kingdom.

DEFICIENCY IN MAN

Only a brief description of scurvy will be given here but the reader is referred to the chapter on "Clinical Manifestations of Certain Vitamin Deficiencies." The onset of adult scurvy can be detected between 60 and 90 days after the beginning of ascorbic acid deficiency. The earliest manifestations, which would almost certainly escape casual observation, are the appearance of a few petechial spots and small ecchymoses. These fade within a few days but are replaced by others. Somewhat later, larger ecchymoses appear and are accompanied by petechiae which become perifollicular in location. At the same time follicular hyperkeratosis develops, especially on the buttocks, thighs, and calves. Many hyperkeratotic lesions contain frag-

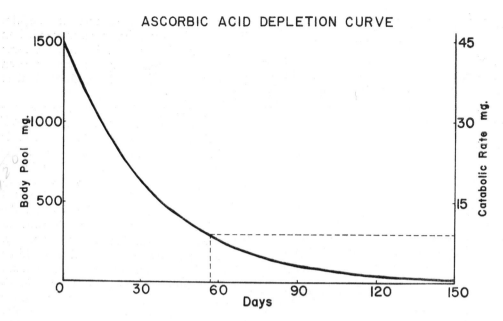

Fig. 5K-1. Curve of ascorbate pool derived from data of nine men whose body pool of ascorbate was labeled with ^{14}C L-ascorbic acid. They were then fed a diet devoid of vitamin C.

Initially the body pool averaged 1500 mg. The average daily rate of catabolism was 3 per cent of the existing body pool. Thus, the maximal rate of catabolism approximated 45 mg/day.

When the body pool fell below 300 mg total and the catabolic rate below 9 mg/day, signs of scurvy began to appear (about 55 days).

From this curve one can estimate the approximate body pool size from the dose. Thus, with a daily intake of 30 mg, the pool size should be about 1000 mg.

mented or coiled hairs and some demonstrate the classic lesion of scurvy; *the hyperkeratotic follicle with a red hemorrhagic halo.* A little later the gums become swollen and bleed easily. It is noteworthy that the gums do not become involved in the absence of teeth and that the gum lesions are most severe where dental hygiene is the poorest. Ocular hemorrhages appear in the bulbar conjunctiva but seldom, if ever, in the fundi.[88] A unique characteristic of scurvy is the development of Sjögren's (sicca) syndrome,[89] which consists of dryness of the mouth and eyes, loss of hair, dry itchy skin, and loosening of teeth and fillings. Near the end of the third month of deprivation, patients develop profound fatigue, weakness, and lethargy. They complain of aching of their legs and soon develop arthralgia followed by joint effusions. A peculiar form of vasomotor instability develops and may be accompanied by pitting edema of the feet and ankles. Oliguria has

been observed in severe scurvy. Psychological changes are common and have been characterized as the "neurotic triad,"[66] which consists of hysteria, depression, and hypochondriasis. Peripheral neuropathy was observed in one scorbutic subject who had hemorrhages into the femoral nerve sheaths of both legs.[90] In infants, scurvy is most apt to occur a short time after they are removed from the breast, unless ascorbic acid supplements are fed. Subperiosteal hemorrhages result in pain in the legs and arms. The lower end of the femur and the upper end of the humerus are most tender. Epiphyseal separations occur, resulting in chest deformities.

THERAPY

Although a great deal has been written about the therapy of scurvy, much of it is conjectural or purely arbitrary. As we have seen from the accounts of scurvy in ancient times, even small quantities of ascorbic acid are sufficient to result in prompt alleviation of the symptoms and signs of scurvy. This was the experience of the British Medical Research Council and it was our experience in treating nine subjects who participated in the Iowa City studies. Daily doses of between 10 and 60 mg of ascorbic acid caused rapid and sustained improvement in signs and symptoms of severely scorbutic subjects. Accordingly, we feel it is reasonable to recommend therapy of scurvy with doses in the neighborhood of 100 mg of ascorbic acid 3 times daily. Only if patients are unable to eat should they be given parenteral ascorbate. Massive amounts of ascorbic acid may cause gastrointestinal distress or electrolyte disturbances. A total intake of 300 mg daily should result in replenishment of body pools within about 5 days, since this dose is almost completely absorbed and, in the deficient state, virtually none is lost in the urine. One word of caution should, however, be given; scurvy can result in sudden death and should be treated promptly.

TOXICITY

Thus far in this chapter we have dealt with a discussion of the manifestations of ascorbic acid deficiency and the daily dose of this vitamin necessary to prevent or cure deficiency. We have shown that about 45 mg of ascorbic acid daily are sufficient to maintain the body pool at or near maximum and that much smaller amounts will prevent or cure scurvy. Any discussion of the hypothetical protective or curative effects of huge doses of vitamin C (in the neighborhood of 100 to 1,000 times the physiologic dose) is outside the scope of this chapter. We can say that we have not seen evidence which convinced us that large doses of vitamin C serve any useful purpose, aside from acidifying the urine—a device employed in certain urinary infections.

We can also conjecture that harmful or undesirable consequences may follow prolonged ingestion of massive doses of ascorbic acid (doses in the range of 5,000 to 15,000 mg daily). The first effect may be nausea, followed by diarrhea. A large amount of ascorbic acid will also be excreted in the urine, where it may interfere with simple tests for glycosuria, giving a false positive with the copper-containing reagents and a false negative with the glucose oxidase methods used in the popular (glucose oxidase-peroxidase) dip stick tests.[91,92] Ascorbate can markedly enhance iron absorption; a result far from desirable in non-anemic men.[93,94] It can also "mobilize" the minerals of the bony skeleton, but the consequences of this action are not yet known.[95-97] Some ascorbate is converted to oxalate[98,99] and fear has been expressed that this may lead to urinary tract stones. Although a low pH should protect against calcium oxalate stones, it would favor the formation of uric acid stones and cystine stones.[100]

Animal studies have demonstrated that large doses of ascorbic acid can cause infertility or abortion,[101,102] or have adverse effects on the fetus.[103] In one clinical study human pregnancies were interrupted by ascorbic acid.[104]

In rats, huge doses of an analogue of vitamin C, dehydroascorbic acid, can, like alloxan, produce permanent diabetes;[105] and L-ascorbic acid itself can potentiate the diabetogenic effect of alloxan in rats.[106] There is as yet no evidence that massive doses of vitamin C can damage the islets of the human pancreas, but definitive tests have not yet been reported.

Ascorbic acid in massive doses may interfere with anticoagulant therapy, both with heparin and with coumadin drugs.[107-109]

Excessive amounts of ascorbic acid, given to chicks, can interfere with intestinal absorption of certain trace minerals.[110]

Vitamin C is an essential nutrient. In proper doses, it prevents scurvy. At the present time there is little reason to prescribe it for any other purpose.

Finally, overdoses of any essential nutrient may result in a "conditioned deficiency," i.e., a relative lack of responsiveness to normal doses.[103]

BIBLIOGRAPHY

1. Papyrus Ebers—Medical Writings ca 1550 B.C. (Quoted in Encyclopedia Britannica), Chicago, 1964.

2. Hippocrates—*The Genuine Works of Hippocrates* ca 600 B.C. Edited by Francis Adams. London Sydenham Society, *1*:196, 267, 1849; Pliny, Compages in Genubers Solverentur ca 63 A.D. Major, R. H. *Classic Descriptions of Disease with Biographical Sketches of the Authors*, Springfield, Charles C Thomas, 1945.

3. Anson, George (Lord). *A Voyage Around the World in the Years 1740, 1, 2, 3, 4.* Compiled by Richard Walter, M.A., Chaplain of H.M.S. Centurion, 3rd Ed. London, the author. 1748.

4. Hess, A. F.: *Scurvy, Past and Present.* Philadelphia, Lea & Febiger, 1920.

5. *Encyclopedia Britannica* (1771). First Edition, Vol. III, 106–110.

6. *Encyclopedia Britannica* (1964). Admiral George A. Anson, 1:1027, James Lind, 14:150, 15:204, Captain James Cook, 10:148.

7. Lind, James: *A Treatise on the Scurvy.* London, A. Millar, 1753. Republished Edinburgh University Press; Edinburgh, R. & R. Clark Ltd., 1953.

8. Cartier, Jacques: "La Grosse Maladie." Reproduction photographique de son 'Brief Recit et Succincte Narration, 1545, suive d'une traduction en langue anglaise du chapitre traitant des aventures de Cartier aux prises avec le scorbut et d'une nouvelle analyse du Mystère de l'Anneda;' B. L. Frank and Others, Montreal, XIX Congrès International de Physiologie, Montreal, The Ronald Printing Co., Ltd., 1953.

9. Åberg: J. Chem. Educ., *27*, 334, 1950.

10. Villiers: Nutr. Today, *4*, 8, 1969.

11. Kodicek and Young: Notes and Records of the Royal Society of London, *24*, 43, 1969.

12. Priestley: Nutr. Today, *4*, 18, 1969.

13. Hunt: Chapt. 6 in *Contributions Relating to the Causation and Prevention of Disease* (Edited by Austin Flint). New York, Published for the U.S. Sanitary Commission by Hurd and Houghton, 1867.

14. Zilva and Wells: Proc. Roy. Soc. (London) Series *B-90*, 505, 1917–19.

15. Svirbely and Szent-Györgyi: Biochem. J., *26*, 865, 1932.

16. King and Waugh: Science, *75*, 357, 1932.

17. Haworth and Hirst: J. Soc. Chem. & Indust., *52*, 645, 1933.

18. Reichstein, Grüssner and Oppenhauer: Helv. Chim. Acta, *16*, 565, 1933.

19. Holst: J. Hyg., *7*, 619, 1907 and Holst, and Frölich, (ibid) p. 634.

20. Burns: Am. J. Med., *26*, 740, 1959.

21. Mumma: Biochim. Biophys. Acta, *165*, 571, 1968.

22. Mead and Finamore: Biochemistry, *8*, 2652, 1969.

23. Baker, Hammer, March, Tolbert, and Canham: Science, *173*, 826, 1971.

24. Mumma and Verlangieri: (Abstract) Fed. Proc., *30*, 370, 1971.

25. Bessey: J. Biol. Chem., *126*, 771, 1938.

26. Schaffert and Kingsley: J. Biol. Chem. *212*, 59, 1955.

27. Srikantia, Mohanram and Krishnaswamy: Am. J. Clin. Nutr., *23*, 59, 1970.

28. Baker, Hodges, Hood, Sauberlich, March and Canham: Am. J. Clin. Nutr. *24*, 444, 1971.

29. Martin: Ann. N.Y. Acad. Sci., *92*, 141, 1961.

30. Kuether, Telford, and Roe: J. Nutr., *28*, 347, 1944.

31. Johnson, Hammer, Halver and Baker: (Abstract) Fed. Proc., *30*, 521, 1971.

32. Wolbach and Howe: Arch. Path., *1*, 1, 1926.

33. Gould: Ann. N. Y. Acad. Sci., *92*, 168, 1961.

34. Morris, Harpur and Goldbloom: J. Clin. Invest., *29*, 325, 1950.

35. Rogers and Gardner: J. Lab. & Clin. Med., *34*, 1491, 1949.

36. Pirani and Catchpole: Arch. Path., *51*, 597, 1951.

37. Antonowicz and Kodicek: Biochem. J., *110*, 609, 1968.

38. Mussini, Hutton and Udenfriend: Science, *169*, 927, 1967.

39. Barnes, Constable and Kodicek: Biochem. J., *113*, 387, 1969.

40. Barnes, Constable and Kodicek: Biochim. Biophys. Acta, *184*, 358, 1969.

41. Pirani, Bly and Sutherland: Arch. Path., *49*, 710, 1950.

42. Kodicek: In: Jackson, *et al.* Ed. Structure and Function of Connective and Skeletal Tissue. Proceedings of a Conference held at Univ. of St. Andrews, Scotland. Sponsored by NATO. London, Butterworth, 1965.

43. Crandon, Lund and Dill: New Eng. J. Med., *223*, 353, 1940.

44. Bartley, Krebs and O'Brien: Medical Research Council Special Report Series 280. London: Her Majesty's Stationery Office 1953.

45. Hodges, Baker, Hood, Sauberlich and March: Am. J. Clin. Nutr., *22*, 535, 1969.

46. Hodges, Hood, Canham, Sauberlich and Baker: Am. J. Clin. Nutr., *24*, 432, 1971.

47. Bourne: Proc. Nutr. Soc. (Engl. and Scot.), *4*, 204, 1946.

48. Edwards and Dunphy: New Eng. J. Med., *259*, 224, 1958.

49. Hess: *Scurvy, Past and Present.* Philadelphia, J. B. Lippincott Co., 1920.

50. Scrimshaw, Taylor and Gordon: Interactions of Nutrition and Infection. World Health Organization, Geneva 1968, pp. 97–100.

51. Honjo, Takasaka, Fujiwara, Imaizumi and Ogawa: Jap. J. Med. Sci. & Biol., *22*, 149, 1969.

52. Kumar and Axelrod: J. Nutr., *98*, 41, 1969.

53. Stepto, Pirani, Consolazio and Bell: Endocr., *49*, 755, 1951.

54. Banerjee and Singh: Am. J. Physiol., *190*, 265, 1957.

55. Morgan: *Vitamins and Hormones.* New York, Academic Press, Vol. IX, p. 168, 1951.

56. Beyer: J. Pharmacol. and Exper. Therapy, *76*, 149, 1942.

57. Lee and Lee: Amer. J. Physiol., *149*, 465, 1947.

58. Lee: Ann. N.Y. Acad. Sci., *92*, 295, 1961.

59. Abboud, Hood, Hodges and Mayer: J. Clin. Invest., *49*, 298, 1970.
60. Goldberg: Brit. J. Haematol., *5*, 150, 1959.
61. Staudinger, Krisch and Leonhäuser: Ann. N.Y. Acad. Sci., *92*, 195, 1961.
62. Peterkofsky and Udenfriend: Proc. Nat. Acad. Sci., *53*, 335, 1965.
63. Cooper: Ann. N.Y. Acad. Sci., *91*, 208, 1961.
64. Levin, Levenberg and Kaufman: J. Biol. Chem., *235*, 2080, 1960.
65. Friedman and Kaufman: J. Biol. Chem., *240*, PC552, 1965.
66. Kinsman and Hood: Am. J. Clin. Nutr., *24*, 455, 1971.
67. Avery, Clow, Menkes, Ramos, Scriver, Stern and Wasserman: Pediatrics, *39*, 378, 1967.
68. Sealock and Silberstein: Science, *90*, 517, 1939.
69. Faulkner and Taylor: J. Clin. Invest., *17*, 69, 1938.
70. Ralli and Sherry: Medicine, *20*, 251, 1941.
71. Nichol and Welch: Proc. Soc. Exper. Biol. & Med., *74*, 52, 1950.
72. May, Hamilton and Stewart: Blood 7, 978, 1952.
73. Sundberg, Schaar and May: Blood, *7*, 1143, 1952.
74. Vilter, Woolford and Spies: J. Lab. & Clin. Med., *31*, 609, 1946.
75. Herbert: New Eng. J. Med., *268*, 201 and 368, 1963.
76. Cox, Meynell, Northam and Cooke: Am. J. Med., *42*, 220, 1967.
77. Hart, Ploem, Panders and Verloop: Acta Med. Scandinav., *176*, 497, 1946.
78. Torre and Green: J. Nutr., *97*, 61, 1969.
79. Bronte-Stewart, Roberts and Wells: Brit. J. Nutr., *17*, 61, 1963.
80. Simonson and Keys: Circulation, *24*, 1239, 1961.
81. Fox and Dangerfield: Proc. of the Transvaal Mine Medical Officer's Assn., *19*, 267, 1940.
82. Chu and Slaunwhite: Steroids, 12:309, 1968.
83. Hammarström: Acta Physiol. Scand. 70(Suppl. 289), 1, 1966.
84. Blaschke and Hertting: Naunyn-Schmiedebergs Arch. Exp. Pathol. Pharmakol., *266*, 296, 1970.
85. Kiss and Neukom: Helv. Chim. Acta, *49*, 989, 1966.
86. Recommended Dietary Allowances, 7th Revised Ed. Publication 1694, National Academy of Sciences, Washington, D.C., 1968.
87. Baker, Hodges, Hood, Sauberlich and March: Am. J. Clin. Nutr., *22*, 549, 1969.
88. Hood and Hodges: Am. J. Clin. Nutr., *22*, 559, 1969.
89. Hood, Burns and Hodges: New Eng. J. Med., *282*, 1120, 1970.
90. Hood: New Eng. J. Med., *281*, 1292, 1969.
91. Präuer: New Eng. J. Med., *284*, 1328, 1971.
92. Glatzel and Rüberg-Sehweer: Med. Klin., *61*, 1249, 1966.
93. Moore: Am. J. Clin. Nutr., *3*, 3, 1955.
94. Pirzio-Biroli, Bothwell and Finch: J. Lab. & Clin. Med., *51*, 37, 1958.
95. Thornton: J. Nutr., *100*, 1479, 1970.
96. Thornton and Omdahl: Proc. Soc. Exper. Biol and Med., *132*, 618, 1969.
97. Ramp and Thornton: Proc. Soc. Exper. Biol. and Med., *137*, 273, 1971.
98. Lamden and Chrystowski: Proc. Soc. Exper. Biol. and Med., *85*, 190, 1954.
99. Lamden: New Eng. J. Med., *284*, 336, 1971.
100. Anon.: The Medical Letter *12*(No. 26), 105, 1970.
101. Neuwiler: Internat. Ztschr. Vitaminforsch., *22*, 392, 1951.
102. Mouriquand and Edel: Compt. Rend. Soc. Biol., *147*, 1432, 1953.
103. Cochrane: Canad. Med. Assoc. J., *93*, 893, 1965.
104. Samborskaja and Ferdman: Bjull. eksp. Biol. Med., No. 8, 96, 1966.
105. Patterson: J. Biol. Chem., *183*, 81, 1950.
106. Levy and Suter: Proc. Soc. Exper. Biol. & Med., *63*, 341, 1946.
107. Owen, Tyce, Flock and McCall. Mayo Clin. Proc., *45*, 140, 1970.
108. Sigell and Flessa: J.A.M.A., *214*, 2035, 1970.
109. Rosenthal: J.A.M.A., *215*, 1671, 1971.
110. Hunt, Landesman and Newberne: Brit. J. Nutr., *24*, 607, 1970.

Chapter

5

Section L   Biotin

ROBERT S. GOODHART

Biotin—which is present in the soil, in lake bottom deposits, in bacteria, and in nearly all foods—is one of the B-complex vitamins. It is inactivated by a carbohydrate-containing protein, avidin, present in egg white. Biotin is synthesized by many microorganisms. A common pathway of biosynthesis appears to be: pimelic acid→7,8-diketopelargonate→7-keto-8-aminopelargonate→7,8-diaminopelargonate→dethiobiotin→biotin.[1]

CHEMISTRY AND METABOLISM

Biotin is a fairly simple organic ring compound. Its empirical formula, $C_{10}H_{16}O_3N_2S$, and structure have been proposed by Kögl and his colleagues who crystallized small quantities from egg yolk.[2] In natural products biotin occurs mainly in bound form. An enzyme, biotinidase, capable of liberating biotin from simple biotin esters and amides is widely distributed in animal tissues.[3] Biologic assays for biotin are done using a number of yeast and bacterial growth techniques. Other organisms, such as *Neurospora crassa* and *Candida guillermondia*, have also been used. Using *Ochromonas danica*, Baker and associates[4] found the biotin content of the blood, serum and urine of 12 normal subjects to fall into the range observed for vitamin B_{12}: blood = 170–279 $\mu\mu g/ml$; serum = 213–404 $\mu\mu g/ml$; urine = 6,260–32,700 $\mu\mu g/ml$. According to these workers, all of the biotin in urine is in the free form.

Biotin enzymes appear to function in carboxylation reactions by a two-step mechanism involving the binding of CO_2 to the biotin moiety of the enzyme with simultaneous hydrolysis of ATP and subsequent transfer of the "high energy" CO_2 to an acceptor.[5] In biotin deficiency there is a reduction in amino acid incorporation into protein, apparently due to a reduction in the synthesis of dicarboxylic acids.[6] Biotin administered to biotin-deficient rats causes an increase in liver ribonucleic acid, which is followed by enhanced protein synthesis *in vivo*.[7] Also, in biotin-deficient rats there seems to be a specific impairment in the utilization of glucose.[8,9] Deficiency also has been reported to retard fatty acid synthesis.[10] Biotin has been shown to participate in the conversion of folic acid to activated reduced and formylated forms; however, it is unknown whether or not this is a direct coenzymatic effect.[11] A biotin-sparing effect of vitamin B_{12}, associated with impaired utilization of vitamin B_{12} in biotin-deficient rats, has been claimed.[12,13] It may be that not only vitamin B_{12} and folate but also biotin participate in one-carbon metabolism.[14] Also, a high level of biotin in a zinc-deficient diet has been reported to alleviate symptoms of zinc deficiency in the rat, and zinc-biotin interrelationships appear to have an effect upon iron metabolism.[15] Biotin, in large doses, increases liver glucokinase activity in the diabetic rat. In this regard, it resembles closely the effect of insulin in terms of the magnitude of its effect, its specificity for certain key glycolytic enzymes, and the inhibition of its action by protein or RNA synthesis inhibitors. It may act either directly on the synthesis of glucokinase or indirectly through an effect on the synthesis or secretion of insulin.[16]

Biotin has the biologic activity previously ascribed to vitamin H (the egg-white injury factor). When rats consume diets containing large amounts of uncooked egg white, they develop a syndrome known as egg-white injury. This is characterized by an eczema-like dermatitis, spasticity or paralysis of the hind legs, and the development of the so-called "spectacle eye" due to circumocular loss of hair. The lesions produced by the diet are not due to a direct toxic action of raw egg white, but result from consumption of the protein, avidin, in egg white, which interacts with, and "neutralizes," biotin in the food as well as the biotin produced in the gut of the experimental animal by bacterial synthesis. Pure avidin is just as effective as raw egg white in producing the lesions in rats or mice.

Daft[17] showed that therapy with crystalline biotin would prevent dermatitis, myocardial necrosis, and other lesions produced in rats by sulfaguanidine or sulfasuxadine. Apparently these compounds interfere with intestinal bacterial growth and synthesis of biotin. Oppel[18] and others also have obtained data which indicate that biotin is synthesized by organisms in the gut of man. Ham and Scott[19] found that biotin synthesis in the intestinal tract of the rat was inhibited by terramycin in the diet and almost completely so by a combination of terramycin and sulfasuxadine. Biotin synthesis was found to be diminished when the diet was free of riboflavin, niacin and pantothenic acid. When starch replaced sucrose in the diet, there was an increased synthesis of biotin in the intestinal tract. A dietary source of biotin is required by germ-free rats.[20]

Biotin deficiency has been produced by feeding chicks and turkeys a diet of sucrose and acid-washed, alcohol-extracted casein. The animals developed dermatitis and perosis. Experimental biotin deficiency has also been produced in fish, cows, pigs, dogs, monkeys, and man.

Boyd and Sargeant[21] reported that rats on a biotin-deficient diet are highly susceptible to the toxic effects of large oral doses of benzylpenicillin.

Sydenstricker and his colleagues[22] fed 4 volunteers a diet rich in egg whites and low in biotin-containing foods. Within 5 weeks the volunteers developed: a fine, non-pruritic dermatitis; a grayish pallor of their skin and mucosa, and depression, lassitude, somnolence, muscle pains, and hyperesthesia. Later, anorexia, nausea, reticulation of the skin, anemia, hypercholesterolemia and changes in the electrocardiograph were observed. All signs and symptoms disappeared within 5 days of therapy with parenteral biotin.

The mean biotin content of the blood of pregnant women has been found to be lower than that of non-pregnant normal adults, and there is a progressive fall in the biotin content of the blood during the course of gestation.[23]

Treatment of a 2-year-old child suffering from propionicacidemia with biotin, 5 mg twice daily by mouth for 5 days, reduced both the resting plasma propionate concentration and the response to isoleucine: also, the child was reported to show slight improvement in alertness and muscle tone while on biotin.[24]

Beneficial effects from the treatment of seborrheic dermatitis of infants and Leiner's disease (a widespread form of seborrheic dermatitis in infants) with biotin have been reported both in this country and in Europe.[25]

BIBLIOGRAPHY

1. Anon.: Nutr. Rev., 28, 189, 1970.
2. Kögl and Tönnis: Z. Physiol. Chem., 242, 43, 1936.
3. Koivusalo, Elorriaga, Kaziro and Ochoa: J. Biol. Chem., 238, 1038, 1963.
4. Baker, Frank, Matovitch, Pasher, Aaronson, Hutner and Sobotka: Analytical Biochem., 3, 31, 1962.
5. Anon.: Nutrition Rev., 21, 310, 1963.
6. Dakshinamurti and Mistry: J. Biol. Chem., 238, 297, 1963.
7. Dakshinamurti and Litvak: J. Biol. Chem., 245, 5600, 1970.
8. Mistry, Dakshinamurti and Modi: Arch. Biochem. Biophys., 96, 674, 1962.
9. Bhagavan, Coursin and Dakshinamurti: Arch. Biochem. Biophys., 110, 422, 1965.
10. Oxman and Ball: Arch. Biochem. Biophys., 95, 99, 1961.
11. Marchetti, Landi and Pasquali: J. Nutrition, 89, 422, 1966.
12. Marchetti and Testoni: J. Nutrition, 84, 249, 1964.
13. Puddu and Marchetti: J. Nutrition, 84, 255, 1964.
14. Bridgers: Nutr. Rev., 25, 65, 1967.

15. Chu, Schlicker and Cox: Nutr. Reports Internat., *7*, 11, 1970.
16. Anon.: Nutr. Rev., *28*, 242, 1970.
17. Daft, Ashburn and Sebrell: Science, *96*, 321, 1942.
18. Oppel: Amer. J. Med. Sci., *204*, 886, 1942.
19. Ham and Scott: J. Nutrition, *51*, 423, 1953.
20. Luckey, Pleasants, Wagner, Gordon and Reyniers: J. Nutrition, *57*, 169, 1955.
21. Boyd and Sargeant: J. New Drugs. *2*, 283, 1962.
22. Sydenstricker, Singal, Briggs, De Vaughn and Isbell: Science, *95*, 176, 1942; J.A.M.A., *118*, 1199, 1942.
23. Bhagavan: Internat. J. Vit. Res., *39*, 235, 1969.
24. Barnes, Hull, Balgobin and Gompertz: The Lancet, *II*, 244, 1970.
25. Nisenson: J. Pediatrics, *51*, 537, 1957.

Chapter

5

Section M   Miscellany

ROBERT S. GOODHART

Bioflavonoids

In 1936, Szent-Györgyi[1] observed what he interpreted to be synergistic potentiation of the antiscorbutic effect of vitamin C by extracts of red pepper and lemon. The active materials in these extracts, later shown to be flavones or flavonols, were reported to decrease capillary bleeding and prolong life in scorbutic guinea pigs, and to overcome vascular purpura of human beings due to many different causes.[2] This group of substances was called vitamin P to denote its effect on capillary permeability. None of these substances has been shown to have a true vitamin effect, however, so this designation was dropped in 1950 upon the recommendation of the American Society of Biological Chemists and the American Institute of Nutrition.[3] The term "bioflavonoids" has been used instead, but the biologic activity of these compounds has not been conclusively demonstrated, though Z. Zloch of Charles University, Plzen, Czechoslovakia,[4] has reported that treatment of vitamin C-deficient, long-term "factor P"-deficient guinea pigs with both bioflavonoids (quercetin or epicatechin) and ascorbic acid showed a significantly favorable influence of the bioflavonoids as compared with results obtained with treatment with ascorbic acid alone. According to Zloch, there was a more rapid restitution of the body weight and a decrease in the proportion of ascorbic acid present in the liver, kidney and adrenals as dehydroascorbic acid, a manifestation, perhaps, of an antioxidant effect of the flavonoids. Reported also were a decrease in serum cholesterol and an increase in serum albumin, as compared to findings in animals treated with ascorbic acid alone.

CHEMISTRY OF THE BIOFLAVONOIDS

The basic structure of a flavone is given in Figure 5M-1 as well as some of its substitution and reduction products in common use. These compounds can combine with sugars to form glycosides, and with metals to form chelates. Quinones with reducing properties can be formed from them also. Pharmacologic effects may be dependent upon such reactions or on direct vasoconstrictor effects.

BIOLOGIC AND CLINICAL INVESTIGATIONS

Though a tremendous amount of work has been done with these compounds, no deficiency state has been induced in animals nor discovered in man. The flavonoid quercetin is reported to have an inhibitory effect on the specific and nonspecific histidine decarboxylase *in vivo* and *in vitro*[5] and to activate Hageman factor.[6] In another study, the bioflavonoids did not alter the inflammatory response or the production of collagen.[7] There is no proof of clinical usefulness at this time. Claims and counterclaims have been made but, unfortunately, there are few well-controlled studies, and these, for the most

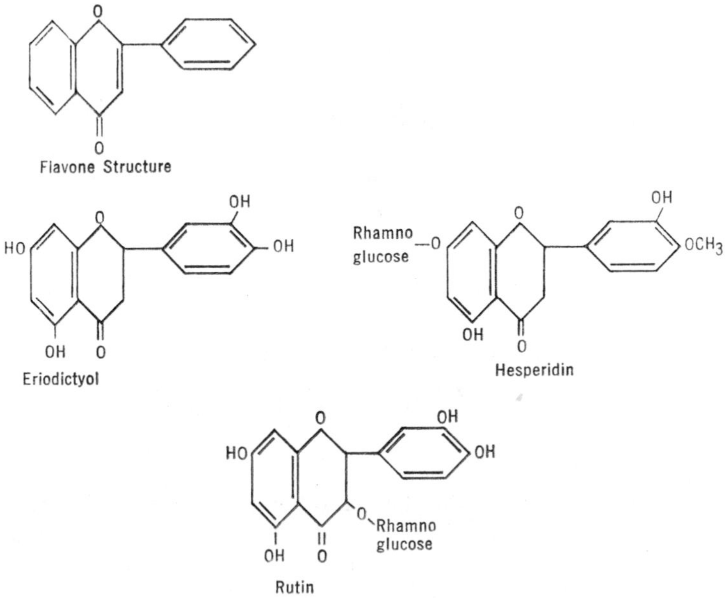

Fig. 5M-1.   Structure of the bioflavonoids.

part, have given negative results.   In the case of some of the compounds in common use, it is doubtful that a significant amount is absorbed from the G.I. tract.

There is no proof that vascular purpura, retinal hemorrhages and cerebrovascular accidents associated with hypertension have been influenced by the administration of the bioflavonoids,[8] though there have been many reports of such benefit.[9]   Similar claims have been made for the purpura and retinopathy of diabetic patients,[10] also without confirmation.   There is no proof that the flavonoids, with or without vitamin C, have any beneficial effect in rheumatic fever, rheumatoid arthritis, habitual abortion, erythroblastosis fetalis, arteriosclerosis, radiation injury, or the common cold.   A monograph, *The Flavonoids in Biology and Medicine*, presents the pros and cons of the problem.[11]

BIBLIOGRAPHY

1. Rusznyak and Szent-Györgyi: Nature, *138*, 27, 1936.
2. Armentano, Bentsath, Beres, Rusznyak, and Szent-Györgyi: Deut. Med. Wchnschr., *62*, 1325, 1936.
3. Joint Committee on Nomenclature: Science, *112*, 628, 1950.
4. Zloch: Internat. J. Vit. Res., *39*, 269, 1969.
5. Smyth, Lambert, and Martin: Proc. Soc. Exp. Biol. & Med., *116*, 593, 1964.
6. Ratnoff: J. Lab. & Clin. Med., *63*, 359, 1964.
7. Bavetta *et al.*:   Am. J. Phys., *206*, 179, 1964.
8. Schweppe, Lindberg, and Barker: Am. Heart J., *35*, 393, 1948.
9. Griffith, Krewson and Naghski: *Rutin and Related Flavonoids*, Easton, Pa., Mack Publishing Co., 1955.
10. Beardwood, Roberts and Trueman: Proc. Am. Diabetes Assoc., *8*, 243, 1948.
11. Shils and Goodhart: *The Flavonoids in Biology and Medicine*, Nutrition Monograph Series No. 2, The National Vitamin Foundation, Inc., New York, 1956.

Choline

Choline is the basic constituent of lecithin and sphingomyelin, the precursor of acetylcholine, an important methyl donor in metabolic processes and an essential nutrient for rats, chicks, turkeys, and other beasts.   Deficiency of choline produces both renal and hepatic disorders in the rat, but it has never been shown to be associated with a specific deficiency disease in man. It has been used all over the world to treat cirrhosis, hepatitis, and fatty liver. Yet there are no data in the literature which demonstrate conclusively that it has therapeutic value. The role of choline and of methyl groups in nutrition has been reviewed by Griffith and Dyer[1] and in a Nutrition Society Symposium published in the Federation Proceedings, *30*, 130–176, 1971, the "Evolution of Present Concepts Concerning The Action of Lipotropic Agents."

STRUCTURE, ANALYSIS AND METABOLISM

Choline was first isolated from the bile by Strecker in 1862. Its chemical name is (β-hydroxyethyl)trimethylammonium hydroxide, and it is widely distributed in nature.

$$(CH_3)_3N \cdot CH_2CH_2OH$$
$$|$$
$$OH$$

Choline

The chemical methods used for estimation of choline rely on its ability to form a colored reineckate salt, soluble in acetone. Ackerman and Salmon[2] have reported an improved method in which preliminary extraction is replaced by hydrolysis with 25 per cent nitric acid. Ackerman and Chou[3] further improved upon its sensitivity by photometric determination of the choline reineckate in alkaline solution at 303 mμ. Microbiologic assays can also be used to measure choline by studying the growth of a mutant strain of *Neurospora crassa*. A fluorometric assay, dependent upon enzymatically coupling choline phosphorylation to the oxidation of niacinamide adenine dinucleotide, has also been reported.[4]

Large amounts of choline are present in most foods consumed by man—especially egg yolks (1.7 gm/100 gm), meat (600 mg/100 gm), fish (200 mg/100 gm), and cereals and cereal products (100 mg/100 gm). Most fruits and soft vegetables contain little or no choline, but quite large amounts are present in legumes.

In the 1930's Best and his colleagues[5-8] began to study the genesis of the fatty livers which developed in dogs made diabetic after pancreatectomy. Eventually they were able to show that choline or betaine prevented the deposition of fat in rats fed diets which were high in beef fat or cholesterol or sucrose. Later it became evident that, in rats, diets deficient in choline produced fatty livers. Hemorrhagic renal lesions which were made worse by pyridoxine were also observed to develop. Other abnormalities which appeared were cirrhosis; anemia; atrophy of the thymus; enlargement of the adrenal cortex, and hypertension. Hamsters, pigs, dogs and chickens[9] also develop fatty livers when placed on choline-deficient diets. Chickens and turkeys also develop perosis.

In 1937, Tucker and Eckstein[10] showed that methionine could cure the fatty livers of rats fed diets deficient in choline. This lipotropic effect was not shared by the closely allied, sulfur-containing amino acids, cysteine and homocysteine. These results indicated that the action of methionine was due to the presence in the molecule of a labile methyl group which was not present in the other two amino acids. Later, Du Vigneaud[11-13] showed that one of the functions of the labile methyl group of methionine was to make possible the synthesis of choline by the body. Out of this work arose his concept of transmethylation reactions, now known to be of considerable importance in metabolic reactions. It soon became apparent that a number of substances exist which are capable of donating a methyl group to acceptor compounds. Examples of such reactions are the formation of creatine and choline from methionine, and of N^1-methylnicotinamide from niacin.

In addition to its role in N-methyltransferase reactions, choline and metabolic products derived from it are involved in the cytidinediphosphocholine:diglyceride cholinephosphotransferase system. Both of these enzyme systems are involved in the synthesis of lecithin. Fewster, Nyc and Griffith[14] have presented evidence that the turnover of fatty acids in phospholipids may be involved in the development of the hemorrhagic kidney of choline deficiency. French[15] found that rats fed ethanol while deficient in choline had more marked fatty changes in the liver than did animals given the choline-deficient diet only. There is some evidence of an increased need for choline at a higher environmental temperature and a reduced need at lower temperatures.[16]

A dietary deficiency of choline can be largely, if not completely, alleviated by providing in the diet sources of labile methyl groups such as betaine or methionine, which permit choline synthesis in the body. Also, choline deficiency is made less severe if folic acid and vitamin B_{12}, which are involved in the synthesis of ethanolamine and methyl groups, are included in the diet.[17,18] Guinea pigs, like the chick and unlike the rat, are unable to methylate ethanolamine directly.[1] Betaine can replace that aspect of the function of vitamin B_{12} which is concerned with the synthesis de novo of methyl groups.[19]

Although labile methyl groups are made available to the body by the consumption of foods containing methionine, choline, betaine and other allied substances, present data indicate that labile methyl groups are also synthesized in the body by fragmentation of large organic molecules, such as dimethyl glycine, to synthetically useful single carbon fragments.[20] The discovery of "active formaldehyde" and of a one-carbon cycle which can synthesize choline in the body casts further doubts on the concept of Sure[21] and others that choline should be regarded as a member of the B-complex vitamins.

BIBLIOGRAPHY

1. Griffith and Dyer: Nutrition Reviews, *26*, 1, 1968.
2. Ackerman and Salmon: Anal. Biochem., *1*, 327, 1960.
3. Ackerman and Chou: Anal. Biochem., *1*, 337, 1960.
4. Browning: Fed. Proc., *30*, 271 Abs., 1971.
5. Best and Huntsman: J. Physiol., *75*, 405, 1932.
6. Best and Ridout: J. Physiol., *78*, 415, 1933.
7. Best, Channon, and Ridout: J. Physiol., *81*, 409, 1934.
8. Best and Huntsman: J. Physiol., *83*, 255, 1935.
9. Couch and Smith: Fed. Proc., *30*, 522 Abs., 1971.
10. Tucker and Eckstein: J. Biol. Chem., *121*, 479, 1937.
11. Du Vigneaud, Dyer, and Kies: J. Biol. Chem., *130*, 325, 1939.
12. Du Vigneaud, Chandler, Moyer, and Keppel: J. Biol. Chem., *131*, 57, 1939.
13. Du Vigneaud: Harvey Lecture, *38*, 39, 1942–43.
14. Fewster, Nyc and Griffith: J. Nutrition, *90*, 252, 1966.
15. French: J. Nutrition, *88*, 291, 1966.
16. Anon: Nutrition Rev., *24*, 335, 1966.
17. Hegsted, Roach and McCombs: J. Nutrition, *92*, 403, 1967.
18. György, Langer, Hirooka, Cardi, Ehrich and Goldblatt: J. Nutrition, *92*, 443, 1967.
19. Young, Lucas, Patterson and Best: J. Biol. Chem., *224*, 341, 1957.
20. Symposium on the Mode of Action of Lipotropic Factors in Nutrition: Am. J. Clin. Nutrit., *6*, 197–331, 1958.
21. Sure: J. Nutrition, *19*, 71, 1940.

Inositol

More than 100 years ago Scherrer[1] found that patients with diabetes, unlike healthy individuals, excreted large quantities of inositol in the urine. Unfortunately, despite this significant finding and despite the fact that it is an essential nutrient for yeasts and rodents, little is known about its metabolism or biologic functions in man.

STRUCTURE, ANALYSIS, AND PRESENCE IN BIOLOGIC MATERIALS

Theoretically there are 9 possible isomers of inositol, but the only one with any biologic or nutritional action is "meso-inositol" (muscle sugar or myo-inositol) which is configuratively related to d-glucose.

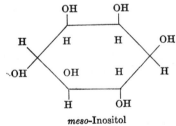

meso-Inositol

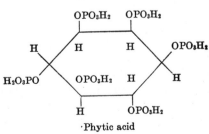

·Phytic acid

It occurs widely in bacteria, yeasts, fruits, plants, and grains. In the latter especially, it occurs as phytic acid, a substance which Mellanby showed many years ago could form stable, unabsorbable calcium salts in the gastrointestinal tracts of mammals and which he believed contributed to the production of rickets in children living on marginal diets high in roughly milled grains.

In 1940 Rapoport[15] found appreciable amounts in chicken and turtle erythrocytes; however, since then, meso-inositol has been isolated from many animal tissues. In 1947 Sonne and Sobotka[16] established the range in fresh, normal, human plasma to be from 0.37 to 0.76 mg/100 ml blood. Slightly higher figures were obtained from pooled plasma. With regard to tissues, Woolley[17] determined free and combined inositol in a variety of organs and dejecta of animals. Large amounts were found in heart muscle (1.6 gm/100 gm), in brain (0.9 gm/100 gm), and in skeletal muscle (0.4 gm/100 gm). It is present in animal tissues largely as the phospholipid, but also as part of more complex water-soluble compounds, as the free form, and in an unidentified complex not readily extracted by repeated treatments with fat solvents and with water.[18] Analyses of inositol by gravimetric or volumetric techniques are tedious and inexact. At present, most analyses are done by specific microbiologic assay, using yeast growth. Details can be found in György's book on vitamin analysis.[19]

BIOLOGIC SIGNIFICANCE AND METABOLISM OF INOSITOL

While the biologic significance of inositol is almost totally unknown, its ubiquitous occurrence in nature, its synthesis in the body, and its presence in large amounts in the heart, brain, and skeletal muscle suggest that it must have some function.

Woolley[2,3] demonstrated that meso-inositol cured alopecia in mice living on deficient diets. The anti-alopecia effects of meso-inositol were specific, and other isomers of inositol were not effective. Later it was shown to cure dietary alopecia in rats. Eagle[4] and his co-workers found *myo*-inositol to be an essential growth factor for the *in vitro* survival and multiplication of all eighteen normal and malignant human cell lines examined by them and for one of two mouse lines. Charalampous, Wahl and Ferguson[5] have reported that inositol deficiency causes a marked decrease of the acid-soluble nucleotides and the ribonucleic acid of mammalian cells in tissue culture. Lembach and Charalampous[6] found that the inability of inositol-deficient KB cells to synthesize nucleotides and RNA at a normal rate precedes all other observed changes and suggest that "observed changes in the levels of various enzymes could reflect the derangement of regulatory mechanisms which, in the normal cell, control the turnover rates of these enzymes in relation to the pace of cell multiplication." Charalampous has further reported that one of the earliest manifestations of inositol deprivation (*in vitro*, in KB cells) is impairment of plasma membrane functions concerned with concentrative amino acid transport and the translocation of K^+ and Na^+.[20,21]

The interrelationship with p-aminobenzoic acid was studied by Martin[7] who showed that the addition of inositol to diets of rats precipitated a syndrome which could be prevented by feeding p-aminobenzoic acid. Contrariwise, addition of p-aminobenzoic acid to the diets precipitated a syndrome which was prevented by feeding inositol. These phenomena were thought to be related to a reciprocal action by these substances on the synthesis of vitamins by intestinal bacteria.

McHenry and his colleagues suggested that inositol acts like lipocaic, since it prevented development of fatty liver caused by feeding biotin or beef liver extract to rats. This has been denied by a number of workers, including Best.[9] Anderson, Coots and Halliday[10] have failed to confirm the claim that inositol prevented the neuromuscular symptoms of scurvy and retarded the loss of ascorbic acid from the organs of guinea pigs on a scorbutigenic diet. Not only did they fail to detect any antiscorbutic effect of inositol, but they also confirmed the observation that the guinea pig does not require a dietary source of inositol.

The consumption of inositol by man is around 1 gm/day, but only a few mg appear in the urine. About 7 per cent of ingested inositol is converted to glucose: inositol is only one-third as effective as glucose in alleviating starvation ketosis. After inositol feeding there is an increase in its concentration in the body, but, when rats are kept on an inositol-free diet for as long as eight months, there is no decrease in the normal total body content of inositol, which remains constant at about 14 mg/100 gm tissue. Needham,[11] who did these experiments, deduced from the data that the body can synthesize inositol. Halliday and Anderson[12] have shown that the rat can synthesize sufficient inositol to meet its needs. By injecting glucose-l-^{14}C and recovering *myo*-inositol-^{14}C from the rat carcasses, they excluded bacterial synthesis in the intestine as a source of this inositol. Hauser and Finelli[13] demonstrated that slices of mammalian kidney, brain and liver, incubated with labeled glucose, were able to utilize glucose carbon for *myo*-inositol synthesis. Kidney incorporated the largest amount of radioactivity into free inositol.

Daughaday and his colleagues[14] studied inositol excretion in diabetes mellitus in man and rats. They found that in healthy men the average daily excretion was 37 mg/day, with a range of from 8 to 144 mg/day. This excretion of inositol was not affected by hydration or dehydration. Increased output of inositol could be produced by intravenous glucose feeding and also by the consumption of 3 gm of inositol per day. In healthy subjects the endogenous renal clearance of inositol was low, but, at high plasma levels resulting from infusions, its clearance rose to levels comparable to creatinine clearance. In 7 diabetic patients the average excretion was abnormally high, ranging from 280 to 850 mg/day. When these patients were treated with insulin, there was a sharp fall to normal levels (30 mg/day). Clearance studies with intravenous plasma loading were

found to be the same in diabetics as in non-diabetics. These findings indicate that inositol is filtered through the glomeruli and reabsorbed by the tubules. Presumably inositol competes with glucose for reabsorption by the tubular cells. In diabetes mellitus and during glycosuria resulting from intravenous infusions of glucose, the reabsorption mechanism for inositol is flooded by the tubular spate of glucose, and large amounts of inositol pass out of the body with the urine. Whether this is harmful is not known.

BIBLIOGRAPHY

1. Neukomm: *Ueber das Vorkommen von Leucin, Tyrosin und Andered Umsatzstoffe in Menschlichen Korper bei Krankheiten.* Zurich, Orell, Füssli u. Comp., 1859.
2. Woolley: J. Biol. Chem., *139*, 29, 1941.
3. ——: J. Biol. Chem., *140*, 461, 1941.
4. Eagle, Lyama, Levy and Freeman: J. Biol. Chem., *226*, 191, 1957.
5. Charalampous, Wahl and Ferguson: J. Biol. Chem., *236*, 2552, 1961.
6. Lembach and Charalampous: J. Biol. Chem., *241*, 395, 1966.
7. Martin: Amer. J. Physiol., *136*, 124, 1942.
8. Gavin and McHenry: J. Biol. Chem., *139*, 485, 1941.
9. Best: Fed. Proc., *9*, 506, 1950.
10. Anderson, Coots, and Halliday: J. Nutrition, *64*, 167, 1958.
11. Needham: Biochem. J., *18*, 891, 1924.
12. Halliday and Anderson: J. Biol. Chem., *217*, 797, 1955.
13. Hauser and Finelli: J. Biol. Chem., *238*, 3224, 1963.
14. Daughaday and Larner: J. Clin. Invest., *33*, 326, 1954.
15. Rapoport: J. Biol. Chem., *135*, 403, 1940.
16. Sonne and Sobotka: Arch. Biochem., *14*, 93, 1947.
17. Woolley: J. Nutrition, *28*, 305, 1944.
18. Anderson, Halliday and Coots: Fed. Proc., *14*, 173, 1955.
19. György (Editor): *Vitamin Methods*, New York, Academic Press, Inc., 1950.
20. Charalampous: J. Biol. Chem., *246*, 455, 1971.
21. Charalampous: J. Biol. Chem., *246*, 461, 1971.

Carnitine (Vitamin B$_T$) Metabolism

In 1947, Fraenkel, while investigating folic acid in the nutrition of insects, found that the meal worm (*Tenebrio molitor*) required a factor, present in the charcoal filtrate of yeast, which had not previously been recognized.[1] To this factor he gave the name "Vitamin

B$_T$." If the meal worms were fed on a synthetic diet deficient only in vitamin B$_T$, they died in 4 to 5 weeks. If this factor was added to the diet in very small amounts, they grew normally. So constant was this finding that he was able to develop a technique for bioassay of vitamin B$_T$ based on the rate of growth of larvae of *Tenebrio molitor*.[2] Using this technique, he found there was a wide distribution of vitamin B$_T$ in yeast, milk, liver, and whey, with particularly large quantities in muscle and meat extracts,[3] which since have proven to be the most potent natural sources of vitamin B$_T$. Although other insects, such as *Palorus ratseburgi*, could not synthesize vitamin B$_T$, Fraenkel and his co-workers found that most insects they studied, as well as higher animals, synthesized the vitamin in their tissues. For example, he found that hen's eggs contained little or no vitamin B$_T$, but substantial amounts occurred in the chicken embryo.

Fraenkel concentrated large amounts of crystalline vitamin B$_T$ in 1948. In studies with Carter,[4] he proved that vitamin B$_T$ was identical with carnitine, a quaternary ammonium compound, which had been discovered in muscle, in 1905, by Gulewitsch and Krimberg.[5] Carnitine is beta-hydroxy-gamma-trimethylaminobutyrate[6] and its formula is

$$\text{OH}$$
$$|$$
$$(CH_2)_3N \cdot CH_2 \cdot CH \cdot CH_2 \cdot COOH$$

Up until Fraenkel's discovery, the most intensive and valuable work on carnitine was done by Strack[7,8,9] between 1935 and 1937. In studies on muscles from cattle and dogs, he found he could not isolate or detect choline or acetylcholine by either chemical or biologic methods. However, he found that the carnitine content of bovine muscle varied between 0.02 and 0.2 per cent. Although the isolation procedure was cumbersome he was able to obtain a pure substance which was a quaternary ammonium compound. He then investigated its chemical properties and from biologic experiments, consisting mainly of perfusion of smooth and striated muscle strips, suggested that carnitine might take the place of choline in the metabolism of muscle.

The importance of creatinine, creatine, and phosphocreatine in the metabolism of muscle is well known. In 1941, Du Vigneaud[10] found that the labile methyl group of methionine was required for the synthesis of creatine from arginine and glycine. More recent work has shown that in the presence of homocysteine the labile methyl groups of choline and betaine can also be used in the synthesis of creatine from its precursor amino acids. The similarity between betaine and carnitine is apparent in Figure 5M-2 and indicates that one metabolic function of carnitine may be that of methyl donation. That this might be true is suggested by the fact that beta-hydroxy-gamma-aminobutyric acid can replace carnitine in the diet of *Tenebrio molitor*, but crotonobetaine and similar compounds are not able to do so. Data have been presented also suggesting the possibility that carnitine in muscle in some manner serves the function of facilitating fatty acid transfer from blood

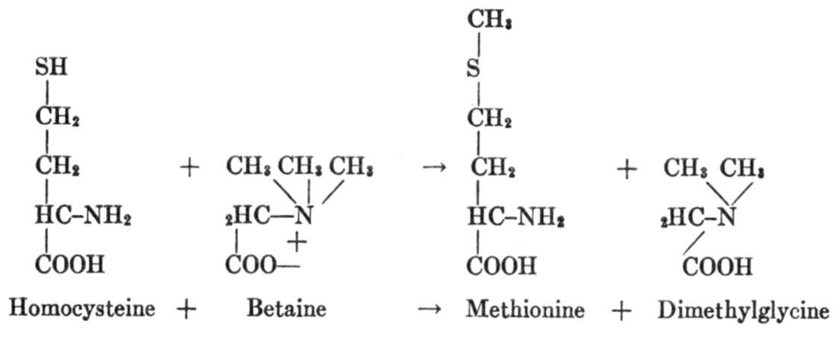

Fig. 5M-2. Methyl donation by betaine. This substance is very similar in structure to carnitine, and presumably carnitine could replace betaine in the above formula to act as a methyl donor in muscle.

vessels to the active sites of fatty acid oxidation within the muscle cells.[12]

Bremer[13] has suggested that carnitine functions as a carrier of active acetyl groups through the mitochondrial membrane and has shown that fatty acyl carnitines represent activated fatty acids that are efficiently utilized by mitochondria from several tissues of the rat. Snoswell and Henderson[14] and Yates and Garland[15] have found that carnitine stimulates the oxidation of long-chain fatty acids. Bressler and Katz[16] have presented data suggesting that carnitine plays a central role in acetoacetate production and long-chain fatty acid synthesis. These workers[17] have reported that the stimulatory effect of carnitine was seen only with those substrates which gave rise to acetyl CoA within the mitochondria. Bressler and Brendel[18] have suggested that carnitine and acetyl CoA-carnitine acyltransferase play an important role in the translocation of acetyl CoA for biologic acetylations, rather than for fatty acid synthesis. Khairallah and Wolf[19] found that, in rats, carnitine has a methionine-sparing action and may thus be considered a food factor required in marginal diets.

The original efforts to study carnitine metabolism in man, and especially in patients with muscular and nutritional diseases, were hampered by methodologic difficulties. Fraenkel, using the bioassay technique mentioned above, had found that in mammals the carnitine content of skeletal muscle was 1 mg/gm dry weight; of heart muscle, 560 mcg/gm; of kidney, 412 mcg/gm and of liver, 280 mcg/gm. Small amounts were present in the blood (7 to 14 mcg/ml), while the 24-hour urine contained 50 to 100 mcg/ml. In animal studies, the urine content of carnitine increased on a high-protein diet and was reduced during starvation and by consumption of a low-protein diet.

Early in 1954, Ansell et al.[11] developed a chemical method for the measurement of carnitine in small amounts of body tissue and fluids. This is based on the degradation of carnitine to trimethylamine by heat in the presence of a strong alkali. In healthy individuals, the range for serum and plasma was found to lie between 860 and 1330 mcg/100 ml, and the urinary excretion ranged from 80 to 130 mg/24 hours. Muscle obtained either through biopsy or at autopsy contained 800 to 2000 mg/gm dry weight. These results compare favorably with those of Fraenkel's bioassay data. Using their carnitine acetyltransferase assay method, Marquis and Fritz[20,21] found spermatozoa (rat) to have the highest specific activities of transferase thus far observed in tissues. They reported that both testosterone and a source of sperm cells were required to maintain high carnitine acetyltransferase levels in epididymal tissue, while only androgens were required to maintain maximal carnitine concentrations in this tissue.

Studies of healthy individuals consuming fixed diets in a metabolic unit[9] indicate that fluctuations of carnitine excretion and of blood levels in man are related to the carnitine content of the diet. On diets low in carnitine or on protein-free diets (which were also very low in carnitine) the urinary excretion fell to 70 mg/24 hours, while it rose to 200 mg/24 hours with high-protein (high carnitine) diets. When the protein content of the diet was reduced from 190 to 153 gm/day, the urinary excretion of carnitine fell from approximately 200 to 150 mg/24 hours. The serum carnitine levels also changed with the dietary intake of protein (and of carnitine), so that high levels were found when large amounts of carnitine were excreted in the urine, and vice versa.

From the data available, there seems to be, in health, a close parallelism between creatinine and creatine excretion and carnitine excretion.

BIBLIOGRAPHY

1. Fraenkel: Nature, *161*, 891, 1948.
2. ———: Fed. Proc. *10*, 183, 1951.
3. ———: Arch. Biochem., *34*, 457, 1951.
4a.———: Arch. Biochem., *34*, 468, 1951.
4b.Carter, Bhattacharyya and Fraenkel: Fed. Proc., *10*, 170, 1951.
4c.———: Arch. Biochem. Biophys., *35*, 241, 1952.
4d.Carter, Bhattacharyya, Weidman and Fraenkel: Arch. Biochem. Biophys., *38*, 405, 1952.
5. Gulewitsch and Krimberg: Ztschr. f. Physiol. Chem., *45*, 326, 1905.
6. Olson: Ann. Rev. Biochem., *35*, 579, 1966.
7. Strack, Wordehoff, Neubaur and Geisendorfur: Ztschr. Physiol. Chem., *233*, 189, 1935.

8. Strack and Schwaneberg: Ztschr. f. Physiol. Chem., *245*, 11, 1939.
9. Strack and Forsterling: Arch. f. Exper. Path. U. Pharmakol., *185*, 612, 1937.
10 Du Vigneaud: *A Trail of Research in Sulfur Chemistry and Metabolism and Rel. Fields,* Ithaca, Cornell University Press, 1952.
11. Ansell, Bhattacharyya, Rix and Kark: Clin. Research Proc., *2*, 79, 1954.
12. Fritz and McEwen: Science, *129*, 334, 1959.
13. Bremer: J. Biol. Chem., *237*, 3628, 1962.
14. Snoswell and Henderson: Biochem. J., *119*, 59, 1970.
15. Yates and Garland: Biochem. J., *119*, 547, 1970.
16. Bressler and Katz: J. Biol. Chem., *240*, 622, 1965.
17. ———: J. Clin. Invest., *44*, 840, 1965.
18. Bressler and Brendel: J. Biol. Chem., *241*, 4092, 1966.
19. Khairallah and Wolf: J. Nutrition, *87*, 469, 1965.
20. Marquis and Fritz: J. Biol. Chem., *240*, 2193, 1965.
21. ———: J. Biol. Chem., *240*, 2197, 1965.

Chapter

6

Major Minerals

Section A   Calcium and Phosphorus

D. M. HEGSTED

Calcium and phosphorus are considered together since they constitute the major part of the mineral content of the skeleton. Over 99 per cent of the total body calcium and approximately 80 per cent of the phosphorus are in the bones. The ratio of calcium to phosphorus in the bone is a little over 2:1 and is approximately constant. Thus, marked changes in the body content of one of these minerals will be reflected in changes in the other.

Many phosphorus compounds occur in the body and phosphorylated compounds are involved in a large number of metabolic pathways. No attempt is made in this chapter to discuss these functions of phosphorus since they are considered in standard textbooks of biochemistry. Attention is directed primarily toward the nutritional requirement of calcium and phosphorus and, since phosphorus is ordinarily considered to occur in adequate amounts in most diets consumed by man, primary discussion is given to calcium requirements. It is remarkable that in spite of the prominence given to calcium in the nutrition literature there is much argument as to the nutritional significance of calcium in most diets. Increasing knowledge has served primarily to emphasize how little is known of calcium requirements and the need for additional criteria to estimate requirements and the adequacy of calcium intakes.

THE BONE MINERAL

It is now generally agreed that the bone salt belongs to a class of minerals called apatites. It is primarily hydroxyapatite which has the composition $Ca_{10}(PO_4)_6(OH)_2$.[1] Most of the apatites form very small or poorly formed crystals which are not well suited for crystallographic study. Thus, much of the data on the bone salt is based upon fluoro-apatite which does occur in well-formed crystals. Ions of similar size are to a variable degree interchangeable in the crystal lattice, fluoride for hydroxyl or strontium for calcium, as examples. Also, the enormous surface area exposed by the small crystals permits extensive adsorption of materials on the surface of the crystals. Bone also contains considerable water.[2] Much of this simply fills the open spaces in the bone and presumably has a composition similar to that of the extracellular fluid. The remainder is tightly bound to the crystals, the so-called "hydration shell." Apparently, only certain ions can enter the hydration shell.[1] Thus, bone always contains a large variety of materials other than those which compose hydroxyapatite. It is difficult if not impossible to determine just where they occur and the extent to which they should be considered a part of the bone mineral or simply as contaminants derived from the extracellular fluid.

It should be noted, however, that the amounts of some of the constituents which are not considered an integral part of the bone mineral are, nevertheless, important. It has been estimated that as much as 60 per cent of the total body magnesium, 25 per cent of the sodium, 80 per cent of the carbonate, and 90 per cent of the citrate may occur in bone[2] and will depend in part upon the nature of the diet. Bone formed with a normal magnesium content, for example, may provide a considerable reserve in time of need, whereas if the bone were formed with limited magnesium, much less would be available.[3] The so-called "bone-seeking elements" such as strontium, lead, radium, uranium, etc. are selectively concentrated in bone. Depending upon the ion, these may replace calcium in the crystal lattice, adsorbed on the surface or present in the hydration shell.[1]

It is clear that the bone serves as a large reserve of buffer. Sodium, magnesium, and carbonate can contribute to the regulation of acid-base balance, and if the bone crystals are sacrificed, phosphate is made available to neutralize hydrogen ions. Acidosis is associated with an increased excretion of urinary calcium and phosphate[4,5] indicating that bone mineral has indeed been mobilized. The mechanisms by which this is achieved, however, are unclear.

BONE FORMATION

The formation of bone and the factors which control its formation and dissolution are only partially understood. For many years[6] it was thought that the extracellular fluid was slightly undersaturated with respect to bone mineral. It was suggested that phosphatase, acting upon some unknown phosphate ester, might elevate the phosphate concentration so that precipitation of a calcium-phosphate salt could occur. However, it is now concluded[1] that normal serum is supersaturated with respect to bone mineral and thus the fluid bathing the crystals cannot have the composition of the extracellular fluid. The bone mineral does not have a fixed solubility product and formation or dissolution of bone cannot be related to the concentrations of calcium and phosphate alone.

Bone is formed by osteoblasts and removed by osteoclasts. These cells form a lining over the bone surface. Thus, although physical-chemical laws obviously hold, it is presumably the local environment controlled by these cells which is responsible for the formation, maintenance and dissolution of bone. What has to be explained eventually is why

bone is continually being formed at many sites and removed at others, both at varying rates depending upon many nutritional, hormonal or other factors. Although calcium and phosphorus are required for the formation of bone, illogical conclusions are drawn from attempting to view bone as the net result of mass effects of the concentration of calcium and phosphate in the serum or from intakes of calcium and phosphorus.

Bone is formed on an organic matrix. The collagen fibers appear to be responsible for the initial seeding.[7] Whatever the original precipiate may be, it is hydrolyzed to form hydroxyapatite. The mineral of young bone contains much more amorphous material which becomes more crystalline as the bone matures. The incorporation of appropriate amounts of fluoride in the bone increases the size of the crystals.[8] These larger crystals with less surface area are thought to be more resistant to erosion and may explain the well-known effect of fluoride in producing a tooth mineral more resistant to dental caries.

There have been many efforts to measure the rates of bone formation through the use of radioisotopes, especially ^{45}Ca and ^{47}Ca. The early studies were misinterpreted since the deposition of the radioisotope in the bone was equated with bone formation. As has already been explained, much of the isotope which appears in the bone does so by adsorption on the surface, by exchange with non-labeled calcium on the surface of the crystal and through recrystalization and diffusion into the crystals. All of these occur without a net increase in the bone or actual formation of new bone salt. The problem, of course, is to distinguish these processes from actual bone formation.

Theoretically, at least, it should be possible from a kinetic analysis of the rate of change of the specific activity of the serum calcium after the injection of an isotope, together with metabolic balance data, to estimate the rates of ebb and flow of calcium into different parts of the body compartments and the rates of bone formation and bone resorption. Figure 6A–1, slightly modified from Heaney,[9] indicates some of the compartments which become labeled and estimates of their size. Within a few minutes to a few hours the

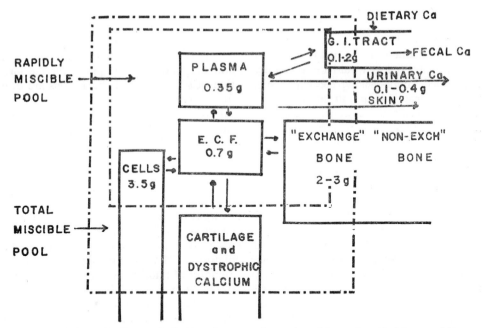

Fig. 6A-1. Schematic diagram indicating the approximate size of the various "calcium pools" and routes of calcium exchange. Modified from Heaney.[9]

"rapidly miscible pool" becomes labeled and additional compartments are labeled as time proceeds. Since the total body calcium of an adult is of the order of a kilogram or so, most of the calcium in the body is in relatively inert parts of the skeleton which are not labeled. Although the concepts of a "rapidly miscible pool" and a "total miscible pool" are useful, it will be apparent that these are not well-defined entities. Rather, there is nearly a gradient of "pools" which come into equilibrium with the extracellular fluid at varying rates. The rates of exchange presumably depend largely upon the degree of exposure to the extracellular fluid.

The figure indicates that some 100 to 200 mg of calcium are secreted into the gut daily where they will partially mix with the calcium of dietary origin. Some will be excreted, some will be reabsorbed. The amount which is reabsorbed will depend in part upon the amount of calcium in the diet and the efficiency with which it is absorbed. It will presumably be affected by the level at which the calcium enters the gut. If it enters the gut at a high level, it will presumably mix more thoroughly with the calcium in the

food than it will if it enters the gut at a lower level. Whether more or less will be reabsorbed will probably depend upon the level of dietary calcium. These kinds of uncertainties emphasize the difficulties of deriving absolute data on the rates of bone accretion or dissolution, especially if it be noted that the amount of calcium flux into and from the gut of endogenous origin may be of the same order as the amount entering new bone.

Obviously, the interpretation of the kinetic data is complex and difficult. The results may depend primarily upon the model used and the assumptions which have, of necessity, to be made.[9-12] It should also be recognized that, at best, the estimates represent an overall average which encompasses substantially different rates in different parts of the skeleton. There is also serious question as to whether "exchange" can be distinguished from "formation." In diseases such as osteomalacia, where histological evidence indicates very little bone formation, the rate of disappearance of the isotopes from the serum is high, suggesting increased rates of bone formation.

In young animals it has been estimated

that the "exchangeable fraction" of the body calcium may be about 5 per cent of the total calcium and that this is substantially decreased in older animals.[1] Also, calcium deficiency appears to increase the exchangeable fraction. This would appear to be an adaptive response to make the utilization of calcium more efficient and may be achieved by increasing the surface area exposed to the extracellular fluid. Similar responses may occur in various diseases and may not be distinguishable from increased rates of true bone formation.

HORMONAL INFLUENCES

Parathyroid Hormone. The central role of the parathyroid hormone on calcium metabolism has long been recognized but the exact mechanisms involved are still the subject of research and debate. As has already been indicated, the bone is viewed increasingly as a vital tissue rather than as a mass of mineral under the influence of physical-chemical laws. The metabolism of bone is controlled by the osteocytes, osteoblasts and osteoclasts—the metabolism of which is under hormonal control. Earlier theories[13] assigned a primary role of the parathyroid hormone to increasing the excretion of urinary phosphate, the mobilization of bone being secondary to this effect. It is now generally agreed that parathormone acts directly upon bone maintaining serum calcium levels at the expense of bone. Although the voluminous literature and conflicting opinions on this hormone cannot be reviewed here, in a recent summary Talmage et al.[14] propose that the primary function is to enhance the entry of calcium into cells. This is presumed to have two somewhat divergent effects. By increasing the intracellular calcium, the hormone stimulates the transcellular movement of calcium in various target cells. In the gut it would aid in the absorption of calcium, in the kidney the transport from lumen to extracellular fluid, and in the bone cells the movement of calcium from the bone to extracellular fluid and thus maintain the calcium level of the extracellular fluid. The second effect proposed for an increased level of cellular calcium, in bone cells only, is a

stimulation of various metabolic activities including mitotic activity, changes in RNA synthesis, suppression of collagen synthesis, increased organic acid production and stimulation of lysosomal activities. These changes would mediate and reflect the influence of parathormone on bone remodeling and the classic effects of the hormone on bone formation and resorption. Thus, Talmage et al. postulate that the increase in the number and activity of the osteoclasts which results from parathormone administration is mediated through the change in intracellular calcium.

Calcitonin. For many years it was held that variation in the secretion of parathyroid hormone, controlled by feedback regulation, was responsible for the precision with which plasma calcium is regulated. The experimental evidence supporting the conclusion was relatively weak and, in perfusion studies of the thyroid-parathyroid with solutions of varying calcium content, Copp et al.[15] concluded that it was necessary to postulate the existence of a new hormone which lowered serum calcium, to account for the results obtained. The hormone, calcitonin,[16,17] is formed by the thyroid gland apparently by the C cells of ultimobranchial origin. In contrast to the parathyroid hormone, its secretion is stimulated by elevation of the plasma calcium level and injections of calcitonin cause a rapid lowering of the plasma calcium and phosphorus. The lowering of these levels might be achieved either by stimulating the return of the minerals to bone or by diminishing loss of mineral from bone. Since in bone culture and in in vivo studies the loss of hydroxyproline is diminished (a measure of breakdown of bone matrix) by calcitonin, it is concluded that the action of the hormone is to diminish bone resorption. Thus, in many ways, the overall effects of calcitonin appear to be the reverse of those of the parathyroid hormone.

FUNCTIONS OF CALCIUM OTHER THAN IN BONE FORMATION

The level of calcium in the blood serum is maintained with rather remarkable precision, considering the large content of the bones, and is ordinarily about 10 mg/100 ml. This is presumably achieved primarily by the effects of the parathyroid hormone and calcitonin on bone. As will be evident later, there is control over absorption from the gut. Markedly different intakes usually have, at most, only transient effects upon the level of circulating calcium.

Approximately 60 per cent of the calcium in the serum is ionized, a very small amount chelated with materials such as citrate, and the remainder bound to serum proteins. The calcium proteinate acts as a weak electrolyte and dissociation approximates the mass law equation[18]

$$\frac{(Ca^{++}) \times (Protein^{--})}{Ca\ Proteinate} = K$$

which is affected also by the pH. The level of ionized calcium is important in the maintenance of the functional integrity of many cells, especially the normal neuromuscular irritability. Any substantial decrease results in tetany while an increase may lead to respiratory or cardiac failure.[19]

Calcium is involved in the clotting of blood and has been shown to activate several enzymes such as adenosine triphosphatase, succinic dehydrogenase, etc. The integrity of the intracellular cement substance and of various membranes is apparently dependent upon the presence of calcium. Although these and other functions of calcium are extremely important in the overall economy of the body, they are rarely influenced by the level of intake. Thus, they are not considered in any detail here.

It has been reported that the level of serum calcium in the Bantu, who consume diets relatively low in calcium, may be approximately 1 mg lower than that usually considered normal.[20] If so, the significance is unknown and has apparently not been reported in other populations who consume similarly low levels of calcium.

Urinary Calcium. The amount of calcium excreted in the urine varies rather widely between individuals but appears to be relatively constant for an individual. Knapp[21] concluded from data collected on over 600

individuals that "the quantity of urine calcium is dependent upon an endogenous factor or factors, presumably endocrine, and to a lesser extent upon the intake of calcium." Values for a 70-kg man with an intake of approximately 700 mg of calcium per day ranged from 85 to 420 mg/day, with an average value of 175 mg/day. In Peruvians accustomed to low calcium intakes, Hegsted et al.[22] observed a mean increase of about 100 mg/day in the urine when the intake was raised approximately 500 mg/day. Malm[23] studied 22 men at intakes of 940 mg/day and 463 mg/day. The mean urinary calcium fell only 30 mg/day, an insignificant change. In 20 men adapted to the lower level of intake, the mean urinary calcium was $200 \doteq 10$ mg/day and, on the high intake, $210 \doteq 13$ mg/day.

Assuming that 90 liters of plasma containing 5 mg of Ca^{++}/100 ml are filtered by the glomerular apparatus each day, some 4.5 gm of calcium are available for excretion by the kidney. The efficiency of the conservation of calcium by the kidney is apparent. It is perhaps remarkable that there is any relationship between intake and urinary excretion. Soluble forms of non-ionized calcium are largely excreted by the kidney as is shown by the administration of EDTA which chelates calcium. A better understanding of the nature of the non-ionized non-protein-bound calcium might provide an explanation of the factors controlling urinary excretion. The point to be made here, however, is that the measurement of urinary calcium appears to offer little as a means of evaluating calcium intake or nutritional status.

Fecal Calcium. The slight changes in urinary calcium associated with major changes in intake and the high correlation of fecal calcium with intake demonstrate that the gut must exercise considerable control over the absorption or excretion of calcium. Much of the fecal calcium represents unabsorbed dietary calcium. As has been indicated earlier, considerable calcium enters the gut from the extracellular fluid either by active secretion or passively with the digestive juices. Estimates of the amount have varied widely. Figure 6A–1 suggested values in the range of 100 to 200 mg/day but estimates based upon assumptions as to the amount and composition of gastrointestinal fluids have ranged as high as 1100 mg/day.[23] If one injects radio-calcium and assumes that the calcium entering the gut will have the same specific activity as that in the serum or urine; that it will mix thoroughly with the dietary calcium; and that it will be absorbed to the same extent as the dietary calcium, one can estimate the contribution of the endogenous calcium to the total fecal output and thus the total input into the gut. Various methods of estimating the endogenous excretion into the gut and the absorption of dietary calcium have been discussed by Lutwak.[24]

A particularly interesting experience was reported by Malm[23] which requires further documentation but may indicate the important role that the gut may play in the control over calcium hemostasis. One of the subjects on an intake of 574 mg of calcium per day was in positive balance of 60 mg/day over a 6-month period. During a 10-month period of increasing worry and stress, he was in negative balance, reaching at one point a net loss of over 900 mg/day and with a fecal excretion of 1250 mg/day—all at the same intake of 560 mg. The total fecal excretion was thus more than twice the dietary intake. With removal of the tension, the balance rapidly improved. If these data are a true representation, there must have been not only a very marked inhibition of absorption but also an outpouring of calcium into the gut. Others[25,26] have recorded unfavorable effects of emotional stress upon calcium balance.

CALCIUM ABSORPTION

In vitro studies with gut loops[27,28] have demonstrated that calcium is absorbed from the gut against a concentration gradient by an energy-requiring process, *i.e.*, there is an active transport of calcium. This is vitamin D dependent (see Chapter 5 Section B) and is most active in animals fed a low calcium diet. In the rat this active transport is found only in the first few centimeters of the duodenum and, strangely enough, is reported to occur in the lower end of the ileum in the hamster. Throughout the remainder of the intestine, calcium is apparently absorbed by passive diffusion which,

however, is also reported to be vitamin D dependent.[29] The uptake is a two-stage process involving uptake at the mucosal surface and transfer to or toward the serosal surface.[30] Apparently, the latter is rate-limiting, although both are vitamin D dependent. As already mentioned, the uptake is also dependent upon parathormone.

There is abundant evidence in animals and man that calcium absorption is dependent upon calcium needs or level in the diet. Efficiency improves with lower intakes or higher calcium needs. Just how this is achieved is unknown but it is possible that the active transport is a reserve mechanism which is called into more active play in time of need.

Much has been written about dietary factors which influence calcium absorption and which are demonstrable in animal studies and sometimes in man. High levels of phosphate, phytate and oxalate in the diet raise the level of fecal calcium and this is usually attributed to the fact that they may form insoluble salts which lower the concentration of ionizable calcium in the gut. Large amounts of phytates have been used therapeutically to inhibit calcium absorption in man.[31] However, it appears most likely that the effects in man are not of primary importance under usual conditions. Large doses of phosphates have been given without effect.[32] Walker *et al.*[33] observed that subjects fed diets high in whole wheat (which contains considerable amounts of phytate) were temporarily in negative balance but "adapted" to the diet and absorbed normal amounts of calcium within a short time. The FAO/WHO report[34] points out that some of the high vegetable diets consumed in various parts of the world contain sufficient phytate to precipitate all of the calcium in the diet, at least theoretically. Yet habitual consumers of such diets are not known to suffer from calcium deficiency. Studies with radiocalcium administered with whole cereals did not indicate marked effects upon calcium balance.[35]

The absorption of phosphorus present as phytate and possibly the release of calcium bound as calcium phytate present unsolved problems. Presumably, the enzyme phytase is required. Whether the enzyme is derived from dietary sources or is of endogenous origin and, indeed, its importance are not clearly known.

Oxalates form a very insoluble salt and can undoubtedly inhibit calcium absorption. Again, it appears that the level in human diets is rarely of real significance.

Severe depletion of the skeleton of mineral does occur in the steatorrheas. This is presumably explained by the formation of insoluble calcium soaps in the gut, in the presence of large amounts of free fatty acids, which are not utilizable. The possibility that there are other more direct effects upon calcium or bone metabolism cannot be entirely excluded.

The intestinal absorption of calcium is often depressed in patients with chronic renal insufficiency, which presumably explains the osteodystrophy which occurs with renal disease. The defect is resistant to vitamin D. Transport of calcium by the duodenum of rats made uremic is also impaired.[36] This defect was not reversed by physiologic doses of vitamin D but did respond to massive doses. Recent evidence indicates that 25-hydroxycholecalciferol must be hydroxylated by the kidney to the 1,25-dihydroxy compound before it can induce either calcium transport from the gut or mobilization of calcium from the bone. The lesion in uremia is presumably a failure to metabolize vitamin D to the active form.

There is evidence in experiments with animals that protein or certain amino acids, citric acid, and lactose may enhance calcium absorption. The lactose effect[37] is intriguing since this sugar occurs only in milk, a food presumably designed for young animals with a high calcium requirement. It has most often been explained[38] that lactose is relatively slowly absorbed and the free sugar in the lower gut may modify the flora and produce a lower pH in the gut, which is favorable for calcium absorption. There is, however, evidence that lactose may form a chelate of calcium,[39] which may protect it from precipitation or otherwise assist in absorption. Work[40] with intestinal segments in vitro also suggests that lactose may have effects distinct from glucose on calcium absorption.

Citrate and amino acids may also act by forming soluble chelates. Again, there is little evidence that indicates a major practical role of these factors in human nutrition as far as calcium absorption is concerned.

CALCIUM REQUIREMENTS

Determination. It must be emphasized that, in contrast to most essential nutrients, clear-cut calcium deficiency of dietary origin is unknown in man. Thus, it is not possible to estimate requirements from the level of dietary intake which cures or prevents deficiency. Because calcium intakes are generally higher in the developed countries than in the developing countries and stature is generally large in the affluent countries, there has been a general reluctance to accept the lower intakes as adequate. However, as will be apparent, there are as yet no definitive studies which associate health with the higher levels of intake.

Most evidence presumably related to calcium needs has been developed by calcium balance studies. Intake and excretion are measured and it is assumed that, in the adult whose skeleton has reached maximum size, the requirement will be that amount of intake which is equivalent to the excretion. However, because it is now clear that individuals can adapt to varying levels of intake, especially by varying the efficiency with which they absorb calcium, this seemingly straightforward approach is now subject to considerable doubt.

During growth, when new skeleton is being deposited, the intake must exceed the excretion, i.e., the balance must be positive. Relatively little direct data are available upon the body calcium content at various ages. Thus, indirect methods have been used to estimate the amount of calcium which should be deposited at various ages for the two sexes.

The Balance Method. It is worthwhile to discuss some of the difficulties in the determination of calcium balance since these appear not to be generally appreciated. At best, the calcium balance must be considered to yield relatively inaccurate values, since it represents the difference between two large values, the intake and the total excretion.

Modest errors in either the intake or excretion will produce large errors in the apparent retention or loss. There is reason to believe[41] that the usual error is to overestimate the intake (the subject may not consume all of the food placed before him) and to underestimate the excretion (failure to collect all of the excreta). Consider the following situation where the subject is in balance but it is assumed that the estimate of intake is 2 per cent too high and the estimated excretion 2 per cent too low.

	Intake mg	Excretion mg	Balance mg
Actual	400	400	0
Determined	408	392	+16
Actual	1500	1500	0
Determined	1530	1470	+60

In actual practice it would be difficult to limit errors to as small as 2 per cent. However, the point to be made is that, especially when intakes are high, apparently large retention values may be obtained, even when the determination is as accurate as at low intakes. A retention of 60 mg/day appears to be large, especially if it is calculated over any

extended period of time. In most studies the finding that the higher the intake is raised, the more positive the balance becomes indicates that there is a bias which leads to abnormal positive retentions. Furthermore, in animal studies,[42] where the animals have been killed for carcass analysis after an extended balance trial, the calcium which was presumably retained cannot be recovered in the carcass. Thus, it seems certain that in many studies the degree of positive balance is overestimated. Unfortunately, there is no independent method which permits an estimate of the accuracy of balance trials.

Requirements for Growth. Holmes[43] summarized most of the balance data on children of different ages which were available in 1945. Most of these studies, perhaps for the reasons just mentioned, yielded calcium retentions which appear too high, since reasonable estimates of skeletal size could not accommodate the calcium presumably being deposited. They do not appear to offer reasonable estimates of calcium needs of the growing child.

Since there are no analyses of normal bodies except of infants and a few adults, estimates of skeletal size must be derived in-

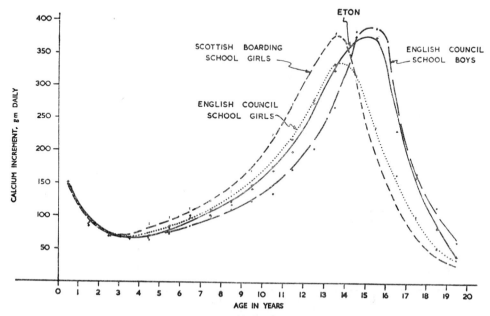

Fig. 6A-2. Estimates of daily increments in body calcium required for the growth of the skeleton derived by Leitch and Aitken.[44]

directly. Several estimates have been made based upon various assumptions as to how the skeleton grows relative to total body weight. The most recent of these by Leitch and Aitken[44] assumes that a normal infant contains about 28 gm of calcium (0.9 per cent calcium) and the adult body from 1.75 to 1.83 per cent calcium. Their estimates yield an eventual total calcium content of an adult male of about 1200 gm and about 1100 gm in the female. The increments required per day if the skeleton grows in proportion to body weight are shown for several English groups in Figure 6A–2. It must be recognized that there is no compelling reason to believe that growth of the skeleton and body weight does occur in parallel, but this is the simplest assumption that can be made.

A different approach has been used by Garn, in his recent book,[45] based upon measurements of the second metacarpal from x-rays pictures taken at intervals in a fairly large group of children in a longitudinal study and in cross-sectional data upon several populations. Total skeleton weights of a rather large number of normal men obtained from Korean War dead[46] yielded an average skeleton of 4290 gm. From measurements of the total width of the bone and the width of the medullary cavity, the volume of cortical bone in the second metacarpal was estimated. In the adult, the ratio—the volume of cortical bone in the metacarpal in mm^3 to total skeletal weight in gm—is estimated to be 0.969. Thus, the total weight of the skeleton at different ages was estimated, assuming that this ratio holds at all ages. It was further considered that the skeleton at all ages would contain 25 per cent calcium. The estimated weight of the skeleton throughout the life span of the two sexes thus derived is shown in Figure 6A–3. The daily incre-

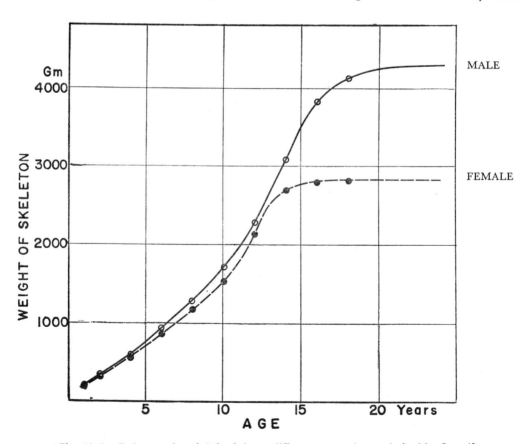

Fig. 6A-3. Estimates of total skeletal size at different ages and sexes derived by Garn.[45]

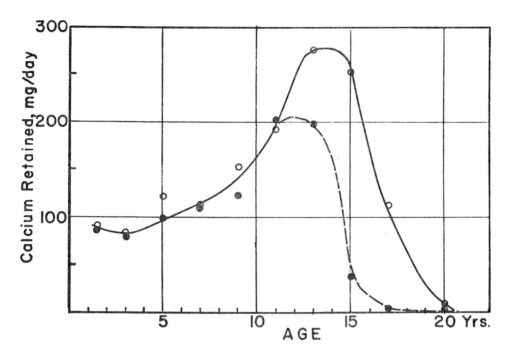

Fig. 6A-4. Daily increments in body calcium required to provide the skeletal sizes shown in Figure 6A-3.

ments in calcium required to form the skeleton are shown in Figure 6A-4. These values are substantially less than those derived by Leitch and Aitken[44] especially for females. The data of Garn may be considered to have a more factual basis than those based simply upon body weight.

These values must be considered as the approximate limits of the rate at which body calcium can be deposited at various ages. Thus, as already mentioned, apparent retentions[47] of 300 mg/day in children 3 to 4 years of age and as high as 800 mg in a 12-year-old must be considered erroneous, or values which could occur for only a limited period of time.

To convert estimates of calcium deposition into dietary needs, two factors must be considered: How much dietary calcium does it take to maintain the skeleton already present and how efficient is the dietary calcium utilized? Again, one is faced with either such limited or variable data that no definitive solutions are in sight.

In rapidly growing animals, such as the rat which has very high calcium requirements

relative to body weight, the maintenance requirement is so low that it cannot be measured. That is, when a low calcium diet is fed the urinary and fecal losses are essentially nil.[48] In young children the excretion of calcium may be also very low.[49] Thus, it is commonly held that there is no real maintenance need in children. Leitch and Aitken consider this somewhat unlikely for a normal child and suggest, from an inspection of the balance data available at different levels of intake, that one might allow 60 mg/day for young children, 160 mg/day for adolescents and 200 to 260 mg/day for adults.

Data upon the absorption of dietary calcium (dietary calcium not recovered in the feces) are also highly variable. Values in various experiments range upward to 70 per cent,[43,44] with many values in the range of 25 to 35 per cent absorption. As has already been indicated, there is abundant evidence that absorptive efficiency varies with calcium need. Indeed, if the estimates of Garn are approximately correct, the overall utilization of the high calcium diets ordinarily consumed by children in the United States must be between 10 and 25 per cent of that eaten. Most data upon efficiency of utilization must reflect the prior diet rather than an inherent limitation in ability to absorb calcium.

Studies on populations who ordinarily consumed lower levels of calcium should be instructive. Limited data indicate, as expected, that efficiency of utilization is indeed higher.[50-52] In addition, cross-sectional data from the Central American countries, in which relatively high levels of calcium intakes are consumed in the north—Guatemala and El Salvador—gradually decreasing toward the south with rather low levels being consumed in Panama, show no significant differences in the size of the second metacarpal which can be related to calcium intake.[45]

Requirements for Adults. The original estimates of calcium need in adults were based upon estimates of the amount of calcium re-

quired in the diet to achieve calcium balance. The literature was summarized by Mitchell and Curzon[53] who produced Figure 6A-5. From this figure it was concluded that approximately 10 mg of calcium/kg/day were required in the average adult to reach equilibrium, or about 0.7 gm/day for a 70-kg man. When similar studies were done with Peruvians[22] who were accustomed to relatively low calcium diets, much lower estimates were obtained. Figure 6A-6 compares the regression of excretion on intake for the data considered by Mitchell and Curzon and those obtained by Hegsted et al.[22] on Peruvians. These data confirm what is obvious on a priori grounds, namely, that people who live on relatively low calcium diets must adjust their metabolism so that balance is approximately achieved at the level they habitually consume. Thus, we reject calcium

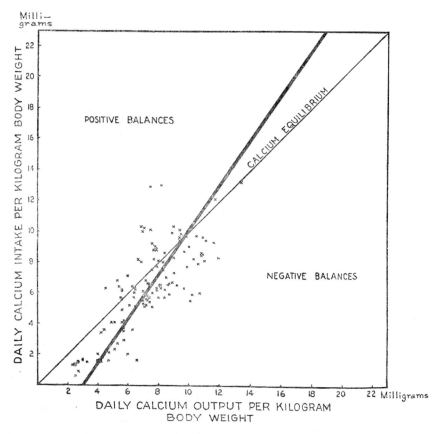

Fig. 6A-5. Calcium balance data summarized by Mitchell and Curzon.[53] The calcium requirement was estimated as the mean value at which intake is equal to excretion, approximately 10 mg/kg/day.

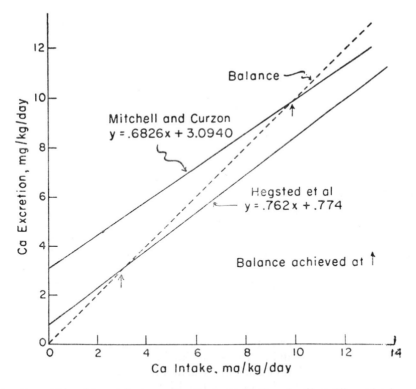

Fig. 6A-6. Comparison of the calcium excretion obtained with Peruvians[22] at different intakes with the data summarized by Mitchell and Curzon.[53]

balance data as an estimate of calcium need. Whether individuals "adapted" to a high calcium intake or a low calcium intake are in better health cannot be determined from balance data alone[54,55] (or indeed, as yet, from any other data). We would also emphasize that "adaptation" should not be considered as a requirement of those who consume low calcium diets. It is equally necessary for those who consume high calcium diets since, otherwise, excessive calcium would be absorbed.

Other than the probability that parathyroid hormone and calcitonin are involved, there are no indications as to how adaptation is achieved. Malm[23] studied 26 men at two levels of intake over rather long periods. When the diet was reduced to 450 mg of calcium per day after a period when they received 940 mg/day, three of the men adjusted immediately; 20 experienced a negative balance for 60 to 140 days but then adjusted their excretion; 3 did not adapt within

the period of study. From these data he estimated that 9 subjects required from 335 to 400 mg/day; 12 required 410 to 500 mg/day; 4 required 540 to 620 mg/day; 1 required 890 mg/day to maintain calcium balance. Whether these data do, in fact, reflect varying need, only time required to adapt, some other factors, or even erroneous balance data is unknown. Radiologic evidence indicated some moderate demineralization in some of the men, but it could not be shown that such men had either higher needs or lesser ability to adapt.

The question as to whether or not any individual can adapt to relatively small calcium intakes is an interesting and important one. It has been argued that those who are unable to adapt may be the individuals who eventually develop osteoporosis. There is also the possibility that adaptation can only be readily achieved over very long periods, perhaps requiring low intakes during childhood. There are few data, but the experiments of Henry and Kon[56] are interesting. These authors reared rats on low and high calcium diets. The animals eventually reached the same level of body calcium, but more slowly in those on the low calcium diet. However, even in old age, when there was no difference in the total body calcium, the animals adapted to the low calcium diet retained calcium more efficiently when given a calcium-free diet. The authors suggest that a more stable skeleton might be formed by animals reared on low calcium intakes.

High producing dairy cattle may develop a tetany called milk fever after parturition, when milk production begins at a high rate. Apparently, the animals are unable to mobilize calcium from the skeleton or absorb sufficient calcium to maintain the serum calcium in the face of the large need for milk formation. Interestingly enough, Boda and Cole[57] reported that the occurrence of milk fever was reduced by feeding a *lower* calcium level prior to parturition. Whatever mechanism the animal utilizes to maintain an efficient mobilization and utilization of calcium is apparently activated by the feeding of the lower level of calcium.

The data summarized by Garn[45] show that, in the male, the pattern of growth in the metacarpal, and presumably other long bones, is a continuing deposition of bone on the subperiosteal surface, continuing at a very slow rate even after age 30, a modest deposition of calcium on the endosteal surface during adolescence and early adulthood, and then continuing loss from the endosteal surface. The net effect is a marked increase in cortical volume up to about age 20. At about age 40 the cortex begins to thin because of an acceleration of loss from the endosteal surface. In the female the pattern is similar except that the deposition upon the endosteal surface is greater, so that the medullary cavity becomes actually smaller than that in young children. Removal of bone from the endosteal surface also begins at about age 40 but at a faster rate than in men. In summarizing data[58] upon the cortical loss between ages 25 to 45 and 45 to 85 in 14 different populations from various parts of the world, Garn found the losses to be similar and not related to the usual calcium intake.

From these data Garn also selected the upper and lower 15 percentiles with regard to calcium intake and compared cortical thickness. In the females between age 25 and 45 the high consumers averaged 1245 mg calcium per day and the low consumers 373 mg calcium per day. No difference in cortical thickness was found. Similarly, individuals with the widest and thinnest cortical thicknesses could not be shown to relate to their calcium intake.

Calcium in Sweat. Balance studies have traditionally ignored the quantity of calcium in sweat, the assumption being made that this is insignificant. However, Mitchell and Hamilton[59] reported the concentration in sweat to vary from 8 to 265 mg/liter. Consolazio *et al.*[60] have calculated losses as high as 1 gm/day in individuals working at high temperatures, who sweated profusely. It must be stressed that, whatever the losses in sweat may be, it is perfectly clear that people in many parts of the world grow and maintain normal skeletons on relatively low calcium intakes. Losses such as those calculated by Consolazio *et al.* simply cannot occur under most conditions. Thus, it must be noted that the data are apparently available only on individuals consuming generous quantities of calcium, in some of Consolazio's subjects apparently as high as 3.5 gm of calcium per day. One must assume that excretion through the skin adapts to intakes, even though excretion in sweat might account for some of the high apparent retentions of calcium seen in balance studies.

Old Age and Osteoporosis. Osteoporosis is an important disease of elderly people. Based upon x-ray films of the spine of a sample of Michigan women, Frame and Smith[61] estimate that something on the order of 14 million women in the United States have a clinically significant degree of osteoporosis. Albright and Reifenstein[13] originally classified osteoporosis as a disease of the bone matrix. It was assumed to be related to a deficiency of sex hormones and unrelated to calcium intake. Sex hormone therapy is apparently not capable of reversing bone loss, although it may be beneficial. The role of the sex hormones is also suggested by the fact that osteoporosis occurs earlier in young women subjected to ovariectomy. Cortical loss (evaluated by measurement of the thickness of the cortex of the metacarpal[45]) also is accentuated after the artificial menopause, indicating again that measurements of the cortex of the metacarpal have a predictive relationship to total bone.

On the other hand, loss of bone may begin before menopause in women and similar loss of bone, albeit to a lesser degree, occurs in men.[45] A variety of other factors have been suggested as possible causal factors, including calcium deficiency and lack of physical exercise. Little convincing evidence is available and the evidence is conflicting. On the one hand, it has been reported that the feeding of high calcium diets results in large retentions of calcium in subjects with osteoporosis.[62–64] Indeed, the retentions reported are so high that, since they are not supported by evidence of a change in skeletal density, they must be erroneous. They were not confirmed by Rose[65] who considers osteoporosis as a nearly irreversible phenomenon. The data of Garn[45] and Smith and Rizek[66] from various populations fail to demonstrate any relationship between calcium intake and rates of bone loss. It is often found, as would be expected, that calcium intakes fall with age and are lower in women than men, but this is primarily due to a lower food intake in women and a decreasing food intake with age. When correction for this trend is made,[67] relationships between calcium intake and degree of osteoporosis cannot be demonstrated. Data obtained from the use of radiocalcium[24,68] do not indicate that osteoporotics are necessarily less efficient utilizers of dietary calcium. Thus, although osteoporosis can be produced in animals by calcium depletion,[69] there is currently no convincing evidence that calcium intake is an etiologic factor in the disease or that high calcium intakes are necessarily beneficial.

It has been reported that there is a relationship to fluoride consumption, high intakes being associated with a lower prevalence of osteoporosis[70,71] and that the administration of relatively large amounts of fluoride is therapeutically beneficial.[72,73] This is consistent with a higher degree of crystallinity of the bone mineral in the presence of fluoride,[8] which may produce a more stable bone mineral. The data available to date, however, suggest that the level of fluoride ordinarily recommended for the control of dental decay has minimal or no effects upon osteoporosis.[74]

Pregnancy and Lactation. The full-term infant body contains about 28 gm of calcium. Analyses of fetuses[44,75] indicate that most of this calcium must be deposited during the last 2 or 3 months of pregnancy, amounting to between 200 and 300 mg daily. Estimates of the calcium content of breast milk yield values in the same range, of the order of 250 mg during early lactation and about 300 mg after 3 months of lactation.[3,34] If it be assumed that the dietary calcium is 30 per cent utilized, then 600 to 900 mg of additional calcium over and above that required for maintenance would be needed if the woman's body is not to lose calcium.

These relatively large amounts of calcium obviously are not consumed by many women who go through a normal pregnancy and who lactate normally. In contrast to these calculations of theoretical need, there is evidence of increased deposition of bone on the endosteal surface during pregnancy and there is a positive correlation between cortical thickness of bone and parity.[45] Thus, as Garn says "the more babies, the more bone left in later life." Although longitudinal data are apparently not available outside the United States, the similarity of the pattern in cross-sectional data on adult women in Central America indicates that, even when diets relatively low in calcium are consumed, there is also deposition of bone during pregnancy. These changes must be hormonally induced and must be associated with an increased utilization of dietary calcium.

The effect of lactation is less clear. Garn states "The implications are that C (cortical thickness) adds during pregnancy normally, that it loses during lactation normally, but that pregnancy without lactation results in a permanent gain in C. Since long lactation with a daily loss of circa 300 mg of calcium is less and less in fashion, the net implication is that pregnancy without lactation will result in a continuing gain in C, of benefit after sixty and through the ninth decade, from a bone mechanical point of view." "In theory, prolonged and repeated lactations lead to premature bone loss as metered by C. This we have not yet shown." In this regard, it is of interest that it has been clearly shown that, in high producing dairy cattle, the loss of body calcium during lactation does occur and this is replaced as the rate of milk production falls. Thus, a temporary mobilization of body calcium cannot necessarily be considered detrimental or permanent. Objective data are not available which support either the large need for calcium during lactation or that lactation on low calcium diets is impaired or detrimental to the mother. The reserve capacity to adapt by increasing absorption or limiting excretion must be presumed to be called into play and to be adequate in the long run on usual diets.

Vitamin D. Vitamin D is discussed elsewhere (Chapter 5 Section B). We would only point out that the normal metabolism of calcium is obviously dependent upon the presence of vitamin D in adequate amounts. Although not well documented in human subjects, in experimental animals the requirements of vitamin D and calcium and phosphorus are mutually dependent. The need for vitamin D can be minimized by high calcium-phosphorus diets and the effects of a low calcium-phosphorus diet are not evident if sufficient vitamin D is supplied. It has been claimed that many elderly people with osteoporosis also show evidence of osteomalacia, presumably representing vitamin D deficiency.[76]

Excessive Calcium Intakes. A number of clinical conditions are associated with excessively high levels of calcium in the serum and urine or calcification of the soft tissues. These would include such various conditions as idiopathic hypercalcemia of infancy, the "milk alkali syndrome," hypercalciuria, and renal stones. These are discussed elsewhere (Chapter 5 Section B and Chapter 30). There appears to be no adequate evidence that high calcium intakes *per se* are a primary causal factor, but it is logical that high intakes may contribute, since low intakes are an integral part of therapy.

PHOSPHORUS

Phosphorus has received relatively little attention in human nutrition since the phosphorus intake is almost always, if not invariably, higher than that of calcium and thought to be entirely adequate. On the other hand, since grasses and hays usually contain more calcium than phosphorus, especially where soils are depleted of phosphorus, phosphorus deficiency is known to occur in grazing animals. The disease, "aphosphorosis," is characterized by a perverted appetite and chewing of bones, wood dirt, etc. As the disease progresses the animals lose their appetites, the general appearance becomes poor, the joints stiff, and the bones become fragile and easily broken.

Phosphorus compounds play a central role in the energy transformations in the body whether derived from fats, carbohydrates or protein; the nucleoproteins responsible for the processes of cell division, reproduction, and the transmission of hereditary characteristics are phosphoproteins; a variety of phospholipids occur in all cells, and so forth. There is no evidence that the intake of phosphorus in man is ever sufficiently low to influence these vital processes and, indeed, the biochemical effects of limitations of phosphorus intakes in animals have been little studied.

The plasma inorganic phosphate level in adults is normally about 3 to 4 mg/100 ml and is 1 to 2 mg higher in children, gradually decreasing to adult levels. Larger amounts are present in the plasma as phospholipids and these vary considerably, depending upon the type and amount of circulating lipoproteins.

ABSORPTION AND EXCRETION

Unlike calcium, most of the dietary phosphorus is absorbed from the intestine, so that the fecal phosphorus is usually about 30 per cent of the intake. Since there is relatively little control over phosphorus absorption, the body content is regulated primarily by urinary excretion which will, therefore, in the normal adult contain phosphorus equivalent to about 70 per cent of the intake. It is likely that most, if not all, of the dietary phosphorus is absorbed as free phosphate. The various phosphate esters must be hydrolyzed by phosphatases prior to absorption. As has been previously discussed, in animals the absorption of phosphate can be decreased by excessive levels of dietary calcium and vice versa, but this does not appear to be a major influence in human nutrition. Similarly, in animals at least, excessive iron and other materials which form insoluble phosphates in the gut can be shown to inhibit absorption.

PHOSPHORUS REQUIREMENTS

Little direct experimental evidence is available upon the phosphorus requirements of man. In the studies of Sherman many years ago,[77] he concluded that approximately 0.88 gm of phosphorus was required to maintain balance, compared to a value of approximately 0.5 gm of calcium. Thus, the impression that the phosphorus requirements of adults are higher than the calcium requirements and a recommended allowance of 1.5 times that of calcium.[78] Since these are practically the only data available on adult man, one can only speculate on whether the values represent something approaching requirements or, as in the case of calcium, an adaptation to the dietary levels usually consumed.

In extensive work with rats, particularly with rachitogenic diets, the data suggest that the calcium:phosphorus ratio in the diet should be approximately 1. It is also argued, upon a teleological basis, that since milk has a Ca:P ratio of a little over 1 that this is an appropriate ratio for infants and children.

Calcium depletion in animals[79,80] is apparently accentuated by high phosphorus intakes. It must be noted, however, that in most human dietaries the phosphorus intakes are high even though calcium intakes are low. No adverse effects or advantages of lowering phosphorus intakes have yet been shown. In fact, the administration of large amounts of phosphate[81] has been reported to improve mineralization and reduce the time required for clinical union in patients with fractures.

The syndrome of phosphate depletion in man after the long-continued use of antacids, which render phosphate nonabsorbable in the gastrointestinal tract, has been described.[82,83] It is characterized by weakness, anorexia, malaise and bone pain, with demineralization of bone and marked negative calcium balance caused mainly by an increase in urinary calcium. Similar metabolic changes occur in phosphate-depleted animals.[84]

RECOMMENDED DIETARY INTAKES OF CALCIUM AND PHOSPHORUS

As will be obvious to the reader of this chapter, recommendations for appropriate intakes of calcium and phosphorus are based upon dubious and controversial data. The basic difficulty is that, even in areas of the world where intakes of calcium are very low by western standards, evidence that calcium deficiency occurs or that higher intakes of calcium will be beneficial is simply not available. It is possible, of course, that appropriate studies have not been done. Nutritionists in the western or more affluent countries, where milk is generally available, where calcium intakes are high, where most of the studies have been done, and where great emphasis has been placed upon the "need of calcium to form good bones and teeth," have been loath to accept that the data available have been misinterpreted and much of the effort has been mistaken.

Comparative values of the recommendations made by several groups[34,78,86] are shown in Table 6A–1. These have been modified somewhat from the original, since the age groups are not the same. However, the wide variation in interpretation of the information available is clear. The basic point made by the FAO/WHO group is that, when one is dealing with countries which have a low calcium intake, an overestimation of the calcium (or other nutrient) needs inevitably leads to expensive nutrition programs which may be useless in terms of health benefits and thus detract from more useful efforts. Countries with more liberal supplies of milk and other high calcium foods can afford to be more generous in their allowance for calcium, even though the higher recommendations may yield no benefits.

I would comment that the intake during

Table 6A-1.   Recommended Intakes of Calcium

Age	FAO/WHO[1] mg/day	Canada[2] mg/day	National Research Council[3] mg/day
0–12 months	500–600	500	400–600
1–9 years	400–500	700–1000	700–1000
10–15 years	600–700	1200	1200–1400
16–19 years	500–600	900	800
Adult	400–500	500	800
Pregnancy and Lactation	1000–1200	1200	1300

[1] Taken from World Health Organization: *Calcium Requirements*, WHO Tech. Report Series No. 230, Geneva, 1962.

[2] Taken from The Canadian Council on Nutrition: *Dietary Standard for Canada*, Canadian Bull. on Nutr., *6*, No. 1, 1964.

[3] Taken from Food and Nutrition Board: Recommended Dietary Allowances, 7th Revised Edition, National Research Council Publ. 1694, Washington, D.C., 1968.

pregnancy and lactation recommended by the FAO/WHO group is unrealistic in public health practice. It is unreasonable to expect the calcium intake to double during pregnancy and lactation in most countries and, if this were to be achieved, calcium in the form of special supplements would be required. There is no evidence that these would be useful. Thus, if the calcium needs during pregnancy and lactation are substantially higher than in the non-pregnant woman, a general elevation of the usual level of intake of adults, *i.e.*, an increase in the recommended level for the normal adult, would be more meaningful as a public health measure.

Due to the high levels of calcium recommended by the Food and Nutrition Board for all age groups, which exceed the usual intakes of many people in the United States and Canada, dietary data are commonly interpreted as showing that a large percentage of the United States population is deficient in calcium[87] and the impression is given that increased intakes of calcium would be beneficial. There is simply no evidence that this is true and, as discussed in this chapter, a great deal of evidence that it is not true. The Recommended Dietary Allowance for calcium in the United States should at least be lowered, so that the recommendations are more in line with usual intakes in much of the population.

BIBLIOGRAPHY

1. Neuman and Neuman: *The Chemical Dynamics of Bone Mineral*, Chicago, Univ. Chicago Press, 1958.
2. Robinson: J. Bone & Joint Surg., *34A*, 389, 1952.
3. Leitch: in *Nutrition: A Comprehensive Treatise*, Vol. I, New York, Academic Press, 1964.
4. Aub: Harvey Lectures, 115, 1928–29.
5. Bogert and Kirkpatrick: J. Biol. Chem., *54*, 375, 1922.
6. Robinson: Biochem. J., *77*, 286, 1923.
7. Gross: J. Biophys. Biochem. Cytology, *2*, 261, 1956.
8. Posner: Fed. Proc., *26*, 1717, 1967.
9. Heaney: Clin. Orthopaedics, *37*, 153, 1963.
10. Bauer, Carlsson, and Lindquist: in *Mineral Metabolism*, Vol. I, New York, Academic Press, 1961, p. 609.
11. Bronner: in *Mineral Metabolism*, Vol. II, New York, Academic Press, 1964, p. 341.
12. McLean and Budy: *Radioisotopes and Bone*, New York, Academic Press, 1964.
13. Albright and Reifenstein: *The Parathyroid Glands and Metabolic Bone Disease*, Baltimore, Williams & Wilkins, 1948.
14. Talmage, Cooper, and Park: Vitamins & Hormones, *28*, 103, 1970.
15. Copp, Cameron, Cheney, Davidson, and Henze: Endocrinology, *70*, 638, 1962.
16. Proceedings of a Symposium, *Calcitonin*: London, William Heinemann Medical Books, Ltd., 1967.

Major Minerals 285

17. Catt: Lancet, *2*, 255, 1970.
18. McLean and Hastings: Amer. J. Med. Sci., *189*, 601, 1935.
19. Edelman: Ann. Rev. Physiol., *23*, 37, 1961.
20. Walker, Arvidsson, and Politzer: S. Afr. Med. J., *28*, 48, 1954.
21. Knapp: J. Clin. Invest., *26*, 182, 1947.
22. Hegsted, Moscoso, and Collazos: J. Nutr., *46*, 181, 1952.
23. Malm: *Calcium Requirements and Adaptation in Adult Men*, Oslo, Oslo Univ. Press, 1958.
24. Lutwak: Amer. J. Clin. Nutr., *22*, 771, 1969.
25. Roberts, Kerr, and Ohlson: J. Amer. Dietet. Assoc., *24*, 292, 1948.
26. Ohlson and Stearns: Fed. Proc., *18*, 1076, 1959.
27. Schachter and Rosen: Amer. J. Physiol., *196*, 357, 1959.
28. Schachter, Dowdle, and Schenker: Amer. J. Physiol., *198*, 263, 1960.
29. Harrison and Harrison: Amer. J. Physiol., *199*, 265, 1960.
30. Schachter, Kimberg, and Schenker: Amer. J. Physiol., *200*, 1263, 1961.
31. Henneman, Carroll, and Albright: Ann. N.Y. Acad. Sci., *64*, 343, 1956.
32. Malm: Scand. J. Clin. Lab. Invest., *5*, 75, 1953.
33. Walker, Fox, and Irving: Biochem. J., *42*, 452, 1948.
34. World Health Organization: *Calcium Requirements*, WHO Tech. Report Series No. 230, Geneva, 1962.
35. Bronner, Harris, Maletskos, and Benda: J. Nutr., *54*, 523, 1954.
36. Baerg, Kimberg, and Gershon: J. Clin. Invest., *49*, 1288, 1970.
36a.Fraser and Kodicek: Nature, *228*, 764, 1970.
36b.Gray, Boyle and DeLuca: Science, *172*, 1232, 1971.
36c.Boyle, Miravet, Gray, Holick and DeLuca: Endocrinology, *90*, 605, 1972.
37. Atkinson, Kratzer, and Stewart: J. Dairy Sci., *40*, 1114, 1957.
38. Vaughan and Filer: J. Nutr., *71*, 10, 1960.
39. Charley and Saltman: Science, *139*, 1205, 1963.
40. Chang and Hegsted: J. Nutr., *82*, 297, 1964.
41. Wallace: Fed. Proc., *18*, 1125, 1959.
42. Duncan: Nutr. Abstr. & Rev., *28*, 695, 1958.
43. Holmes: Nutr. Abstr. & Rev., *14*, 597, 1945.
44. Leitch and Aitken: Nutr. Abstr. & Rev., *29*, 393, 1959.
45. Garn: *The Earlier Gain and the Later Loss of Cortical Bone*, Springfield, Charles C Thomas, 1970.
46. Baker and Newman: Amer. J. Phys. Anthropol., *15*, 601, 1957.
47. Sherman and Hawley: J. Biol. Chem., *53*, 375, 1922.
48. Ellis and Mitchell: Amer. J. Physiol., *104*, 1, 1933.
49. Kinsman, Sheldon, Jensen, Bernds, Outhouse, and Mitchell: J. Nutr., *11*, 429, 1939.
50. Nicholls and Nimalasuriya: J. Nutr., *18*, 563, 1939.
51. Joseph, Kurien, Swaminathan, and Subrahmanyan: Brit. J. Nutr., *13*, 213, 1959.
52. Kurien, Narayanarao, Swaminathan, and Subrahmanyan: Brit. J. Nutr., *14*, 339, 1960.
53. Mitchell and Curzon: Actualities Scientifique et Industrielles, No. 771, Herman & Cie., 1939.
54. Walker: Ann. N.Y. Acad. Sci., *69*, 989, 1958.
55. Walker, Walker, Richardson, and Christ: Amer. J. Clin. Nutr., *23*, 244, 1970.
56. Henry and Kon: Brit. J. Nutr., *7*, 147, 1953.
57. Boda and Cole: Ann. N.Y. Acad. Sci., *64*, 370, 1956.
58. Garn: *The Earlier Gain and the Later Loss of Cortical Bone*, Springfield, Charles C Thomas, 1970, p. 49.
59. Mitchell and Hamilton: J. Biol. Chem., *178*, 345, 1959.
60. Consolazio, Matouch, Nelson, Hackler, and Preston: J. Nutr., *78*, 78, 1962.
61. Smith and Frame: New Eng. J. Med., *273*, 73, 1965.
62. Nordin: Lancet, *1*, 1011, 1961.
63. Nordin: Amer. J. Clin. Nutr., *10*, 384, 1962.
64. Whedon: Fed. Proc., *18*, 1112, 1959.
65. Rose: Postgrad. Med., *40*, 158, 1964.
66. Smith and Rizek: Clin. Orthopaedics, *45*, 31, 1966.
67. Guggenheim, Menczel, Reshef, Schwartz, Ben-Menachem, Bernstein, Hegsted, and Stare: Arch. Environ. Health, *22*, 259, 1971.
68. Spencer, Lewin, Fowler, and Samachson: Amer. J. Med., *46*, 197, 1969.
69. Jowsey and Gershon-Cohen: Proc. Soc. Exp. Biol. Med., *116*, 437, 1964.
70. Leone, Stevenson, Besse, Hawes, and Dawber: Arch. Industrial Health, *21*, 326, 1960.
71. Bernstein, Sadowsky, Hegsted, Guri, and Stare: J.A.M.A., *198*, 499, 1966.
72. Rich and Ensinck: Nature, *191*, 184, 1961.
73. Purves: Lancet, *2*, 1188, 1962.
74. Korns: Public Health Reports, *84*, 815, 1969.
75. Widdowson and Spray: Arch. Dis. Child., *26*, 205, 1951.
76. Exton-Smith, Hodkinson, and Stanton: Lancet, *2*, 999, 1966.
77. Sherman: J. Biol. Chem., *41*, 173, 1920.
78. Food and Nutrition Board: Recommended Dietary Allowances, 7th Revised Edition, National Research Council Publ. 1694, Washington, D.C., 1968.
79. Henrikson, Lutwak, Krook, Skogerboe, Kallfelz, Belanger, Marier, Sheffy, Romanus, and Hirsch: J. Nutr., *100*, 631, 1970.
80. Krook, Lutwak, Henrikson, Kallfelz, Hirsch, Romanus, Belanger, Marier, and Sheffy: J. Nutr., *101*, 233, 1971.
81. Goldsmith, Woodhouse, Ingbar, and Segal: Lancet, *1*, 687, 1967.
82. Lotz, Ney, and Bartter: Trans. Assoc. Amer. Phys. (Philadelphia), *77*, 281, 1964.
83. Lotz, Zisman, and Bartter: New Eng. J. Med., *278*, 409, 1968.
84. Day and McCollum: J. Biol. Chem., *130*, 269, 1939.

85. Young, Lofgreen, and Luick: Brit. J. Nutr., *20*, 795, 1966.
86. The Canadian Council on Nutrition: *Dietary Standard for Canada*, Canadian Bull. on Nutr., *6*, No. 1, 1964.
87. U.S. Department of Agriculture: Food Intake and Nutritive Value of Diets of Men, Women, and Children in the United States, Spring 1965, Agricultural Research Service 162–18, Washington, D.C., 1969.

Chapter

6

Section B   Magnesium

Maurice E. Shils

Human magnesium deficiency was first described in a small number of patients in 1934.[1] Understanding of the prevalence of this deficiency, its symptomatology, relationships to other electrolytes and association with various disease states has come slowly. The observations of Flink and co-workers indicating depletion of this ion in alcoholics[2] were an important step forward. Beginning 5 years later, a series of clinical case reports began to focus attention on hypomagnesemia in malabsorptive states. Endocrine disorders, abnormalities in the newborn, renal tubular defects and iatrogenic influences have been added to the list. With increasing ease and frequency of measurement of magnesium in body fluids,[3] it has become obvious that human depletion occurs much more commonly than had been assumed previously.

NORMAL METABOLISM

Body Partition. Magnesium shares some of the attributes of calcium in its characteristics of absorption and storage in bone, a similarity to potassium in being an important intracellular constituent and a resemblance to sodium in the efficiency with which the normal kidney retains the ion when serum levels fall. This eclectic state is of additional interest, since it is now apparent that a deficiency of magnesium affects the metabolism of each of the other three ions in some manner.

The adult human weighing 70 kg contains approximately 20 to 28 gm of magnesium,[4-6] equaling 1667 to 2400 mEq of this ion (1 mEq = 0.5 mM = 12 mg). About 55 per cent is present in bone and about 27 per cent

in muscle. Muscle, liver, heart and pancreas contain about the same amount (approximately 16 mEq per kg wet weight).[6,7] Erythrocyte content varies from 4.3 to 6.2 mEq per liter depending on method.[7] Normal serum levels also vary depending on method but, with atomic absorption methods, the range is usually 1.5 to 2.1 mEq/L.[8] Magnesium ion in erythrocytes and plasma exists in free, complexed and protein-bound forms: in plasma the approximate percentages are 55, 13 and 32, respectively.[7] Cerebrospinal fluid magnesium is greater than that of plasma (approximately 2.5 mEq/L) despite the absence of protein; about 55 per cent is free and the remainder is complexed.[7] Magnesium in sweat averages 0.6 mEq per liter in man in a hot environment.[9]

Intake, Excretion and Homeostasis. Magnesium intake varies greatly because of the widely variable content of different foods.[6] Fifteen to 40 mEq per day are probably an average range for healthy individuals in the United States and Western Europe.[10] Of this intake approximately 60 to 70 per cent is excreted in the stools by most individuals.[7,10] The remainder (other than that retained in new tissue or lost in sweat or desquamated skin) is excreted in the urine. A number of physiologic factors influence normal absorption. These include total magnesium intake, intestinal transit time, rate of water absorption and resultant luminal magnesium concentration, and the amounts of calcium, phosphate and lactose in the diet.[7] When radioactive magnesium (^{28}Mg) was given intravenously only 2 per cent[11] or less[12] was excreted in the stool. With a high magnesium intake (47 mEq/day) absorption of the ingested radioisotope (used as a tracer) was 23.7 per cent; at the more usual intake of 20 mEq/day, absorption was 44.3 per cent; with a very low intake (1.9 mEq/day), it was 75.8 per cent.[12]

When magnesium intake is severely restricted, output becomes very small. On intakes of less than 1 mEq per day, daily urinary and fecal losses each averaged less than 1 mEq after an initial adjustment period.[13,14] As magnesium intake increases after a period of deficiency urinary excretion increases markedly as serum levels approach the lower normal range.[13] Supplementing a normal intake increases urinary excretion without altering normal serum levels.[15] The efficient intestinal and renal conservation and excretory mechanisms in normal individuals permit homeostasis over a wide intake of dietary magnesium, just as they do for sodium. However, unlike the control of sodium, there does not appear to be an efficient hormonal homeostatic mechanism for regulating serum magnesium. The normal range is the resultant of a balance between gastrointestinal absorption and renal excretion. Since gastrointestinal mechanisms of magnesium transport are not very efficient, the renal threshold is presumably the critical factor in determining that level. Summaries of data on renal handling of magnesium have been published recently.[7,15] Reabsorption probably occurs in a manner similar to that for calcium and sodium and there is interdependence in the clearance of these three ions.[7] Heaton has suggested that, in the rat at least, magnesium filtered from serum with concentrations below the lower limit of normal is reabsorbed, and the magnesium appearing in the urine at higher serum concentrations is derived from tubular secretion.[15]

Since parathyroid hormone (PTH) mobilizes bone salts, its administration to normal animals may be expected to affect serum and urinary magnesium. The hormone in moderate doses caused little or no rise in plasma magnesium in normal rats,[16] dogs,[17,18] or man.[19,20] In hypoparathyroid subjects[20] an early fall in urinary magnesium excretion occurs following PTH; this is followed by an increased excretion of magnesium and calcium. The magnesium excretory response in normal subjects is variable.[7,20,21a,21b] Calcitonin derived from pig causes hypocalcemia but no significant change in serum magnesium in the dog,[22,23] monkey[24] or normal man.[24,25] Urinary magnesium in the dog may be decreased[22] or unchanged[23] under various experimental conditions. The effects of other hormones on magnesium metabolism have been summarized by Walser.[7]

Biochemistry. Magnesium plays a key role as a prosthetic group in many essential enzymatic reactions. The enzymes include those that hydrolyze and transfer phosphate groups (phosphokinases). Thus, magnesium is involved in reactions involving ATP and in those, at almost every step, in the phosphorylation of glucose in its anaerobic metabolism and in its oxidative decarboxylations in the citric acid cycle requiring thiamine pyrophosphate, in the activities of alkaline phosphatase and of pyrophosphatase, in the activation of amino acids and in the formation and multiple actions of cyclic AMP. It is further involved in protein synthesis through its action on ribosomal aggregation, its roles in binding messenger RNA to 70S ribosomes and in the synthesis and degradation of DNA. Documentation of these and other enzymatic functions is given elsewhere.[7,8,26,27] Magnesium plays an important role in neuromuscular transmission and activity: it acts at some points synergistically with calcium, while at others it is antagonistic. This complex area has been reviewed elsewhere.[7,8,28,29]

MAGNESIUM DEFICIENCY

Experimental Animals. Acute and near-total deprivation of this cation in diets fed to growing animals produces one of the most rapidly developing, and, in the rat, one of the most dramatic of all deficiencies. After 3 to 5 days of acute deficiency young rats develop peripheral vasodilatation which increases for approximately 1 week and then gradually subsides; concomitantly the animals become progressively hyperkinetic when disturbed and then develop tonic-clonic convulsions which are often fatal.[30] This study estabished the association between magnesium depletion and neuromuscular changes. Other signs of deficiency in rats include reduced growth, alopecia, skin lesions and edema, and hypertropic gums. Calcification and degenerative changes in various organs, especially the kidney, have been prominent on the usual diets, which tend to be fairly high in calcium. Calcification begins in the kidney as luminal concretions in the ascending loop of Henle. Studies in the kidney[31] and heart[32] permit understanding of the sequence of changes from subcellular organelles to gross alterations. Although the rat has been, by far, the most widely used animal, many other species have been studied, including various fowl,[33] guinea pig,[34] mouse,[35] pigs,[36] sheep and cattle,[37–39] dogs,[40–43] monkeys[44,45] and man.

Human Deficiency. The symptomatology and biochemical abnormalities ascribable to this deficiency are still not completely defined and there exist areas of disagreement despite (or because of) numerous clinical case reports. This situation is attributable to two major factors: first, experimentally induced symptomatic human deficiency has been induced to date in only one study,[13,46,47] and, second, symptomatic human deficiency observed in patients has always developed in a setting of predisposing and complicating disease states. The latter have included severe malabsorption of various etiologies,[48–58] chronic alcoholism with malnutrition,[2,48,49,] [59–62] prolonged magnesium-free parenteral feeding, usually in association with prolonged losses of gastrointestinal secretions,[2,48,49,55,63] burns,[64] acute or chronic renal disease, involving tubular dysfunction,[1,65] lactation losses,[66] childhood malnutrition,[67,68] post-natal tetany syndromes,[69–71,79,80,97] familial disorders of renal[72] or intestinal conservation[80,97] and parathyroid disorders, especially in the immediate post-parathyroidectomy period.[73,75] In such clinical circumstances, associated complex and uncontrolled variables—such as multiple dietary inadequacies, changes in oral and parenteral nutrients and medications, metabolic abnormalities, manifestations of basic disease and severe infection occurring in close proximity to the magnesium therapy—often

make it difficult and potentially misleading to ascribe certain clinical manifestation specifically to magnesium deficiency.

There are four recorded efforts to induce magnesium deficiency experimentally in human volunteers.[13,76–78] In the study in which symptomatic depletion occurred,[13,46,47] plasma magnesium fell progressively on the magnesium-deficient diet (< 0.8 mEq per day), to levels which were 10 to 30 per cent those of control periods (Fig. 6B–1). Erythrocyte magnesium declined more slowly and to a lesser degree. Urine and fecal magnesium decreased to extremely low levels within 7 days. Hypocalcemia occurred in 6 of the 7 subjects, despite adequate calcium intake and absorption and no prior evidence of gastrointestinal or parathyroid abnormalities. Hypocalciuria was noted early in the depletion in all cases (Fig. 6B–2). Serum phosphate was normal or slightly low in all but one subject and urinary excretion was usually

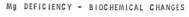

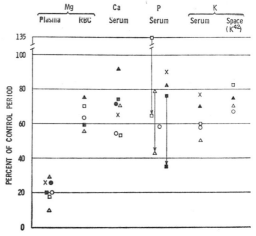

Fig. 6B–1. Biochemical changes observed in the course of experimental human magnesium depletion. The maximum deviation observed in the course of the depletion is indicated as a percentage of the average control levels for each subject for magnesium, calcium, inorganic phosphate, and potassium. K[42] space indicates the estimate of exchangeable body potassium using [42]K. The transient decrease in serum inorganic phosphate noted in 3 individuals immediately following magnesium repletion is indicated by a line connecting values observed in the late depletion period with those observed in early repletion (from Shils,[13] courtesy Williams and Wilkins Co.).

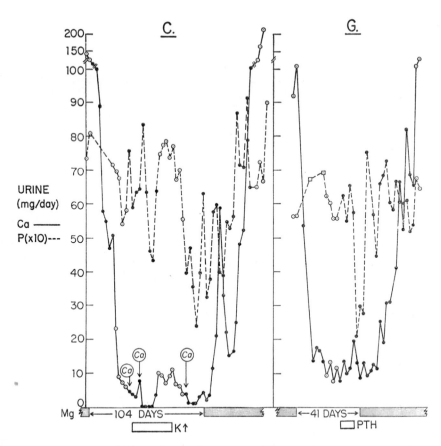

Fig. 6B-2. Urinary calcium (Ca) and inorganic phosphate (P) excretion in two subjects prior to, during and after magnesium depletion. Note that the P value is ten times the ordinate figure, that there is a change in the ordinate scale above 100 mg and that the time axis is not to scale. Average daily excretions for a 2-week period are indicated as squares, weekly averages as open circles and individual daily values as solid circles. In the lefthand graph of C, Ca↓ indicates an infusion of 5 gm of Ca gluconate; no effect was noted on Ca excretion. In subject G Ca excretion and serum Ca values were not affected by parathyroid hormone (PTH) injection (750 U over a 5-day period); urinary P did not change consistently during deficiency or in response to PTH but there was an abrupt fall for 3 days immediately after PTH with an equally abrupt rise several days after instituting Mg. The marked hypocalciuria occurring with Mg depletion was noted in all depleted subjects (from Shils,[13] courtesy Williams and Wilkins Co.).

unaffected. Most deficient subjects developed hypokalemia and negative potassium balance; serum sodium remained normal and the subjects were in positive sodium balance.

Neurologic signs occurred in 5 of the 7 after deficiency periods ranging from 25 to 110 days. Hypomagnesemia, hypocalcemia and hypokalemia were present in all consistently symptomatic patients (Figs. 6B–1 and 6B–3). Despite the hypocalcemia, deep tendon reflexes were either normal or decreased. The electromyogram revealed rapid-firing high-

pitched potentials during the deficiency period in the 5 patients tested. The electro-encephalogram showed no changes related to the deficiency. Anorexia, nausea and apathy occurred frequently and heralded exacerbation of the neurologic changes. When electrocardiographic changes occurred, they were compatible with coexisting hypo-calcemia or hypokalemia. All abnormalities reverted to normal with reinstitution of magnesium. Strongly positive potassium balances associated with negative sodium balances

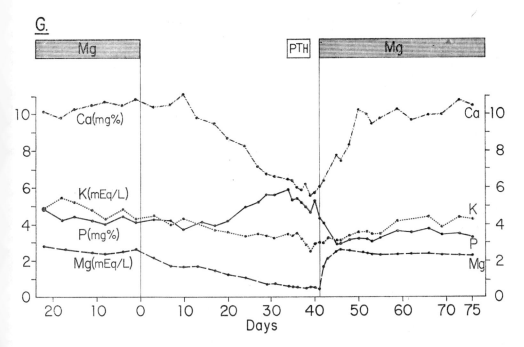

Fig. 6B-3. Blood chemistries in subject on experimental magnesium (Mg) depletion. Mg was omitted after a month on the control diet. The rise in serum inorganic phosphate (P) with Mg depletion in this patient was unique among the depleted subjects. On depletion day 25 Trousseau and Chvostek signs first occurred and the former became progressively stronger as plasma calcium (Ca), Mg and potassium (K) continued to decline. On depletion day 35, parathyroid hormone (PTH) was given i.m. at 50 units t.i.d. for 5 days; this had no effect on plasma Ca but appeared to decrease P. On day 41, anorexia, nausea, paresthesias and generalized muscle spasticity developed; 17 mEq of Mg i.v. was then given with rapid improvement; this was followed by similar amounts of Mg i.m. 12 and 15 hours later. Dietary Mg (40 mEq daily) was resumed on the third repletion day (from Shils,[13] courtesy Williams and Wilkins Co.).

occurred as magnesium was retained, electrolytes returned to normal and urine magnesium and calcium rose.

It is concluded from this study that magnesium is essential for the normal metabolism of potassium and calcium in adult man, that magnesium is essential for the mobilization of calcium from bone, that the signs and symptoms are associated with complex electrolyte changes occurring secondarily to magnesium deficiency, that the alterations in various electrolytes in blood and tissues and their relative intakes influence the development and manifestation of clinical and biochemical changes, and that the occurrence in clinical situations of otherwise unexplained hypokalemia and hypocalcemia should suggest the possibility of significant magnesium depletion.

Hypomagnesemia occurred with hypo-

calciuria, but without hypocalcemia or symptoms of deficiency, in 2 subjects ingesting 2 to 5 mEq of magnesium per day in another study.[78] The four subjects in the remaining two experimental studies did not become hypomagnesemic within the 20 to 38 days of deficiency.[76,77] The numerous differences in types of subjects and diet composition in these experimental studies have been discussed.[13]

The signs and symptoms noted in the experimental depletion[13,46,47] covered a wide spectrum, including personality change, spontaneous generalized muscle spasm, tremor, fasciculations and Trousseau and Chvostek signs. These have been described separately or in various combinations in clinical cases of hypomagnesemia.[2,49,51,55,57,58,65,66,70] The subjects in the experimental study[13] had no coma, convulsions, significant myoclonic jerks or athetoid movements, which have been reported to occur in certain cases.[2,49,55,58,67,69-71,79,80] Convulsions with or without coma seem to occur much more frequently in acutely deficient infants than in adults. Normoreflexia or hyporeflexia was noted in association with hypocalcemia and positive Trousseau signs in the experimental depletion; hyperreflexia was never seen.[13] The clinical literature on this point is contradictory: hyperreflexia has been reported frequently in symptomatic cases with hypomagnesemia, while others have noted normal or depressed reflexes.[2,50,51,54] Our experience and that of others are not in accord with statements that the Chvostek sign, but not the Trousseau sign, is elicited in magnesium deficiency.[55,81] The development of anorexia, nausea and vomiting, heralding exacerbation of neurologic symptoms, has been one of the more striking observations in experimental depletion.[13,46]

A striking change in the hypomagnesemic subjects becoming symptomatic in the experimental study was the development of hypocalcemia and hypokalemia.[13,46] The clinical literature is also in disagreement about the relationship of magnesium deficiency to hypocalcemia and to latent or overt tetany (defined here as a positive Trousseau sign or spontaneous carpopedal spasm). Some investigators have expressed the opinion that tetany is not a manifestation of magnesium deficiency per se.[2,50,55,82-84] However, there is increasing evidence that the hypocalcemia, developing with marked magnesium deficiency, does not respond satisfactorily and persistently to calcium administration alone: it does improve with magnesium administration.[48,51,52,54,56-58,70,80,85-87,97] It is worth emphasizing that parenteral administration of large amounts of calcium, parathyroid hormone or vitamin D is potentially dangerous in the magnesium-depleted individual, because of the predisposition towards soft tissue calcification in this deficiency. Another type of clinical picture has been noted in which hyperirritability, tetany and other neuromuscular abnormalities occurred in a setting of hypomagnesemia and *normocalcemia*; these responded to magnesium but not to calcium salts.[49,67,68,71,88]

There is increasing support for the view that hypokalemia and total body depletion of this ion occur in serious magnesium depletion in adults.[13,45,58,78] However, the majority of cases of neonatal tetany associated with hypomagnesemia and hypocalcemia presented with normal serum potassium; no data are given on potassium balance or body stores. In malnourished children with magnesium depletion hypokalemia is often present.[67,68]

Treatment of Magnesium Depletion. The amount and route of magnesium administration will depend upon the severity of depletion and its etiology. Symptomatic deficiency is best treated by the intravenous or intramuscular route. It is our practice to initiate treatment in older children and adults with relatively small amounts of magnesium sulfate intravenously (*i.e.* 2 gm [17 mEq]) over 1 or 2 hours in saline or dextrose solutions, with other nutrients as required. In the presence of cardiac arrhythmias and electrolyte abnormalities, the patient is monitored during the initial infusion. Another 2 to 4 gm are then given by continuous infusion over the remaining 24 hours or by periodic intramuscular injections. This administration is given daily for 2 or more days and the situation reassessed. An estimate of the degree of depletion may be obtained by measuring daily urinary magnesium levels during repletion. When a sudden increase in urine levels occurs, serum magnesium levels usually have become persistently normal and immediate repletion has been achieved.[13] A program of longer-term oral or, if necessary, periodic intravenous or intramuscular administration should then be established to maintain normal serum levels. Supplementary magnesium may be given as tablets of milk of magnesia or as gelatin capsules packed with powdered magnesium sulfate (Epsom salts), -chloride or -oxide; one is given 3 to 6 times per day. Improvement of existing steatorrhea will decrease fecal magnesium losses. Treatment of other underlying disease, replacement of potassium deficits, and avoidance of alcohol are essential where indicated. Calcium administration in the treatment of hypocalcemia secondary to magnesium deficiency usually is unnecessary: serum calcium usually will return to normal levels within a week of initiating magnesium repletion. Alternative programs of magnesium replacement in adults have been utilized, usually with higher doses than advocated here.[89] Asymptomatic hypomagnesemia may be treated with smaller or less frequent doses. Reported experience in the treatment of symptomatic magnesium depletion in infants is unanimous concerning the rapid efficacy of relatively small amounts of intravenous or intramuscular magnesium in controlling neurological signs and restoring serum levels.[69-71,79,80,97] Administration of 0.5 to 1.0 ml of 50 per cent magnesium sulfate solution (2 to 4 mEq of magnesium ion) 2 or 3 times per day appears adequate. The duration and follow-up of treatment will depend upon the etiology of the depletion.

Interrelationships Among Magnesium, Calcium, Parathyroid Hormone and Bone Metabolism. The present status of this important subject may be summarized as follows:

1. Rats deficient in magnesium often develop hypercalcemia, hypophosphatemia, hypocalciuria and hyperphosphaturia. These and other findings have led various investigators to postulate the development of a hyperparathyroid state resulting from the deficiency,[16,90,91] although contrary evidence exists (*vide infra*).

2. Variations in magnesium concentration have the same directional effects on parathyroid gland secretion as do variations in calcium. Thus, perfusion of isolated parathyroid glands of goats and sheep with hypomagnesemic blood leads to an increased concentration of parathyroid hormone in the effluent blood, whereas hypermagnesemia causes a decreased hormone production.[92] Parathyroid hormone secretion by bovine glands cultured *in vitro* was affected in the same general way by varying the magnesium concentration as it was by varying the calcium.[93]

3. It is necessary to reconcile the findings in the preceding paragraphs with the hypocalcemia which occurs in many magnesium-deficient species, including man, monkey, ruminants and the dog. The apparent contradiction with the rat now appears to be partially explained. Traditionally, the calcium content of the diets used in almost all studies of the rat has been relatively high. When the calcium fed to rats is reduced appropriately, then the magnesium-deficient animals become hypocalcemic while the magnesium-fed controls are normocalcemic.[45,94] This finding suggests that the hypercalcemia so often noted in the deficient rat is, at least in part, secondary to a dietary and intestinal effect rather than to one based entirely on increased bone resorption.

4. The etiology of the hypocalcemia occurring in almost all magnesium-deficient species is presently unsettled. Impaired intestinal absorption and severe depletion secondary to urinary losses have been ruled out as explanations since they are not supported by balance data. Hypocalcemia as the result of impaired parathyroid hormone production and secretion is a possible mechanism. This is supported by the excellent responses to parenteral parathyroid hormone administration which have occurred in magnesium-deficient infants,[80] rats,[16,45,94,95] dogs[16,96] and monkeys.[16,98] However, there are data supporting an alternative mechanism, namely, that parathyroid hormone production is normal or even increased in deficiency but that bone is refractory to normal hormonal action. Patients with hypomagnesemia and hypocalcemia associated with alcoholism[99] or malabsorptive states[57] were noted to be initially unresponsive to parathyroid extract; following magnesium repletion, they responded to repeat doses of hormone preparation. Increased parathyroid hormone secretion in response to perfusion of isolated parathyroid glands with hypomagnesemic blood[92] has been mentioned. Furthermore, *in vitro* studies of rat bone support the concept of a permissive role for magnesium in the resorptive response of bone to parathyroid extract.[100,101] Final proof of the nature of the sequence of events leading to hypocalcemia awaits serial measurements of serum parathyroid hormone levels and of bone calcium kinetics in magnesium-deficient patients before and during repletion. There has recently appeared a report on the levels of serum immunoreactive parathyroid hormone (IPTH) in one patient with hypomagnesemia secondary to an isolated defect in the in-

testinal transport of magnesium.[101a] In the presence of hypomagnesemia and hypocalcemia, serum IPTH levels were in the undetectable to low range. After 24 hours of magnesium repletion, as serum magnesium and calcium were rising, there was a striking increase in serum IPTH above the upper limits of normal. As serum calcium rose to normal with further magnesium therapy, the IPTH decreased. Cessation of therapy resulted in recurrent hypomagnesemia and hypocalcemia and a return of IPTH to undetectable level. Confirmation of this finding in cases of magnesium depletion with hypocalcemia induced by this and other etiologies will permit the conclusion that the hypocalcemia is secondary to impaired synthesis or secretion of parathyroid hormone.

Requirements. Establishment of firm data for adequate intake of magnesium for individuals of different ages and physiological status is difficult because of the complex dietary and physiologic interrelationships of magnesium with calories, calcium, phosphate, protein, lactose, potassium and probably other nutritional factors. A large number of balance studies have been performed on adults to obtain data on magnesium requirements (reviewed by Seelig[10]). However, some reservations about much of these data are indicated, either because of the short duration of the study or the inadequacy of the analytical procedures.

The Recommended Dietary Allowances for magnesium of the National Research Council suggest about 5 mg per kg body weight for adult men and women, up to 10 mg per kg for adolescents, up to 12 mg per kg for growing children and 8 to 10 mg per kg for infants up to a year.[101] Seelig recommends 6 mg per kg especially for adult males.[10] These amounts appear to be more than adequate for normal individuals; they may be grossly inadequate for those with serious intestinal and renal absorptive defects.

Hypermagnesemia and Magnesium Toxicity. The normal kidney is capable of excreting absorbed or injected magnesium ion so rapidly that serum levels do not rise to clinically significant levels. In the treatment of preeclampsia and eclampsia with magnesium, relatively massive doses have been given with the objective of maintaining the serum level at 5 to 8 mEq/L and patients with normal kidneys were able to excrete 40 to 60 gm of magnesium sulfate per day.[89] Hypermagnesemia may develop in other clinical situations where magnesium-containing drugs, usually antacids, are given to individuals with renal insufficiency.[1,102,103] The pharmacology of magnesium has been reviewed by Walser.[7] It has been reported that central depression begins to appear at levels above 8 mEq/L and pronounced anesthesia occurs at about 20 mEq/L. Infusion of magnesium sulfate, raising plasma concentrations of magnesium to approximately 15 mEq/L, induced profound paralysis of skeletal muscle (with the exception of the diaphragm and a few other muscles) in two human subjects; there was no evidence of anesthesia and the authors question the previous literature suggesting this.[104] In addition to paralysis, very high blood levels are associated with respiratory depression, coma and death in experimental animals. Calcium infusion counteracts magnesium toxicity. While such dangerously high serum levels are unlikely in the usual clinical situations, avoidance of magnesium-containing medications in patients with significant renal disease is recommended, unless otherwise indicated and monitored.

BIBLIOGRAPHY

1. Hirschfelder: J.A.M.A., *102*, 1138, 1934.
2. Flink, Stutzman, Anderson *et al.*: J. Lab. Clin. Med., *43*, 169, 1954.
3. Alcock: Ann. N.Y. Acad. Sci., *162*, 707, 1969.
4. Duckworth and Warnock: Nutr. Abstr. Rev., *12*, 167, 1942–43.
5. Widdowson, McCance and Spray: Clin. Sci., *10*, 113, 1951.
6. Schroeder, Nason and Tipton: J. Chron. Dis., *21*, 815, 1969.
7. Walser: Rev. Physiol. Biochem. Exp. Pharmacol. (Erg. Physiol.) *59*, 185, 1967.
8. Wacker and Parisi: New Eng. J. Med., *278*, 658, 1968.
9. Consolazio, Matoush, Nelson, *et al.*: J. Nutrition, *79*, 407, 1963.
10. Seelig: Am. J. Clin. Nutrition, *14*, 342, 1964.
11. Avioli, Lynch and Blastomsky: Clin. Res., *11*, 40, 1963.
12. Graham, Caesar and Burgen: Metabolism, *9*, 646, 1960.
13. Shils: Medicine, *48*, 61, 1969.

14. Barnes, Cope and Gordon: Ann. Surg., *152*, 518, 1960.
15. Heaton: Ann. N.Y. Acad. Sci., *162*, 775, 1969.
16. Heaton: Clin. Sci., *28*, 543, 1965.
17. Greenberg and Mackey: J. Biol. Chem., *98*, 765, 1932.
18. Roberts, Murphy, Miller and Rosenthal: Surg. Forum, *5*, 509, 1954.
19. Gill, Bell and Bartter: Clin. Res., *10*, 405, 1962.
20. Bethune, Turpin and Inoue: J. Clin. Endocrin. Metab., *28*, 673, 1968.
21a. Shelp, Steele and Rieselbach: Metabolism, *18*, 63, 1969.
21b. Paunier, Ray and Wyss: Hel. Med. Acta, *35*, 504, 1969–70.
22. Cramer, Parkes and Copp: Canad. J. Physiol. Pharmacol., *47*, 181, 1969.
23. Clark and Kenny: Endocrinol., *84*, 1199, 1969.
24. Bell, Barrett and Patterson: Proc. Soc. Exp. Biol. Med., *123*, 114, 1966.
25. Foster, Joplin, MacIntyre et al.: Lancet, *1*, 107, 1966.
26. Sutherland: J A.M.A., *214*, 1281, 1970.
27. Wacker and Vallee: In *Mineral Metabolism*, eds. Comar and Bronner, Vol. 2 Pt. A, New York, Academic Press, 1964, Chap. 23, pp. 490–493.
28. Thesleff and Quastel: Ann. Rev. Pharmacol., *5*, 263, 1965.
29. Hubbard, Llinas, and Quastel: *Electrophysiologic Analysis of Synaptic Transmission*, Monog 19, Physiol. Soc., London, Edward Arnold, 1969.
30. Kruse, Orent and McCollum: J. Biol. Chem., *96*, 519, 1932.
31. Schneeberger and Morrison: Lab. Invest., *14*, 674, 1965.
32. Heggtveit: Ann. N.Y. Acad. Sci., *162*, 758, 1969.
33. Van Reen and Pearson: J. Nutrition, *51*, 191, 1953.
34. Grace and O'Dell: J. Nutrition, *100*, 37, 1970.
35. Hamuro: J. Nutrition, *101*, 635, 1971.
36. Miller, Ullrey, Zutaut, et al.: J. Nutrition, *85*, 13, 1965.
37. Rook and Storey: Nutrition Absts. Rev., *32*, 1055, 1962.
38. Girard, Brochart, Parodi and Sevestre: Ann. Biol. Anim., Biochem. Biophys., *4*, 345, 1964.
39. Rook: Ann. N.Y. Acad. Sci., *162*, 727, 1969.
40. Syllm-Rapoport and Strassburger: Acta Biol. Med. Germ., *1*, 141, 1958.
41. Vitale, Hellerstein, Nakamura and Lown: Circ. Res., *9*, 387, 1961.
42. Bunce, Jenkins and Phillips: J. Nutrition, *76*, 17, 1962.
43. Wener, Pintar, Simon et al.: Am. Heart J., *67*, 221, 1964.
44. Vitale, Velez, Guzman and Correa: Circ. Res., *12*, 642, 1963.
45. Shils: Unpublished Data.
46. Shils: Am. J. Clin. Nutrition, *15*, 133, 1964.
47. Shils: Ann. N.Y. Acad. Sci., *162*, 847, 1969.
48. Randall, Rossmeisl and Bleifer: Ann. Intern. Med., *50*, 257, 1959.

49. Vallee, Wacker and Ulmer: New Eng. J. Med., *262*, 155, 1960.
50. Hanna, Harrison, MacIntyre and Fraser: Lancet, *2*, 172, 1960.
51. Fletcher, Henly, Sammons and Squire: Lancet, *1*, 522, 1960.
52. Balint and Hirschowitz: New Eng. J. Med., *265*, 631, 1961.
53. Booth, Babouris, Hanna and MacIntyre: Brit. J. Med., *2*, 141, 1963.
54. Petersen: Acta Med. Scand., *173*, 285, 1963.
55. Gerst, Porter and Fishman: Ann. Surg., *159*, 402, 1964.
56. Heaton and Fourman: Lancet, *2*, 50, 1965.
57. Muldowney, McKenna, Kyle et al.: New Eng. J. Med., *281*, 61, 1970.
58. Gerlach, Morowitz and Kirsner: Gastroent., *59*, 567, 1970.
59. Mendelson, Ogato and Mello: Ann. N.Y. Acad. Sci., *162*, 918, 1969.
60. Jones, Shane, Jacobs and Flink: Ann. N.Y. Acad. Sci., *162*, 934, 1969.
61. Sullivan, Wolpert, Williams and Egan: Ann. N.Y. Acad. Sci., *162*, 947, 1969.
62. Wolfe and Victor: Ann. N.Y. Acad. Sci., *162*, 973, 1969.
63. Baron: Brit. J. Surg., *48*, 344, 1960–1961.
64. Broughton, Anderson and Bowden: Lancet, *2*, 1156, 1968.
65. Randall: Ann. N.Y. Acad. Sci., *162*, 831, 1969.
66. Greenwald, Dubin and Cardon: Am. J. Med., *35*, 854, 1963.
67. Back, Montgomery and Ward: Arch. Dis. Child., *37*, 106, 1962.
68. Cadell: New Eng. J. Med., *276*, 535, 1967.
69. Davis, Harvey and Yu: Arch. Dis. Child., *40*, 289, 1965.
70. Dooling and Stern: Canad. Med. Assn. J., *97*, 827, 1967.
71. Wong and Teh: Lancet, *2*, 18, 1968.
72. Gitelman, Graham and Welt: Ann. N.Y. Acad. Sci., *162*, 856, 1969.
73. Agna and Goldsmith: New Eng. J. Med., *259*, 222, 1958.
74. Potts and Roberts: Am. J. Med. Sci., *235*, 206, 1958.
75. Hanna, North, MacIntyre and Fraser: Brit. Med. J., *2*, 1253, 1961.
76. Fitzgerald and Fourman: Clin. Sci., *15*, 635, 1956.
77. Barnes, Cope and Gordon: Ann. Surg., *152*, 518, 1960.
78. Dunn and Walser: Metabolism, *15*, 884, 1966.
79. Clarke and Carre: J. Pediat., *70*, 806, 1967.
80. Paunier, Radde, Kooh et al.: Ped., *41*, 385, 1968.
81. Fishman: Arch. Neurol., *12*, 562, 1965.
82. Booth, Babouris, Hanna and MacIntyre: Brit. Med. J., *2*, 141, 1963.
83. MacIntyre, Hanna, Booth and Read: Clin. Sci., *20*, 297, 1961.
84. Smith, Hammarsten and Eliel: J.A.M.A., *174*, 77, 1960.

85. Fourman and Morgan: Proc. Nutrition Soc., *21*, 34, 1962.
86. Friedman, Hatcher and Watson: Lancet, *1*, 703, 1967.
87. George and Chambers: Texas J. Med., *58* 812, 1962.
88. Miller: Ann. J. Dis. Child., *67*, 117, 1944.
89. Flink: Ann. N.Y. Acad. Sci., *162*, 901, 1969.
90. MacIntyre, Boss and Troughton: Nature, *198*, 1058, 1963.
91. Lifshitz, Harrison, Bull and Harrison: Metabolism, *16*, 345, 1967.
92. Buckle, Care, Cooper and Gitelman: J. Endocrinol., *42*, 529, 1968.
93. Targovnik, Rodman and Sherwood: Endocrinol., *88*, 1477, 1971.
94. MacManus and Heaton: Clin. Sci., *36*, 297, 1969.
95. Chase and Hahn: Clin. Res., *18*, 622, 1970.

96. Suh, Csima, and Fraser: J. Clin. Invest., *50*, 2668, 1971.
97. Friedman, Hatcher, and Watson: Lancet, *1*, 703, 1967.
98. Dunn: Clin. Sci., *41*, 333, 1971.
99. Estep, Shaw, Watlington *et al.*: J. Clin. Endocrinol. Metab., *29*, 842, 1969.
100. MacManus, Heaton and Lucas: J. Endocrinol., *49*, 253, 1971.
101. Nat. Res. Council: Recommended Dietary Allowances—7th ed., 1968, Nat. Acad. Sci. Publ. 1694, Washington, D.C.
101a. Anast, Mohs, Kaplan and Burns: Science, *177*, 606, 1972.
102. Randall, Cohen, Spray, and Rossmeisl: Ann. Intern. Med., *61*, 73, 1964.
103. Freeman, Lawton and Chamberlain: New Eng. J. Med., *276*, 113, 1967.
104. Somjen, Hilmy and Stephens: J. Pharmacol. Exp. Therap., *154*, 652, 1966.

Chapter

6

Section C Iron

Carl V. Moore*

Iron is essential to higher forms of life because its central role in the heme molecule permits oxygen and electron transport. Total body iron varies with weight, hemoglobin concentration, sex and size of the storage compartment. It amounts normally to about 50 mg/kg of body weight in adult men and to about 35 mg/kg in adult women.[1] The tabulation in Table 6C–1 emphasizes the wide range, from less than 2 gm in small women to more than 6 gm in large men.[2] The amount of iron that must be assimilated from food in order to maintain this supply is determined by the amount excreted, the loss in menstrual flow or from hemorrhage, the demands of pregnancy and by the needs related to growth in children.

Two functional compartments of body iron are recognized: (1) an essential component

(roughly 70 per cent) contained in hemoglobin, myoglobin, heme enzymes, cofactor and transport iron; and (2) non-essential storage iron found predominantly in liver, spleen and bone marrow as ferritin and hemosiderin (roughly 30 per cent). Quantitative distribution of the essential fraction is approximately: 85 per cent in hemoglobin; 5 per cent in myoglobin (has one iron atom per molecule, found in concentration of 2 to 3 mg per gm wet weight of human muscle; serves as a reservoir of oxygen for muscle metabolism); 10 per cent in the ubiquitous intracellular heme enzymes (cytochromes, cytochrome oxidase, peroxidase, catalase, etc.) plus iron serving as a cofactor in other enzyme systems; and 4 mg as transport iron bound to transferrin in the plasma.[1,3]

When iron deficiency is well developed, not enough iron is avilable to sustain normal

* Deceased

Table 6C-1. Estimates of Total Body Iron in Adults to Emphasize the Wide Variations Produced by Body Size and Normal Range of Hemoglobin Values

	Male, 70 kg Hb 16 gm/100 ml	Male, 100 kg Hb 18 gm/100 ml	Female, 45 kg Hb 12 gm/100 ml
"Essential" iron			
Hb Fe	2.67 mg	4.2 gm	1.26 gm
Functional tissue iron†	~.45	~.64	~.29
Transport iron	~.005	~.007	~.003
Storage iron	0.5 – 1.5	0.5 – 1.5	0.3 – 1.0
Total: as low as			<2 gm
as high as		>6 gm	

† Myoglobin, metalloenzymes.

hemoglobin production and an anemia characterized by hypochromic microcytic red blood cells results: defective synthesis of the other heme complexes and iron-containing metalloenzymes has been difficult to demonstrate but may be partly responsible for the fatigue, epithelial changes and other associated clinical manifestations. Iron deficiency anemia is a medical and public health problem of prime importance, causing few deaths, but contributing seriously to the weakness, ill-health and substandard performance of millions of people. Milder degrees of iron deficiency—too mild to produce anemia—can now be detected with reasonable accuracy and appear to have a relatively high incidence among children and young women; whether they impair performance or cause symptoms is still not certain. Iron excess or overload is of increasing clinical concern: it occurs in hemochromatosis, transfusion hemosiderosis, or as a consequence of prolonged, excessive oral iron intake.

METABOLISM[4,5]

The main metabolic pathways of iron can be defined in terms that are at least semiquantitative (Fig. 6C–1). As a result, the factors involved in the pathogenesis of iron deficiency and of iron overload are more clearly understood.

Intake. Information about the iron in the diets of different people is still fragmentary. Most published figures, obtained from dietary surveys rather than from actual analysis, indicate that the average daily intake is between 10 and 30 mg.[6] A convenient figure to remember is that the diets of people who live in so-called Western countries contain about 5 to 7 mg of iron per 1,000 calories.[1] A weight-conscious young woman, therefore, who limits her intake to 1,000 to 1,500 calories per day will consume only 6 to 9 mg of food iron. These estimates, however, ignore the iron in drinking fluids or added or lost during food preparation. The high iron content in the diet of the Bantu is derived

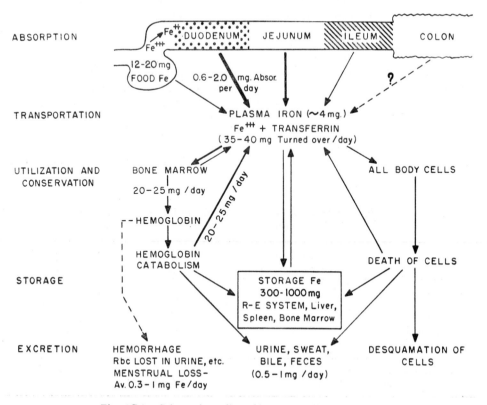

Fig. 6C-1. Schematic outline of iron metabolism in adults.

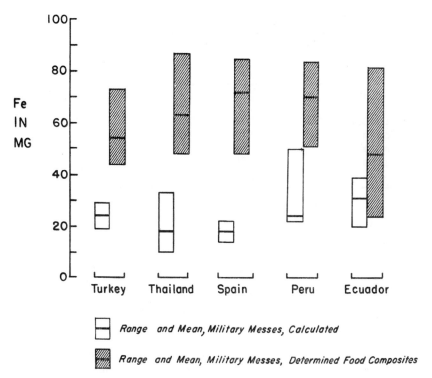

Fig. 6C-2. Iron intake (mg) per man per day in military messes. Note that in each case the values are much higher when determined on food composite than when calculated from food composition tables.

largely from the iron pots used in cooking and for the preparation of fermented beverages.[4]

The U.S. Committee on Nutrition for National Defense has published a series of studies[7] made in a number of countries. Some of these results are illustrated in Figure 6C–2 and contain two surprises: (a) the *calculated* mean iron intake was comparatively high (20 to 30 mg per day); but (b) the values *determined* by analysis of the food as served were even higher in every instance. The food had been prepared in iron cooking utensils. This experience caused us to explore the effect of cooking in castiron skillets or Dutch ovens, utensils that are commonly found in American kitchens (Table 6C–2). The iron utensil contributed significantly to the iron content of each cooked food, but did so particularly in the case of spaghetti sauce and apple butter, the two foods cooked for the longest period of time and having an acid reaction. The gradual substitution of aluminum and stainless steel in the manufacture of cooking equipment has almost certainly had an adverse effect on dietary iron intake. The iron content of canned or tinned food may increase significantly when the cans are stored for a matter of months.

Failure to consider the iron content of drinking fluids introduces another source of error in dietary surveys, of varying significance in different areas. Cider and wine made in Europe or in the United States may have as much as 2 to 16 mg of iron or more per liter.[8] The iron in city water supplies is usually low, but amounts greater than 5 mg per liter may be found in the water from some deep wells or bore holes.[9]

Absorption. *Mechanism and Regulating Factors.* Since the body has a limited ability to excrete iron except by hemorrhage, normal iron balance is maintained largely by regulation of the iron absorbed. Ingested iron tends to be solubilized and ionized by the acid gastric juice, reduced to the ferrous state, and chelated; substances like ascorbic

Table 6C-2.   Effect of Cooking in Iron Skillet (Dutch Oven) on Fe Content of Foods

Food	Cooking time min.	Iron content, mg/100 gm	
		Glass dish	Dutch oven
Spaghetti sauce	180	3.0	87.5
Gravy	20	0.43	5.9
Potatoes, fried	30	0.45	3.8
Rice, casserole	45	1.4	5.2
Beef hash	45	1.52	5.2
Apple butter	120	0.47	52.5
Scrambled eggs	3	1.7	4.1

acid, sugars and amino acids which form low molecular chelates tend to promote absorption (Fig. 6C–1). The concept that only ferrous forms of iron traverse the brush border of intestinal mucosal cells may be an oversimplification. The much greater solubility of ferrous than of ferric hydroxide at the neutral to alkaline pH of the duodenum may be a critical factor in determining the greater solubility of ferrous iron, providing greater opportunity for chelation, and greater exposure of the mucosa to solubilized forms of iron before precipitation occurs. There is some evidence that normal gastric secretions contain a chemically unidentified stabilizing factor, probably an endogenous chelate, which helps slow the precipitation of ingested iron at the alkaline pH of the small intestine. In achlorhydria and gastrectomized subjects, impaired absorption is presumably related to the decreased solubilization and chelation of the ferric iron in food.[10] Absorption may occur at any level of the small intestine, but is most efficient in the upper portion. The chemical form(s) of iron that enters mucosal cells, the nature of receptor sites, and the transmucosal transport system are unknown. The entry of iron at the brush border seems to be by passive diffusion; exit from the serosal surface of cells to the plasma transferrin probably requires metabolic energy. Direct entry into lymphatic channels is insignificant. Most of the iron absorbed into the blood stream seems to pass rapidly through the mucosal cells in the form of small molecules; that portion taken up in excess of the rapid transport capacity combines with apoferritin to form ferritin. Some of the ferritin iron may later be released for uptake into the blood stream, but most of it seems to remain in the mucosal cells until they are desquamated at the end of their 2 to 3 day life span. *Intraluminal influences* that decrease absorption include: rapid transit time; achylia; malabsorption syndromes; precipitation by alkalinization, phosphates, phytates, and ingested alkaline clays[11] or antacid preparations. A gastric absorption-retarding chelate of high molecular weight (gastroferrin) has also been described;[12] it is said to bind iron and prevent absorption. Low concentration of this factor in hemochromatosis and iron deficiency is postulated to be one of the causes for augmented absorption in these conditions. Its existence is disputed.[5] As the intraluminal concentration of iron is increased, the per cent absorbed decreases, but the total retained by the body rises steadily (Table 6C–3). Uptake is increased by reducing substances (ascorbic acid), chelating agents

Table 6C-3.   Absorption of Iron from Graded Doses of Ferrous Sulfate; Normal Subjects*

Dose of iron (mg)	Mean iron absorption	
	% + S.E.	mg
0.1	33.1 ± 4.59	0.033
1.0	29.8 ± 3.87	0.30
10.0	17.8 ± 4.9	1.8
100.0	12.6 ± 1.75	12.6

* From Smith, M. D., and Pannacciulli, I. M.: Absorption of inorganic iron from graded doses. Brit. J. Haemat. *4*, 428, 1958.

(*e.g.*, ascorbic acid, succinic acid, sugars, sulfur-containing amino acids), and possibly by the stabilizing gastric factor previously mentioned. Alcohol and deficiency of pancreatic exocrine secretions have been reported to stimulate absorption, but not all workers are in agreement.

The *systemic regulatory mechanisms* which influence iron absorption have never been identified in spite of intensive search;[2,4,5] they operate to:

(1) Increase absorption in iron deficiency, during the latter half of pregnancy, usually whenever erythropoiesis is stimulated (including ineffective erythropoiesis), and in patients with hemochromatosis;

(2) Decrease absorption in iron overload, and when erythropoiesis is depressed.

Various possibilities investigated include low levels of plasma transferrin saturation, local hypoxia, possible humoral factors, and mucosal iron concentration. For several decades, the concept of a "mucosal block" of iron absorption dominated the literature. Ferritin was regarded as the mediator of absorption; uptake was thought to continue until the intracellular concentration of ferritin blocked further assimilation. Compelling reasons for rejecting the theory have been documented,[2,5] but a recently proposed variant has attracted considerable attention.[10,13] It is postulated: (a) that the columnar mucosal cells formed in crypts at the base of villi contain a variable amount of transferrin-derived iron; (b) that this intracellular deposit regulates, within limits, the quantity of intraluminal iron which enters cells; (c) that the cellular iron may enter the body according to need or remain within the cells to limit absorption and be lost when the cells are sloughed from the tips of villi at the end of their brief life span. According to this concept, little iron is incorporated from transferrin into mucosal cells of iron-deficient subjects and absorption is enhanced. Conversely, in iron-loaded subjects, the mucosal cells formed are well endowed with iron, absorption is limited, and the cellular iron is excreted when desquamation occurs.

Of considerable nutritional importance is the fact that heme iron, an important dietary form of iron, is absorbed by a different mechanism from that described above for inorganic and non-heme forms of food iron. Some investigators believe that heme is taken up by mucosal cells after it has been released from its globin combination by proteolytic duodenal enzymes, while others believe that the protein portion is removed largely within the mucosal epithelium.[10,14] In either case, iron is liberated by a heme-splitting substance, presumably an intracellular enzyme, and is transferred to plasma in a form that can be bound by transferrin. Only a small portion of the heme absorbed by mucosal cells is delivered to the portal blood as the iron-porphyrin complex.[15] Absorption of heme iron is increased in iron deficiency, but to a lesser extent than occurs with inorganic ferrous salts. Other differences between the absorption of heme and of non-heme forms of iron include: failure of ascorbic acid to increase the uptake of hemoglobin iron; failure of substances like phytates and desferrioxamine to depress the absorption of hemoglobin iron; slower rate of appearance in plasma; and lesser diminution of hemoglobin iron absorption when inorganic iron is administered simultaneously.[16-18]

Absorption from Foods. Information about the absorption of iron from foods has been difficult to obtain and is, therefore, still meager.[6,18,19] The best current estimate is that healthy subjects absorb 5 to 10 per cent and iron-deficient subjects 10 to 20 per cent. The maximum amount of iron that one can expect to be absorbed from an average diet in the United States is probably about 1 to 2 mg in normal adults and 3 to 6 mg in iron-deficient patients.

The earliest measurements were made with balance techniques. Even though several of these studies were done with meticulous care, the difference between oral intake and fecal loss was small and difficult to measure with precision; furthermore, differentiation between excreted and unabsorbed iron was not possible. They have the merit of having been done on mixed diets fed over a period of several weeks so that the effect of daily variation on results was minimized. Absorption, calculated on the basis of positive balance, ranged from 7.3 to 21 per cent.[2,18]

Major Minerals

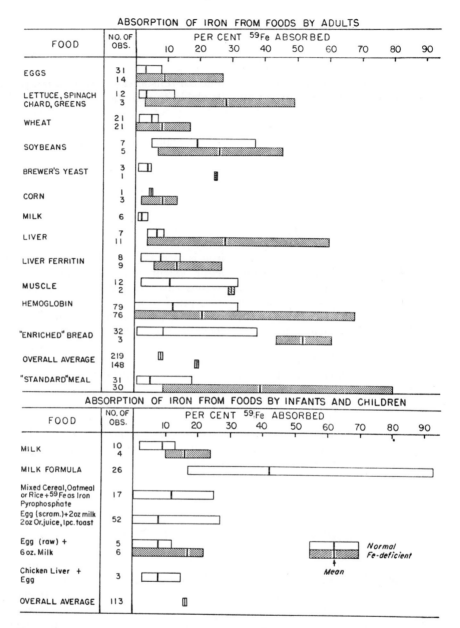

Fig. 6C-3. Radioiron measurements of the absorption of iron from foods by adults, infants, and children. The length of the bars indicates the variation among different subjects for each food; the heavy vertical line across each bar indicates the average value. The amount of iron in each feeding varied from 1 to 17 mg. *Clear bars:* normal subjects; *cross-hatched bars:* iron-deficient patients.

Most data have been obtained by measuring the absorption of iron from single foods prepared or grown so as to contain radioactive iron so that isotopic methods could be used to measure absorption after the food was pre-pared and fed as it would be in a normal diet. The earlier published results are summarized in Figure 6C–3.[18] The overall average for 219 observations on normal subjects approxi-mated 10 per cent and for 148 observations on iron-deficient patients 20 per cent. Note that variations in absorption from any given food are often wide; that assimilation by children tends to be better than by adults; and that absorption from liver, muscle, hemoglobin and soybeans is better than from eggs, milk and cereals.

These data have been extensively augmented, particularly as the result of a collaborative effort between investigators in Venezuela and Seattle.[19] Figure 6C–4 records results obtained on 520 subjects; seven foods of vegetable and five foods of animal origin were examined. Absorption exceeded 10 per cent from animal foods, was poor from rice and spinach, and tended to be better from soybeans than from other vegetable sources. All results obtained with radioiron-tagged foods suffer from several important deficiencies: food was given as a single test dose so that daily variations in absorption resulting from emotional or other factors that may influence function and motility of the gastrointestinal tract were not measured;

the possible interaction of various foods on iron absorption was not determined. Ascorbic acid, for instance, will increase the uptake of iron from some foods[2] while eggs have been reported to decrease assimilation.[20] The Venezuelan and Seattle workers have made an impressive start at studying these interactions.[21,22] One vegetable (maize or black beans) and one animal food (fish or veal muscle) tagged with different isotopes (^{55}Fe and ^{59}Fe) were fed to the same subjects separately and mixed in the same meal. Veal iron absorption was diminished about 20 per cent when veal was combined with vegetable foods; iron absorption from either corn or black beans was almost doubled when these foods were mixed with animal food. It was further demonstrated: (1) that the enhancing effect of fish muscle could be duplicated by feeding amino acids in the same composition as is found in fish muscle, and (2) that cysteine seemed to be the amino acid primarily responsible for the enhancing effect.

These results emphasize how difficult it will

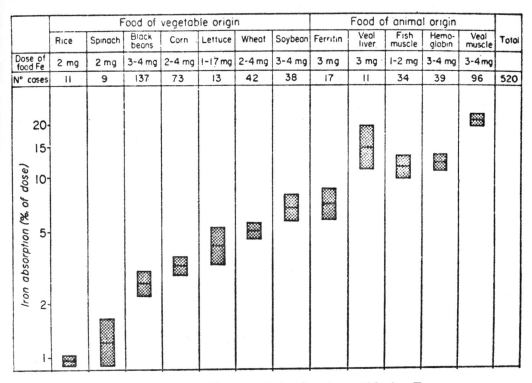

	Food of vegetable origin							Food of animal origin					
---	Rice	Spinach	Black beans	Corn	Lettuce	Wheat	Soybean	Ferritin	Veal liver	Fish muscle	Hemo-globin	Veal muscle	Total
Dose of food Fe	2 mg	2 mg	3-4 mg	2-4 mg	1-17 mg	2-4 mg	3-4 mg	3 mg	3 mg	1-2 mg	3-4 mg	3-4 mg	
N° cases	11	9	137	73	13	42	38	17	11	34	39	96	520

Fig. 6C-4. Absorption of iron from foods. (Layrisse and Martinez-Torres: *Progress in Hematology,* courtesy of Grune and Stratton.)

be to obtain composite data on the absorption of iron from a complete diet, and have re-stimulated interest in the use of "standard" or mixed meals[18,23] to which a tracer dose of inorganic radioiron is added as an external tag. Evidence is accumulating to indicate that the non-heme iron in food is converted during cooking and digestion into a common pool, and that absorption of the external tag will probably provide a measure of the iron absorbed from this pool.[78] If this is true, information will be accumulated more rapidly, because the laborious and difficult isotopic labeling of individual foods will be circumvented and the interaction of different foods can more easily be studied. It appears that radioiron-tagged hemoglobin will similarly serve as an external tag for measuring the absorption of heme iron in food. Absorption from a complete diet, therefore, can be determined by using both an inorganic and a hemoglobin external tag.

Transportation. Iron is transported in plasma bound to transferrin, a beta$_1$ globulin carrier protein with a molecular weight of 86,000 and a biological half-life of 8 to 10.5 days.[24] Formed in the liver, the 7 to 15 gm of transferrin present in the normal adult are equally distributed in the intra- and extra-vascular space. Transferrin has two separate binding sites each capable of binding one atom of ferric iron.[25,26] It serves a complex function since it must both *accept* iron that is being absorbed from the intestinal tract or being released from sites of storage and of hemoglobin destruction, and *deliver* it to the bone marrow for hemoglobin synthesis, to reticuloendothetial cells for storage, to the placenta for fetal needs, and to all cells for iron-containing enzymes. The metal is slightly bound at physiological pH; exchange occurs at specific cellular receptor sites. The best studied are the receptor sites on developing red blood cells; they gradually diminish in number as the cells mature.[27] Transferrin apparently attaches itself to the receptors on the erythroblast or reticulocyte, gives up one or both atoms of iron, and then recirculates as a carrier protein (Fig. 6C–5). The rate of uptake by reticulocytes from transferrin containing two atoms of iron is roughly 10 times the rate from molecules with only one atom. This and related observations have given rise to the postulate that one of the iron-binding sites on transferrin is "erythroblast oriented" while the other is concerned with storage iron. At least 19 genetic variants have been recognized; all seem to function in the same way. The average transferrin content of normal plasma varies from 215 to 350 mg per 100 ml, but concentration is ordinarily expressed in physiological terms as total iron-binding capacity (TIBC): roughly 300 to 450 μg per 100 ml. The amount of iron in plasma (90 to 180 μg per 100 ml in males and 70 to 150 μg in women) is sufficient to bind only about one-third; the remaining two-thirds represent a latent or un-

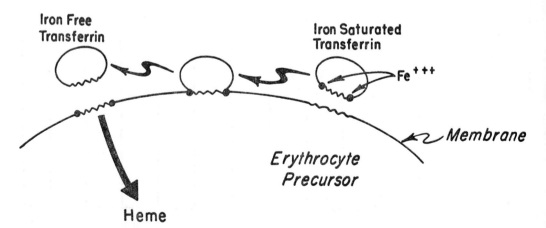

Fig. 6C-5. Schematic representation of the transfer of iron from transferrin to an erythrocyte precursor.

bound reserve (UIBC). The plasma iron undergoes a diurnal variation, with morning values being about 30 per cent higher than those in the evening; it is not influenced by season, exercise, or normal meals.

Although the total circulating plasma iron is only 3 or 4 mg, the turnover rate is rapid.[3,13] About 70 to 90 per cent of the amount transported goes to the bone marrow where it is transferred to developing red blood cells to support hemoglobin synthesis: the remainder is exchanged largely with reticulo-endothelial and hepatic parenchymal cells: only a small fraction is used for myoglobin and cellular metalloenzymes. One can determine the plasma iron turnover rate (PITR) with reasonable accuracy. After the intravenous injection of trace amounts of radioiron (as ^{59}Fe-citrate or ^{59}Fe Cl$_3$) the disappearance of radioactivity is followed for 2 or 3 hours and plotted semilogarithmically (Fig. 6C–6). The time required for the activity to reach half that initially present (T/2 time) varies in normal subjects from 60 to 120 minutes. More rapid clearance rates are found in iron deficiency and in the presence of accelerated erythropoiesis; slower rates occur with erythroid hypoplasia. Using the T/2 time and plasma iron values, one can calculate the PITR from the following formula:[4,28]

$$\text{PITR (mg/day)} = \frac{0.693}{^{59}\text{Fe T/2 (hrs.)}} \times \text{mg Fe/ml}$$

plasma $\times$ plasma vol. (ml) $\times$ 24 hrs.

Normal values for PITR range from 25 to 40 mg per day. The PITR is increased when erythropoiesis is stimulated and decreased when erythropoiesis is depressed. In iron deficiency where the T/2 time is rapid and the plasma iron value is low, the PITR is usually normal.

Changes of differential diagnostic value occur in the iron-binding capacity and plasma iron in various diseases (Fig. 6C–7). Increased total iron-binding capacity is found in iron deficiency, the third trimester of pregnancy, and in response to hypoxia; decreased levels occur in infection, protein malnutrition, many types of iron overload and in conditions where protein is lost, as in nephrosis or pro-

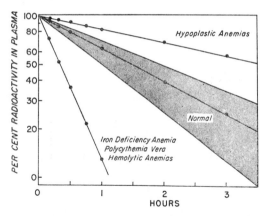

Fig. 6C-6. Plasma radioiron clearance curves for normal subjects and patients with increased and decreased erythropoiesis.

tein-losing enteropathies. The level of plasma iron is determined by the balance between iron extracted from the blood by organs of utilization or storage and that being delivered to the blood by absorption, hemolysis, or release from storage sites. Consequently, it is low in iron deficiency, with accelerated erythropoiesis, and in inflammatory states where release from reticuloendothelial (R. E.) cells is impaired; it tends to be high in iron overload, with hemolysis, or in patients with depressed rates of red blood cell formation.

Utilization. The amount of iron utilized for hemoglobin synthesis per day in a normal adult is approximately 20 to 25 mg. This value can be calculated as follows:

(a) A man with a blood volume of 5,000 ml and a hemoglobin level of 15 gm per 100 ml has 750 gm of circulating hemoglobin or 2.55 gm of circulating hemoglobin iron (Hb multiplied by 0.34 per cent).

(b) The normal life span of the red cell is about 120 days, so 2.55 gm/120 or 21 mg of iron would be required daily to replace the catabolized hemoglobin. The amount can also be determined: after a tracer dose of radioiron is given intravenously, the percentage of the injected radioactivity which is utilized for hemoglobin synthesis and delivered to the peripheral blood in newly formed erythrocytes is measured. Normally the radioactivity rises for 7 to 14 days and then plateaus at 70 to 90 per cent of the injected

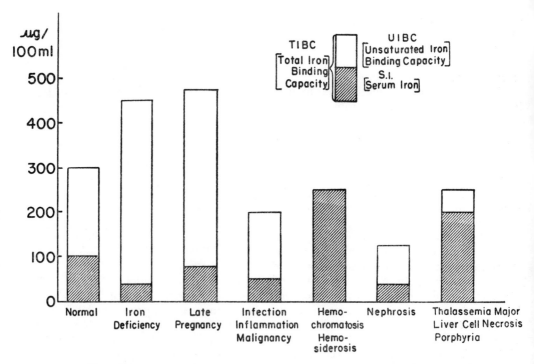

Fig. 6C-7. Relationships of serum iron, unsaturated iron-binding capacity, and total iron-binding capacity in various clinical conditions.

amount. The PITR in mg/24 hours is multiplied by the maximum per cent radioactivity found in circulating hemoglobin to give the amount of iron used per day for hemoglobin formation. For instance,

    if the PITR is 35 mg/day, *and*
    if 80 per cent of the injected dose appears in circulating hemoglobin, then
    35 × 80% = 24 mg Fe used for hemoglobin synthesis/day.

For a detailed discussion of these ferrokinetic considerations, see references 4 and 28.

A normally functioning marrow can increase its production of red blood cells and of hemoglobin by a factor of approximately 6 times: under maximal stimulation, therefore, as much as 100 to 125 mg of iron could be used for hemoglobin synthesis per day. Turnover rates for the iron in myoglobin and the iron-containing respiratory enzymes are unknown.

Ferrokinetic data indicate that most of the iron used by developing red cells for hemo-globin synthesis comes from the transferrin in plasma. Bessis and Breton-Gorius, however, have demonstrated an alternative pathway.[29] When histiocytes in the marrow digest phagocyted erythrocytes, the released iron is converted within the cytoplasm of the phagocyte to ferritin and is transferred by a process of pinocytosis (or "ropheocytosis") to the cytoplasm of surrounding erythroblasts. The ferritin then finds its way to the mitochondria of the nucleated red cell where the iron is presumably changed to a form in which it can combine with protoporphyrin to make heme.

Storage and Tissue Iron. Iron in excess of need is stored intracellularly as ferritin and as hemosiderin. Ferritin consists of a shell of 24 chemically identical protein subunits surrounding a micelle of ferric hydroxyphosphate.[30] The amount of iron varies but those molecules that are completely filled with iron have a molecular weight of 900,000, and contain approximately 5,000 ferric atoms per molecule—enough to form 1,200 hemoglobin molecules. Recent work has established at least a limited organ specificity for ferritin: liver and spleen ferritins have different electrophoretic mobilities and some differences in the amino acid structure of the protein subunits. Ferritin can be identified by electron but not by light microscopy; the iron visible by light microscopy of appropriately stained cells is hemosiderin, a compound composed of aggregated ferritin molecules together with other structural elements.[4,29] In these two forms, iron is segregated and apparently less toxic to cells than when present in a more reactive state. The major sites of storage are the hepatic parenchymal cells and R. E. cells of the bone marrow, liver, and spleen. The immediate source of most R. E. iron stores is hemoglobin iron released from erythrocytes phagocyted at the end of their life span. Hepatic parenchymal iron probably comes primarily from plasma transferrin. In the liver and spleen of normal animals, there is a slight preponderance of ferritin over hemosiderin iron. With increasing concentrations of tissue iron, this ratio is reversed and at high levels the additional storage iron is deposited as hemosiderin. Of great physiologic importance is the fact that both forms are capable of being mobilized for hemoglobin synthesis when the need for iron exists. The mechanism by which ferritin iron is released to the plasma is obscure.[30]

Quantitative measurement of normal iron stores has proved difficult, but reasonable estimates derived from available data are 300 to 1000 mg for adult women and 500 to 1500 mg for adult men. More recent studies suggest that more people fall into the lower half of these ranges than into the upper half. For instance, Scott and Pritchard[31] measured the iron actually available for hemoglobin synthesis in 11 healthy college women with normal hemoglobin values who had never bled abnormally nor been pregnant: systematic phlebotomy was done over a period of weeks to determine how much hemoglobin their iron stores could regenerate. In 3 subjects, the iron converted into hemoglobin was less than 100 mg, in 5 more it ranged from 112 to 348 mg, in only 3 did it amount to more than 500 mg (606 to 743 mg).

Increased iron stores may be brought about in two ways:

(a) Without actual increase in total body iron. When an anemia develops because of hemolysis or aplasia of the marrow, there is less iron in circulating hemoglobin, more in tissue stores.

(b) A true increase in total body iron is found in patients with hemochromatosis, transfusion hemosiderosis, after excessive and prolonged iron therapy, and in cytosiderosis. The amount in tissues may exceed 30 gm, depending on the cause and duration of the metabolic defect.

A rough estimation as to whether iron stores are deficient or excessive may be made from the serum iron, total iron-binding capacity, and stainable iron in bone marrow aspirates.[4,5,32–34]

	Serum Fe	Total iron-binding capacity	Stainable iron in marrow
Normal	70 – 180 μg/100 ml	300 – 450 μg/100 ml	+
Iron deficiency	<50 μg/100 ml	often >450 μg/100 ml	0
Iron overload	>180 μg/100 ml	Normal or diminished, and completely or almost completely saturated	+++

Not much is known about the changes which occur in myoglobin and the various metalloenzymes of iron. Conflicting results have been reported about decreases in myoglobin in experimentally induced deficiency. While the hepatic and renal cytochrome C decreases in rats made iron deficient by a combination of bleeding and an iron-poor diet, the only enzymatic change detected in iron-deficient patients has been a decrease in the cytochrome oxidase activity of buccal mucosal tissue: these relationships have been reviewed in detail by Beutler et al.[5]

Conservation. The avid way in which the body conserves and reutilizes iron is an important characteristic of iron metabolism. Mention has already been made of the fact that a normal adult catabolizes enough hemoglobin each day to release 20 to 25 mg of iron. If this amount were excreted, the iron requirement would be enormously increased and would far exceed the dietary iron absorbed. Actually, more than 90 per cent is conserved so that it can be used over and over again. Iron released from cells that die anywhere in the body is presumably handled and conserved in a similar manner.

Iron Transfer to the Fetus. The fetus has a highly effective acceptor system for assimilating iron. Iron from the maternal transferrin is transferred to the placental tissue, to the fetal transferrin, and then to the fetal tissues. This pathway seems to be a one-way street, capable of operating effectively against increased maternal requirements for iron and even in the face of maternal iron deficiency. During the last trimester of pregnancy, it may account for a transfer of 3 to 4 mg of iron per day to the fetus.[35,36]

Excretion. The body has a limited capacity to excrete iron except by hemorrhage. The best estimates of daily iron turnover in adult men have been calculated to average between 0.90 and 1.05 mg or approximately 13 μg per kg of body weight in subjects studied in Seattle, Venezuela, and South Africa.[37] The external loss is distributed roughly as follows:

	mg
Gastrointestinal	
Blood	0.35
Mucosal	0.10
Biliary	0.20
Urinary	0.08
Skin	0.20

Urinary iron excretion may be increased significantly in patients with proteinuria, hematuria, hemoglobinuria, and hemosiderinuria; the etiological role of hemosiderinuria in the iron deficiency associated with cardiac anemia (*e.g.*, implanted artificial heart valves, calcific aortic stenosis) is of considerable clinical importance. The iron excreted in feces is derived from blood lost into the alimentary canal (1.2 ± 0.5 ml whole blood per day)[38] from unabsorbed biliary iron and from desquamated intestinal mucosal cells. Disagreement has existed about the magnitude of dermal loss with some workers claiming that it may be particularly high among people living in hot, moist climates. One of the South African groups in the above study was made up of Durban Indians who worked in a laundry where both temperature and humidity were very high; their computed daily losses were not significantly greater than those in sedentary, white office workers who lived in a temperate climate.[37,39]

When discussion of iron excretion is extended to a consideration of normal menstrual loss or the iron "cost" of a normal pregnancy, difficulty is encountered because of the wide normal variation. While the menstrual blood loss for any individual normal woman tends to be quite constant from month to month, the difference among women is considerable.[40] In an extensive study[41,42] among Swedish women, the mean menstrual loss was found to be 43 ± 2.3 ml, equivalent to an average of about 0.6 to 0.7 mg of iron per day. Several other important generalizations were made: (*a*) no great difference was found among the several age groups except the smallest mean value occurred among the 15-year-old girls and the largest among women in the 50-year group; (*b*) the upper normal limit of menstrual loss is somewhere between 60 to 80 ml per period; (*c*) in 95 per cent of women, loss was found to average less than 1.4 mg Fe per day; and (*d*) women who consider their menses normal may lose more than 100 ml and occasionally more than 200 ml per period.

Pathologic blood loss from any site constitutes an important form of iron excretion: 1 ml of blood with a hemoglobin value of 15 gm per 100 ml contains 0.5 mg of iron. The chronic loss of only a small volume of blood, therefore, may significantly increase iron requirements. Recognition must also be given to the fact that each 500 ml of blood removed for transfusion purposes removes from the donor between 200 and 250 mg of iron, depending on the hemoglobin value. Spread equally over a year, that amounts to roughly 0.6 to 0.7 mg per day. The effect of multiple donations is obvious.

The iron "cost" of pregnancy is high.[1,43] The external loss in urine, feces and sweat continues and amounts to about 170 mg for the gestational period. About 270 mg (200 to 370 mg) are contributed to the fetus, and another 90 mg (30 to 170 mg) are contained in the placenta and cord. The amount of iron lost in hemorrhage at delivery has been underestimated in the past and averages about 150 mg (range 90 to 300 mg). Iron is required for the expansion of the red blood cell mass that occurs during the last half of pregnancy, but this amount is largely conserved when the circulating red blood cell volume is returned to normal after delivery. Lactation causes an additional drain of approximately 0.5 to 1 mg per day. If one ignores the external loss, since it would have occurred anyway, plus the iron needed for the expanded blood volume and the enlarging uterus, since it is largely conserved, then the total iron "cost" of a normal pregnancy can be estimated to vary from about 420 to 1030 mg (Table 6C–4), or 1 to 2.5 mg per day spread over a 15-month period (pregnancy 9 months, lactation 6 months).

Iron Required for Growth. The iron required for growth and its attendant increase in circulating hemoglobin mass has not been studied in detail but is obviously influenced by the rate of growth, *i.e.* the rapid growth during infancy and the growth spurt of adolescent males. The calculations in Table 6C–5 provide a rough estimate of 0.35 to 0.7 mg per day on the average for boys, and 0.3 to 0.45 mg for girls.

Iron Requirements and Nutritional Allowances. The foregoing discussion has emphasized the limitations of our information about iron loss, the dietary intake of iron and the efficiency of iron absorption from the gastrointestinal tract. In addition, the variations from person to person are relatively large. Enough data are available, however, to permit reasonable estimates of the amount of iron required to maintain a positive balance at various age levels of the population. These approximations are good enough to serve as a guide to physicians and health organizations in their attempts to decrease the high incidence of iron deficiency. They are summarized in Table 6C–6. Calculations of the daily food iron requirement are based on an average absorption of 10 per cent—an assumption that seems reasonable since assimilation tends to become more efficient as need

Table 6C-4. Iron "Cost" of a Normal Pregnancy

Iron contributed to fetus	200–370 mg
In placenta and cord	30–170
In blood loss at delivery	90–310
In milk, lactation 6 months	100–180
	420–1030 mg*
Average per day (pregnancy 9 mo., lactation 6 mo.)	1–2.5

* These figures are in addition to the normal excretory loss of 0.5 to 1 mg/day and ignore the demand during the second half of pregnancy for iron to support the expansion of red blood cell mass. This latter amount (200 to 600 mg) is not included as an iron "cost" because it is largely conserved (and not lost to the body) when the red blood cell mass returns to normal after delivery.

Table 6C-5. Estimates of Average Daily Iron Requirements for Growth

	Boys	*Girls*
Adult wt. greater than birth wt. by	50–100 kg	45–70 kg
Normal body iron per kg	50 mg	35 mg
Iron in total wt. gained	2,500–5,000 mg	1,575–2,450 mg
Years of growth	20 yr.	15 yr.
Estimated iron required for growth: Av. per year	125–250 mg	100–163 mg
Av. per day	0.35–0.70 mg	0.3–0.45 mg

Table 6C-6. Estimated Iron Requirements in Mg/Day

	External Loss*	Menses	Pregnancy "Cost"	Growth	Fe Requirement	Daily Food Intake Requirement‡
Adult males (50–100 kg)	0.65–1.3				0.65–1.3	6.5–13
Non-menstruating Women (45–70 kg)	0.6 –0.9				0.6 –0.9	6–9
Menstruating Women (45–70 kg)	0.6 –0.9	0.1–1.4			0.7 –2.3	7–23
Pregnancy (50–80 kg)	0.65–1.0		1.0–2.5		1.65–3.5	16.5–35
Adolescent Boys (50–100 kg)	0.65–1.3			0.35–0.7	1–2	10–20
Adolescent Girls (45–70 kg)	0.6 –0.9	0.1–1.4		0.3–0.45	1–2.7	10–27
Children†					0.4 –1.0	4–10
Infants†					0.5 –1.5	5–15

* 0.013 mg/kg.
† Estimates taken from Reference 1.
‡ Assuming 10 per cent absorption.

increases. It is evident that men and non-menstruating women, in the absence of pathologic bleeding, should have little difficulty obtaining the iron they need from diets prevalent in the United States (12 to 18 mg Fe/day). The balance may be precarious, however, in many menstruating women and adolescent girls who, because of concern about their weight, restrict their diets and not infrequently have a low iron intake of 10 mg or less per day. The requirements during pregnancy are frequently so large that they are greater than the amount available from diet alone. Particularly in women with depleted stores, supplemental iron therapy is necessary during the latter half of pregnancy if iron deficiency is to be prevented. The estimates for infants are based on the work of Moe[44] and Sturgeon;[45,46] iron requirements in relation to food intake are high because of the rapid rate of growth.

IRON DEFICIENCY AND IRON-DEFICIENCY ANEMIA

The anemia of iron deficiency is characterized by small, pale erythrocytes, depleted iron stores, a plasma iron of less than 40 μg per 100 ml, an elevated iron-binding capacity and less than 15 per cent saturation of the transferrin. Hypochromia, however, is a relatively late manifestation of iron deficiency and milder degrees can now be recognized. Because of the limited ability of the body to excrete iron except as shed blood, iron depletion occurs slowly in the absence of frank hemorrhage. When the balance becomes negative, the tissue stores of ferritin and hemosiderin are called on to meet daily needs and consequently begin to shrink (Fig. 6C-8). Concurrently, iron absorption becomes more efficient in an attempt to compensate, and the plasma iron-binding protein increases. When iron stores are nearly depleted the plasma iron falls to subnormal levels and erythropoiesis slows. Progressively fewer erythroblasts in the marrow contain siderotic (cytoplasmic non-heme iron) granules. Erythrocytes formed at this stage are probably hypochromic, but hypochromia only gradually becomes evident while pre-existing corpuscles live out their normal life span. During this period, the anemia is mild and normocytic, normochromic; hypochromia and more severe anemia develop as the iron depletion becomes more complete. The time required for this sequence of changes may vary from months to years, depending on the

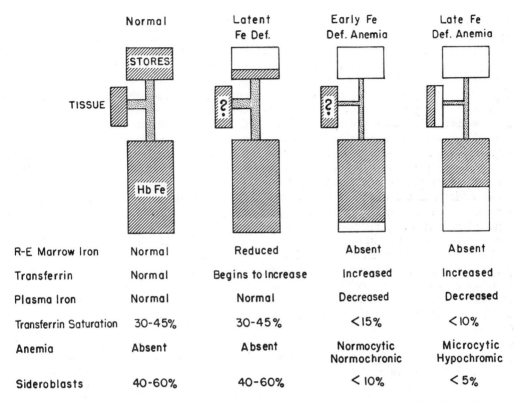

	Normal	Latent Fe Def.	Early Fe Def. Anemia	Late Fe Def. Anemia
R-E Marrow Iron	Normal	Reduced	Absent	Absent
Transferrin	Normal	Begins to Increase	Increased	Increased
Plasma Iron	Normal	Normal	Decreased	Decreased
Transferrin Saturation	30-45%	30-45%	<15%	<10%
Anemia	Absent	Absent	Normocytic Normochronic	Microcytic Hypochromic
Sideroblasts	40-60%	40-60%	<10%	<5%

Fig. 6C-8. Schematic representation of the development of iron-deficiency anemia. The "?" in the tissue iron blocks indicates the uncertainty about when depletion occurs.

initial level of iron stores and the size of the negative balance. For instance, if the negative balance is only 1 mg a day and stored iron is initially 1,000 mg, roughly 3 years would be required to deplete the ferritin and hemosiderin. The sequence just described would be altered if blood loss initiating the iron-deficient state were large. In that case, anemia would be produced early as a result of the hemorrhage; serum iron would decrease early in response to the accelerated erythropoiesis; the rise in iron-binding protein would occur after the hyposideremia; and depletion of iron stores would follow rather than precede these other changes. The sequence schematically represented in Figure 6C–8, however, illustrates the more usual course and the way in which mild degrees of iron deficiency can be recognized before hypochromic anemia appears. The clinical significance of mild (non-anemic) iron deficiency is not clear: it causes no recognized disturbance in a sense af well-being. If diet improves or blood loss diminishes so that balance is restored, the patient may live for years with nearly depleted iron stores without any apparent interference with health.

Incidence. No information currently exists about the prevalence of iron deficiency without anemia.[5] Incidence figures usually relate to the prevalence of anemia and assume, probably correctly, that iron deficiency is the principal cause. The anemia is most frequent in those areas of the world where dietary intake, particularly of animal protein, is low, where infection with intestinal parasites is common and where medical care is inadequate. Survey studies indicate that in certain parts of India and Africa nearly half the population may be affected. Frequency is greatest among the poorer classes and at those times in life when iron requirements are highest, during growth and during the reproductive years in women. In the United

States, incidence figures are as high as 20 per cent for young children[5] and 5 to 10 per cent for women between the ages of 15 and 45. Garby and his associates obtained convincing evidence that 10 to 24 per cent of the female population of Uppsala have iron-deficiency anemia.[47] The percentage of normal pregnant women who enter pregnancy with a normal hemoglobin concentration and subsequently have a decrease in hemoglobin below 10 gm per 100 ml varies greatly in different geographic areas.[48] In Australia, South Africa and parts of the United States, the incidence has been reported to be 4 per cent or less, whereas an incidence of 10 to 16 per cent has been found in other areas of the United States and in Scotland, and of 24 to 36 per cent in Ireland, India, and among a clinic population in Montreal. Adequate data do not exist to define the true incidence of iron-deficiency anemia in the United States; the estimate of 18,000,000 has been called conservative.[5] More than 90 per cent of cases among adults are found in women. Occurrence in adult males and postmenopausal women is much less common and, with few exceptions, is primarily the consequence of blood loss.

Pathogenesis. Iron deficiency results from one or a combination of the following: inadequate diet, impaired absorption, blood loss, or repeated pregnancies. If an individual reaches adult weight with normal body stores of iron, deficiency caused solely by poor diet or poor absorption takes years to develop, in the absence of blood loss or pregnancy, because iron excretion is so limited; these factors are more frequently contributory rather than primary causes. In temperate zones, the two most common causes of iron deficiency among adults are increased menstrual bleeding and hemorrhage from the alimentary canal.[49] The development of iron deficiency in an adult man or a postmenopausal woman means blood loss until proved otherwise.

Defective assimilation can be caused by diets that are grossly deficient or high in cereal content and low in animal protein. Geophagia interferes with the absorption of iron, probably because the ingested clay chelates or precipitates iron as insoluble compounds in the lumen of the gut.[11] Clay-eating is practiced particularly by children and adult women; among the poorer classes, its prevalence is probably much greater than is generally realized. Poor uptake of iron occurs in malabsorption syndromes and in chronic diarrhea from any cause. After partial or total gastrectomy two defects in iron absorption are observed: assimilation of food is subnormal, and the increase in absorption that usually accompanies iron deficiency does not take place.[50,51] When patients with atrophic gastritis and achlorhydria develop a negative balance they also are not able to increase the uptake of iron as much as are comparable individuals with normal gastric function.

Except for pregnancy, *high output* of iron is caused by blood loss. Hemorrhage from wounds, from the nose or mouth, genitourinary tract and from hemorrhoids is obvious. Bleeding from the gastrointestinal canal is often occult and amounts up to 30 ml, if lost by adults high in the tract, may not cause guaiac-positive stools. Hiatus hernia, peptic ulcers, varices, *salicylate ingestion*, diverticuli, benign or malignant tumors, intestinal parasitic infestation (particularly hookworm disease) and regional enteritis or ulcerative colitis are the most common causes of occult hemorrhage. Occult gastrointestinal blood loss may be detected in nearly 50 per cent of affected infants; usually no discrete lesions can be identified. The effect of normal menstrual loss on iron requirements has been discussed. Women frequently, however, fail to recognize an abnormal flow. The following suggest that menstrual volume is excessive: the need to wear double pads because one soaks through; duration of periods greater than 5 days; passage of large clots, and use of more than 12 pads per period. The admirable and necessary donation of blood for transfusions must be regarded as a form of hemorrhage, as must also the collection of large amounts of blood withdrawn for diagnostic study.

Not infrequently, patients are observed in whom the cause for iron deficiency is not found during the course of careful clinical evaluation: their diets seem adequate; no absorptive defect can be recognized, no blood loss can be detected. In the careful clinical study of patients seen at the Radcliffe Infirmary at Oxford, 17 per cent of 371 patients fell in this category.[49] No distinctive features could be found. In all probability, blood loss is unrecognized because it is intermittent or small enough in amount to be detected only with isotopic techniques.

Under four conditions, iron-deficient erythropoiesis may be found even though body iron is normal or greater than normal: (a) hereditary absence of transferrin; (b) congenital pulmonary hemosiderosis; (c) paroxysmal nocturnal hemoglobinuria, and (d) patients with inflammation who are unable to mobilize iron from R. E. cell depots. Increased amounts of iron are found in these conditions in the liver, lungs, kidneys and R. E. systems, respectively, but not enough are made available to the bone marrow to support normal hemoglobin synthesis.

Much interest has been focused on the fact that iron-deficient patients often feel tired, develop epithelial changes, and frequently experience a sense of well-being soon after iron therapy has been started. A causative decrease in one of the cellular metalloenzymes has been suspected and sought for, but no consistent defect has been found.

Diagnosis. Iron deficiency without anemia can be recognized by: a plasma iron level less than 40 μg per 100 ml, an iron-binding capacity greater than 400 μg per 100 ml, and only 5 to 15 per cent saturation of the iron-binding capacity.[32] Further confirmation can be obtained by demonstrating that fewer than 5 per cent of the nucleated red blood cell precursors contain cytoplasmic siderotic granules (sideroblasts), and that there is little or no stainable iron (hemosiderin) in slides prepared from aspirated bone marrow. Other methods have been used experimentally to estimate storage iron (phlebotomy to determine how much iron can be mobilized to compensate for the controlled hemorrhage, by a radioiron dilution technique[52] and by measuring urinary iron excretion after parenteral injection of desferrioxamine), but histologic evaluation of bone marrow slides stained with Prussian blue is the only practical clinical method.[5] Fortunately, the concentrations of iron in liver and hematopoietically active marrow are approximately equal:[52] these two organs are the principal sites of iron storage, an estimate of the iron content in either site provides a reasonable guide for the total reserves. As with most procedures, the method has certain limitations: if iron has recently been administered parenterally, stainable iron particles may be found even if the patient is deficient, because of slow release from the injected iron complexes.

Of greater practical importance is the diagnosis of iron deficiency advanced enough to impaire erythropoiesis. The anemia is at first mild, and may be normocytic, normochromic in type. As the deficiency state becomes more advanced the erythrocytes become hypochromic (mean corpuscular hemoglobin concentration less than 30 per cent), vary moderately in size and shape and decrease to a mean corpuscular volume of less than 80 cubic microns. The red blood cell count is only rarely less than 3 million cells per cu mm and may even be within the normal range: the hemoglobin is reduced to a proportionately greater degree and may be less than 5 gm per 100 ml. Reticulocytes are usually normal or reduced in number, but may rise temporarily following sudden increase in blood loss. The leukocyte count is normal or may be slightly low. Platelets are frequently elevated to levels about twice that of normal subjects, but mild thrombocytopenia is observed rarely; under both circumstances, the platelet count returns to normal when iron deficiency is corrected. The marrow is cellular and tends to be hyperplastic, particularly for normoblasts, most of which are fairly mature. The erythrocyte life span is usually normal, but instances of moderately shortened survival have been reported. Hypochlorhydria and achlorhydria occur more commonly than in comparable population groups; their incidence varies with the methods used for stimulating gastric secretion, with the age of the patient and with the cause of the iron deficiency. For instance, achlorhydria is unusual in chronic iron deficiency of hookworm disease.[53] In the Oxford series, the incidence was about 40 per cent by the single dose histamine test, but only 16 per cent with the augmented histamine test.[49]

The anemias that are most likely to be confused with iron-deficiency anemia are those in which hypochromia results from infection or a block or defect in porphyrin or globin synthesis (thalassemia, hemoglobinopathies, lead intoxication, pyridoxine-responsive anemias, sideroblastic refractory anemia). Differentiation can be made, however, because the marrow iron is not depleted and transferrin saturation, except in the anemia of infection, is not low; even in that instance, however, the stainable bone marrow iron serves to differentiate.

Study of patients with iron-deficiency anemia is never complete until the cause for the deficiency is recognized. Both the fact and the source of any blood loss must be identified. Carcinomas, particularly of the gastrointestinal tract, may be detected in this search long before other manifestations would have appeared. At times it is helpful to tag a sample of the patient's red blood cells with radioactive chromium, readminister the blood, and then measure the radioactivity that will be found in the feces if blood is oozing from a gastrointestinal lesion. The same technique may be used to provide a quantitative measure of menstrual loss.

Clinical Manifestations. Patients with laboratory evidence of iron deficiency but with normal erythrocyte values or only a mild normocytic, normochromic anemia may complain of weakness, fatigue and lassitude. These vague symptoms are difficult to relate specifically to iron deficiency: iron therapy in some instances is attended by an increased sense of well-being, but administration of placebos occasionally accomplishes a similar result. The possibility exists that iron therapy replenishes a still unidentified tissue iron compound that causes the improvement.

Some patients with iron-deficiency anemia have no sense of ill health; the abnormality may be discovered during the course of a medical examination for other reasons. The anemia may develop so gradually that it interferes only moderately with work efficiency, even when the hemoglobin is as low as 9 gm per 100 ml. Most of the complaints are common to all anemias: weakness, fatigability, pallor, dyspnea on exertion, palpitation and a sense of "dead-tiredness." When

standardized exercise is carried out on a bicycle ergometer, it can be shown that the time needed to restore cardio-respiratory functions to pre-exercise resting values is markedly prolonged.[54] Coldness and paresthesia of the hands and feet are not infrequent. Only a minority complain of the abnormality causing the anemia, *i.e.* hiatus hernia, peptic ulcer, hemorrhoids. Symptoms are usually so insidious in onset that their duration cannot be dated with accuracy.

Manifestations related to the oral cavity and the gastrointestinal tract have attracted attention both because of their frequency and because of uncertainty as to their pathogenesis. Vague gastrointestinal complaints, such as a capricious appetite, flatulence, epigastric distress with eructation, constipation or diarrhea and nausea, are fairly common. Pica is practiced by some patients with iron-deficiency: geophagia, starch-eating and pagophagia. The latter is a craving for an ingestion of large amounts of ice.[55] Geophagia is often but not always corrected by iron therapy. The suggestion has been made that severe degrees of iron-lack may cause secondary malabsorption phenomena, possibly related to a decrease in iron-containing or iron-dependent enzymes in intestinal mucosal cells.[56] Glossitis characterized by varying degrees of papillary atrophy and soreness is found more often in patients over the age of 40 years and with greater frequency in women than in men. Angular stomatitis occurs in 10 to 15 per cent of patients, particularly among those who are edentulous. Dysphagia, hypochromic anemia and post-cricoid esophageal stricture, often accompanied by a web at this site, constitute an interesting triad (Paterson-Kelly or Plummer-Vinson syndrome) found particularly but not exclusively in middle-aged women. It has been regarded as a precancerous lesion, but that relationship has been doubted.[57] Gastroscopic examination with gastric biopsy done on northern Europeans has demonstrated gastritis with varying degrees of glandular damage in about 80 per cent of cases and atrophic gastritis in a few. It is by no means certain that these oral and gastrointestinal manifestations are the direct result of iron deficiency. For instance, the incidence of glossitis, angular stomatitis and dysphagia varies greatly among patients in different population groups and seems to be decreasing in communities where iron deficiency remains prevalent. The varying incidence of these epithelial changes plus the fact that they seem to occur more frequently in "low input" than in "high output" (blood loss) iron deficiency suggest that they may be caused by associated deficiencies. In patients with achlorhydria the secretion of acid often returns after treatment with iron, particularly in younger patients, but the histologic appearance of the gastric mucosa has only rarely been observed to improve.[49]

The fingernails, and sometimes the toenails as well, often become lusterless, thin, brittle, flattened and then spoon-shaped (koilonychia). When the hemoglobin falls below 8 gm per 100 ml the heart may become dilated and hemic murmurs may be heard. The spleen is enlarged enough to be palpable at the costal margin in about 10 per cent of cases. Mild degrees of vitiligo and of dependent edema are not infrequent. Neurologic examination is normal in spite of paresthesias. Rarely, papilledema, visual disturbances and elevated cerebral spinal fluid pressure, simulating intracranial tumors, may be found in iron-deficient women; these unusual manifestations are corrected by iron therapy.[5] Another interesting syndrome occurs among young males in Iran: dwarfism, iron-deficiency anemia, hepatosplenomegaly, hypogonadism and geophagia.[58] A similar syndrome without geophagia has been observed in Egypt: coexistent zinc deficiency has been claimed.[59]

Treatment. Adequate therapy must not only correct the deficiency, but also treat its cause. Increased menstrual flow, occult loss of blood from the urinary or gastrointestinal tracts or defective absorption must be searched for and corrected if possible. Wise selection of a therapeutic agent requires knowledge of what the maximum hematologic response might be, the amount of iron required to produce this maximum effect and the absorption that can be expected from a given iron compound. The physician should observe the patient to make certain that a response is obtained: a satisfactory rise in the hemoglobin level attributable to the iron therapy constitutes the final proof confirming the diagnosis.

Hematologic Response and Amount of Iron Required for Maximum Effect. The pattern of response to iron therapy by a patient with iron-deficiency anemia is schematically summarized in Figure 6C–9. About 5 to 7 days after therapy is begun, the reticulocyte level begins to rise, reaches a peak of 10 to 15 per cent between 10 to 14 days, and then falls during the next week to normal levels; the height of the reticulocyte peak is inversely proportional to the original hemoglobin value. The hemoglobin begins to increase in about 7 to 10 days; it rises at a rate of 0.2 to 0.3 gm per 100 ml per day when the anemia is severe and at 0.1 to 0.2 gm per 100 ml when the initial hemoglobin level is greater than 7.5 gm per 100 ml. As the hemoglobin concentration approaches normal, the rate of increase slows: from 4 to 8 weeks are required before normal values are attained. Return of the plasma iron to normal may take another month or two.

The *daily* dose of iron should ideally be great enough to support a maximum hemoglobin increase: 0.3 gm per 100 ml per day or 15 gm of new circulating hemoglobin in a patient with a blood volume of 5 liters. It requires 50 mg of iron. This value would obviously vary with the blood volume but is a reasonable average figure to provide for adults. The comparable figure for children varies with body weight and can be calculated by estimating the blood volume to be 70 ml per kg.

The *total* amount of iron that must be absorbed or injected to correct the deficiency can also be estimated. Assume, for instance, that a woman with severe iron-deficiency anemia has only 5 gm of hemoglobin per 100 ml. If the normal hemoglobin level is 14 gm and her blood volume is 4 liters, she must increase her circulating hemoglobin 360 gm; this amount contains about 1.2 gm of iron (360 × 0.34 per cent). One should also provide 0.5 to 1 gm of storage iron. The total amount needed to correct the deficiency in this instance, therefore, would be 1.7 to 2.2 gm.

Oral Therapy. The ideal iron preparation for oral therapy should be well absorbed,

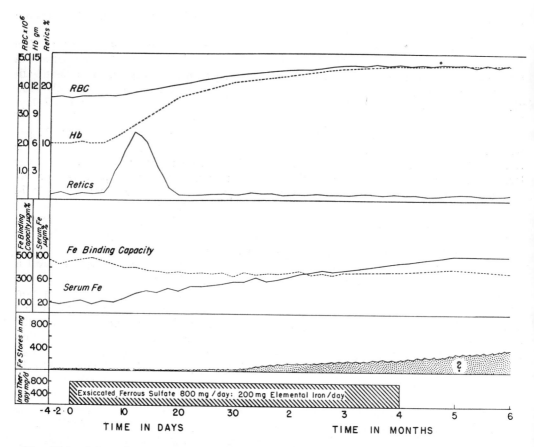

Fig. 6C-9. Schematic representation of hematologic response to iron therapy. No accurate data are available to describe the reappearance of storage iron; its reaccumulation may be slower than shown—hence the question mark.

well tolerated by the gastrointestinal tract in therapeutic doses, and inexpensive. Since ferrous iron is so much more efficiently absorbed than the ferric form, simple highly soluble ferrous salts come closest to approaching the ideal—and ferrous sulfate is recognized as the standard against which all other compounds must be evaluated. The most elegant job of comparing the absorption from different iron compounds has been done by Brise and Hallberg with a double isotope technique:[60] 30 mg of iron as ferrous sulfate and 30 mg as the preparation under study were given on alternate days for a total of 10 days: the two preparations were labeled with two different isotopes of iron so that absorption from the preparation under study could be compared with that from ferrous

sulfate (Fig. 6C–10). A number of compounds were absorbed about as well as ferrous sulfate: ferrous succinate, ferrous lactate, ferrous fumarate, ferrous glycine sulfate, ferrous glutamate, and ferrous gluconate; none was superior. Relatively large amounts of ascorbic acid given along with ferrous sulfate increased absorption slightly, but not enough either to justify the added cost or to permit significant reduction in the daily dose of ferrous sulfate.

Each of the preparations listed in Table 6C-7 is thoroughly acceptable. An iron-deficient patient will absorb approximately 20 per cent of the iron in these tablets. Since the recommended daily dose provides roughly 200 to 240 mg of iron, the desired 40 or 50 mg should be assimilated. Iron salts are all irritating to the gastric and intestinal mucosa. In those patients who complain of severe epigastric distress, tolerance can frequently be induced by reducing the dose to one tablet per day and then gradually adding one tablet per day until the full therapeutic dose is reached. Alternatively, other preparations may be tried until one is found that can be tolerated. Children tend to have less gastrointestinal distress from iron therapy

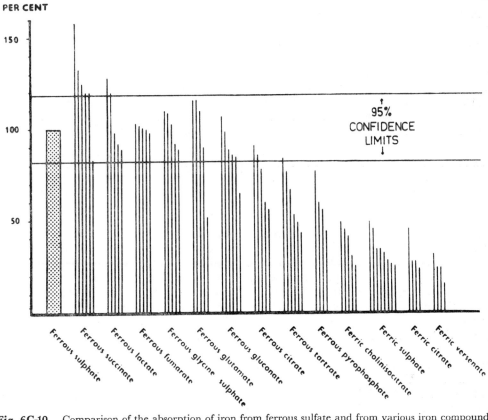

Fig. 6C-10. Comparison of the absorption of iron from ferrous sulfate and from various iron compounds. Daily dose equivalent to 30 mg elemental iron. Ferrous sulfate and the other compounds under study were tagged with different isotopes of iron and given on alternate days for 10 days. (From Brise and Hallberg, Acta Med. Scandinav. Suppl.)

Table 6C-7.   Recommended Oral Iron Preparations

Preparation	gm/tablet	Iron content %	Iron content mg Fe/tablet	Acceptable adult dose tablets/day
Ferrous sulfate, 7H$_2$O	0.32	20	60	4
Ferrous sulfate, exsiccated	0.2	29	60	4
Ferrous gluconate	0.32	12	40	4 or 5
Ferrous fumarate	0.2	33	66	4
	0.32	33	105	2 or 3
Ferroglycine sulfate	0.25	16	40	5

than do adults. A satisfactory schedule is to give half the adult dose to children who weigh from 15 to 35 kg, and the full dose to those heavier than 35 kg. For smaller children and those unable to take tablets, liquid preparations are available.

A common error is to discontinue iron therapy after the 2 or 3 months required for correction of the anemia. Replenishment of iron stores occurs slowly when iron is given orally because absorption falls off as the hemoglobin rises toward normal; consequently, oral therapy must be continued for 6 to 12 months if stores are to be repleted. If the chronic bleeding responsible for iron de-

ing from brisk hemorrhage, whose hemoglobin level is critical, or who have serious complications demanding immediate correction of the anemia.

Parenteral Therapy. Parenteral administration of iron should be reserved for those subjects who are unable to tolerate or absorb orally administered iron: (1) patients with ulcerative colitis, regional enteritis, intestinal shunts, colostomy or ileostomy; (2) patients with malabsorption syndromes; and (3) the rare person who is unable or unwilling to cooperate or who has severe intolerance to oral therapy. The three best preparations available for parenteral use are:

Preparation	Fe in mg/ml	Route	Recommended daily dose
Iron dextran	50	I.M.	2 ml
Iron sorbitol	50	I.M.	2 ml
Dextriferron	20	I.V.	1.5 ml increasing to 5 ml

ficiency cannot be corrected or controlled, continuous iron therapy is required.

Preparations which, in addition to iron, contain molybdenum, copper, cobalt, ascorbic acid, the various vitamins including folic acid and B_{12}, liver, or bone marrow extracts, etc., are more expensive, and no more effective in correcting iron deficiency and in some instances have distinct disadvantages. Fortunately most are being withdrawn in the United States by order of the Food and Drug Administration. Injections of folic acid and of vitamin B_{12} do not increase the response to iron. Also to be deplored is the recent practice of packaging ferrous sulfate in enteric coated tablets or in capsules containing delayed release granules: the per cent of iron absorbed is distinctly less because iron is released more distally in the small intestine where absorption is less efficient.

Oral iron therapy may fail in patients with malabsorption syndromes, with diarrhea, or in those who have had a gastrectomy. In the latter two instances, iron tablets may move so quickly through the small intestine that they reach the cecum before disintegrating; x-ray films of the abdomen may demonstrate the radiopaque pellets in the large bowel. Blood transfusions are rarely necessary in the treatment of iron-deficiency anemia and should be reserved for patients who are suffer-

In each instance, one half the recommended dose should first be given to establish the patient's ability to tolerate the material. The total dose should be carefully calculated to correct the hemoglobin deficit and to provide an additional 500 mg for storage, but should not be greater than 2 gm per course. Intramuscular injections should be given via a zigzag needle tract to avoid unsightly staining of the skin. Systemic reactions are unusual but may be severe: headache, fever, arthralgia, back pain, and rarely peripheral vascular collapse. Rates of hemoglobin increase do not differ significantly from those produced by proper oral therapy.

Prognosis. When patients with iron-deficiency anemia die, they do so because of other disease responsible for the depletion, *e.g.*, gastrointestinal or other types of malignant neoplasm, peptic ulcer, regional enteritis, ulcerative colitis, etc. Recurrence of the anemia is common because the precipitating cause is not recognized, continues, or recurs.[49] Patients with severe gastritis tend to develop achylia gastrica and have a higher incidence of subsequent pernicious anemia. Those with chronic severe epithelial changes in the oral cavity have a somewhat higher attack rate of carcinoma of the upper gastrointestinal tract. In affected children whose growth and development are retarded, iron therapy frequently produces at least partial correction of the defect.

Supplements to Prevent Development of Iron Deficiency. In the United States and several other countries, the cereal most commonly eaten, usually wheat flour or rice, is being fortified with iron. Flour in the United States is enriched with 12 mg iron per pound (460 gm): bread baked under commercial conditions contains about 0.022 to 0.037 mg Fe per gm of wet weight. That the iron can be absorbed was proved in experiments where bread fortified with radioactive iron was fed: normal subjects absorbed from 1 to 12 per cent, while iron-deficient subjects assimilated several times as much.[61] Recent evidence indicates that soluble inorganic iron added to food is absorbed to the same extent as is the intrinsic iron in that food.[78] Since iron in rice and corn is poorly absorbed,[19] these cereals are poor vehicles for fortification. Under current consideration in the United States is a contested proposal by the Food and Drug Administration to increase iron enrichment to 40 mg per pound of wheat flour and to 25 mg per pound loaf of bread. Approximately 10 per cent of the iron is absorbed from iron-fortified cereals prepared for infants.[62] These kinds of enrichment seem highly desirable, but they are expensive, fraught with technical difficulties, and are difficult to provide on a world-wide basis. Their effectiveness, however, has been vigorously challenged by Elwood in a series of publications,[63,64] and is currently being reevaluated in several countries.

There are two times in life when iron supplementation is recommended: during infancy and pregnancy. A daily dietary allowance of 1.0 to 1.5 mg dietary iron/kg/day achieves optimal iron nutrition for a substantial majority of the infant population.[44-46] In an infant of average weight, dosages of 6 to 9 mg/day at 3 months of age, gradually increased to 8 to 12 mg/day at 6 months of age, and to 10 to 15 mg/day by 12 months of age will satisfy this allowance, according to Sturgeon's data: he believes that no further increase is necessary in later infancy. Supplementation by iron-enriched cereals or by iron salts is usually required if an intake of 15 mg is to be achieved. In a careful study from Montreal, de Leeuw and her associates found that 78 mg (but not 39 mg) of elemental ferrous iron daily for 24 weeks to normal pregnant women in the McGill University Clinic were adequate to achieve optimal hemoglobin mass and to maintain iron stores.[48] This amount is surprisingly high. While private patients may eat more meat and have a higher natural intake of iron, supplementation for them would also seem to be an advisable prophylactic measure.

IRON OVERLOAD

An excessive body load of iron can be produced by greater than normal absorption from the alimentary canal, by parenteral injection, or by a combination of both mechanisms. The excess iron is deposited largely as hemosiderin in R. E. cells, or in the parenchymal cells of certain tissues. The site of deposition is in part dependent on the portal of entry. When excess iron is derived from intestinal absorption, it is carried to tissues bound by plasma transferrin and transferred to parenchymal and R. E. cells as well as to developing erythroblasts. On the other hand, parenterally administered iron, given usually as transfused blood, ends up largely in R. E. cells where the transfused erythrocytes are eventually destroyed and their hemoglobin degraded. In iron overload the plasma iron and transferrin saturation are usually increased, the total iron-binding capacity somewhat depressed (Fig. 6C–7). A simple classification based on mechanism of production is:

A. Excessive absorption of iron
   1. "Idiopathic" hemochromatosis.
   2. Excessive intake (siderosis in the Bantu; prolonged therapeutic administration of iron to subjects not iron deficient).
   3. In patients with chronic alcoholism, chronic liver disease (usually portal cirrhosis), and possibly pancreatic insufficiency.
   4. In patients with certain types of refractory anemia, usually associated with ineffective erythropoiesis and increased hemolysis.
B. Transfusional hemosiderosis.

The term "hemosiderosis" has been used to designate an increase in iron storage without associated tissue damage: hemochromatosis indicates that such damage is present, particularly in the liver, that the iron is widely dispersed, and that the amount of iron is greatly increased (usually 20 to 40 gm).[4,65]

Difference of opinion exists about the designation of idiopathic hemochromatosis as a distinct entity. The dominant view regards it as a rare but specific disease: (a) produced by a genetically controlled unidentified inborn error of metabolism which causes increased absorption of iron and the slow accumulation throughout life of excessive quantities of parenchymally distributed hemosiderin, (b) characterized clinically by the development during adult life of portal cirrhosis, bronze pigmentation, diabetes mellitus, a tendency to hypofunction of endocrine glands (the gonads, the anterior pituitary), and myocardial failure.[66] MacDonald, on the other hand, questions the validity of the evidence favoring a genetic defect as responsible for increased absorption and tissue avidity for iron, and argues vigorously that hemochromatosis is always secondary to environmental factors responsible for increased retention of iron (diet or disease associated with greater than normal assimilation).[67] Another question for which no final answer can yet be given is the following: Are the high concentrations of iron responsible *per se* for tissue injury or does damage to tissues occur only when some other abnormality (*e.g.*, nutritional, metabolic, toxic, infectious) is superimposed? The failure of animal experiments to provide a definitive solution may be related to the fact that iron overload has usually been induced by injecting forms of iron which are taken up primarily by R. E. cells and are not readily redistributed to parenchymal sites; furthermore, induction of tissue damage may take longer than the animals can usually be kept alive.[68] Those who do believe that iron has a noxious effect point out that cirrhosis, fibrosis, and disturbance of organ function are particularly likely to occur when excessive amounts of iron are absorbed from the alimentary canal and deposited primarily in parenchymal rather than (or in addition to) R. E. cells. In the Bantu, a positive correlation exists between the concentration of iron in the liver and the incidence of portal

cirrhosis: with concentrations greater than 2 gm per 100 gm dry weight, most of the patients have portal cirrhosis.[69] The large amount of intracellular iron may cause progressive destruction of parenchymal cells and replacement by fibrous tissue.[70] The relationship between diabetes mellitus and cardiomyopathies in iron overload and deposition of hemosiderin in the pancreas and myocardium have also been cited as evidence favoring toxicity of the iron. The improvement reported in patients with idiopathic hemochromatosis after removal of a large fraction of their excess iron by therapeutic phlebotomy would seem to argue strongly for a noxious effect of iron overload.

Of greatest nutritional interest are the forms of secondary iron overload due to increased alimentary uptake.

Siderosis in the Bantu.[4,66,71] Iron overload in the Bantu results from long-continued exposure to diets containing too much iron, derived largely from cooking pots and from the drums used in the preparation of fermented alcoholic beverages. In adult males, the intake may exceed 100 mg of iron per day. The condition frequently becomes manifest in late adolescence, reaches its greatest severity between the ages of 40 and 60 years, and is usually more severe in males whose alcoholic consumption tends to be greater. The pathologic pattern of the iron overload is one of hepatic and reticuloendothelial involvement. Portal cirrhosis becomes evident in the majority of patients (but not in all) when the hepatic concentration of iron reaches 2 gm or more per 100 gm of dry weight,[69] a redistribution of iron takes place so that parenchymal deposits of hemosiderin are found in the epithelial cells of many organs, particularly the pancreas and the myocardium. Approximately 20 per cent of these subjects develop clinical diabetes, but myocardial failure has not been described. To what extent these changes are due to the iron alone, to the chronic alcoholism, or to the associated nutritional disturbances is unknown.

Portal Cirrhosis, Chronic Alcoholism, and Pancreatic Insufficiency. Patients with alcoholic or nutritional portal cirrhosis of the liver frequently have increased amounts of stainable iron in their livers, although the total amount present is rarely greater than 1 gm.[72] With the larger amounts, hemosiderin deposits are found in parenchymal cells of the liver, pancreas, heart, and adrenal glands. Clinical similarity to hemochromatosis is accentuated by the occurrence in portal cirrhosis of increased skin pigmentation, a greater than normal incidence of diabetes mellitus, and testicular atrophy. Cardiac failure, when it occurs, can usually be accounted for on other grounds. More males than females are affected and clinical manifestations are most prominent in late middle life. A number of possible explanations for the iron overload have been cited. Patients with portal cirrhosis are frequently wine drinkers, consuming several liters daily: American and European wines contain significant quantities of iron and several milligrams per day may be derived from that source alone.[8] Alcohol increases the absorption of ferric iron.[73] Patients with chronic liver disease or chronic pancreatitis absorb iron excessively from the gut.[74,75] Whether these patients should be regarded as having hemochromatosis or portal cirrhosis with hemosiderosis is difficult to determine. Their body load of excess iron is usually distinctly less than that reported for hemochromatosis. Some workers, however, contend that no sharp distinction is possible; they believe that hemosiderosis may progress, with increasing and more widespread distribution of iron, to the complete picture of hemochromatosis without any sharp dividing line.

Prolonged Iron Therapy. In a few instances, the prolonged administration of iron to patients who did not need it has been responsible for iron overload; manifestations indistinguishable from hemochromatosis were presumably secondary.[76,77] Since iron preparations are advertised widely in the United States, are available without prescription, and are consumed in large quantities, it is surprising that more examples have not been reported.

Refractory Anemia.[4,5] The amount of iron found in the tissues of patients with refractory anemia, particularly those with a hypercellular marrow and ineffective erythropoiesis, is occasionally greater than can be accounted for by the transfusions they have received. In some cases, little blood has been given during the course of the illness yet excess iron was present. Not all of these subjects have erroneously been treated with iron, although that has happened in some instances. Excessive absorption of dietary iron from the gut must have occurred, supposedly because of the accelerated but ineffective erythropoiesis. Bothwell and Finch found 31 such patients reported in the literature: the anemias included refractory anemia, what would now be called sideroblastic achrestic anemia, thalassemia major, and paroxysmal nocturnal hemoglobinuria: all had a cellular erythroid marrow.[4] Twenty-six had portal cirrhosis and an additional 4 had increased portal tract fibrosis; 5 had diabetes, and 6 more had impaired glucose tolerance; at least 15 showed increased pigmentation of the skin. In patients like these, the distribution of hemosiderin is parenchymal as well as in R. E. cells. Why they develop the changes of hemochromatosis, whereas transfusional hemosiderosis is found in most multi-transfused subjects with similar loads of body iron, remains a mystery. Nutritional differences between the two groups cannot clearly be identified. Factors of possible significance are these: (1) cirrhosis may result from serum hepatitis; (2) parenchymal distribution of iron may be related to the gastrointestinal portal of entry of a significant portion of the excess body iron.

BIBLIOGRAPHY

1. Committee on Iron Deficiency: J.A.M.A., *203*, 407, 1968.
2. Moore: Harvey Lectures, *55*, 67, 1959–1960.
3. Moore and Dubach: in *Mineral Metabolism*, Vol. 2, Part 13, New York, Academic Press, 1962. Chapter 30, p. 288.
4. Bothwell and Finch: *Iron Metabolism*, Boston, Little, Brown & Co., 1962.
5. Fairbanks, Fahey, and Beutler: *Clinical Disorders of Iron Metabolism*, 2nd Ed., New York, Grune & Stratton, 1971.
6. Moore: Scandinavian J. Haemat., Series Haematologica, *6*, 1, 1965.
7. U. S. Interdepartmental Committee for National Defense: "Nutrition Survey of the Armed Forces." Iran (1956), Turkey (1958), Spain (1958), Ethiopia (1959), Peru (1959), Ecuador (1960), The Kingdom of Thailand (1961).

8. MacDonald: Arch. Int. Med., *112*, 82, 1963.
9. Taylor: *The Examination of Water and Water Supplies* (Tresh, Beale, and Suckling), 7th Ed., Boston, Little, Brown & Co., p. 699, 1958.
10. Conrad: in *Iron Deficiency*. Ed. by Hallberg, Harwerth, and Vannotti, London and New York, Academic Press, p. 87–114, 1970.
11. Minnich, Okcuoglu, Tarcon, Arcasoy, Cin, Yorukoglu, Renda, and Demirag: Am. J. Clin. Nutr., *21*, 78, 1968.
12. Luke, Davis, and Deller: Lancet 2, 844, 1968.
13. Conrad and Crosby: Blood, *22*, 406, 1963.
14. Weintraub, Weinstein, Huser, and Rafal: J. Clin. Invest., *47*, 531, 1968.
15. Brown, Hwang, Nicol, and Ternberg: J. Lab. & Clin. Med., *72*, 58, 1968.
16. Turnbull, Cleton, and Finch: J. Clin. Invest., *41*, 1897, 1962.
17. Hallberg and Solvell: Acta Med. Scand. *181*, 335, 1967.
18. Moore: in *Occurrence, Causes and Prevention of Nutritional Anaemia*, Ed. by Blix, Symposia of the Swedish Nutrition Foundation VI, Stockholm, Alquist & Wiksell, p. 92, 1968.
19. Layrisse and Martinez-Torres: in *Progress in Hematology*, New York, Grune & Stratton, Vol. VII, p. 134, 1971.
20. Elwood: Lancet, 2, 516, 1968.
21. Layrisse, Cook, Martinez-Torres, Roche, Kuhn, and Finch: Blood, *33*, 430, 1969.
22. Martinez-Torres and Layrisse: Blood, *35*, 669, 1970.
23. Pirzio-Biroli, Bothwell, and Finch: J. Lab. & Clin. Med., *51*, 37, 1958.
24. Awai and Brown: J. Lab. & Clin. Med., *61*, 363, 1963.
25. Laurell: Pharmacol. Rev., *4*, 371, 1952.
26. Fletcher and Huehns: Nature, *218*, 1211, 1968.
27. Jandl and Katz: J. Clin. Invest., *42*, 314, 1963.
28. Finch, Deubelbeiss, Cook, Eschbach, Harker, Funk, Marsaglia, Hillman, Slichter, Adamson, Ganzoni, and Giblett: Medicine, *49*, 17, 1970.
29. Bessis and Breton-Gorius: Blood, *14*, 423, 1959.
30. Crichton: New Eng. J. Med., *284*, 1413, 1971.
31. Scott and Pritchard: J.A.M.A., *199*, 147, 1967.
32. Bainton and Finch: Am. J. Med., *37*, 62, 1964.
33. Beutler, Robson, and Buttenwieser: Ann. Int. Med., *48*, 60, 1958.
34. Weinfeld: Acta Med. Scandinav. Suppl., *427*, 1, 1965.
35. Bothwell, Pirbella, Mebust, and Finch: Am. J. Physiol., *193*, 615, 1958.
36. Davies, Brown, Stewart, Terry, and Sisson: Am. J. Physiol., *197*, 87, 1959.
37. Green, Charlton, Seftel, Bothwell, Mayet, Adams, Finch, and Layrisse: Am. J. Med., *45*, 336, 1968.
38. Ebaugh, Clemens, Rodman, and Peterson: Am. J. Med., *25*, 169, 1958.
39. Bothwell: in *Iron Deficiency*. Ed. by Hallberg, Harwerth, and Vannotti, London and New York, Academic Press, p. 151, 1970.
40. Hallberg and Nilsson: Acta obst. et gynec. scandinav., *43*, 352, 1964.
41. Hallberg, Högdahl, Nilsson, and Rybo: Acta obst. et gynec. scandinav., *45*, 320, 1966.
42. Rybo: in *Iron Deficiency*. Ed. by Hallberg, Harwerth, and Vannotti, London and New York, Academic Press, p. 163, 1970.
43. Moore: in *Iron Metabolism, an International Symposium*, Ed. by Gross, Berlin, Springer-Verlag, p. 241, 1964.
44. Moe: Acta paediatrica, Suppl. 150, 1963.
45. Sturgeon: Pediatrics, *17*, 341, 1956.
46. Sturgeon: in *Iron in Clinical Medicine*, Berkeley, University of California Press, p. 183, 1958.
47. Garby, Irnell, and Werner: Acta Med. Scand., *185*, 107 and 113, 1969.
48. deLeeuw, Lowenstein, and Hseih: Medicine, *45*, 291, 1966.
49. Beveridge, Bannerman, Evanson, and Witts: Quart. J. Med., *34*, 145, 1965.
50. Baird and Wilson: Quart. J. Med., *28*, 35, 1959.
51. Stevens, Pirzio-Biroli, Harkins, Nyhus, and Finch: Ann. Surg., *149*, 534, 1959.
52. Gale, Torrance, and Bothwell: J. Clin. Invest., *42*, 1076, 1963.
53. Foy and Kondi: Trans. roy. Soc. trop. Med. & Hygn., *54*, 419, 1960.
54. Andersen and Barkve: Scand. J. Clin. Lab. Invest., *25*, Suppl. 114, 1970.
55. Coltman: J.A.M.A., *207*, 513, 1969.
56. Kimber and Weintraub: New Eng. J. Med., *279*, 453, 1968.
57. Jacobs: Brit. J. Cancer, *15*, 736, 1961.
58. Halsted, Prasad, and Nadimi: Arch. Int. Med., *116*, 253, 1956.
59. Prasad, Miale, Farid, Sandstead, and Schulert: J. Lab. & Clin. Med., *61*, 537, 1963.
60. Brise and Hallberg: Acta Med. Scandinav. Suppl., *376*, 23, 1962.
61. Steinkamp, Dubach, and Moore: Arch. Int. Med., *95*, 181, 1955.
62. Schulz and Smith: Am. J. Dis. Child., *93*, 30, 1957.
63. Elwood: Lancet, 2, 516, 1968.
64. Elwood: Am. J. Clin. Nutrition, *23*, 1267, 1970.
65. Finch and Finch: Medicine, *34*, 381, 1959.
66. Charlton and Bothwell: in *Progress in Hematology*, New York, Grune & Stratton, Vol. V, p. 298, 1966.
67. MacDonald: in *Progress in Hematology*, New York, Grune & Stratton, Vol. V, p. 324, 1966.
68. Brown, Dubach, Smith, Reynafarje, and Moore: J. Lab. & Clin. Med., *50*, 862, 1957.
69. Isaacson, Seftel, Keeley, and Bothwell: J. Lab. & Clin. Med., *58*, 845, 1961.
70. Block, Moore, Wasi, and Haiby: Am. J. Path., *47*, 89, 1965.
71. Bothwell: Scandinavian J. Haemat., Series Haematologica, *6*, 56, 1965.
72. MacDonald and Pechet: Arch. Int. Med., *116*, 381, 1965.
73. Charlton, Jacobs, Seftel, and Bothwell: Brit. Med. J., 2, 1425, 1964.
74. Challender and Malpas: Brit. Med. J., 2, 1516, 1963.

75. Davis and Badenoch: Lancet, *2*, 6, 1962.
76. Case Records of the Mass. Gen. Hosp. Case 38512, New Eng. J. Med., *247*, 992, 1952; Case 44131, ibid *258*, 652, 1958.

77. Wallerstein and Robbins: Am. J. Med., *14*, 256, 1953.
78. Cook, Layrisse, Martinez-Torres, Walker, Monsen, and Finch: J. Clin. Invest., *51*, 805, 1972.

Chapter

7

Water, Electrolytes and Acid-Base Balance

H. T. Randall

INTRODUCTION

Water is an essential and major component of all life on earth. Not just a passive solvent in which inorganic salts, organic compounds and dissolved gases interact, water participates actively in forming the building blocks for cells and is a component of most of them, as well as being the environment in which cells live and from which they obtain their nutrition.

Electrolytes comprise a wide variety of compounds, from simple inorganic salts of sodium, potassium and magnesium, to complex organic molecules often synthesized by and unique to the individual. Electrolytes share the phenomenon with water itself of dissociating into positively and negatively charged ions, and have the additional property of variably affecting the concentration of hydrogen ion in a solution; this effect depends both on individual ion characteristics and on interaction with other ionized and partially ionized substances in the solution. Major differences in specific ion concentrations exist between cell fluid and extracellular fluid; these differences are maintained by a substantial expenditure of energy by cells and are critical to cell metabolism and survival.

The hydrogen ion concentration of intracellular fluid and extracellular fluid differs. Both are held within very narrow ranges by a complex series of reactions within the organism, and by the ability selectively to excrete excessive acid or base loads by the kidneys. Diets vary in the effective amount of acid and base they contain. Metabolic processes of the body create an additional acid load which must be excreted to maintain optimum concentration.

The term *balance* implies a state of equilibrium which is dynamic for intakes of water, electrolytes and other nutrients, the conversion and utilization of metabolizable nutrients, and the excretion of ingested substances or their end products of metabolism. The net result is that the stable individual remains in energy balance, and in equilibrium of water, electrolytes and hydrogen ion concentration. Growth requires a positive balance. However, fluid, electrolyte and acid-base balance constitute far more than just a consideration of intake and output of water and electrolytes and of the differences between them. This discussion considers body composition including body cell mass and supporting and protecting tissues; fluid compartments and their size, composition and function; metabolism of water and electrolytes, and the regulatory mechanisms that defend the volume, content, and acid-base balance of the body. With these as background, alterations in water balance, in electrolyte composition and distribution, and acidosis and alkalosis are analyzed. Parenteral fluid and electrolyte therapy are discussed as an alternative and often necessary means of maintaining or correcting abnormalities in fluid, electrolyte and acid-base balances.

NORMAL BODY COMPOSITION

Essential to an understanding of the requirements of normal man for water and electrolytes as a part of nutrition, is knowledge of what constitutes normal body composition.

The reader is referred to Chapter 1 of this book for a detailed description of body composition, variations with age and by sex and body habitus, and the methods used for analysis.

For purposes of this chapter, the studies and terminology of Moore and his associates[1] are used. By isotopic dilutional techniques and chemical analysis they have determined not only the major chemical composition of the body, but, more importantly, its functional compartments. The range of normal body composition in both males and females over a wide span of age has been established, and abnormal changes in body composition resulting from disease or injury have been evaluated.

Total Body Water. The largest single component of the body is water. Body water is distributed throughout the cells, the extracellular fluids, and the solid supporting structures. The highest concentration of water is present in metabolically active cells of muscle and viscera, the lowest in relatively inert and inactive supporting structures such as the skeleton. Isotope dilution studies using either heavy water (^2H_2O, or D_2O) or tritiated water (^3H_2O) have shown that in the normal adult male, under the age of forty, approximately 60 per cent of body weight is water. In young women the exchangeable body water averages about 50

per cent of body weight, chiefly because the percentage of fat is higher than in men and the percentage of skeletal muscle is lower. In both sexes there is considerable normal variation of total body water content which makes accurate prediction of total body water difficult in a given individual. In the studies of Moore and his associates,[1] total body water is expressed as regression equations based on total body weight. Table 7–1 presents data from studies of 132 normal males and 88 normal females. Each series is divided to show differences due to age. Significant differences in regression equations exist for each group. There is a gradual and significant decline with age in total body water as a percentage of body weight.

Hume and Weyers[2] have suggested that total body water is closely correlated with body surface area. Table 7–2 presents a summary of their data; the regression equations and correlation coefficients are based on data from analysis of body water composition of 30 male and 30 female hospitalized patients using ^3H_2O isotope dilution measured at 2 and 3 hours after injection. Figures for 11 obese and 19 non-obese females are expressed as regressions of predicted surface area on measured body water using the DuBois formula for prediction of surface area (Fig. 7–1). A very high correlation is noted between predicted body surface and pre-

Table 7-1. Total Body Water (TBW) by Sex and Age[1]

Sex	Age Group (years)	Subjects	Mean Body Wt. (kg)	Mean TBW (liters)	95% Confidence Limits of Mean as % of Mean	Ratio(%) TBW(L) to Weight (Kg)
Male	16–30	63	71.75	42.26	±16	58.9
Male	31–60	56	73.57	40.24	±17	54.7
Male	61–90	13	69.42	35.82	±16	51.6
Female	16–30	54	60.89	30.99	±13	50.9
Female	31–90	34	62.62	28.36	±21	45.2

Predicted normal:

Males: $\dfrac{\text{TBW in L}}{\text{body wt in kg}} \times 100 = 79.45 - 0.24 \,(\text{Wt}) - 0.15 \,(\text{age})$

Females: $\dfrac{\text{TBW in L}}{\text{body wt in kg}} \times 100 = 69.81 - 0.2 \,(\text{Wt}) - 0.12 \,(\text{age})$

Table 7-2. Relationship Between Measured Total Body Water and Height, Weight and Predicted Body Surface Area in Adults*

Sex	Number	Age Group	Regression Equation: TBW on H and W**	Multiple Correlation Coefficient TBW, H and W	95% Confidence Limit—1 Patient H and W Known
M	30	35–71, x̄ 54.5	TBW=0.194781H + 0.296785W − 14.012934 r,H and W = 0.547(P<0.01);r, − H + TBW = 0.711 (P<0.001);r, W+TBW=0.920(P<0.001)	r=0.953	±27.5%
F	30	33–84, x̄ 53.7	TBW+0.344547H+0.183809W−35.270121 r,H and W = 0.589(P<0.001);r, H and TBW = 0.770(P<0.001) r,W and TBW = 0.913(P<0.001)	r = 0.957	±27.5%

Sex	Number	Age Group	Regression Equation on Surface Area Predicted on TBW Measured***	Correlation Coefficient	
M Non-obese	25	40–71, x̄ 57.2	Y = 0.5244 + 0.03193X	r = 0.916 P < 0.001	Although not stated, 95% confidence limits for predicting TBW in one individual would be of the order of ± 25%.
F Non-obese	19	41–84, x̄ 56.4	Y = 0.4172 + 0.03831X	r = 0.826 P < 0.001	
F Obese >10% over x̄ for adults	11	33–63, x̄ 50.2	Y = 0.9013 + 0.02811X	r = 0.813 P < 0.001	

* Data taken from Hume and Weyers[2] showing regression equations for total body water based on height, weight, and predicted body surface area Figures are based on a hospitalized patient population.
** Where TBW is in liters, H (Height) in cm. and W (Weight) in kg.
*** Y = Body surface area in meters², X = TBW in liters.

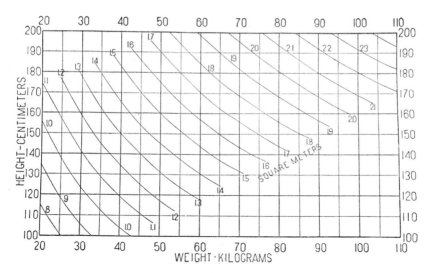

Fig. 7-1. Graph showing the relationship of height in centimeters and weight in kilograms to body surface area in square meters.[3]

dicted total body water in their male and female populations, as might be expected when linear regression of body water is based on height and weight. They suggest that estimates of surface area and of total body water are essentially interchangeable in defining predicted normal lean body mass, total body potassium, normal red cell volume, and cardiac output.

A comparison of predicted total body water between Moore's data[1] and those of Hume and Weyer[2] indicates a somewhat higher percentage of total body water by the Hume and Weyer method for both males and females of middle age. For example, an average height, average weight 55-year-old male (177 cm, 79 kg) would have a predicted body surface area of 1.97 M[2] (see Fig. 7–1) and a total body water of 45.3 liters, while the expected total body water of males in this age group from Moore's data is 54.7 per cent of body weight or 43.2 liters, and 41.3 liters from the prediction formula in Table 7–1. Similarly, a 162-cm, 67.3-kg, 55-year-old female with a body surface area of 1.72 M[2] would have a total body water of 34.0 liters, compared to 47.2 per cent of body weight or 31.8 liters from Moore's group average, and 30.7 liters from the prediction formula. Individual variation is so great, with 95% confidence limits for total body

water of the order of ± 16% of the mean in Moore's series, and ± 25% of the calculated individual value in Hume and Weyers' series, that such differences have no statistical significance. The differences might be predicted, however, on the basis that Hume and Weyers' patients were recovering in hospital, many from such stressful states as myocardial infarction, cardiovascular accident, acute bronchitis, and peptic ulcer, and they might be expected to have a somewhat expanded total body water under these circumstances.

Because of the relative simplicity of determining body surface area using the graph devised by DuBois[3] and the close correlation between predicted surface area and predicted total body water shown by Hume and Weyers,[2] Figures 7–1, 7–2, and 7–3 are provided for guidance in making estimates of predicted total body water. Wide normal individual variation must be expected.

Total body water, as a percentage of body weight, is higher in children and in adults who are lean or who have larger than normal skeletal muscle mass. It tends to decrease as body weight increases with obesity. Body water as a percentage of body weight also declines slowly with age in both sexes. Figure 7–4, utilizing Widdowson's data on growth and composition of the fetus and newborn[4] and Moore's studies of adults,[1] illustrates the

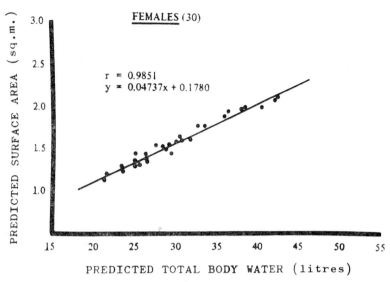

Fig. 7-2. Relationship between predicted body surface and predicted body water for women of middle age.[2]

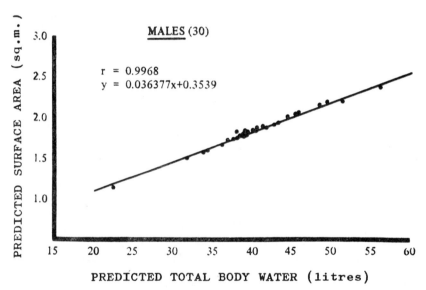

Fig. 7-3. Relationship between predicted body surface area and predicted body water for men of middle age.[2]

extremely high total body water content of the fetus and newborn infant, with progressive decrease in both total body water and the relative proportion of extracellular fluid to body weight and to total water with growth and maturation.

Body water constitutes a higher percentage of body weight in athletes than in non-athletes. Novak, Hyatt and Alexander[5]

found an average of 70 per cent of body weight as water in 21 college gymnasts, track men and swimmers; these men had remarkably lean bodies (95 to 96 per cent of body weight was estimated to be fat-free). Sixteen football and 10 baseball players of the same age group (19 to 22 years) averaged 14 per cent of body weight as fat and 63 per cent of weight as water.

BODY COMPOSITION BY AGE

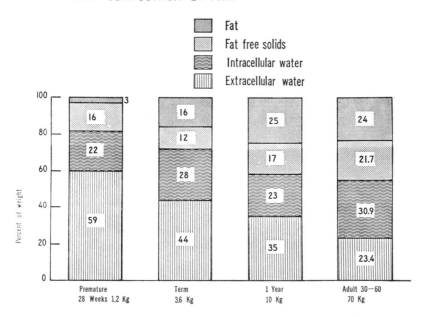

Fig. 7-4. Comparison of water content as per cent of total weight of premature and term infants, a child of 1 year, and normal adult 70-kg male. Total water decreases progressively as does extracellular water, while intracellular water increases with increase in body cell mass. Data taken from Widdowson[4] and Moore *et al.*[1]

Brill *et al.*[6] have measured total body water in markedly obese patients (260 to 440 pounds) in preparation for small bowel bypass operation. Such patients have a 21.3 ± 12.4 per cent greater total body water content than was anticipated on the basis of ^{40}K estimates of lean body mass and have a relatively expanded extracellular fluid space. They were also noted to have a much increased insensible water loss, averaging a daily evaporative loss of 2.4 to 2.9 liters as compared to a normal value of 0.9 liters.

Total body water may be considered as being distributed in two major compartments or spaces, based on differential concentration of the two major cations, sodium and potassium, and by the volume represented by dilution of radioactive isotopes, or other substances which appear to reach equilibrium in a portion of the total water pool.[1] The two major compartments are intracellular water (ICW) and extracellular water (ECW). *Intracellular water* is that portion of TBW within cells. Body composi-

tion studies indicate that from 50 to 58 per cent (average 55 per cent) of TBW is intracellular in normal healthy adults. Lean individuals with a relatively large skeletal muscle mass, such as trained young male athletes, have a higher percentage of TBW within cells, while females tend to have a more nearly equal distribution of TBW between ICW and ECW. *Extracellular water* consists of the water component of the extracellular fluids, plasma, interstitial fluid, and the water component of extracellular solids including tendon, fascia, dermis, collagen, elastin and skeleton. Since there is no way of distinguishing *in vivo* among the various areas of distribution of ECW, except for measurement of plasma volume and total ECW, ECW is usually considered as a two subcompartmental distribution of interstitial fluid and plasma.

The size of the ECW compartment as a volume or space depends upon methods used for measurements, and varies from 15 to 16 per cent of body weight when inulin, sucrose or mannitol is the indicator; it is as high as 27 per cent of body weight if ^{24}Na is assumed to be distributed entirely extracellularly, which it is not. Measurement of other small ions, such as $^{35}SO_4^=$ and $^{82}Br^-$, gives equilibration values of distribution of from 21 to 26 per cent of body weight for ECW; these data suffer from the fact that these ions enter into cells to some degree with time. As a practical matter, ECW can be considered as 23 per cent of body weight in normal adults, or even as 20 per cent of body weight as is commonly used clinically for extracellular fluid estimation in water and electrolyte balance problems.

Figure 7–5 illustrates the proportions of body weight as total body water in normal adult men and women, and its distribution as ICW, interstitial fluid, and plasma. Comparison of this Figure with Figure 7–4 indicates the major differences in water content and distribution that exist between adults and infants and emphasizes a reason for the special problem of water and electrolyte balance in infants.

TOTAL BODY SOLIDS: FAT AND FAT-FREE SOLIDS

Total body solids (*TBS*) are the remainder of body weight when total body water is subtracted:

$$TBS(kg) = Body\ Wt\ (kg) - TBW(L).$$

Total body solids are divided into body fat and fat-free solids.

Total body fat (*TBF*) is a derived figure in body composition analysis and is discussed in more detail in Chapter 1. In normal individuals, the assumption is made that body fat is anhydrous, and that the fat-free body is 73.2 per cent water, as determined by simultaneous multiple isotope dilution:

$$\%\ Body\ Fat = 100 - \frac{\%\ Body\ Water}{0.732}$$

$$Body\ Fat\ (kg) = \%\ Body\ Fat \times \frac{Body\ Wt.\ (kg)}{100}$$

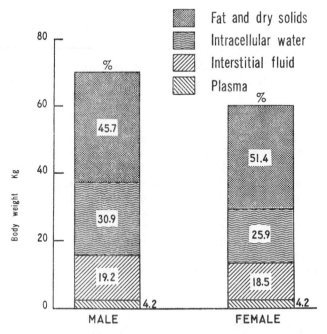

Fig. 7-5. Body water as percentage of body weight, with approximate distribution as intracellular water, interstitial water and plasma water for adult men and adult women. Data from Moore *et al.*[1]

This estimate depends heavily on the state of hydration of the fat-free body, which may vary from 0.67 to 0.85 or so. Moore has prepared a nomogram based on the ratio $\dfrac{\text{Intracellular Water}}{\text{Total Body Water}}$, which should be consulted for greater accuracy in predicting or estimating TBF.[1]

Fat-free solids (FFS) is another derived

administration of the isotope. It is about 65 per cent of total body sodium and does not change significantly with age or sex in normal adults. Na_e/kg is lower in females than in males since the former have a higher percentage of body fat. Individual variation in Na_e is considerable and is a function of body composition. Average Na_e in normal adult males and females is given by Moore et al.[1] as:

	Age Group (Yrs.)	Number	Na_e (mEq/Kg.)	95% C.L.* (% of mean)
Males	16–84	149	40.5	±21%
Females	16–90	78	37.1	±17%

* Confidence Limits

Table 7–3 gives prediction values for normal Na_e.

value, obtained by subtracting total body fat from total body solids:

$$FFS(Kg.) = TBS_{Kg.} - TBF_{Kg.}$$

The relative proportion of total body solids to body weight in men and women is shown in Figure 7–5.

THE MAJOR ELECTROLYTES OF BODY WATER: SODIUM, CHLORIDE AND POTASSIUM

Total Body Sodium. The sodium ion content of the normal human body is stated to be from 52 to 60 mEq/kg in the adult male, and 48 to 55 mEq/kg in the female. A 70-kg man would therefore have from 3600 to 4200 mEq (83 to 97 grams) of sodium. From 35 to 40 per cent of the total body sodium is in the skeleton, and 65 to 75 per cent of skeletal sodium is unexchangeable or

Residual Sodium. The portion of exchangeable sodium not accounted for by the product of extracellular water volume (ECW) and extracellular water sodium concentration in mEq/L is residual sodium. This averages 10–15% of Na_e.

Total Body Chloride. This averages about 33 mEq/kg in a normal adult male[8] so that a 70-kg man contains about 2300 mEq or 81.7 grams. Predominantly an extracellular ion, chloride is found in low concentration in bone and is probably loosely bound, but exchangeable, in connective tissue. Chloride is in part intracellular; the erythrocytes have the highest cellular concentration with gastric mucosa, gonads and skin containing lesser amounts.

Exchangeable Chloride (Cl_e). This is usually determined by equilibration with $^{82}Br^-$, although $^{36}Cl^-$ has been reported recently as a useful tracer.[9] Data for exchangeable chloride are as follows[1]:

	Age Group (Yrs.)	Number	Cl_e mEq/Kg.	95% C.L.* (% of mean)
Males	16–90	67	29.4	±23%
Females	16–90	60	26.4	±21%

* Confidence Limits

very slowly exchanged with that in body fluids and isotope tracers.[1,7]

Total Exchangeable Sodium (Na_e). Na_e is the pool of sodium within the body with which $^{24}Na^+$ or $^{22}Na^+$ comes into equilibrium, as usually measured at 24 hours after

Cl_e bears a specific relationship to Na_e such that $Cl_e = 0.7315\ (Na_e) - 16$.

Total body potassium in the healthy young adult male is stated to be from 42 to 48 mEq per kilogram body weight.[1] A 70-kg man would contain from 2940 to 3360 mEq

Table 7-3. Formulas for Predicting Normal Values in Body Composition
For the Adult[1]

1. *Total Body Water* (*TBW*)

    Males $\dfrac{TBW\ (L)}{Body\ Wt.\ (kg)} \times 100 = 79.45 - 0.24\ (Body\ Wt.) - 0.15\ age$

    Females $\dfrac{TBW\ (L)}{Body\ Wt.\ (kg)} \times 100 = 69.81 - 0.26\ (Body\ Wt.) - 0.12\ age$

2. *Intracellular Water* (*ICW*)

    Males $\dfrac{ICW}{TBW} \times 100 = 62.3 - 0.16\ age$

    Females $\dfrac{ICW}{TBW} \times 100 = 52.3 - 0.07\ age$

3. *Exchangeable Potassium* (K_e)

    Using ICW for males or females as appropriate

    $K_e(mEq) = 150\ (ICW_L) + 4(TBW - ICW)$

4. *Exchangeable Sodium* (Na_e)

    $Na_e(mEq) = 163.2(TBW_L) - 69 - K_e(mEq)$

5. *Exchangeable Chloride* (Cl_e)

    $Cl_e(mEq) = 0.7315(Na_e) - 16$

6. *Regression Equation for $Na_e + K_e$ on TBW*

    $Na_e(mEq) + K_e(mEq) = 163.19(TBW_L) - 69$

7. *Extracellular Water* (*ECW*)

    $ECW = TBW - ICW$

    $ECW = Plasma\ Volume \times 0.93 + Interstitial\ Fluid\ Vol. \times 0.98$

8. *Extracellular Fluid* (*ECF*)

    $ECF = Plasma\ Volume + Interstitial\ Fluid$

    $ECF = ECW \times 1.03$

9. *Osmolar Balance*

    $\dfrac{Na_e(mEq) + K_e(mEq)}{TBW\ (L)} = 150$

(115 to 131 grams) of potassium. In trained athletes with larger than normal muscle mass, total body counting of ^{40}K gives values of 60 and 65 mEq per kilogram body weight.[5] Virtually all of body potassium appears to be exchangeable with ^{42}K in the normal adult in 24 hours. The only exceptions are erythrocyte potassium which is slowly exchanging, and the skeleton where the small amount present may not exchange fully. For practical use total body potassium and exchangeable potassium (K_e) are the same.

Total exchangeable potassium (K_e) is the pool of potassium within the body which comes into equilibrium with ^{42}K in 24 hours. Approximately 98% of K_e is considered to be intracellular. Since the potassium concentration of extracellular fluids averages 3.5 to 5.0 mEq/L, the total extracellular potassium in a 70-kg adult male is about 60 mEq.

Exchangeable potassium differs in males and females and declines in both sexes as a function of age as indicated below[1]:

	Age Group (yrs.)	Number	K_e (mEq/Kg.)	95% C.L.* (% of mean)
Males	16–30	97	48.1	±23%
	31–60	34	45.1	±20%
	61–90	20	37.3	±16%
Females	16–30	59	38.3	±20%
	31–60	28	34.2	±23%
	61–90	21	29.7	±29%

* Confidence Limits

Total Body Potassium by ⁴⁰K Counting. Brill et al.[6] and Novak et al.[5] have determined total body potassium by whole body counting of naturally occurring ^{40}K, which emits gamma rays of 1.46 Mev maximal energy, and occurs as a small fraction (0.0119%) of the stable potassium pool of ^{39}K (93.08%) and ^{41}K (6.91%). When calibrated with known amounts of ^{40}K in properly distributed geometry, body counts can be directly interpreted in terms of mEq potassium. Normal values for K_e can be predicted from body weight, sex, and age (Table 7–3).

Na_e, K_e, and TBW. The sum of K_e and Na_e, called "total base" by Moore et al.,[1] has a very high correlation with TBW when each of the three variables are measured independently by isotope dilution techniques. The regression equation for this relationship is:

$$Na_e \text{ (mEq)} + K_e \text{ (mEq)} = 163.19 \text{ TBW(L)} - 69$$
$$r = 0.99 \ (P < 0.001)$$

Unaffected by age groups or sex, this relationship permits close estimation of the third factor, when any two are known. Na_e bears a close relationship to extracellular water in both males and females, as does Cl_e. K_e bears an even closer relationship to intracellular water, since the concentrations of K are very low in all extracellular fluids (4 mEq/L) as compared to the intracellular value which averages 150 mEq/L.

In healthy individuals, Na_e/K_e ratios approximate 0.85 in males and 1.0 in females. In a wide variety of illness, such as trauma, sepsis, cardiac or renal insufficiency, and prolonged inadequate nutrition whether due to failure of intake or to malabsorption, the Na_e/K_e ratio rises; values of 1.5 or higher are not unusual in debilitated edematous individuals.

BODY CELL MASS AND EXTRACELLULAR TISSUES

A functional consideration of normal body composition involves division of the body into its living cells, and their fluid and solid extracellular supporting structures (Figure 7–6).

Body cell mass (BCM), a concept defined and developed by Moore et al.,[1] consists of all of the cells of the body, regardless of their location. All have a high intracellular potassium concentration, and all utilize chemical energy from food, or tissue catabolism, to perform thermal, chemical, and sometimes mechanical work. The body cell mass is not uniform in metabolic rate, in chemical, mechanical, or thermal work done, or in fuel requirements, since these vary from one cell type and location to another, and with the activity of the body.

Chemical analysis of representative samples of cellular tissues from man indicate a K/N ratio of very close to 3 mEq of potassium for each gram of nitrogen. Virtually all the potassium and a very high percentage of protein are intracellular. Assuming an average K/N ratio of 3 mEq/gram N, and a total net weight of average cells (excluding extracellular fluid) of N × 25,[1] body cell mass can then be calculated:

$$BCM = \frac{(K_e - ECK) \times 25}{3}$$

Since extracellular potassium (ECK) is relatively very small it can be ignored and

$$BCM_{gm} = K_e(mEq) \times 8.33$$

Intracellular water (ICW) can be calculated from K_e on the basis of $\dfrac{K_e(mEq)}{150} = ICW\ (L)$ in normals, since potassium concentration intracellularly is approximately 150 mEq/L (149.7 ± 7.2). Intracellular K concentration can be adjusted for changes in extracellular fluid tonicity by adjustment of the equation $\dfrac{Na_e + K_e}{TBW} = 150$, a ratio which is an expression of the osmolar equilibrium between cells and extracellular fluids. As noted previously, ICW is normally 50 to 58 per cent of TBW, with males tending to have a higher percentage of TBW as ICW. The ratio $\dfrac{ICW}{TBW}$ is altered in a variety of diseases, almost all of which result in a decreased ratio by expansion of both TBW and ECW as a percentage of body weight, with or without loss of BCM as well.

Oxygen consumption and caloric expenditure are closely correlated with BCM. Kinney *et al.*[10] have measured oxygen consumption as 8 to 10 ml/min/kgBCM, and caloric expenditure as 2.7 to 3.6 calories/hour/kgBCM. Novak *et al.*[5] measured basal oxygen consumption of young athletes as 6.6 to 7.58 ml O_2/min/kgBCM.

Creatinine excretions have been reported of 60 to 80 mgm/kgBCM/day[10] and of 47 to 51 mgm/kgBCM/day.[5] This author has become doubtful of the value of daily creatinine excretion as a measure of skeletal muscle mass in seriously ill patients, having observed in many patients a striking fall in total creatinine excretion and in plasma creatinine levels following introduction of a high caloric-amino acid nutritional regimen.

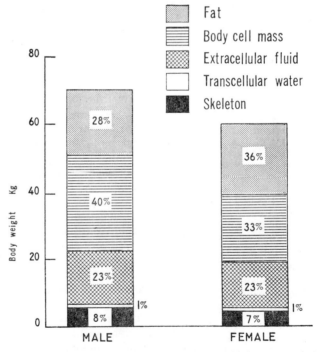

Fig. 7-6. Body cell mass and its proportional relationship to supporting structures. Extracellular fluid includes non-cellular elements of connective tissue and tendons, as well as interstitial fluid and plasma. Transcellular fluid is fluid of joints, cerebrospinal fluid, and the content of the resting gastrointestinal tract. Based on data from Moore *et al.*[1]

This occurred whether the high caloric material was given intravenously or as chemically defined diets. Plasma creatinine levels of 0.4 mgm per cent and total creatinine excretion in the urine of less than 0.5 gram a day in adults accompanied a positive nitrogen balance. These data suggest that some part of creatinine production is related to muscle catabolism.

Extracellular tissues (ECT) are those fluids and solids of the body that are wholly outside of cells. Even though some of these have extremely small cell components, only the extracellular part of such tissues is considered as ECT. *Extracellular fluid (ECF)* has been discussed. The extracellular solids include the skeleton, tendons, fascia, dermis, collagen and elastin. *Interstitial fluid* comprises about three-fourths of total extracellular fluid and 15 to 18 per cent of body weight. Interstitial fluid is in intimate communication with plasma, being separated only by capillary walls which permit easy diffusion of all but large protein molecules. Its protein content is much lower and therefore its water content is higher than that of plasma, as are concentrations of chloride and bicarbonate as required by the Gibbs-Donnan distribution equilibrium. The plasma component of extracellular fluid varies between 3.5 and 5 per cent of body weight and averages 4.2 per cent. Normal protein concentration is approximately 7 gm/100 ml, and therefore plasma is about 93 per cent water. Because of the lower water content of plasma and the presence of protein molecules which behave as nondiffusible anions, the concentration of cations in plasma water is higher than that in interstitial fluid, and the concentration of inorganic anions is somewhat lower.

Extracellular Solids. No measurement of extracellular water takes accurately into account the extracellular solids, of which the skeleton is the largest component. The skeleton is estimated to be 10.5 per cent of the normally hydrated fat-free body weight in health, which makes it of the order of 8 per cent of total body weight in males and 7 per cent total body weight in females of normal body composition (Fig. 7-6). Skeletal bone contains about 30 per cent water. It also contains a substantial amount of sodium,

230–288 mEq/kg in fat-free dry cortical bone, of which 65–75 per cent is unexchangeable, and as much as 85 per cent not associated with chloride. Potassium content of bone is low.[1] A nomogram of skeletal weight based on K_e and K_e/FFS has been prepared by Moore and associates which is useful for more precisely estimating skeletal weight.[1] In wasting diseases, in which there is substantial loss of both BCM and fat, the skeleton becomes a much larger percentage of body weight.

Dense connective tissue of fascial sheaths and tendons together with other collagen in the body has been estimated to comprise 6 per cent of body weight in dogs and 2–3 per cent in man. Subcutaneously equilibrated, fat-free collagen of fascia in the dog has been shown by Fulton to contain 70 per cent water, and 57 mEq Na^+ per kg, suggesting that 45 per cent of the water content is bound in such a way as to exclude sodium.[11]

Extracellular solids are, therefore, not chemically homogeneous with extracellular fluids. Equilibria for water, sodium, chloride and probably hydrogen ion within extracellular solids appear to be rather specific for the solid tissue considered. These observations are of importance when considering the behavior of ECF, particularly interstitial fluid, in the derangements of acid-base balance and, particularly, with hypoxic hypoperfusion.

ELECTROLYTE CONCENTRATION OF BODY FLUIDS

Figure 7-7, modified from the famous diagrams of Gamble,[12] illustrates the approximate composition of interstitial fluid and intracellular water in comparison with that of plasma with its more precisely known values. Table 7-4 gives the range of normal and the analytic error of laboratory determinations for the major electrolytes of plasma as usually determined in serum. Values in this table are from the literature and from our laboratories.[13,14,15] It should be remembered that there is both a range of values present in normal individuals and an error present in any laboratory determination. The ranges shown take into considera-

Table 7-4. Normal Electrolyte Concentration of Serum

Electrolytes	Range of normal including laboratory-method variance	Reliability of laboratory test-95% confidence limits
Cations		
Sodium	136–145 mEq/L	± 3 mEq.
Potassium	3.5–5.0 mEq/L	± 0.2 mEq
Calcium	4.5–5.5 mEq/L (9.0–11.0 mgm%)	± 0.1 mEq
Magnesium	1.5–2.5 mEq/L (1.8–3.0 mgm%)	± 0.04 mEq
Anions		
Chloride	96–106 mEq/L	± 2.0 mEq
CO_2(content)TCO_2	24 – 28.8 mEq/L	± 0.2 mEq
Phosphorus (inorganic)	3.0–4.5 mg% (1.9 to 3.25 as $H PO_4 =$)	Considerable variance due to analytic problem
Sulfate (as S)	0.8–1.2 mgm% (0.5–0.75 mEq/L as $SO_4 =$)	Method dependent
Lactate	0.7–1.8 mEq/L (6 to 16 mgm%)	Method dependent
Protein	6.0–7.6 gm% (14–18 mEq/L) Depends on albumin	Method dependent

tion both the normal variation, and the 95% confidence limits of the laboratory procedure in a well-run clinical laboratory. Repeating any laboratory test will reduce the probability of error due to the test. When laboratory reports do not help to confirm the clinical diagnosis or course, it is wise both to repeat the test and to re-examine and re-evaluate the patient.

An approximation of the accuracy of determination of the sodium, chloride, and bicarbonate concentrations of the plasma or serum or the determination of the existence of a major electrolyte abnormality in the patient can be made by equating the serum sodium concentration (in mEq) with the sum of the chloride and bicarbonate concentrations (in mEq) plus 10 mEq:

$$\text{mEq Na} = \text{mEq HCO}_3 + \text{mEq Cl} + 10$$

Since the sum of the cations and the anions in any biologic system must be equal and since sodium ion is the major cation of extra-cellular fluid and of serum or plasma, most of the anions balance sodium. The anionic structure of serum or plasma is somewhat more complex than that of the cations, because of the presence of substantial amount of plasma protein, the molecules of which behave primarily as anions at the pH of plasma. The sum of bicarbonate (27 mEq) and chloride (105 mEq) equals all but 10 mEq of the normal sodium concentration. The relationship between the sum of the two anions and the serum sodium concentration normally remains constant. If the sum of bicarbonate plus chloride plus 10 mEq is *less* than ± 5 mEq of the sodium concentration on repeated determinations, one of two conditions exist: either there has been the addition of substantial amounts of another anion or there is a major error in the laboratory determination of one or more of the three components. Conversely, if $HCO_3 + Cl + 10$ is greater than sodium by more than 3 to 5 mEq, hypoproteinemia is the likely cause if laboratory error is ruled out.

Much less is known about intracellular fluid (ICF) than about plasma and interstitial fluid. Muscle cells, liver cells and erythrocytes obviously contain different functional proteins within them and their electrolyte content is different as well. However, the body cell mass has certain characteristics which all its cells share in common and many of these are different from extracellular fluid. The major intracellular cations are potassium and magnesium and there is relatively little sodium. Bicarbonate ion is present within cells in less than one half the concentration in ECF. The predominating intracellular anions are organic phosphates, and protein in substantial amounts (Figure 7–7). Approximately 23 per cent of BCM is protein.

The osmolality of intracellular fluid is generally considered to be about the same as ECF, since water diffuses freely into and out of cells as shown by isotope dilution. The only exception in man would appear to be the medullary area of the kidney, where an osmotic gradient nearly 4 times that of ECF, and presumably of renal tubular cells, is maintained.

FORCES CONTROLLING THE WATER AND ELECTROLYTE BALANCE BETWEEN CELLS AND EXTRACELLULAR FLUID

Osmolality and Osmotic Pressure. A substance in solution in water on one side of a semipermeable membrane which is freely permeable to water but through which the solute cannot pass exerts an effect such that water molecules tend to diffuse in larger numbers *toward* the solution side where the water molecule concentration (or activity) is less. Osmotic pressure is the physical force necessary on the solution side of the membrane to *prevent* the net movement of water across the membrane toward the solution and to maintain equilibrium. One gram molecular weight of a substance which does not dissociate into ions, such as glucose or urea, contains 6.06×10^{23} molecules and is termed 1 osmole; dissolved in 1 liter of water 1 osmole will require a pressure equal to 17004 mm Hg on the solution side to maintain equilibrium across a membrane permeable only to water. One milliosmole (mOsm

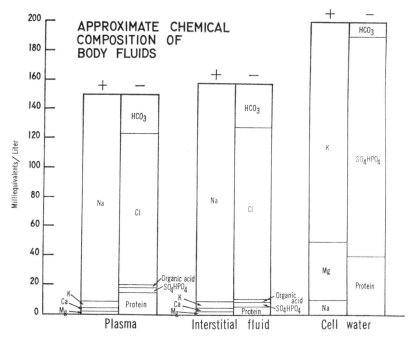

Fig. 7-7. The electrolyte concentrations of plasma and interstitial fluid are compared with an approximation of the electrolytes in cell water. Cell membranes separate and maintain striking concentration and electrolyte differences between intracellular and extracellular fluids. Modified from Gamble.[12]

or mO) is 1/1000th of an osmole and when dissolved in 1 liter of water has an osmotic pressure of 17 mm Hg.

Since the number of particles determines osmotic pressure, substances which ionize affect osmotic pressure according to the degree of dissociation. For example, sodium chloride dissociates into Na^+ and Cl^- in such fashion that at 0.154 molar concentration (that of body fluid) there are about 1.85 particles for each original molecule and exert a pressure of 286 mO, rather than 308 mO.[16]

Osmolality of a solution can be determined on the basis that 1 osmole dissolved in 1 liter of water will depress the freezing point of water by 1.86° centigrade. Normal plasma or serum (fibrinogen molecules are very large so their absence makes virtually no difference) freezes at $-0.533°$ C and osmolality is therefore $\dfrac{0.553}{1.86}$ or 297 mO. Freezing point depression osmometers are widely available in clinical laboratories today and are of great value in determining not only plasma osmolality but that of urine and other biological fluids, thereby assisting the clinician in evaluation of fluid and electrolyte balance in his patient.

With such large forces present even with small differences in osmolality, and the fact that cell membranes, with very limited exceptions such as the distal nephron of the kidney, are quite freely permeable to water, osmolality must be nearly if not exactly equal within cells and their surrounding extracellular fluids. Such is almost certainly the case despite substantial differences in individual ion content and protein concentration between cells and ECF (Fig. 7–7). In order to permit such ionic discrepancies to exist, other forces must be at work and energy must be expended. *The Gibbs-Donnan Equilibrium Rule* provides that under equilibrium conditions, the *product* of concentration of any pair of diffusible cations and anions on one side of a membrane will equal the *product* of the same pair of ions on the other side. When a non-diffusible ion is present on one side of a membrane, the situation is altered, so that while the products of the concentration of the pairs of diffusible ions are equal, the concentrations on the two sides

are unequal, and remain so. Within cells, organic phosphates and protein are non-diffusible, and hold an excess of the cations K and Mg (Fig. 7–7). These forces are balanced by the remarkable property of living cells of keeping sodium out of the cell by continuous pumping. This counter osmotic gradient together with the probability that not all the ions and protein molecules are active (some being "bound" in large protein aggregates) provides the best current explanation of the ability of the body cell mass to maintain the transmembrane differences that are essential to life.

Osmotic Pressure, Diffusion and Reabsorption in Tissue Nutrition. Starling[17] observed that 1% saline solution was rapidly absorbed from subcutaneous tissue and measured the protein oncotic pressure (colloid osmotic pressure) of dog serum against 1.03% of saline as 30 to 41 mm Hg. His hypothesis of filtration of plasma against this gradient at the high pressure end of a capillary and the return of the filtrate at the low pressure end is well known, but accounts for a very small fraction of the total extracellular circulation according to Pitts.[16]

The major exchanges of water, electrolytes, nutrient substances, oxygen, carbon dioxide, and other end products of metabolism occur by diffusion. Water and plasma electrolytes, which are very small ions, diffuse rapidly back and forth across capillary membranes. Capillary water exchanges with interstitial water several times a second. Sodium, chloride, glucose and urea diffuse at different rates exchanging at rates of twice a second to 40 times a minute. *Net* transfer by diffusion depends on diffusion down a gradient with glucose and oxygen moving toward cells and carbon dioxide, organic acids and new water toward the capillary. Oxygen and carbon dioxide, because of their lipid solubility, are free to diffuse across all of the capillary membrane while water and electrolytes are believed to pass through minute pores in the endothelial membrane.[18]

The electrolyte diffusion mechanism across capillary membranes is in contrast with cell membranes where the sequence of cation selectivity resembles narrow-pore fixed-site systems, as described by Eisenman *et al.*,[19] including active transport mechanisms, such as that associated with Na-K activated ATPase for sodium and potassium.

The distribution of fluid volume between plasma and the interstitial fluid compartments is controlled by a balance of hydrostatic forces. Capillary hydrostatic pressure, including both blood pressure and gravity, and high capillary flow rates result in net flow from capillaries to the interstitial fluid. Colloid osmotic pressure of plasma protein, tissue elasticity, and slow capillary flow rates result in a net return flow into capillaries. Anything which alters capillary permeability, such as injury due to heat, toxins, or prolonged hypoxia with acidosis, results in varying degrees of loss of plasma protein into the interstitial fluid. Loss of colloid osmotic pressure reduces return flow to the capillary, with resulting local expansion of the intracellular fluid space. Edema becomes clinically evident when the interstitial fluid volume increases above approximately 50 per cent.

Cells are compound structures, with organelles that in complexion appear to be related to cell metabolism and function. As pointed out by Leaf,[20] the regulation of intracellular volume and ionic concentration is a function *primarily of each individual cell*, with some assistance from neighboring cells in organ systems. The concentration of water, ions, protein, nucleic acids and even hydrogen ion probably varies from site to site within cells. Gross averages do not reflect these important gradients.

Regulation of cell volume and concentration of ions within cells is an energy-requiring process involving active transport of sodium and potassium across cell membranes. The source of energy for this active transport system, as it is for practically every kind of energy expenditure by cells, is the metabolism of adenosine triphosphate. Katz and Epstein[21] have reviewed the substantial evidence developed in the last few years that, in addition to ATP, an enzyme, sodium-potassium activated ATPase, is always present in cells that pump sodium and potassium. This enzyme has an absolute requirement for magnesium, but also requires that both sodium and potassium be present together for maximal activity. It has one site with a high affinity for K^+, and another quite separate for Na^+. The enzyme is present on cell membranes and their extensions. It is inhibited by the presence of cardiac glycosides on the outside of the cell membrane, as is active transmembrane transport of sodium. Changes in Na-K activated ATPase in the kidney appear to be correlated with work of Na and K transport, adding further evidence that the enzyme has something to do with the "sodium pump" that enables cells to maintain their intracellular ionic integrity.

One of the effects of differing concentrations of potassium and of other ions on opposite sides of a cell membrane is the development of an electrical potential across the membrane. A potential of -90 mV exists within muscle cells when compared to the ECF surrounding them. This negative potential may help to explain the rejection of Cl^- ion by most cells not involved in chloride transport.

Leaf[20] has postulated that a balance of solutes stabilizes cell volume; extracellular sodium balances the effects of intracellular colloids, and a dynamic steady state results. As much as one third of the total resting energy of skeletal muscle cells may be directed to the sodium pump. When metabolism of cells is interfered with by hypoxia or any other metabolic inhibitor, cells swell. The mechanism appears to be the entrance of Na^+ and Cl^- ions into the cell producing increased intracellular osmolality, and results in increased water content as water follows solute. At the same time, K^+ is lost, but not equivalently to sodium, so that the result is a net gain in water. Figure 7–8 illustrates schematically the processes involved. If the cell survives a new equilibrium appears to be established with time in which the intracellular Na^+ concentration, and probably Cl^-, is higher than normal while the total water content of the tissue returns approximately to control levels. Analysis of the potassium, sodium, chloride, water and magnesium content by wet weight of fascia and gross fat-free abdominal rectus muscle of rats has been made following a standard surgical incision through the muscle and its repair as compared to untraumatized mus-

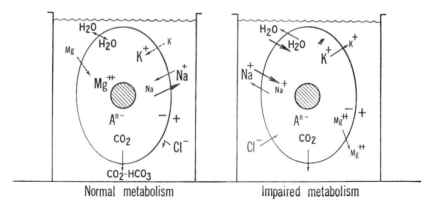

Normal metabolism   Impaired metabolism

Fig. 7-8. The effect of injury, including hypoxia, on the electrolyte and water content of cells. Inhibition of normal metabolism results in depression of the cell membrane sodium pump. Sodium, chloride and water enter the cell, while potassium and magnesium are lost. Water influx results in swelling of the cell. Modified from Leaf.[20]

cle.[22] The injured muscle shows a rapid and significant increase in water, sodium and chloride content by the time of completion of the operation. Water content reaches its peak by day 2 and decreases slowly thereafter, reaching control level by day 20. Sodium content, however, continues to rise, and potassium content to fall independent of change in total water content until day 10, following which there is a slow fall in sodium and chloride content of muscle matched by a progressive rise in potassium content over the next 50 days to the end of the experiment. These observations suggest that there is a range of dynamic equilibria in skeletal muscle with different ratios of intracellular and extracellular ions that is compatible with survival. Repair by replacement of sodium by potassium and magnesium within the cells proceeds slowly and is relatively independent of changes in water content.

Similar processes may occur in severe debilitating illness as well as with the hypoxia of hypoperfusion and acidosis of shock. Intracellular sodium may be higher than normal and intracellular potassium lower per unit of intracellular water in severe illness; in addition there is a substantial expansion of the ECF, and an increase in TBW with Na_e/K_e ratios substantially greater than 1.0 as has been demonstrated.[1]

THE METABOLISM OF WATER AND ELECTROLYTES

Water Balance

Man requires free water to maintain water balance. Even with maximum concentration of urine solutes, the water contained in the foods of a normal diet and the water produced by oxidation of food are inadequate to provide for urinary excretion of the end products of metabolism, and for losses of water from the bowel and vaporizing from the respiratory tract and skin. The amount of water and dilute liquids ingested daily varies widely with habit and climate, but in temperate climates averages 1000 to 2500 ml a day. Water in semi-solid and solid foods averages 1000 to 1500 ml. Water of oxidation adds 200 to 400 ml. a day. The average adult therefore adds a total of 2500 to 4500 ml of water daily to a body pool of 30 to 50 liters.

Loss takes place by four different routes: urinary output and the water content of stool, both of which are measurable, and by evaporation from the respiratory tract and from the skin; the latter are measured only with great difficulty and are termed "insensible losses." In the normal individual water intake and loss balance very closely, and daily body weight fluctuates less than 2 per cent, and usually less than 1 per cent if determined at the same time of day. Insensible losses depend on body size, physical exertion, and on environmental temperature and humidity. In an environment of moderate temperature and humidity losses are substantially less than in a warm humid environment where sweat loss becomes large. Respiratory insensible loss averages 300–500 ml/day in females and up to 750 ml/day in males. Surface evaporation and sweat together average 400 to 600 ml a day. Total insensible water loss is between 300 and 500 ml/meter^2 of body surface area/day, with minimal activity in a temperate environment.[13,14,23] Sweat volume is small in a temperate climate except with vigorous activity, but may reach several liters a day, with serious losses of both water and sodium chloride, in warm humid environments with exposure to the sun.

Daily or more frequent *weighing* of the individual is the only reliable method of keeping track of insensible losses. Combined with a record of measured intake and of urinary volume and bowel output, body weight permits reasonably accurate accounting of water balance on a day to day basis.

Urinary volume represents the difference between total water intake plus water of oxidation and the sum of insensible losses plus the water in stool (normally 100 to 200 ml per day). Normal adults excrete from 1000 to 2500 ml of urine a day. Minimal urine volume with normal kidney function in a young adult is 400 to 600 ml/day. This requires the ability to concentrate the urine to a specific gravity of above 1.030 and with an osmolality of 1000 to 1400 mO. Urea represents more than one half of total solutes from a normal diet. Urea excretion is increased by high protein intake, and by trauma or sepsis which produces increased catabolism of body cell mass. A large protein intake or illness may substantially increase minimal urine volume. Renal disease increases the minimal volume required to clear a given solute load since the ability to concentrate the urine is diminished or lost.

Thirst is the mechanism for stimulating ingestion of water. Physiological stimuli produce a sensation of dryness of the mouth and hypopharynx and the desire to drink. They result from a decrease in volume of body fluids without change in osmolality or an increase in osmolality without change in volume and are usually a combination of both. A 1 to 2 per cent decrease in total body water is the usual stimulus, and represents a change of 350 to 700 ml in the normal adult. A decrease in intravascular volume as seen with acute hemorrhage, and the infusion or ingestion of hypertonic solutions are also effective stimuli to the sensation of thirst. The centers for control of thirst are located in the ventromedial and anterior hypothalamus, and are in close relationship to or overlap the centers of the neurohypophysis which regulate antidiuretic hormone (ADH).[16,24]

Thirst may occur in spite of a normal or even over-expanded total body water, if intracellular fluid is decreased by infusion of hypertonic extracellular fluids, or if effective interstitial and intravascular fluid volume are decreased by rapid sequestration of a part of the volumes into an area of injury, such as a burn or an area of infection, or by rapid accumulation of ascitic fluid or peripheral edema. Thirst is inhibited by expansion of total body water, by reduction of osmolality, or by isotonic expansion of body fluids. Experimental and accidental traumatic lesions of the ventromedial and anterior hypothalamus and tumors of this region may affect both thirst mechanism and ADH secretion.[24]

Antidiuretic Hormone (ADH). As thirst is the regulator of input of water in man, so antidiuretic hormone has a fundamental role in the regulation of water balance and in control of water excretion. By altering the permeability to water of the cells of distal renal tubules and collecting ducts, ADH controls the amount of water reabsorbed and the volume of urine excreted. When ADH level is high in the plasma, the epithelium of the distal tubules and collecting ducts is more permeable to water which diffuses from the tubules into the hypertonic medullary interstitium of the kidney and is thus returned to the circulation. When ADH levels are low, the distal nephron is relatively impermeable to water and a larger volume of urine of a lower osmolality is excreted. With severe reduction in plasma ADH, as occurs with injury to the neurohypophysis, very large volumes of very dilute urine are excreted necessitating ingestion of many liters of water a day to prevent dehydration from this state of diabetes insipidus.

The tracts responsible for the synthesis, storage and release of ADH consist of para-ventricular hypothalamic and supra-optic nuclei, and the neurohypophyseal tract of axons arising from cells in these nuclei which pass down the stalk of the pituitary into the posterior lobe of the gland. The hormone must be stored within the hypothalamic course of these axons as well as in the neuro-hypophysis, since, following hypophysec-tomy or pituitary stalk section for such conditions as metastatic breast cancer, only a minor fraction of the patients have per-manent diabetes insipidus.

Table 7–5 summarizes the factors which are known to stimulate or inhibit ADH secretion. The normal half-life of ADH in the circulation is about 15 to 20 minutes. The length of time necessary for a water load to shut off ADH is 90–120 minutes. Most of the ADH in the circulation is deactivated by the liver and kidneys, while about 10 per cent is excreted in the urine.[24,25]

Inappropriate secretion of ADH results in major alteration of body fluid balance through water retention. The clinical find-ings, as discussed by Bartter and Schwartz,[25] are: 1. Hyponatremia with hypo-osmolality of the plasma. 2. Continued renal excretion of Na+ despite hyponatremia. 3. Absence of clinical evidence of volume depletion. 4. Urine less than maximally dilute. 5. Normal renal function and adrenal function.

The primary causes of the syndrome of inappropriate secretion of ADH include tumors (particularly cancer of the lung or pancreas which synthesize ectopic ADH); injury, infection, trauma or tumors of the brain or its meninges; pulmonary infection of severe degree, often with cavity formation; the postoperative state with anesthesia and sepsis; and, most commonly, injudicious overloading of patients with parenteral dex-trose and water.

Symptoms appear to be related to the rate of change of the sodium concentration and osmolality of the plasma. If these fall slowly, over several days or weeks, there are essen-tially no complaints until the sodium concen-tration falls to approximately 120 mEq/L. With a rapid dilution by water ingestion or infusion or when the serum sodium is below 120 mEq/L, loss of appetite, nausea, vomiting and weakness are the chief complaints. Patients become drowsy, irritable, confused and sometimes hostile. Muscle weakness is

Table 7-5. Factors Which Stimulate or Inhibit Release of ADH[24]

	Stimulate	*Inhibit*
Osmotic—	Hyperosmolar extracellular fluid	Hypo-osmolar extracellular fluid
Non-osmotic—	Decreased carotid artery and aortic blood pressure via baroreceptors	Elevated blood pressure
	Decreased tension in left atrial wall and pulmonary veins	Increased left auricular pressure
	Emotional stress or pain	
	Quiet standing	Supine position
	Elevated temperature of blood	Cold, ↓ Blood temperature
	Drugs: Acetylcholine, morphine, meperidine, barbiturates, nicotine	Alcohol, diphenyl-hydantoin, epinephrine? atropine?
	? low oxygen saturation via carotid body	
	Low plasma volume or ECF	

pronounced, deep tendon reflexes are diminished or absent, and neurologic signs resembling bulbar palsy may be seen. Coma, convulsions, and death may occur. Edema is rare, except with water overloading in excess of 3 to 4 liters.

Plasma sodium and chloride concentrations tend to fall together in patients with inappropriate ADH release. Bicarbonate concentration of the plasma remains nearly normal as does blood pH. The urine volume is not increased, and a relative oliguria may exist. The characteristic finding of substantial amounts of sodium in the urine (30 to 50 mEq/L or more) in the face of hyponatremia is characteristic, and is seen only with inappropriate ADH, adrenal insufficiency, or severe renal disease.

Treatment consists of water restriction. A maximum intake of 500 to 700 ml a day in the adult, with 150 grams of carbohydrate either orally, or as 25% dextrose in the limited volume of water given slowly intravenously into the superior vena cava will result in a progressive rise in plasma sodium and osmolality. Urine volume tends to rise. If water intoxication from excessive water by infusion is the cause, a brisk diuresis may occur, while urine sodium excretion diminishes. Unless sodium depletion is known to exist concurrently, sodium salts usually should not be administered.

The inappropriate ADH syndrome may persist for a long period of time. Nolph's study of such a case[26] suggests that water retention is independent of sodium intake. With an expanding volume on a constant sodium intake, sodium loss in the urine increased, while potassium was retained. The sodium loss, however, was insufficient to explain the resulting hyponatremia without substantial water retention. Neither an increase in glomerular filtration rate nor a decrease in aldosterone secretion explained the sodium loss which accompanied volume expansion. Nolph postuated a decrease in proximal renal tubular sodium reabsorption, possibly triggered by the expansion of ECF volume to explain the phenomenon. Water restriction resulted in a markedly positive sodium balance in his patient, while increasing sodium intake merely resulted in isotonic expansion.

An excellent review of regulation of body fluids by Shore and Claybaugh[27] is recommended as a resource for greater detail.

Electrolyte Metabolism

In this section consideration is given to the metabolism of sodium, potassium and chloride. Calcium, magnesium, phosphate, iron, iodine and other trace elements have been considered in other chapters.

Sodium Balance. *Sodium Intake.* The value of salt, sodium chloride in relatively pure state, has been recognized as not only a pleasurable but also essential component of man's diet since early recorded history. In most of the world today intake of sodium salts is regulated more by taste, custom and habit than by need. Careful planning of diets is necessary to reduce sodium intake below 1 gram a day, which is approximately the minimal requirement for an active normal adult in a temperate climate. Diets containing less than 0.3 gram of sodium are unpalatable and not well tolerated by most patients.

Normal sodium intake varies from 2 grams to as much as 10 grams a day. A group of 28 adults who volunteered to undergo metabolic balance studies for two weeks prior to elective surgery for gallbladder disease or inguinal hernia were permitted to select their own diet and seasoning, the only limitation being moderate fat restriction for those with gallstones and a total caloric intake of 30 to 40 calories per kilogram body weight a day. Thirty-five diet weeks yielded an average sodium intake in food and added salt of 98.9 mEq (2.28 grams) a day, with two-thirds of the group selecting an intake of from 76 to 120 mEq (1.75 to 2.75 grams) of sodium. Potassium intake ranged from 65 to 88 mEq (2.5 to 3.4 grams) and chloride from 85 to 145 mEq (2.4 to 4.1 grams).[23] All but 6 to 10 mEq of the ingested sodium, and 4 to 6 mEq of potassium were recovered from urine and stool in these patients. Since the patients neither gained nor lost significant weight, and were in nitrogen balance, the missing sodium and potassium were interpreted as "insensible loss," probably losses from the skin surfaces, and by desquamation of skin cells. Streeten, Rapaport and Conn[7] found a mean surface loss of 3.3 mEq of sodium a day in normal volunteers bathed in distilled water whose clothes were also analyzed for sodium loss, so our estimates may be somewhat high.

Renal Regulation of Electrolyte Balance. With an adequate intake of sodium, regulation of sodium concentration of body fluids and of sodium balance is renal. However, sodium balance is not merely a matter of glomerular filtration and of the secretion of sufficient aldosterone to control distal renal tubular reabsorption of sodium. Sodium salts are the primary determinant of the volume and composition of extracellular fluid, and indirectly of the osmolality and composition of cells as well. Extra renal factors are important in renal regulation of sodium balance.

In a normal adult of average size, approximately 125 ml of plasma are filtered through glomerular membranes each minute. This filtrate contains not only the electrolytes of plasma in their normal concentration in plasma water, but also glucose, urea, uric acid, amino acids and creatinine. In 180 liters of glomerular filtrate, taking the Donnan factor of 0.95 for univalent cations, and 1.05 for univalent anions into consideration, almost 24,000 mEq of sodium (552 grams), along with nearly 20,000 mEq of chloride, 5,100 mEq of bicarbonate, and 684 mEq of potassium are filtered each day![16] This represents more than 8 times the total body sodium content and 250 times the average daily intake. In order to maintain balance about 99.5 per cent of the filtered sodium and chloride, virtually all of the bicarbonate, and 92 per cent of the potassium must be reabsorbed, along with all of the glucose, most of the amino acids, and a substantial portion of urea and uric acid. Only creatinine is excreted without reabsorption. It is obvious, therefore, that regulation of sodium balance by the kidneys depends upon perception of small changes in extracellular fluid and plasma volume. Regulation is both intra-renal and extra-renal.[28,29]

Intra-Renal Factors Controlling Sodium Balance. 1. Glomerular Filtration Rate. When the glomerular filtration rate falls, the fall in sodium excretion is proportionately much larger than the decrease in the glomerular filtration rate. Since 99.5 per cent of filtered sodium is normally reabsorbed, a small change in filtration rate represents a substantial reduction in the total amount of sodium filtered. With a rise in GFR there is relatively little increase in sodium excreted. 2. Tubular reabsorption. The proximal renal tubule is probably responsible for much of the "balance" changes in proximal tubular absorption which occur very rapidly with change in GFR and are probably not humorally controlled. Aldosterone controls distal tubular sodium reabsorption and potassium secretion. Changes in dietary sodium intake induce reciprocal levels of aldosterone secretion by the adrenals, and by this mechanism balance is maintained under normal conditions.

However, patients adrenalectomized for advanced breast cancer, or adrenal hyperplasia, can maintain sodium balance on varied intakes of sodium and a constant intake of cortisone, provided sodium intake is not extremely low. Also, escape from administered aldosterone occurs by excretion of sodium in the urine after excessive (300 mEq) sodium loading by saline infusion. While aldosterone takes about one hour to produce an effect, decrease in blood volume produces an almost immediate effect on renal sodium excretion. These facts have led to postulation of the existence of a "third factor" in renal control of sodium which is released by volume expansion and which decreases sodium reabsorption by the proximal nephron.[28]

Extra-Renal Factors Controlling Sodium Balance. VOLUME RECEPTORS. A decrease in left auricular pressure results in increased renal sodium retention as does a decrease in blood volume. Conversely, an increase in left auricular pressure results in increased sodium output as does isotonic volume loading unless cardiac output is decreased.

SALT DEPLETION OR EXCESS. Salt depletion enhances renin output, activating aldosterone through angiotensin mediators and resulting in sodium retention. Salt loading increases renal blood flow and decreases renin output with a resultant increase in sodium excretion.

EDEMA. Edema, whether due to right-sided heart failure, liver disease, the nephrotic syndrome, or hypovolemia and hypoproteinemia on a nutritional basis, results in decreased renal excretion of sodium and in an expansion of the ECF. Because of decreased GFR and renal blood flow, the kidneys behave as if the blood volume was decreased. Renal control of sodium balance is based on "effective" or "functional" blood volume and ECF, rather than absolute values of either.

The common causes of hyponatremia and of hypernatremia are listed in Table 7–6. Absolute deficiency or excess of sodium, which determines treatment, depends not only on *concentration*, but also on total *volume* of plasma and ECF, which must be assessed on the basis of history and physical examination of the patient.

Potassium Balance. Daily potassium intake in food usually varies from 60 to 100 mEq; almost all of this is excreted in the urine with a small component in feces in the absence of diarrhea. Intracellular potassium is lost with debilitating diseases with loss of body cell mass, and is lost in substantial amounts with diuretics and as the result of steroid administration. Immediately following surgical operations or other trauma, potassium is lost in excess of that expected from nitrogen loss, and appears in high concentration in the urine. There is often a transient rise in plasma potassium concentration during and immediately after surgical treatment, a rise that is accentuated in the debilitated, hyponatremic patient with an expanded extracellular fluid. Potassium is retained, and a positive balance is achieved a day or two before nitrogen balance becomes positive in early convalescence following illness.

Plasma or Serum Potassium Concentration. This is *not* a reliable index of total body potassium, nor is it *per se* an indication for the administration or withholding of potassium. Only the

---

Table 7-6. Causes of Hyponatremia and Hypernatremia

1. *Hyponatremia* = plasma sodium concentration less than 135 mEq/L:
   a. In patients with chronic wasting illnesses, e.g. cancer; chronic infection; liver disease; semi-starvation; ulcerative colitis; congestive heart failure; ascites and edema.
   b. Following major surgical treatment or extensive trauma, e.g. extensive soft tissue injury; burns; major fractures; severe infection; fluid sequestration in a third space of tissue injury; transcellular pooling, anesthesia, morphine, and meperidine.
   c. With excessive water intake, usually iatrogenic, e.g. patients with antidiuresis of trauma or chronic debility; excessive intravenous glucose and water; retained water from irrigations or hypotonic wet dressings; excessive oral intake; acute renal insufficiency without adequate water restriction; inappropriate ADH syndrome.
   d. As the result of abnormal external loss of sodium with inadequate replacement, e.g. gastrointestinal losses through diarrhea or vomiting or intestinal intubation; bowel, biliary or pancreatic fistulae; following decompression of incompletely obstructed distal urinary tract; osmotic diuresis from glucose, mannitol, or urea; excessive sweating; adrenal insufficiency.
   e. As the result of dietary restriction or drugs, e.g. chlorothiazide, mercurial diuretics, ethacrynic acid or furosamide diuresis; low sodium diets for prolonged periods, particularly in chronic heart, liver, or kidney disease, and for hypertension.
   f. Factitious, e.g. laboratory error or sampling error with dilution by glucose infusion or other sodium-free sources of water.

2. *Hypernatremia* = plasma sodium more than 150 mEq/L:
   a. Dehydration by loss of hypotonic fluid (desiccation) without adequate water replacement, e.g. respiratory loss with fever, dry oxygen, tracheotomy, hyperventilation of dyspnea and metabolic acidosis; skin losses with burns, fever of various etiologies; prolonged exposure to dry heat.
   b. Excessive solute loading: Concentrated tube feedings of all types high in protein and salts without adequate supplemental water intake; electrolyte solutions as the total source of water intake.
   c. Large volume of dilute urine, e.g. ineffective antidiuretic hormone level; diabetes insipidus, brain stem injury, and post-hypophysectomy state.

extremes of high and low concentration are of themselves important. Potassium concentration in excess of 6 mEq/L with no hemolysis in the specimen requires an explanation and appropriate treatment. Levels of potassium of 7 mEq/L or higher constitute an emergency requiring immediate action for the patient who is threatened with cardiac arrest.

Respiratory or metabolic acidosis, hypoxia, dehydration, renal insufficiency and extensive trauma all tend to raise the plasma potassium concentration by transfer of potassium from cells to extracellular fluid. Patients with chronic debilitating illnesses are likely to have an exaggerated rise in potassium concentration in the immediate postoperative period, and particular attention should be paid to the risk of hyperkalemia in such patients, despite the fact that their total body potassium may be diminished by as much as 50 per cent.

Significantly low potassium concentrations begin with values below 3.5 mEq/L. Values of 2.5 mEq or lower are serious, particularly if accompanied by a metabolic alkalosis, as is usually the case. Infusions of dextrose in water will lower the plasma potassium in a fasting patient by about 0.5 mEq/L below resting levels, since potassium is withdrawn from the plasma in the process of glycogen synthesis. Alkalosis, both metabolic and respiratory, lowers plasma potassium concentration as the result of both an intracellular shift and increased renal excretion of potassium.

Hypokalemia. A plasma potassium level of less than 3.5 mEq/L is often accompanied by disordered smooth muscle function, with production or prolongation of paralytic ileus. Sensitivity to digitalis is one of the most important hazards of hypokalemia, with digitalis toxicity appearing with otherwise normal doses. The electrocardiogram in hypokalemia is frequently associated with depressed RST, flattened or inverted T waves, prolonged QT interval and U waves; various arrhythmias may develop. Marked weakness and lethargy are common events. Occasionally the usual hyporeflexia progresses to ascending skeletal muscle paralysis, and interference with function of the muscles of respiration and swallowing becomes a serious and sometimes fatal event. Common causes of hypokalemia are listed in Table 7-7.

Hypokalemic alkalosis is commonly seen in patients who have lost chloride, hydrogen

Table 7-7. Common Causes of Hypokalemia

Hypokalemia = plasma potassium levels less than 3.5 mEq/L:

1. Loss of chloride as acid gastric juice leading to metabolic alkalosis and potassium loss by vomiting or aspiration of the stomach.

2. Administration of diuretics, particularly the chlorothiazide types, with a metabolic alkalosis and marked renal potassium loss.

3. Following trauma, surgical treatment, or anesthesia, with antidiuresis and sodium conservation, and major urinary loss of potassium in excess of nitrogen; usually potassium intake is markedly reduced in these situations. (Often a transient hyperkalemia precedes postoperative hypokalemia.)

4. Administration of adrenal steroids or the presence of Cushing's disease.

5. In the rehydration phase, following dehydration, particularly in patients with dehydration due to diabetic acidosis, where severe hypokalemia may occur during rehydration, insulin therapy and treatment of acidosis.

6. In chronic renal diseases where there is tubular wastage of potassium.

7. With prolonged acidosis or alkalosis, of whatever cause, due to renal wastage of potassium.

8. In patients on prolonged parenteral fluid therapy with inadequate potassium replacement, particularly those with small bowel fistulae or prolonged suction drainage of the gastrointestinal tract.

N.B. All of the above are enhanced by a preexisting deficit of total body potassium due to wasting diseases with loss of body cell mass and expansion of extracellular fluid.

ion, and potassium from the gastrointestinal tract by vomiting or gastric suction. In the early phases a fall in potassium concentration is related to alkalosis as bicarbonate rises to compensate for chloride loss. Laboratory values show a plasma chloride below 95 mEq/L and total carbon dioxide in excess of 30 mEq/L. Plasma sodium concentration may be low, particularly with inadequate replacement. Plasma potassium will be in the range of 2.5 to 3.2 mEq/L and pH will be 7.45 to 7.52 if P_{CO_2} is normal. Urine pH is initially alkaline but becomes acid, despite elevated plasma total carbon dioxide, bicarbonate, and pH levels. Recent work has shown that both chloride ion and potassium must be administered to correct the alkalosis, which begins with loss of chloride and hydrogen ion, is increased in severity by renal wastage of potassium in the presence of an alkalosis, and is perpetuated by an increased renal tubular reabsorption of bicarbonate, which continues the alkalosis and results in the paradoxical aciduria.

TREATMENT. The treatment of hypokalemia is the administration of potassium chloride. Intravenous solutions should not exceed 40 mEq/L of potassium ion per liter, and the salt must therefore be given in 5% glucose in water or other isotonic solutions. The rate of intravenous administration of potassium salts should not normally exceed 30 mEq/hour in the average size adult, except in emergency situations such as digitalis toxicity or skeletal muscle paralysis, when constant electrocardiogram monitoring is essential. Therapeutic doses of potassium chloride are 50 to 150 mEq/day, and 40 mEq/day is indicated in baseline parenteral fluids. Potassium can be given by mouth in the form either of high potassium fluids such as orange or grapefruit juice, or as solutions of KCl (7.5-10%). High concentrations of potassium salts are irritating to the stomach, and should be diluted before administration.

Hyperkalemia. Plasma levels of potassium above 6 mEq/L must be considered abnormally elevated and potentially dangerous, and levels of 7 mEq/L or higher are emergencies. The biochemistry laboratory should notify the patient floor staff and the responsible physician at once when plasma potassium levels of 6.5 mEq/L or more are found. The electrocardiogram changes include peaking of T waves and widening of the QRS complex and various arrhythmias may develop. The chief danger is death due to cardiac arrest. Causes of this condition are listed in Table 7-8. The commonest cause is renal insufficiency; and some degree of renal insufficiency exists with hypovolemia in most patients with hyperkalemia, except when it is due to acute hypoxia.

TREATMENT. Immediate treatment of hyperkalemia consists of measures to decrease the plasma concentration rapidly, including:

1. The administration of sodium bicarbonate intravenously to combat acidosis and shift potassium intracellularly; 44

Table 7-8. Common Causes of Hyperkalemia

Hyperkalemia = plasma potassium 6.0 mEq/L or more; emergency level 7.0 mEq/L or more:

1. Acute or chronic renal failure, whether due to parenchymal disease, perfusion, deficiency, or obstruction.
2. In acute dehydration, adrenal insufficiency, diabetic acidosis.
3. Immediately following massive injury, burns, major operations. Potentiated by preexisting body cell wasting disease and increased by the presence of devitalized tissue and of extravascular blood.
4. In severe metabolic or respiratory acidosis and with prolonged inadequate perfusion of tissues (shock).
5. With major infection, hemorrhage into the gastrointestinal tract, or other causes of rapid and massive catabolic use of protein, in the presence of some degree of renal insufficiency.
6. With overly rapid infusion of high concentrations of potassium salts.
7. Factitious—due to hemolysis of blood specimen or laboratory error in measurement.

mEq in 200 ml of 5% glucose in water can be used as a test dose, with electrocardiogram monitoring. Decreases in the amplitude and spiking of T waves are favorable signs.

2. The administration of glucose with insulin intravenously to utilize potassium for glycogen synthesis. One unit of regular insulin for each 5 gm of glucose is usually safe. If mixed with the glucose, thorough initial mixing and frequent agitation of the flask to assure uniform distribution of the insulin are important.

3. The intravenous use of calcium gluconate for temporary alleviation by calcium of the effects of hyperkalemia on the heart.

Further treatment includes the elimination of potassium intake in food and parenterally, and the use of sodium-charged polystyrene sulfonate resins (Kayexalate®) either orally or by enema. In patients with renal failure, peritoneal dialysis or hemodialysis is often necessary to control hyperkalemia. Such measures are essential when plasma potassium levels of 7 mEq/L persist or recur after the emergency treatment outlined.

Chloride. Normal plasma chloride concentration is 100 to 106 mEq/L, a value which, like plasma sodium, is subject to very little normal variation. Dietary intake is usually in excess of sodium, and virtually all of the intake is excreted in the urine, the excess constituting, with phosphate, sulfate, and uric acid, a titratable acidity of 40 to 60 mEq of hydrogen ion a day. Changes in chloride ion concentration in the plasma follow those of sodium in dilutional hypotonicity and in desiccation dehydration. Deviation from the normal plasma sodium/chloride ratio of slightly less than 3:2 is usually due to excessive chloride loss from the gastrointestinal tract or kidneys, or to chloride retention with renal disease or ureterointestinal anastomoses (Table 7–9).

Acid-Base Balance

L. J. Henderson in 1909 pointed out the significance of bicarbonate as a reserve of

Table 7-9. Common Causes of Hypochloremia and Hyperchloremia

Hypochloremia = plasma chloride level less than 98 mEq/L:

1. Dilutional hypochloremia with hyponatremia in an expanded extracellular fluid following trauma, with wasting diseases, in water retention with overloading, with sequestration of extracellular fluid in a third space of injury.

2. Chloride loss from the gastrointestinal tract, particularly from vomiting or gastric suction, but common with salt loss from all levels without adequate replacement.

3. As the result of diuretics, with a loss of chloride in excess of sodium, and with high loss of potassium in urine.

4. Following administration of adrenal steroids, with sodium retention and potassium and chloride loss in urine.

5. As a compensating mechanism in chronic respiratory acidosis; with high plasma carbon dioxide level and normal or low pH.

6. Combined with an elevated plasma carbon dioxide level and pH and a low plasma potassium level in hypokalemic hypochloremic alkalosis.

7. In chronic renal disease and in acute renal failure.

Hyperchloremia = plasma chloride above 110 mEq/L:

1. Combined with hypernatremia in desiccation dehydration, with excess solute loading, or in diabetes insipidus or brain stem injury.

2. With ureterointestinal anastomoses due to reabsorption of chloride by the bowel; potentiated by renal insufficiency and by prolonged exposure of bowel mucosa to urine.

3. Iatrogenic—with excessive administration of ammonium chloride or hydrochloric acid.

alkali in excess of acids other than carbonic, and developed the "Henderson equation." Hasselbalch devised a hydrogen electrode which would function in the presence of carbon dioxide, demonstrated the influence of respiration on blood pH, and suggested the logarithmic form of Henderson's equation, now known as the Henderson-Hasselbalch equation (vide infra). D. D. Van Slyke, who recounted these facts in *Summary of Acid Base History in Physiology and Medicine*,[30] developed volumetric apparatus for measuring the total CO_2 content of plasma, and demonstrated that the Gibbs-Donnan theory, as applied to the distribution of electrolytes across membranes, fitted chloride and bicarbonate distribution with oxidation and reduction of hemoglobin in the erythrocyte-plasma system. He also defined buffers as ". . . substances which by their presence in a solution increase the amount of acid or alkali that must be added to cause a unit change in pH." Peters and Van Slyke in 1931 introduced the terms metabolic acidosis and alkalosis and respiratory acidosis and alkalosis referring to those conditions in the body which produced changes primarily in the plasma bicarbonate concentration as *metabolic* and to those primarily affecting CO_2 tension as *respiratory*.[31]

This physiological language has persisted in clinical medical practice where acidosis and alkalosis are defined as abnormal conditions caused by the accumulation or loss of acid or base.

With rapidly increasing use of pH determination of the blood by clinicians and clinical laboratories in recent years, greater emphasis is being placed on the state of the blood in which pH deviates from normal. In this laboratory language, acidosis and alkalosis are defined in terms of change in pH of the blood, and as changes in whole blood buffering systems in terms of base excess, or negative base excess, depending upon the amount of strong acid or strong alkali necessary to return a sample of blood to normal pH under standard conditions of temperature, O_2 saturation and P_{CO_2}.

Definitions of Acid-Base. Because of the differences in physiological (clinical) and laboratory terminology in definition of acidosis and alkalosis and the confusion that resulted, an international conference was held in 1966 to attempt to develop common definitions. The following definitions are those agreed upon by an ad hoc committee of the conference[32] and are used in the clinical discussion which follows.

Acid-Base Terminology. The Brønsted-Lowery System. *Acid.* An acid is a substance which is a proton donor. *Base.* A base is a substance which is a proton recipient. The general form for acid-base relationship is given as:

$$A_1 + B_2 \rightleftharpoons A_2 + B_1$$

where A_1, B_1 represent one conjugate acid-base pair and A_2, B_2 represent a second conjugate acid-base pair. This takes into consideration the active role of water in solutions.

$$A_1 + B_2 \rightleftharpoons A_2 + B_1$$
$$CH_3COOH + H_2O \rightleftharpoons [H_3O^+] + [CH_3COO^-]$$
$$H_2CO_3 + H_2O \rightleftharpoons [H_3O^+] + [HCO_3^-]$$

Water and H_3O^+ represent one conjugate pair in both systems, acetic acid and the acetate ion, and carbonic acid and bicarbonate ion the second conjugate pairs, respectively.

Buffers. Under Van Slykes' definition of buffers, carbonic, phosphoric, organic acids, and the acidic portions of protein molecules (proton donor sites) together with their conjugate bases are buffers. Sodium, potassium, magnesium, calcium and chloride *ions* as such do not function as buffers and are neither acids nor bases. They are "aprotes" since they neither donate nor receive protons.

pH. Hydrogen Ion Concentration and Activity. pH is the logarithm of the reciprocal of the hydrogen ion concentration:

$$pH = \log \frac{1}{[H^+]}$$

In thermodynamic terms, pH defines the hydrogen ion activity:

$$pH = \log \frac{1}{a_{H^+}} = -\log {}^a H^+$$

Since the activity coefficient for hydrogen ion is not precisely known, it is assumed to be 1, therefore:

$$aH^+ = cH^+$$

where cH is hydrogen ion concentration expressed as nanomoles/L (10^{-9} moles). At pH values of whole blood compatible with survival, the concentration of hydrogen ion at 37° C is:

pH	cH(nanomoles/L)
7.0	100
7.1	80
7.2	63
7.3	50
7.4	40
7.5	32
7.6	25
7.7	20

It is essential that the temperature and whether whole blood or plasma is examined be stated in reporting both pH and hydrogen ion content or activity.

The Carbon Dioxide System. *Total Carbon Dioxide Concentration* (TCO_2). The total carbon dioxide extractable from a biologic fluid with strong acid. This includes dissolved carbon dioxide, carbonic acid, bicarbonate ion, and carbamino compounds. This is the usual value reported by clinical laboratories as total CO_2 or CO_2 content of plasma.

Partial Pressure of Carbon Dioxide, or Carbon Dioxide Tension (P_{CO_2}). The partial pressure of carbon dioxide in gas phase in equilibrium with a biological fluid is usually reported in mm Hg. While P_{CO_2} can be directly measured by diffusion through a specially prepared Teflon membrane standardized with gas of known CO_2 concentration, the value is often calculated from pH and TCO_2 by use of a nomogram based on the Henderson-Hasselbalch equation.

Carbonic Acid Concentration ($HHCO_3$). In biological fluids, this quantity is very small in comparison to dissolved carbon dioxide concentration. The usual units are mmol/L or mEq/L.

Dissolved Carbon Dioxide Concentration. Strictly speaking, this is the quantity of dissolved carbon dioxide gas in a specified volume; usually $HHCO_3$ is included. The sum of the two is designated as $S \times P_{CO_2}$ where S is the solubility coefficient relating the sum of the concentrations of dissolved CO_2 and H_2CO_3 in mmol/L to P_{CO_2} in mm Hg. This value is temperature dependent;

at 37° centigrade for blood or plasma, S = 0.0306.

Bicarbonate Ion Concentration (HCO_3^-). The chemical definition is the concentration of HCO_3^- in biological fluids. However, in physiological studies and clinical use, it is calculated as total $CO_2 - S \times P_{CO_2}$. This value includes carbamino compounds and carbonate ion in addition to bicarbonate ion, which makes very little difference in plasma or interstitial fluid, but introduces large errors for intracellular fluid:

$$[HCO_3^-] = TCO_2 - S \times P_{CO_2}$$

Standard Bicarbonate Concentration. The plasma bicarbonate ion concentration of plasma equilibrated at P_{CO_2} of 40 mm Hg and 37° C. Units are mEq/L.

Bicarbonate Concentration at Standard pH. This is similar to standard bicarbonate concentration except that pH is set at 7.40 and P_{CO_2} is the variable. Units are mEq/L.

Carbon Dioxide Combining Power. The total carbon dioxide concentration of plasma, anaerobically drawn and separated from blood, and equilibrated to P_{CO_2} of 40 mm Hg at room temperature. Units are mmol/L. This value is rarely used because of dependence on conditions in the blood when the plasma is separated, and because it is dependent on uncontrolled room temperature.

Buffer Base. The sum of the concentration of buffer ions of whole blood bicarbonate, plasma proteins, and hemoglobin. Units are mEq/L. This value and base excess, which is derived from it, are determined on whole blood, and are hemoglobin dependent.

Base Excess. As defined by Astrup and Siggard-Anderson[32,33]: "The base concentration (*of whole blood*) as measured by titration with strong acid to pH 7.40 at a P_{CO_2} of 40 mm Hg at 37° centigrade. For negative base excess, the titration must be carried out with strong base." Units are mEq/L. Negative base excess is sometimes termed base deficit.

Henderson-Hasselbalch Equation.

$$pH = pK_i + \log \frac{[\text{total } CO_2 - S \times P_{CO_2}]}{[S \times P_{CO_2}]}$$

$$pH = pK_i + \log \frac{[HCO_3^-]}{[S \times P_{CO_2}]} \quad \text{where } pK_i = 6.11$$

The Henderson-Hasselbalch equation is for serum or plasma. Calculation of one value (usually P_{CO_2}) from the other two is frequently done in clinical laboratories.

Acid-Base Status of the Blood. *Definitions for Clinical Evaluation and Treatment.* Two methods of reporting and evaluating the acid-base status of whole blood and plasma are in current use. Both have strong advocates and each method has both advantages and disadvantages.

The CO_2-Bicarbonate Buffer System Method. The older and more commonly used method in the United States characterizes the acid-base status of the *blood* (and by inference, of the patient) in terms of the CO_2-bicarbonate buffer system of the plasma. Clinically the most useful measurements are: plasma bicarbonate, $[HCO_3^-]$; blood or plasma P_{CO_2}; and plasma pH. Plasma bicarbonate is determined from total CO_2 content of plasma and the pH from the Henderson-Hasselbalch equation. P_{CO_2} is either directly measured with one of several instruments that depend on diffusion of CO_2 through a special CO_2 membrane or it is calculated from total CO_2 and pH. Plasma pH is measured directly from plasma protected against CO_2 loss to air, using a glass electrode pH meter which is standardized against precisely prepared buffer solutions of known pH. The measurement is made at 37° C.

Plasma bicarbonate concentration is used as a measure of the *metabolic* component of acid-base abnormalities, recognizing that alternations in plasma bicarbonate concentration may be manifestations of a primary metabolic derangement or may reflect compensatory changes secondary to a respiratory P_{CO_2} derangement. Similarly, P_{CO_2} is regarded as a measure of the *respiratory component* of acid-base disequilibria, recognizing that such changes may represent either the primary derangement, or be due to secondary compensatory changes.

The Whole Blood Base Excess, or Δ Buffer Base Method. Proponents of this system, based on the work of Siggard-Anderson and Astrup,[33] hold that the metabolic component of acid-base equilibrium can be most precisely determined by titrating to pH 7.40 with strong acid the base excess of *whole blood* which is equilibrated at P_{CO_2} at 40 mm Hg at 37° C. The determination of the number of mEq of base lost or gained by 1 liter of whole blood under these circumstances is independent of respiratory function and represents nonvolatile acid or base accumulation. It is stated that the two most valuable parameters for clinical evaluation of acid-base metabolism are P_{CO_2} and the accumulation of nonvolatile acids or bases.

Values that are determined include: Whole blood base excess or ΔBb; blood or plasma P_{CO_2}; plasma pH.

Base excess is not independent of P_{CO_2} *in vivo.* The titration curve of blood *in vivo* is slightly different than *in vitro.* As with any system of analysis of acid-base status, a careful assessment of the patient is essential for clinical interpretation and for determination of therapy.

In the discussion which follows, the first of the two methods will be used. Interconversion is possible with a graph, if both oxygen saturation and hemoglobin concentration of whole blood are known, as is often the case with seriously ill patients. Regardless of which method of acid-base terminology and analysis is used, it must be remembered that there are very few independent acid-base variables in blood and that pH, total CO_2, $[HCO_3^-]$, $[H^+]$, $[OH^-]$ and $[hemoglobin^-]$ are *dependent* variables. Stewart[34] has shown that independent variables constitute only 3 groups: **1.** The partial pressure of CO_2, P_{CO_2}, which is under respiratory control. **2.** The difference between the sum of the inorganic cations (excluding H^+) and the anions of strong acids. This component is under renal control through renal regulation of both cation and anion concentrations. **3.** The total buffer present per liter, including protein, and hemoglobin in the case of blood. With knowledge of these 3 independent variables, the concentration of all the dependent variables, including pH and $[HCO_3^-]$ can be calculated from computer-derived nomograms.

There are two main causes of acid-base disturbance, *respiratory*, due to abnormalities of CO_2 excretion, and *metabolic*, due to abnormalities of production, ingestion, or excretion of hydrogen ion.[31,35] Disturbances in one of the two categories usually provoke compensation by the other system. Most patients have a primary defect in one system, with a secondary compensating change in the other. However 41 per cent of 139 patients studied in detail had mixed primary types of derangements due to a wide variety of diseases.

Acidosis and alkalosis should be referred to as conditions which would result in alteration of the pH of blood and plasma, *if there were no secondary compensating changes* and may result in pH changes even with compensation. Acidosis or alkalosis can be further defined as respiratory, metabolic, or mixed as the laboratory findings and the clinical pattern indicate. More specific descriptive adjectives, such as renal, diabetic, lactic, or respiratory, can be used, without necessarily indicating a change in pH *per se.*

The Ad Hoc Committee on Acid Base Terminology[32] strongly advised that secondary compensatory mechanisms are *not* and should *not* be considered as acidosis or alkalosis. Rather the primary etiologic factor should be described, and compensation indicated, such as "metabolic acidosis with compensatory fall in Pco_2" or better still, simply give the laboratory numbers as observed.

Mixed disturbances exist when there are two or more distinct etiologic factors present. These should be described clearly to differentiate them from a single factor with compensation, *e.g.*, "mixed disturbance—metabolic acidosis and respiratory alkalosis," or "mixed disturbance—diabetic and renal acidosis."

Table 7–10 gives the range of normal values found for the set of determinations commonly used in acid-base evaluation. A Siggard-Anderson curve nomogram (Radiometer A/S, Copenhagen, Denmark) is used in determining buffer base and base excess after equilibrating arterial blood (90 per cent saturated with oxygen or more) at 37° C at two standard Pco_2 values, one higher and one lower than Pco_2 40 mm Hg.

A wide variety of nomograms relating pH, total CO_2 and Pco_2 are in use today. One variant developed by R. V. Stephens in our laboratory from the nomogram devised by Poppell[36] has proved useful clinically because it relates the two most commonly measured factors in acid-base determination, pH and total CO_2, to acidosis and alkalosis of both metabolic and respiratory origin. The pH is plotted in such a fashion that Pco_2 values are straight lines, thus making determination simpler.[37] Its use is demonstrated in later figures.

Metabolic Acidosis

Metabolic acidosis is a set of conditions that without compensatory changes would tend toward a decrease in the pH of blood.

Table 7-10. Whole Blood and Plasma Values for Acid-Base Evaluation

	Range of Normal	*95% Confidence Limits of Laboratory Method*
Hemoglobin	12.5–16.0 gm.%	± 5% of value
pH (arterial)	7.35–7.45	± 0.02 pH units
Pco_2 (arterial)	35–45 mm Hg	± 3% of value
Plasma total CO_2	24–28.8 mmol/L	± 0.2 mmol/L
[HCO_3^-] plasma	22.85–27.45 mEq/L	Calculated value, see text.
Buffer Base	43–47 mEq/L whole blood	See text
Base Excess	—3 to +3 mEq/L	See text

Usually compensation is incomplete. The pH of arterial blood is less than 7.38, total CO₂ less than 24 mEq and Pco₂ less than 35 mm Hg. The common causes of metabolic acidosis may be divided into 4 major groups.

1. Increased production of organic acids.
   a. Ketosis—with increased fat metabolism. This occurs in diabetes mellitus; starvation; hypermetabolism of thyrotoxicosis, fever and sepsis; high fat-low carbohydrate diets; following trauma and major operations, often combined with relative starvation and acute dehydration, particularly in infants.
   b. Cellular hypoxia including lactic acidosis resulting from prolonged inadequate oxygenation of tissues; pulmonary insufficiency, acute or chronic; hypermetabolism due to exertion, seizures, fever; congestive heart failure; shock, whether due to hemorrhage or sepsis; anesthesia—cardiopulmonary bypass and acute adrenal insufficiency.
2. Decreased excretion of hydrogen ion due to renal dysfunction, with retention of [SO₄⁼] and [HPO₄⁼] ions. This occurs with decreased renal blood flow in shock, cardiac failure, hypovolemia, and vascular disease, intrinsic renal disease, acute or chronic; obstructive uropathy; renal disease plus a high protein diet, MgSO₄, NH₄Cl or methionine and ureterosigmoidostomy with renal disease.
3. Loss of base in excess of chloride and sulfate ions resulting from dehydration with sodium loss from diarrhea, biliary or pancreatic fistulae, long tube drainage or small bowel fistula and diuretics that inhibit carbonic anhydrase.
4. Increased intake of acid, *e.g.* acidifying salts such as NH₄Cl and CaCl₂; amino acid solutions given parenterally or in elemental diets, particularly if the amino acids are present as hydrochlorides or sodium chloride in the presence of reduced renal function.

Compensation for metabolic acidosis is both respiratory and renal. Respiration is increased in rate and particularly in depth with a lowering of Pco₂ and a partial return of pH toward normal. Renal adjustment, if renal function permits, is a slower process involving an increase in both ammonium ion production and titratable acidity with increased hydrogen ion excretion and conservation of base to restore plasma bicarbonate toward normal. High correlation exists between plasma Pco₂ and plasma [HCO₃⁻], r = .97, and between blood pH and plasma Pco₂ r = .83 in a series of 60 children with uncomplicated metabolic acidosis.[38] Respiratory compensation by marked and sustained hyperventilation is characteristic of metabolic acidosis and a very useful clinical sign of its presence.

Treatment of metabolic acidosis is directed toward the cause of acidosis. In addition, therapy must be planned to reinforce the diminished bicarbonate reserve and combat the hyperkalemia, which may become a serious threat. Efforts should be made to keep the CO₂ content of the plasma at or above 15 mEq/L, and the best drug for this purpose is sodium bicarbonate, which provides sodium without the anion of a strong acid. Experience has demonstrated that it takes 2 mEq of NaHCO₃/L of extracellular fluid to raise the plasma CO₂ by 1 mEq/L. Thus, a patient who has a CO₂ content of 10 mEq/L and who weighs 70 kg will require 140 mEq of NaHCO₃ to restore the CO₂ to 15 mEq/L (70 × 0.2 × 5 × 2 = 140). This may be administered as an isotonic solution (1.2%) or in critically ill patients as a 5% solution given intravenously very slowly. Serum potassium level may fall markedly and, hence, must be carefully monitored. Potassium must be administered if this occurs. It is not necessary to give enough NaHCO₃ to bring the plasma CO₂ to normal levels, and the amount of sodium required to do so may be excessive. Titration of the patient to maintain a CO₂ somewhere above 15 mEq/L is usually adequate in the short-term management of metabolic acidosis.

Figure 7–9 summarizes the primary changes that occur in pH, Pco₂ and total CO₂ in metabolic and respiratory acidosis and alkalosis, together with the early compensatory changes that are induced by the primary condition.

STATE	Δ pH	ΔPCo_2	ΔTCo_2	EARLY SECONDARY COMPENSATION
Metabolic Alkalosis	↑	± TO ↑	↑ *	Variable ΔPCo_2 within O_2 limits, Renal excretion $[HCo_3]^-$
Respiratory Alkalosis	↑	↓ *	± TO ↓	Renal ? $[HCo_3]^-$ excretion ↑ Organic acid c̄ Hypoxia
Metabolic Acidosis	↓	↓	↓ *	Hyperventilation, Renal $[H]^+$ excretion
Respiratory Acidosis	↓	↑ *	↑	Renal excretion of Cl^- and $[H]$

* INITIAL AND PRIMARY CHANGE

Fig. 7-9. Primary changes in pH, PCo_2 and total CO_2 resulting from metabolic or respiratory alkalosis and acidosis. Compensatory changes are also indicated.

Respiratory Acidosis

Retention of carbon dioxide is a condition which, if compensating mechanisms were not available, would produce a fall in the pH of blood. Although complete compensation is seen in mild cases, compensation is usually incomplete, with a fall in pH of the blood, accompanied by a compensatory increase in total CO_2 of the plasma. There is an increase of hydrogen ion and a decrease in pH of the blood caused by an increase in PCo_2 and in H_2CO_3. The pH of blood is usually less than 7.38, and the PCo_2 is more than 47 and usually more than 50 mm Hg. The CO_2 content of the plasma is not altered in the acute phase but rises with compensation and is elevated in the chronic form. Arterial blood gas and pH determinations are diagnostic.

Common causes of respiratory acidosis are: 1. Hypoventilation, which may be due to airway obstruction, pneumothorax, pleural effusion, atelectasis, pneumonitis, thoracotomy, upper abdominal incisions or skeletal muscle weakness. Carbon dioxide retention often occurs acutely as the result of medications which depress respiration, e.g. anesthesia, narcotics, barbiturates and other sedatives or muscle relaxants. 2. Arteriovenous shunting in poorly ventilated segments of the lungs due to atelectasis or pneumonitis or inter-stitial edema, resulting in elevation of systemic arterial PCo_2. 3. Inadequate ventilation with respirators.

Compensation for respiratory acidosis is renal with increased tubular reabsorption of sodium and bicarbonate and increased secretion of chloride and hydrogen ion. The result is a rise in plasma bicarbonate which partially or completely restores pH to normal.

Acute respiratory acidosis requires emergency treatment, the success of which rests on recognition of inadequate ventilation long prior to the development of cyanosis. Restlessness and a rise in blood pressure and pulse rate may be the first signs of hypercapnea and hypoxia. Hypotension follows. The use of narcotics only increases the problem through suppression of the respiratory center. Making certain of the airway, administering oxygen cautiously, and assisting respiration are indicated.

Figure 7–10 demonstrates on the Stephens nomogram the changes that occur with respiratory acidosis and with metabolic acidosis. Line A-A, from Elkinton,[35] represents the effect of inhalation of 7.5 per cent CO_2 on normal individuals with resultant acute respiratory acidosis. There is no change in total CO_2 beyond that due to dissolved CO_2 with the increased PCo_2. Lines B-B and C-C represent two different groups

···ACID-BASE PATTERN-ANALYSIS DIAGRAM···

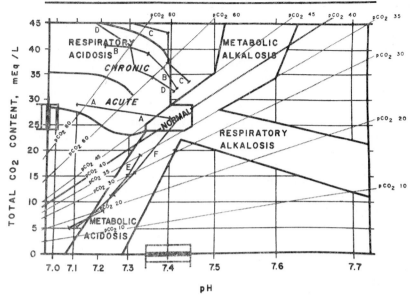

Fig. 7-10. Patient data from the literature showing acute and chronic respiratory acidosis and metabolic acidosis. These data are plotted on the Stephens nomogram relating pH and total CO_2 of plasma to P_{CO_2} and indicating the zone of values usually seen in primary disturbances.[37] A-A, acute respiratory acidosis;[35] B-B, chronic respiratory acidosis;[40] C-C, mixed disturbance, chronic respiratory acidosis and metabolic alkalosis;[40] D-D, linear regression, respiratory acidosis;[35] E-E, metabolic acidosis, adults;[35] F-F, metabolic acidosis, children.[38] Plots are corrected to reflect total CO_2.

of patients with respiratory acidosis from the study of Eichenholz et al.[40] Group I (line B-B) were patients not treated with factors likely to produce metabolic alkalosis, while Group II patients (line C-C) had received diuretics, steroid therapy, or had vomited or been on gastric suction, all factors known to produce metabolic alkalosis. The increased levels of bicarbonate at several levels of P_{CO_2} in the second group of patients are evident. This group constitutes a mixed disturbance of respiratory acidosis and metabolic alkalosis, while Group I is relatively pure respiratory acidosis with compensation by an increase in total CO_2 and in bicarbonate. Line D-D, also from Elkinton,[35] is a plot of the regression $[HCO_3^-] = 20.6 + 0.20 \, P_{CO_2}$. Elkinton points out that the relationship of the rising bicarbonate to rising P_{CO_2} is curvilinear and would better fit a curvilinear regression as is suggested by the curves of B-B and C-C.

Metabolic acidosis with compensation by hyperventilation with reduction of P_{CO_2} is illustrated by lines E-E and F-F. E-E is a plot of data on 27 patients with metabolic acidosis.[35] The regression equation for this series is $P_{CO_2} = 8.8 + 1.51 \, [HCO_3^-] \pm 4.0$. Data on 60 children with uncomplicated metabolic acidosis observed by Albert et al.[38] (F-F) have the regression equation of $P_{CO_2} = 1.54 \, [HCO_3^-] + 8.36$. The similarity of response of the adults and the children is striking and would appear to indicate an essentially normal response.

Metabolic Alkalosis

Metabolic alkalosis is a condition which would tend to elevate the pH of blood or plasma in the absence of compensatory changes and which does so when compensation is incomplete. The common causes of metabolic alkalosis are a loss of body acid, particularly loss of chloride ion, an excess of base, usually sodium, and the loss of significant amounts of potassium.

1. Loss of acid results from vomiting; gastric intubation with loss of acid gastric secretion; gastrocolic fistula or aciduria with potassium and chloride depletion.

2. **Excess** of base results from absorbable antiacids—particularly $NaHCO_3$; sodium salts of weak acids, particularly lactate, citrate, blood transfusions with ACD anticoagulant; Ringer's lactate solution to replace acid or neutral losses from the gastrointestinal tract; or with vegetable diets.

3. Potassium depletion results from the use of diuretics, particularly thiazides and furosamide; gastrointestinal losses, particularly lower G.I. tract, diarrhea; prolonged unreplaced loss of chloride ion with alkalosis and enhanced renal secretion of potassium; lack of potassium intake, particularly in intravenous fluids and with vomiting; adrenal steroid administration, or Cushing's disease or potassium-losing renal tubular disease.

Compensation for metabolic alkalosis is also respiratory and renal. In some patients there is diminished ventilation, with some increase in Pco_2, particularly when the CO_2 content of the plasma rises above 35 mEq/L. However, respiratory compensation is small and cannot be detected in the majority of patients.

Goldring *et al.*[39] studied normal volunteers made alkalotic under controlled conditions by administration of buffers, diuretics, and aldosterone. Alkalosis induced by sodium bicarbonate, THAM, and ethacrynic acid was associated with high values of arterial Pco_2 (Pco_2 values of 46 to 48 mm Hg) while alkalosis induced by thiazide diuretics and aldosterone was associated with normal arterial blood Pco_2 values despite comparable increase in HCO_3^- values to a range of 30 to 34 mEq/L.

Figure 7–10 indicates that some patients have an increase in Pco_2 values at 35 mEq total CO_2 to compensate in this range. However, Figure 7–11, plotted from Elkinton's data[35] on patients with simple metabolic alkalosis (line G-G), suggests relatively little

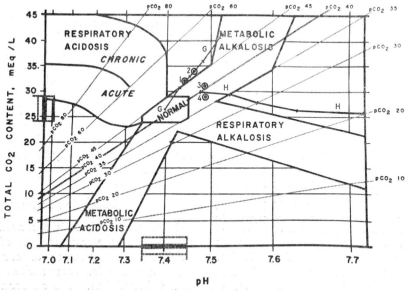

...ACID-BASE PATTERN-ANALYSIS DIAGRAM...

Fig. 7-11. Patient data from the literature showing metabolic alkalosis and respiratory alkalosis. G-G, regression of Pco_2 on $[HCO_3^-]$, $Pco_2 = 42.1 + .18 \, [HCO_3^-]$, suggesting only slight respiratory compensation[35]; H-H, respiratory alkalosis, $[HCO_4^-] = 20.6 + 0.20 \, Pco_2$[35]; points 1 and 2 and 3 and 4 from Goldring *et al.*[39] Plots corrected to reflect total CO_2.

compensation for rising HCO_3^- by inhibition of CO_2 loss through hypoventilation.

Initial renal compensation following the loss of chloride ion occurs by excretion of sodium bicarbonate resulting in an alkaline urine. Unless adequate amounts of sodium, potassium, chloride, and water are made available, this soon leads to dehydration. Metabolic alkalosis increases renal excretion of potassium, and as depletion of this ion develops, renal tubular reabsorption of bicarbonate increases, leading to the paradox of an acid urine in an alkalotic patient and helping to perpetuate the alkalosis.

Treatment of metabolic alkalosis is directed to correction of the cause. Alkalosis caused by sodium retention (steroids or exogenous administration) will correct itself on cessation of therapy. Alkalosis caused by chloride and potassium loss responds to the administration of chloride and potassium. Both ions are required, and potassium chloride is the drug of choice. Isotonic saline solution also provides additional chloride.

Respiratory Alkalosis

Respiratory alkalosis is a primary decrease in Pco_2 and in $HHCO_3$ and is reflected in an increase in pH of the blood. The cause is increased ventilation, in both rate and depth, with a reduction of the normal alveolar Pco_2 below 35 mm. Hg. Initially there is no change in the CO_2 content of the plasma.

The causes of hyperventilation and respiratory alkalosis are multiple and include: 1. Apprehension and pain. 2. Fever, particularly if associated with some lung infection or atelectasis. 3. Hepatic failure with elevated blood ammonia. 4. Central nervous system injury. 5. Respirators with hyperventilation. 6. Septicemia, particularly gram-negative sepsis. 7. Salicylate intoxication.

A mild degree of respiratory alkalosis is a common finding in a high percentage of postoperative patients and is often associated with some degree of metabolic alkalosis as well.[41]

Severe respiratory alkalosis produces hypocapneic vasoconstriction (which reduces cerebral circulation) and hypoxia by decreasing the release of oxygen from hemoglobin and decreasing arterial Po_2, with the production of excess lactic acid. In addition, depression of the ionization of calcium may lead to tetany, and the fall in plasma potassium leads to cardiac arrhythmias and digitalis intoxication. With circulatory failure, there is rapid conversion to a severe and often lethal metabolic acidosis.

The *compensation for respiratory alkalosis* is renal with the excretion of sodium bicarbonate in the urine. However, sodium retention and antidiuresis following trauma substantially or completely block this compensation and, as a result, an alkaline urine is seldom seen.

Treatment of respiratory alkalosis depends on its severity. A mild degree of alkalosis, partially respiratory in origin, is seen in a large percentage of postoperative patients upon whom blood-gas analysis is performed. In general, these patients have good cardiac, pulmonary, and renal function and will recover without treatment. The development of respiratory alkalosis may be an early clinical indication of the presence of septicemia and should lead the observant physician to institute vigorous antibiotic therapy. Severe respiratory alkalosis has a poor prognosis owing to the underlying causes of the hyperventilation. Within the limits imposed by oxygen demand, narcotics have proved effective in reducing ventilation. Theoretically, the inhalation of an oxygen-carbon dioxide mixture, with sufficient CO_2 to raise the Pco_2 to normal, should be effective. In the few instances tried, patients have tolerated this procedure poorly.

The Effect of Diet on Water, Electrolyte and Acid-Base Balance. In relating water, electrolyte, and acid-base balance to nutrition, this chapter is not complete without examining the results of normal body metabolism, and the effects of variations in dietary intake, including total starvation.

Cellular metabolism of neutral dietary or tissue content results in the production of hydrogen ion, and of fixed acid anions, both of which require excretion if acid-base balance is to be preserved. For example, a neutral substance such as glucose, in the process of metabolism, is converted into lactic and pyruvic acids, with the production of hydrogen ion. Unless there is interference with the normal metabolic sequence, however, these intermediary products of metabolism are then promptly oxidized to neutral end products, CO_2 and water. Other organic anions, such as citrate and acetoacetate, are

glomerular filtrate are transformed by exchange of hydrogen ion for sodium or potassium into acid salts, and inorganic cation is also preserved by combining inorganic anion with ammonium ions derived from amino acids. These processes are schematically illustrated by Pitts[16] as follows:

$$Na_2HPO_4 + H_2CO_3 \longrightarrow NaH_2PO_4 \text{ (excreted)} + NaHCO_3 \text{ (reabsorbed)}$$
$$Na_2SO_4 + 2 H_2CO_3 + 2 NH_3 \longrightarrow (NH_4)_2SO_4 \text{ (excreted)} + 2 NaHCO_3 \text{ (reabsorbed)}$$

metabolized to CO_2. When P_{CO_2} is constant, as is the case with normal respiratory function, the amount of CO_2 lost by respiration is equal to the amount produced. Of the order of 15 to 20,000 mM of CO_2 are produced by the average adult per day.

Nonvolatile acids are also produced as the result of digestion of dietary intake and normal cellular metabolism. Strong inorganic acid anions include (Cl^-) and (SO_4^-), the latter resulting from the metabolism of the sulfur-containing amino acids, cysteine and methionine, as well as from ingested sulfate. In addition, phosphate (HPO_4^-) is produced from the metabolism of proteins and phospholipids. While phosphate behaves as a buffer salt, it cannot be excreted in the form H_3PO_4 in the urine because the pH required is too low; in effect, it too behaves as a strong acid anion. Uric acid, the end product of metabolism of purine bases in man and other primates, is also excreted in the urine, representing about 5 per cent of the normal acid load.

The average North American diet contains an excess of cations of approximately one mEq per kg of body weight per day.[42] This excess is partially balanced by the excretion in stool of an average excess of cations over inorganic anions of 35 mEq per day, so that in healthy individuals nonvolatile acid production is equal to renal acid excretion plus 25 to 35 mEq neutralized by the dietary cation excess. However, dietary intake is highly variable. Fruit, vegetables, milk and coffee contain more inorganic cation than anion, while meat and eggs contain more inorganic anion than cation.

Renal mechanisms for disposal of nonvolatile acid anions involve two processes. Buffer salts which enter the renal tubule in the

Titratable acidity of the urine is defined as the amount of strong base necessary to return urine to the pH of plasma. The total acid load excreted in the urine is the sum of the titratable acidity (buffer effect) plus the strong acid anions combined with ammonium ion. According to Pitts,[16] titratable acid in the urine is 10 to 30 mEq per day in normal man, while acid combined with ammonia is 30 to 50 mEq per day. Thus, 40 to 80 mEq of strong acid anions in excess of fixed base—in effect 40 to 80 mEq (H^+)—are excreted daily in the urine.

Both of the above mechanisms are utilized in renal compensation for respiratory and non-renal metabolic acidosis as previously discussed. When organic acid anions such as lactate and the keto acid ions, acetoacetate and beta hydroxybutyrate, are presented to the kidneys in very large amounts and require excretion, fixed base, largely sodium, and water are both excreted in abnormal amounts, resulting in dehydration and loss of plasma bicarbonate. When an excess of sodium is filtered in the presence of an elevated plasma bicarbonate, sodium and bicarbonate ions are excreted in an alkaline urine; this is a situation often seen in persons who are strict vegetarians.

Starvation. Starvation induces major changes in both water and electrolyte balance. Initially, weight loss is substantially greater than can be accounted for on the basis of endogenous protein and fat metabolism. While weight loss in starvation is to some extent conditioned by the pre-fasting diet, and particularly by previous levels of sodium intake in obese patients, Weinsier[43] reported that an initial weight loss of 800 to 1500 grams occurs in the first 24 hours, followed by an average loss of 1 kilogram a day for about 10 days. There is then a progressive fall in weight loss to 300 grams a day in the second month of fasting.

Initial weight loss is largely water and salt. The sodium loss exceeds that produced by simple dietary sodium restriction. Initially it is about 150 to 250 mEq a day, and slowly declines to 1 to 15 mEq a day with prolonged fasting. Even if the patient is on a sodium-restricted diet before fasting, sodium excretion is still elevated by fasting. Administration of a sodium supplement with water[43,44] or a balanced salt solution containing sodium and potassium[45] fails to prevent sodium and water loss. Since sodium is the major extracellular cation, reduction in extracellular fluid volume as the result of water and sodium loss may be reflected in a decrease in blood volume. An average reduction in 10 days of 14 per cent was observed by Maagøe[46] in a series of patients who were 51 to 61 per cent overweight. The decrease in blood volume was significantly reduced to 5 per cent or less when fasting patients were given 90 mEq of sodium as sodium chloride a day. Bloom[47] has shown that the sodium loss in starvation is not due to ketosis but, rather, to an abrupt decrease in available carbohydrate. This confirms the observations of Gamble[12] that the mild ketoacidosis of starvation does not in itself produce loss of fixed base and that ketones in the urine in starvation can be substantially reduced by the administration of small amounts of carbohydrate.

Potassium is also lost in starvation. Initial losses of 40 to 45 mEq a day gradually diminishing to a level of 10 to 15 mEq a day after the tenth day were reported by Cahill.[48] The plasma potassium concentration usually remains at a low normal level. The potassium and nitrogen losses in starvation are the result of mobilization of body protein for gluconeogenesis from the glucogenic amino acids.[48] About 75 grams of protein (representing 12 grams of nitrogen and 35 to 40 mEq of potassium) are required, together with 16 grams of glycerol and 36 grams of lactate and pyruvate recycled through the Cori cycle, to provide about 150 grams of glucose a day which appear to be essential in early starvation as a substrate for energy requirements of the central nervous system and bone marrow.

Some glucose is regularly required by red blood cells for their metabolism.

Amino acid metabolism in starvation has also been studied. Felig *et al.* have shown that if amino acids are determined as a group, there is a slight but significant fall in serum levels; individual amino acids behave differently, however.[49] Some, including glycine, increase in starvation; valine, leucine and isoleucine increase transiently and then fall while arginine levels decrease progressively. Alanine behaves uniquely; it is extracted by the splanchnic circulation to a greater extent than all other amino acids combined, and it appears to be the regulatory mechanism which controls hepatic gluconeogenesis. Infusion of small amounts of alanine results in a rapid increase in blood glucose concentration offering further confirmation of the hypothesis.[48,49]

The Effects of Carbohydrate. Bloom[47] observed that placing obese starving patients on a 600 kcal diet promptly prevented excessive loss of sodium and water in the urine. Individual tests with salt, protein, fat, and carbohydrate showed that only carbohydrate produced sodium retention and associated water retention in the fasted then refed patient. Diet mixtures containing 1500 and 2000 kcal composed of protein and fat, with or without salt, failed to prevent a starvation type of sodium and water excretion. The addition of as little as 50 grams of glucose, isocalorically in exchange for fat in these diets, resulted in prompt sodium and water retention. Subsequent studies[43,44,45] have shown that sodium retention associated with carbohydrate feeding is not related to significant changes in aldosterone excretion, nor is it blocked by spironolactone. It does not appear to be a result of or influenced by glucocorticoids or by changes in catecholamine excretion. It is of interest that glucose administration inhibits furosamide induction of natriuresis and that insulin appears to be necessary for the sodium retention effect of glucose to be apparent in diabetics.[44,45]

The exact nature of the mechanism by which carbohydrate affects sodium and water balance remains unknown. However, this effect must be kept in mind whenever seriously ill patients are being treated. We have observed that a weight gain of 2 to 4 per cent of body weight occurs promptly (within one to two days) when patients are placed either on high caloric parenteral nutrition, or when placed on purified diets which consist largely of amino acids and either glucose or sucrose. A prompt loss of 2 to 4 per cent of body weight occurs when either the parenteral regimen or the "elemental" diet is stopped, even if the patient is immediately able to tolerate a diet of reasonably normal composition. This suggests that the effect of carbohydrate on sodium and water balance is not confined to starvation and refeeding; it may occur with substantial carbohydrate loading. The role of insulin in this phenomenon merits further investigation.

Prolonged Meat and Fat Diets. McClellan and DuBois[50,51] more than forty years ago studied the effects of a diet of meat and animal fat on two Arctic explorers who lived in New York City for one year exclusively on a diet composed of beef, veal, lamb, pork and chicken. The carbohydrate intake was very small consisting solely of the glycogen of the meat. Protein content of the diet ranged from 100 to 140 grams, the fat from 200 to 300 grams, and carbohydrate from 7 to 12 grams a day. Both explorers, and DuBois himself who tried the diet for ten days, lost weight during the first week. Weight loss ranged from 1.8 to 3.6 per cent of body weight, and this loss was explained as a "shift in the water content of the body while adjusting itself to the low carbohydrate diet."

The two explorers remained mentally alert, physically active, and showed no specific changes in any body system. While on the diet both men consistently excreted "acetone bodies" in the urine. Urine volume was higher when carbohydrate was first omitted, and was at its lowest level when carbohydrate was first added. A persistently negative calcium balance was the only potentially serious abnormality, amounting to about 0.3 Gm/day.[50]

High urine specific gravity, 1.020 to 1.030 in urine volumes of 1500 ml or more a day, was observed and reflects the 40 to 50 grams of urea excreted together with substantial amounts of phosphate, sulfate and potassium.

Modern high protein, low carbohydrate diets sometimes used for weight reduction require a substantial fluid intake to provide sufficient urine volume to avoid prerenal azotemia.

BIBLIOGRAPHY

1. Moore, Olsen, McMurray, Parker, Ball, and Boyden: Body Cell Mass and its Supporting Environment: Body Composition in Health and Disease, Phila., Saunders, 1963.
2. Hume, and Weyers: J. Clin. Path., 24, 234, 1971.
3. DuBois: Basal Metabolism in Health and Disease, 3rd ed., Phila., Lea and Febiger, 1936.
4. Widdowson: Growth and Composition of the Fetus and Newborn In Biology of Gestation, Vol. II, The Neonate, (N. S. Assali, Ed.), New York, Academic Press, 1968.
5. Novak, Hyatt, and Alexander: J.A.M.A., 205, 764, 1968.
6. Brill, Sandstead, Price et al: Am. J. Surg., 123, 49, 1972.
7. Streeten, Rapaport, Abraham, and Conn: J. Clin. Endocrinol. Metab., 23, 928, 1963.
8. Boling, Taylor, Entenman, and Behnke: J. Clin. Invest., 41, 1840, 1962.
9. Swan, Nelson, and Hankes: Ann. Surg., 174, 287, 1971.
10. Kinney, Lister, and Moore: Ann. N.Y. Acad. Sci., 110, 711, 1963.
11. Fulton: Ann. Surg., 172, 861, 1970.
12. Gamble: Chemical Anatomy, Physiology, and Pathology of Extracellular Fluid: A Lecture Syllabus, 5th ed., Cambridge, Harvard University Press, 1947.
13. Bland: Clinical Metabolism of Body Water and Electrolytes, Phila., Saunders, 1963.
14. Randall: Fluid and Electrolyte Therapy in Surgery Chap. 2 In Principles of Surgery (S. I. Schwartz, Ed.), New York, Blakiston, McGraw-Hill, 1969.
15. Kinney, J. M. (Ed). Manual of Preoperative and Postoperative Care, 2nd ed. Comm. on Preoperative and Postoperative Care, Am. College Surg. Phila., Saunders, 1971.
16. Pitts: Physiology of the Kidney and Body Fluids, Chicago, Year Book Medical Publishers, Inc., 1963.
17. Starling: J. Physiol., 19, 312, 1895–96.
18. Pappenheimer: Physiol. Rev., 33, 387, 1963.
19. Eisenman, Sandblom, and Walker: Science, 155, 965, 1967.
20. Leaf: Am. J. Med., 49, 291, 1970.
21. Katz and Epstein: New Engl. J. Med., 278, 253, 1968.
22. Rocchio and Randall: Am. J. Surg., 121, 460, 1971.
23. Randall: Surg. Clin. N.A., 32, 3, 1952.
24. Kleeman and Fichman: New Eng. J. Med., 277, 1300, 1967:
25. Bartter and Schwartz: Am. J. Med., 42, 790, 1967.

6. Nolph: Am. J. Med., *49*, 534, 1970.

7. Shore and Claybaugh: Ann. Rev. Physiol., *34*, 235, 1972.

28. Earley and Daugharty: New Engl. J. Med., *281*, 72, 1969.

29. Ulbrich and Marsh: Ann. Rev. Physiol., *25*, 91, 1963.

30. Van Slyke: Ann. N.Y. Acad. Med., *133*, 5, 1966.

31. Peters and Van Slyke: Quantitative Clinical Chemistry—Interpretations, Baltimore, Williams and Wilkins, 1931.

32. Siggard-Anderson: Scand. J. Clin. Lab. Invest., *12*, 311, 1960.

33. Rept. Ad Hoc Comm. on Acid-Base Terminology *In* Current Concepts of Acid-Base Measurement (E. M. Weyer, Ed.), Ann. N.Y. Acad. Sci., *133*, 1–274, 1966.

34. Stewart: Personal communication.

35. Elkinton: Med. Clin. N.A., *50*, 1325, 1966.

36. Poppell, Vanamee, Roberts, and Randall: J. Lab. Clin. Med., *47*, 885, 1956.

37. Randall: Postoperative Oliguira, Acid-Base Imbalance and Fluid Disequilibrium *In* Critical Surgical Illness (J. D. Hardy, Ed.), Phila., Saunders, 1971.

38. Albert, Dell, and Winters: Ann. Intern. Med., *66*, 312, 1967.

39. Goldring, Cannon, Heinemann, and Fishman: J. Clin. Invest., *47*, 188, 1968.

40. Eichenholz, Blumentals, and Walker: J. Lab. Clin. Med., *68*, 265, 1966.

41. Lyons and Moore: Surgery, *60*, 93, 1966.

42. Harrington and Lemann: Med. Clin. N.A., *54*, 1543, 1970.

43. Weinsier: Am. J. Med., *50*, 233, 1971.

44. Gozansky and Herman: Am. J. Clin. Nutr., *24*, 869, 1971.

45. Vervebrants and Arky: J. Clin. Endocr., *29*, 55, 1969.

46. Maagøe: Metabolism, *17*, 133, 1968.

47. Bloom: Am. J. Clin. Nutr., *20*, 157, 1967.

48. Cahill: New Engl. J. Med., *282*, 668, 1970.

49. Felig, Owen, Wahren, and Cahill: J. Clin. Invest., *48*, 584, 1969.

50. McClellan and DuBois: J. Biol. Chem., *87*, 651, 1930.

51. McClellan, Rupp, and Toscani: J. Biol. Chem., *87*, 669, 1930.

Chapter

8

Trace Elements

Section A Iodine

RALPH R. CAVALIERI

HISTORICAL ASPECTS

Although scientific knowledge of the role of iodine in human nutrition has been accumulated entirely within the past 150 years, the use of iodine-containing medicaments for the treatment of goiter goes back into antiquity. This disorder was certainly known to the ancients. Seaweed and burnt sponge, which we now know to be rich in iodine, were employed in the treatment of goiter by the ancient Chinese, the Egyptians, and the Incas of South America. The first true milestone of modern times was the discovery of elemental iodine by Courtois in 1811 in the mother-liquor of saltpeter from which he isolated a violet crystalline substance. Within 3 years, Gay-Lussac named the substance "Iode" (from the Greek for violet-colored) and Davey proved its elemental nature. Credit for the introduction of iodine into medical use and its popularization is usually given to two Geneva physicians, Coindet and Straub (1820). However, the first recorded therapeutic use of the newly discovered element was by Prout, an English physician, who prescribed solution of potassium iodate for simple goiter (1816). By 1819, iodine was on the formulary of London's St. Thomas' Hospital.[1]

The first suggestion that endemic goiter might be due to iodine deficiency was made in 1830–31 by Prevost in Switzerland and Baussingault in France. Prevost and Maffoni in 1846 actually stated that the cause of endemic goiter and cretinism is the absence of iodine in the drinking water and air of those regions affected. Between 1859 and 1876, a French chemist Chatin undertook the ambitious task of measuring the iodine content of samples of soil, water, and air from various regions. He concluded from his studies that iodine lack caused goiter and that iodine is a specific in the treatment of the disorder. Unfortunately, Chatin's chemical methods were not adequate, and his conclusions came under criticism. In addition, the widespread, indiscriminate use of iodine for the treatment of all sorts of thyroid disorders with uneven success led to a reaction against Chatin's views.[2]

It was not until 1896 that iodine was identified in the thyroid gland by Baumann, although Kocher, the famous Swiss pioneer in the surgery of goiter, had suggested years earlier that iodine might be a physiologically important constituent of the gland. The chemical studies of Baumann and Oswald led to the next important milestone, the isolation by Kendall in 1914–15 of the first of the two active principles of the thyroid, thyroxine. Harington, in the 1920's, characterized the structure of thyroxine and proved it definitively by synthesizing the hormone.[3] When radioactive iodine became available as a tracer, further advances in the field followed rapidly. Gross and Pitt-Rivers (1952) identified the second thyroid hormone, triiodothyronine.[4]

In parallel with early chemical studies investigation was proceeding at the clinical level. Although cretinism had been known since ancient times, it remained for Gull (1874) to describe adult hypothyroidism and Ord (1878) to give it the name, myxedema. Within a decade, it became apparent that myxedema is the result of thyroid failure, mainly through the experimental work of Schiff, Hofmeester, and Horseley, and the astute clinical observations of Kocher and the Reverdins on patients who had undergone total thyroidectomy. In what now seems a logical next step, patients suffering from spontaneous myxedema were given thyroid replacement therapy (Murray, 1891). The results were dramatic and rewarding. The modern era of clinical thyroidology had begun.[3] The credit for awakening interest in the importance of iodine in the prevention of simple goiter must go to David Marine and his co-workers in the United States.[5] Their classic studies among schoolchildren of Ohio in 1917–18 demonstrated conclusively that iodine supplementation greatly reduced the incidence of goiter in that region. The importance of adequate dietary iodine is now well accepted by the health-science community. Effective public health measures have finally been instituted in most of the regions of the world affected.

METABOLISM OF IODINE IN MAN

Dietary iodine is converted largely to iodide in the gastrointestinal tract. Absorption of iodide is rapid and complete. Once it enters the circulation, iodide ion is distributed throughout the extracellular fluid.[6] There is no significant binding of iodide ion in plasma. Certain tissues possess the ability to concentrate iodide: salivary glands, gastric mucosa, lactating mammary glands, the choroid plexus, and, most importantly, the thyroid gland. Of these tissues, only the thyroid is capable of utilizing iodine in the synthesis of the thyroid hormones (Fig. 8A–1).

The kidneys are responsible for nearly all of the excretion of iodide from the body.[7] The urinary clearance rate of iodide in man is about 30 ml plasma per minute; there is no renal mechanism for conserving iodide in the face of dietary deficiency of the element.

Normally, little inorganic iodine is excreted in the feces. Impairment of renal function, if severe, will diminish urinary excretion of iodide and thereby cause an elevation in the plasma iodide level (if dietary intake is unchanged). On the other hand, an osmotic diuresis will increase urinary iodide loss and thereby lower the plasma level.

The initial step in the biosynthesis of the thyroid hormones is the transport of iodide from the blood into the follicular cells of the thyroid gland by the concentrating mechanism already mentioned. This thyroidal iodide "trap" is dependent upon metabolic energy generated within the thyroid cells by aerobic processes. Certain monovalent anions, *e.g.*, perchlorate, thiocyanate, and nitrate, inhibit the trap by competing with iodide. Perchlorate is the most potent of these inhibitors. Once within the thyroid gland, iodide is rapidly oxidized to a higher oxidation state, perhaps I° or I^+, by a specific enzyme, iodide peroxidase, which is located within the follicular cells. This active form of iodine reacts with tyrosine residues within thyroglobulin to form mono- and diiodo-tyrosine residues. The latter iodotyrosines then react in a coupling process to yield the active hormones, thyroxine (T_4) and triiodothyronine (T_3). All of these reactions, from the initial organic binding of iodine to the coupling reaction, are believed to occur within the thyroglobulin molecule. This protein is a large (MW = 670,000) glycoprotein synthesized only in the thyroid gland and stored in the colloid. It contains 120 tyrosine residues, about $\frac{2}{3}$ of which are available for iodination. The iodine content of thyroglobulin from normal human glands varies widely depending in part on the iodine supply, though many factors influence the degree to which thyroglobulin is iodinated.[8]

Secretion of Hormones. In order for the hormones to be released from the thyroid into the blood, thyroglobulin must be broken down by proteolytic enzymes into its constituent amino acids. In the process, free hormones, T_4 and T_3, and free iodotyrosines are released inside the follicular cells. The iodotyrosines are normally stripped of iodine by a specific iodotyrosine deiodinase; the iodide which is released is available for re-utilization by the gland. This intrathyroidal mechanism for recycling iodine serves the important function of conserving iodine in the face of a low dietary supply.[8]

The release of T_4 and T_3 into the blood probably occurs by passive diffusion, although the thyroid hormone-binding protein in plasma may play a role in facilitating the process of release from the gland. About 4 molecules of T_4 are secreted for every molecule of T_3, but the ratio of the two hormones varies under various conditions (see below).

Distribution and Metabolism of the Hormones. In normal humans approximately one-third of the total quantity of T_4 in the blood (excluding that within the thyroid) is in the plasma, one-third is in the liver, and the remainder is distributed among other tissues.[9] Both the circulating pool and hepatic pool of T_4 probably serve both as a reservoir of the hormone and as a buffer to modulate abrupt changes in the level of T_4 at sensitive sites in the body, *e.g.*, the heart. Both T_4 and T_3 are reversibly bound to a specific plasma "carrier," thyroxine-binding globulin (TBG).[10] Because of the strong binding between T_4 and TBG, the level of free T_4 is only a small fraction (about 1/2000) of the level of total T_4 in plasma. It is this free (unbound) fraction of circulating T_4 which is believed to be the form which is available for entry into most tissues (particularly the liver) and which ultimately exerts the multiple effects of the hormone. The distribution of T_3 in man is quite different than that of T_4. Most of the extrathyroidal pool of T_3 is in tissues, predominantly skeletal muscle, and relatively little is in the circulation.[11] T_3 is bound much less strongly to TBG than is T_4, which explains the more rapid onset and duration of action of the former hormone. The intrinsic biological potency of T_3 is about three times greater than that of T_4, a difference which is not due to differences in binding to plasma proteins. Recently evidence has been accumulating in support of the notion, originally put forward by Gross and Pitt-Rivers in 1952, that T_4 is converted to T_3 in extrathyroidal tissues of man.[12] The magnitude and significance of this conversion remain to be established. Both hormones are metabolized by liver and other tissues. The major pathway of metabolism involves deiodination; the iodide formed in this process returns to the iodide pool and is handled like any other iodide in the body. A less prominent pathway in man is the conjugation of T_4 and T_3 in the liver, excretion of the conjugated hormones in the bile, and ultimate elimination in the feces. A large proportion of the hormone conjugates is recovered by deconjugation in the intestinal lumen and absorption into the blood (enterohepatic cycle).[13]

The effects of thyroid hormone on the body are complex and far-reaching. Their profound influences on growth and development, protein synthesis, differentiation, and energy metabolism have been studied extensively.[14] Still, it is not known whether all of the effects of these hormones are mediated via a single mechanism.

Regulation of Iodine Metabolism. The most important single regulator of the activity of the thyroid gland is thyrotopic hormone (TSH), a protein secreted by the anterior pituitary. TSH stimulates every step in the biosynthesis and secretion of the thyroid hormones, from the initial "trapping" of iodide ion to the proteolysis of thyroglobulin. In the absence of TSH, for example, in hypopituitarism, thyroid gland activity slows to a small fraction of the normal level. Administration of TSH in this situation restores full activity to normal. TSH also stimulates growth of the thyroid by increasing the size and number of follicular cells. There is a sensitive feedback mechanism between the pituitary and the thyroid which serves to maintain an adequate level of thyroid hormone. A fall in output of hormone from the thyroid, for example, evokes an increase in TSH secretion. Contrariwise, an increase in the circulating level of thyroid hormone causes a lowering in TSH. The pituitary-thyroid axis is influenced in turn by the centers in the hypothalamus. Recently a potent hypothalamic hormone (TRF) has been identified and synthesized.[15] This factor causes the release of TSH from the pituitary. Undoubtedly, much future research will be concerned with the relationships involving the central nervous system, the pituitary, and the thyroid.

The supply of iodine influences thyroid

IODINE METABOLISM

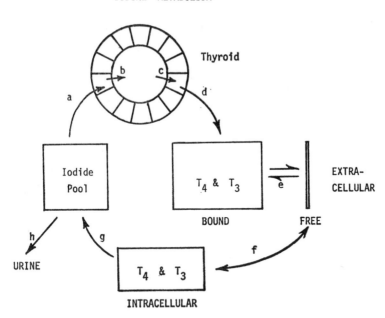

Fig. 8A-1. Simplified schema of iodine metabolism. (a) Iodide ion is actively concentrated by the thyroid follicular cells. (b) Multiple reactions including oxidation and organification of iodide into thyroglobulin, to form iodotyrosines and iodothyronines. (c) Proteolysis of thyroglobulin. (d) Release of the iodothyronines, thyroxine (T_4) and triiodothyronine (T_3), the active hormones. (e) Reversible equilibrium between free and bound hormones in extracellular fluid. (f) Interaction of free hormone with cellular binding sites, also a reversible process. (g) Enzymatic degradation of hormones with release of iodine to the body iodide pool, from which iodide is either excreted via the kidney (h) or returned to the thyroid gland.

activity in several ways.[7] Under conditions of iodine lack, the iodide transport process is stimulated, with the result that an increased proportion of the circulating iodide pool becomes available to the gland.[16] The individual follicular cells increase in size (hypertrophy) and number (hyperplasia). Thyroglobulin is synthesized more rapidly. Proportionately more T_3 and less T_4 are formed and secreted.[17] These alterations in function induced by iodine lack are for the most part mediated by an increase in TSH. The effect of these changes is to enable the normal individual to maintain a normal metabolic state (euthyroidism) in the face of a limited supply of iodine.[18]

Pharmacologic Effects of Excess Iodide. An excellent review of the diverse effects of excessive amounts of iodide in humans has appeared recently.[19] Small to moderate increments in iodide intake, i.e., up to 10 times the "normal" requirement of about 100 µg per day, lead to little or no chemical effects in individuals with normal thyroids. The gland for a time takes up more iodine than it releases (positive iodine balance), but within a few weeks the absolute amount of I^- taken up by the thyroid is reduced toward normal. During the entire period of excess iodide ingestion, the rate of hormonal secretion remains normal. In patients with hyperthyroidism, in contrast, the effects are quite different. Small doses of iodide, as little as 1 mg per day, cause a prompt inhibition of hormone release and marked amelioration of the symptoms of thyrotoxicosis.[20] This effect appears to be a direct one on the hyperactive gland itself and not an effect on the pituitary, as it occurs both in cases of toxic nodular goiter and in untreated Graves' disease, disorders in which blood levels of TSH are low.[13] Administration of exogenous TSH has been shown to reverse the iodide-induced inhibition of hormone release. This particular effect of iodide has been used with advantage in the treatment of hyperthyroidism, especially in the period before the advent of the thionamide class of anti-thyroid drugs. The actual mechanism is not well understood, but the result of treatment with iodides ("Lugolization") is a diminution in the vascularity of the gland, an increase in colloid deposits, and a decrease in the size of the follicular cells. Unfortunately, the inhibitory effect is often short-lived; many cases "escape" after a period of a few weeks, and thyroid hyperfunction returns full-blown in spite of continuation of iodide therapy. Once they have escaped, such cases are resistant to attempts at re-induction of iodide inhibition.

The acute effects of large doses of iodide in experimental animals and in humans without hyperthyroidism include an inhibition of thyroid hormone synthesis. This phenomenon was discovered in rats by Wolff and Chaikoff.[21] Elevation of the plasma level of iodide above 20 to 35 μg per 100 ml caused a prompt cessation of thyroxine synthesis. However, the animals escaped from this acute inhibition within a day or two. This escape has been termed "adaptation" and apparently is due to a diminution of the iodide-transport process. The biochemical mechanism of the Wolff-Chaikoff effect is not well understood. The effect also occurs in humans, but most individuals appear to "adapt" to excessive doses of iodide and thyroid hormone synthesis proceeds unimpaired. Some are unable to adapt, however.[22] In such cases, most of whom have a history of some pre-existing thyroid disorder, prolonged ingestion of iodide (200 mg or more daily for weeks to months) leads eventually to hypothyroidism and usually some degree of thyroid enlargment (iodide goiter). Such iodide-induced hypothyroidism is usually rapidly reversed on withdrawal of the iodide. Either iodide itself (*e.g.*, KI) or any drug which contains iodine (*e.g.*, iodopyrine, an anti-asthmatic medication) has been shown to cause iodide myxedema and/or goiter.

In addition to the sporadic cases of iodide goiter, an interesting endemic form has been studied.[19] Along the coast of the Northern Island of Japan, a relatively common form of simple goiter affecting nearly 10 per cent of the population has been traced to an extremely high dietary intake of iodine in the form of seaweed ("kombu"). Studies of iodine metabolism in such cases show evidence of the Wolff-Chaikoff type of block in thyroid hormone synthesis, an effect which could be reversed on withdrawal of seaweed from the diet and re-established with administration of potassium iodide. Typically, the goitrous individuals in this endemic area are euthyroid, perhaps because ingestion of the seaweed is intermittent throughout the year. The fact that only a minority of all persons exposed do develop obvious goiters suggests a pre-existing partial biochemical defect in the thyroids of these individuals.

Still another effect of excess iodine was noted almost as soon as the element came into widespread use in the treatment of goiter in iodine-deficient areas. A few euthyroid patients with long-standing goiter developed hyperthyroidism of iodine therapy. This phenomenon, termed "Jod-Basedow" (literally, Basedow's disease secondary to iodine), occurred often enough to lead to a reaction against the use of this treatment for goiter. The most likely explanation for Jod-Basedow is that such goitrous thyroids contain autonomous areas which are only poorly functioning until supplied with a sufficient supply of iodide, at which point hyperthyroidism ensues.

Estimation of Dietary Iodine. Table 8A–1 lists the iodine content of each of several categories of food determined by direct chemical analysis of samples of diets

Table 8A-1. Iodine Content of Composites of Food Categories[23]

Food Categories	No. of Samples	Iodine (μg/wet kg) Mean ± S.E.	Median
Seafoods	7	660 ± 180	540
Vegetables	13	320 ± 100	280
Meat Products	12	260 ± 70	175
Eggs	11	260 ± 80	145
Dairy Products	18	130 ± 10	139
Bread & Cereal	18	100 ± 20	105
Fruits	18	40 ± 20	18

employed at the Clinical Center, National Institutes of Health.[23] The authors of this study emphasize that these data apply to this institution and are not necessarily applicable to foods available elsewhere and prepared under other conditions. The iodine content of a given food varies widely, depending on the types of soil, fertilizers, animal feed, and on the method of processing the foods. For example, in some regions of the U.S. bread may account for a large proportion of iodine intake (150 μg per slice) because certain bakeries add iodate to dough as a stabilizing agent.[24,25] The consumption of iodized salt is another important variable. An individual may add as much as 8 gm of table salt to his food per day. If iodized, this would provide up to 600 μg iodine.[23] The average is about 2 gm salt (150 μg I). In view of the difficulties in estimating dietary iodine, many workers have employed total urinary iodine excretion to estimate iodine intake. This assumes, of course, the subject is in iodine balance, i.e., intake equals excretion, during the period of the study. It has been demonstrated, however, that normal and goitrous individuals may be in positive or negative balance for prolonged periods of time.[26,27] It follows, then, that the only certain method of determining iodine intake, short of using formula diets, is to perform analyses on samples of the actual diet consumed or of food categories.

Tests of Thyroid Function in Man. The most widely used method of measuring the activity of the thyroid gland is the radio-iodine uptake test.[28] The procedure involves oral administration of a tracer dose (5 to 10 microcuries) of radioactive iodide, usually ^{131}I, and determination of the fraction of the dose in the gland at a given interval, usually 24 hours after the dose. The normal range is 10 to 40 per cent, but these values vary from one region to another, depending on the techniques of counting radioactivity and on the iodine supply in the locality. This test is of particular value in the diagnosis of hyperthyroidism. In this condition, the radioiodine uptake is usually higher than 40 per cent at 24 hours. When this diagnosis is suspected, it is advisable to determine the uptake value at a shorter interval (e.g., at 2 hours) as well

as at 24 hours after the tracer dose. This test is not very helpful in the diagnosis of hypothyroidism; there is considerable overlap between normal and hypothyroid values at all intervals. The thyroid suppression test has proved useful in confirming the diagnosis of hyperthyroidism (Graves' disease) and in following the course of this disease. In this test, the thyroid radioiodine uptake is determined before and after the administration of thyroid hormone. Patients with active Graves' disease typically show no decline in the uptake value (thyroid autonomy), whereas those without this disorder exhibit a decrease in uptake due to suppression of TSH secretion by the administered thyroid hormone.

Thyroid scanning is often performed in conjunction with the thyroid uptake test. The scan shows the distribution of radioiodine within the gland thereby providing an estimate of gland size and permitting the detection of areas of hyperfunction ("hot" nodules) and areas of relative hypofunction ("cold" foci).

The most useful screening tests to determine thyroid status of an individual involve the measurement of the effective concentration of thyroid hormone in the blood. Until recently, the level of serum protein-bound iodine (PBI) was the most widely employed test of this type. The PBI measures total precipitable iodine in serum, and therefore includes some iodinated proteins which are not active as thyroid hormone. Furthermore, the common x-ray contrast materials and many iodine-containing medications cause spurious elevations in serum PBI. The widespread recent availability of methods which measure serum thyroxine (T_4) concentration has made the less specific serum PBI nearly obsolete. Some of the T_4 methods utilize column chromatographic separation prior to chemical T_4 iodine measurement; others employ a principle known as competitive-binding, which involves the progressive displacement of labeled T_4 from specific binding sites on TBG as the concentration of unlabeled T_4 is increased.

A reversible equilibrium exists in plasma between the free and the protein-bound forms of the thyroid hormones.[10] In the case of T_4, the equilibrium is normally far in favor of the bound form. Thus, about 99.97 per cent of the total T_4 is bound; only 0.03 per cent is free (diffusible). It is generally held that the level of free hormone, rather than that of the bound form, determines an individual's metabolic status. With rare exceptions, the concentration of free T_4 is abnormally high in cases of hyperthyroidism and low in patients with hypothyroidism. Since the concentration of free T_4 in plasma is too low to measure directly (even in hyperthyroidism), various methods have been devised to estimate this quantity by indirect means. The most common such method is the free thyroxine index, which is the calculated product of the concentration of total T_4 in serum (measured by any of several methods as discussed above) and the ratio of free over total T_4. The latter may be estimated from either the T_3 resin uptake or T_4 resin uptake values, both of which involve the addition of a tracer amount of labeled hormone to serum in order to determine the proportion of label which is not bound to serum protein. Other ways of estimating the free-to-bound ratio of T_4 include equilibrium dialysis, ultrafiltration, or dextran-gel separation. One of the reasons why the free thyroxine index has become so widely used as a diagnostic screening test of thyroid status is that the plasma protein (TBG) which binds T_4 (and T_3) is altered in a large number of non-thyroidal disorders and by various medications. Among the latter, the most common are oral contraceptives containing estrogens. Euthyroid women taking such birth-control agents show elevated serum T_4 levels due to high TBG but a normal free T_4 index. (The same combination of results is seen during normal pregnancy.) Thus, the free T_4 index is presently the most reliable laboratory indicator of thyroid status.[28]

The measurement of TSH levels in blood has recently become another useful clinical test.[29] Patients with hypothyroidism due to primary thyroid failure exhibit abnormally high levels of TSH in plasma, by virtue of the activity of the hypothalamus-pituitary feedback mechanism. On the other hand, cases of secondary hypothyroidism, due to hypothalamic or pituitary disease, show low levels of TSH. Prior to the availability of sensitive methods of measuring TSH, the differential diagnosis of these two types of hypothyroidism was sometimes difficult.

SIMPLE GOITER

Simple goiter may be defined as an enlargement of the thyroid gland with hypertrophy and/or hyperplasia of the follicular epithelial cells, not primarily due to inflammatory or neoplastic processes. There may be excessive accumulation of colloid as well. The goiter is usually diffuse and, in its early stages, at least partially reversible with the administration of thyroid hormone. In long-standing cases, the goiter may become multi-nodular and does not completely regress with hormone replacement. The pathogenesis of simple goiter is not completely understood. However, most authorities regard the condition as a compensatory response, via the TSH mechanism, to inadequate supply of thyroid hormones by the thyroid gland.

Iodine Deficiency. The once widely accepted view that iodine deficiency is *the* cause of all cases of goiter in endemic areas has now been modified. Administration of iodine in large-scale prophylactic programs in endemic goiter areas, such as the Congo, New Guinea, and the Andean regions of South America, has markedly reduced the formerly high incidence of goiter. This response supports the thesis that iodine deficiency in these regions was one causative factor in these areas.[30] On the other hand, there are several reasons to implicate other factors operating at the same time: Before iodine administration, the incidence of goiter, although high in certain deficient localities, never reached 100 per cent; some individuals in these areas escaped goiter even though they were exposed to severely iodine-deficient diets. Iodine replacement does not prevent goiter completely.[31] Within a given endemic area, the incidence of goiter does not correlate with the iodine intake (as estimated from daily urinary excretion of iodine). For example, on Idjwi Island (Lake Kivu) in the Congo, the incidence of goiter is 54 per cent in the north and only 5 per cent in the southern part of the island. Yet the average

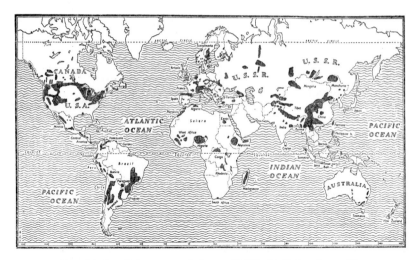

Fig. 8A-2. Goiter areas of the world (World Goiter Survey[2]).

urinary excretion of iodine was found to be similar in both locales (less than 20 μg I per 24 hours).[32] These considerations and others have led workers to conclude that factors other than iodine deficiency may be important, at least in some endemic areas.[33,34] Such factors might include genetically determined defects in the enzymes responsible for thyroid hormone biosynthesis, dietary goitrogens, and infectious agents. Bacterial goitrogens have been detected in the water supply of certain districts.[35] According to this view, iodine deficiency plays a permissive role by "uncovering" borderline or subtle biochemical defects (genetic or acquired) in hormone synthesis.[32] One may imagine that in a given population a continuum of varying degrees of susceptibility to goiter exists. In areas where plenty of iodine is available, the incidence of "iodine-deficiency" goiter is relatively low since only those individuals with severe biochemical defects are affected. Under conditions of more limited iodine supply, an increasing proportion of the susceptible group develops goiter, until in extreme iodine deficiency, an endemic situation prevails. (Fig. 8A–2).

Anti-Thyroid Drugs. Many types of external agents are capable of inducing simple goiter in man.[36] Common to all of these is their ability to inhibit the synthesis, the secretion, or the effectiveness of thyroid hormones. The most common anti-thyroid drugs are the thiocarbamides, or thionamides. Propylthiouracil and methimazole (Fig. 8A–3), the most potent of this class, block hormone synthesis within the thyroid by inhibiting coupling of iodotyrosines and, to a lesser extent, by inhibiting formation of iodotyrosines. A number of agents used in medicine for other pur-

6-n-propylthiouracil

1-methyl-2-mercaptoimidazole (Methimazole, Tapazole®)

Goitrin

Fig. 8A-3. Chemical formulas of some anti-thyroid compounds. Propylthiouracil and methimazole are used in the treatment of hyperthyroidism. Goitrin is a potent anti-thyroid substance which is present in rutabaga and other members of the cabbage family.

possess incidental anti-thyroid activity. For example, para-aminosalicylic acid, used in treatment of tuberculosis, can induce goiter by virtue of its propylthiouracil-like action. Other drugs with similar effects, but less potent, include sulfonamides, tolbutamide, resorcinol, and iodide itself (see above). Another class of agents induces goiter (and hypothyroidism) by interfering with the thyroidal iodide transport mechanism. Thiocyanate and perchlorate are of this type.

Dietary Goitrogens. Certain foods have been shown to contain substances which induce goiter in experimental animals. In a series of painstaking studies, Greer and his associates isolated from rutabaga and turnips a substance which has anti-thyroid activity (similar in potency to thiouracil).[37] They named the material "goitrin" (Fig. 8A-3). Subsequently, goitrin was detected in other vegetables of the cabbage family. Certain other foods also exhibit some degree of anti-thyroid activity, but the active substance in them has not been identified. Goiter due solely to dietary goitrogens is probably uncommon. However, if such foods were consumed in large quantities, especially in an iodine-deficient environment, goiter might develop.

Biochemical Defects in Thyroid Hormone Synthesis. In areas of the world outside of recognized "goiter-belts," simple goiter sometimes occurs in certain families. There may or may not be hypothyroidism or cretinism coexisting. When such familial cases have been investigated, selective defects in one or another of the steps in thyroid iodine metabolism have usually been found presumably on a genetic basis.[30] The commonest form of defect involves the process by which iodide is oxidized and incorporated into tyrosyl residues, probably due to deficient thyroidal iodide peroxidase activity. Another form of defect consists of a lack of the thyroidal iodotyrosine deiodinase enzyme. It is interesting that patients with the latter defect are successfully treated by daily administration of a few mg of iodide. The latter observation supports the idea that some cases of iodine-deficiency goiter may represent instances of a partial thyroid enzyme defect which has been brought out by a relative iodine lack.

The dietary requirement for iodine must therefore be different for different regions, depending upon the presence or absence of goitrogens in the diet, and for different individuals within each region depending upon genetic and acquired factors which influence the ability to adapt to limited iodine supply. Nevertheless, as a general guide, a daily intake of 100 μg iodine is considered adequate for most adults, assuming there is no exposure to goitrogenic agents. The iodine requirement is probably somewhat greater in childhood, during the growth spurt of adolescence, and during pregnancy and lactation.

Treatment of Simple Goiter. There is no question that wide-scale supplementation of the diet with iodine has reduced significantly the incidence of goiter in those areas where goiter was once highly prevalent. In the United States, iodized salt contains 76 μg iodine per gm. On a reasonably varied diet and with an average consumption of added iodized salt (2 to 6 gm per day), the typical American takes in somewhat more than 500 μg iodine per day.[23] In most countries of Europe, salt is iodized to approximately one-tenth the U.S. level. In those areas of the world where iodine deficiency continues to be a problem and where socioeconomic conditions preclude widespread use of dietary supplementation, administration of iodized oil by intramuscular injection in mass-inoculation programs promises to be an effective means of preventing endemic goiter.[38]

Simple goiters often regress somewhat in size under treatment with iodides, to the degree that iodine deficiency contributes to its causation. The response of large, long-standing goiters to iodides is often disappointing. The preferred treatment in such cases is thyroid hormone. In fact, the most effective means of obtaining regression of almost any type of non-toxic goiter, regardless of the cause, is to administer thyroid hormone. Thyroxine, 0.1 to 0.3 mg daily, is the form most commonly used.

BIBLIOGRAPHY

1. Iason: *The Thyroid Gland in Medical History*, New York, Forben Press, 1946.

2. *Iodine Facts*. World Goiter Survey. Facts 271–380. London, Iodine Educational Bureau, 1946.
3. Harington: *The Thyroid Gland: Its Chemistry and Physiology*, London, Oxford University Press, 1933.
4. Gross and Pitt-Rivers: Lancet, *1*, 439, 1952.
5. Kimball and Marine: Arch. Int. Med., *22*, 41, 1918.
6. Berson: Am. J. Med., *20*, 653, 1956.
7. Wayne, Koutras, and Alexander: *Clinical Aspects of Iodine Metabolism*, Philadelphia, F. A. Davis Co., 1964.
8. Pitt-Rivers and Cavalieri: Thyroid Hormone Biosynthesis. In: *The Thyroid Gland*, vol. 1, ed. by Pitt-Rivers and Trotter, Washington, Butterworth, 1964.
9. Cavalieri and Searle: J. Clin. Invest., *45*, 939, 1966.
10. Robbins and Rall: The Iodine-Containing Hormones. In: *Hormones in Blood*, 2nd Ed., ed. by Gray and Bacharach, Vol. 1, London, Academic Press, 1967.
11. Cavalieri, Steinberg, and Searle: J. Clin. Invest., *49*, 1041, 1970.
12. Sterling: Recent Progress in Hormone Research, *26*, 249, 1970.
13. Ingbar and Woeber: The Thyroid Gland. In: *Textbook of Endocrinology*, 4th Edition, ed. by Williams, Philadelphia, W. B. Saunders Co., 1968.
14. Tata: Biological action of thyroid hormone at the cellular and molecule levels. In: *Actions of Hormones on Molecular Processes*, ed. by Litwack and Kritchevsky, New York, John Wiley & Sons, 1964.
15. Schally, Arimura, Bowers *et al.*: Recent Progress in Hormone Research, *24*, 497, 1968.
16. Stanbury, Brownell, Riggs *et al.*: *Endemic Goiter*, Cambridge, Harvard University Press, 1954.
17. Choufoer, van Rhijn, Kassenaar, and Querido: J. Clin. Endocrinol. and Metab., *23*, 1203, 1963.
18. Studer and Greer: *The Regulation of Thyroid Function in Iodine Deficiency*, Bern, Hans Huber, 1968.

19. Wolff: Am. J. Med., *47*, 101, 1969.
20. Volpe and Johnston: Ann. Int. Med., *56*, 577, 1962.
21. Wolff and Chaikoff: J. Biol. Chem., *172*, 855, 1948.
22. Braverman, Woeber, and Ingbar: New Eng. J. Med., *281*, 816, 1969.
23. Vought and London: Am. J. Clin. Nutrition, *14*, 186, 1964.
24. London, Vought, and Brown: New Eng. J. Med., *273*, 381, 1965.
25. Pittman, Dailey, and Beschi: New Eng. J. Med., *280*, 1431, 1969.
26. Malmos, *et al.*: J. Clin. Endocrinol. and Metab., *27*, 1372, 1967.
27. Vought, Maisterrana, Tovar, and London: J. Clin. Endocrinol. and Metab., *25*, 551, 1965.
28. Cavalieri: Radioisotopes in the Diagnosis of Thyroid Disease. In *Atomic Medicine*, 5th Ed, ed. by Behrens, King, and Carpender, Baltimore, Williams & Wilkins Co., 1969.
29. Odell, Wilber, and Paul: J. Clin. Endocrinol. and Metab., *25*, 1179, 1965.
30. Stanbury: Familial Goiter. In: *The Metabolic Basis of Inherited Disease*, 2nd Ed., 1966, ed. by Stanbury, Wyngaarden, and Fredrickson, New York, McGraw-Hill Book Co., 1966.
31. Gaitan, Wahner, Correa, Bernal, Jubiz, Gaitan, and Llanos: J. Clin. Endocrinol. and Metab., *28*, 1730, 1968.
32. Beckers: Pathophysiology of Nontoxic Goiter. In: *Endemic Goiter*, Pan-American Health Organiz. Scientific Publication No. 193, 1968.
33. Roche and Lissitzky: Etiology of Endemic Goiter. In: *Endemic Goiter*, World Health Organization Monograph No. 44, 1960.
34. Wahner, Mayberry, Gaitan, and Gaitan: J. Clin. Endocrinol. and Metab., *32*, 491, 1971.
35. Gaitan, Island, and Liddle: Trans. Assoc. Amer. Physicians, *82*, 141, 1969.
36. Greer: Recent Progress in Hormone Research, *18*, 187, 1962.
37. Greer: J. Clin. Endocrinol. and Metab., *12*, 1259, 1952.
38. Kevany, Fierro-Benitez, Pretell, and Stanbury: Am. J. Clin. Nutrition, *22*, 1597, 1969.

Chapter

8

Section B   The Biochemical and Nutritional Role of Trace Elements

TING-KAI LI

AND

BERT L. VALLEE

The importance of inorganic elements in biochemical and physiologic processes is now well established at all levels of cellular complexity. Although more than 60 elements have been discovered in bacteria, fungi, higher plants, animals and man, few of them have been studied intensively. Investigations have necessarily been restricted to those occurring in amounts large enough to be measurable, even if not always precisely, by available techniques. Calcium, carbon, chlorine, hydrogen, iodine, iron, nitrogen, magnesium, oxygen, phosphorus, potassium, sodium, and sulfur comprise this group.

Trace elements, micronutrient elements, or *minor elements* are terms applied to the remaining elements occurring constantly in biologic systems. The following are generally included among the trace elements: aluminum, antimony, arsenic, barium, boron, bromine, cadmium, chromium, cobalt, copper, gallium, lead, lithium, manganese, mercury, molybdenum, nickel, rubidium, selenium, silver, strontium, tin, titanium, vanadium and zinc. They have been grouped together quite arbitrarily but have in common the uncertainty of assigning to them definite physiologic functions and difficulty in measuring their concentration in biologic fluids which varies from 1×10^{-6} to less than 1×10^{-12} grams/gram wet weight of tissue. Thus, these designations often have implied reference both to the total amounts and to the problems in qualitative and quantitative detection of the elements, but they are also sometimes inferred to denote uncertainty as to biologic significance.

Perhaps for the latter reason *iron, iodine,* and *fluorine,* though occurring in these concentration ranges, are generally considered as distinct from the trace element group because their established importance to health, and their medical significance is no longer questioned. The roles of these elements are discussed in separate chapters.

Criteria for the essentiality of any element in nutrition have been stated:[1] in the absence of a specific element, a deficiency state develops on diets otherwise adequate and satisfactory, *i.e.,* containing all other dietary essentials in adequate amounts and proportions and free from toxic properties. Dietary supplementation of this specific element and this element alone reverses the deficiency state, resulting in repeated and significant responses in growth and health.

With some elements, the deficiency state has been correlated further with the finding of subnormal concentrations of the element in the blood, tissues and organs of the deficient animals and of altered metabolism. At the present time, chromium, copper, cobalt, manganese, molybdenum, selenium and zinc are classified as *essential* trace elements in animal nutrition. There are recent reports that nickel[2] and tin[3] may be essential nutrient elements for fowl and rats, respectively. The essentiality of bromine, barium, and strontium is less certain, and others, such as cadmium and vanadium, have suspected functions of significance because of their consistent presence in tissues and cellular components and association with specific macromolecules. No doubt, many of the elements of currently unknown physiologic activity will be found to participate in vital processes and, as analytical techniques improve, the exact loci of these trace elements and their metabolic functions may be expected to be identified.

Trace elements and the many avenues of approach to medical problems which they seem to offer have generated much speculation and many hypotheses in regard to their role in human diseases. The obvious experimental difficulties in appraising the functional significance of trace elements in normal and disease states (*vide infra*) have often led to confusion as to their true role and to skepticism among serious investigators. As a consequence, there has been much debate occasioned by the observation of the decrease or increase of a given metal ion concentration in the blood of patients with a given disease and efforts to relate such data to the etiology of the disease have not been uniformly successful. Trace metals have been invoked as mechanistic factors to "explain" disease states as diverse as cancer, arteriosclerosis, hypertension, arthritis, porphyria, lupus erythematosus, multiple sclerosis and amyotrophic lateral sclerosis, but the evidence has often not stood the test of time. Even though variations in metal ion concentrations of tissues and body fluids are commonly observed in many disease states, such findings do not necessarily have etiologic significance.

HISTORICAL DEVELOPMENT AND PRESENT PERSPECTIVE

Awareness of the presence and functional significance of trace elements in living systems began about a century ago when iron, copper and zinc were found to be essential to the growth of plants and microorganisms and to be constituents of certain respiratory and blood pigments in snails and molluscs. Later, vanadium was discovered to function in the respiration of tunicates.

Investigations of cellular respiration and the involvement of iron in oxidative processes first suggested that metals may be an essential part of enzymatic reactions and pointed the way to the eventual discovery of metalloenzymes. However, the idea of a generalized function for the trace elements was slow to emerge and most of the experimental work leading to the presently more secure basis of understanding has been performed within the last 40 years.

Knowledge of the essentiality of trace metals to animal nutrition emerged principally through two approaches: basic studies of the effects on animals of highly purified or specially constituted diets designed to be low or high in the trace elements in question and applied studies of a number of naturally occurring endemic diseases of man or animals that were found to be due to a deficiency or an excess of one or more trace elements. During the last 25 years, there have been intensive investigations of the metabolic dynamics of metals within the body and their mode of action within the tissues. This development was greatly assisted and stimulated by the advent of isotopes and other concurrent developments in analytical chemistry and enzymology. Radioactive isotopes permitted studies of the absorption, retention, and excretion of various elements. It became possible to measure the ranges of normal concentrations of a variety of trace elements in plant and animal tissues and to relate such data to age, sex, geography and disease.[4-6] The discovery of *metalloenzymes* and *metalenzyme complexes* demonstrated conclusively that trace metals served critical roles in enzymic processes. These advances have directed particular attention in recent years to the basic biochemical lesions associated with the diverse manifestations of trace element deficiencies and excesses in the animal body.

Classically, the appearance of specific lesions or abnormalities in the animal was used to define the limiting factors in diseases of nutritional origin. Clinical and pathologic studies have served as essential diagnostic tools in the investigation of all trace element deficiencies and toxicities. It is important, nevertheless, to recognize their limitations.

Not all trace element disorders result in specific and characteristic clinical signs or pathologic changes which are recognized readily, especially if the disorder is mild. Symptomatology and histopathology may vary depending upon a variety of factors including the species, its sex and age, the timing, duration and severity of deprivation, the nature of the element itself and its relation to other elements or constituents in the diet. Bone deformities, anemia, reproductive failure, neurologic dysfunction and defective development of the integument and its appendages are common. Mild micronutrient imbalances are often indistinguishable from primary dietary deficiency due to starvation or simply the loss of appetite. Moreover, the clinically or pathologically obvious functional or structural abnormality may be merely the final expression of a defect arising earlier in a chain of metabolic events and may bear no simple relationship to the limiting element. Because trace elements are biologically active at very low concentrations, rigidly controlled experimental conditions are essential. Failure to observe appropriate precautionary measures has often led to erroneous conclusions. Moreover, a given nutrient element may have multiple modes of action and the specific biologic response to this element may occur within a relatively narrow concentration range. At concentrations above this range, the element may actually become inhibitory or deleterious to the organism, a toxic or pharmacologic manifestation resulting from interaction of the element at other sites.

A further difficulty in the interpretation of many studies results from the frequent occurrence of abnormalities in metal metabolism brought about by *metal ion antagonism* or *conditioned deficiencies* occurring when the normal intake of a nutrient does not meet the needs of an organism due to unusual secondary circumstances or factors. Failure to absorb a metabolite, the inability to synthesize it into a biologically active intermediate and excessive excretion are among the simplest examples of such conditioning factors. The antagonistic action of zinc and molybdenum with copper may serve to illustrate the type of problem encountered

frequently: the anemia, subnormal growth and reproductive failure in rats induced by excess zinc in diets and the severe diarrhea and loss of condition in cattle attributed to molybdenum intoxication in a disease known as *teart* were both later found to be due to conditioned copper deficiency.

Another problem in assessing the function of trace metals in biological processes arises from the fact that their roles are frequently indirect. Thus, cobalt alone is completely ineffective in the treatment of patients with pernicious anemia; it is therapeutically significant largely as a constituent of the vitamin B_{12} molecule. These and similar problems underlie the difficulties encountered in establishing meaningful relationships between disease and alterations in trace metal metabolism.

For these reasons and because the determination of concentrations of trace elements, like that of other metabolites, in tissues, cells, subcellular components and body fluids is a corollary to the elucidation of their role in health and disease, the attention of present-day investigators has centered upon the *distribution* and *function* of metals at the subcellular, enzymatic and molecular levels. Moreover, the advances in analytical chemistry, biochemistry, and molecular biology have permitted the formulation of new hypotheses and their experimental evaluation by means previously unavailable.

Presently, reliable measurements of small concentrations of trace elements present in tissues, cells, subcellular particles, body fluids, proteins and nucleic acids can be performed by colorimetry, fluorimetry, polarography, emission spectrography, flame spectrophotometry, neutron activation analysis, x-ray fluorescence and atomic absorption spectrometry. The last method, recently developed, is particularly sensitive for the measurement of certain metals.[7] Thus, it is possible, for example, to detect zinc, cadmium, magnesium, copper, nickel, and cobalt in concentrations of a few parts per billion or less.[8]

Such studies are becoming indispensable in detecting and defining trace element disorders and in delineating the environmental limits under which they are likely to occur. As understanding of the sites and modes of action of micronutrient elements grows, it seems likely that chemical analyses or enzyme assays of particular parts of tissues or cell components will become ever more effective diagnostic aids. When these criteria are used jointly and the combined evidence is assessed by the discerning investigator, rapid and revealing data for the recognition and prediction of both deficiency and toxicity states may be obtained even when these are mild.

SOIL-PLANT-ANIMAL RELATIONSHIPS

The natural occurrence of deficiency or intoxication of a trace element in animals and man depends ultimately upon the plant, soil and water for their supply of mineral nutrients. Deficiency and intoxication states in plants and farm animals which depend upon a limited area for grazing and upon fodder or regulated feedings usually are recognized readily and the responsible element can be identified. Trace element deficiencies, toxicities and imbalances in man are usually milder, more restricted and more difficult to diagnose and trace to their natural source due to a variety of factors.[1] Human mineral requirements are low as compared with those of modern breeds of animals because of a slower growth rate and lower rate of reproduction. The sources of human foods and beverages usually comprise minerals derived from a range of soil types. Modern human dietaries contain a great variety of types of foods so that trace element abnormalities which may be present in particular parts of plants, animal tissues, or fluids can be offset by the consumption of other types of food not affected by deficiencies. The industrial treatment of various foods provides the opportunity both for gains and for losses of trace elements during storage, transport, preservation and processing. Thus, the impact of these influences upon the qualitative adequacy of human diets combines to render the nutritional abnormalities in man far more likely to be associated with a poor choice of foods rather than with their source and, more commonly, the deficiency or intoxication states occur as a *conditioned imbalance* brought about by other factors, *e.g.*, poor absorption. However, when the choice and quality of foods are poor and the dependence on locally grown foods is high, local soil deficiencies or excesses may accentuate the dietary abnormalities and adversely affect human health and nutrition.

BIOCHEMISTRY AND PHYSICAL CHEMISTRY

The search for an explanation of the physiologic role of trace elements has emphasized their association with enzyme systems in living cells. For operational purposes, the enzymes which are affected by metals can be considered in two groups: metalloenzymes and metal-enzyme complexes.[9]

A *metalloenzyme* contains a metal as an integral part of the molecule in a fixed amount per molecule of protein. The small number of metal atoms are bound firmly to a limited number of apparently specific sites and are not removed from the protein by mild procedures. When the element is dissociated from the protein moiety by more vigorous manipulation, all measurable biologic activity is lost and is not readily restored by the readdition of this or any other metal. The specific and unique chemical nature of the metal-protein interactions apparently confers both stability and reactivity on the molecule. In some metalloenzymes the metal atom serves primarily as a component of the active site and participates directly in the catalytic process. In other instances, the metal may serve to maintain the tertiary and quaternary structures of the protein, and its loss affects catalytic function indirectly by causing structural changes. In some enzymes, the metals appear to play both catalytic and structural roles. The elucidation of the physical and chemical basis of metal-protein interactions and their relationship to biologic function constitutes a rapidly advancing and widening area of modern biochemistry.

A large number of metalloproteins, with and without known enzymatic function have now been isolated from a variety of sources ranging from bacteria to man and are characterized sufficiently to be considered "pure."

Copper, cadmium, iron, cobalt, manganese, molybdenum, and zinc may be mentioned in this group. Although relatively few of these metalloproteins have been obtained from human sources, their significance with respect to the biochemistry, physiology, and pathology of man is becoming increasingly clear, since their function in different phyla constitutes a common biologic denominator. Structurally, chemically, and catalytically similar metalloenzymes are found in species of widely diversified evolutionary histories, thereby indicating their general metabolic importance.

Metalloenzymes may be contrasted with *metal-enzyme complexes*, which compose a far larger group of enzymes which are more loosely associated with metals, the criteron of association being the *activation* of catalysis. In this group, specificity of association cited above is lacking. The metals may be removed quite readily and different ones may substitute for one another in many instances. The metals which have been found to activate metal-enzyme complexes include magnesium, manganese, cobalt, zinc, cadmium, chromium, nickel, calcium and other alkaline earths, iron, copper, and mercury. Some of the rare earths have also been found to activate a few enzymes. The metal ion is not an integral part of the molecule when isolated and in many instances the enzymes may be active in the absence of the metal ion. These circumstances increase the difficulties of assessing the biologic significance of these *in vitro* findings.

Some investigators have considered the differences between these two groups of metal-enzyme systems to be a matter only of degree rather than of kind. A continuous spectrum of the firmness of association between metal and protein has been postulated, with metalloenzymes at one end and metal-enzyme complexes at the other, but both having similar biochemical function. Other workers have emphasized the dissimilarities. Whatever the hypothesis, metalloenzymes operationally lend themselves more readily to a definitive assessment of the physiologic role of a metal in enzyme systems at this time, since the element and the enzyme may be studied jointly *in vitro* and *in vivo*, the inherent specificity of their association lending

biologic significance to the results and providing a chemical basis for the biological manifestations. While metal-enzyme complexes have been of great theoretical importance in the understanding of catalytic phenomena and general mechanisms of metalloenzyme function, it has been more difficult to establish the nature of the underlying chemistry.

Delineation of the role of trace metals in the function and structure of enzymes represents a significant advance in our understanding of the manner in which metals participate in biologic processes and provides a fundamental basis in relating trace elements to health and disease. The discovery of substantial quantities of firmly bound metals including nickel, chromium, cobalt, and manganese in ribonucleic acids[10] constitutes another potentially important new avenue for the investigation of the role of metals in biology. These metals apparently stabilize the secondary and tertiary structure of RNA[11] and may play an important role in protein synthesis. The following sections deal with the individual trace elements currently thought to be important for the health and nutrition of man. With a few exceptions, most of the references point to authoritative reviews and pertinent studies published in more recent years.

COPPER

Copper is a constituent and essential nutrient of most if not all animals and plants and its deficiency can lead to severe derangement of growth and metabolism. It has been known to be an essential component of respiratory pigments for over a century and is being detected in an increasing number of proteins and enzymes. It serves as an oxygen carrier in the hemolymph of molluscs and arthropods. In plants, cuproenzymes serve as oxidoreductants of phenols and, in animals, they additionally participate in melanin formation. In animals copper is involved in activities as diverse as hemoglobin synthesis, bone and elastic tissue development, and the normal function of the central nervous system.[12,13]

Physiology and Metabolism. The average copper concentration of an adult vertebrate is of the order of 1.5 to 2.5 μg per gm fat-free tissue. A total of 100 to 150 mg of copper is found in normal man. In general, the liver (10 to 15 mg), kidney, heart, hair and brain (10 mg) contain the highest concentrations of copper. Spleen, lung, muscle and bone contain intermediate, while pituitary, thyroid and thymus have the lowest concentrations. There are about 45 μg of copper per gm dry weight of adult human liver, while there may be 5 to 10 times as much in fetal liver. During growth, the highest concentrations of copper appear in the rapidly developing structures. Over 90 per cent of the copper in mammalian plasma is associated with the α_2-globulin, ceruloplasmin, while over 60 per cent of the copper in erythrocytes is presumed to be associated with erythrocuprein, now known to have superoxide dismutase activity. A small amount of the plasma copper is bound to amino acids, i.e. histidine, threonine, and glutamine, apparently in equilibrium with that bound to albumin.[14] In other tissues and fluids the biochemical substances with which the major part of the copper is associated are largely undefined.

On a normal diet copper is not accumulated preferentially by any tissue. About 25 per cent of the ingested copper is absorbed from the upper alimentary tract, enhanced by acid and prevented by calcium. Copper complexed with neutral or anionic organic substances may be absorbed more readily than the free ion. A mechanism for the regulation of the absorption of copper from the gastrointestinal tract according to demand, similar to that for iron, has not been established. The bile is the major pathway of copper excretion and a small amount, usually less than 30 μg per 24 hour volume, is excreted in the urine independent of the intake. Less than 5 per cent of the ingested copper is retained.

Human whole blood contains about 100 μg per 100 ml of copper distributed about equally between erythrocytes and plasma. The concentration of serum copper in normal individuals is constant and is independent of age, sex, the menstrual cycle, food intake, diurnal or seasonal influences and tissue stores. Compared with that of adults, serum copper concentration in newborn infants is low, primarily owing to the low concentration of ceruloplasmin. The transport of copper, absorbed either gastrointestinally or administered intravenously has been studied with radioactive copper, ^{64}Cu. There is a transient initial rise in serum copper associated with the albumin fraction, followed by a slower secondary rise associated with the α_2-globulin fraction, ceruloplasmin. Ingested copper, loosely bound to serum albumin, is transported rapidly to the liver, bone marrow, and other organs where it is stored and becomes incorporated into cuproproteins. The slow secondary rise of serum radioactivity associated with ceruloplasmin can be taken to represent the incorporation of copper into this protein by synthesis and, perhaps, by exchange. The amino acid-bound fraction in serum may be involved with the transport of copper across cell membranes.[15]

Administration of estrogens markedly increases both serum copper and ceruloplasmin concentrations. Increased serum copper concentrations are found in pregnancy and in hepatic cirrhosis due to hyperestrogenism. Serum copper concentrations tend to be elevated in severe thyrotoxicosis.

The subcellular distribution of copper in rat liver has been studied: ^{64}Cu distributes differentially between the nucleus and cytoplasm, the uptake in the cytoplasm being much greater than that of the nucleus. The supernatant fractions contain the highest concentrations and about 65 per cent of the total liver copper as compared to 27 per cent of the total liver nitrogen. Whether this soluble protein is relatively free or is bound tightly to proteins is, as yet, unknown. Factors which influence the concentrations in the liver include diet, age, hormones, and pregnancy. Diets abnormally high or low in copper content generally cause corresponding changes in the concentrations of the liver and, frequently, of the blood. Sheep and cattle are extremely sensitive to the copper content of the diet, and in these species the copper concentration of the liver varies directly as a function of the intake.

Biochemistry. The growing number of biochemical systems with which copper is associated specifically suggest its involvement in a broad range of biologic functions.[16] Some of the purified cuproenzymes and copper-containing proteins are shown in Table 8B–1. Importantly, copper is a constituent of cytochrome oxidase, the terminal oxidase

Table 8 B-1. Cuproenzymes and Cuproproteins

Enzyme or Protein	*Source*
Hemocyanin	Molluscs, arthropods
Mitochondrocuprein	Neonatal bovine and human liver
Pink copper protein	Human erythrocytes
Ceruloplasmin	Human plasma
Uricase	Porcine liver
Cytochrome c oxidase	Bovine heart
Monoamine and diamine oxidase	Bovine plasma and liver, porcine kidney, pea seedlings
Dopamine β-hydroxylase	Adrenal glands
Ascorbic acid oxidase	Squash, cucumber
Laccase	Latex of lacquer tree
D-galactose oxidase	Dactylium dendroides
Phenolase (tyrosinase)	Neurospora crassa, mushrooms, mammalian tissues, melanomas
Ribulose diphosphate carboxylase	Spinach
Quercetinase (Dioxygenase)	Aspergillus flavus
Azurin	Pseudomonas aeruginosa and Bordetella pertussis
Stellacyanin	Latex of lacquer tree
Plastacyanin	Spinach, Phaseolus vulgaris, Chemopodium album
Mung bean pigment	Mung bean seedlings
Umecyanin	Horseradish root
Proteins Containing both Copper and Zinc	
Superoxide dismutase (cytocuprein, cerulocuprein, erythrocuprein, hepatocuprein)	Brain, erythrocyte and human, equine and bovine liver

of the electron transport mechanism from which ATP is synthesized oxidatively. This enzyme also contains heme as a prosthetic group. Cuproenzymes catalyze oxidation reactions, including phenolic amine substrates such as the catecholamines. Ceruloplasmin also exhibits phenol oxidase activity, and there is a good correlation between the copper content of the serum and its capacity to oxidize substances such as para-phenylenediamine, benzidine and other phenols including catecholamine. It also has ferro-oxidase activity, i.e., it oxidizes ferrous iron to ferric iron.[17] Ceruloplasmin has a molecular weight of 150,000 and contains 8 gm atoms of copper per mole which can be removed in the presence of ascorbic acid.[18] The copper-free, colorless, apoceruloplasmin can be recombined with cuprous ions to form ceruloplasmin. The copper atoms of ascorbate oxidase can also be reversibly restored and appear to serve both catalytic and structural roles in the molecule. Dopamine β-hydroxylase from adrenal medulla converts dopamine to norepinephrine.[19] Tyrosinase or phenoloxidase activity, present in plants such as potatoes and mushrooms, is also found in melanocytes and melanoma tissue of animals and man. The enzymatic activity is associated with the mitochondrial fractions of cells and is responsible for melanin formation. The skin of human albinos has no detectable tyrosinase activity indicating a deficiency of this enzyme as the basis for the absence of pigment in the skin and uveal tract. Enzymes involved in the oxidation of mono- and diamines, uric acid, cytochrome c, and galactose are all copper proteins. Amine oxidase apparently is also involved in the oxidative deamination of ε-amino groups of lysyl residues forming desmosine, the cross-linking group of elastin.[20] Crosslinking of collagen is similarly dependent upon a cuproenzyme. In addition to these cuproenzymes a number of enzymes such as ureidosuccinase, lecithinase and oxaloacetic decarboxylase are activated by copper, i.e., they form metal-enzyme complexes.

Cerebrocuprein, erythrocuprein and hepatocuprein, collectively called cytocuprein, are identical bluish-green soluble proteins containing about 0.35 per cent copper.[21] They contain 2 atoms each of copper and zinc per molecule of protein.[22] Their physiologic function is uncertain although they are thought to represent important steps in copper metabolism. Erythrocuprein has been shown to have superoxide dismutase activity, *i.e.*, it catalyzes the breakdown of superoxide radicals to oxygen and hydrogen peroxide.[23] Extracts of brain from patients with hepatolenticular degeneration (Wilson's disease) contain an abnormal copper protein which is isolated together with cerebrocuprein. A protein with high copper affinity has also been demonstrated in the liver of such patients. Mitochondrocuprein isolated from the mitochondria of neonatal liver contains 3 per cent copper and is insoluble.[21] Its amino acid composition is remarkably similar to that of metallothionein, a cadmium- and zinc-containing protein from kidney. It does not have cytochrome c oxidase activity and its function is presently unknown. Recently, a low molecular weight protein, claimed to be similar to metallothionein, has been identified in the cytosol of bovine duodenum and liver and human liver which binds copper.[24] However, the characteristics of the protein moiety have not been reported. A transport function for this protein has been postulated.

Ribonucleic acid isolated from a number of biologic sources contains significant amounts of firmly bound copper in addition to other metals. Significant concentrations of copper have also been shown to be present in isolated and purified viruses, perhaps through association with nucleic acid.

Copper influences erythropoiesis; its deficiency impairs iron absorption and transport and decreases hemoglobin synthesis. Concomitant with the decrease in plasma ceruloplasmin concentration, there is reduced transport of iron from the intestine and from the iron stores in tissues and liver to the plasma. The oxidation of ferrous iron to ferric iron by ceruloplasmin is apparently important for the formation of transferrin.[25] Utilization of iron for hemoglobin synthesis is also impaired and abnormal erythrocytes with shortened life span are produced.

Nutrition. The necessity of copper for animal nutrition has now been recognized for more than 30 years although chemical and clinical evidence of primary copper deficiency in man has not been reported.[1] Because copper is widely distributed in foods and cooking utensils, it seems improbable that copper deficiency would occur in man except under extreme conditions. Dietary sources of copper are similar to those of iron. Milk products are relatively poor sources. The normal copper intake of man is estimated to be 2.5 to 5 mg per day, an amount adequate for the maintenance of positive copper balance.[26] Children require about 0.05 to 0.1 mg per kg body weight daily.

Copper deprivation leading to hypochromic anemia has been demonstrated in rats, rabbits, chickens, pigs, dogs, sheep, goats, and cattle. The absorption of iron from the gastrointestinal tract is decreased and there is a reduction in the survival time of red blood cells. Total body iron stores are reduced, and the capacity of bone marrow to produce erythrocytes is limited. Malnourished prisoners of war and mentally defective infants placed on diets identical to those producing copper deficiency in swine do not develop hypocupremia or any other evidence of copper deficiency. However, anemia responding to the administration of copper has been reported to occur in infants fed a milk diet for several months following their recovery from kwashiorkor.[27]

Copper is essential for the normal development of bone, the central nervous system, and connective tissue. Lambs born of copper-deficient ewes develop *enzootic ataxia* or swayback characterized by an incoordination of gait. A similar disease has been observed in calves and piglets. Histologic examination shows diffuse symmetrical cerebral demyelinization with secondary degeneration of the motor tracts in the spinal cord. Cerebellar folia are absent or deformed. Deficiencies in sheep and cattle lead to osteoporosis and spontaneous fractures. Growing animals develop a rickets-like disease and osteoblastic activity is impaired. Bone collagen from copper-deficient animals show increased solubility and decreased crosslinking. Bone amine oxidase and cytochrome oxidase activities are decreased. Abnormalities in pigmentation and crimp of hair and wool, the former presumably related to decreased activity of the phenol oxidases, have also been found in a number of species. Alopecia and dermatoses as well as alterations in the texture and quality of hair and wool have been observed.

Severe copper deprivation in cows leads to myocardial fibrosis and a seasonal incidence of sudden death known as "falling disease." Cardiac hypertrophy has been observed in pigs. It has been suggested that the reduction of cytochrome oxidase activity in copper deprivation may lead to the observed cardiac hypertrophy in an effort to compensate for the reduction in respiratory activity. Cardiac and aortic aneurysms and rupture have also been observed in copper-deficient pigs and chicks. Studies of the aorta have shown decreased tensile strength and elastin content and striking pathologic change of the elastic fibers. There is an increased amount of a soluble protein which appears to be an elastin precursor. The lysine content of elastin is markedly increased, due to the failure of conversion of lysine to desmosine, the cross-linking residues of elastin.[28] This reaction is catalyzed by amine oxidase, which is decreased in activity in the serum, aorta, heart and kidney of copper-deficient animals.[29] The close similarity of these findings to those observed in lathyrism produced by β-aminopropionitrile, a chelating agent and inhibitor of amine oxidase, suggests that they share common mechanisms in generating the observed abnormalities of bone and connective tissue.

Several *conditioned* copper intoxication or deficiency diseases in animals have been observed. In cattle, a disease known as *teart* characterized by severe diarrhea and loss of condition was initially attributed to molybdenum intoxication. The resemblance of this disease to that exhibited by cattle in certain copper-deficient areas led to the empirical and successful use of copper sulfate in the treatment of "teart." It soon became apparent that molybdenum in the diet of ruminants could exert a profound effect on copper metabolism. Conversely sheep grazing on pastures with low molybdenum content rapidly accumulated toxic quantities of copper whereas a surfeit of molybdenum led to signs of copper deficiency and depletion of tissue copper stores. Furthermore, the "tox-

icity" of molybdenum is greatly enhanced by an increased intake of inorganic sulfate and perhaps reduced by an increased intake of manganese. Neither molybdenum nor sulfate alone interferes with copper retention and the effectiveness of either increases to a maximum as the intake of the other is increased. Apparently molybdenum plus sulfate interferes with the availability of copper by blocking tissue utilization or promoting copper excretion or both.

The copper deficiency caused by excess dietary zinc in rats resulting in anemia, subnormal growth and reproductive failure is another example of a conditioned copper deficiency. Feeding of excess dietary zinc reduces the liver cytochrome oxidase and catalase activities of rats markedly while the administration of small amounts of copper sulfate restores the enzymatic activities to normal. In addition, the excess zinc in the diet suppresses liver copper concentrations if the copper intake is marginal. On the other hand, an excess intake of copper also reduces the zinc concentrations of the liver.

Other biochemical studies have shown that copper deprivation leads to decreased tyrosinase, polyphenol oxidase and ascorbic acid oxidase activities in plants. In copper-deficient rats, cytochrome oxidase and amine oxidase activities and ceruloplasmin and hemoglobin concentrations are reduced. Extreme copper deficiency leads to the loss of oxidative capacity in mitochondria due to a decrease of cytochrome oxidase activity. ATP synthesis is decreased and phospholipid synthesis is depressed.[30] Mitochondria become fragile and more susceptible to aging. A reduction in DPN cytochrome c reductase and increased isocitric dehydrogenase activities have also been observed.

Copper Metabolism and Human Disease. Serum copper concentrations are increased in a number of acute and chronic pathologic conditions.[13] Viral and microbial infections, rheumatoid arthritis, rheumatic fever, lupus erythematosus, myocardial infarction, severe thyrotoxicosis, acute and chronic leukemia, a variety of malignant neoplasm, hemochromatosis, portal and biliary cirrhosis may be listed. In general the concentration in red blood cells is unaffected. In infections and myocardial infarction the ceruloplasmin concentration rises concomitant with the increase in copper concentration. A parallel increase in serum oxidase activity is observed. These increases in copper and ceruloplasmin content are unexplained and are not correlated with the change in sedimentation rate. In patients with portal and biliary cirrhosis the copper content of liver is increased.

Hypocupremia has been observed in a variety of states. In the nephrotic syndrome the urinary excretion of copper is increased in direct proportion to the amount of protein lost in the urine. Ceruloplasmin, not normally detected in the urine, is excreted and serum ceruloplasmin concentrations are decreased. Low serum copper concentrations have been observed also in kwashiorkor, sprue, celiac disease and idiopathic hypoproteinemia, presumably due to an imbalance in the rate of synthesis and breakdown of ceruloplasmin.

An uncommon malady of infants is characterized by edema, hypoproteinemia, anemia, hypoferremia and hypocupremia and decreased serum ceruloplasmin concentrations. These manifestations are similar to the copper- and iron-deficiency anemias produced in swine on milk diets, and are corrected by administration of iron and copper. The administration of copper to experimental animals has been noted to induce the synthesis of ceruloplasmin which, in turn, participates in regulating iron absorption and transport.

Hepatolenticular degeneration or Wilson's disease is a rare, genetic disease transmitted as a recessive trait and is the condition best known to be associated with hypocupremia.[31] The cardinal manifestations are the neurologic abnormalities arising from dysfunction of the lenticular region of the brain, signs of hepatic cirrhosis and the demonstration of a brown or gray-green (Kayser-Fleischer) ring at the limbus of the cornea. Renal abnormalities characterized by amino aciduria, glucosuria, phosphaturia, uricosuria, proteinuria and polypeptiduria may be present along with hypophosphatemia and hypouricemia. The serum copper concentration is generally depressed while urinary excretion is markedly increased. Ceruloplasmin concentration is generally decreased, and cytochrome oxidase activity of leukocytes is decreased. The liver, basal ganglia, cerebral cortex, kidney and Kayser-Fleischer corneal rings of patients with Wilson's disease contain excessive quantities of copper. In liver the largest amount of copper is present in a subfraction of liver cells corresponding to neonatal hepatic mitochondrocuprein. Variations in serum copper concentration are due to a high and variable content of the loosely bound copper associated with albumin. Studies with radioactive copper indicate that absorption is increased in individuals with hepatolenticular degeneration: up to 0.56 mg per day per mg of ingested copper or 20 to 50 times normal is retained. It appears that incorporation of copper into ceruloplasmin is deranged and that most of the plasma copper is associated loosely with serum albumin. The pathogenesis of the disease remains unknown. It has been suggested that patients with this disease may synthesize abnormal proteins having an increased affinity for copper, although evidence that the soluble brain proteins are unchanged electrophoretically in Wilson's disease has been thought not to favor this hypothesis. At present a hypothesis favored by many is that a combination of factors, including decreased incorporation of copper by ceruloplasmin due to abnormalities of its synthesis and increased and differential tissue affinity, may jointly determine the increased deposition of copper in certain critical loci. The neurologic manifestations have been attributed to the inhibition in brain tissues by copper of a number of enzymes, in particular membrane-bound ATPase and pyruvate oxidase.

Attempts to eliminate excessive copper in body tissues and to prevent reaccumulation are the most promising modes of therapy. Various copper chelating agents which are excreted in the urine have been employed, including 2,3-dimercaptopropanol (BAL), ethylenediamine tetraacetate (Versene) and β,β-dimethylcysteine (penicillamine). The latter, when given orally, has given the most encouraging clinical results.[32]

Copper Intoxication. Chronic ingestion of excess copper in fodder of sheep leads to accumulations 10 to 20 times the normal concentration of copper in the liver. The animals suffer no apparent ill effects until suddenly a large amount of excess copper is liberated into the blood stream producing a hemolytic anemia, hemoglobinuria and jaundice. Over 60 per cent of the circulating red cells may be destroyed during the crisis and atrophy of the liver may occur. A similar type of hemolytic jaundice has been observed in cattle. Acute copper intoxication in man due to ingestion of copper produces nausea, vomiting, epigastric pain, diarrhea, ptyalism, headache, dizziness, weakness and a metallic taste. In more severe cases tachycardia, hypertension and coma may ensue, followed by jaundice and hemolytic anemia, hemoglobinuria, uremia and death. Serum ceruloplasmin concentrations are increased as is loosely bound serum copper.[33]

ZINC

The presence of zinc in living organisms and its role as an essential nutrient have been recognized for almost a century, but difficulties in analysis limited early investigations to qualitative efforts. It was not until 1934 that conclusive evidence was adduced that zinc is essential to the normal growth and development of animals. The isolation and purification by Keilin and Mann in 1940 of carbonic anhydrase, found to contain zinc as a component of the molecule and essential for its enzymatic functions, offered the first concrete basis for an explanation of a mode of action of this element. Since then zinc has been found in many highly purified enzymes revealing the diversity of its function in protein and carbohydrate metabolism. Zinc-deficiency states in mammals as well as in man have been described.[34,35]

Physiology and Metabolism. The total amount of zinc in the human body has been estimated to be between 2 and 3 gm. Zinc is found in all human tissues varying from 10 to 200 μg per gm wet weight. Most organs, including the pancreas, contain 20 to 30 μg, while liver, voluntary muscle and bone contain 60 to 180 μg per gm. Larger quantities of zinc are found in the tissues of the eye, in particular the iris, retina and choroid. Zinc is not accumulated preferentially by any

tissue though the prostate, prostatic secretions and spermatozoa are remarkably high in their content of zinc (860 μg per gm for normal human prostate) which is not accounted for by the content of either carbonic anhydrase or alkaline phosphatase. To date there is no functional explanation for the high concentration of zinc in the male reproductive tract. Differences in organ content from species to species are not remarkable in most instances. Human whole blood contains about 900 μg of zinc per 100 ml. Normal serum zinc concentrations average 121 $\pm$ 19 μg/100 ml.[36] Normal erythrocytes contain 1.44 mg per ml of packed red blood cells. Three per cent of all the blood zinc is found in leukocytes which contain 3.2 $\times$ 10^{-2} μg zinc per million cells, about 25 times more than is found in a comparable number of erythrocytes. Blood zinc concentrations do not exhibit seasonal or diurnal variations and there is no difference in concentration between the sexes. Practically all zinc in serum is protein bound and is distributed in at least two and possibly more fractions.[37] Globulins bind zinc most firmly and an α-2-macroglobulin has been isolated and shown to be a zinc metalloprotein.[38] Most of the remainder is probably bound loosely to albumin which appears to be concerned primarily with transport. A large percentage of the erythrocyte zinc appears to be associated with carbonic anhydrase and that in leukocytes with alkaline phosphatase. Serum zinc decreases during pregnancy and with estrogen administration.

The distribution of ^{65}Zn injected in the mouse and the dog indicates that the liver accumulates the largest fraction of the total dose, and the most rapid turnover of ^{65}Zn was observed to occur in liver, pancreas, kidney and pituitary. About 10 per cent of the total ^{65}Zn given was excreted in the pancreatic juice within the first few days. Bone and red blood cells accumulated ^{65}Zn.

Zinc is widely distributed in a variety of foods. Foodstuffs from animal sources, and in particular shellfish, are rich in this element. The average human dietary intake is about 10 to 15 mg per day of which about 5 mg are retained. The site and mechanism of absorption of zinc from the intestine are not known with certainty. The availability of zinc for absorption is decreased by phytic acid, a phosphorus storage compound of plant seeds, which forms insoluble zinc-phytate complexes. Calcium can further decrease its availability by forming the more insoluble mixed zinc-calcium-phytate complex.[39] Once absorbed zinc is excreted primarily in gastrointestinal and pancreatic secretions. Urine contains about 0.5 mg per day, an amount apparently independent of intake and urinary volume. Studies in the rat indicate that, in contrast to iron, the body stores of zinc are not readily mobilized and, hence, there is an unusual dependence upon a regular, exogenous supply of the element, particularly during periods of growth.

Biochemistry. Zinc is closely associated with various proteins. Since many different zinc proteins may be present in most organs, the total zinc content of tissues is an inadequate guide to the manifold functions of the metal. The large number of zinc metalloenzymes which have been isolated point to the wide importance of this metal in metabolism (Table 8B–2). A number of pyridine nucleotide-dependent dehydrogenases from diverse sources and species have been characterized, which depend upon zinc for their activity and/or structural integrity. The detection of zinc in such enzymes which are critical for cellular oxidation may explain the high concentrations of this element in the liver. Alcohol dehydrogenase, which is present in liver as well as other organs, oxidizes ethanol and other primary and secondary alcohols as well as vitamin A alcohol and reduces retinene. Retinene reductase of the retina is apparently identical or very similar to this enzyme from liver. Horse liver alcohol dehydrogenase contains 4 atoms of zinc per molecule of protein and zinc is essential not only to the catalytic function of the enzyme, but also to maintain the subunit structure.[40,41] In addition to ethanol, alcohol dehydrogenase from *human* liver also oxidizes methanol and ethylene glycol, serving as the primary mechanism of detoxification of these and other similar compounds.[42] Thus far no other metals have been identified with certainty in similar dehydrogenases other than those listed in the table, although there is presumptive evidence

Table 8B-2.
Zinc Metalloenzymes and Metalloproteins

Enzyme	Source
Alcohol dehydrogenase	Yeast, equine and human liver
Lactate dehydrogenase	Rabbit muscle
D-Lactate-cytochrome c reductase	Yeast
Glyceraldehyde-3-phosphate dehydrogenase	Bovine and porcine muscle, yeast
Glutamate dehydrogenase	Bovine liver
Aldolase	Yeast, Aspergillus niger, E. coli
Carbonic anhydrase	Bovine, simian, human and porcine erythrocytes, rat prostate, shark, parsley
Alkaline phosphatase	E. coli, porcine kidney, human placenta and leukocytes
Procarboxypeptidase A and B	Bovine, porcine and Pacific spiny dogfish pancreas
Carboxypeptidase A and B	Bovine, porcine and Pacific spiny dogfish pancreas
Neutral protease	Bacillus subtilis, Bacillus megatherium, Aeromonas proteolyticum, Serratia
Thermolysin	Bacillus thermoproteolyticus
Leucine aminopeptidase	Porcine kidney
Pyruvate carboxylase	Yeast
Phosphomannose Isomerase	Yeast
AMP-aminohydrolase	Rabbit muscle
Dipeptidase	Porcine kidney, mouse ascites tumor cells
Aspartate transcarboxylase	E. coli
DNA-polymerase	E. coli, sea urchin
Proteinase	Cotton mouth or water moccasin
α-Macroglobulin	Human serum
Proteins Containing Both Zinc and Cadmium	
Metallothionein	Equine kidney and liver, human kidney and liver, rabbit liver
Metalloenzymes Containing Both Calcium and Zinc	
Amylase	B. subtilis
Metalloenzymes Containing Both Zinc and Manganese	
Superoxide dismutase	E. coli

that many other pyridine nucleotide-dependent dehydrogenases may contain metals.

Carbonic anhydrase which catalyzes the reaction $CO_2 + H_2O = H_2CO_3$ is present in erythrocytes in high concentrations and many tissues exhibit activity catalyzing this reaction. Without this enzyme carbon dioxide elimination cannot take place with sufficient -rapidity to sustain life and, hence, this enzyme is as important to carbon dioxide transport as is hemoglobin to oxygen transport. Carbonic anhydrases from ox, monkey and human erythrocytes all contain 1 gm atom of zinc per mole of enzyme, and correlations have been obtained between the zinc content and enzyme activity in red blood cells under both normal and pathologic conditions. Substitution of cobalt for zinc results in an enzymatically active carbonic anhydrase.[43]

Both carboxypeptidase A and B from pancreatic juice contain 1 atom of zinc per molecule of protein. The single zinc atom is indispensable for the catalytic activities of the enzymes which hydrolyze peptide bonds to liberate the amino acids from the carboxy-terminals of proteins and peptides. The zinc in carboxypeptidase A can be replaced *in vitro* by other metals, *e.g.*, Co, Mn, Ni, Fe, Cd, Hg, and Pb, with consequent dramatic alterations in catalytic activity and substrate specificity.[44] Both carboxypeptidase A and B are excreted into the gastrointestinal tract and are implicated in proteolysis and digestive processes.

The zinc atoms of alkaline phosphatase from E. coli appear to be essential for both catalytic function and subunit structure of the enzyme. A decrease in alkaline phosphatase activity has long been noted in zinc-deficient experimental animals, a change which may now be attributed to a failure of synthesis of the active holoenzyme. The alkaline phosphatase of leukocytes may well be identical with the zinc-containing protein of human leukocytes which contains 0.3 per cent of zinc per gm dry weight of protein, and is responsible for 80 per cent of all zinc found in human leukocytes.

In addition to the enzymes listed in Table 8B–2, there are many other enzymes whose activities are increased by the addition of zinc. This effect may not be specific since other metal ions also activate most of these systems. The zinc-activated metal-enzyme complexes include a number of dipeptidases and tripeptidases, carnosinase, histidine deaminase, enolase, dinucleotide pyrophosphatase, α-D-mannosidase, phosphoenolpyruvate carboxylase, pyridoxal kinase and others.[45]

In addition to the critical role of zinc in the mechanism of action of these many enzymes, this element may be associated with other important biologic systems. Zinc is firmly bound to RNA stabilizing secondary and tertiary structure, and thus relates to both protein and RNA metabolism. Indeed impaired synthesis of both protein and RNA has been observed in zinc-deficient microorganisms, particularly *Euglena gracilis* and *Mycobacterium smegmatis*. Consequently, growth is impaired, and the DNA content of the deficient organisms doubles as does also their cellular size. Amino acids and other organic acids, nucleotides and phosphates accumulate as a result of their inability to synthesize protein and RNA.[46] Similar features have also been reported in plants. In zinc-deficient animals, there is also impaired DNA synthesis and administration of zinc stimulates DNA synthesis as well as polyribosome formation.[47] Tumor growth in rats is inhibited by dietary zinc deficiency.

A relationship between zinc and porphyrins has long been known and the excretion of zinc complexes of uroporphyrin and coproporphyrin in urine has been described in human diseases such as porphyria. However, the significance of these compounds is uncertain since zinc porphyrins are known to form nonenzymatically. The enzymatic incorporation of zinc into porphyrins by an enzyme, zinc chelatase, present in chromatophores of *Rhodopseudomonas spheroides*[48] and also found in mammalian organs has recently been demonstrated. At present, however, there are no known biologically active zinc porphyrins.

A relationship of zinc to the action of insulin, glucagon, corticotropin and other hormones has been postulated. Despite much study and circumstantial evidence, however, a role for zinc in hormonal function has not been established with certainty. The crystallization of insulin at pH values near 6 may be accomplished only in the presence of zinc ions or other metals such as cadmium, cobalt or nickel. Two atoms of zinc associate with 6 molecules of insulin to form a hexamer of MW 36,000. Porcine proinsulin also reacts with zinc.[49] However, physiologically active insulin can be prepared in both amorphous and crystalline form, entirely free of zinc and other metals. Thus the physical-chemical association of zinc with insulin *in vitro* has not been shown to be a compositional or structural feature essential for function. It cannot be judged from available evidence whether an insulin-zinc complex forms *in vivo* and is necessary for biological activity.

Nutrition. On the basis of the current knowledge of the biochemical role of zinc in enzymatic processes and in protein and RNA synthesis, a model predicting the metabolic alterations and clinical manifestations to be expected owing to a zinc-deficiency state can be formulated. The salient features of such a model are shown in Table 8B-3, many of which have indeed been seen in experimental zinc deficiency in swine, lamb, rats, chicken, Japanese quail and other animals, as well as in man.

Table 8B-3. Manifestations of Zinc Deficiency Expected on the Basis of the Known Roles of the Element in Protein Formation and Metalloenzyme Function

Protein Synthesis	Metalloenzymes
Abnormal growth of hair and nails	Increased organic acids
Deformed bone formation	(*e.g.*, Components of TCA cycle)
Defective wound healing	Decreased ethanol tolerance
Decreased pancreatic enzyme synthesis	Decreased proteolysis
Decreased peptide hormone synthesis	Altered phosphate metabolism
Sterility	Imbalance between aerobic and anaerobic metabolism
Anemia	
Abnormal serum protein pattern	Acid-base imbalance
Increased amino acids	
Increased phosphates	
Increased uric acid	

Zinc deficiency in animals is characterized by failure to grow, anorexia, testicular atrophy, decreased size of the accessory sex glands and skin lesions. A decrease in food intake is an early sign of the deficiency state and force-feeding produces signs of ill health. Zinc supplementation promptly restores appetite. In rats hypoplasia of the coagulating and prostate glands, seminal vesicles and hypospermia occur, reversed by the administration of zinc. Testicular degeneration when it occurs is not reversible. Notably, cadmium also destroys testicular tissue when administered subcutaneously to rats, but when it is injected together with a large excess of zinc acetate testicular degeneration is prevented. This metal ion antagonism between cadmium and zinc is not limited to the testes, since zinc deficiency in chickens becomes more severe when cadmium is administered simultaneously and higher concentrations of zinc are required to overcome the deficiency state. Zinc-deficient rats characteristically develop hyperuricemia and the activities of pancreatic enzymes are decreased as are intestinal and kidney alkaline phosphatase activities. *In vitro* addition of zinc to homogenates of the intestine and kidney from zinc-deficient animals fully restores alkaline phosphatase activity.[50] Synthesis of the apoenzyme apparently is unimpaired, but enzyme activity is lacking due entirely to inadequate concentrations of zinc to form the active holoenzyme. Pancreatic carboxypeptidase activity has been shown to decrease quite specifically and rapidly in response to zinc deficiency and return to normal on repletion.[51] Changes in the activities of a number of dehydrogenases in the bone, kidney, intestine, esophagus and testes of zinc-deficient rats and swine have been noted.[52] Apparently these tissues are most sensitive to zinc depletion. Lowering of carbonic anhydrase activity is not usually encountered although there is slight anemia. The most striking histological finding in zinc-deficient rats is hyperkeratinization of the epidermis and parakeratosis of the esophagus, as is found also in other animal species.[53] This may relate in part to the strikingly abnormal sulfur metabolism which has been found to occur in zinc-deficient animals.[54]

Offsprings of rats made zinc deficient for even short periods of time during their pregnancy develop major congenital malformations involving the skeleton, brain, heart, eyes, gastrointestinal tract and lungs, emphasizing the importance of zinc to normal growth and development.[55] Fetal mortality is also increased. Abnormalities and decrease in plasma proteins have been reported in zinc-deficient rats, chicks, swine and the Japanese quail. Table 8B–4 summarizes and compares the chemical and enzymatic alterations which have been observed in zinc-deficient animals with those in plants and microorganisms.

In hogs zinc deficiency may occur spontaneously or be induced experimentally and is called porcine parakeratosis. This disease is characterized by dermatitis, diarrhea, vomiting, anorexia, severe weight loss and eventual death. The spontaneous disease has occurred in animals fed specialized diets and has been attributed to the practice of adding bone meal to the diet to accelerate growth and ossification. The experimental disease is aggravated by large amounts of dietary calcium, and, thus, parakeratosis in hogs is a conditioned zinc deficiency. The mechanism of the Ca-Zn antagonism is unknown. Supplements of zinc carbonate in the diets of hogs with either spontaneous or experimentally induced parakeratosis result in prompt recovery. A similar disease has been reported in cattle.

In recent years a syndrome of severe iron deficiency, anemia, hepatosplenomegaly, hypogonadism, hyperpigmentation and dwarfism in Iranian and Egyptian dwarfs has been attributed to primary zinc deficiency.[56] Geophagia is common in the Iranian dwarfs, and it was suggested that zinc deficiency may have resulted from excessive consumption of a cereal diet containing large amounts of phytate which inhibits iron and zinc absorption. A similar syndrome in Egyptian dwarfs studied in greater detail showed, in addition, evidence of primary pituitary hypofunction associated with reduced activities of gonadotrophic and growth hormones. Their plasma zinc content and that of their red blood cells and hair were decreased as was the 24-hour exchangeable zinc pool, while plasma turnover of zinc was increased. Sweat and urinary zinc excretion and serum alkaline phosphatase activity were decreased. Upon treatment with supplemental zinc salts a

Table 8B–4.   Chemical and Enzymatic Consequences of Zinc Deficiency in Different Phyla

	Chemical Composition		Enzymatic Activity
	Decrease	Increase	Decrease
Microorganisms	Protein RNA (ribosomal) Pyridine nucleotides	DNA Amino acids Polyphosphates Phospholipids ATP Organic acids	Alkaline phosphatase Alcohol dehydrogenase D-Lactate dehydrogenase Tryptophan desmolase
Plants	Protein Auxin Ethanolamine	Amino acids	Tryptophan desmolase Carbonic anhydrase Aldolase Pyruvic carboxylase
Animals	Red blood cells serum proteins	Uric acid	Alkaline phosphatase Pancreatic proteases Malate dehydrogenase Lactic dehydrogenase NADH diaphorase Alcohol dehydrogenase Carboxypeptidase A

striking response in growth and development and of secondary sex characteristics was observed, exceeding that seen on treatment with a balanced diet alone. Serum zinc concentrations rose to normal. The anemia which was attributed to the concomitant iron deficiency of these patients due to parasitic infestations was not reversed by the administration of zinc. The zinc-deficiency syndrome is now being recognized, particularly in young individuals with intestinal malabsorption of prolonged duration during their adolescence.[57,58]

Zinc in Human Disease States. Serum zinc concentrations are decreased below the range of normal values in acute and chronic infections such as pneumonia, bronchitis, erysipelas and pyelonephritis and are restored upon recovery. They are decreased in untreated pernicious anemia and reversed by vitamin B_{12} therapy. Serum zinc concentrations are also decreased in myocardial infarction and accompany the well-known changes in a variety of enzyme activities and increase in the copper concentration of serum. Decreased serum zinc values have also been reported in various malignancies, although a uniform pattern is not discernible. This has also been seen in kwashiorkor, nephrosis, uremia, intestinal malabsorption, and in Laennec's cirrhosis. Increase in leukocyte zinc has been observed in patients with refractory anemia accompanied by leukopenia, while the zinc concentration of leukocytes in acute and chronic lymphatic and myelogenous leukemia is decreased to 10 per cent of the normal value. This phenomenon is apparently independent of the maturity of the cells but may be related to the decreased leukocyte alkaline phosphatase activities in some of these conditions. Excessive zinc excretion has been noted in leukemia and Hodgkin's disease though no cause is immediately apparent. The zinc content and carbonic anhydrase activity of red cells parallel each other and are significantly correlated in normal individuals as well as in those afflicted with anemia, polycythemia vera, secondary polycythemia, leukemia and congestive failure. Both parameters vary directly with the hematocrit level and the hemoglobin concentration. In untreated pernicious anemia, how-

ever, the erythrocyte zinc concentration and carbonic anhydrase activity are close to normal though the hematocrit, erythrocyte count and hemoglobin levels are markedly decreased. The mean corpuscular zinc concentration and carbonic anhydrase activity are increased several times more than the high mean corpuscular hemoglobin and out of proportion to the increase in cell size. Upon remission zinc concentration and carbonic anhydrase activities return to normal values. Zinc has also been noted to promote wound healing both in man and in animals.[59]

Zinc and Post-alcoholic Cirrhosis. The discovery of zinc in such mammalian enzymes as liver alcohol dehydrogenase and glutamic dehydrogenase stimulated the study of zinc metabolism in human liver disease. Marked abnormalities in the metabolism of this metal were found to occur in post-alcoholic cirrhosis.[36] The concentration of zinc in the serum of patients with a severe degree of this disease was decreased to 66 ± 19 μg per 100 ml as compared to the normal of 121 ± 19 μg per 100 ml. Greatest depressions were noted in patients in hepatic coma and concentrations of less than 30 μg per 100 ml signified an ominous prognosis. Among tests on liver function the zinc data correlated best with studies of BSP retention. Analyses of liver tissue from patients who died of post-alcoholic cirrhosis revealed only half the normal content of zinc and iron, while calcium, magnesium, aluminum, manganese and copper concentrations were normal. Significantly, patients with post-alcoholic cirrhosis excreted abnormally large quantities of zinc in their urine, 1000 ± 200 μg per 24 hours. Administration of zinc sulfate in physiologic quantities to such patients tended to restore the normal excretory pattern in urine. A tendency toward restoration of normal liver function was often noted.[60] Apparently a conditioned zinc deficiency may be a feature of post-alcoholic cirrhosis in man. It has been suggested that the low serum zinc concentration in cirrhosis may reflect a change in the synthesis, degradation, metal content, or specific activity of the zinc-containing dehydrogenases which are cardinally involved in intermediary carbohydrate and protein metabolism. It cannot be stated, however, whether these abnormalities of zinc metabolism constitute primary or secondary manifestations of the disease though they emphasize the significance of the metal to this nosologic entity. Human liver alcohol dehydrogenase has recently been isolated and identified as a zinc metalloenzyme.[61] Studies of this protein in patients with post-alcoholic cirrhosis should be of special interest in furthering understanding of the subcellular pathology and etiology of this disease.

Zinc Toxicity. Compared to copper, lead, mercury and arsenic, zinc is relatively nontoxic. However, *inhalation* of zinc oxide fumes in high concentration, as may occur in industrial settings, produces an acute illness of relatively short duration characterized by chills, fever, cough, salivation, headache, leukocytosis and pulmonary infiltrates. Constant exposure produces tolerance, but intermittent exposure results in recurrence of the illness.

Poisoning due to *ingestion* of zinc may occur when foods have been stored in galvanized containers. Signs and symptoms of toxicity are nausea, vomiting, abdominal cramps, diarrhea and fever. In experimental animals, feeding of massive doses of zinc produces anemia, retarded growth and eventual death.

MANGANESE

A considerable amount of evidence has accumulated that manganese is essential in animal nutrition.[62,63] Although its essentiality for man has never been demonstrated clearly, functions similar to those in other mammals are assumed.

Physiology and Metabolism. Manganese is widely distributed in mammalian tissues, the highest concentrations (about 2 to 3 μg per gm) occurring in bone, pituitary, liver, pineal, and lactating mammary glands and the lowest in lung, connective tissue and muscle. The total manganese content of an adult human has been estimated to be about 20 mg, and the concentrations in individual organs tend to remain relatively constant throughout life. Within cells, manganese is located both in the nucleus and in cytoplasmic organelles. The turnover rate and concentration are relatively high in mito-chondria and relatively low in the nucleus. Injected ^{56}Mn tends to localize preferentially in liver and pancreatic tissues and in cytoplasm rather than in nuclei.

Like iron, manganese is absorbed rather poorly from the intestinal tract. High dietary concentrations of calcium and phosphorus decrease absorption but information about the factors that control assimilation from foods is meager. It is presumably transported in plasma by binding to a β-1 globulin designated "transmanganin." It is not entirely clear, however, that transmanganin differs from transferrin since the latter protein has been shown to bind manganese and copper as well as iron. In normal persons the plasma concentration is about 2.5 μg per 100 ml, distributed approximately equally between cells and plasma. Manganese is excreted largely via the intestinal tract with much of it excreted in the bile and pancreatic juice. Urinary excretion is very small. It has been reported that estrogen increases the concentration of manganese in serum, and glucocorticoids alter its body distribution.[63,67]

The average daily intake of manganese in adult man has been estimated to be 3 to 9 mg; about 40 per cent is absorbed. Children presumably require at least 200 μg per kg of body weight. The element is widely distributed in foodstuffs, particularly in wheat germs, seeds, nuts, leafy vegetables, and meat. Animal tissues, seafoods, poultry and dairy products are relatively poor sources of manganese. A nutritional requirement for manganese has not been demonstrated in man.

Biochemistry. Manganese has been shown to activate a large number of metal-enzyme complexes involving transferase, hydrolase, lyase, isomerase, and ligase reactions. This effect is not specific since other metals, in particular magnesium, may substitute for manganese in most instances.[45] Arginase, cysteine desulfhydrase, prolinase, thiaminase, dipeptidases, phosphoglucomutase, glucokinase, leucine aminopeptidase, isocitric dehydrogenase, carnosinase, glutamine synthetase, acetyl CoA synthetase, and enolase are examples. Fully active arginase binds 4 atoms of manganese per molecule of enzyme. Two of the manganese atoms are bound strongly and cannot be removed without significant protein denaturation. Manganese is required for the enzymatic incorporation of xylose and galactose[64] into glycoproteins. These sugars are present in the mucopolysaccharides, heparin, chondroitin sulfate and dermatan sulfate, which are joined to the protein by a xylosyl-serine bond. Manganese, present in high concentrations in melanocytes, also appears to participate in the final auto-oxidation of melanin granules.

The biotin-dependent *pyruvate carboxylase* of chicken liver was the first manganese metalloenzyme to have been identified; it contains 4 gm atoms of manganese per mole of protein.[65] More recently, a superoxide dismutase from E. coli has been identified as a manganese enzyme containing 2 atoms of manganese and two atoms of zinc per molecule.[66] L-arabinose isomerase, a manganese-dependent enzyme from Lactobacillus gayonii, has been reported to be specific for this metal, and hence may be another manganese metalloenzyme.

Manganese also replaces the native zinc atoms of carboxypeptidase A of bovine pancreas and the neutral protease of B. subtilis, giving rise to enzymatically active products. In addition to chromium, nickel and other metals, manganese has been found to be firmly associated with ribonucleic acids isolated from diverse sources, presumably serving a role as an important determinant of the native structure.[11] It may also function in protein synthesis by stimulating RNA polymerase activity. A manganese porphyrin in the erythrocytes of man, rabbits, and birds has been reported.[67] Manganese ions have been postulated to play a role in oxidative phosphorylation and in the metabolism of fatty acids and cholesterol synthesis.

Nutrition. In both mammals and birds, manganese deficiency is characterized by defective growth, bone abnormalities, reproductive dysfunction, central nervous system manifestations, in particular ataxia, and disturbances in lipid metabolism.[1,63] Manganese deficiency has been induced in rats, mice, rabbits, pigs, and in cattle. Liver arginase activity and manganese concentration are reduced in manganese-deficient rabbits. Manganese-deficient guinea pigs exhibit impaired glucose tolerance and de-

creased granulation of the beta cells of the pancreatic islets. In rats, manganese is essential for lactation, and maternal manganese deficiency results in abnormal otic labyrinth development in the offspring. In this regard, there exists an interesting relationship between manganese and a genetic disease of rats (pallid strain). Pallid rats have an inherited defect in the formation of otoliths and lack postural orientation when blindfolded or placed in water. Feeding pregnant pallid rats manganese will prevent the phenotypic expression of this disease in their offspring.[68] Birds develop spontaneous manganese deficiency of two forms: *chondrodystrophy*, characterized by defective growth, edema and generalized bone disease occurring in embryonic life and associated with a high mortality, and *perosis*, evidenced by shortening and thickening of the bones, accompanied by slipping of the epiphyses and of the Achilles tendon, occurring in post-embryonic life. The biochemical mechanisms in which manganese is involved for proper osteogenesis are unknown but do not appear to relate to its calcification. Skeletal maturation is retarded due to a depression or suppression of endochondral bone growth at the epiphyseal cartilages, including matrix formation and cell proliferation. A reduction in mucopolysaccharide and hexosamine content of the epiphyseal cartilage occurs,[69,70] and the galactotransferase enzyme activity of cartilage is decreased.[71] The cartilage of newborn manganese-deficient guinea pigs, which exhibit widespread skeletal defects, has a decreased content of hyaluronic acid, chondroitin sulfate and heparin.[72] Bone and blood phosphatase activities are lowered. In addition to perosis and chondrodystrophy, deficient chicks frequently exhibit neurologic symptoms, particularly ataxia. Susceptibility to manganese deficiency in chickens appears to be genetically controlled and is aggravated by a diet high in calcium, phosphorus or ferrous citrate. In borderline cases the deficiency is improved or prevented entirely by the additional intake of inositol or choline.

Deficiency states attributable specifically to manganese have not been identified in humans and no human diseases have been proved to be causally related. On the basis of the protective effects of manganese against chronic hydralazine poisoning in animals, it has been suggested that lupus erythematosus and the "hydralazine syndrome" in man may be related to manganese deficiency.[73] The possible interrelations between manganese metabolism and aspects of certain diseases and their therapy, in particular the extra-pyramidal syndromes, have been considered.[63,67]

Toxicology. Chronic manganese poisoning occurs primarily in miners who inhale large quantities of manganese dust over prolonged periods. The disease is characterized by an encephalitis-like picture with manifestations of extrapyramidal disease. In mild cases, symptoms are reversed by withdrawal from exposure or treatment with disodium dicalcium ethylene diamine tetraacetate.[74] Increased concentrations of the metal are found particularly in the lung. Pulmonary changes similar to pneumoconiosis may occur. Clinical changes begin insidiously with asthenia, anorexia, apathy, headache, impotence, leg cramps and speech disturbances. Eventually, the syndrome simulates a progressive hepatolenticular degeneration and in some aspects resembles Parkinson's disease. Facial expression is mask-like, the voice monotonous, and intention tremor, muscle rigidity and spastic gait appear. Tendon reflexes are exaggerated and clonus may develop.

Ingestion of potassium permanganate results in acute poisoning. A strong oxidizing agent, it causes irritation and necrosis of gastric mucosa, hemolytic jaundice and capillary damage. Protracted ingestion of large amounts of manganese results in elevated concentrations in the liver, but no other ill effects, such as extrapyramidal symptoms, develop.

COBALT

Cobalt serves its paramount, known biologic function as a component of vitamin B_{12}. The biochemistry, physiology, nutrition and metabolism of this vitamin are discussed in Chapter 5 Section J. Hence, this section will concern other aspects of the biochemical and nutritional role of this element, which, however, are still closely related to vitamin B_{12} in some instances. The chemistry and biochem-

istry of vitamin B_{12} and related corrinoids have been reviewed recently.[75] Cobalt is widely distributed in nature, prompting a search for other biologic functions. The first non-vitamin B_{12} cobalt enzyme, the biotin-dependent oxalacetate transcarboxylase containing about 2 atoms of cobalt and 4 of zinc per molecule, has been isolated very recently from Proprionbacterium shermanii.[76] Experimentally, cobalt can replace zinc in a number of zinc enzymes, *e.g.*, carboxypeptidase A and B, bovine, human and monkey carbonic anhydrases, the neutral protease of B. subtilis and horse liver alcohol dehydrogenase, resulting in active enzymes whose catalytic functions are modified in characteristic fashion. Cobalt activates a number of enzymes, among them a variety of phosphotransferases and lyases although these are active in the complete absence of metals or in the presence of other metals.[45] In pharmacologic doses cobalt stimulates erythropoiesis.

Metabolism. The synthesis of vitamin B_{12} by bacteria requires cobalt. In ruminants this occurs in the proximal portion of the intestine from which the vitamin is then absorbed. The total ingestion of 0.07 to 0.08 mg of cobalt per day is sufficient for the bacterial synthesis of the vitamin required by sheep, and probably by cattle as well.[1] In other animals and man, however, where bacterial formation of vitamin B_{12} takes place only in the colon, absorption is minimal. Therefore, to be of nutritional value for the human, cobalt must be ingested or injected as vitamin B_{12}. Humans obtain their requirement of this nutrient largely from animal tissues. If man has a need for cobalt other than vitamin B_{12}, the requirement is unknown, although about 0.1 μg of cobalt per day would be sufficient to supply the amount needed to synthesize an adequate amount of vitamin B_{12}. The normal diet supplies about 5 to 8 μg per day.[77]

In view of the small quantities of cobalt present in tissues and body fluids, its quantification has been a major problem and much of the analytical data on record is of dubious value. In animals, orally absorbed or intravenously administered cobalt is excreted primarily in the urine. The greater part of ingested cobalt is not absorbed and is excreted in the stool; the fraction retained is concentrated mostly in the liver and kidneys, which contains about 0.2 parts per million based on the dry weight of the organs. The mode of storage, however, is uncertain. The cobalt concentration of human plasma is about 60 to 80 $\mu\mu$g per ml and that of whole blood 80 to 300 $\mu\mu$g per ml. Its estimation by bio-assay as part of vitamin B_{12} has become a clinical test, since the determination of cobalt itself at these concentrations is difficult.

Nutrition. Cobalt deficiency in ruminants, variously called enzootic marasmus, pine or bush sickness in essence is a vitamin B_{12} deficiency, which manifests by impaired growth, listlessness, anorexia, progressive emaciation and varying degrees of anemia.[1,77] The livers of affected animals are deficient in cobalt but contain excessive amounts of iron. Feeding of cobalt both prevents and cures it, but injected cobalt is ineffective. Therapeutic response to liver extract or vitamin B_{12} in amounts comparable to those used for treatment of pernicious anemia in man has been disappointing. About 300 μg of vitamin B_{12} per week is the dose required to alleviate the symptoms. Ruminants apparently have a much higher requirement for the vitamin than do man and other animals. High concentrations of molybdenum in the forage interferes with and may actually arrest the synthesis of vitamin B_{12} in the rumen of cattle, presumably because of its effect on the metabolism of the microorganisms in the rumen.

The Erythropoietic Stimulating Effect of Cobalt. Administration of pharmacologic amounts of cobalt, either orally or parenterally, will induce polycythemia in rats, mice, guinea pigs, rabbits, dogs, pigs, chickens, ducks, hogs and man. The development of polycythemia is apparently independent of other metals but is inhibited or prevented by cystine, methionine, cysteine, histidine, choline, nicotinamide and ascorbic acid. Reticulocytosis, elevated erythrocyte and hemoglobin levels, increased total red blood cell mass and normoblastic hyperplasia in the marrow occur. This effect is not mediated through vitamin B_{12}. Cobalt may induce polycythemia by increasing the formation or

inhibiting the destruction of erythropoietin, the erythropoietic stimulating hormone secreted primarily by the kidney,[78] but it does so in pharmacologic, not physiologic, doses. There is as yet no evidence that cobalt is a part of erythropoietin, a glycoprotein, or that it is essential to the maintenance of a normal concentration of the hormone under physiologic conditions. Cobalt administration apparently also increases iron absorption as well as globin synthesis. The value of cobalt therapy of human anemias has been studied extensively[79] but is beyond the scope of this chapter.

Toxicity. Congestive heart failure due to cardiomyopathy has been reported in individuals who consumed large quantities of beer which had 1.2 ppm of cobalt, added during processing as a foam stabilizer. In addition, the afflicted individuals developed polycythemia, pericardial effusion, thyroid hyperplasia, and neurological abnormalities. On autopsy, the heart contained 10 times the normal amount of cobalt, and showed vacuolar degeneration of the muscle and degenerative changes in the myofilaments, mitochondria and sarcoplasmic reticulum. In experimentally induced cobalt cardiomyopathy, the metabolism of pyruvate and fatty acids is impaired. Cobalt is known to bind to lipoic acid and may perhaps interfere with critical decarboxylation reactions in this manner.[80] The anatomic and metabolic changes induced by cobalt in myocardium, however, are not specific and the toxic effects of cobalt and ethanol may be synergistic in beer-drinkers' cardiomyopathy.

SELENIUM

The physical and chemical properties of selenium closely resemble those of sulfur. Information about the metabolism of selenium is fragmentary and little is known about its participation in biochemical reactions.[81] However, within the last decade, selenium has been recognized to be an essential nutrient element in certain species, and its metabolism appears to differ in some aspects from that of sulfur.[82] It prevents dietary liver necrosis in the rat and pig, a fatal exudative diathesis in chicks and turkeys, nutritional muscular dystrophy in lambs, calves and chicks and multiple necrotic degeneration of heart, liver, muscle, and kidney in the mouse.[1,83,84]

These diseases result from diets multiply deficient in vitamin E and selenium. In other studies selenium by itself has been shown to be required for the optimal growth of chicks. Chicks fed a diet deficient in selenium alone also show poor feathering and atrophy of the pancreas. The latter lesion leads to impaired absorption of fats as well as of vitamin E, and serum vitamin E concentrations of these chicks become abnormally low.[85] A recent report has shown that children with kwashiorkor have decreased selenium stores, suggesting that human selenium deficiency may occur with protein-calorie malnutrition.[86]

Present evidence indicates that the metabolically active form of selenium may be combined with a specific organic substance (Factor 3) possessing several times the potency of inorganic and other known organic selenium compounds. Sodium selenite, selenium-containing amino acids, and several other selenium compounds may replace Factor 3 at slightly higher concentrations in the diet. Monoselenocarboxylic acids have been reported to be very potent.[87] Sodium selenite is 500 times more effective in treating the deficiency disease states than is vitamin E which, when given alone, is not entirely or consistently effective. However, selenium cannot replace all the functions of vitamin E and the relationship of selenium to vitamin E remains to be elucidated. Organic selenium compounds have been noted to inhibit lipid peroxidation, and in this manner it is similar to and may replace some of the functions of vitamin E.

The highest concentrations of selenium are found in liver, kidney, heart and spleen. There are about 0.22 μg of selenium per ml of blood in man. It is excreted in the urine. Absorption seems to depend on the solubility of the selenium compound ingested and on the dietary ratio of selenium to sulfur. At least part of selenium toxicity may be due to the interference with absorption by sulfur, e.g., selenate with sulfate and seleno-amino acids with the sulfur-containing amino acids. Once absorbed, selenium is deposited in various amounts in all tissues of the body, except fat. In ruminants, a large percentage of the ingested selenium is incorporated by the bacteria of the rumen into seleno-analogs of cysteine and methionine which are absorbed and deposited in tissues as seleno-amino acids and then incorporated into proteins.[88] Selenium has been found in many highly purified proteins, e.g., aldolase, cytochrome c, hemoglobin, myoglobin, myosin and ribonucleoproteins.[89] Even in nonruminants much of the ingested selenium is incorporated in body tissues as selenocysteine and selenomethionine.

The precise biochemical function of selenium and seleno-organic compounds is still poorly understood. They have been regarded as cofactors at specific sites of intermediary metabolism, while others have ascribed to them a more nonspecific function as biologic antoxidants. Dietary supplementation with either vitamin E or selenium compounds prevents "respiratory decline" in liver slices, a metabolic phenomenon characteristic of incipient liver necrosis. In this regard, vitamin E is more effective and it would appear that this vitamin and selenium function at different stages in the oxidation of α-ketoglutarate to succinate. It has been suggested that selenium is involved in the first step of the reaction sequence, i.e., the decarboxylation of α-ketoglutarate, since, by analogy, selenium-selnite is a potent inorganic catalyst for the dehydration of carbonic acid, whereas vitamin E functions in the succeeding step involving lipoyl dehydrogenase.[90] Like vitamin E, selenium and selenium-containing amino acids are potent inhibitors of lipid peroxidation. They also decompose hydrogen peroxide and scavenge free radicals, protecting against radiation damage. Thus, they may function in maintaining the stability of biologic membranes of structures such as mitochondria, microsomes and lysosomes.[91]

Toxic amounts may act as antagonists of sulfur metabolism and are known to inhibit certain enzymes, such as succinic dehydrogenase, urease, choline oxidase, tyramine oxidase and proline oxidase. The element also adversely affects embryonic development: it inhibits mitosis at metaphase, and bone and cartilage develop abnormally.[84]

Selenium poisoning occurs in animals grazing on alkali (high salt) pastures.[1,84] The acute toxicity syndrome, "blind staggers," is characterized by blindness, abdominal pain, salivation, muscle paralysis and death from respiratory failure. Chronic toxicity, "alkali disease," produces dullness and roughness of coat, loss of hair, sore hoofs, erosion of the joints of long bones, cardiac atrophy, cirrhosis of the liver and anemia in cattle. Some of these signs may be attributed to the replacement of cystine by selenocystine in keratin. Poisoning occurs owing to the ingestion of certain plant species which accumulate selenium from the soil. A diet high in protein affords some protection, as does sulfate. More importantly, arsenic given at low levels of 5 parts per million in the drinking water prevents selenosis. The mechanism of its action is not known. However, there is no evidence that humans living in seleniferous areas develop symptoms attributable to selenium intoxication, although their urinary excretion of the element is above normal levels.

CHROMIUM

In recent years evidence has been adduced that chromium may have an important role in the carbohydrate and lipid metabolism of animals and their utilization of glucose. Thus far its involvement in glucose metabolism and insulin action has been explored most extensively in rats.[92] Deficiency syndromes have also been produced in mice and squirrel monkeys.

The amount of chromium present in animal tissues is not well defined, largely owing to difficulties in analysis. Concentrations ranging between ten and several hundred parts per billion have been reported. This discrepancy may be partly methodologic and also may reflect geographic variation. The total body content of chromium is low, less than 6 mg. Highest concentrations are found in skin, fat, adrenal glands, brain and muscle. Geographic variations are large, and a progressive decline in tissue concentrations with age has been reported in the United States.[93]

Knowledge of the metabolic movements of chromium is sparse. Only a few per cent of ingested chromium is absorbed. It is excreted mainly by way of the kidney. Trivalent chromium is bound to transferrin in serum, whereas hexavalent chromium has a selective affinity for red blood cells. These properties have enabled the use of radioactive chromium isotopes for the study of mass and turnover of erythrocytes and plasma proteins. Neither the oxidation state nor the physiologic function of chromium in tissues is known at present.

In vitro chromium has been found to react with biologic macromolecules and enzymes similar to other transition elements. Its use for the tanning of skins is well known. Chromium has been found associated with RNA isolated from many different species, together with Ni, Fe, Mn and other elements. It activates several enzymes, including the succinate-cytochrome dehydrogenase system and phosphoglucomutase and has been noted to stimulate fatty acid and cholesterol synthesis.[94]

The effect of trivalent chromium in reversing a diet-induced mild glucose intolerance in rats was discovered in 1959. Rats raised on a Torula-yeast diet developed a mild impairment of glucose utilization as measured by intravenous glucose tolerance testing. When given trivalent chromium in amounts not much above the estimated daily intake, glucose tolerance returned to the normal range within 24 hours, whereas 40 other elements were ineffective.[95] When great care was taken to minimize extraneous metal contamination, rats eventually developed more severe symptoms of chromium deficiency. Depression of growth rates, severe impairment of glucose metabolism approaching frank diabetes and increased incidence of atheromatous lesions in the aorta were observed.[92] Corneal opacification has been noted to develop in rats fed a diet low in both protein and chromium, but not in protein alone.[93]

The mode of action of trivalent chromium in regulating glucose metabolism has been studied, using chromium-deficient epididymal adipose tissue. Chromium itself does not stimulate the incorporation of glucose into lipids and CO_2, but it enhances the stimulatory effects of insulin.[96] It has been suggested that, among other factors, chromium facilitates the binding of insulin to cell membranes by forming a "bridge" between the insulin molecule and the membrane.[92] The concentration range within which chromium is stimulatory is very narrow and excess amounts of chromium depress insulin activity.

The above findings have naturally raised the question whether chromium metabolism is related to diabetes. To date, the evidence correlating impaired chromium metabolism with glucose intolerance in man is still incomplete. However, in certain instances, chromium supplementation of maturity-onset diabetic patients improves glucose utilization.[97,98] Improvement of glucose tolerance in some children with kwashiorkor has also been reported.[99] While such studies may serve to further document the functional role of trace metals in metabolism and biochemical pathways, the effect of chromium can be expected to alter only one aspect of the many facets of this complex disease On the basis of current data, it appears that the biologically active form of chromium may potentiate insulin action, but it is not a hypoglycemic agent *per se*.

MOLYBDENUM

Molybdenum began to attract attention as a trace element of nutritional importance when it was demonstrated some 30 or 40 years ago that the growth of azotobacter was increased several times by the addition of minute amounts of molybdate, if gaseous nitrogen served as the only source of nitrogen. Subsequent work showed that traces of molybdenum are present in all plants and animal tissues. The functional significance of molybdenum in normal animal metabolism gained credence when the addition of molybdenum to the diet of rats increased the xanthine oxidase activity of tissues.[100] Subsequently the element was found to be a constituent of various flavin-dependent enzymes, *e.g.*, xanthine and aldehyde oxidases in animal tissues and hydrogenase and nitrate reductases in plant tissues. However, an unequivocal requirement of molybdenum for the growth and maintenance of normal life cycles of experimental animals remains to be demonstrated. While great strides in the biochemistry of this element have been made, no

syndrome characteristic of molybdenum deficiency has been recognized in animals.[101] Similarly its nutritional role is uncertain. The subsequent discussion will emphasize the rather impressive biochemical evidence for a presumed nutritional role.

Animal tissues contain small amounts of molybdenum, 0.1 to 3 parts per million, based on the dry weight of tissues.[1,101] The largest amounts are found in the liver, kidney, bone and skin. It is absorbed readily from the intestinal tract and is excreted rapidly in the urine. A small amount is also excreted in bile. Especially in liver, kidney and bone, the concentrations of tissue molybdenum can be increased or decreased by raising or lowering dietary intake. Diets deficient in molybdenum decrease the intestinal and liver xanthine oxidase activities which can be corrected by additions of small amounts of molybdate to the diet. Increase in dietary sulfate and copper is accompanied by an increase in urinary excretion of molybdenum and its depletion in blood and tissues.

The chemical forms in which molybdenum exists in tissues have not yet been proven unequivocally, though it seems probable that, during oxidation and reduction, molybdenum cycles between Mo(V) and Mo(VI).[102] At least part is bound to the various molybdoproteins. The protein donor groups which bind molybdenum are also uncertain, though the weight of evidence at present favors binding to sulfur. Xanthine oxidases from milk and animal tissues catalyze the oxidation of a number of substrates, among which are purines, aldehydes, pteridines, DPNH, certain pyrimidines and other heterocyclic compounds. They contain both molybdenum and iron as well as the flavin coenzyme, FAD.[103] Present evidence indicates the presence of 2 molecules of FAD, 2 atoms of molybdenum and 8 atoms of iron per molecule of highly purified preparations of xanthine oxidase of milk. Xanthine oxidase from mammalian livers also contains 4 gm atoms of iron and 1 gm atom of molybdenum per mole of FAD but that from bird livers contains 8 gm atoms of molybdenum per mole of bound FAD. Aldehyde oxidase from mammalian liver in addition contains 1 to 2 moles of coenzyme Q_{10}. The iron in these enzymes appears to be associated with a stoichiometric quantity of acid-labile sulfur such as is found in the ferredoxins. These enzymes therefore are complex metalloflavoproteins containing at least two metals, *i.e.*, iron and molybdenum, which are necessary for their catalytic activity; whether the metals are required solely for electron transport or whether they participate in maintaining the structural integrity of the enzymes as well is poorly understood. It is generally agreed that, in oxidation-reduction, hydrogen from the donor is transferred sequentially to the oxygen acceptor through Mo, FAD and Fe.[102] Recently, a molybdohemeprotein, sulfite oxidase, has been isolated from bovine liver.[104] This enzyme catalyzes the oxidation of sulfite to sulfate. Its physiologic importance is emphasized by the recognition in a child of the lack of hepatic sulfite oxidase activity. In this instance, the urine contained sulfite and thiosulfate and severe pathophysiological sequelae were fatal.[105]

Molybdenum is also essential for nitrogen fixation of leguminous plants and for the biologic conversion of nitrate to ammonia or amino acids by fungi and higher plants, as well as other processes in plant metabolism.[102] Nitrate reductase isolated from plants and bacteria contains FAD, heme and molybdenum, but their stoichiometric relationship has not been defined. Recently, molybdoferredoxins from Azotobacter vinelandii and Clostridium pasteurianum have been purified. They contain Mo, Fe and acid-labile sulfur and are required for the ATP-dependent reductive assimilation of nitrogen.[106] Molybdoferredoxin is a component of the nitrogenase enzyme complex, which also contains ferredoxin.[107]

The nearest approximation to an induced deficiency state has been produced by feeding tungsten, a specific inhibitor of molybdenum, to chickens.[108] This results in depletion of tissue xanthine oxidase, increased excretion of xanthine and hypoxanthine, decreased excretion of uric acid, growth retardation and death. These effects can be overcome by the administration of sufficient amounts of molybdenum. A growth-promoting effect of molybdenum in the growing lamb has been reported. A stimulating effect on cellulose-

degrading microorganisms was suggested as the mechanism, with subsequent increase in ruminal cellulose degradation.

Chronic ingestion of excess amounts of molybdenum produces a disease state called "teart" in several animal species. Its interrelationship with copper and sulfate in nutrition has been the subject of intensive investigation (*vide supra*).

CADMIUM

Minute concentrations of cadmium have been found in tissues and fluids of most animals but no biologic function for this element has as yet been demonstrated.[1] The isolation and characterization of a cadmium-containing protein from horse, rabbit and human kidneys demonstrate that this element can be a normal constituent of biologic matter, rather than a contaminant.[109] These findings have awakened interest in the possible biochemical and physiologic role of the element, since the specific association of an element with a native biologic macromolecule represents an important first step toward the eventual definition of its biologic function.

Metabolism. In most animal tissues cadmium concentrations are of the order of less than 1 μg per gm wet tissue. The total body concentration of cadmium in man increases with age and varies in different areas of the world.[6] The cadmium content of the liver and the kidney is significantly higher than that of other tissues. Equine and human kidneys may contain amounts varying from 10 to 100 μg per gm wet weight.

Recent studies suggest that both in liver and in kidney cadmium is bound specifically to metallothionein.[110] The protein has not as yet been identified in other tissues. Cadmium localizes predominantly in the renal cortex, in regions corresponding to the proximal tubules. Deposits in the glomeruli or blood vessels have not been detected.

There is no conclusive evidence for a physiologic regulation of cadmium absorption or excretion. The element is absorbed poorly from the gastrointestinal tract and is excreted slowly. In dogs the total excretion of injected cadmium proceeds at a rate equivalent to a half-life of approximately 1 year and mainly through the intestinal tract. In man the average daily net uptake of cadmium is between 15 and 35 μg and urinary excretion is approximately 10 μg per liter.[111]

The physiologic function of cadmium is unknown. It has been suggested that cadmium is a toxic element and an etiologic factor in essential hypertension.[112] Cadmium given orally or parenterally to rats induces hypertension, reversed by chelating agents,[113] but in other animal species the effect may be hypotension.[114] Analyses of kidney cortex containing the major fraction of the renal cadmium content do not reveal large differences between normal material and that obtained from individuals succumbing from hypertension or a variety of renal disorders, but the ratio of cadmium to zinc appears higher in the hypertensive group. However, it is significant to note that there is *no* increased incidence of essential hypertension in patients suffering from chronic cadmium poisoning.[115] Hence, evidence that cadmium exposure may lead to hypertension in man is largely inferential, and experimental proof is lacking.

Biochemistry. Cadmium is specifically associated with a protein of molecular weight close to 10,000, first isolated from horse kidney cortex and named metallothionein.[116] It represents 1 to 2 per cent of the total weight of soluble proteins in horse renal cortex. Electrophoretically and ultracentrifugally homogeneous preparations contain as much as 5.9 per cent cadmium, 2.2 per cent zinc, and 9 per cent sulfur. Cadmium and zinc compete for the same binding sites and may be isomorphic in metallothionein. Most of the sulfur is accounted for by cysteine which constitutes 30 per cent of the amino acids in the protein, and one atom of cadmium or zinc is apparently bound to three sulfhydryl groups. The unique physical and chemical properties of this protein suggest a distinctive physiologic and biochemical role in homeostatic mechanisms, *e.g.*, in catalysis, storage, transport, immune phenomena or detoxification, although efforts to identify its biologic function have not been successful thus far. Similar proteins have also been isolated from human and rabbit kidneys and from the livers of horses and cadmium-exposed rabbits.[117,118]

It is of interest that substantial quantities of mercury were found in metallothionein, displacing cadmium and zinc, when it was isolated from kidneys of patients who had received mercurial diuretics.

Cadmium activates a considerable number of enzymes among them carnosinase, arginase, histidase, tryptophan oxygenase and formylglutamic acid deformylase. This action is not specific, since several of these enzymes are also activated by other metals. Cadmium can replace the native zinc atom of carboxypeptidases A and B, resulting in a change of the substrate specificity of these enzymes.

Toxicity. Pulmonary emphysema occurring in workers manufacturing alkaline accumulators and castings of copper-cadmium alloys has been described, a syndrome thought to be due to chronic long-term exposure to cadmium.[119] Proteinuria occurs in about 80 per cent of the individuals exposed in this manner for 8 years and more, and aminoaciduria especially of serine and threonine is frequent. Renal damage ranges from mild and scattered tubular degeneration to severe tubular and glomerular lesions. Anemia has also been described in some cases of human cadmium toxicity. The livers and kidneys of these patients accumulate 10 to 100 times more cadmium than that found in the organs of healthy unexposed individuals. These high tissue cadmium concentrations remain for many years after cessation of exposure, indicating that excretion is slow. However, death usually results from progressive pulmonary decompensation rather than from kidney damage.

Recently a syndrome of osteomalacia and nephropathy (Ouch-Ouch disease or Itai-Itai Byo) has been described in Japanese women and thought to be due to chronic cadmium poisoning.[120] The patients develop extreme bone pain due to osteomalacia and pseudofractures (hence the name of the disease) and have proteinuria, amino-aciduria, glucosuria and hypercalciuria. The syndrome is largely confined to women who have had multiple pregnancies or who are postmenopausal and whose urinary and tissue concentrations of cadmium are increased. The incidence of hypertension may be higher than in the normal population. The epidemiology has been traced to contamination of river water by waste products from a cadmium mine. Cadmium concentrations of crops in that area were increased. Ingestion of water and produce from this region over long periods gave rise to the disease.

Prolonged administration of large amounts of cadmium to rabbits produces tubular lesions similar to those observed in man.[121] However, chronic ingestion of 0.1 to 10 parts per million of cadmium has no discernible adverse effects on rats as judged by general health, growth rate, and pathologic examination, although large amounts of the metal are retained in liver and kidney. Higher doses, however, cause stunted growth, accompanied by hypochromic-microcytic anemia and tubular atrophy and interstitial fibrosis of the kidneys.

The parenteral administration of a single dose of cadmium chloride to rats results in necrosis and atrophy of the testis and placental necrosis, without permanent damage to other organs.[122,123] Cadmium sterilization, apparently brought about through interference with testicular circulation, also occurs in mice, rabbits, guinea pigs and hamsters. Strikingly, the toxic action of cadmium on the testis and placenta is prevented by previous administration of zinc, suggesting these two metals compete for the same binding site of some critical biologic molecule in these tissues. Chronic cadmium intoxication in cattle results in stunted growth, liver and kidney damage, abnormal testicular growth and sperm production. These effects are also partially offset by the concomitant administration of zinc.

Cadmium is known to interact with the sulfhydryl groups of certain enzymes, resulting in inactivation. This circumstance may be pertinent to its toxic effects which have led to its classification as a "toxic" element. Most transition and group IIB metals will exert such toxic effects when administered in excess or by an unusual route.

BIBLIOGRAPHY

1. Underwood: *Trace Elements in Human and Animal Nutrition*, 3rd Ed. New York, Academic Press, 1971.
2. Nielsen and Sauberlich: Proc. Soc. Exp. Biol. Med., *134*, 845, 1970.
3. Schwarz, Milne and Vinard: Biochem. Biophys. Res. Commun., *40*, 23, 1970.
4. Bowen: *Trace Elements in Biochemistry*, New York, Academic Press, 1966, p. 61.
5. Tipton and Cook: Health Phys., *9*, 103, 1963.
6. Tipton, Schroeder, Perry and Cook: Health Phys., *11*, 403, 1965.
7. Walsh: Advan. Spectr., *2*, 1, 1961.
8. Fuwa and Vallee: Anal. Chem., *35*, 942, 1963.
9. Vallee: *Enzymes*, Vol. 3B, eds., Boyer, Lardy and Myrbäck, 2nd ed., New York, Academic Press, 1960, p. 225.
10. Wacker and Vallee: J. Biol. Chem., *234*, 3257, 1959.
11. Fuwa, Wacker, Druyan, Bartholomay and Vallee: Proc. Natl. Acad. Sci. U.S., *46*, 1298, 1960.
12. Scheinberg and Sternlieb: Pharmacol. Rev., *12*, 355, 1960.
13. Adelstein and Vallee: *Mineral Metabolism*, Vol. 2B, eds. Comar and Bronner, New York, Academic Press, 1962, p. 370.
14. Sarkar and Kruck: *Biochemistry of Copper*, eds. Peisach, Aisen and Blumberg, New York, Academic Press, 1966, p. 183.
15. Neumann and Suss-Kortsak: J. Clin. Invest., *46*, 646, 1967.
16. Peisach, Aisen and Blumberg: *Biochemistry of Copper*, New York, Academic Press, 1966.
17. Osaki, Johnson and Frieden: J. Biol. Chem., *241*, 2746, 1966.
18. Scheinberg: *Biochemistry of Copper*, eds. Peisach, Aisen and Blumberg, New York, Academic Press, 1966, p. 513.
19. Blumberg, Goldstein, Lauber and Peisach: Biochim. Biophys. Acta, *99*, 187, 1965.
20. Hill, Starcher and Kim: Federation Proc., *26*, 129, 1967.
21. Porter: *Biochemistry of Copper*, eds. Peisach, Aisen and Blumberg, New York, Academic Press, 1966, p. 159.
22. Carrico and Deutsch: J. Biol. Chem., *245*, 723, 1970.
23. McCord and Fridovich: J. Biol. Chem., *244*, 6049, 1969.
24. Evans, Majors and Cornatzer: Biochem. Biophys. Res. Commun., *40*, 1142, 1970.
25. Roeser, Lee, Nacht and Cartwright: J. Clin. Invest., *49*, 2408, 1970.
26. Gubler: J.A.M.A., *161*, 530, 1956.
27. Graham, Cordano and Baertl: Proc. 6th Intern. Congr. Nutr., Edinburgh, E. & S. Livingstone, Ltd., 1964, p. 523.
28. O'Dell, Elsden, Thomas, Partridge, Smith and Palmer: Nature, *209*, 401, 1966.
29. Bird, Savage, and O'Dell: Proc. Soc. Exp. Biol. Med., *123*, 250, 1966.
30. Gallagher and Reeve: Aust. J. Exp. Biol. Med. Sci., *49*, 21, 1971.
31. Bearn: *The Metabolic Basis of Inherited Disease*, eds. Stanbury, Wyngaarden and Fredrickson, 2nd ed., New York, McGraw-Hill Book Co., 1966, p. 61.

32. Sternlieb and Scheinberg: J.A.M.A., *189*, 748, 1964.
33. Holtzman, Eliott, and Heller: New Eng. J. Med., *275*, 347, 1966.
34. Vallee: Physiol. Rev., *39*, 443, 1959.
35. ———: *Mineral Metabolism*, Vol. 2B, eds. Comar and Bronner, New York, Academic Press, 1962, p. 443.
36. Vallee, Wacker, Bartholomay and Robin: New Eng. J. Med., *255*, 403, 1956.
37. Himmelhoch, Sober, Vallee, Peterson and Fuwa: Biochemistry, *5*, 2523, 1966.
38. Parisi and Vallee: Biochemistry, *9*, 2421, 1970.
39. Oberleas, Muhrer and O'Dell: *Zinc Metabolism*, ed. Prasad. A. S., Springfield, Charles C Thomas, 1966, p. 225.
40. Li: *Zinc Metabolism*, ed. Prasad, A. S., Springfield, Charles C Thomas, 1966, p. 48.
41. Drum, Harrison, Li, Bethune and Vallee: Proc. Natl. Acad. Sci. U.S., *57*, 1434, 1967.
42. Blair and Vallee: Biochemistry, *5*, 2026, 1966.
43. Lindskog and Malmstrom: J. Biol. Chem., *237*, 1129, 1962.
44. Valle, Riordan and Coleman: Proc. Natl. Acad. Sci. U.S., *49*, 109, 1963.
45. Vallee and Coleman: *Comprehensive Biochemistry*, Vol. 12, eds. Florkin and Stotz, Amsterdam, Elsevier Publishing Co., 1964, p. 165.
46. Wacker: Biochemistry, *1*, 859, 1962.
47. Weser, Seeber and Warnecke: Biochim. Biophys. Acta, *179*, 422, 1969.
48. Neuberger and Tait: Biochem. J., *90*, 607, 1964.
49. Grant and Coombs: Essays in Biochem., *6*, 69, 1970.
50. Iqbal: Enzymol. Biol. Clin., *11*, 412, 1970.
51. Mills, Quarterman, Williams, Dalgarno and Panic: Biochem. J., *102*, 712, 1967.
52. Prasad, Oberleas, Wolf and Horwitz: J. Clin. Invest., *46*, 549, 1967.
53. Follis: *Zinc Metabolism*, ed. Prasad, Springfield, Charles C Thomas, 1966, p. 129.
54. Hsu and Anthony: J. Nutr., *100*, 1189, 1970.
55. Hurley: Amer. J. Clin. Nutr., *22*, 1332, 1969.
56. Prasad: Federation Proc., *26*, 181, 1967.
57. Caggiano, Schnitzler, Strauss, Baker, Josephson and Wallack: Am. J. Med. Sci., *257*, 305, 1969.
58. MacMahon, Parker and McKinnon: Med. J. Austr., *II*, 210, 1968.
59. Pories and Strain: *Zinc Metabolism*, ed. Prasad, Springfield, Charles C Thomas, 1966, p. 378.
60. Vallee, Wacker, Bartholomay and Hoch: New Eng. J. Med., *257*, 1055, 1957.
61. von Wartburg, Bethune and Vallee: Biochemistry, *3*, 1775, 1964.
62. Cotzias, G. C.: Physiol. Rev., *38*, 503, 1958.
63. ———: *Mineral Metabolism*, Vol. IIB, eds. Comar and Bronner, New York, Academic Press, Inc., 1962, p. 403.
64. Robinson, Telser and Dorfman: Proc. Natl. Acad. Sci. U.S., *56*, 1859, 1966.
65. Scrutton, Utter, and Mildvan: J. Biol. Chem., *241*, 3480, 1966.

66. Keck, McCord and Fridovich: J. Biol. Chem., *245*, 6176, 1970.
67. Cotzias: Proc. 6th Internl. Congr. Nutr., Edinburgh, E. & S. Livingstone, Ltd., 1964, p. 252.
68. Hurley: Federation Proc., *27*, 193, 1968.
69. Leach and Meunster: J. Nutr., *78*, 51, 1962:
70. Leach: Federation Proc., *26*, 118, 1967.
71. Leach, Muenster and Wein: Arch. Biochem., *133*, 22, 1969.
72. Tsai and Everson: J. Nutr., *91*, 447, 1967.
73. Comens: *Metal Binding in Medicine*, ed. Seven, Philadelphia, J. B. Lippincott Co., 1960, p. 312.
74. Penalver: Arch. Ind. Health, *16*, 64, 1957.
75. Hill: *Inorganic Biochemistry*, ed. Eichhorn, Amsterdam, Elsevier, in press.
76. Northrop and Wood: J. Biol. Chem., *244*, 5801, 1969.
77. Smith: *Mineral Metabolism*, Vol. IIB, eds., Comar and Bronner, New York, Academic Press, Inc., 1962, p. 349.
78. Jacobson, Gurney and Goldwasser: Advan. Internal Med., *10*, 297, 1960.
79. Wintrobe: *Clinical Hematology*, 5th ed. Philadelphia, Lea & Febiger, 1961, p. 142.
80. Alexander: Ann. Intern. Med., *70*, 411, 1969.
81. Rosenfeld and Beath: *Selenium*, New York, Academic Press, Inc., 1964.
82. Nissen and Benson: Biochim. Biophys. Acta, *82*, 400, 1964.
83. Schwarz: Federation Proc., *20*, 665, 1961.
84. Scott: *Mineral Metabolism*, Vol. IIB, eds., Comar and Bronner, New York, Academic Press, 1962, p. 543.
85. Thompson and Scott: J. Nutr., *100*, 797, 1970.
86. Burk, Pearson, Wood and Viteri: Amer. J. Clin. Nutr., *20*, 723, 1967.
87. Schwarz and Fredga: J. Biol. Chem., *244*, 2103, 1969.
88. Shrift and Virupaksha: Biochim. Biophys. Acta, *100*, 65, 1965.
89. McConnell and Roth: Biochim. Biophys. Acta, *62*, 503, 1962; and Proc. Soc. Exp. Biol. Med., *120*, 88, 1965.
90. Schwarz: Federation Proc., *24*, 58, 1965.
91. Tappel: Federation Proc., *24*, 73, 1965.
92. Mertz: Federation Proc., *26*, 186, 1967.
93. Mertz: Physiol. Rev., *49*, 163, 1969.
94. Curran: J. Biol. Chem., *210*, 765, 1954.
95. Schwarz and Mertz: Arch. Biochem. Biophys., *85*, 292, 1959.
96. Mertz, Roginski and Schwarz: J. Biol. Chem., *236*, 318, 1961.
97. Glinsmann and Mertz: Metab. Clin. Exptl., *15*, 510, 1966.
98. Levine, Streeten, and Doisy: Metabolism, *17*, 114, 1968.
99. Hopkins, Ransome-Kuti and Majaj: Amer. J. Clin. Nutr., *21*, 203, 1968.
100. Richert and Westerfeld: J. Biol. Chem., *203*, 915, 1953.
101. deRenzo: *Mineral Metabolism*, Vol. 2B, eds. Comar and Bronner, New York, Academic Press, 1962, p. 483.

102. Bray, Palmer and Beinert: J. Biol. Chem., *239*, 2667, 1964.
103. Bray: *Enzymes*, Vol. 7A, eds. Boyer, Lardy and Myrbäck, 2nd ed., New York, Academic Press, 1963, p. 533.
104. Cohen and Fridovich: J. Biol. Chem., *246*, 359, 1971.
105. Irreverre, Mudd, Heizer and Laster: Biochem. Med., *1*, 187, 1967.
106. Bui and Mortenson: Proc. Nat. Acad. Sci. U.S., *61*, 1021, 1968.
107. Vandecasteele and Burris: J. Bact., *101*, 794, 1970.
108. Higgins, Richert and Westerfeld: J. Nutr., *59*, 539, 1956.
109. Margoshes and Vallee: J. Am. Chem. Soc., *79*, 4813, 1957.
110. Piscator: Nord. Hyg. Tidskr., *45*, 76, 1964.
111. Pulido, Fuwa and Vallee: Anal. Biochem., *14*, 393, 1966.
112. Schroeder: J. Chronic Diseases, *18*, 647, 1965.
113. Schroeder and Buckman: Arch. Environ. Health, *14*, 693, 1967.
114. Dalhamn and Friberg: Acta Pharmacol. Toxicol., *10*, 199, 1954.
115. Friberg: Acta Med. Scand. Suppl., *240*, 1, 1950.
116. Kägi and Vallee: J. Biol. Chem., *235*, 3460, 1960; and *236*, 2435, 1961.
117. Pulido, Kägi and Vallee: Biochemistry, *5*, 1768, 1966.
118. Piscator: Nord. Hyg. Tidskr., *45*, 76, 1964.
119. Friberg: Arch. Ind. Health, *20*, 401, 1959.
120. Emmerson: Ann. Intern. Med., *73*, 854, 1970.
121. Axelsson and Piscator: Arch. Environ. Health, *12*, 360, 1966.
122. Parizek: J. Endocrinol., *15*, 56, 1957.
123. Chiquoine: J. Reprod. Fertility, *10*, 263, 1965.

PART II

Safety and Adequacy of the Food Supply

Chapter

9

Criteria of an Adequate Diet

ROBERT S. GOODHART

Diet patterns and food habits vary not only from one nation to another, but also from individual to individual. There is no single pattern of diet which must be followed to insure good nutrition. No single food can be designated essential for life or health. The animal body does require calories, certain fatty acids, amino acids, vitamins, minerals and water in sufficient amounts and in proper combinations to permit optimum growth and maintenance and repair of tissues under the environmental conditions to which the particular individual is exposed. The essential nutrients are widely dispersed in nature and can be obtained from many combinations of foods with varying ease. Some people depend upon beef and pork as sources of amino acids, others prefer horse, fish, dogs, rats, snails, locusts, snakes, or venison. These are all good sources of high-quality protein.

Not only do diet patterns and food values vary but so also do requirements for specific nutrients, depending on genetic and environmental factors, diet patterns, severity and nature of stress situations, age, sex, rate of growth, etc. Largely because of these two factors—differences in nutritional needs of individuals and variation in nutritive value of foods—it is impossible to devise a general food plan that will be just right for everyone.[1] There are other influences of major importance in determining the dietary requirements either of the individual or of groups of persons. These include the organism's ability to adapt to its diet, to adjust to its environment, and the aspirations of the individual and of the society in which he lives. It is not at all certain, for example, that the nutritional requirements for maximum size, early maturity, active sex life and maximum muscular development are identical with those for maximum longevity. Diets designed to protect the individual against bacterial infections, *e.g.* tuberculosis, may lower resistance to certain viral infections and predispose the individual to obesity and coronary artery disease in later years. Thus, statements such as "An adequate diet is one which meets in full all the nutritional needs of the person"[2] have little meaning unless they can be interpreted in terms of either the person's ambitions for himself or the community's designs for or on him.

How these various considerations may influence dietary recommendations can be illustrated by comparing the standards of different United States agencies with each other and with those of other countries. Table 9–1 gives the recommendations for certain nutrients, for the young, healthy, moderately active, adult male made by two American agencies and by Canada and Japan. Although all the committees which formulated these recommendations had access to the same basic information, there are some considerable differences among their conclusions.

It should be apparent that the recommendations of national or international bodies on dietary intakes cannot be used, by themselves, as standards for the assessment of nutritional status of either individuals or population groups. Their practical uses are three: (1) in the planning of food production and distribution programs; (2) in the planning of mass feeding or food rationing pro-

Table 9-1. United States, Canadian and Japanese Recommended Dietary Intakes for Young, Healthy, Normally Active, Male Adults**

Standard	Wt. in lbs.	Calories	Protein gm	Calcium gm	Vitamin A I.U.	Iron mg	Thiamin mg	Riboflavin mg	Niacin mg	Ascorbic Acid mg	Vitamin D I.U.
National Research Council, United States[3]	154	2800	65	0.8	5000*	10	1.4	1.7	18 (equiv.)	60	0
I.C.N.N.D., United States[4]	154	2900	70	0.4	3500	9	0.96	1.2	10	30	
Dietary Standard for Canada[5]	158	2850	48	0.5	3700†	6	0.9	1.4	9	30	0
Standard Nutritional Requirements for Japanese[6] (light work)	123	2500	70	0.6	2000‡	10	1.3	1.3	13	65	400

* Assuming two-thirds of the total vitamin A activity as carotene and one-third as the preformed vitamin. If the sole source were preformed vitamin A, the allowance would be 3000 I.U.

† Based on the mixed Canadian diet supplying both vitamin A and carotene. As the preformed vitamin A, the suggested intake would be about two-thirds of that indicated.

‡ All as preformed vitamin A.

** The figures given in this table, and elsewhere in this chapter, for agency-recommended dietary intakes are those which were current at the time of revision of this chapter (March 1972). The Food and Nutrition Board of the National Research Council, in common with the other mentioned agencies, periodically revises its recommendations, a fact which emphasizes, of course, the tentative nature of the recommendations.

grams; (3) as a useful starting point for nutrition therapy.

The N.R.C.[3] places the minimum daily nitrogen loss of adults at 3.2 mg, equivalent to 20 mg of protein, per basal calorie (2 mg N for endogenous urinary loss, 0.4 mg for minimum fecal loss, and 0.8 mg N lost through the skin and integumental growths). On this basis, the requirement of adult males for protein with a biological value of 100 may have a range as great as or greater than from 0.43 to 0.51 gm per kg of body weight, depending upon the body weight and the associated basal metabolism. Allowing an additional 30 per cent, as the N.R.C. does, "for individual variability within a large population" these figures become 0.56 and 0.66 respectively. Since the N.R.C. attaches a biologic value of 70 to the protein in the American diet, the figures must be further corrected to 0.80 gm and 0.94 gm. For the 70-kg "reference man" the protein allowance amounts to 0.928 gm per kg of body weight, or a total of 65 gm per day. This is probably about twice the minimum requirement.

The Dietary Standard for Canada[5] also includes an additional 30 per cent for individual variability and estimates the NPU (net protein utilization value) of Canadian dietary protein at 70 (NPU of the reference protein equals 100). However, the obligatory nitrogen losses are calculated in terms of body weight to the 0.75 power, which correlates with basal energy metabolism. The figures for adults are: urinary loss 125 mg $N/kg^{0.75}$, fecal loss 25 mg $N/kg^{0.75}$, skin loss 15 mg $N/kg^{0.75}$. Thus, the protein requirement for a 70-kg adult male is approximately 47 gm per day, or about 72 per cent of the recommended allowance of the Food and Nutrition Board, N.R.C., U.S.A. The moral is clear. If meat prices are too high for you in the United States, move to Canada. True, meat may be just as expensive there, but you can get along on less.

The I.C.N.N.D.[4] recommends 1 gm of protein per kg of body weight as a practical and realistic minimum when dealing with populations where a high proportion of protein will come from non-animal sources and considers an intake of 1.0 to 1.5 gm of protein per kg of body weight to be "acceptable"

under these conditions. In Japan, where dietary protein from animal sources supplies, on the average, about 33 to 35 per cent of the total dietary protein[6] (in the United States $\frac{2}{3}$ of the dietary protein is from animal sources), the recommendation for a young, normally active male amounts to 1.25 gm per kg of body weight, which appears generous but reasonable. The Japanese, however, increase this allowance to approximately 1.7 gm per kg of body weight for men engaged in "heavy" and "very heavy" work, for reasons not explained in the 1960 report of the Ministry of Health and Welfare.[6]

Swaminathan (Central Food Technological Research Institute, Mysore, India)[7] estimates the obligatory nitrogen loss in the urine and sweat to be 2.0 mg/basal calorie, that in the feces to be 0.6 mg/basal calorie and integumental losses to be 0.1 mg/basal calorie, for a total of 2.7 mg/basal calorie, equivalent to 17 (16.875) mg of protein. If we use these figures, add 30 per cent for individual variability and take the biological value of the dietary protein to be 70, we find that the healthy 70-kg adult male on an American- or Canadian-type diet has a dietary requirement for 55 gm of protein daily.

An FAO/WHO Expert group concluded that intakes of 400 to 500 mg per day of calcium represented a practical allowance for adults.[8] This conclusion appears to be concurred with by Canada and the I.C.N.N.D. (for use in evaluating diets in relatively underprivileged areas of the world). The recommendations of the N.R.C. (Table 9–1) appear to be conditioned by our past dietary practices (see Chapter 6A) and the results of calcium balance studies. Hegsted[9] points out that "although most of the people of the world do not consume enough calcium to meet dietary recommendations, and thus are often said to be calcium deficient, there is no convincing evidence that this is true. We do not even know what calcium deficiency looks like in man."

Japan's relatively high allowance may be related to the belief that "Perhaps one of the essential reasons for [the] present unsatisfactory physiques of the Japanese may be found in the shortage of this nutrient."[6] The 1960 Japanese recommendations for calcium do represent a decrease from previous recommendations, "Because no deficiency symptoms of calcium have been found by the present in spite of [the fact that] calcium intake of the population [did not attain] the level of the requirement."[6]

Differences exist in regard to practically every other nutrient for which requirements or allowances have been recommended by more than one agency. It is impossible, at least for me, to avoid the conclusion that the primary reasons for these differences are to be found in the milieu in which the various recommendations are drawn.

The Recommended Dietary Allowances of the Food and Nutrition Board, U.S.A. are designed to afford a margin of sufficiency above average physiological requirements to cover variations among essentially all individuals in the general population. They provide a buffer against the increased needs during common stresses and permit full realization of growth and productive potential; but they are not to be considered adequate to meet additional requirements of persons depleted by disease, traumatic stresses, or prior dietary inadequacies. On the other hand, the allowances are generous with respect to temporary emergency feeding of large groups under conditions of limited food supply and physical disaster.[3]

The I.C.N.N.D.[4] has recommended standards only for active young adult men, living in a temperate climate and consuming a varied diet, to be used in association with biochemical and physical examination data to estimate the incidence of nutritional inadequacies in large groups of such men.

"The Canadian Dietary Standard was designed to fulfill certain functions. It may be used for planning diets and food supplies for groups of healthy people. It may also be used as a guide in the planning of diets and food supplies for individuals. The figures do not represent average requirements, but rather the recommended intakes are proposed as adequate for the maintenance of health among the majority of Canadians. The figures for calories more closely resemble average requirements than do those for other nutrients. This has been done because of the recognized problem of the harm of an excessive caloric intake.

"The figures suggested in the standard are, in every case, in excess of known minimal requirements. This excess has been included to take into account the individual variation in nutrient requirement imposed by differences in biochemical and biophysical constitution. The excess recommended above minimal requirement is also included in recognition of the belief that an intake somewhat above minimal may confer added benefits to health. Were suitable methods available, it might be possible to express the recommendations as optimal requirements. In the absence of suitable criteria of optimal health, the margin of safety, as the excess has been termed, is a measure of our ignorance and the figure given is the best estimate of a suitable intake. There is no evidence that intakes above those recommended will confer any added benefit to health."[5]

Again, the Japanese standard has still a different objective as indicated in the following quotations from the 1960 report of the Ministry of Health and Welfare on Nutrition in Japan.[6] "As a whole, therefore, nutrition of the nation is still more to be improved. It is not enough to meet all the requirements as the standard is based on the physiques of the Japanese of today, and we are not satisfied to be in the present physiques, which are, compared to many other nations, rather dwarfish." . . . "We are not satisfied, however, as we said before, with just the recovery to the prewar state but aim to become one of the healthy, able-bodied and able-minded peoples of the world and in a well-grown size, too."

The Recommended Dietary Allowances of the National Research Council and the Dietary Standard for Canada are summarized in Tables A–1 and A–2 in the Appendix.

CALORIES

The calorie used in the study of metabolism is the large calorie, which is the amount of heat required to raise 1 kg of water from $15°$ to $16°$ C. Energy (calories) is required for all body processes and all the individual's activities. The need is the sum of the basal metabolism + the energy liberated in exercise + the increment of energy due to the specific dynamic action of food. The first two are of determining influence; the third is of importance only when great precision in dietary arrangement is demanded.

Calorie standards have been published by the Food and Agricultural Organization of the United Nations.[10,11] The recommendations on calories contained in the 1968 revision of the Recommended Dietary Allowances represent a modification of the FAO standards made to conform more closely to the average sizes and activities of young men and women in the United States and to our mean annual temperature. In the 1968 revision the "reference man," age 22, weighs 70 kg and the "reference woman," age 22, weighs 58 kg. The mean annual temperature is taken as 20° C. These standard persons are presumed to be lightly active physically, being neither sedentary nor engaged in hard physical labor. Light activity is defined as that requiring the expenditure of 120 to 240 calories per hour.[3]

The N.R.C. suggests that calorie allowances be reduced by 5 per cent between ages 22 and 35, by 3 per cent per decade between ages 35 and 55, and by 5 per cent per decade from ages 55 to 75. A further decrement of 7 per cent is recommended for age 75 and beyond.

There does not appear to be any reason to increase calorie allowances for activity in the cold, except to compensate for the relatively small (2 to 5 per cent) increase in expenditure associated with carrying the extra weight of cold weather clothing. Such clothing also increases energy expenditure slightly by its "hobbling" effect. Of course, if the body is inadequately clothed, body cooling will occur and calorie needs will increase because of the increased metabolic rate associated with shivering and other involuntary movement. It also should be remembered that there is a tendency to increase activity in the cold, while in the heat activity tends to be avoided.

"Energy requirements are increased in men performing prescribed work at a high temperature (37.8° C). Under such conditions, body temperature and metabolic rate increase and the body expends extra energy in its efforts to maintain thermal balance. Thus, while little adjustment appears to be necessary for change in environmental temperature between 20° and 30° C, it would seem desirable, when men are physically active (rate of energy expenditure over 3,000 k cal/day), to increase calorie allowances by at least 0.5 per cent for every degree of temperature rise between 30° and 40° C."[3]

The National Research Council[3] also suggests adjustment for body size by the following formulae:

Calories for Men (RMR* + 13W†) × (per cent adjustment for age)

Calories for Women (RMR + 7W) × (per cent adjustment for age)

* RMR = resting metabolic rate
† W = desirable body weight in kg

The Canadian Council on Nutrition[5] recognizes that caloric requirements are related to "metabolic body size," which it defines as $Wt_{kg}^{0.75}$. The basal metabolic rate, young adults, is taken as 70 ($Wt_{kg}^{0.75}$) calories per day.

Maintenance activity is described as that of an unemployed person engaged only in waiting upon himself and this is estimated to be 133 per cent of the basal metabolic rate; thus, the maintenance requirements are 93 ($Wt_{kg}^{0.75}$) calories per day.

Work calories also are computed in terms of metabolic size by the formula b ($Wt_{kg}^{0.75}$). The numerical value of b varies with the degree of activity. Thus the caloric requirements of a young adult, male or female, are equal to 93 ($Wt_{kg}^{0.75}$) + b ($Wt_{kg}^{0.75}$). Values of b for four general categories of activity have been calculated, Table 9–2.

As people grow older their general activity decreases. This was recognized in the F.A.O. report,[11] and reductions in the caloric allowances with advancing age were proposed. These reductions were made in the total calories. Such a correction would not apply in the case of the Canadian standard, because, in it, the various estimates for energy expenditure are calculated separately from the *maintenance* requirement.

The energy requirement for any particular

Criteria of an Adequate Diet

Table 9-2. Caloric Expenditures for Various Degrees of Activity by a 65-kg Man: b × (Wt. $^{0.75}_{kg}$) Canada[5]

Category of Activity	Calories per Minute		Calories per 8 Hours		b Applicable to 8 Hours' Work	
	Range	Av.	Range	Av.	Range	Av.
A	0.1–2.1	1.1	50–1010	530	2–44	23
B	2.1–3.1	2.6	1010–1490	1250	44–65	55
C	3.1–4.5	3.8	1490–2160	1825	65–94	80
D	4.5–5.8	5.1	2160–2785	2450	94–122	107

activity must be in the same range among people of the same body size, regardless of age. The difference would be in the maintenance activity. Not only does the basal metabolic rate decrease with advancing age, but the more active components of *maintenance* living are gradually dropped, and the person becomes more sedentary. In recognition of this, in this standard the decrements in the energy allowances with advancing age are made in the *maintenance* fraction. In degree they are the same as those proposed in the F.A.O. report[11] to be applied to the total caloric allowances.

It is considered that the total maintenance requirement decreases by the following amounts with age: 25 to 35 years, 3 per cent of requirements at 25; 35 to 45 years, 5 per cent; 45 to 55 years, 9 per cent; 55 to 65 years, 13 per cent; and over 65 years, 17 per cent. These decrements, applied only to the maintenance recommendations, are based on the known decreases in basal metabolic rate and the suggested decrements in total energy requirements (FAO report[11]).[5]

For practical purposes, in handling the individual adult patient, it is quite satisfactory to assume the calorie requirement of the average woman to be 35 calories per kg of desirable body weight, and that of the average man to be 40 calories per kg of desirable body weight, with a range from 30, for the sedentary, to 55 calories per kg of desirable body weight for men habitually engaged in strenuous physical exertion. On follow-up, adjustments to meet actual individual requirements can be made.

Adjustments in calorie allowances are also necessary for pregnancy, lactation, growth, physical activity and metabolic aberrations. To provide a table or formulae by which these adjustments could be calculated with any degree of accuracy for the individual person would be to pretend to knowledge which we do not possess. In the last analysis, calorie allowances must be adjusted to meet specific needs. "The proper allowance for an individual is that which over an extended period will maintain body weight or rate of growth at the level most conducive to well-being."[3] Height and weight tables are given in the Appendix.

Calorie allowances for infants and children are discussed in Chapter 24.

CARBOHYDRATES

In the United States carbohydrates provide from 40 to 50 per cent of the calories in the diet. Since carbohydrates provide a relatively cheap source of calories, the proportion is higher in the diet of the lower economic groups than in that of the upper income brackets. In general, throughout the world the proportion of carbohydrate in the diet appears to be determined by the availability or non-availability of other foods. Refined sucrose probably represents an exception to this rule, since the consumption of this source of vitamin-free calories appears to be inordinately high wherever it is readily available. Adaptation to diets very low in carbohydrate is possible, but, in individuals accustomed to diets in which 40 per cent or more of the calories come from carbohydrate, at least 100 gm of carbohydrate per day appear to be needed to avoid ketosis, excessive protein breakdown, and other undesirable metabolic responses.[3]

The more indigestible complex carbohydrates, such as cellulose, have an important function in providing bulk for the intestinal contents.

FATS

The lack of certain fatty acids results in genuine nutritional deficiency; a small amount of fat is therefore essential in man's diet. At first this requirement was believed to be extremely small, so small in fact as to be negligible; but this is probably an error; however, it is not yet possible to state definitely a reasonable allowance for fat in the diet or to indicate the characteristics of a fatty acid mixture most favorable for the support of health, beyond the general recommendation that prudence would seem to dictate a diet in which at least one-half of the fat calories come from unhydrogenated vegetable oils (see Chapter 31). Approximately 40 per cent of the calories in the average American diet are provided by fat.

PROTEIN

Recommendations for healthy young adults have been discussed. The protein requirement is increased during pregnancy and lactation, and during recovery from disease and injury; but it is not increased by muscular activity, provided that the calorie requirement is satisfied. Protein requirements are relatively high for the periods of rapid growth and lower during periods of slow growth. They range from about 2.5 to 3 gm per kg of body weight in early childhood to 1.5 to 2 gm in late childhood and adolescence, to something less than 1 gm for adults, depending upon individual variations and the biological value of the dietary protein. The recommended allowances for protein assume adequate calorie intakes. For requirements during pregnancy and childhood see Chapters 23 and 24.

Actually the requirement is for amino acids, rather than for protein as such, thus accounting for the higher biologic value of animal proteins as compared to vegetable proteins, the latter being incomplete in amino acid composition for animal tissue synthesis. It is recommended that a variety of foods be included in the diet and especially foods of animal origin.

VITAMINS

The vitamins are organic substances required in minute amounts for the metabolism of foodstuffs and the discharge of important body functions. They are useless without substrata upon which to act or media in which to operate, without carbohydrates, protein, fat, water, oxygen and certain minerals. The proper foods are essential for health and the vitamins, either natural or synthetic, are essential for the efficient and optimum utilization of ingested foodstuff by the body.

In Tables A–1 and A–2 in the Appendix are listed the National Research Council's Recommended Dietary Allowances (and the Canadian recommendations) for vitamins A, E, folacin, B_6, B_{12}, thiamin, riboflavin, niacin, ascorbic acid and vitamin D. It must be emphasized that these recommendations are *designed for the maintenance of good nutrition of most healthy persons in the United States of America and Canada*. Many healthy individuals require less than the recommended allowances and some apparently healthy persons may require more. None of these recommendations applies to persons suffering from disease, metabolic disorders and injury, and they are *not* to be used as standards for hospital diets.

Other vitamins known to be essential for man include pantothenic acid (daily requirement probably around 10 mg[3]), biotin (perhaps 150 to 300 μg, considerable intestinal synthesis[12]) and vitamin K, for which the requirement of healthy adults is around 1 mg daily, probably met almost entirely, if not completely so, by intestinal synthesis.

In June 1970, a comprehensive annotated bibliography on biotin, by F. L. Billings, was published by Hoffman-La Roche Limited, Montreal, Canada.

Vitamin activity in man has not been demonstrated for either para-aminobenzoic acid (PABA) or pangamic acid (vitamin B_{15})

and further discussion of them in this context, at this time, is not indicated. A chromium-containing micronutrient, "the glucose tolerance factor," required for optimal utilization of blood sugar in the experimental animal "and probably also in man" has been reported to have been found in brewer's yeast and in whole wheat.[13]

MINERALS

In selecting diets, calcium, iron and iodine are the minerals requiring most consideration. Generally, if the calcium and protein needs are met through common foods, the phosphorus requirements also will be met.

In the absence of growth, pregnancy or blood loss, the iron requirement is readily met by the customary mixed diet; however, during the period of active growth and during the active sexual period of the female special attention must be given to the iron content of the diet and supplementary iron may be indicated; iron deficiency anemia is common (see Chapters 6C and 23).

The requirement for iodine is small, probably about 0.001 mg per day per kg of body weight,[3] or a total of 0.07 mg daily for a 70-kg adult. To insure a margin of safety for adults, the National Research Council recommends a daily intake of 0.08 to 0.15 mg[3] (see Table A–1 in Appendix). This need can be met by the regular use of iodized salt. During adolescence and pregnancy it is of special importance that an adequate intake of iodine be assured.

Potassium is especially abundant in both plant and animal tissues and does not need particular consideration. The average intake of sodium chloride (salt) by the normal adult is 7 to 15 gm daily. This includes sodium and chlorides contained in foods as well as those added to food as salt. It more than meets the normal requirements. Under unusual conditions, such as doing heavy work in a hot climate, 10 to 15 gm daily, or even more, may be required with meals and in drinking water. However, after acclimatization to heat, the sodium content of sweat is greatly reduced and the allowance for salt can be near to normal.

The adult requirement for magnesium has been estimated at 300 to 450 mg daily.[3] (Also see Chapter 6B.)

The requirement for copper by adults is about 2 mg daily. Infants and children require approximately 0.05 to 0.10 mg for each kg of body weight. The requirement for copper is approximately one-tenth that for iron. A good diet normally will supply sufficient copper.

Man's average dietary intake of 10 to 15 mg of zinc daily appears to be adequate. A mixed diet containing recommended amounts of animal protein apparently satisfies the requirements, but diets strictly limited to vegetable sources of protein may be inadequate.[3]

Certain trace elements, in addition to copper and iodine, commonly found qualitatively in biological organisms have functional significance most frequently associated with enzyme systems. Other than that the amounts are exceedingly small, relatively little is known about the quantitative levels necessary for essential physiologic function of these elements in human nutrition, and less is known about desirable levels. Included are chromium, manganese, molybdenum, and selenium.

WATER

A suitable allowance of water for adults is 2.5 liters daily in most instances. An ordinary standard is 1 ml for each calorie of food. Much of this quantity is contained in prepared foods. Water should be allowed *ad libitum*. Sensations of thirst usually serve as adequate guides to intake, except for infants and sick persons. Under conditions of extreme heat or excessive sweating, the sensation of thirst may not keep pace with the actual water requirements, and forced intakes up to 1 liter per hour may be indicated for a short time.

In closing this chapter, I again remind the reader that all estimates of nutrient requirements arrived at by committees represent the results of accommodation and, in some instances, may not even approximate the actual requirements of an individual or group. (At its best, applied human nutrition is far from an exact science.) Also, I bring to your attention the fact that the Food and Nutrition Board of the National Research Council promises us another revision of the Recommended Dietary Allowances sometime in 1973.[14]

To better understand and interpret the quotations of nutritional requirements and allowances contained in this chapter, the reader is urged to study the preceding chapters on the specific nutrients.

BIBLIOGRAPHY

1. Page and Phipard: U.S. Dept. of Agriculture, Home Eco. Res. Rep. No. 3, Washington, D.C., 1957.
2. Maynard: J.A.M.A., *170*, 457, 1959.
3. National Research Council, Food and Nutrition Board: *Recommended Dietary Allowances*, Revised 1968, NRC Publication 1694, Washington, D.C., 1968.
4. Interdepartmental Committee on Nutrition for National Defense: *Manual for Nutrition Surveys*, Second Edition, 1963, U.S. Government Printing Office, Washington, D.C.
5. Canadian Council on Nutrition: *Dietary Standards for Canada 1963:* March 1964 (Protein revised 1968), Department of Public Printing and Stationery, Ottawa.
6. Ministry of Health and Welfare, Japan: *Nutrition in Japan 1960*, Tokyo, November, 1960.
7. Swaminathan: Nutrition Reports International, *3*, 277, 1971.
8. World Health Organization: *Calcium Requirements*, WHO Tech. Report Series No. 230, Geneva, 1962.
9. Hegsted: J. Am. Dietet. A., *50*, 105, 1967.
10. Food and Agriculture Organization of the United Nations: FAO Nutritional Studies No. 5, *Calorie Requirements*, Washington, D.C., 1950.
11. Food and Agriculture Organization of the United Nations: FAO Nutritional Studies No. 15, *Calorie Requirements*, Rome, 1957.
12. Sebrell and Harris: *The Vitamins*, Vol. 1, New York, Academic Press, 1954.
13. Progress Report, Human Nutrition Research Division, Agricultural Research Service, USDA, Beltsville, Md., July 1, 1971, page 2.
14. Activities Report—1971, Food and Nutrition Board, National Research Council, Washington, D.C., 1972.

Chapter

10

Naturally Occurring Toxic Foods

O. MICKELSEN,

M. G. YANG,

AND

ROBERT S. GOODHART

According to a commonly accepted definition, nutrition is devoted to the study of those substances that promote growth and facilitate repair of body tissues and processes. On this basis, most nutrition scientists exclude toxic foods from their consideration. By so doing, they often ignore the fact that most toxic foods were discovered primarily when an attempt was made to use the food for nutritional purposes. The people who had only limited food resources early recognized the toxicity of their native foods and developed means of making the foods safe. Examples of such foods are the cycad kernels which, on Guam, are soaked in water for about 10 days before being dried and ground into flour.[1] By this means, the toxic glycoside in the cycad kernel is destroyed. Of more practical importance is the processing of soybean meal which inactivates the various toxic substances present in the original plant. The proper control of time and temperature during the processing of soybeans produces a meal of high nutritive value. This accounts for its phenomenal increase in animal-feeding practices.[2]

One problem that arises in a discussion of naturally occurring toxic foods is the definition of "naturally occurring." Selenized wheat is a case in point. Only when the wheat is raised on land where the selenium indicator plants have transformed this metal into compounds that can be absorbed by wheat roots is the cereal likely to be toxic.[3] Shellfish,

which are normally non-toxic, become highly injurious after feeding on *Gonyaulax catanella*. The paralytic poison produced by this species of dinoflagellates is present in mussels and clams harvested from the area where these organisms abound.[4]

Another problem revolves around the fact that many foods become toxic if consumed in too large amounts. On this score, some individuals even would include carbohydrates since an excessive intake produces obesity with its concomitant complications. The validity of such a statement can be argued equally well by proponents of both views but since obesity *per se* will be discussed in other sections, we shall say no more about it here. Vitamins A and D, however, do fall within the realm of potentially toxic substances which are present in naturally occurring foods.[13-33] Seal and polar bear livers, with their high concentration of vitamin A, have been associated with severe disturbances among Arctic explorers who have eaten them.[5] As little as three-fourths of a pound of this liver contains 7,500,000 I.U. of vitamin A. This is sufficient to produce symptoms of acute toxicity.* The toxicity of vitamins A and D is discussed in Chapter 5, Sections A and B respectively.

At the other end of the spectrum are such readily recognized toxic substances as sele-

* The liver of polar bears contains 20,000 I.U. vitamin A per gm,[6] whereas beef and pork liver contain only 100 to 500 I.U. per gm.[7]

412

nium and chromium. Both these elements were initially considered only as toxic substances because of the effects produced either in animals[8] or in fish.[9] Within the past few years, both selenium[10] and chromium[11] have been associated with essential biologic reactions. The amount of these elements needed by animals is only a small fraction of that associated with their toxic manifestations.

The importance and significance of naturally occurring toxic foods are difficult to evaluate. This stems from the fact that their significance may be grossly exaggerated since many individuals attribute their minor illnesses or even indispositions to foods that they ate. If the illness involves enough individuals or becomes serious, a study may be initiated which frequently provides a more definitive answer to the problem. On the other hand, the minor illnesses may not be reported, with the result that the incidence of such toxicities may be greatly underestimated. Some indication of the magnitude of the problem comes from a survey of the 1959–1960 reports submitted to the National Clearing House for Poison Control Centers.[12] These reports from 50 states, the District of Columbia, Puerto Rico and the Canal Zone indicated that, in the one year surveyed, 1,051 cases were reported that were due supposedly to the eating of poisonous plants. These involved "175 plants in addition to mushrooms." There were no fatalities in this series and, in most cases, the symptoms were of a minor nature.

TOXICITY FROM METALS

The largest part of the total body burden of most metals in biologic species is traceable to diet: sources of which include constituents of rocks and minerals that weathered to produce the soil; water erosion of soil particles; metals as added ingredients or impurities in fertilizers; pesticides containing metals, such as arsenic, lead, copper, mercury, manganese and zinc; metals in manure and sludge; and those present in airborne dust (industrial and mining wastes, fossil fuel combustion products, wind-eroded soil particles, radioactive fallout, pollen, sea spray, meteoric and volcanic material). Plants may grow normally but contain levels of selenium, cadmium, molybdenum or lead that are toxic to animals. Plants exclude arsenic, beryllium, nickel, zinc and mercury by only minimal absorption of these metals from soil.[34]

The toxic action of metals believed to be most important is enzyme poisoning. Mercury, lead, copper, beryllium, cadmium and silver have been found to inhibit alkaline phosphatase, catalase, xanthine oxidase, and ribonuclease in fish. Some metals act as antimetabolites, e.g., arsenate substituting for phosphate: metals may form precipitates or chelates with essential metabolites: they may catalyze the degradation of essential metabolites: metals, such as gold, cadmium, copper, mercury, lead and uranium, may react with cell membranes and alter their permeability or even rupture them: some metals may replace structurally or electrochemically important elements in cells and then not function, such as lithium substituting for sodium, calcium for potassium, and strontium for cadmium.[34] An excellent review of the ecological aspects of metals has been written by Dr. J. Lisk.[34]

Perhaps the two naturally occurring toxic metals in foods of most practical importance are mercury and selenium, although mercury, lead, and cadmium are the most serious environmental pollutants. Mercury is extremely toxic, very volatile and widely distributed over the surface of the earth. It undergoes methylation which increases its toxicity and mobility in aquatic and animal circulatory systems. Mercury poisoning in man resulting from the eating of contaminated fish is described later in this chapter under the title of *Minamata Disease*.

Selenium. Toxicity associated with the ingestion of seleniferous foods has been limited largely to grazing animals. Although the condition was described sporadically from the time of Marco Polo,[3] it was not until the early part of this century when parts of South Dakota and Wyoming were opened to grazing that the toxicity now recognized as due to selenium became a problem. In the summers of 1907 and 1908, as many as 15,000 sheep died in parts of Wyoming with the cause of death attributed to the ingestion of woody aster and Gray's vetch, both known to accumulate large amounts of selenium.

Although selenium toxicity has been important among a variety of animals, there is little evidence that man has suffered from this poisoning as a result of eating foods. Following extensive studies of people living in the seleniferous areas of South Dakota, Wyoming, and Nebraska, M. I. Smith[35] concluded that he could not establish the presence of selenium poisoning among these individuals. There were no symptoms of toxicity despite the fact that some people excreted enough selenium in their urine to make it comparable to that of experimental animals receiving toxic levels of selenium in their rations. Physical examinations of the 111 individuals included in the study[36,37] indicated a high incidence of dental caries. Selenium at levels below those that produce toxicity has been reported as an agent facilitating the development of carious lesions among school children in certain areas of Oregon.[38]

During the past few years, the emphasis on selenium has changed from its role as a toxic substance to that of a nutritionally important element. Its intimate relationship to vitamin E and its action in curing or preventing white muscle disease in sheep and cattle have given it an importance never dreamed of when its toxic properties were first recognized (see Chapter 8, Section B on Trace Elements).

SUBSTANCES THAT INTERFERE WITH NUTRIENT UTILIZATION

Citral. While attempting to produce glaucoma in experimental animals, Leach and Lloyd[39] reported that a single subcutaneous dose of 10 μg of citral (an unsaturated aldehyde) raised the ocular tension of an adult rabbit. A similar effect was produced in monkeys by the oral administration of 2 to 5 μg a day for two weeks. At the same time, they fed some monkeys orange peel which is a good source of citral. Both the citral and the orange peel diets were reported to produce changes in the eyes of the monkeys similar to those seen in vitamin A deficiency. Large doses of vitamin A or sulthydryl-containing substances such as "cystein hydro-

chloride" were reported to reverse the action of citral. On this basis, they suggested that citral is an antagonist to vitamin A.[40]

The significance of these findings, if valid, would be far reaching since Leach and Lloyd point out that extrapolating from their animal studies to man gives a toxic dose of citral "in 2 gm of uncooked orange peel." With the large amounts of marmalade used in certain countries, some cases of vitamin A deficiency resulting from the ingestion of this food might be anticipated.

Subsequent work of two other groups has not clarified the relationship of citral to vitamin A. Moore[17] in his monograph on vitamin A points out the similarity in the structures of the vitamin and citral. On that basis he suggests that citral might function as an antimetabolite. Evidence to support this suggestion came from work with tissue cultures of chick embryo trachea, esophagus, cornea and skin. Aydelotte[41] showed an antagonistic action between citral and vitamin A. However, no attempt was made to overcome completely the citral effect by adding large doses of vitamin A, and for this reason it is impossible to accept the investigator's conclusion "that citral may be a competitive inhibitor of vitamin A." Finally, it should be pointed out that the effect of citral on the intraocular pressure of rabbits could not be duplicated by another group of investigators.[42] They used doses as high as 26 mg of citral per rabbit without finding any effect on the eyes of these animals.

For these reasons, it would appear that the English can still enjoy their daily tea with muffins and marmalade without any fear of developing a vitamin A deficiency.

Pyridoxine Antagonist. The presence of a growth-depressing factor in linseed meal was recognized as early as 1928. This inhibitory factor could be destroyed by autoclaving or incubating the meal after it was moistened with water or 50 per cent ethyl alcohol. That the growth inhibitor was a pyridoxine antagonist became evident when extra amounts of this vitamin added to the raw linseed meal ration produced normal growth in chicks.[2]

The isolation of this inhibitor has been achieved by Klosterman, Lamoureux and

Parsons[43] who showed that the compound exists in flaxseed. The name of the compound is: 1-[N-γ-L-glutamyl)amino]-D-proline. The active part of the molecule appears to be 1-amino-D-proline which forms a stable derivative with pyridoxal phosphate. Linatine was the name given to this compound. It is present in linseed meal at a concentration of about 100 ppm.

Thiaminase. The initial interest in this enzyme stemmed from the thiamin deficiency which appeared among foxes fed frozen carp as part of their ration.[2] With the recognition that this enzyme was distributed in a wide variety of fishes,[44-47] there was a possibility that some individuals consuming large amounts of seafood might develop a thiamin deficiency. The closest approach to such a condition is Haff or Yuksov disease. This disease has been reported from a number of areas in northern Europe among people consuming such fish as perch, bream, and lake trout.[48] Although some investigators have suggested a relation between Haff disease and thiaminase present in the fish consumed by these individuals,[48] such a relationship may be more apparent than real. The reasons for this are: (1) the symptoms appear within 24 hours after eating the fish; (2) the urine has a brownish-black color; and (3) recovery is usually complete 24 hours after eating the fish.[49] A deficiency of thiamin would not be associated with any of these characteristics.

A more direct association between the consumption of a food containing thiaminase and a consequent deficiency involves bracken fern. This plant (*Pteridium aquilinum*), which grows in upland pastures or open woods, remains green even when most forage crops have succumbed to drought. If, at such times, monogastric animals consume considerable amounts of this plant over a period of a few weeks, they show symptoms of thiamin deficiency about four weeks after first eating the fern.[50] Most of the reported cases involved horses and, even with animals of that size, only four weeks were required for a deficiency to become manifest. Complete recovery occurs if supplemental thiamin is given before the condition becomes terminal.

Bracken fern is known to be carcinogenic for cattle, guinea pigs, rats, and mice. In a study to determine whether this activity was related to its thiaminase content, Pamukcu, Yalciner, Price, and Bryan fed the fern to two groups of rats, one of which received, in addition to the common diet, once weekly subcutaneous injections of 2 mg thiamin hydrochloride.[51] Interestingly, both male and female rats receiving the supplemental thiamin "developed a statistically significant higher incidence of bladder tumors" compared to those which had not received the thiamin supplement. There was no difference in the incidence of intestinal tumors, which was extremely high in both groups. The authors suggest that thiamin administration perhaps altered the absorption, distribution, metabolism, or excretion of the bracken fern carcinogen by the host.

Thiamin-destroying factors are being found in ever greater numbers of plants that are normally used as food by human subjects, but the significance of these observations has still to be established. In one study, antithiamin activity was found in 31 vegetables and 18 fruits, with the highest activity in blackberries, black currants, red beets, Brussels sprouts and red cabbage.[52] A report from Japan[53] points out that some ferns, including bracken, have "enjoyed a popularity as edible" foods in various parts of the Orient. This report states that it is commonly recognized that dimness of vision results from eating large amounts of bracken fern in the early spring. How this disturbance might relate to a thiamin deficiency is not clear.

The potentially disturbing feature about the thiaminases present in many plant products is the fact that there appear to be at least two different types—one heat labile, the other heat stable.[53] The latter appears to be resistant to drying, is probably of small molecular weight, requires oxygen for its action and has an activity optimum at pH 8. Under present dietary practices, these thiamin-destroying factors are primarily of theoretical interest. Should the individuals in any area be forced, through unusual circumstances, to consume large amounts of such foods as spinach, cabbage and blackberries then a thiamin deficiency may become a reality.

The ingestion of large amounts of bracken fern by ruminants produces an acute hemorrhagic condition which is not related to a thiamin deficiency.[50] The toxic principle for cattle appears to be heat labile and water soluble; an extract freed of protein by precipitation at *p*H 3 produced a reduction of leukocytes in sheep.[2]

Goitrogens. The nature and distribution of goitrin, the antithyroid compound present in various members of the cabbage family, have been described elsewhere in this volume (see Chapter 8, Section A on Iodine). For this reason, the present discussion will be limited to the reported transmission of goitrogenic compounds through milk.

The recent attention this problem has received stems largely from the 1954 report of Clements[54] that children in certain parts of Australia and Tasmania developed goiters which were not prevented by potassium iodide administration. These children drank milk from cows fed marrowstem kale (choumoellier, *Brassica oleracea* var. *acephala*), a good source of the L-5-vinyl-2-thiooxazolidone isolated by Greer and co-workers from a number of goitrogenic plants.[55] This and a number of compounds structurally related to it inhibit the incorporation of iodine into the thyroid hormone.[56]

Clements' suggestion that a goitrogenic compound is transmitted through milk[57] stimulated two different groups in Finland to explore this problem. Peltola[58] initiated his study in an effort "to show that the goitre endemic in the eastern, southeastern and central parts of Finland may not be caused by iodine deficiency in the food as has been suggested . . . , but by a goitrogenic factor contained in cattle fodder and in cow's milk. . . ." For his studies, rats were fed *ad libitum* a "standard diet" (composition not given) that provided each rat with 150 μg of iodine per day (about 50 times the daily requirement) and milk secured from a dairy in a goitrous area. The thyroid glands from these rats were 1.5 to 2.0 times heavier than those in the animals fed the same standard diet but milk from a non-goitrous area. The one discordant finding was the reversal in ^{131}I uptake by the thyroids. Through the eleventh week of the study, the uptake was

less by the thyroids of the rats receiving milk from the goitrous area. However, the next determination at the end of one year showed a reversal in ^{131}I uptake. The difference in weights of the thyroid glands was reportedly confirmed in another study utilizing a ration that provided each rat with 14 μg of iodine per day.[59]

The other group working with Virtanen developed a sensitive analytical method for L-5-vinyl-2-thiooxazolidone.[60] By this procedure, they found 3 μg per ml of press juice from the green parts of marrowstem kale which, according to Clements and Wishart,[57] was the source of the goitrogen in the Tasmanian and Australian milk. Winter rape and Swede turnips contained 33 and 32 μg per ml respectively. Further study showed that the goitrogen was unstable in fresh milk. Heating, which destroyed peroxidases, preserved the compound. The highest concentration of the goitrogen in milk when cows were fed marrowstem kale, winter rape, or Swede turnips was 20 μg per liter. According to the Finnish investigators, this concentration is too low to produce any goitrogenic action.[61]

The work of Clements and Wishart, involving a determination of ^{131}I uptake by the thyroids of two subjects after ingesting milk from the goitrous areas of Tasmania, was repeated by the second group of Finnish workers.[62] They had 22 normal subjects drink, at one time, 1.5 to 2.2 liters of milk from cows fed large amounts of turnip or rape greens. This did not change the accumulation of ^{131}I by the thyroids of these normal subjects. Approximately 100 times the amount of L-5-vinyl-2-thiooxazolidone and thiocyanate present in the milk had to be given before any effect could be demonstrated on the ^{131}I uptake by the thyroids of these subjects.

The rat-feeding studies of Peltola were repeated by Virtanen and co-workers.[61] Although they received milk from the same dairy in the goitrous area as Peltola, they found no enlargement of the thyroid glands of their rats. From these studies, it would appear that the goitrogens present in natural products play a minor role, if any, in the development of human endemic goiter. Even the possibility that these compounds may influence the cattle feeding directly on the plants seems remote, since the preceding papers from Finland make no reference to the presence of enlarged thyroids among dairy cows in the goitrous areas.

Oxalates. An upsurge of interest in oxalates occurred in the 1930's when spinach was considered a valuable addition to the diet of children.[63] As a result of this, extensive analyses of foods were made for oxalic acid. One of the more comprehensive of these indicated that oxalic acid made up about 10 per cent of the dry weight of such foods as spinach, New Zealand spinach, Swiss chard, beet tops, lamb's-quarters, poke, purslane, and rhubarb.[64] This acid is present "primarily in the form of insoluble calcium oxalate crystals which can be demonstrated in microscopic sections of the leaves."[65] Foodstuffs of animal origin contain only small amounts of oxalates.[66] Both animal studies[63,64] and clinical trials with children[67] indicated that the calcium in spinach was not available, especially when the calcium content of the diet was close to the minimum requirement. The presence of soluble oxalates in foods may decrease the absorption of calcium from other foods.[67]

When the diet was adequate in the nutrients required by the rat (e.g., 0.61 per cent calcium, 0.71 per cent phosphorus, 20 per cent casein, 8 per cent yeast), the addition of 0.9 per cent potassium oxalate did not influence growth rate of weanling rats nor their bone ash level during the 10 weeks of the study.[68] When the level of potassium oxalate was raised to 2.5 per cent, bone ash was reduced slightly without any change in growth rate. On the basis of Kohman's analyses,[64] the 2.5 per cent potassium oxalate would be equivalent to about 13 per cent dried spinach. Similar results were secured when 10 children (5 to 8 years of age) were fed "simply prepared common foods" to which 100 gm canned spinach was added.[69] Over a period of 60 to 85 days, the retention of calcium, phosphorus, and nitrogen was not influenced by the spinach added to the diet, when compared to the preceding control period.

A more direct toxic effect has been associated with the ingestion of rhubarb leaves. The leaves contain about three to four times as much oxalic acid as the stalks.[65] A number of cases of poisoning, reportedly due to this food, have appeared, most of them during World War I,[63] but others more recently. One of the more recent involved four 3- to 6-year old children who ate the raw leaves and stalks.[70] One of these children had convulsions. Individuals who develop mild symptoms of oxalic acid poisoning following the ingestion of rhubarb complain of gastroenteritis with abdominal pain, diarrhea and vomiting —occasionally with hematemesis. In severe cases, hemorrhagic diathesis, dysuria, hematuria, convulsions, collapse, noncoagulability of blood, and coma are seen.[65]

Certain household plants may prove potentially more dangerous a poison than rhubarb. One woman who supposedly took only one bite of the stalk of a *Dieffenbachia sequine* plant developed severe edema of the face, tongue, palate, and buccal mucosa. Since she was unable to swallow, she was given fluids intravenously. The report[71] indicated that the corrosive burns were due to the presence of calcium oxalate and certain unidentified glycosides. However, the symptoms exhibited by this patient do not fit those usually associated with oxalate poisoning. Since the Dieffenbachia plant is so commonly displayed in homes and offices, it may pose a danger to small children.

The problem of oxalate poisoning is even more acute and severe in certain western states where a range crop, the halogeton, may contain as much as 37 per cent oxalic acid on a dry weight basis.[72] The use of this plant as fodder by sheep has resulted in large numbers of deaths. According to one report, the most effective means of preventing the mortality is to provide another source of feed, such as alfalfa pellets containing 15 per cent calcium carbonate, when sheep are grazing in areas heavily infested with the halogeton plant.[73]

Although the most apparent action of oxalates would appear to be on calcium metabolism, it is still not certain that this is the primary locus of action. As far as calcium absorption is concerned, there is evidence that animals become adapted to the presence of oxalates in the ration. This was shown by the change in the negative calcium balance during the first few days after the ration fed to cattle was supplemented with small amounts of soluble oxalate. Thereafter, the calcium balance gradually became positive.[74] The improvement in the calcium balance was associated with the metabolism of the oxalate to carbonate. Some pharmacologists[75] claim that the toxicity of oxalates can be overcome completely by administering calcium salts. Other investigators[73] claim that sheep given large amounts of oxalates did not recover when infused with calcium gluconate; the calcium merely prolonged life for a few days.

Fish and Iron Deficiency. A report from Norway[76] indicated that when mink were fed certain species of raw fish (coal fish, *Gadus virens*, or whiting, *Gadus merlangus*), they became severely anemic and died. Parenteral iron therapy cured this anemia. Additional work by another group[77] suggested that the substance making the dietary iron unavailable was located primarily in the viscera. This substance was inactivated by cooking.[78]

That more than a simple sequestering of iron is involved in this problem is suggested by the finding that, when the young of mink that had developed anemia while consuming the raw-fish ration were fed the same ration as their parents, they all developed anemia.[77] On the other hand, when young from "anemia-resistant" parents were fed the raw-fish ration, few, if any, developed anemia.

Not only may genetic factors be involved in this condition, but species differences may also exist. This was shown by the fact that weanling rats, when fed a ration containing 90 per cent of "gutted, raw coal fish (heads included)," showed no anemia and were able to reproduce.[79] When the young were continued on the raw-fish ration, they developed a severe hypochromic type of anemia. A statement is made by these Norwegian investigators that they "have fed 'raw fish diet' to female rats continuously through 10 generations. None of the parturient rats died during this 10-generation experiment."

LEGUMES

Soybeans. Although the major emphasis on the toxic factors in soybeans has centered around its antitryptic activity, this may be of only minor significance in explaining the poor growth of animals fed unheated soybean meal.[80] The antitryptic factor in soybeans was described by Read and Haas in 1938[81] and independently discovered by Ham and Sandstedt in 1944.[82] When this factor was described, it appeared to offer an explanation for the experimental findings with raw soybeans. However, shortly thereafter, various studies using amino acid rations to which crude soybean trypsin inhibitors were added indicated that some other factor was responsible for the poor growth-promoting properties of raw soybeans.[2]

The effect of heat in improving the nutritional value of soy proteins was recognized as early as 1917 when Osborne and Mendel[83] showed that rats grew better after the soybean meal had been heated. One of the early explanations for the effect of heat involved a change in the protein so that the sulfur amino acids became more available.[2,84] The metabolic explanation for this observation is still not clear. Recent work has shifted from an emphasis on the poor absorption of the sulfur amino acids in raw soybeans to a disturbance in the metabolism of cystine and methionine when raw soybeans are fed to rats. This involves an increase in the percentage of labeled carbon dioxide expired by rats given a dose of labeled methionine.[85,86]

The hemagglutinating factor in soybeans has also been eliminated as a possible factor responsible for growth inhibition. A part of the evidence for its inactivity came from Liener's work wherein he showed there was no relation between the hemagglutinating activity of his preparations and their growth-depressing activity.[87]

At present, there is no valid explanation for the growth-inhibiting action of raw soybeans. It is likely that the growth inhibition may be due to a number of factors. Most of the harmful effects seen when raw soybeans are fed largely disappear when the meal is properly toasted.

Even properly heated soybean meal may produce a zinc deficiency when this meal is the primary protein in rations fed various species of animals. The explanation for the appearance of this deficiency is related to the phytic acid content of soybean meal.[88] Especially when an excess of calcium is present in the ration, the binding of the zinc by the phytic acid in the soybean produces symptoms of a severe zinc deficiency.[89,90]

The development of a zinc deficiency is not limited to rations containing soybeans as the source of protein; a similar deficiency develops when sesame meal is used in rations fed to chicks.[91] In all these cases, the addition of extra zinc to the soybean or sesame meal ration restored the growth rate of the animals to normal.

Iodine is another mineral deficiency associated with the ingestion of soybean meal. The work of McCarrison[92] led him to suggest the presence of a goitrogenic substance in soybean meal, since large amounts of iodine in the diet did not prevent the development of this condition. Subsequent work with rats[93,94] and chicks[95] indicated that the iodine requirement is increased when soybeans are included in the ration and that heating the soybeans does not completely eliminate this effect.

With the wider use of soybean milk as a liquid formula for infants, a few reports have appeared describing enlarged thyroids in a few infants fed this formula.[96-100] In all of these cases, the heat treatment used in processing the soybean meal was adequate to destroy its "goitrogenic" property.[96] Not all soy products used in infant formulas are "goitrogenic."[101] The addition of iodine to the previously offending liquid soy formula has apparently eliminated the thyroid enlargement previously seen.[102]

Lathyrism. Lathyrism is a neurologic disease seen only in human subjects who have consumed fairly large amounts of *Lathyrus sativus* (chickling vetch), *L. cicera* (flat-podded vetch), or *L. clymenum* (Spanish vetchling).[103] *L. sativus* is cultivated in India and grows wild in the Tian Shian mountains (in western China); *L. cicera* is used as cattle fodder in France, Italy and Algeria and is used in making bread when wheat is difficult to get; *L. clymenum* is grown in Spain, North Africa and the Orient.[104] The symptoms seen in human subjects were described by Cantani in 1873 who gave the disease its

current name.[104] However, the condition has been recognized for many centuries, with one of the earliest descriptions provided by Hippocrates.[105] This disease has occurred in the countries bordering the Mediterranean, with Algeria having more cases than the other countries; it is endemic in India where as many as 7 per cent of the people in certain villages are afflicted with lathyrism.[103,106]* The lathyrus plants grow when severe drought reduces the regular food supply. Under such conditions or during famines associated with high food prices, these legumes may make up as much as one-third to one-half the total diet.[103] If the high consumption of these legumes continues for six months or more, lathyrism frequently follows.[106]

Human lathyrism is frequently referred to as neurolathyrism as suggested by Selye.[105] This condition usually develops in individuals between the ages of 15 and 30 years and occurs 12 to 20 times more frequently in men than in women.[104,108] The first symptoms are a feeling of heaviness of the legs with weakness setting in shortly thereafter. While standing, the leg muscles become tremulous and when the individual starts to walk, he may drag his feet. The leg muscles may become spastic and rigid. The gait becomes jerky; short steps are taken with the subject walking on the balls of his feet. Tingling sensations are felt in various parts of the body. There may be complete loss of sensation to heat and pain.[108] Most of these symptoms are associated with lesions in the spinal cord. The lateral pyramidal tracts are usually degenerate with sclerosis of the spinal cord and funiculi of Goll.[104]

Although a number of attempts have been made to associate lathyrism with dietary deficiencies,[107,109] there is ample evidence that the consumption of the seeds of various lathyrus plants is responsible for the disease. This relationship was apparent from the time

* No cases of lathyrism were reported in Russia prior to 1890. At that time, the cultivation of *L. sativus* was started. The workers on a government estate at Saratoff received corn bread which contained a large amount of ground *L. sativus* seeds. Within six months, 33 men and 1 woman showed signs of lathyrism. Clinical descriptions of these cases are reviewed by Gardner and Sakiewicz.[104]

of Hippocrates and was especially evident in the sixteenth century. At that time, Prince George of Wurtenberg forbade the use of bread containing lathyrus (*L. sativus*) in his principality. An edict to that effect was promulgated when a number of his subjects developed lathyrism.[104,106]

More recently, many attempts have been made to isolate the toxic factor from lathyrus seeds. In most cases, the relevance of these compounds to human lathyrism remains obscure. Ressler and associates[110] isolated L-α,γ-diaminobutyric acid from seeds of *L. latifolius* (perennial sweet peas) and *L. sylvestris* (flat pea) and β-cyano-L-alanine from the seeds of *Vicia sativa*.[111] When given by stomach tube to rats, both these compounds produced hyperirritability, tremors, convulsions and, within two to three days, death. Subcutaneous administration produced less obvious neurologic symptoms. The concentration of these compounds in the pea and vetch seeds varied but ranged from about 0.1 to 1.5 per cent.

The cyanoalanine compound theoretically is related to the aminopropionitriles responsible for the development of osteolathyrism. Decarboxylation of the alanine compound should lead directly to the parent nitrile compound.[110] Whether this reaction occurs under natural conditions is unknown. The cyanoalanine and diaminobutyric acid, which were reported to produce neurotoxic symptoms in rats, have not been isolated from *L. sativus* and, for this reason, the significance of their physiologic reactions has been open to some question. The primary basis for this concern is the claim that "this syndrome is not an equivalent of the spontaneous neurolathryrism of man."[112]

A neurotoxic substance has been isolated from *L. sativus*. The first suggestion for such a substance came from a report that an alcoholic extract of the seeds, when injected into day-old chicks, produced retraction of the head and twisting and stiffening of the neck.[113] After a single injection, the symptoms disappeared in about 11 to 12 hours. The injection of small doses of the extract each day into the chicks maintained the symptoms permanently. One of the compounds isolated from the alcoholic extract

and associated with these symptoms was (β-N-oxalyl)-α,β-diaminopropionic acid.[114] Injection of 20 mg of this compound into day-old chicks produced neurologic disturbances with recovery after a few hours. Injection of 48 mg produced death. The susceptibility of different species to this compound varies as shown by the fact that when mice were injected intraperitoneally (48 mg per mouse), they showed no immediate symptoms but did drag their hind legs. That the oxalic acid present in the compound was not responsible for the symptoms became evident when an equivalent amount of that acid was injected into day-old chicks with no untoward results. That the oxalic acid is an integral part of the molecule was shown when the free diaminopropionic acid proved innocuous after injection into chicks.[115]

Much of the early experimental work with lathyrus seeds involved osteolathyrism or odoratism.[105] Both these terms are used to describe the condition produced in rats fed rations containing considerable amounts of the legume *L. odoratus*. When the ration contained 25 per cent ground seeds of this species, weanling rats developed deformities of the spinal cord in three to four weeks. These abnormalities were readily detected by means of x rays.[116] Similar skeletal abnormalities were seen when the ration contained *L. hirsutus* (caley pea) or *L. tingitanus* or *L. pusillus* (Singletary pea).[107,109,117]

The compound initially isolated from *L. odoratus* and shown to produce odoratism was β-(-N-γ-L-glutamyl)-aminopropionitrile.[117–119] This compound was present in five different varieties of *L. odoratus* at levels ranging from 58 to 160 mg per 100 gm, whereas in *L. pusillus* and *L. hirsutus*, its concentration was 62 and 21 mg per 100 gm respectively.[103] Shortly after the announcement of its structure, three different laboratories showed that the gamma glutamyl group was not essential for its action.[103]

The incorporation of the active compound, β-aminopropionitrile, in a ration at a level of 0.1 to 0.2 per cent reproduces all the symptoms seen when *L. odoratus* is fed. The symptoms include skeletal abnormalities involving kyphosis, scoliosis, increased shaft diameter, exostoses and rib cage deformities; hernias, which are otherwise rare in rats; reproductive failure; and dissecting aneurysms of the aorta.[103,109] All these changes are traceable to alterations in collagen. The collagen of rats with odoratism is "abnormal both in form and distribution"[112] resulting in a reduction in its tensile strength. Studies with isotopic sulfur indicate that the primary change is a failure in the formation of chondroitin sulfates A and C and their complexes with proteins resulting in a defect in fibrogenesis.[112]

The defect in odoratism involving primarily collagen formation is in contrast to the human disease or lathyrism in which the essential lesion involves the nervous tissue.

Intriguing results have been secured in the isolation of toxic compounds from both the *L. odoratus* and *L. sativus* groups of peas. However, the substance responsible for the development of human lathyrism still appears to be unknown. The oxalyl diaminopropionic acid, which on intraperitoneal injection produces neurologic alterations in chicks, ducklings, and pigeons, has no visible effect when injected into monkeys (C. Gopalan, personal communication).

Favism. Sensitivity to fava or broad beans appears to be an example of an inherited metabolic disturbance. In sensitive individuals, the inhalation of pollen from these plants or ingestion of the bean in either the cooked or raw state produces a hemolytic anemia. Sensitive individuals show a deficiency of glucose-6-phosphate dehydrogenase in their blood and consequently a reduction in glutathione blood levels.[120] The glutathione level in the red blood cells of these individuals is still further reduced following the eating of fava beans. Hemolysis of the older red cells follows. Why the younger red cells are resistant to this action is unknown. This explains why, except under peculiar conditions, the individuals recover once the hemolysis ceases.[121] The means whereby the toxic substance in fava beans lowers the glutathione content of the blood are unknown.

Most of the sensitive individuals are children of parents who originated from the Mediterranean area, Asia, or Taiwan.[122] Since the enzymatic deficiency in favism appears to be common to a number of other disturbances, it is assumed to be transmitted in the same way, *i.e.*, sex linked. It is the mother of the affected males who carries the genetic defect.[121] Favism may be more complicated than is suggested by the enzymatic deficiency seen in individuals with this disease. This is evident from the fact that not everyone who is deficient in this enzyme develops hemolysis of the blood after eating fava or broad beans. There are many Negroes who have this enzymatic defect, but favism is seen rarely in these individuals. They do, however, exhibit hemolysis when treated with the antimalarial compound, primaquine, certain sulfonamides, and a number of other compounds, but not by broad beans.[121]

In some areas of the world, the sensitivity to fava or broad beans affects a fair proportion of the people. In June 1965, along the Caspian Sea in Iran, there were 1143 individuals who developed hemolysis following the ingestion of broad beans; of these, 16 died.[123] In that area, the hemolytic condition routinely affects a large number of people especially during spring, with a peak load in June when broad beans are harvested. In Iran, the hemolysis is reported to occur to a greater extent among adults than children. Nothing is said as to whether this unusual age distribution is associated with the exclusion of the bean from the diets of the children. It was also stated that the incidence of favism was almost five times greater among men than women.

From a nutritional standpoint, it is important to bear in mind the widespread occurrence of favism. This admonition is especially important for individuals making agricultural recommendations in various parts of the world. On Taiwan, where a fair proportion of the population has favism, the Joint Commission on Rural Reconstruction has been advocating the cultivation of fava beans as a dietary staple and as a green fertilizer.[124]

The toxic substance in fava beans does not appear to have been isolated. Reports from Taiwan[124–126] claim that the toxic substance is vicine (2,4-diamino-6-hydroxypyrimidine-β-D-glycopyranose). This is present in fava beans to the extent of about 0.5 per cent of their dry weight.

FOODS THAT ARE TOXIC
UNDER SPECIAL CIRCUMSTANCES

Cheese. The presence of various symptoms in patients receiving monoamine oxidase inhibitors is an illustration of a food toxicity seen in special groups of people. These individuals complained of hypertension with its resulting crises—severe headache and palpitation. Initially, these disturbances were considered side effects of the monoamine oxidase inhibitors. It was almost 10 years after the introduction of these drugs that the "side effects" became associated with the consumption of cheese.[127]

The monoamine oxidase inhibitors are used to treat patients with depressive states. These drugs inhibit the enzyme that "destroys" serotonin, norepinephrine, and related neurohormonal compounds. As a result of this and possibly other reactions, the drugs produce a euphoric state.

The tyramine in cheese is a potent vasopressor substance. Under normal circumstances, it would be metabolized through the action of the monoamine oxidases. When the activity of these enzymes is inhibited by any of the drugs used in treating patients with various depression states, then the tyramine from the cheese can act on the blood vessels producing severe hypertension and its sequelae. They may include a painful stiff neck and sometimes nausea and vomiting in addition to headaches and palpitation.[127-130] A few fatalities have occurred in patients treated with one of the monoamine oxidase inhibitors after eating cheese.[131-135]

Tyramine in cheese is formed by the decarboxylation of tyrosine. This and other amino acids are liberated during the ripening of cheese by bacteria acting on the peptides formed from the action of renin on casein.[127] Other foods normally contain pressor amines without the intervention of bacterial action. One of these is broad beans (*Vicia faba L.*) which also precipitates headaches, palpitation, and hypertensive crises in patients treated with monoamine oxidase inhibitors.[128,129] In this case, the pressor amine responsible for the difficulties is 3,4-dihydroxyphenylalanine (dopa).

The concentration of tyramine in cheese is related to the ripening or maturation time, bacterial flora, and manufacturing process. Cheddar cheese is reported to contain sufficient tyramine to produce a hypertensive crisis in patients treated with a monoamine oxidase inhibitor. Different samples of cheese vary considerably in their tyramine content.[127] Only limited information is available as to the dose of pressor amines that is dangerous for patients being treated with the monoamine oxidase inhibitors. Tyramine is 1/20 to 1/50 as active as adrenalin in producing hypertension.[136] It has been proposed that 25 mg of tyramine are a dangerous dose for patients treated with monoamine oxidase inhibitors. On this basis, 4 of 22 samples of cheese approached that value in an average serving of 50 gm. The concentration of tyramine in these cheeses ranged from 0 to 1 mg per gm.[127] Another group reported that only 6 mg of tyramine by mouth were sufficient to produce a blood pressure increase in patients treated with monoamine oxidase inhibitors. This amount of tyramine could be secured by eating 20 gm of ordinary cheddar cheese or a glass of Chianti wine.[137]

In normal individuals, there is a dramatic rise in the urinary excretion of p-hydroxyphenylacetic acid after eating cheese. This acid is probably derived from tyramine by oxidation with monoamine oxidase and aldehyde oxidase.[136] Unfortunately, this work was not extended to include patients treated with monoamine oxidase inhibitors. It was reported that after two weeks of receiving one of these inhibitors, the concentration of 5-hydroxytryptamine in the brain was twice that in the brain of patients not receiving the inhibitor.[138]

Wheat Gluten. Patients with celiac disease are now recognized as being sensitive to certain fractions of wheat gluten. This disease has many of the symptoms seen in patients with idiopathic and tropical sprue.[139] A number of early investigators reported that the elimination of wheat from the diet produced an improvement in the condition of celiac patients. Even the so-called banana diet, as originally proposed by Haas,[140] was one that completely eliminated wheat.[141] Despite these early suggestions of a dietary involvement in celiac disease, the treatment continued to be primarily symptomatic. However, the dramatic response secured by the Dutch investigators with one of their pediatric patients when wheat gluten was added to or removed from the diet was enough to establish this protein as the dietary factor associated with the symptoms seen. When wheat gluten is removed from the diet of these patients, improvement occurs in all aspects of the disease, but it may require as long as a year before the individual is completely restored to normal functioning.[139]

The observation of the Dutch investigators[142] that the removal of wheat from the diet of these patients improved their condition immediately focused attention on the proteins in that cereal.[143] Since gluten contains fairly large amounts of glutamine, this compound was given to patients with celiac disease, but it had no effect on the patients' condition.[144] An extension of these studies showed that following the ingestion of wheat, patients with celiac disease showed a greater increase of bound glutamine in their blood than normal children.[145,146] According to Frazer,[139] these glutamine-containing peptides have no deleterious effects, but they "provide some evidence for a faulty barrier function of the intestinal mucosa of these patients."

The exact fraction of wheat gluten responsible for the syndrome is unknown. A number of investigators have shown that predigesting wheat gluten with either pancreatin or pepsin or trypsin did not destroy the factor toxic to celiac patients.[147] Earlier, Frazer[148] showed that an enzyme extract from hog intestinal mucosa destroyed the toxic substance. The same happened when wheat gluten was hydrolyzed with crude papain.[147] The latter enzyme preparation contained a deamidase which liberated ammonia during the conversion of N-L-glutamic peptides to the corresponding pyrrolidone carboxyl peptides. On this basis, it was suggested that the offending agent is a peptide that has L-glutamine as its N-terminal amino acid.

A complication has been introduced to this problem with the suggestion that precipitins to the antigens of wheat gliadin "are readily detected in approximately 50 per cent of sub-jects with well-documented gliadin-induced celiac disease."[149] On this basis, the precipitin reaction was proposed as presumptive evidence for the presence of the disease. This proposal would imply that either the intact gliadin protein crossed the intestinal mucosa or the antigenic portion of the molecule remained intact during digestion.

Inky Cap Mushrooms. Under ordinary circumstances, the consumption of the inky cap mushroom *Coprinus atramentarius* produces no unpleasant reactions. However, if an alcoholic beverage is drunk during or shortly after a meal that included this mushroom, the face of the drinker and perhaps other parts of his body soon become purplish-red.[150] Apparently, this mushroom contains a compound related to antabuse. So far, the compound has not been isolated. Indirect evidence suggests it is not antabuse.[151]

MUSHROOMS

Poisoning due to the ingestion of mushrooms has occurred for many centuries. One of the early incidents involved the deaths of the wife and three children of the Greek poet Euripides in the fifth century B.C.[152] A fair number of cases have occurred in France with a mortality rate of over 40 per cent.[153] In England, between 1920 and 1945, 38 fatalities from eating mushrooms were reported.[153] In the United States, less than 2 per cent of the cases reported to the National Clearinghouse for Poison Control Center involved mushrooms.[154] A partial explanation for the few cases of mushroom toxicity stems from the fact that only a few species are toxic. For instance, although there are over 800 species of these plants in New England, only 53 are considered poisonous (see reference 155 for a list of the toxic mushrooms and colored photographs of the more poisonous varieties).

In the 37-year period following 1924, there were 24 deaths in the United States attributable to mushroom poisoning.[155] Half these were associated with the eating of mushrooms of the *Amanita* species and the others to *Gyromitra esculenta* and unidentified mushrooms. These fatalities resulted from mushrooms that were collected by the individual or someone other than a commercial producer. There is one nonfatal epidemic in which canned mushrooms imported from Taiwan produced headaches and varied neurologic disturbances in 55 of 80 women who ate a soup prepared with these mushrooms.[156] In the latter cases, the symptoms appeared within minutes after eating the soup containing mushrooms. The symptoms resembled those attributable to *Amanita muscaria*.

Apparently there is considerable variability among individuals to mushroom toxicity. Part of this results from: (1) Difficulty in classifying the mushrooms. The Amanita, among which are some of the more poisonous mushrooms, pose the greatest taxonomic problesm.[50] For many years, the white, yellow, green, gray, brown, and black mushrooms that resembled *A. phalloides* were believed to be variants of the same species. More recently, it has been recognized that these are different species and that they differ markedly in their content of toxins.[157] (2) Development of sensitivity to the mushroom or variation in its toxicity. For the same mushroom, *Gyromitra esculenta*, there are reports that it can be eaten once without any disturbances, but frequently on the second or third occasion, toxic manifestations follow its consumption.[158] Another report states that this same "mushroom has caused poisoning in persons who had eaten it for years without ill-effect, and small, localized groups of cases have occurred more frequently in some years than others."[155] Presumably, this variability in toxicity was due to "climatic or other undetermined factors." Recent studies of the same species of mushrooms collected in the same park show a variability in toxin concentration from none to a high value.[157] (3) Individual predilection to mushroom toxicity. Some people are able to eat mushrooms with impunity, while others develop severe toxicity when eating the same kind.[156,159,160]

In the United States, two of the more toxic mushrooms are *Amanita phalloides* and *A. muscaria*.[50] The toxic principles in these two differ in that the former contains cyclopeptides and the latter alkaloid-like compounds. The ingestion of *A. phalloides* and its close

relatives accounts for most of the fatal cases of mushroom poisoning.[50]

Most of the toxic mushrooms contain more than one toxic compound. For instance, the *A. phalloides* mushrooms contain at least five toxins that are related biochemically since they are all cyclopeptides that have only a few amino acids, some of which do not occur in proteins.[161] Each of the toxins contains one sulfur atom which is not present as a sulfhydryl group. At least two of these toxins (α- and β-amanitine) are heat-stable and for them there is no effective antidote.[154] Treatment of patients with severe poisoning after eating these mushrooms involves careful fluid and electrolyte therapy.[153] Although an antitoxin against *A. phalloides* was reportedly prepared at the Pasteur Institute in France as far back as 1925, its use in other countries appears to have been extremely limited since the best that can be said for it is that "There is no clear record of its effectiveness in man."[153,162]

The symptoms associated with the ingestion of the toxic *A. phalloides* mushroom do not appear for 10 to 20 hours. At that time, the individual suddenly experiences severe abdominal pain, vomiting, and diarrhea. Excessive thirst develops with anuria. Hemoglobinuria is absent. The severe pain may be accompanied by screams alternating with periods of temporary remission. The patient rapidly loses strength and may die within 48 hours after eating large quantities of the mushrooms. In less severe cases, jaundice, cyanosis, and marked coldness of the skin may appear after two to three days, with death occurring on the sixth to eighth day. Death is frequently preceded by coma and occasionally by convulsions. Autopsy reveals fatty degeneration and necrosis of the liver and kidney, degeneration of areas in the central nervous system, and hemorrhagic areas in various organs.[49,152] Animal studies have shown that one of the major disturbances following the ingestion of these mushrooms involves a reduction in liver glycogen level and the failure of this to be restored following glucose therapy.[161] Despite these biochemical studies, the mechanism whereby the toxins of *A. phalloides* produce their effects is obscure.

The other important mushroom toxicant is muscarine which is found in *Amanita muscaria*, from which it was isolated in 1869,[162] *Amanita pantherina* and certain species of the *Boletus*, *Russula*, and *Clitocybe* genera.[154] Muscarine is a heat-stable quaternary ammonium base which resembles choline esters in some of its actions. Most of its effects are attributable to stimulation of the parasympathetic postganglionic nerves.[162] Frequently within minutes to, at most, a few hours after eating these mushrooms, the individual exhibits excessive salivation and lacrimation; contracted pupils that do not respond to light; nausea and frequent vomiting; excruciating abdominal pains with severe diarrhea; dizziness and confusion may appear, with convulsions in the more advanced state.[152] In one group of women, who presumably had consumed mushrooms containing muscarine, the symptoms were limited to headache, malaise, and muscular tingling, especially of the facial muscles.[156] Atropine is the specific antidote and must be given in sufficiently large doses (0.5 to 15.0 mg subcutaneously every four hours) to dilate the pupils and inhibit sweating.[162]

For the peace of mind of the reader who may be a gourmet and enjoys mushrooms with his meals, it should be pointed out that the domestically cultivated varieties (*Agaricus bisporus*) are free of any toxic substance and that the more poisonous species are not amenable to cultivation.[156]

FISH

Allergic Reactions. This problem is subject to a great deal of conflicting testimony, partly because of the psychoneurotic factor in many allergic reactions[163] and the confusion in classifying fish by the lay public. The problems arising from the former difficulty are illustrated by the report of a man who developed asthma after eating salmon croquettes. The cook put the croquettes in the refrigerator near the butter. The next day, the butter had a slight flavor reminiscent of salmon. When the man used the butter, he promptly developed asthma.[164] The commercial classification of fish frequently differs from that recognized by the ichthyologists.

For instance, weak fish is often called sea bass and perch may be bass, a true perch, or a sea bass.[164] A related problem exists among the solutions used in testing for food sensitivity. Antigenically, the same preparation from a variety of sources showed "a marked lack" of uniformity in antigenic components.[165]

It has been stated that "fish and shellfish are known to serve as powerful allergens which in some persons may produce almost explosive reactions."[166] These reactions include urticaria, angioneurotic edema, gastrointestinal disturbances, and migraine, with asthma and coryza seen less frequently. Attempts have been made to classify fish on the basis of those to which an allergic individual might be sensitive, *e.g.* those allergic to cod might also react to trout, carp, herring, and sardines. Whether such a classification will survive is doubtful since there are reported cases of allergies to one specific type of seafood with no reactions to other closely related species.[164,166]

Biotoxins. *Mollusks—Paralytic Shellfish Poisoning.* Mussels and clams and occasionally scallops and oysters from both the Atlantic and Pacific coastal areas as well as such other areas as South Africa, New Zealand, Belgium, Germany, France, England, and Ireland have produced poisoning in man.[166] This poisoning is associated with the growth in the water of the dinoflagellate (unicellular organisms with a cell wall composed of cellulose, and with two or more flagella arranged transversely and longitudinally to facilitate a whirling motion as they advance), *Gonyaulax catenella*, and, perhaps, *G. tamarensis* and *Pyrodinium phoneus*. These organisms produce a poison that is retained in the dark gland or hepatopancreas of the mussel or other shellfish feeding on these organisms. The shellfish show no disturbance as a result of the toxin. However, should the contaminated seafood be eaten by man, symptoms of toxicity usually develop in from one half to three hours after eating.[4]

The symptoms associated with paralytic shellfish poisoning include a numbness of the lips and fingertips with an ascending paralysis and finally death from respiratory paralysis. Death may occur in 3 to 20 hours after eating the shellfish. Should the person survive the first 24 hours, the prognosis for his complete recovery is good.[4] Mortality among the individuals who develop paralytic shellfish poisoning is reported to be about 8.5 per cent.[166] In most areas, the poisoning is confined to local residents who dig for their own shellfish. In the Alaskan coastal area, the problem becomes of more importance to general public health, since the shellfish from this area are canned or frozen with a wide distribution.

As a protective measure along United States and Canadian coastal waters, a quarantine is posted whenever the toxicity of the shellfish becomes dangerous. The toxicity is determined by injecting an aqueous extract of the shellfish into mice. The time elapsing from the intraperitoneal injection of the extract until death occurs is a measure of the toxicity.[166,167] Even this measure is not completely adequate, since sampling of shellfish from various areas in the same region may suggest low levels of toxicity while other areas nearby may have highly toxic shellfish. This was evident when 32 persons in one region became ill "before sampling techniques indicated that a quarantine should have been established."[166]

Ordinary cooking procedures reduce the toxicity but not enough to make the seafood safe for eating. Since about 95 per cent of the poison is concentrated in the digestive organs or dark meat,[167] removal of those tissues would make the seafood safe; the white meat contains no poison.[166] The toxicity disappears from mussels once the dinoflagellates leave the water. This was evident when mussels were removed from contaminated water and placed in water free of dinoflagellates; they lost their toxicity in a few days.[168] The Alaskan butter clams, on the other hand, retain their toxicity for long periods of time. The source of the poison in the Alaskan clams is not known for certain, since the water where these clams grow contains large numbers of plankton but none of these appears to be toxic.[167] That an organism comparable to the dinoflagellates is probably responsible is suggested by the isolation of the same toxic compound from butter clams and the dinoflagellates.[169]

The compound isolated from both the Alaskan butter clams and axenic cultures of the dinoflagellates has been given the name "saxitoxin."[169] This word comes from the scientific name for the butter clams, *Saxidomus giganeus*. The compound has the formula $C_{10}H_{17}N_7O_4$. The toxin appears to block nerve transmission in the motor axon and not at the end-plate. This is presumably brought about by blocking the increase of sodium conductance normally associated with excitation. On the basis of experiments with cats, it was estimated that the lethal dose of this toxin for an adult would be 0.4 mg administered intravenously.[170] By the oral route, the toxic dose has been suggested as 8 mg.[171]

Squid and Octopus. Fresh squid and octopus have produced a seasonally occurring toxicity among the inhabitants of certain areas in Japan. This toxicity involves primarily the gastrointestinal tract and recovery usually occurs within 48 hours. The nature of the toxin appears to be unknown.[166]

Minamata Disease. The toxicity associated with the consumption of fish from Minamata Bay on the island of Kyushu in Japan illustrates some of the problems that occur in the field of fish poisons. The first recognition of any disturbance among the people who lived along the shores of Minamata Bay was in 1953. These individuals complained of numbness of the extremities, slurred speech, unsteady gait, deafness, and visual disturbances. Mental confusion and muscular incoordination were apparent in all patients. The mortality rate was 33 per cent. Since all patients had eaten fish caught in the bay, fishing there was prohibited.[172]

A few years prior to the appearance of this disease, a large chemical plant in that area had dug a new drainage ditch. From then on, the effluent from the factory was poured into the bay rather than into the ocean where it had gone previously.[173]

Shellfish gathered from the shores of the bay proved toxic when fed to cats, which showed a variety of neurologic disturbances.[172,174] Although selenium was suggested as the most likely toxin,[172] ashing the shellfish so as to retain this element produced a nontoxic residue when incorporated into the ration of cats at the same level as the intact shellfish.[174]

Reports from Japanese investigators indicated that organic mercury compounds in the fish were responsible for the toxicity.[175] This seemed plausible since the mercury catalyst used by the chemical plant in the manufacture of vinyl polymers was discarded through the drainage ditch into the bay. One report suggested that the toxic compound was dimethyl mercuric sulfide.[176]

That the problem has not been closed is suggested by a report claiming that mercury toxicity is not responsible for the Minamata episode.[177] It was stated that the concentration of mercury in the silt at the mouth of the stream carrying the effluent from the vinyl plant is no greater than that in silt secured from comparable bays near which other chemical plants are located. Furthermore, it was claimed that the mercury content of fish from Minamata Bay is no greater than that in fish from many other places where no symptoms of toxicity have been seen.

Poisonous Fishes. A large number of fish have been reported to be poisonous when eaten.[166,178] Many of these are found in tropical waters in the regions around coral reefs with most of the deep-sea fish being nontoxic except for the barracuda.[179] Most of the cases of poisoning associated with the eating of poisonous fishes have come from Japan.[180] For most of these, the compound responsible for the poisoning has not been isolated or at best has been only sketchily characterized.[178] A large number of the poisonous fish, when eaten, produce neurologic symptoms for which there are no palliative measures.[181]

Fish containing the ciguatera toxin are distributed in a global belt extending from latitude 35° N to 35° S.[182,183] Within this belt, the toxicity of fish varies insofar as both geographic and species distribution are concerned. For instance, about half the fish caught to the north of the lagoon entrance to Christmas Island one year were toxic, while only one-fifth of those caught to the south of the entrance about 6 miles away were toxic. Furthermore, in the same area of the Pacific, the toxicity of the same species

of fish varies from year to year. This toxin appears in such fish as the snapper, grouper, sturgeon, jack, and moray eel.[183]

Ciguatera toxin has not been isolated in pure form. There was some discrepancy as to the solubility of the toxin in water,[184] but there now appears to be agreement that it is insoluble in water and perhaps absolute ethanol. Ether and other fat solvents appear best adapted for the extraction of the toxin from fish.[182]

Different species of animals vary in their response to the toxin. Mice appear weakly sensitive to the intraperitoneal injection of an aqueous suspension of toxic fish muscle, but when given a larger dose by mouth, the material was nontoxic.[184] On the other hand, the cat and mongoose are susceptible to orally administered fish containing ciguatera toxin.[183]

The puffer fish toxin was at one time believed identical with the paralytic shellfish toxin but more complete studies indicate certain differences in their actions.[185] For one thing, the shellfish poison is more toxic for dogs and cats than the compound from puffer fish. They also differed in their effects on ECG of the dog and cat, with the greatest difference in the isolated rabbit heart where the puffer poison had no effect, while the shellfish poison had marked cardiotoxic effects.

Final evidence for the difference in these compounds was provided by the group working with Mosher.[186,187] These investigators found that the crystalline compound isolated from the puffer fish (*Sphoeroides rubripes*) is the same as a compound present in the eggs of the California newt (*Taricha torosa*). Both compounds were nontoxic when large amounts were injected into newts, while much smaller amounts killed rats, mice, frogs, goldfish, and tiger salamanders within a few minutes. This toxin "appears to occur only in one family of Amphibia (the Salamandridae) and one suborder of fishes (the Tetraodontoidae). This extremely limited distribution is a remarkable biogenic finding."[187] The historical development of the research that led to the identification of these two compounds is described by Mosher *et al.*[187]

The puffer fish is a delicacy among many

groups of people. Special skill is required to remove all the viscera completely when preparing it for serving. Mosher *et al.*[187] record that four soldiers came upon a bonfire where native fishermen had roasted some of these fish. They had left the livers of the fish on shells. Despite the dire warnings of a native, the soldiers ate a little of the liver—some of them only chewing one bite without swallowing any. The first soldier who ate a little of the liver died in half an hour, the others at varying intervals during the next 24 hours. Recent data from Japan indicate that in 1956 to 1958, there were 715 individuals who were poisoned from eating this fish and that 59 per cent of them died.[187]

The highest concentration of toxin occurs in the ovaries of the fish; this varies through the year, with the highest concentration occurring just before spawning in the spring.[187] Lesser amounts are found in the liver and skin. The formula for the toxin is $C_{11}H_{17}N_3O_8$ and the structure proposed for it is that of a spirane-type compound.

CYCAD

Cycads are palm-like trees consisting of nine species growing mainly in the tropics and subtropics. The use of cycads by the peoples on various southwest Pacific islands stems from the fact that this is one of the few plants capable of surviving adverse climatic conditions. Prior to and during World War II, it provided a source of calories during droughts and following severe typhoons as well as being a supplement when food supplies became low because of military action.[1]

Widespread interest in cycad toxicity developed when amyotrophic lateral sclerosis was suspected of being associated with the ingestion of flour prepared from cycad nuts. The incidence of amyotrophic lateral sclerosis is 100 times greater among the Chamoro Guamanians than among the inhabitants of the United States or Europe. Human patients suffering from amyotrophic lateral sclerosis progressively become paralyzed in their extremities and die about five years after the onset of symptoms. There is presently no known cure for this disease. In an attempt to determine the etiology of

amyotrophic lateral sclerosis, investigators at the National Institutes of Health were impressed by the reported similarity of this disease to the paralytic symptoms seen in cattle and sheep that had eaten cycads.[1] The people on Guam use the seeds of the cycad both as an emergency source of food and to a lesser extent as a regular part of their diet. The starchy center or the kernels of the seeds are used in thickening various dishes (soups, tortillas, fruit desserts), while the outer husk of the seed is used as a confection.

For many years, the Guamanians recognized that the kernels of *Cycas circinalis* are toxic. They attempt to eliminate the toxin by soaking pieces of the kernel in vats of water. The water may be changed several times during a soaking period of 7 to 10 days. After soaking, the kernels are dried in the sun and then ground to a powder which is stored in a convenient place. The composition of this powder is similar to that of wheat flour.[188]

The recent work in this area was initiated by the assumption that the soaking process might not always completely remove the toxic agents from the cycad kernel. To evaluate this possibility, cycad kernels were obtained from Guam. These had been processed by the Guamanians and were purchased at their local markets. This material was ground and then incorporated into diets fed to rats over a period of almost two years. The results of that study indicated that the processed kernel was relatively safe for the rats. Nevertheless, the experimental animals lost more body weight under adverse laboratory conditions than the control rats. This occurred when the temperature in the animal room fell rapidly in conjunction with a sudden and severe drop in the external temperature. During the study, 6 of 45 experimental rats died and another 7 rats were sacrificed because they were moribund. None of the 15 control rats died or became moribund during this time.[189]

In contrast to the processed kernel, the unprocessed kernel is toxic when fed to rats at high levels, and carcinogenic when fed at lower levels over a five- to seven-month period. Benign and malignant tumors developed, mainly in the liver and kidneys of the latter animals. None of these rats or any of those fed the processed kernel developed any neurologic symptoms.[190] Furthermore, other animals, including cows, horses, swine, and guinea pigs, when fed the unprocessed kernel, did not develop neurologic disturbances. Microscopic examination of the brain and spinal cord of these animals revealed no lesions that could be traced to cycad kernels.[191]

The neurologic disturbances originally described by Australian investigators as occurring in cattle grazing on cycad leaves[1,192] have also been described among cattle grazing in the highlands of the Dominican Republic.[193] These cattle exhibited a "goose-stepping" gait with posterior weakness and ataxia. By means of the Marchi stain, it was possible to "demonstrate destruction of myelin around single nerve fibers" in the fasciculus gracilis, dorsal spinocerebellar, lateral corticospinal, ventral corticospinal, and medial longitudinal fasciculus tracts. A preliminary report suggests that a compound isolated from the cycad kernel produces neurologic disturbances when injected into chicks. The compound presumably responsible for this is "a new amino acid, α-amino-β-methylaminoproprionic acid."[194] The relationship of this observation to the conditions observed in animals fed cycad products will require further study. The amounts of the compound needed to produce neurologic changes in chicks appear to be much larger than the animals would secure when consuming rations containing toxic levels of cycad kernel.

Current findings suggest that the neurologic symptoms associated with the ingestion of cycad by experimental animals occur especially when the leaves of these plants are eaten. There also may be a neurotoxic compound in the seeds to which chicks are more susceptible than are rats.

Another part of the cycad (*Cycas circinalis*), the husk, is chewed fresh by the Guamanians to relieve thirst, or, when dried, eaten as candies. The husk is not processed except for drying.[1] When the dried husk was fed to rats, acute toxicity symptoms appeared within a few days. The rats showed an increase in hemoglobin and hematocrit con-

centrations. Those rats fed rations containing 6 per cent or more of husk in the diet died in about 10 days. Autopsy revealed massive hemorrhages in the gastrointestinal tracts which were probably the immediate cause of death. Other symptoms included ascites, an intense yellow color of the urine, and edema under the skin near the sternum. The pancreas of these rats was white and edematous and resembled curdled milk.[195] Rats fed lower concentrations (0.5 to 1.0 per cent of husks) developed tumors in the liver, kidneys, and other internal organs much like those fed unwashed cycad kernels.

The identification of the toxic substance in cycad stems from the simultaneous isolation of a crystalline substance, cycasin, from cycad seeds (*Cycas revoluta*) by the Australian[197] and Japanese workers.[196] This compound was identified as methylazoxymethanol-β-glucoside. The aglycone of this glucoside, methylazoxymethanol, is common to the glycosides present in other species of cycad.[197,198] The latter glycosides have sugars other than glucose linked to the aglycone.

The beta glycoside linkage in cycasin explains why the glycoside is nontoxic when injected into conventional animals[199] or fed to germ-free animals.[200] To liberate the active aglycone requires a beta glucosidase and these enzymes are present only in bacteria and not in mammalian cells. When the bacterial action in the gastrointestinal tract is circumvented by injection or when no bacteria are present, as in germ-free animals, cycasin remains intact and, as such, is nontoxic. A possible exception to the absence of beta glucosidases in mammalian tissues comes from the observation that cycasin injected into day-old rat pups was toxic.[201] After a single injection, these animals developed kidney tumors when they were about five months old. It is possible that another explanation besides the presence of beta glucosidases in newborn rats may cover this situation. After the injection, the pups may have excreted all the cycasin in their urine and this may have been consumed by their dam in whose gastrointestinal tract hydrolysis of the cycasin may have occurred. The aglycone may then have been secreted in the milk, thus producing the tumors.

Evidence for the preceding suggestion comes from the finding that when pregnant rats are fed either unprocessed kernel or cycasin, the fetuses show typical toxic effects.[191,202] The transplacental transfer of the toxic agent was sufficient to produce liver tumors at a later date in the progeny of the pregnant rats. The toxic factor can also be transferred from dam to young through the milk. This is true for lactating rats, cows, and pigs.[191]

The public health implications of these findings are difficult to evaluate. For one thing, there is considerable variation in species susceptibility to the carcinogenic effects resulting from cycad feeding. Even if human beings are susceptible to the carcinogenic agents in the cycad, it is possible that most of these compounds have been removed during the processing to which the kernels are subjected by the Guamanians. It should, however, be recognized that there is a possibility that these compounds (in the unprocessed husk) may be consumed by both pregnant and lactating women. Under such circumstances, the compounds may be transferred to the fetuses or nursing infants who, presumably, are especially susceptible to such toxicities. The dangers may be enhanced by the transmission of these compounds through cows' milk which may be used by the infants and children where cycad plants are endemic.

MISCELLANEOUS AGENTS

Kuru. This is a degenerative disorder of the central nervous system restricted to Melanesian natives of one region of the eastern highlands of New Guinea. Death occurs in less than one year in most patients. It is transmitted by eating the brains of close relatives.[203]

Cyanide Poisoning. In many areas of the tropics persons who consume large amounts of foods rich in cyanogenic glycosides (*e.g.* cassava) develop a slowly progressive ataxic neuropathy which often includes bilateral nerve deafness and optic atrophy. Thiocyanate is found in high concentration in the blood of patients with this disease, probably as a result of detoxification of cyanide. Clinical improvement results from a reduction of the amount of cassava in the diet and

the substitution of noncyanogenic foods.[203] Cycasin, the toxic substance in cycad, also is a cyanogenic glycoside.

Chattos. Monstrous lambs with midfacial malformations (cyclopian sheep, chattos) have been born to ewes in certain Rocky Mountain herds which have fed on *Veratrum californicum*, an herb that grows only in the high altitude ranges grazed by the affected herds. The active teratogens in *V. californicum* have been found to be cyclopamine, cycloposine, and jervine, all steroids with a rigidly positioned tetrahydrofurylpiperidine side chain at C–17.[204]

Aflatoxin. In the summer of 1960 there was an outbreak of a new disease in turkeys in farms within a 100-mile radius of London, England. The loss of poults was estimated to be over 100,000, with death due to acute liver necrosis. Shortly thereafter there was an outbreak of this "turkey X disease" in Cheshire. The common factor between these two outbreaks was Brazilian groundnut meal in the food. A similar disease was found to have occurred in Brazil and Africa: all had in common groundnuts in the food. Most toxic samples of groundnuts were found to be heavily contaminated with *Aspergillus flavus*, and toxic material was obtained from cultures of the fungus grown on heat-sterilized, nontoxic nuts.[205] It was named "aflatoxin."

Subsequently aflatoxin was found to be made up of four substances, B_1, B_2, G_1, and G_2, with B_1 being the most toxic. It apparently interacts with DNA and prevents the DNA polymerase transcribing the DNA, and thereby inhibits DNA synthesis and RNA polymerase.[205] Thus protein synthesis is inhibited and cell death ultimately results.[205] Aflatoxins are toxic to every animal species tested, and aflatoxin B_1 is the most potent hepatocarcinogen known.[206] It has been demonstrated that aflatoxin B_1 produces cytological changes in human embryonic lung cell cultures[207] and inhibits the growth of human liver cells.[208] *Aspergillus flavus* has been shown to contaminate and grow on stored cassava, beans, peas, and cereals, as well as groundnuts.[206]

Alpert *et al.*[206] determined the aflatoxin levels in 480 food samples stored for consumption between harvests and collected from different parts of Uganda, in 1966–1967. They found that 29.6 per cent of their samples contained detectable levels of aflatoxins and that 3.7 per cent contained more than 1 μg/kg. The frequency of aflatoxin contamination was particularly high in provinces with a high hepatoma incidence, or where cultural and economic factors favored the ingestion of moldy foods. The authors suggest that aflatoxin exposure may account for the high incidence of hepatoma in Uganda and perhaps elsewhere.

BIBLIOGRAPHY

1. Whiting: Econ. Botany, *17*, 271, 1963.
2. Mickelsen and Yang: Fed. Proc., *25*, 104, 1966.
3. Rosenfeld and Beath: *Selenium, Geobotany, Biochemistry, Toxicity and Nutrition*. New York, Academic Press, 1964.
4. Schantz: In *Venomous and Poisonous Animals and Noxious Plants of the Pacific Region*, ed. by Keegan and McFarlane. New York, Pergamon Press, 1963, p. 75.
5. Rodahl: *Hypervitaminosis A*. Norsk Polarinstitutt Skrifter Nr. 95, Oslo, 1950.
6. Rodahl and Moore: Biochem. J., *37*, 166, 1943.
7. *Composition of Foods*, Agric. Handbook No. 8, 1963 ed., U.S. Dept. Agric.
8. Moxon: *Alkali Disease or Selenium Poisoning*, S. Dakota Agric. Exp. Sta. Bull. 311, Brookings, S. Dakota, May 1937.
9. Fromm and Stokes: J. Water Pollut. Cont. Fed., *34*, 1151, 1962.
10. Schwarz and Foltz: J. Amer. Chem. Soc., *79*, 3292, 1957.
11. Mertz: Fed. Proc., *26*, 186, 1967.
12. O'Leary: Arch. Environ. Health, *9*, 216, 1964.
13. Persson, Tunnell and Ekengren: Acta Pediat. Scand., *54*, 49, 1965.
14. Soler-Bechara and Soscia: Arch. Int. Med., *112*, 462, 1963.
15. Gerber, Raab and Sobel: Amer. J. Med., *16*, 729, 1954.
16. ———: Nutr. Rev., *12*, 370, 1954.
17. Moore: *Vitamin A*. Amsterdam, Elsevier Pub. Co., 1957.
18. Light, Alscher and Frey: Science, *100*, 225, 1944.
19. Walker, Eylenberg and Moore: Biochem. J., *41*, 575, 1947.
20. Friend and Crampton: J. Nutr., *73*, 317, 1961.
21. Stitt: Nutr. Rev., *21*, 257, 1963.
22. Roe: New York J. Med., *66*, 869, 1966.
23. Lightwood: Arch. Dis. Child., *27*, 302, 1952.
24. Scott: *Vitamin D in Nutrition*. Madison, Wis., Wis. Alumni Res: Fdn., 1965.
25. Stapleton, MacDonald and Lightwood: Amer. J. Clin. Nutr., *5*, 533, 1957.
26. Roe: New York J. Med., *66*, 679, 1966.
27. Stewart, Mitchell, Morgan and Lowe: Lancet, *1*, 679, 1964.
28. Forfar, Balf, Maxwell and Tompsett: Lancet, *1*, 981, 1956.
29. Cuthbertson: Brit. J. Nutr., *17*, 627, 1963.
30. Feller: New Eng. J. Med., *259*, 1050, 1958.
31. Clark and Bassett: J. Exp. Med., *115*, 147, 1962.
32. Bicknell and Prescott: *Vitamins in Medicine*, London, Wm. Heinemann Med. Books Ltd., 1942, p. 598.
33. Meyer and Angus: Arch. Dis. Child., *31*, 212, 1956.
34. Lisk: New York J. Med., *71*, 2541, 1971.
35. Smith: J.A.M.A., *116*, 562, 1941.
36. Smith, Franke and Westfall: Pub. Health Reports, *51*, 1496, 1936.
37. Smith and Westfall: Public Health Rep., *52*, 1375, 1937.
38. Hadjimarkos and Bonhorst: J. Pediat., *52*, 274, 1958:
39. Leach and Lloyd: Trans. Ophthal. Soc. U.K., *76*, 453, 1956.
40. ———: Proc. Nutr. Soc., *15*, XV, 1956.
41. Aydelotte: J. Embryol. Exp. Morph., *11*, 279 and 621, 1963.
42. Rodger, Saiduzzafar and Grover: Amer. J. Ophthal., *50*, 309, 1960.
43. Klosterman, Lamoureux and Parsons: Biochemistry, *6*, 170, 1967.
44. Deutsch and Hasler: Proc. Soc. Exp. Biol. Med., *53*, 63, 1943.
45. Melnick, Hochberg and Oser: J. Nutr., *30*, 81, 1945.
46. Jacobsohn and Azevedo: Arch. Biochem., *14*, 83, 1947.
47. Hilker and Peter: J. Nutr., *89*, 419, 1966.
48. Shewan: In *Fish as Food*, ed. by Borgstrom. New York, Academic Press, 1962, Vol. 2.
49. Berlin: Acta Med. Scand., *129*, 560, 1948.
50. Kingsbury: *Poisonous Plants of the United States and Canada*. Englewood Cliffs, N.J., Prentice-Hall, Inc., 1964.
51. Pamukcu, Yalciner, Price and Bryan: Cancer Res., *30*, 2671, 1970.
52. Kundig and Somogyi: Int. Z. Vitaminforsch., *34*, 135, 1964.
53. Fujiwara and Matui: J. Biochem., *40*, 427, 1953.
54. Clements: Med. J. Austral., *2*, 894, 1954.
55. Greer: Borden Rev. Nutr. Res., *21*, 61, 1960.
56. Roche and Lissitsky: In *Endemic Goitre*. Geneva, WHO, 1960, p. 351.
57. Clements and Wishart: Metabolism, *5*, 623, 1956.
58. Peltola and Krusius: Acta Endocrinol., *33*, 603, 1960.
59. Peltola: Acta Endocr., *34*, 121, 1960.
60. Kreula and Kiesvaara: Acta Chem. Scand., *13*, 1375, 1959.
61. Virtanen, Kreula and Kiesvaara: Z. Ernährungswiss., Suppl. 3, 23, 1963.
62. Vilkki, Kreula and Piironen: Ann. Acad. Sci. Fenn., Ser. A. II. Chem. 110, 1962.

63. Tisdall, Drake, Summerfeldt and Jackson: J. Pediat., *11*, 374, 1937.
64. Kohman: J. Nutr., *18*, 233, 1939.
65. Jeghers and Murphy: New Eng. J. Med., *233*, 208, 1945.
66. Zarembski and Hodgkinson: Brit. J. Nutr., *77*, 627, 1962.
67. Editorial: J.A.M.A., *109*, 1907, 1937.
68. MacKenzie and McCollum: Amer. J. Hyg., *25*, 1, 1937.
69. Bonner, Bates, Horton, Hunscher and Macy: J. Pediat., *12*, 188, 1938.
70. Kalliala and Kauste: Nutr. Abstr. Rev., *35*, 485, 1965.
71. Drach and Maloney: J.A.M.A., *184*, 1047, 1963.
72. Cook and Gates: J. Range Manage., *13*, 97, 1961.
73. Cook and Stoddart: Utah Agr. Exp. Sta. Bull. 364, 1953.
74. Telapatra, Ray and Sen: J. Agric. Science, *38*, 163, 1948.
75. Sollmann: *Manual of Pharmacology.* Philadelphia, W. B. Saunders Co., 1948.
76. Helgebostad and Martinsons: Nature, *181*, 1660, 1958.
77. Stout, Oldfield and Adair: J. Nutr., *70*, 421, 1960.
78. ———: J. Nutr., *72*, 46, 1960.
79. Gjönnes and Helgebostad: Acta Vet. Scand., *6*, 239, 1965.
80. Pusztai: Nutr. Abstr. Rev., *37*, 1, 1967.
81. Read and Haas: Cereal Chem., *15*, 59, 1938.
82. Ham and Sandstedt: J. Biol. Chem., *154*, 505, 1944.
83. Osborne and Mendel: J. Biol. Chem., *32*, 369, 1917.
84. Mitchell and Smuts: J. Biol. Chem., *95*, 263, 1932.
85. Barnes and Kwong: J. Nutr., *86*, 245, 1965.
86. Kwong and Barnes: J. Nutr., *81*, 392, 1963.
87. Liener and Pallansch: J. Biol. Chem., *197*, 29, 1952.
88. O'Dell and Savage: Proc. Soc. Exp. Biol. Med., *103*, 304, 1960.
89. Oberleas, Muhrer and O'Dell: J. Anim. Sci., *21*, 57, 1962.
90. Forbes: J. Nutr., *83*, 225, 1964.
91. Lease, Barnett, Lease and Turk: J. Nutr., *72*, 66, 1960.
92. McCarrison: Indian J. Med. Res., *21*, 179, 1933.
93. Sharpless, Pearsons and Prato: J. Nutr., *77*, 545, 1939.
94. Halvorson, Zepplin and Hart: J. Nutr., *38*, 115, 1949.
95. Wilgus, Gassner, Patton and Gustavson: J. Nutr., *22*, 43, 1941.
96. Van Wyk, Arnold, Wynn and Pepper: Pediatrics, *24*, 752, 1959.
97. Shepard: Pediatrics, *24*, 854, 1959.
98. Shepard, Pyne, Kirschvink and McLean: New Eng. J. Med., *262*, 1099, 1960.
99. Hydovitz: New Eng. J. Med., *262*, 351, 1960.
100. Ripp: Amer. J. Dis. Child., *102*, 106, 1961.
101. Sarett: Pediatrics, *24*, 855, 1959.
102. Anderson and Howard: Pediatrics, *24*, 854, 1959.
103. Strong: Nutr. Rev., *14*, 65, 1956.
104. Gardner and Sakiewicz: Exp. Med. Surg., *21*, 164, 1963.
105. Selye: Rev. Canad. Biol., *16*, 1, 1957.
106. Dastur and Iyer: Nutr. Rev., *17*, 33, 1959.
107. Lewis, Fajans, Esterer, Shen and Oliphant: J. Nutr., *36*, 537, 1948.
108. Stockman: J. Pharmacol. Exp. Ther., *37*, 43, 1929.
109. Geiger, Steenbock and Parsons: J. Nutr., *6*, 427, 1933.
110. Ressler, Redstone and Erenberg: Science, *135*, 188, 1961.
111. Ressler: J. Biol. Chem., *237*, 733, 1962.
112. Weaver and Spittel: Proc. Staff Meet. Mayo Clin., *39*, 485, 1964.
113. Roy, Nagdrajan and Gopalan: Current Sci. (India), *32*, 116, 1963.
114. Murti, Seshadri and Venkitasubramanian: Phytochem., *3*, 73, 1964.
115. Adie, Rao and Sarma: Current Sci. (India), *32*, 153, 1963.
116. McKay, Lalich, Schilling and Strong: Arch. Biochem. Biophys., *52*, 313, 1954.
117. Duprey and Lee: J. Amer. Pharm. Ass., *43*, 61, 1954.
118. ———: Nutr. Rev., *21*, 28, 1963.
119. Schilling and Strong: J. Amer. Chem. Soc., *77*, 2843, 1955.
120. Zinkham *et al.*: Bull Johns Hopkins Hosp., *102*, 169, 1958.
121. Beutler: In *The Metabolic Basis of Inherited Disease*, ed. by Stanbury, Wyngaarden and Fredrickson. New York, McGraw-Hill Book Co., 1966.
122. ———: Brit. Med. J., *2*, 1140, 1965.
123. Iranian Institute Nutrition, First Report of the Symposium on Research Relating to Favism in Iran, August 1965, Teheran, Iran.
124. Lin and Ling: J. Formosan Med. Ass., *61*, 484, 1962.
125. ———: J. Formosan Med. Ass., *61*, 490, 1962.
126. ———: J. Formosan Med. Ass., *61*, 579, 1962.
127. Blackwell and Mabbitt: Lancet, *1*, 938, 1965.
128. Blomley: Lancet, *2*, 1181, 1964.
129. Hodge, Nye and Emerson: Lancet, *1*, 1108, 1964.
130. ———: Nutr. Rev., *23*, 326, 1965.
131. Read and Arora: Lancet, *2*, 587, 1963.
132. Mann: Lancet, *2*, 639, 1963.
133. Foster: Lancet, *2*, 587, 1963.
134. Womack: Lancet, *2*, 463, 1963.
135. Blackwell: Lancet, *2*, 414, 1963.
136. Asatoor, Levi and Milne: Lancet, *2*, 733, 1963.
137. Horwitz, Lovenberg, Engelman and Sjoerdsma: J.A.M.A., *188*, 1108, 1964.
138. MacLean, Nicholson, Pare and Stacey: Lancet, *2*, 205, 1965.

139. Frazer: Advances Clin. Chem., *5*, 69, 1962.
140. Haas: Amer. J. Dis. Child., *28*, 421, 1924.
141. Weijers and Van de Kamer: Amer. J. Clin. Nutr., *11*, 51, 1965.
142. Dicke, Weijers and Van de Kamer: Acta Paediat., *42*, 34, 1953.
143. Weijers, Van de Kamer and Dicke: Advances Pediat., *9*, 277, 1957.
144. Van de Kamer and Weijers: Acta Paediat., *44*, 465, 1955.
145. Weijers and Van de Kamer: Acta Paediat., *44*, 536, 1955.
146. ———: Acta Paediat., *48*, 17, 1959.
147. Messer, Anderson and Hubbard: Gut, *15*, 259, 1964.
148. Frazer: Proc. Roy. Soc. Med., *49*, 1009, 1956.
149. Heiner, Lahey and Wilson: Amer. J. Dig. Dis., *9*, 786, 1964.
150. Kingsburgy: *Poisonous Plants of the United States and Canada*. Englewood Cliffs, N.J., Prentice-Hall, Inc., 1964, p. 96.
151. Weir and Tyler: J. Amer. Pharm. Assoc. Sci. Ed., *49*, 426, 1960.
152. Van der Veer and Farley: Arch. Int. Med., *55*, 773, 1935.
153. Grossman and Malbin: Ann. Int. Med., *40*, 249, 1954.
154. Cann and Verhulst: Amer. J. Dis. Child., *101*, 127, 1961.
155. Buck: New Eng. J. Med., *265*, 681, 1961.
156. Rose and Rieder: Ann. Int. Med., *64*, 372, 1966.
157. Tyler, Benedict, Brady and Robbers: J. Pharm. Sci., *55*, 590, 1966.
158. Smith: *Mushrooms in Their Natural Habitat*. Portland, Oregon, Sawyer's Inc., 1949, p. 152.
159. Murrill: Mycologia, *2*, 255, 1910.
160. Deerness: Mycologia, *3*, 75, 1911.
161. Wieland and Wieland: Pharmacol. Rev., *11*, 87, 1959.
162. Grollman: *Pharmacology and Therapeutics*. Philadelphia, Lea & Febiger, 1962.
163. Burden: Ann. Int. Med., *43*, 1283, 1955.
164. Fenton: In *Practice of Allergy*, by Vaughn and and Black. St. Louis, C. V. Mosby Co., 1948.
165. Cohen: J. Allerg., *30*, 267, 1959.
166. Halstead: In *Fish as Food*, ed. by Borgstrom. New York, Academic Press, 1962, Vol. 2.
167. Schantz: Ann. N.Y. Acad. Sci., *90*, 834, 1960.
168. Sommers, Whedon, Kofoid and Stohler: Arch. Pathol., *24*, 537, 1937.
169. Schantz, Lynch, Vayvada, Matsumoto and Rapoport: Biochemistry, *5*, 1191, 1966.
170. Kao and Nishiyama: J. Physiol., *180*, 50, 1965.
171. Meyer: New Eng. J. Med., *249*, 843, 1953.
172. McAlpine and Araki: Lancet, *2*, 629, 1958.
173. Kurland, Faro and Siedler: World Neurol., *1*, 370, 1960.
174. Mickelsen and Laqueur: Unpublished data.
175. Irukayama, Kondo, Kai and Fujiki: Kumamoto Med. J., *14*, 157, 1961.
176. Uchida, Hirakawa and Inoue: Kumamoto Med. J., *14*, 181, 1961.
177. Kiyoura: Air Water Pollut., *7*, 459, 1963.
178. Courville, Halstead and Hessel: Chem. Rev., *58*, 235, 1958.
179. Davidson and Passmore: *Human Nutrition and Dietetics*, 3rd ed. Baltimore, The Williams & Wilkins Co., 1966.
180. Kawabata: In *Fish as Food*, ed. by Borgstrom. New York, Academic Press, 1962, Vol. 2, p. 467.
181. Halstead: *Dangerous Marine Animals*. Cambridge, Maryland, Cornell Maritime Press, 1959.
182. Hessel, Halstead and Peckham: Ann. N.Y. Acad. Sci., *90*, 788, 1961.
183. Banner, Scheuer, Susaki, Helfrich and Alendar: Ann. N.Y. Acad. Sci., *90*, 770, 1961.
184. Banner and Buroughs: Proc. Soc. Exp. Biol. Med., *98*, 776, 1958.
185. Murtha: Ann. N.Y. Acad. Sci., *90*, 820, 1961.
186. Buchwald, Durham, Fisher, Harada, Mosher, Kao and Fuhrman: Science, *143*, 474, 1963.
187. Mosher, Fuhrman, Buckwald and Fischer: Science, *144*, 1100, 1964.
188. Campbell, Mickelsen, Yang, Laqueur and Keresztesy: J. Nutr., *88*, 115, 1966.
189. Yang, Mickelsen, Campbell, Laqueur and Keresztesy: J. Nutr., *90*, 153, 1966.
190. Laqueur, Mickelsen, Whiting and Kurland: J. Nat. Cancer Inst., *31*, 919, 1963.
191. Mickelsen, Campbell, Yang, Mugera and Whitehair: Fed. Proc., *23*, 1363, 1964.
192. Edwards: J. Bur. Agr. W. Austral., *1*, 225, 1894.
193. Mason and Whiting: Fed. Proc., *25*, 533, 1966 (abst.).
194. Bell and Vega: Fed. Proc., *26*, 322, 1967 (abst.).
195. Yang, Campbell, Keresztesy, Laqueur and Mickelsen: Fed. Proc., *24*, 626, 1965.
196. Nishida, Kobayashi and Nagahama: Bull. Agr. Chem. Soc. Japan, *19*, 77, 1955.
197. Riggs: Chem. Industr., *35*, 926, 1956.
198. Cooper: J. Proc. Royal Soc. (New South Wales), *74*, 450, 1941.
199. Nishida, Kobayashi, Nagahama, Kojima and Yamane: Seikagaku (Biochemistry), *28*, 218, 1956 (in Japanese). See ref. 1.
200. Laqueur: Fed. Proc., *23*, 1386, 1964.
201. Magee: *Fourth Conference on the Toxicity of Cycads*, ed. by Whiting. Bethesda, Maryland, National Institutes of Health, 1965.
202. Spatz and Laqueur: Fed. Proc., *25*, 662, 1966 (abst.).
203. Anon: Brit. Med. J., *2*, 481, 1972.
204. Mulvihill: Science, *176*, 132, 1972.
205. Rees: Gut, *7*, 205, 1966.
206. Alpert, Hutt, Wogan and Davidson: Cancer, *28*, 253, 1971.
207. Legator, Zuffante and Harp: Nature, *208*, 345, 1965.
208. Gabliks: Fed. Proc., *24*, 626, 1965.

Chapter

11

Additives and Pesticides in Foods

BERNARD L. OSER

CHEMICAL ADDITIVES TO FOOD

The complexities of modern urbanized society have placed increasing demands on growers and processors of food for products of uniform composition with organoleptic appeal, of good keeping quality, in sanitary, packaged form, and convenient to prepare in the home. To achieve these objectives, it is necessary to exercise a high degree of technological skill and quality control at all stages, and entails the judicious use of chemicals. Scientists are well aware of the fact that all natural foods are complex mixtures of chemicals, many of which can be demonstrated to be toxic in excessive dosage. The deliberate addition of chemicals to food, however, is often looked upon with concern by the laity. It is not unreasonable, therefore, that strict legislative controls be adopted to insure protection of the public health. Even such traditional methods of chemical preservation as the use of salt, smoke, spices, etc. have come under regulatory scrutiny in the light of modern methods for the toxicological assessment of safety.

The avenues by which chemicals may enter the food supply are best illustrated by the definition of food additives in the Federal Food, Drug and Cosmetic Act: ". . . any substance the intended use of which results or may reasonably be expected to result, directly or indirectly, in its becoming a component or otherwise affecting the characteristics of any food (including any substance intended for use in producing, manufacturing, packing, processing, preparing, treating, packaging, transporting, or holding food; and including

any source of radiation intended for any such use . . ."[1] Under the law, all such additives must be safe for use, including even those classes of substances exempt from certain of the regulatory requirements for prior approval as defined in the Act.

This broad definition thus includes not only substances introduced intentionally into food to achieve desired purposes, but those which become components of foods indirectly and unintentionally, such as through contact with equipment or containers. It is important to recognize that incidental or accidental chemical contaminants are not food additives, although in rare cases, where they are considered to be unavoidable, tolerances or guidelines have been established limiting their presence in foods. Under Federal law, additives to food are not permitted if their use is unsafe, deceptive, or not in accord with good manufacturing practice. The legal definition makes no distinction between natural substances, such as spices and essential oils, and synthetic chemicals, even though the latter may be identical in composition with naturally occurring substances.

The basic purpose of the food additive amendment to the Food, Drug and Cosmetic Act is to require approval by the Food and Drug Administration of the evidence establishing the safety of use of a food chemical prior to its introduction into interstate commerce. Several classes of substances, as indicated above, are not included in the category of food additives as defined in the statute, because their regulatory control is exercised under other sections of the Act. For example, to the extent that pesticide chemicals are used in production, storage and transportation of raw agricultural commodities, they are defined as "economic poisons" under the Federal Insecticide, Fungicide and Rodenticide Act.[2] When pesticide residues are present in processed foods, as ready to eat, at levels not greater than those permitted in the raw agricultural commodities they are exempt from the category of food additives. However, when the concentration of pesticide residue in a processed food exceeds the tolerance set for the raw agricultural commodity the food is adulterated, unless it conforms to a specific food additive regulation. A similar exemption applies in the case of a dye, pigment or other coloring substance, provided that, when added or applied to a food, it conforms to the color additive regulations prescribed for its safe use.

Not included in the statutory definition of food additives are those substances which are used in accordance with sanctions or approvals granted prior to enactment of the food additives amendment. This exemption includes substances permitted in foods for which definitions and standards of identity have been established by the Food and Drug Administration and those permitted by the Department of Agriculture under the Poultry Products Inspection Act or the Meat Inspection Act. Also included under the "prior sanction" exemption are substances granted specific approval for use by FDA through direct communication with individual firms before enactment of the food additives amendment.

A major category of substances not encompassed under the food additives definition is those which are deemed to be generally recognized as safe, under the conditions of intended use, by scientists qualified by training and experience to evaluate food safety. The law provides that these scientists base their judgments upon "scientific procedures" and, in the case of substances used prior to 1958, upon "experience based on common use in food." The necessary expertise specified under the regulations is "sufficient training and experience in biology, medicine, pharmacology, physiology, toxicology, veterinary medicine, or other appropriate science to recognize and evaluate the behavior and effects of chemical substances in the diet of man and of animals." General recognition of safety is not the prerogative of any special group of scientists, in government or out, so long as these qualifications are met. For example, the Flavor and Extract Manufacturers' Association has published long lists of substances used in food flavors which a panel of independent scientists has evaluated as GRAS (generally recognized as safe).[3,4]

Publication of a "complete" GRAS list by the Food and Drug Administration is not mandatory. Shortly after enactment of the food additives amendment, the Food and Drug Administration promulgated a partial list of substances and their respective uses for review by appropriately qualified scientists. This was eventually published (and dubbed the "white list") as Section 121.101 of the food additive regulations.[5] In accordance with the recommendation made at the White House Conference on Food, Nutrition and Health in 1969, this list, as well as other substances believed to have prior sanction, is being reviewed at the present writing from the standpoint of current usage and criteria for safety evaluation. When this review and assessment will have been completed, it is expected that a revised GRAS list will be published by the Food and Drug Administration and substances not included thereon either will be subject to specific food additive regulations or will be dropped from use.

In accordance with a recent pronouncement of the Food and Drug Administration, certain restrictions have been imposed on the eligibility of substances for classification as GRAS.[6] In order to qualify, they must meet the following criteria: (1) Substances of natural biological origin must have been widely consumed for their nutrient properties prior to 1958 without detrimental effect; (2) Such substances would qualify also if modified only by "conventional processing" as practiced prior to 1958. No announcement will be promulgated in the Federal Register in cases falling under (1) and (2) above. However, affirmation by Food and Drug Administration and notice in the Federal Register will be required (3) "Where processing may reasonably be expected to significantly alter the composition of the substance"; or (4) where breeding or selection may alter the composition to a degree sufficient to affect the nutritive value or concentration of toxic constituents, or in the case of (5) distillates, isolates, extracts, concentrates, or reaction products of GRAS substances, or (6) substances of natural biological origin intended for consumption for other than their nutrient properties, or (7) substances not of natural biological origin but identical with a natural GRAS component. GRAS classification will not be assigned if a substance has no history of food use or if its safe use requires setting a limitation. Any substance not meeting the criteria paraphrased briefly in (3) to (7) above will require a food additive regulation.

This new interpretation of the statutory requirements for GRAS status raises a number of questions which will doubtless have to be resolved in the coming years.

Pesticides. Under the Food, Drug and Cosmetic Act, a pesticide chemical is an economic poison as defined under the Federal Insecticide, Fungicide, Rodenticide Act, *viz.*:

"... (1) any substance or mixture of substances intended for preventing, destroying, repelling, or mitigating any insects, rodents, nematodes, fungi, weeds, and other forms of plant or animal life or viruses, except viruses on or in living man or other animals, which the Secretary shall declare to be a pest, and (2) any substance or mixture of substances intended for use as a plant regulator, defoliant or desiccant."

Each type of pesticide is more explicitly defined in that Act.

The production of an adequate food supply and its protection against predators and spoilage would not be possible without the use of pesticides. It has been estimated that man has been deprived of a fifth to a half of the total world food production through infestation and spoilage. A great variety of pesticidal chemicals is used, each with its own particular spectrum of activity against specific insects, mites, blights, weeds, or other agricultural pests. Legal tolerances have been established which limit the concentration of residue that may remain in or on a food crop, after allowing appropriate inter-

vals between the last application and harvesting and other "good agricultural practices" such as washing, stripping of outer leaves, etc. The practical efficacy of pesticides from the standpoint of the protection of agricultural productivity and the safety of applicators and farm workers is subject to approval by the U.S. Department of Agriculture which issues regulations governing their use. In the event that residues may remain after harvesting, the determination of safety and the setting of tolerance limits are the prerogative of the Department of Health, Education and Welfare, *i.e.* the Food and Drug Administration. Legal tolerances for pesticide residues on agricultural crops are set at levels far below the experimentally determined "no adverse effect" level in animals and are designed to assure the safety of foods as ready to eat.

Among the major categories (and examples) of pesticides are *chlorinated hydrocarbons* (DDT, dieldrin, aldrin, benzene hexachloride, chlordane, methoxychlor); cholinesterase inhibitors, including *organophosphorus compounds* (parathion, malathion, ethion) and *carbamates* (dithiocarbamates of iron, manganese and zinc, and dimethyl dithiocarbamates of manganese, and sodium); *dinitro compounds*, dinitro-ortho-cyclohexylphenol and its dicyclohexylamine salt; and *inorganic compounds* (arsenites of calcium, sodium, copper, lead and magnesium, and fluorides and bromides). Certain pesticides like pyrethrum, rotenone and piperonyl butoxide are exempt from tolerances when applied to growing crops but not if applied at or after harvest.

A number of pesticides had been approved for use on the ground that no residue remained on the fruits or vegetables, and hence it was not required to establish tolerances. Subsequently, it was found by the use of more sensitive analytical procedures that demonstrable amounts of these substances, albeit only traces, were present. Consequently, the regulations of the Food and Drug Administration requiring prior proof of safety were invoked. Since many of these substances were thought to be present in what was believed to be toxicologically inconsequential amounts, a procedure for establishing "negligible residue" tolerances has been adopted, which generally requires somewhat less extensive animal studies for safety evaluation.[7]

Color Additives. The addition of coloring agents to food is an age-old practice. Natural coloring agents, such as carmine, turmeric, annatto, and saffron, have been superseded to a large extent by synthetic organic compounds. Those in present food use in the United States are eight in number. They belong to the categories of *mono-azo compounds:* amaranth (FD&C Red No. 2), tartrazine (FD&C Yellow No. 5), and sunset yellow FSF (FD&C Yellow No. 6); *triarylmethane compounds:* brilliant blue FSF (FD&C Blue No. 1), fast green FSF (FD&C Green No. 3), and benzyl violet 4B (FD&C Violet No. 1); *erythrosine* (FD&C Red No. 3); and *indigotine* (FD&C Blue No. 2). Ponceau SX (FD&C Red No. 4) is permitted for use only in maraschino cherries and citrus red 2 only for coloring oranges; both are azo colors. The aluminum or calcium lakes of the FD&C colors are also used. In recent years, β-carotene (provitamin A) and several related synthetic carotenoids have found application as food colors.

All of these substances come within the scope of the color additives amendments to the Food, Drug and Cosmetic Act[8] since they are "capable (alone or through reaction with other substances) of imparting color" to foods. Incidentally, color is defined to include "black, white and intermediate grays," thus bringing carbon black and titanium dioxide under regulatory control. Pigments or dyes used in the fabrication of containers or packaging materials which impart chemically, but not visually, detectable traces to foods contained therein are considered to be food additives.

Not only is the usual evidence to demonstrate safety of food colors under the conditions of intended use a prerequisite for listing, but those substances formerly known as the coal-tar colors (designated by FD&C numbers) are required to be certified by the Food and Drug Administration. Accordingly, a sample of each production batch must be sent to Washington to be examined for identity and purity according to published speci-

fications, whereupon it is assigned a certification number, prior to shipment in interstate commerce.

FUNCTIONAL CATEGORIES OF FOOD ADDITIVES

Additives that are purposefully and intentionally introduced into foods to achieve specific effects during production or processing or to impart or retain a desired characteristic are classified as "direct" additives. Many of these have been exempt from food additive regulations on the ground that they are generally recognized as safe under the conditions of intended use. However, since these substances are currently under review and evaluation, no distinction will be made here between those that are GRAS and those subject to specific regulations. The functions of direct additives to foods are discussed and classified in a publication of the Food Protection Committee of the National Academy of Sciences—National Research Council.[9]

Functional effect and examples of substances used to achieve them include:

Acids, alkalies and buffering agents: widely used in food technology for neutralization and regulation of *p*H, particularly of acid foods, and to impart the acidity characteristic of various foods such as soft drinks and confections. *p*H control is essential in the dairy, brewing, baking and other fermentation industries. Among the agents used are: citric, acetic, lactic, phosphoric, malic and fumaric acids, glucono-delta-lactone, sodium, calcium and magnesium hydroxides, carbonates and bicarbonates, and various phosphates, citrates and tartrates.

Preservatives: used to prevent or inhibit spoilage due to bacteria, yeasts or molds, and are essential under modern conditions of storage, packaging and distribution of food. Examples are benzoic acid and benzoates, methyl and propyl parahydroxybenzoates, sulfur dioxide and sulfites, sodium and calcium propionate.

Antioxidants: added to retard rancidity and other oxidative changes in vegetable or animal oils, and fats, and in essential oils. Among the more common are butylated hydroxyanisole (BHA), butylhydroxytoluene

(BHT), propyl gallate, ascorbic and eryth-orbic acids, and thiodipropionic acid.

Sequestrants may be used to bind or chelate trace metals which tend to induce or accelerate changes in flavor, color, or turbidity. In addition to the salts of organic acids, such as the acetates, citrates, gluconates, and tartrates, this group includes various phosphates, pyrophosphates, and especially ethylenediamine tetraacetic acid (EDTA) and its calcium and sodium salts.

Emulsifying agents are employed to effect dispersion of oils in aqueous media, and vice versa, and are essential for the production of margarine, salad dressings, cheese spreads, frozen desserts, and confectionery. They are also used in the baking industry to regulate the volume and texture of bread and other bakery products. Included in this group are mono- and diglycerides of the fatty acids which occur in edible oils and fats, polyoxyethylene and sorbitan esters of these fatty acids (Spans® and Tweens®) and lactylic esters of fatty acids (stearyl-2-lactylic acid and its calcium salt).

Flavoring agents comprise by far the largest single category of direct food additives. They are used not only to impart aromatic and taste properties to foods, but also to mask objectionable organoleptic qualities and to adjust for variations in flavor intensity of natural foods. In addition to the aids and buffering agents mentioned above, they include spices and herbs, essential oils, oleoresins, extracts, gums, balsams, and a large number of chemical substances isolated from natural sources or produced synthetically; in either case, when known by its chemical name a substance is generally classed as "synthetic." Many of the latter are counterparts of naturally occurring components of fruits, berries, and other plant parts used as or in foods. Nearly a thousand natural and "synthetic" flavoring substances have been determined to be safe under the conditions of use.[3,4,10] Among the most common are vanillin, citral, eugenol, diacetal, cinnamic aldehyde, menthol, methyl anthranilate, and methyl salicylate.

Stabilizers such as various vegetable gums are employed for the purpose of imparting texture and body to foods like processed cheese, puddings, soups, confectionery, etc.

They help to prevent the separation of emulsions and the formation of graininess due to ice crystals in frozen desserts. In addition to certain common food components like starches, pectin, and gelatin, they include alginates, carrageen (Irish moss), gums derived from locust bean, karaya, tragacanth, and acacia, and synthetic cellulosic gums. In this functional category belong various chemically modified starches.

Maturing and bleaching agents are required in the milling and baking industries to accelerate the oxidation of flour and thus control the elasticity and stability of dough, *e.g.* during mechanical bread making. Among them are benzoyl peroxide, chlorine dioxide, potassium bromate, acetone peroxide and azodicarbonamide. Dough conditioners and yeast foods include a variety of chemicals essential to modern baking technology.

Anticaking agents are used in powdered foods such as salt, confectioners' sugar, baking powder, etc. to prevent lumping and to permit free flow. They include the silicates and stearates of calcium, magnesium and sodium, and aluminum calcium silicate.

Texturizing agents are used to retain the firmness or crispness of pickled or canned vegetables. Among them are alums (potassium or sodium aluminum sulfate) used in pickling cucumbers and several calcium salts, in canned peas, tomatoes, and potatoes.

Other substances are used for miscellaneous purposes such as to impart clarity or foaming property to beverages, to inhibit foaming during processing or filling operations, and as propellant gases in aerosol containers.

Indirect Additives. Modern methods of distribution of foods from growers and processors to retail outlets demand packaging in containers of great variety and size. The materials of which they are composed include wood, glass, paper, paperboard, metals, plastics, cotton and rubber. The largest single group of indirect additives are the components of food packaging materials which "may reasonably be expected to result . . . in (their) becoming a component . . . of any food."[1] Resins and lacquers are applied as coatings to metallic containers; waxes and synthetic polymeric resins are used to coat paperboard and other types of fiber packaging materials.

A multitude of chemical components are used to impart stability, flexibility, grease resistance, moisture repellency, clarity, color or other physical properties to containers. The components of cap liners and of adhesives employed in the fabrication of food containers also fall within the class of indirect additives.

The passage of the food additives amendment raised the question, for the first time in many instances, of whether or not any of the components of food packaging materials might "reasonably be expected" to become components of food. In certain cases, it was regarded as expedient by the industries concerned to include all substances then in use in the manufacture of food packages as potential food additives, hence a number of regulations of the "omnibus" type were promulgated covering paper and paperboard containers, plastics and resins, rubber, cap lacquers, and adhesives, to cite a few.

Processing aids such as defoaming, wetting, or washing agents may, in some cases, remain or leave residues in foods even though not intended and most of these come under food additive regulations. Fumigants and residues of extraction solvents also belong in this category as do filtration aids (e.g. fuller's earth) and synthetic polymers used as ion exchange resins.

Other types of indirect additives are those contained in foods derived from livestock and poultry whose feed contains growth promoting agents, e.g. coccidiostats, antibiotics, organic arsenicals, etc. The use of veterinary drugs for the prevention or treatment of diseases like mastitis in cows or blackleg and coccidiosis in poultry involves the risk that residues may be transmitted to foods (meat, milk, eggs) derived from animal sources. Regulations for the use of drugs in food-producing animals take into consideration the safety of residues of the drugs or their metabolites in food for man. Where relevant, withdrawal intervals are required prior to the collection of milk or eggs, or the slaughter of cattle, hogs, or poultry for food use.

Legal Aspects. Unless the use of a substance satisfies one of the statutory exemptions from the definition of a food additive, it is subject to the issuance of a regulation by the Food and Drug Administration specifying the permitted conditions of use. Any person may petition for such a regulation but, once issued, anyone may use the substance as identified, in the manner described. It falls upon the petitioner however to supply the required information upon which an appraisal of the safety under conditions of use may be made. The petition must contain:[11]

(A) the name and all pertinent information concerning such food additive, including, where available, its chemical identity and composition;

(B) a statement of the conditions of the proposed use of such additive, including all directions, recommendations, and suggestions proposed for the use of such additive, and including specimens of its proposed labeling;

(C) all relevant data bearing on the physical or other technical effect such additive is intended to produce, and the quantity of such additive required to produce such effect;

(D) a description of practicable methods for determining the quantity of such additive in or on food, and any substance formed in or on food, because of its use; and

(E) full reports of investigations made with respect to the safety for use of such additive, including full information as to the methods and controls used in conducting such investigations.

Difficulties are not infrequently encountered in defining the chemical identity of a substance, particularly if it is of natural origin, sufficiently to insure uniformity and reproducibility. The lack of suitably specific or sensitive analytical methods to detect and determine the presence of minute traces, e.g. of packaging "migrants" or other indirect additives, may present obstacles to the granting of petitions. However, the most critical information, viz. that relating to toxicological evaluation, is more often than any other factor responsible for rejection or delays in approval of petitions. The type of data generally required are:

(a) Acute oral toxicity tests in a minimum of two species of animals one of which should be a non-rodent (excluding rabbits). In addition to mortality data (usually expressed as the LD_{50}) premortal signs of toxicity, and gross post-mortem examinations should be recorded.

(b) Short-term oral toxicity studies (at least 90 days in rodents and 6 months in non-rodents) at multiple dosage levels, with observations of growth, physical appearance and behavior, efficiency of food utilization, hemocytological and hemochemical changes, urine analyses, tests of hepatic and renal function, and, post-mortem, gross autopsies, including the weighing of all major organs, and histopathologic examinations. The short term tests may be extended to provide reproductive or teratogenic data in rodents. The animals may be bred through two pregnancies, some of the females being delivered by cesarian section to permit observation of implantation and resorption sites, corpora lutea, prenatal mortality and teratologic abnormalities, as revealed upon examination of soft and skeletal tissues. In addition, observations are recorded for efficiency of fertilization, gestation, live and still births, postnatal survival to weaning and the number and weight of offspring.

(c) Long term oral toxicity studies in at least two species, one a non-rodent. These are generally run for 2 years, a major part of the life cycle of the rodent (but not, of course, of the dog or primate). In special cases, however, tests with non-rodents may continue for 5 to 10 years. The observations are similar to those made in the short term tests and are repeated entirely or in part, at 1, 3, 6, 9, 12, 18 and 24 months. Premortal signs and days of death or sacrifice of moribund animals are recorded. The study may be designed to yield additional data on reproduction and lactation efficiency by increasing the number of pregnancies in the parent or first generation, and continuing the study into several successive generations. More specific data on teratogenetic potential are obtained by administering test dosages to different groups prior to, during, or after the most critical period of fetal organogenesis, viz. the second trimester of pregnancy.

The main purpose of long-term studies in rodents is to reveal the possibility of a carcinogenic effect particularly in the highest dosage group. This is ideally set at the maximum level which will permit a sufficient number of the animals to survive beyond 1.5 years to permit statistically valid comparison of tumor incidence between the test and control groups. Examinations of microscopic sections for neoplastic changes are made by light microscopy, occasionally supplemented by electron microscopy.

Some investigators are recommending tests for mutagenic potential, particularly where carcinogenic or teratogenic effects are found or suspected. However, methodology cur-

rently available in this field is still under study, and interpretation in relation to human health hazard has not been sufficiently well established. The methods vary widely in principle and, in order to develop a body of data on the subject, it is proposed that at least three basic procedures be employed, viz. in vivo cytogenetic study involving karyotyping for the detection of chromosomal aberrations, the host-mediated assay in which mutagenic changes are observed in neurospora or E. coli injected intraperitoneally into treated animals, and the dominant lethal test in which treated males are mated with untreated females.[12]

A recent report of the Food Protection Committee of the National Academy of Sciences—National Research Council on the "Evaluation of the Safety of Food Chemicals"[13] has stated that:

Proper evaluation of the safety of a food chemical under the conditions of intended use takes into account:

(1) the food consumption pattern of the population concerned with particular reference to the amount, frequency and duration of intake of the substance in question and of chemically and pharmacologically related substances;
(2) the maximum no-adverse-effect level in test animals with particular reference to a species whose metabolic handling of the substance is similar to that in man;
(3) the application of a suitable safety factor, i.e. a fraction of the maximum no-adverse-effect dose in the test animal expressed in terms of mg per kg body weight (or per square meter of body surface) per day.

Where legal tolerances are set, they are based not on the maximum safe levels estimated from animal studies, but on the limits established by good manufacturing (or agricultural) practice, and, of course, at levels not exceeding safe limits in the total diet.

Under the Federal Food, Drug and Cosmetic Act, no food additive is permitted if its use would be considered deceptive or, for whatever reason, unsafe. By statutory definition, a substance is unsafe "if it is found to induce cancer when ingested by man or animal, or if it is found, after tests which are appropriate for the evaluation of the safety of food additives, to induce cancer in man or animal. . . ." (the so-called Delaney Clause). It is this provision that led to the outlawing of safrole, the characteristic flavor ingredient of root beer, and the widely used synthetic sweetener, cyclamate. This legal mandate recognizes no specific experimental conditions for determining the carcinogenic potential of a substance; any dose, no matter how large, administered to any species of animal, no matter how frequently or how long, might condemn a substance as a carcinogen. Literal interpretation of this provision of the law makes no allowance for minute or unavoidable traces of carcinogens. Thus, questions have arisen after the absence of a carcinogen was established by chemical analysis only to have a more sensitive method become available; or when unavoidable traces of aflatoxin or benzo-α-pyrene, both known carcinogens, were revealed in peanut butter or smoked meats, respectively. It is also recognized that various foods naturally contain traces of cancer-inducing substances, but escape legal prohibition because these substances are not "added." These are examples of how the legal concept of "zero tolerance" or "no residue" has been found to be scientifically untenable. The Food and Drug Administration has administratively taken the pragmatic position in certain cases of setting "actionable" limits on the presence of such carcinogens, taking cognizance of the sensitivity of currently available analytical methodology. In the view of many responsible scientists, the Delaney Clause should be amended to permit greater latitude and discretion on the part of those qualified by scientific training and experience to exercise it. On the other hand, some contend that the principle of "zero tolerance" implicit in this statute should be extended to prohibit potential teratogens and mutagens and other agents believed to be etiologically related to chronic or irreversible pathological states. This is one of numerous controversies among scientists and regulatory agencies both here and abroad surrounding the use of food additives which time alone can resolve.

BIBLIOGRAPHY

1. Federal Food, Drug & Cosmetic Act, as amended 1962, Sec. 201(s).
2. Federal Insecticide, Fungicide, and Rodenticide Act 1948; Sec. 2a.
3. Recent Progress in the Consideration of Flavoring Ingredients under the Food Additives Amendment. III GRAS Substances. Food Technol., *19*, 151–197 (1965).
4. Recent Progress in the Consideration of Flavoring Ingredients under the Food Additives Amendment. IV GRAS Substances. Food Technol., *24*, 25–28 (1970).
5. Code of Federal Regulations, Title 21, Chapter 1, Subpart B, Sec. 121.101.
6. Federal Register *36*, 12093–12094, June 25, 1971.
7. Federal Register *37*, 5723–5724, April 13, 1966.
8. Federal Food, Drug & Cosmetic Act. Sec. 201 (t)(1).
9. Chemicals Used in Food Processing. National Academy of Sciences—National Research Council, Publication No. 1274, 1965.
10. Code of Federal Regulations, Title 21, Chapter 1, Sec. 121.1163 and 121.1164.
11. Federal Food, Drug & Cosmetic Act as amended 1962, Title 21, Chapter 1, Subpart B, Sec. 120.7.
12. Food and Drug Administration Advisory Committee on Protocols for Safety Evaluations: Panel on Reproduction Report on Reproduction Studies in the Safety Evaluation of Food Additives and Pesticide Residues, Tox. and Appl. Pharmacol. *16*, 264–296 (1970).
13. Evaluation of the Safety of Food Chemicals, National Academy of Sciences—National Research Council Food Protection Committee, Food and Nutrition Board, 1970.

Chapter

12

Radioactivity in Foods

C. L. Comar

AND

J. C. Thompson, Jr.

There is little doubt that atomic energy will assume an important role in our civilization and it is appropriate that future possible hazards be evaluated. Although present environmental radiocontamination and exposure of the population are due almost entirely to fallout from nuclear weapons, peacetime operations may become increasingly important as sources of radioactive contamination. In addition to fallout, small quantities of radioactive materials may be released into the environment as a result of such operations as mining of uranium and thorium ore; nuclear fuel processing; reactor installations in power plants, submarines, ships, and aircraft (normal operations and accidents); use of nuclear explosions for earth moving; and applications of radioisotopes in medicine, industry, and agriculture. Thus, we now stand at an important crossroad in regard to radioactive contamination of the environment. Over the past years we have developed a great body of information based mainly on experience from the testing of nuclear devices and there has been much thinking about what might happen in nuclear warfare. This preoccupation with fallout was justified on the basis that radiation exposures to the population from peacetime applications were insignificant as compared to those from nuclear explosions. For the future, problems of radioactive contamination, if any, will hopefully come from peacetime applications in which benefits far outweigh any added risks.

Radioactivity from environmental contamination reaches the human population primarily in food. However, at the present time it can be concluded that there is no reason for any change in our nutritional habits or food technology as a result of fallout contamination. Research must continue, nevertheless, so that recommendations can be made to minimize the intake of radioactive contamination should this ever become necessary.

RADIOISOTOPES OF POTENTIAL HAZARD

The relative hazard of radioactive materials will be governed by the amount released into the environment, physical half-life, efficiency of transfer through the food chain to the human diet, degree of absorption by the body, and length of time retained in the body. Because of these factors the list of potentially hazardous radioisotopes is reduced considerably, with those of greatest immediate concern being the radioisotopes of iodine, barium, strontium, and cesium. Extensive data are available on the passage of these radioactive materials through food chains and their metabolism in the human body.[1-4] Table 12-1 summarizes their characteristics from the standpoint of environmental contamination. Other radioisotopes found in peaceful nuclear operations such as ^{3}H, ^{85}Kr, ^{51}Cr, ^{65}Zn, ^{55}Fe, ^{60}Co, ^{54}Mn, etc. may be important under certain conditions but will tend to follow similar contamination patterns. Unique pathways and characteristics might require special consideration under some conditions, but such radioisotopes are intensively studied before releases are permitted.

The radioisotopes of iodine collect in the thyroid gland and those of barium concentrate in bone. Since isotopes of both of these elements have short physical half-lives they can be dangerous only during certain periods, depending on the frequency and nature of production and contamination. Experience has indicated that iodine-131 may be most important shortly after tropospheric and local fallout and releases from reactor accidents. Barium-140 is of much less concern because it is transmitted less efficiently through the food chain. Strontium-89, which is produced in higher activities than strontium-90, may be the more hazardous radioisotope shortly after production, whereas strontium-90 with a much longer half-life becomes more dominant with time. The radioisotopes of strontium are cumulative in bone. Cesium-137, which follows potassium in metabolism, is considered less of a hazard than strontium-90 because cesium is turned over relatively rapidly in the body, is not selectively concentrated in any one part of the body, and does not pass appreciably from soil to plant in the food chain.

Insofar as other radionuclides are concerned, carbon-14 (half-life of about 5700 years) is of greatest interest because carbon is such an important constituent of living matter. Little attention has been given to the movement of carbon-14 in the food chain because the specific activity of carbon-14 in the population can be estimated directly from its specific activity in atmospheric carbon dioxide, which is essentially the sole precursor of carbon in food and body tissues. The extent of carbon-14 contamination is most conveniently expressed in terms of naturally occurring levels of carbon-14, which have always existed as a result of the action of cosmic ray neutrons on nitrogen atoms. It is estimated that the peak excess atmospheric carbon-14 activity occurred during the 1963–1965 period when levels were more than 100 per cent greater than normal

atmospheric levels. Following this peak, which resulted from nuclear testing, the levels have declined to about 70 per cent excess in 1970. This decline will continue so that by the year 2000 the excess levels will be about 3 per cent.[2,3,5] Such large reductions are brought about mainly by movement between reservoirs (*i.e.* exchange between atmosphere, biosphere and ocean-surface layer); further decreases will occur only by radioactive decay.[2] Carbon-14 is expected to produce about the same amount of total harm as strontium-90, but because of its long half-life its effects will be spread over thousands of years.

There are a few radionuclides that are considered potentially more significant in relation to seafoods than in the terrestrial food chain; these include cerium-144, zinc-65, iron-55, iron-59, and cobalt-60. The exposure of the human population to these radionuclides and to others that have been detected in air, rain or tissues, such as sodium-22, manganese-54, tritium and plutonium, is considerably less than exposure to the radionuclides listed in Table 12–1.[2] This pattern is expected to continue with doses from peaceful uses seldom approaching the levels received from fallout testing.

PATHWAYS IN THE FOOD CHAIN

Radioactive contaminants are transferred to man by means of specific pathways through the terrestrial and aquatic food chains. Terrestrial food chains are the main sources of radiocontaminants and their generalized pathways are illustrated in Figure 12–1. Specific pathways for barium, iodine, strontium and cesium are described in Table 12–1. Aquatic food chains follow the same general principles with many interrelationships between water, vegetation, animals and man. However, the aquatic food chains have not contributed significant amounts of radiocontaminants because of normal dilution factors and a limited intake of aquatic food products.

Fallout from the atmosphere can be retained by above-ground plant parts, such as leaves, fruits or seeds, or it can be absorbed

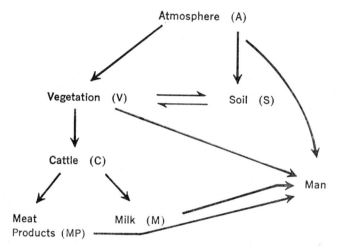

Fig. 12-1. Diagram of main terrestrial food chains by means of which environmental radioactive contaminants reach the human population.

directly by basal parts and surface roots of plants. In addition, radioactive contaminants can enter the soil and pass through the roots into plants just like any soil nutrient. Man ingests the radioactive material both by direct consumption of plant materials and by consumption of products from animals that have eaten contaminated forage.

Radioiodine is deposited from the atmosphere on the surface of vegetation which is grazed by dairy animals and the ingested radionuclide is secreted into milk. Exposure of man to ^{131}I also occurs by consumption of fruits and vegetables; however, such exposure is usually minor because of the time delay. Also, the surface area of these products as consumed by man is very small compared to the surface area grazed by an animal, and most often the surface contamination of fresh fruits and vegetables is removed by washing or skinning before consumption. Man inhales ^{131}I that is present in air, but observations have shown that this route of contamination is relatively unimportant. Thus, only one item of the diet, fresh milk, is by far the most important source of ^{131}I for the human population, although locally grown produce consumed within a short time could be a significant contributor.[6-8]

Radiostrontium reaches man primarily by his consumption of dairy products and foods of plant origin. It reaches man both by

surface contamination of plants (fallout-rate dependent) and via the soil (cumulative dependent). The relative importance of these two routes varies, depending upon the magnitude of the fallout rate, soil reservoir, crop characteristics and the time pattern of contamination. In 1958, for example, surface contamination of cereals was quite evident, and in some areas as much as 80 per cent of the radiostrontium in food had originated as surface contamination. By 1960, the general contribution from surface contamination had declined to approximately 20 per cent.[9] Increased fallout rates from nuclear testing in 1961 and 1962 again raised the contribution from surface contamination to more than 50 per cent.[2,9,10] However, with the cessation of above-ground nuclear testing the fallout rate has dropped and the soil reservoir will become the main source of radioactivity in foods.

The movement of strontium radionuclides from soil to man is interrelated with and, to some extent, governed by the simultaneous movement of calcium. For this reason, levels of ^{90}Sr are often expressed in terms of "strontium units", namely, picocuries of ^{90}Sr per gm of calcium.

It must be emphasized that the important factor is the amount of ^{90}Sr and of calcium in the total diet. For example, if foodstuff A were to contain 10 picocuries of ^{90}Sr per gm

Table 12-1. Comparison of Radioisotopes in Environmental Contamination

	Iodine-131	Barium-140	Strontium-89	Strontium-90	Cesium-137
Physical half-life	8 days	13 days	51 days	28 years	30 years
Metabolic behavior	collects in thyroid	like calcium, collects in bone	like calcium, collects in bone	like calcium, collects in bone	like potassium, collects in muscle
Removal rate from body	fast	slow	slow	slow	relatively fast
Main pathways in food chain*	A→V→C→M→Man	A→V→C→M→Man	A→V, S→V, C→M, Man	A→V, S→V, C→M, Man	A→V→C→MP, V→M→Man
Samples for monitoring radioisotope levels	vegetation, milk, and thyroid	vegetation and milk	soil, vegetation, milk, dairy products, bone, and aquatic food	soil, vegetation, milk, dairy products, bone, and aquatic food	vegetation, milk, dairy products, meat, and whole body

* A = atmosphere, V = vegetation, M = milk, S = soil, C = cattle, MP = meat products.

of calcium and contributed 0.1 gm of calcium, whereas foodstuff B were to contain 1 picocurie of ^{90}Sr per gm of calcium and contribute 1 gm of calcium to the diet, it could be said that both foodstuffs were equally important contributors, even though foodstuff A was 10 times more contaminated than foodstuff B. Thus, one cannot make any judgment from analytical values on a single constituent of the diet, it is necessary to consider the total diet.

In regard to the deposition of ^{90}Sr in the human population two practical generalizations can be made as follows:

1. Calcium is preferentially utilized relative to ^{90}Sr in practically every step of the food chain from vegetation to human bone, thus providing a biological barrier against ^{90}Sr.

2. Food processing that involves washing or discarding of outer layers of plant foods serves as a mechanical barrier.

Were it not for these processes the ^{90}Sr of the human population would be several times higher than it is now.

A word should be said about milk, because in the United States dairy products are the largest single source of dietary calcium. Attention has been focused on milk because it has been the most important single item used for analysis and evaluation of food contamination. This is because milk is produced regularly all year round, is convenient to handle, can be readily sampled so as to represent large or small areas, and does contain the most important radiocontaminants. It must be emphasized that the use of milk as an indicator food does not mean that milk is a major factor in determining total ^{90}Sr intake. As a matter of fact, because the dairy cow secretes, in proportion to the amounts ingested, 10 times as much calcium as strontium into the milk, the calcium originating from the milk will be the least contaminated of all food sources of calcium.

For ^{137}Cs, the direct contamination of plant materials is the most important route of contamination, since this element is fixed in the soil and generally rendered unavailable for root uptake. Aquatic pathways have been a minor contributor because of the dilution factors normally existent in most bodies of water. However, with more widespread peaceful uses of nuclear energy in small confined bodies of water, coupled with a natural tendency for ^{137}Cs to be concentrated in certain tissues, there will be greater need for closer evaluations of ^{137}Cs levels in aquatic organisms. Similar care will have to be exercised for other radionuclides planned for release to the aquatic environment where the ecosystems are not as well defined or characterized as they are for the terrestrial environment.

RADIOISOTOPE LEVELS

The pattern of the levels of radioisotopes in the biosphere (soil-plants-animal products-man) can be understood only in terms of the timing and size of the nuclear explosions that produced them. Table 12-2 presents such data.[11,12,14] Thus, radionuclide levels arising from tests subsequent to the 1958 moratorium would be expected to exceed the highest levels observed in 1959. This is due to the cumulative soil contribution and an increased fallout rate which resulted from the intensity of testing during 1961–1962. An understanding of the pathways, as well as weapons yield, production and distribution patterns, is necessary to estimate accurately future levels of radioactivity.

Because of the transient nature of ^{131}I in milk, very few measurements were made of levels resulting from tests prior to 1957;

Table 12-2. Fission Yields of
Nuclear Explosions[11,12,14]

Period	Total by Period	Cumulative Total
	(megatons)	
1945–1956	52	52
1957–1958	40	92
1959–1960	Test moratorium	
1961	25	117
1962	76	193
1963–1970	Underground tests primarily, except those by France and China which have been less than 5-megaton fission yield.	

limited data were reported during 1957–1959. After the disappearance of the ^{131}I from the 1958 tests, none was observed until the resumption of nuclear testing by Russia in 1961. Monitoring networks began to record ^{131}I in milk by mid-September and continued to detect appreciable levels until late December. Values as high as 730 pCi ^{131}I/liter of milk were observed, with monthly averages of 80, 100, 65 and 14 for the September to December period; values were less than 10 pCi/liter during the next 4 months.[12] Increased testing by both the United States and Russia in the spring of 1962 caused ^{131}I levels in milk to rise again, with monthly averages in the United States rising from 20 in May to 70 pCi/liter of ^{131}I in November.[12] Such averages do not indicate the variability in ^{131}I deposition since milk from some individual collection stations exceeded 700 pCi/liter during the summer of 1962. Daily averages or values from individual dairy herds were even higher in certain locations. However, by February 1963 the average ^{131}I levels in the United States were again below 10 pCi/liter or undetectable except for localized contamination from ventings of underground tests and some limited contamination from the French and Chinese above-ground testing programs.[12]

Dietary levels of ^{90}Sr, which are expressed as picocuries of ^{90}Sr per gm of calcium, have been estimated at approximately 0.4, 2, 4, 5, 7, 12, 18, 11, 7, 11, 22, 26, 21, 15, 12, 12, 11, 8 for each year from 1953 to 1970, respectively.[11–14] Values are predicted to be less

than 10 for the next 3 to 5 years, assuming no large-scale atmospheric testing. An indication of the typical contributions of various foods is given in Table 12–3.[14] No significant differences in ^{90}Sr/Ca values have been found for typical infant, teenage, or adult diets. The breast-feeding of infants, however, should give an appreciable reduction of ^{90}Sr intake during the first few months of life. Based on observations and knowledge of metabolism, it can be assumed that the value of ^{90}Sr per gm of calcium in the human population will fall close to one-fourth of the value of the total diet.[2]

The most extensive data are those on levels of ^{90}Sr in milk. In general, the values for milk are expected to be about 30 to 60 per cent of the values for total diet depending upon the relative importance of the rate-dependent vs. cumulative-dependent pathways.[15] In regard to variability, it appears that in any one month the highest value observed in the country might be 10 times the lowest; however, there is less variation in the total diet and in the levels found in the human population, presumably because the individual consumes food that originates from many areas.

Because the amount of rainfall is an important factor governing the fallout rate, the Federal Radiation Council has considered the country to be divided into "wet" and "dry" areas.[11] The "wet" region includes all states bordering on and extending east of the Mississippi River as well as the Far Northwest. The "dry" region includes the

Table 12-3. Typical Contributions of Various Foods to the Total Strontium-90 of Diet in New York City for 1960-1970[14]

	Picocuries of ^{90}Sr/day		Percentage Contribution	
	Average 1970	Range 1960–1970	Average 1970	Range 1960–1970
Milk	4.8	4.8–18.4	38	35–56
Flour & cereals	1.8	1.7–8.5	14	13–25
Root vegetables	0.9	0.8–1.8	7	4–10
Leafy & other vegetables	2.4	1.0–3.6	19	8–21
Fruits	1.8	0.9–2.9	14	6–20
Meat, fish, eggs	0.4	0.2–1.1	3	2–5
Water	0.6	0.3–1.5	5	3–5
Total daily ^{90}Sr intake	12.7	10.5–33.5		

Great Plains, inter-mountain, and southwest states where average rainfall is generally less than 30 inches per year. As an example, the ^{90}Sr content of milk in the "wet" area is usually $1\frac{1}{2}$ to 2 times higher than in the "dry" area.

Typical values for the contribution of various foodstuffs to the ^{137}Cs in the human diet are as follows (Chicago 1961–70): 32 per cent from milk, 27 per cent from meat, 23 per cent from flour and cereals, 8 per cent from vegetables, and 10 per cent from fruits.[14] Values for ^{137}Cs in picocuries per liter of milk were 65, 10, 10, 44, 114, 94, 52, 29, 11, 12, 8 and 9 for 1959 through 1970, respectively.[12] Levels have declined with time as a result of the cessation of nuclear testing, although the rate of decline has lagged considerably behind the decrease in the fallout rate. It has been suggested that, in permanent pastures, there is an interaction with organic matter that prolongs the availability of ^{137}Cs to plant roots by reduction of binding by clays. Levels in the human population expressed in terms of picocuries per gm of potassium have been 2, 7, 14, 32, 36, 47, 57, 48, 32, 43, 80, 140, 112, 69, and 41 for 1953 to 1968 respectively.[17] In general, it appears that the levels in the body lag behind those in the diet by about 4 months and that the ^{137}Cs/K ratio in the body is about three times the ratio in the diet.

Considerable attention has been given to the situation in some arctic regions where the ^{137}Cs levels in food and man are 100 or more times greater than those in the northern temperate latitudes. This is primarily the result of accumulation of fallout on lichens and other native vegetation which grow slowly and are grazed by reindeer and caribou. The meat from these animals constitutes a large part of the diets of arctic populations.

Recent concerns for radioactive releases from nuclear reactors and nuclear fuel reprocessing facilities have intensified efforts to minimize such releases and expand monitoring programs. These efforts have been instituted because of the one major difference between radioactivity from fallout and peaceful releases: the problem of worldwide fallout distribution as compared to the local distribution problem inherent with reactor releases. The widespread contamination patterns of fallout permitted generalizations to be drawn for wide regions with much less sampling rigor required. Localized peacetime releases may require much more intensive efforts to detect changes that may occur over time and to determine unique critical organisms or pathways that were heretofore relatively unimportant. Operating experiences to date indicate that releases in most instances have been well within authorized levels, usually resulting in dose rates at the boundary zones which are 1 to 5 per cent of the normal background levels in the area. Special consideration is being given to the aquatic environment because of the different pathways and interrelationships to other releases and contaminants in this medium. However, it must be pointed out that these releases are generally much lower than the levels already experienced from fallout releases.[16]

Table 12-4.   Comparison of Levels of Man-Made Radiation and Natural Background Radiation[11]

| Site | Radiation Dose During Next Seventy Years (Roentgens) | | |
	From Background	From 1962 Tests	From Tests through 1962
Bone	9	0.28	0.46
Bone marrow	7	0.13	0.22
Reproductive cells	7	0.06	0.13

BIOLOGICAL CONSEQUENCES OF ENVIRONMENTAL RADIOCONTAMINATION

From knowledge of the amounts of radioactivity present in man's body, reasonable estimates can be made of the radiation dosage that is delivered. Whereas there is a considerable body of information on the effects of radiation on man and animals, it has been impossible to detect any biological effects at levels of radiation and dose rates as low as those resulting so far from nuclear testing. Thus, the best basis for estimating the effect of man-made radiation exposure on man is a comparison with the levels of natural background radiation to which the human population has always been exposed. Such a comparison is presented in Tables 12–4[11] and 12–5.[18]

These dosages take into account exposure from radionuclides of strontium, cesium and carbon, which are the elements of primary concern as potential long-term hazards. Thyroid doses from [131]I (half-life, 8 days) are not included because peak dose rates persist only for a short period of time and these are discussed later. The most authoritative estimates of the consequences of such radiation exposure, in terms of natural incidences and additional cases of gross defects, leukemia and bone cancer, are presented in Table 12–6.[11]

Since ^{131}I is the fallout radionuclide most likely to produce the greatest radiation exposures within short times (up to several weeks) after nuclear detonations it is of interest to consider estimated radiation dosages and possible biological effects. The dose to the thyroid of infants 6 to 18 months was estimated to range from 0.03 to 0.65 roentgens in 1961 and 1962 as determined from high and low individual stations of the Public Health Service Pasteurized Milk Network. It has been estimated that a small number of infants conceivably could have received doses from 10 to 30 times the average.[11] Because the dose is inversely related to the size of the thyroid gland, the exposure of adults would be about one-tenth the values cited previously for infants.

In May 1953, local areas in Utah were reported to have received unusual amounts of fallout from the Nevada test site, with reconstructed estimates of thyroid dose ranging from less than 10 rads to above 400 rads. Examinations in 1965 of school children from the areas in question have revealed no thyroid abnormalities that can be ascribed specifically to radiation. Experience is avail-

Table 12-5. Average Radiation Exposures in 1969[18]

Millirems/Year	
Background	120
Fallout	
Carbon-14	1
Strontium-90	8
Cesium-137	0.8
Tritium	
Prior to 1945	0.0015
At present	0.06
In year 2000	0.005

Table 12-6. Estimated Consequences of Radiation Exposure[11]

	Natural Incidence	From Background Radiation	From Tests through 1962
Estimated number of gross physical and mental defects in children of persons now living in United States	4,000,000 to 6,000,000	—	200 to 500
Estimated number of leukemia cases in next 70 years in United States	840,000	0 to 84,000	0 to 2,000
Estimated number of cases of bone cancer in next 70 years in United States	140,000	0 to 14,000	0 to 700

able on the relatively high exposures (up to 1000 rads or more) of the thyroid gland of human beings by virtue of: (a) diagnostic and therapeutic x-ray treatment, (b) diagnostic and therapeutic use of ^{131}I, (c) exposure of a Marshallese population, and (d) exposures at Hiroshima and Nagasaki. In general, it appears that radioactive iodine, delivering dosages of several hundred rads to the thyroid of infants or young children, will produce a high incidence of thyroid nodules, whereas the incidence of cancer has not been observable and must be extremely low.[6]

On the basis of this and estimates presented in Table 12–6, it is generally agreed that health risks from present and anticipated levels of environmental radiocontamination are probably not zero, but are too small to justify individual anxiety or attempts to modify dietary intakes.

GOVERNMENTAL RESPONSIBILITY AND REMEDIAL MEASURES

Although there need not be individual anxiety about fallout, there must be concern and interest on the part of officials and scientists who have authorized responsibility. There are two interrelated areas of consideration: (1) the establishment of radiation standards or levels as guidelines at which remedial actions should be recommended, and (2) the development of remedial or preventative measures to reduce the exposure of the population to radioactive contamination.

Radiation Standards. It is necessary that an official body stipulate some level or range of radiocontamination at which preventive or remedial action should be given serious consideration. To the Federal Radiation Council falls the crucial and most difficult task of setting radiation standards. This body, which was created in 1959, is comprised of representatives from all the national agencies that have an interest in any aspect of radiation. Its major function is to advise the President with respect to radiation matters directly or indirectly affecting health, including guidance for all Federal agencies in the formulation of radiation standards and in the establishment and execution of programs of cooperation with states.[11] The re-

cent formation of the Environmental Protection Agency (EPA) has resulted in numerous organizational re-alignments within the Federal Government. Among them is the shifting of responsibilities of the Federal Radiation Council to EPA. Although these changes have altered the functional aspects of the Federal Radiation Council, the basic philosophy for radiation protection is still maintained in accord with, and mutually compatible with, guidance from the National Council on Radiation Protection and Measurements (NCRP) and the International Commission on Radiological Protection (ICRP).

In 1960, the Federal Radiation Council provided the general philosophy for radiation protection. The term "Radiation Protection Guide" (RPG) was introduced and defined as "the radiation dose which should not be exceeded without careful consideration of the reasons for doing so; every effort should be made to encourage the maintenance of radiation doses as far below this guide as practicable." RPGs were developed for radiation workers, individuals in the population and for suitable samples of exposed population groups. The RPG for whole body exposure of individuals in the general population (exclusive of natural background and deliberate exposure of patients by practitioners of the healing arts) was established as 0.5 rem per year. The value was set at one-third of this dose, or 0.17 rem per year, for suitable samples of exposed population groups. These guides were considered appropriate for normal peacetime operations and were not to apply to contamination produced by weapons testing.

In 1961, in order to provide guidance for agencies in developing appropriate programs for control of intake of radioactivity from the environment, the Federal Radiation Council described a graded approach for various radionuclides. Three ranges of transient rates of daily intake were determined with various actions outlined for each range. The objective of this approach was to limit the intake of radioactive materials so that the specified RPGs would not be exceeded. Table 12–7 presents an outline of the ranges and recommended actions for ^{89}Sr, ^{90}Sr and

Table 12-7. Federal Radiation Council Recommended Daily Intake Ranges and Action Criteria to Remain Below Radiation Protection Guides[11]

	Daily Intake Levels (picocuries/day)		
	Range I	Range II	Range III
[89]Sr	0–200	200–2000	2000–20,000
[90]Sr	0– 20	20– 200	200– 2000
[131]I (infant)*	0– 10	10– 100	100– 1000

Action Criteria	
Range I	Surveillance adequate to provide reasonable confirmation of calculations.
Range II	Active surveillance and controls so that exposures will not exceed upper limit of Range II.
Range III	Active surveillance and controls designed to return levels of radioactive intake to Range II or lower.

*Ranges designed for the most susceptible group. Adult levels would be increased by a factor of 10.

[131]I. The upper limit of Range II is based on an annual RPG considered as an acceptable risk for a lifetime.

Since ^{131}I is the only radionuclide which has attained levels near the established guidelines, the status in regard to radiation standards is discussed in terms of this radionuclide. In brief, the Federal Radiation Council guidance for ^{131}I is represented by an annual average intake of 100 picocuries per day or an annual intake of 36,500 picocuries as the upper level of so-called Range II, above which the application of control measures is to be considered. Although the guidelines were originally presented with appropriate qualifications, especially restricting their application to normal peacetime industrial operations, there seemed to be an understanding in the minds of most individuals that these standards should also apply to fallout. In the fall of 1962, concentrations in milk in some areas of the country approached the levels at which action appeared to be warranted by the Federal Radia-

tion Council guidelines. As a matter of fact, at least one state undertook to reduce the ^{131}I levels in commercial fresh milk by arranging for farmers to utilize stored feed instead of pasture for dairy herds.[19]

In response to this situation the Federal Radiation Council issued an official statement on September 17, 1962, which affords some clarification and from which the following excerpts are taken:[20]

In some localities in the United States, average annual intake values of radioactive iodine have approached the upper level of Range II, and, in one locality, have slightly exceeded Range II. This had led to actions and proposed actions involving countermeasures or preventive health measures. The Federal Radiation Council does not recommend such actions under present circumstances.

The Council believes, based on competent scientific advice, that any possible health risk which may be associated with exposures even many times above the guide levels would not result in a detectable increase in the incidence of disease.

The Radiation Protection Guides are not a dividing line between safety and danger in actual radiation situations nor are they alone intended to set a limit at which protective action should be taken. As applied to fallout, guides can be used as an indication of when there is need for detailed evaluation of possible exposure risks and when there is need to consider whether any protective action should be taken under all the relevant circumstances.

Radiation exposures anywhere near the guides involve risks so slight that countermeasures may have a net adverse rather than favorable effect on the public well-being. The judgement as to when to take action and what kind of action to take to decrease exposure levels involves consideration of all factors.

In view of the misunderstanding regarding the application of Radiation Protection Guides, the Federal Radiation Council considered the problems of fallout from nuclear tests and in 1964–1965 established "Protective Action Guides" for ^{131}I, ^{89}Sr, ^{90}Sr and [137]Cs. These set forth the projected absorbed doses of individuals in the general population that warrant protective action following a contaminating event. Categories were developed for acute contaminating events and are shown in Table 12–8 along with some of

Table 12-8. Federal Radiation Council Protective Action Guides and Action Criteria— Acute Localized Event[11]

	Annual Projected Dose	
	Individual (rads)	Population (rads)
^{89}Sr, ^{90}Sr, ^{137}Cs		
Category I	10*	3
Category II	5	2
Category III	0.5	0.2
^{131}I		
Category I	30	10

Protective Actions

Category I
  (1) Remove cattle from pasture to stored feed.
  (2) Switch to uncontaminated milk by changes in processing or distributing with diversion or disposal of contaminated milk.

Category II
  (1) Modify animal feed utilization, food processing and marketing practices.
  (2) Diversion of crops to remove radionuclides from food chain areas.
  (3) Destruction of selective food or feed crops.

Category III
  (1) Action to be determined on a case-by-case basis.

* Total dose must not exceed 15 rads.

the protective actions considered appropriate for the given categories. The relationships between the levels of radionuclides in food products and the projected doses to the population are also discussed in the referenced publications but are too complex to be presented here. Similarly complex release criteria are in effect for peaceful uses of nuclear energy. Recent actions of the Atomic Energy Commission will institute special release restrictions on light water cooled nuclear powered reactors that limit effluent releases so that annual whole body dose rates for individuals will not exceed 5 per cent of background levels.[21] Other types of reactors, fuel fabrication plants, or radioisotope processing plants will be covered by subsequent regulations.

It is important to keep clearly in mind the difference between "local" fallout and "world-wide" or stratospheric fallout. The levels for Categories I and II of Table 12–8 are likely and the actions proposed are feasible only for local fallout. Effective protective action to cope with world-wide fallout conditions could only be achieved by long-term changes in: (a) agricultural practices, (b) food processing practices, or (c) basic dietary habits. The Federal Radiation Council concluded that, while surveillance of world-wide contamination should be continued, the health risks therefrom over the next several years would be too small to justify protective action.

Remedial Measures. It is prudent that knowledge be obtained to cope with any foreseeable contingencies and research must be done on preventive measures.[22] The fact that such work is under way, however, should not be interpreted by the lay public to indicate that these measures are needed or desirable under existing conditions. In general, any remedial measure, to be useful, must fulfill certain requirements: (a) it must be effective in removing contamination; (b) it must be safe in that the health risk from its use must be less than that from the radiocontaminant; (c) it must be practical from the standpoint of application; (d) the responsibility for the application must be defined since this cannot be left to the individual but has to be done on a national or on a state basis; (e) the impact on the public must be considered so that there is no panic that could lead to malnutrition having a deleterious effect that might far outweigh the expected benefits from the removal of the radiocontaminant.

Specific comments on remedial measures are limited here to ^{131}I, since this radionuclide, if any, will probably be the first to require action. Remedial measures for ^{131}I are relatively simple because of its short half-life and because it reaches the public primarily in a single identifiable food, milk. Measures that have been proposed are as follows, starting with the most practical.[22]

Use of Stored Feed Instead of Pasture for Dairy Cows. The practicability of this procedure depends first of all upon the availability of stored feed (usually over twenty days old) in a given location at the needed time. Another problem is the time element. The peak of ^{131}I in milk is usually reached within a few days after deposition and, unless animals are transferred to stored feed within that time, the procedure may be of little avail. This means that plans must be made well ahead of time so that they can be put into effect immediately upon notification.

Use of Evaporated or Powdered Milk for Young Children and Pregnant and Lactating Women. This approach would be quite effective but there would undoubtedly be a public relations problem in that many individuals in the rest of the population would also want to stop using fresh milk. The feasibility would depend upon the available stores and production capacity for such products.

Use of Other Stored Milk Products. The feasibility of this measure would depend upon the maintenance and availability of large enough stores of such items as refrigerated, frozen or canned milk.

Pooling of Milk. Theoretically, the ^{131}I level in milk from regions of high contamination can be reduced by pooling with milk from regions of low contamination. Limiting factors would be the necessary assay of milk supplies and logistics.

Addition of Stable Iodine to Human Diet. Increased levels of stable iodine in the diet will reduce the deposition of ingested ^{131}I in the thyroid. However, the consensus of medical opinion is that there would be certain health risks in the use of stable iodine on a population-wide basis.

Strontium-90 decontamination is a much more difficult problem and as yet there are no preventive or remedial measures that fulfill the criteria of effectiveness, safety and feasibility, except possibly the removal of ^{90}Sr from milk by ion exchange. This process has been demonstrated on a commercial scale and could be initiated as a part of most milk plants at costs approaching 1 cent per quart. However, this measure would be regarded as an emergency capability which would have little application under current and expected contamination levels. Similar techniques have also been explored for ^{137}Cs and ^{131}I with comparable results. Other research

is being continued on the possibilities of soil control, liming of soils and addition of stable calcium to dairy rations and human diets.

SUMMARY

In regard to environmental radiocontamination there seems to be general agreement about the following: (1) the behavior of radioactive materials in their movement from the site of production through the atmosphere and the food chain to reach the human population; (2) the levels of radiation exposure of the population from given amounts and patterns of nuclear testing; and (3) the maximum biological effects that can be expected from a given degree of environmental contamination.

There are many areas of uncertainty that require continued research and attention. These include among others: (1) the significance of local regions of high fallout that might result from combinations of circumstances, such as high rainfall, low soil calcium and local distribution from underground bursts; (2) more detailed knowledge on the biological and social consequences of radiation exposure of large populations; for instance, consideration of the possibility that certain segments of the population (*e.g.*, the developing fetus, the sick, the young, the aged) could be more sensitive to radiation than the population at large, and that some individuals in the world population could be unusually sensitive to radiation; and (3) the development of effective and feasible preventive and remedial measures for the reduction of exposure from environmental contamination.

It seems clear that any use of nuclear energy or radiation most probably involves a biological cost to the individual or society, even though the harm may not be observable. There is little question but that the benefits from controlled peacetime applications of nuclear energy more than justify its use. The effects of environmental radiocontamination from nuclear explosions prior to 1970 are small enough so that individual anxiety is not warranted, and any individual action to reduce exposure is likely to be detrimental as well as futile. Nevertheless, in regard to weapons tests, there are too many intangibles to permit a logical evaluation of both sides of the fundamental equation—benefit versus cost.

BIBLIOGRAPHY

1. Comar, Goldblith, Kraybill, Reitemeier and Shank: Health Physics, *9*, 569, 1963.
2. Reports of the United Nations Scientific Committee on the Effects of Atomic Radiation. General Assembly 17th Session, Suppl. No. 16 A/5216, 1962; 19th Session Suppl. No. 14A/5814, 1964; 21st Session, Suppl. No. 14A/6314, 1966; 24th Session, Suppl. No. 13A/7613, 1969.
3. Russell: *Radioactivity and Human Diet*, Oxford, Pergamon Press, 1966.
4. Comar: Annual Review of Nuclear Science, *15*, 175, 1965.
5. Health and Safety Laboratory: United States Atomic Energy Commission, New York Operation Office, HASL Report 243, p. I–3, 1971.
6. Report of the Subcommittee of the National Academy of Sciences, National Research Council Advisory Committe to the Federal Radiation Council on "Pathological Effects of Thyroid Irradiation," 1967.
7. Wasserman, Lengemann, Thompson, and Comar: in *Radioactive Fallout, Soils, Plants, Foods, Man* (E. B. Fowler, Editor) Amsterdam, Elsevier, 236, 1965.
8. Thompson: Health Physics, *13*, 1967 and *14*, 1968.
9. Agricultural Research Council Radiobiological Laboratory: Report for 1964–1965, ARCRL *14*, 75, 1965.
10. Russell: Health Physics, *11*, 1305, 1965.
11. Federal Radiation Council Report No. 1, 1960 through No. 7, 1965. U.S. Government Printing Office, Washington, D.C.
12. Public Health Service: Radiological Health Data, Monthly Reports, *1*, No. 1, 1960 through *12*, No. 5, 1971.
13. Kulp and Schulert: ^{90}Sr *in Man and his Environment*. Vol. III, Publications, Geochemical Laboratory, Columbia University, 1961.
14. Health and Safety Laboratory: United States Atomic Energy Commission, New York Operations Office. HASL Report No. 111, 1961 through No. 243, 1971.
15. Michelson, Thompson, Hess and Comar: J. Nutrition, *78*, 371, 1962.
16. Technical Reports: Northeastern Radiological Health Laboratory BRH/NERHL 70–1, 70–2, 70–3; Division of Environmental Radiation BRH/DER 70–2.
17. Gustafson and Miller: Health Physics, *16*, 167, 1969.
18. Larson: in Environmental Effects of Producing Electric Power. 91st Congress of the United States. Part 1, 254, 1969.
19. Utah State Department of Health: Utah's Experience with Radioactive Milk, 1962.
20. Public Health Service: Radiobiological Health Data, Monthly Reports, *3*, No. 11, 1962.
21. Federal Register, *36*, No. 111, 1962.
22. National Advisory Committee on Radiation: Radioactive Contamination of the Environment: Public Health Action, 1962. Public Health Service, Washington, D.C.

PART III

Interrelations of Nutrients and Metabolism

Chapter

13

Hormonal Control of Nutrient Metabolism

ALBERT B. EISENSTEIN

AND

SANT P. SINGH

The ability of animals to utilize carbohydrate, protein and fat as fuel provides the energy necessary to maintain life. Each of these essential nutrients has a specific and important role as a source of energy which complements that of the others. Carbohydrate (glucose) is used by all tissues as fuel and some, *e.g.*, the brain and the erythrocyte, are almost totally dependent on a constant supply of glucose. Unfortunately, the capacity for storage of carbohydrate is small so that after 24 hours of starvation the depots are exhausted. Protein catabolism begins after only a few hours of food deprivation and yields amino acids which are directed into the pathway of carbohydrate synthesis in liver and kidney. Thus, the supply of glucose is replenished. During starvation, fat tissue is broken down with release of fatty acids, glycerol and ketone bodies. Muscle can use fatty acids and ketone bodies almost exclusively to provide energy. In the chronically starved animal metabolic adjustments occur which are designed to protect protein stores since loss of approximately half the body protein is incompatible with life. The brain develops the capacity to use ketone bodies as fuel hence the need for protein catabolism with conversion of amino acids to glucose is lessened. When the food supply is plentiful protein synthesis occurs as new tissues are formed and old tissues replaced. If caloric intake is greater than energy expenditure, fatty acids are synthesized and stored as triglycerides in fat depots.

The synthesis and catabolism of carbohydrate, protein and fat are influenced by many hormones. These agents control nutrient metabolism in a variety of ways. Certain hormones increase the supply of substrate for synthetic processes while others act on specific enzymatic reactions which regulate the flow of intermediates along biochemical pathways. Transport of substrate across the cell membrane is an important action of several hormones. Some complex metabolic processes are stimulated by one hormone and inhibited by another, thus fine adjustments in the rate or direction of the reactions are possible. In this chapter, the role of hormones in nutrient metabolism is discussed. We have not attempted to consider every hormone that is known to influence these processes but have tried to deal with those that currently appear to have the most significant roles.

PROTEIN METABOLISM

Hormonal Effects on Body Protein Distribution. *Corticosteroids.* A major action of the adrenal glucocorticoids is to induce protein catabolism in peripheral tissues. Cortisone administration results in increased nitrogen excretion due to loss of protein from the carcass whereas the protein content of liver and other viscera increases.[1] Amino acids liberated as a result of protein breakdown in the periphery are transported to the liver where they may be utilized in synthesis of new protein. Not only is there protein synthesis but the total nucleic acid content of the liver also increases. This is due primarily to a rise of RNA content.[2] It is interesting that the responses to cortisone and to protein feeding are similar in that both lead to increased liver protein and RNA.[3]

Insulin. Early evidence that insulin has an important role in protein synthesis was provided by the observation that ingestion of sugar by animals or human subjects produced a prompt but temporary lowering of plasma amino acid concentration. The concentration of all amino acids was not altered to the same extent but they were removed from plasma in the relative proportions needed for protein formation in muscle.[4] In studies utilizing labeled amino acids, carbohydrate-fed animals demonstrated increased incorporation of amino acids into muscle protein but liver protein formation was not affected. The lowering of plasma amino acid concentration which follows glucose administration results in reduced hepatic urea production and a diminished supply of amino acids for protein synthesis in tissues other than muscle.[3] It was soon realized that the influence of carbohydrate feeding on protein synthesis was due to the action of insulin since the effect of sugar ingestion on plasma amino acid concentration was abolished in diabetic animals. Furthermore, insulin causes a rapid fall in blood amino acid level and stimulates *in vitro* uptake of amino acids by muscle, liver and other tissues. Insulin enhances uptake of amino acids *in vivo* within a few minutes after injection, whereas the *in vitro* action of the hormone in liver has a delayed onset and takes several hours to reach its maximum. The rapid uptake of amino acids induced by insulin *in vivo* appears to be due to hormonal action on muscle.

Anabolic Hormones (Androgens and Growth Hormone). The nitrogen-retaining effect of insulin is shared by androgens and growth hormone (GH). Animals receiving a normal diet respond to testosterone with an increase in protein content of muscle, liver and other viscera. If the androgenic steroid is given to animals that are fasting or have been fed a protein-free diet, there is acceleration of protein loss from liver but protein degrada-

tion in muscle is slowed.[5,6] Growth hormone also exerts a preferential effect on protein synthesis in muscle as shown by the finding that the relative size of certain muscles is increased more following administration of the hormone than are the liver, other muscles and viscera. Furthermore, treatment of animals with GH increased the incorporation of labeled amino acids into muscle protein but conversion to liver protein was reduced.

Catabolic Hormones (Thyroid Hormones, Estrogens). Short-term thyroxine (T_4) administration to animals leads to an increase of liver protein and RNA while there is a concomitant loss of protein from muscle. If treatment with T_4 is continued both liver and carcass are reduced in size but the liver is less affected than are peripheral tissues.[3] Thyroid hormones act on the liver to produce increased uptake of amino acids and it has been demonstrated that they enhance incorporation of amino acids into protein by liver microsomes.[7]

Large doses of estrogens cause nitrogen loss from the animal body but their effect seems to be indirect since it is abolished by adrenalectomy.

Hormonal Effects on Protein Metabolism. *Insulin.* Although the profound influence of insulin on glucose utilization was recognized before effects of the hormone on protein metabolism were detected, it is now apparent that the action of insulin on the latter process is as important as its role in carbohydrate metabolism. Insulin affects protein and amino acid metabolism in several ways: (1) it lowers the blood amino acid level in parallel with reduction of blood sugar, (2) incorporation of amino acids into protein of isolated tissues is enhanced, and (3) the hormone acts as an inducer and suppressor of synthesis of certain hepatic enzymes concerned with glycolysis and gluconeogenesis.[8]

Insulin lowers the blood amino acid level in normal as well as diabetic humans and animals. The time required for insulin to lower the blood amino acid level is very similar to that for glucose. Lotspeich[9] reported that insulin lowered the blood level of the 10 essential amino acids in normal, fasted dogs. Leucine, lysine, isoleucine, arginine, valine and threonine showed the largest changes when considered in relation to their concentration in blood. Other investigators found that plasma amino acid levels were higher in diabetic rats than in controls with leucine, isoleucine and valine showing the most striking changes.

Muscle incubated *in vitro* liberates amino acids and the rate of release of amino acids is depressed by addition of insulin to the incubation mixture. Furthermore, a similar effect of insulin on amino acid release from the isolated liver has been observed. Using the perfused human forearm preparation, Pozefsky also found that insulin suppresses release of amino acids from muscle.[10] In addition to reducing amino acid release, insulin also stimulates accumulation of these compounds by muscle as shown by increased uptake of the non-utilizable amino acid, α-aminoisobutyric acid.

Insulin added to isolated muscle preparations promotes incorporation of labeled amino acids into tissue protein. This stimulatory effect of the hormone is not restricted to muscle but also occurs in adipose tissue, mammary gland slices, costal cartilage, bone marrow cells and leukocytes as well as other tissues.[8] Insulin stimulates incorporation of naturally occurring amino acids into protein by tissues of normal animals except for the liver in which action of the hormone is evident only in diabetic preparations. There has been a question as to whether the stimulatory effect of insulin on amino acid incorporation into protein was a consequence of enhanced entry of amino acids into the tissue. Wool and Krahl[11] showed that if amino acids were accumulated by the diaphragm *in vivo*, subsequent exposure to insulin *in vitro* increased their incorporation into protein. Furthermore, there is increased conversion of amino acids which have been synthesized in muscle into tissue protein. Thus, it is clear that insulin stimulates protein synthesis as well as amino acid uptake.

In searching for the primary action of insulin, various investigators have examined the effect of the hormone on RNA synthesis. Wool and others[12,13] have shown that insulin stimulates incorporation of labeled precursors into nucleic acid although Manchester could not completely confirm these observations.[8] Other investigators have found that tissue RNA content declines in diabetes and is raised following replacement therapy with insulin.

Although the effects of insulin in muscle are quite apparent, it has been more difficult to clarify the role of the hormone in hepatic protein metabolism. Liver slices from diabetic rats show decreased capacity to incorporate amino acids into protein, a defect which can be corrected by insulin treatment. However, addition of insulin to liver of diabetic animals *in vitro* does not restore the depressed rate of protein synthesis unless the diabetes is mild and glucose is also present. In microsomes prepared from diabetic liver, amino acid incorporation is impaired and can be restored to normal by prior administration of insulin.[14] There is an increased efflux of amino acids from liver of diabetic animals which is corrected by insulin therapy.

Activities of a number of hepatic enzymes are altered in experimental diabetes. Glucokinase, glycogen synthetase, phosphofructokinase, pyruvate kinase and pentose shunt enzymes are depressed in diabetic liver, whereas glucose-6-phosphatase, fructose-1,6-diphosphatase, phosphoenolpyruvate carboxykinase and pyruvate carboxylase are increased. These abnormalities are corrected by insulin administration. The increase in activity of the first group of enzymes after insulin treatment would facilitate disposition of glucose through oxidation and storage, while reduced activity of the second group would lower the elevated gluconeogenesis found in diabetes. Although there is evidence that insulin acts directly to induce synthesis of certain enzymes (*e.g.*, glucokinase) and to suppress formation of others, it has not been established that the hormone regulates liver carbohydrate metabolism by primary control of enzyme synthesis and degradation. Of added significance are reports which describe insulin stimulation of RNA polymerase activity, of liver cell hyperplasia and DNA synthesis.[15] The relationship of these alterations to the changes in enzyme levels in diabetes and after insulin treatment remains to be elucidated.

Growth Hormone (GH). Many early clinical and experimental observations pointed to an important role for GH in protein metabolism. Hypophysectomy was followed by abrupt cessation of growth in the young animal and by weight loss in the adult. The decline in weight following pituitary removal was accompanied by negative nitrogen balance which persisted for several weeks before nitrogen equilibrium was regained. Force feeding prevented weight loss in hypophysectomized rats, however, carcass analysis revealed that nitrogen storage was slight and there was an abnormal accumulation of fat.[16] Administration of GH to intact or hypophysectomized rats results in increased body weight accompanied by a rise in water and protein content of the body and loss of fat. It has been shown that the increases in tissue protein content brought about by GH treatment result from enhanced protein biosynthesis and not from reduced protein breakdown.

Subsequently, GH was found to stimulate incorporation of labeled amino acids into liver protein while hypophysectomy had the opposite effect. Amino acid conversion to protein in a cell-free system containing liver microsomes and cell sap was less than normal if the tissue was taken from hypophysectomized rats. Treatment of the animals with GH before removal of the liver restored the incorporating activity of this system. Separation of the system into microsomes and cell sap showed that hypophysectomy and GH treatment of rats affected the ability of the microsomal fraction to incorporate amino acids into protein rather than that of the cell sap.[17]

Injection of amino acids into the rat and study of liver cell fractions confirmed the *in vitro* observation that GH increased the amino acid-incorporating capacity of microsomes. GH also enhanced amino acid incorporation into protein by the isolated diaphragm of hypophysectomized rats when the hormone was added to the incubation medium.[17a] Hjalmarson and Ahren investigated the effects of GH on uptake of AIB by diaphragms of normal and hypophysectomized rats.[17b] Their results demonstrated that muscle of hypophysectomized rats was far more responsive to GH than was normal diaphragm. The insensitivity of normal muscle to GH is

due to the fact that this tissue has been exposed to GH secreted *in vivo*.

Efforts to uncover the mechanisms by which GH stimulates protein synthesis have focused on the effects of the hormone on RNA metabolism. Not only is there a fall in protein content and capacity for protein synthesis in the hypophysectomized animal but there is also a decline in RNA content and its rate of synthesis. Treatment with GH returns RNA synthesis to normal. Ribosomes prepared from liver of hypophysectomized rats have an impaired capacity to incorporate amino acids into protein even though they have an RNA content similar to that found in ribosomes from normal rats.[18] Although it was thought that GH might stimulate synthesis of messenger RNA, no such specific effect has been discovered. Instead, GH administration stimulates synthesis of all types of RNA and enhances RNA polymerase activity.[15] The observation that GH promotes amino acid incorporation into protein in the presence of actinomycin D indicates that RNA synthesis may not be required in order for the hormone to exert its characteristic effects.

Adrenal Cortical Steroids. Removal of the adrenals from fasting rats results in prompt reduction of nitrogen excretion and a decline of blood glucose and liver glycogen. Replacement therapy with corticosteroids restores urinary nitrogen to the previous level and corrects abnormalities of carbohydrate metabolism.[19a] These observations demonstrate the important influence of corticosteroid hormones on protein metabolism. Subsequently, many investigations have revealed that cortical steroids promote protein catabolism and interfere with protein synthesis.

MUSCLE PROTEIN. Engel studied the effects of corticosteroids on protein metabolism by determining the rate of urea formation in nephrectomized rats. Urea production was not altered for 2 to 3 hours after hormone administration, then rose and remained elevated for 3 to 6 hours.[19b] Engel believed that increased urea formation was due to accelerated protein catabolism or inhibition of protein anabolism. Similar conclusions were reached by Friedberg and Greenberg who observed decreased plasma amino acids after adrenalectomy and increased plasma, muscle and liver amino acids after administration of a lipid extract of adrenal cortical tissue.[20] More recent data reveal that cortisol or cortisone administration results in increased levels of free amino acids in muscle and reduced capacity of muscle to concentrate amino acids. The accumulation of free amino acids in muscle of corticosteroid-treated animals appears to be due to inhibition of protein synthesis.[21] Other investigators found that the increase of individual amino acids in plasma during ACTH treatment of dogs paralleled the proportions of the same amino acids in muscle, thus, indicating that muscle was their source. Bondy determined the effects of adrenal cortical extract (ACE) and adrenalectomy on accumulation of amino acids in plasma of eviscerated rats.[22] ACE produced a greater increase of plasma amino nitrogen (N) in 3 hours than occurred in saline-treated controls, while adrenalectomy resulted in a much diminished rise of plasma amino N. Of added importance was the finding that glucose administration abolished the extra accumulation of amino acids induced by ACE. Since glucose does not alter amino acid metabolism, its effect appeared to be due to inhibition of ACE-induced protein breakdown. It is now generally recognized that muscle is the chief site of protein breakdown and liberation of amino acids following corticosteroid administration.

Muscle protein formation, as measured by incorporation of radioactive amino acids, is raised soon after adrenalectomy and is reduced when animals are treated with glucocorticoids.[23] Furthermore, steroid treatment diminished uptake of amino acids by muscle. Adrenal cortical hormones also depress amino acid incorporation into protein by spleen, lymphocytes, reticulocytes, bone cells and thymus tissue. Although these findings demonstrate that corticosteroids interfere with protein synthesis in certain tissues, the mechanism by which these agents act is not understood. It is possible that the steroids suppress RNA formation since they reduce RNA polymerase activity in thymus nuclei and, as a result, there is decreased incorporation of labeled precursors into RNA.

LIVER PROTEIN. In contrast to their effects in muscle, adrenal cortical hormones enhance amino acid trapping by the liver though their action is complex. Noall et al.[24] demonstrated that cortisol administration to rats led to a marked increase in hepatic uptake of α-aminoisobutyric acid (AIB) within a few hours after the hormone was given. Weber found that injection of corticosteroids into fed rats produced a rapid increase of the free amino nitrogen level in liver.[25] Others observed elevation of only selected amino acids after cortisol injection into fasting rats, thus, indicating that the nutritional state of the animal influences hormone response. Addition of glucocorticoid to isolated, perfused rat livers stimulates transport of AIB from medium into liver although there is a lag period of about 1 hour before the effect is apparent.[26]

Although glucocorticoid administration causes increased N excretion due to protein loss from the animal carcass, protein content of the liver and other viscera increases.[27] Deposition of protein in liver following adrenal steroid treatment is affected by the amount of energy provided by diet with greater protein synthesis occurring when the caloric content of the diet is high. This finding suggests that the capacity of liver to utilize amino acids derived from peripheral tissue catabolism depends upon a constant and adequate caloric intake. The increase in liver protein synthesis resulting from steroid administration is accompanied by an increase in tissue RNA content.

SYNTHESIS OF LIVER ENZYMES. Tryptophan pyrollase (TP) was the first liver enzyme found to be induced by glucocorticoids. Activity of the enzyme is stimulated by corticoids as well as its substrate tryptophan. The mechanisms by which cortisone and tryptophan elevate tryptophan pyrollase are different since effects of these agents are additive. Using immunochemical methods, Feigelson and Greengard demonstrated that both hormone and substrate increase pyrollase concentration in proportion to the rise of enzyme activity.[28] Cortisol has been shown to increase synthesis of the enzyme, whereas tryptophan has little effect on amino acid incorporation into enzyme protein.

Tryptophan stabilizes the enzyme by causing a great decline in the rate of degradation.[29]

Tyrosine transaminase (TT) concentration in liver is elevated quickly and markedly in response to glucocorticoids. In contrast to TP which is stabilized by tryptophan, TT is not affected in this manner by tyrosine nor does substrate induction of the enzyme occur. Kenney has shown that the rate of TT synthesis is accelerated four- to fivefold by corticosteroids.[29] Increased synthesis is apparent within 1 hour after injection and the elevated rate is maintained for an additional 4 to 5 hours. Induction of TT is due to a direct action of glucocorticoids on the liver since the steroids stimulate enzyme activity in isolated perfused rat liver.

Corticosteroids also cause elevation of glutamic-alanine transaminase (GAT) levels, however, the rise of enzyme activity is much slower than that of TP or TT. Enzyme activity increases about fivefold after several days of steroid treatment.[30] Glucocorticoids increase activity of pyruvate carboxylase (PC), phosphoenolpyruvate carboxykinase (PEPCK), glucose-6-phosphatase (G6Pase) and fructose-1,6-diphosphatase (FDPase), enzymes which are considered to regulate the rate of gluconeogenesis. As Kenney has made clear, even though activity levels rise, there is no direct evidence to demonstrate that enzyme synthesis is responsible for the increases.[29] Furthermore, the enhanced PEPCK activity produced by cortisol can be reproduced by administration of glucagon. The cortisol-induced rise of PEPCK is blocked by administration of glucose or insulin both of which suppress glucagon secretion thus raising the possibility that glucocorticoids do not affect PEPCK directly but act by causing release of glucagon.[29]

Since corticosteroids stimulate synthesis of certain enzymes, intensive investigation to uncover the mechanism by which this effect is mediated has been conducted. It was learned that glucocorticoids influence hepatic RNA metabolism in several ways (see review by Kenney[29]). Synthesis of nuclear RNA occurs prior to the first elevation of induced enzymes. All types of RNA—ribosomal, transfer and "DNA-like"—are elevated by cortisol suggesting that the hormone actually affects precursor pools and not true synthesis of RNA. This question has not been conclusively answered as yet. The activity of RNA polymerase is augmented by corticosteroid treatment thus supporting the concept that all DNA-directed synthesis of RNA is elevated by the hormone. The significance of the increase in RNA synthesis which occurs following cortisol administration is unclear at this time.[29]

CORTICOSTEROIDS AND PROTEIN METABOLISM IN MAN. The catabolic and antianabolic actions of glucocorticoids on protein metabolism are responsible for many of the characteristic clinical features of Cushing's syndrome. Loss of protein leads to wasting of bone matrix and osteoporosis. Atrophy of skin and supporting tissue and increased capillary fragility are evidenced by ecchymoses and cutaneous striae which are commonly present. There is often poor wound healing in hyperadrenocorticism. Muscle wasting and weakness may be so pronounced that the patient has difficulty in rising from a squatting position. A chronic excess of corticoid hormones, whether of endogenous or exogenous origin, inhibits growth in children.

Despite clinical evidence of protein wasting, patients with Cushing's syndrome remain in nitrogen balance if the diet contains 1 gm of protein per kg of body weight. Ingestion of a high-protein diet, whether it contains adequate calories or not, results in positive nitrogen balance, while a low-protein diet is associated with negative nitrogen balance regardless of caloric content.[31] The administration of testosterone to patients with Cushing's syndrome induces positive nitrogen balance and improves skin thickness and strength.

Thyroid Hormones. Short-term administration of thyroxine (T_4) leads to an increase in liver protein and RNA and a loss of protein from the carcass. If hormone treatment is prolonged, protein depletion is general although loss from the liver is less than from peripheral tissues. Foley[32] found an increased amino acid concentration in venous blood draining the forearm of human subjects treated with thyroid hormone. The catabolic effect of T_4 on peripheral protein stores is similar to that of corticosteroids, however, the adrenal steroids reduce amino acid transport into muscle and decrease muscle protein synthesis, whereas T_4 does not have these effects. In the livers of rats receiving T_4 the level of all amino acids was increased but in the carcass only histidine, lysine and tryptophan concentrations were elevated.[33] These changes are different from those observed after corticosteroid administration since the latter hormones increase free amino acids in the carcass rather than in viscera.

An effect of thyroid hormones on protein synthesis was demonstrated by the observation that triiodothyronine (T_3) increased incorporation of amino acids into protein by isolated liver microsomes and mitochondria. This enhancement of protein synthesis could not be demonstrated in the presence of actinomycin suggesting that the hormonal effect was mediated by stimulating RNA formation.[15] This suggestion has been confirmed by Tata[34] who demonstrated increased nuclear RNA synthesis beginning 3 to 4 hours after T_3 adminstration and becoming maximal at 15 hours. Later, there is a rise in RNA polymerase, stimulation of ribosome formation and elevated protein synthesis. Thyroid hormone administration leads to increased formation of specific hepatic proteins, *e.g.*, glycerophosphate dehydrogenase and carbamyl phosphate synthetase.

Androgenic Hormones. A stimulatory effect of androgenic hormones on growth and protein metabolism has been long recognized. The androgens do not have a uniform effect on all organs and tissues but are particularly active on genital structures. In seminal vesicles, testosterone increases the RNA-DNA ratio, the activity of amino acid activating enzymes and incorporation of amino acids into protein.[16] Muscle is also a major site of androgen action although not all muscles respond to the hormones in similar manner. In the guinea pig, masticatory muscles are more sensitive to androgens than are other skeletal muscles. The response of hepatic protein metabolism to androgenic steroids is less clear than that of muscle. Testosterone administration to rats eating a normal diet caused protein retention in liver as well as in other viscera and muscle, however, in fasted, castrated guinea pigs testosterone stimulated

liver protein breakdown while it acted to conserve muscle protein. Some investigators have been unable to detect an effect of androgens on liver protein metabolism.

Many observations demonstrate that androgens stimulate muscle growth. Female animals and castrated males have smaller muscles with reduced content of protein and DNA than do normal males. When androgens are administered to castrated animals, there is protein deposition in muscle. In studies of the mechanism by which androgens exert their anabolic action, it was found that testosterone administration did not elevate muscle DNA content nor were there changes in the number of muscle cells. The increased muscle weight induced by androgenic hormones results from growth of individual muscle fibers and not from formation of new fibers. Furthermore, following castration muscle fiber size is decreased but there is no change in number of fibers (see review by Young[35]). Androgens do not affect all muscles in the same manner as indicated by the increased sensitivity of temporal and masseter muscles in the guinea pig and perineal muscles of the rat.

Androgen administration enhances incorporation of ^{14}C-labeled amino acids into muscle protein in normal or castrated rats and also stimulates amino acid uptake by isolated muscle strips. Breuer and Florini[36] found that muscle ribosomes obtained from castrated animals were less active in protein synthesis than were ribosomes from normal animals or castrated animals treated with androgens. These investigators also observed that actinomycin D prevented androgen stimulation of ribosome activity. Castration reduces the RNA content and ribosome activity and increases nuclear RNA polymerase activity. Liao *et al.* suggested that the RNA synthesized as a result of androgen treatment may be primarily ribosomal.[37] These investigators showed that actinomycin inhibited the hormonal effect on RNA synthesis but did not alter the basal level of nuclear RNA formation.

CARBOHYDRATE METABOLISM

Hormonal Effects on Carbohydrate Metabolism. *Insulin.* The discovery that insulin lowered the blood sugar in man and animals focused attention on the effects of this hormone on carbohydrate metabolism. The ability to control hyperglycemia in patients with diabetes mellitus further emphasized the importance of insulin and the rise in respiratory quotient which followed its administration demonstrated that glucose utilization was enhanced. Although the decline of blood glucose which follows insulin administration has attracted major attention, the hormone also stimulates glycogen synthesis, promotes glucose oxidation and has important influences on metabolism of proteins and lipids.

Many attempts to explain the blood sugar-lowering effects of insulin have been made. It was suggested that action of the hormone was mediated through a direct enzymatic action, however, this could not be substantiated. Levine and associates[1,2] demonstrated that insulin accelerated membrane transport of sugars by determining effects of the hormone on disposition of non-metabolizable analogs of glucose. The most detailed studies of the role of insulin in membrane transport of sugars were conducted utilizing the perfused rat heart preparation. Insulin increases sugar transport fourfold in normal hearts and up to six- or sevenfold in hearts from diabetic animals.[3] The onset of hormone action is rapid with accelerated transport being evident within 1 to 2 minutes after the hormone is introduced into the perfusion fluid and reaching a maximum 15 to 20 minutes later. Insulin not only promotes transport of non-utilizable sugars into the muscle cell but has a similar effect on movement of glucose across the cell membrane.[3] Transport of glucose into skeletal and heart muscle, fat cells and fibroblasts is stimulated by insulin, however, entry of glucose into hepatic cells and the brain does not depend on this hormone. The mechanism by which insulin stimulates glucose transport has not been elucidated but it is believed that it acts on a carrier substance present in the membrane.[4] Cuatrecasas[5] has demonstrated that insulin combines with a specific receptor in fat cells and that action of the hormone on glucose uptake by the adipocyte depends upon this reaction. The combination of hormone

and receptor can be separated with neither insulin nor the cell membrane being irreversibly altered. The stimulation of glucose transport induced by insulin is antagonized by growth hormone, corticosteroids and free fatty acids.

Insulin causes glycogen deposition in the liver, an effect which depends on activation of the enzyme glycogen synthetase. The enzyme exists in two forms: one (D) depends on glucose-6-phosphate for its activity and the other (I) is active in the absence of glucose-6-phosphate. Insulin injection into normal or diabetic rats raises the level of synthetase I in liver.[6] Administration of insulin to normal, fed rats results in a rapid conversion of synthetase D to I in skeletal muscle. Glycogen synthetase is quickly converted from the I to the D form in heart muscle, skeletal muscle and liver by epinephrine, an action which is discussed more fully later.

Insulin not only promotes disposition of intracellular glucose by stimulating glycogen synthesis but the hormone also acts to accelerate glycolysis. Glucokinase which is involved in the initial enzymatic reaction of glycolysis in liver (phosphorylation) depends on insulin for maintenance of activity. In the absence of insulin or in subjects who are fasting or ingesting a carbohydrate-free diet, glucokinase activity drops to low values within 48 hours.[7] When insulin levels are reduced, activity of phosphofructokinase is diminished in both liver and muscle so that glucose utilization is diminished.

Glucagon. Until recently the effects of glucagon on carbohydrate metabolism appeared to be less important than those of insulin, however, it is now evident that the role of glucagon is as significant as that of insulin. Glucagon provides glucose for the organism when there is need for this substance as an energy source. How does the hormone of the pancreatic alpha cell act to make glucose available so that it may be utilized? It has long been known that glucagon is a powerful glycogenolytic agent in liver and a good deal has been learned about its mechanism of action. Glucagon stimulates production of cyclic AMP (CAMP) by activating the enzyme adenyl cyclase. CAMP promotes the conversion of inactive phosphorylase to active phosphorylase, an enzyme which participates in breakdown of glycogen to glucose. Sokal[8] demonstrated that glucagon is a more potent glycogenolytic agent than epinephrine and believes that it is the only humoral factor which could serve as a physiological regulator of hepatic glycogenolysis. The hormone is effective in the liver at a concentration of 3×10^{-11} M, its onset of action is rapid and its duration of action is quite short. In addition to its stimulatory effect on glycogen degradation, glucagon reverses the activation of glycogen synthetase induced in dog liver by administration of glucose and insulin.[9] This action prevents glucose from being stored in liver thus it remains available for use as fuel.

Glucagon also provides glucose for the organism through a powerful stimulation of hepatic gluconeogenesis. Glucagon enhances glucose formation from amino acids, especially alanine, and from lactate and pyruvate.[10] The hormone produces its effect when present in physiological concentration. The action of glucagon on gluconeogenesis can be totally reproduced by CAMP and the evidence indicates that glucagon acts to promote gluconeogenesis by activating adenyl cyclase in the plasma membrane. Insulin causes a reduction of CAMP levels and, thus, gluconeogenesis is inhibited.

Glucagon and insulin are counter-regulatory hormones in control of carbohydrate metabolism. Insulin enables glucose to penetrate into the cell where it may be used to provide immediate energy or where it can be stored for subsequent use. It is also the signal which directs the liver to turn off the glucose-producing machinery (gluconeogenesis). Glucagon is secreted when glucose is in short supply, i.e., during starvation, hypoglycemia and after exercise. It causes prompt release of glucose through hepatic glycogenolysis and stimulates gluconeogenesis. Although it may at first appear paradoxical, glucagon secretion is increased in diabetes mellitus despite elevated blood sugar values.[11] The rise in glucagon secretion probably occurs because glucose utilization is diminished.

Catecholamines. Epinephrine influences carbohydrate metabolism in several ways. The catecholamine stimulates glycogenolysis in muscle through a series of reactions that begins with acceleration of adenyl cyclase activity and increased formation of CAMP. The end result of this action is that phosphorylase *b* is converted to phosphorylase *a* which catalyzes breakdown of muscle glycogen to glucose. Epinephrine also stimulates hepatic adenyl cyclase activity and, as a result, phosphorylase activity is enhanced. The rise of phosphorylase activity results in conversion of liver glycogen to glucose. It appears that rat liver has independent adenyl cyclase systems, one of which responds to epinephrine and the other being controlled by glucagon.[12]

Epinephrine is a potent stimulator of hepatic gluconeogenesis from such substrates as lactate, pyruvate and alanine. Although the catecholamine acts by increasing the CAMP level in liver just as does glucagon, epinephrine is less powerful than the pancreatic hormone.[13] Epinephrine and glucagon appear to act at the same regulatory site since study of levels of the intermediates involved in gluconeogenesis reveals that both hormones accelerate conversion of pyruvate to phosphoenolpyruvate.[14]

Catecholamines impair peripheral utilization of glucose by inhibiting insulin secretion by the pancreas and by causing a rise of the glucose-6-phosphate level. Hexokinase activity is inhibited when glucose-6-phosphate accumulates hence glycolysis is diminished.

Corticosteroid Hormones. For many years the adrenal cortical steroids have been considered to be the hormones most importantly involved in acceleration of gluconeogenesis. Adrenalectomy of rats and dogs results in decreased formation of glucose from pyruvate or lactate, an abnormality which can be corrected by administration of adrenal cortical steroids. In rat liver slices increased glucose and glycogen production from labeled pyruvate and CO_2 occurs if the animal has been treated with corticosteroids. Recently, evidence has been reported which indicates that the steroids act in conjunction with glucagon to augment the rate of glucose synthesis in perfused liver of adrenalectomized rats and that neither hormone alone will stimulate glucose formation.[10] The view that adrenal steroids exert a permissive action on gluco-neogenesis has been expressed.

Adrenal glucocorticoids are also concerned with glycogen synthesis. Administration of cortisol or other active glucocorticoid causes glycogen deposition in liver of normal or adrenalectomized animals. Glycogen synthetase activity is depressed in fasted, adrenalectomized rats and is restored to normal by corticosteroid administration. Adrenal steroid stimulation of glycogen synthetase requires about 4 hours to reach its maximal level, however, in the presence of glucose, activation occurs within several minutes. There is also evidence that glucocorticoid hormones inhibit glucose utilization. *In vitro* uptake of glucose by skin and lymphatic tissue is reduced by the presence of corticosteroids. Fain[15] observed that addition of dexamethasone to incubated rat adipose tissue resulted in diminished uptake of ^{14}C-glucose, decreased oxidation of glucose to CO_2 and diminished conversion of glucose to glyceride-glycerol and fatty acid.

Thyroid Hormones. Thyroid hormones affect glucose synthesis and glycogen degradation as well as glucose oxidation and absorption. Glycogen content of the liver is markedly decreased in thyrotoxicosis or when pharmacological doses of thyroxine (T_4) are administered to animals. Thyroid hormones modify actions of other hormones on carbohydrate metabolism, especially the catecholamines. For example, when the level of T_4 is raised, the glycogenolytic and lipolytic effects of epinephrine and norepinephrine are potentiated. The synergistic action of T_4 and catecholamines is thought to result from their common action of stimulating adenyl cyclase to produce CAMP. As mentioned previously, CAMP activates phosphorylase, an enzyme involved in glycogen degradation.

Thyroid hormones increase the supply of glucose for oxidation by their catabolic action on liver glycogen and, in addition, these agents enhance glucose synthesis by liver.[16] The mechanism of action of thyroid hormones on gluconeogenesis is not fully understood but it is known that the substrate supply to liver is increased because of accelerated peripheral protein breakdown with release of amino acids. There are reports which demonstrate that T_4 administration results in increased activity of hepatic enzymes concerned with gluconeogenesis, however, this is probably a response to the acceleration of gluconeogenesis rather than an initial action of the hormone.

Many patients with hyperthyroidism show a marked rise of blood sugar within the first 60 to 90 minutes following glucose ingestion. Although the incidence of diabetes is increased in hyperthyroidism, the abnormality of glucose tolerance has been attributed to more rapid intestinal absorption of the sugar. In hypothyroidism, absorption of a glucose load from the intestine is delayed. Glucose oxidation is enhanced when the T_4 level is elevated. Disposal of glucose via the Emden-Meyerhof and the hexose monophosphate shunt is augmented.

Growth Hormone. Growth hormone has an anti-insulin action. Insulin promotes entry of glucose into the muscle cell where it is phosphorylated. Growth hormone depresses the phosphorylation of glucose in muscle, an action shared by the corticosteroids. Growth hormone exerts its inhibitory effect on phosphorylation by stimulating release of fatty acids from adipose depots. Fatty acids and ketone bodies impair glucose utilization by skeletal and heart muscle.[17]

Acute administration of growth hormone to normal human subjects is followed by a short-lived fall of plasma free fatty acids and a more prolonged decrease of glucose. The decline of blood sugar is secondary to stimulation of the pancreatic beta cells by the pituitary hormone. Prolonged growth hormone administration produces hyperglycemia in animals and man despite enhanced insulin secretion. It is evident that resistance to the blood sugar-lowering action of insulin has been induced. This is at least partially due to the increased concentration of plasma fatty acids. In patients with acromegaly the incidence of diabetes mellitus may exceed 20 per cent.[18] In many other acromegalics whose blood sugar is within normal limits, plasma insulin values are markedly elevated especially after glucose ingestion. Thus, insulin resistance not only occurs after experimental administration of growth hormone but is a natural phenomenon as well.

The marked elevation of pancreatic insulin secretion which occurs in the acromegalic indicates that growth hormone has a trophic effect on the pancreatic islets.

FAT METABOLISM

Hormonal Effects on Fat Metabolism. Lipids are a major source of energy for the body and their metabolism is influenced by a number of hormones. Recently, it has been recognized that adipose tissue is not an inert depot for fat but is a major site for conversion of carbohydrate to fat and an important control point for the hormonal regulation of energy balance.[1] A consideration of hormonal influences on the mechanisms by which fat is stored and mobilized is important in the understanding of lipid metabolism. The effects of various hormones upon these aspects of fat metabolism will be discussed in this section.

Insulin. A principal effect of insulin on lipid metabolism is to stimulate conversion of glucose carbon into fatty acids and triglyceride. Lipogenesis takes place primarily in adipose tissue and it is generally accepted that this tissue is a major site of insulin action. Winegrad and Renold[2] showed that insulin added *in vitro* to rat adipose tissue increased incorporation of ^{14}C-glucose into fatty acids. Similar effects of insulin on triglyceride synthesis were observed. After an overnight fast, conversion of labeled glucose into glyceride-glycerol of adipose tissue was enhanced severalfold by the addition of a physiological concentration of insulin to the incubation medium.[3] Experiments with *in vivo* administration of insulin have provided similar evidence for insulin facilitation of lipogenesis from carbohydrate in adipose tissue as well as in liver.

Since glucose utilization is essential for lipogenesis, the rate of lipid formation is controlled by the rate of glucose metabolism. Increased glucose utilization can facilitate lipid synthesis in the following manner: (1) by supplying acetyl CoA, a precursor of fatty acids, (2) by providing α-glycerophosphate for esterification of fatty acids to form triglyceride, (3) by generating reduced triphosphopyridine nucleotide (NADPH) which

is mandatory for the crotonyl-CoA-butyryl-CoA hydrogenation, an important step in fatty acid synthesis. Thus, insulin by virtue of its effect on glucose metabolism has a significant influence on fat synthesis in adipose tissue. Insulin also facilitates accumulation of fat by a direct effect on lipid metabolism. The enzyme lipoprotein lipase which is located on the cell membrane is stimulated by insulin.[4] As a result, hydrolysis of chylomicrons arriving from the gut and of pre-beta-lipoproteins synthesized in liver is accelerated with release of fatty acids. Consequently, transport of the released fatty acids into adipose tissue is increased.

In the liver, insulin stimulates lipogenesis in a manner similar to that observed in adipose tissue. During insulin deprivation, hexose monophosphate shunt activity is impaired and, as a result, NADPH is not provided in the amounts needed for fatty acid synthesis. Esterification of fatty acid in liver is also diminished in the absence of insulin. Perfusion of normal rat liver with high concentrations of FFA resulted in conversion of a considerable amount of FFA into triglyceride.[5] Similarly, in normal dogs more than half of the infused FFA was esterified; conversely, insulin deficiency resulted in a significant decrease in conversion of FFA into triglyceride.[6] The impaired capacity for esterification of FFA is due to decreased availability of α-glycerophosphate.[7]

Whether all effects of insulin on lipid metabolism are due to enhanced permeability of the cell membrane to glucose or whether some intracellular actions of insulin also have a significant role is not established. The *in vitro* stimulation of fatty acid synthesis from glucose produced by insulin can be duplicated in the absence of insulin by raising the concentration of glucose in the medium.[8] Gordon and Cherkes[9] have demonstrated that incubated adipose tissue from diabetic animals released FFA and glycerol at a higher than normal rate and the increased rate of lipolysis was inhibited by insulin. The antilipolytic action of insulin results, in part, from stimulation of glucose utilization which provides α-glycerophosphate for esterification of fatty acids. However, Jungas and Ball[10] have shown that insulin also inhibits lipolysis in adipose tissue in the absence of glucose. In fact this tissue is so sensitive to insulin that it is used in a bioassay of the hormone.[11] Although the exact mechanism for the direct antilipolytic action of insulin is not clear, a speculation is that it may be mediated via lowering of the cyclic AMP level in the fat cell. Butcher *et al.*[12] reported that insulin lowered cyclic AMP in isolated fat cells of the rat. Others have demonstrated similar *in vitro* insulin action on cyclic AMP in intact fat pads as well as in homogenates of the same tissue.[10,13] In addition, it has been observed that incubation of fat pad with insulin decreased the level of active phosphorylase and increased the independent form of glycogen synthetase.[14] These effects are expected if cyclic AMP levels are reduced.

The net result of the antilipolytic, lipid synthetic and glycerogenic actions of insulin is to convert energy ingested as carbohydrate to a storage form as lipid.[15] Thus, after a carbohydrate meal with the consequent rise in insulin secretion glucose is utilized in adipose tissue for fatty acid synthesis and, simultaneously, there is a decrease in release of fatty acids due to the antilipolytic action of insulin. Conversely, during insulin deficiency there is decreased ability to store energy as fat since utilization of carbohydrate is impaired. Furthermore, there is mobilization of stored fat which produces a rise in plasma levels of FFA and triglyceride. An increased amount of lipid reaches the liver where it is oxidized to acetyl CoA. Acetyl CoA is converted into ketone bodies which are ultimately released into circulation because fatty acid synthesis is blocked. Accumulation of ketones, elevated levels of total blood lipid, the rise in plasma FFA and occurrence of fatty liver in individuals with insulin deficiency are all reflections of deranged fat metabolism.

Glucagon. Glucagon stimulates lipolysis in adipose tissue and liver. As a result, there is increased release of long- and short-chain fatty acid CoA esters. Intravenous administration of glucagon produces a prompt but transient rise followed by a fall in plasma levels of FFA.[16] The depression of plasma FFA which follows glucagon results from stimulation of insulin secretion since the ef-

fect can be abolished by infusion of anti-insulin serum along with glucagon[17] and by pancreatectomy.[18] *In vitro* data provide similar evidence for an increase in lipolysis by glucagon.[19] The lipolytic action in adipose tissue is mediated via stimulation of cyclic AMP which activates a hormone-sensitive lipase.[20]

In liver, the lipolytic effect of glucagon is powerful and rapid. Several studies have shown that enhanced lipolysis may be responsibile in part for the stimulation of gluconeogenesis and ketogenesis observed after glucagon administration. Carboxylation of pyruvate to oxaloacetate is enhanced by the increased availability of acetyl CoA, thus accounting for the stimulation of gluconeogenesis.[1] In isolated liver perfusions, addition of fatty acid increases the rate of gluconeogenesis from lactate and pyruvate. The effects of glucagon on fat metabolism have been produced with rather large doses of glucagon and it appears that physiological levels of the hormone may not significantly alter lipid metabolism. Furthermore, since glucagon stimulates insulin secretion, the resulting antilipolytic action counteracts glucagon-induced fat mobilization.

Catecholamines. Both norepinephrine and epinephrine are important physiological stimulants of fat mobilization from adipose tissue.[21] Within a few minutes after injection of either catecholamine into humans or animals a significant increase in plasma FFA and glycerol is observed.[22] Epinephrine-induced lipolysis does not persist as long as that due to norepinephrine probably because epinephrine simultaneously increases hepatic production of glucose which inhibits lipolysis from adipose tissue. In addition to mobilization of FFA, catecholamines also stimulate conversion of ^{14}C-labeled glucose into triglyceride-glycerol as well as esterification of FFA to form triglyceride.[23] However, stimulation of lipogenesis is of lesser magnitude than that of lipid mobilization.

Effects of catecholamine-induced lipolysis become readily evident in tissues which normally take up considerable amounts of FFA. Liver, kidney, lung, heart and skeletal muscle utilize FFA as a major source of energy. When lipid mobilization is enhanced, plasma

FFA levels rise and fatty acid uptake by tissues is increased since this, in part, depends upon the blood levels. Fatty acids are oxidized to CO_2 and water but a small proportion is converted into triglyceride for storage. In the liver, FFA are also utilized to form ketone bodies and low-density lipoproteins (LDL). Some of the esterified fatty acid from liver is released into circulation in the form of LDL for ultimate extrahepatic storage or oxidation.

Recent evidence suggests that the lipolytic action of catecholamines is due to an increase in formation of cyclic AMP from ATP.[20,24] Adenyl cyclase enzyme systems catalyze the formation of cyclic AMP from ATP; catecholamines and other lipolytic hormones including ACTH, TSH, and glucagon stimulate adenyl cyclase and, thus, promote cyclic AMP formation. Direct evidence for a role of cyclic AMP in human adipose tissue has been provided by Carlson et al.[25] These workers reported an increased level of the nucleotide in adipose tissue incubated with norepinephrine for a short period of time. Cyclic AMP activates a lipase that induces hydrolysis of triglyceride to fatty acids. The lipolytic action of catecholamines is mediated via a β-adrenergic receptor[26] which when stimulated leads to formation of cyclic AMP. The hormone-sensitive lipase which is activated by CAMP is present not only in adipose tissue, but also in liver, heart and skeletal muscle.[27]

Adrenal Cortical Steroids and Fat Metabolism. Inhibition of lipogenesis by adrenal steroids has been observed by several investigators. Fat synthesis in liver is depressed in the alloxan diabetic rat; however, after adrenalectomy lipid formation returns to near normal levels.[28] When cortisol is administered to adrenalectomized, diabetic animals fatty acid synthesis is depressed. Cortisol inhibition of hepatic fatty acid synthesis is evident within 2 to 6 hours and occurs concomitantly with an increase in glucose formation from pyruvate.

Jeanrenaud and Renold[29] studied metabolism of pyruvate-2-^{14}C and glucose-U-^{14}C by adipose tissue from normal and adrenalectomized rats. Production of $^{14}CO_2$ from these substrates and incorporation of glucose and pyruvate into long-chain fatty acids were similar in epididymal adipose tissue from normal and adrenalectomized rats if the nutritional status of the animals was comparable. Injection of cortisone into fasted, adrenalectomized rats 12 to 24 hours before the epididymal fat pad was removed resulted in decreased conversion of pyruvate to fatty acids. These investigators found that adrenalectomy did not alter glucose metabolism in adipose tissue from diabetic rats, nor was incorporation of glucose carbon into long-chain fatty acids affected. On the other hand, other observations revealed that adrenalectomy increased glucose oxidation and incorporation of the hexose into long-chain fatty acids by epididymal fat tissue from alloxan diabetic rats. Not all investigators agree that corticosteroids depress lipid synthesis. Hays and Hill[30] studied triglyceride-synthesizing activity and acyl-CoA synthetase activity in hepatic microsomes of cortisone-treated rats. Triglyceride synthesizing activity was increased twofold and the level of acyl-CoA synthetase was elevated 30 per cent by chronic cortisone treatment. Nevertheless, the bulk of evidence available indicates that fat synthesis is inhibited by corticosteroids.

Hormonal regulation of lipid mobilization is mainly exerted by controlling the rate of triglyceride hydrolysis in adipose tissue. Catecholamines, which are potent lipolytic agents, rapidly activate lipolysis through a cyclic AMP-mediated activation of lipase. Growth hormone and glucocorticoids cause a marked increase in fatty acid release by adipose tissue from adrenalectomized rats if the animals are treated with the hormones *in vivo*. However, neither hormone alone stimulates fatty acid release.[31] *In vitro* addition of GH to incubated adipose tissue or fat cells will mobilize fatty acids after a 2-hour lag period, an effect which is potentiated by glucocorticoid. Corticosteroids do not alter lipolysis in the absence of GH. The lipolytic effects of GH and glucocorticoids are blocked by inhibitors of protein and RNA synthesis, thus, indicating that RNA and protein synthesis are necessary for their action. These inhibitors do not block the action of rapidly acting lipolytic substances such as catecholamines. GH and dexamethasone also increase sensitivity of fat cells to the lipolytic actions of epinephrine; an effect which is due to increased accumulation of cyclic AMP.

In contrast to their limited effects in adipose tissue corticosteroids exert an important lipolytic action in liver. Klausner and Heimberg[32] reported that triglyceride release by isolated liver of adrenalectomized rats was impaired and that pretreatment of the animal with cortisone or addition of cortisol to the perfused liver restored lipid output to normal. These investigators found that the concentration of cortisol required to stimulate triglyceride release by liver of normal or adrenalectomized rats was quite specific and that at this concentration glucose release was also enhanced. When the critical level of cortisol was exceeded, hepatic triglyceride release was diminished.

In humans, intravenous injection of cortisol is followed first by a 30 per cent decline in blood free fatty acids (FFA) which lasts about 90 minutes. Subsequently, FFA rise progressively until 3 hours after hormone injection the level is about 35 per cent greater than the control value.[33] Other studies have shown that prolonged steroid treatment results in elevated plasma lipids, an effect which may account for the fatty liver which is produced in experimental animals by chronic glucocorticoid administration. When circulating corticosteroid levels are increased in human subjects with Cushing's syndrome or in those treated with steroids, remarkable changes in fat distribution occur. Chronic corticoid excess leads to fat accumulation in the face, supraclavicular areas, over the lower cervical vertebra in the trunk. The explanation of this curious predilection for fat deposits is not known.

Growth Hormone. Administration of growth hormone (GH) to normal or hypophysectomized animals produces a decrease in carcass fat, an increase in plasma FFA and liver lipid. These metabolic alterations reflect stimulation of lipolysis by GH,[34] however, the exact mechanism of this action is not clearly established. Rather than exerting a direct effect, GH appears to potentiate the effect of other lipolytic hormones. Fain *et al.*[31] have shown that when GH and dexamethasone were added to a fat cell suspension, lipolysis was stimulated even with very low concentration of the polypeptide hormone. They also found that GH-induced lipolysis was mediated via the synthesis of new protein since the effect was inhibited by puromycin and actinomycin. A role for cyclic AMP in the lipolytic action of GH has been suggested since insulin inhibits growth hormone-induced lipolysis. The antilipolytic effect of insulin is considered to be due to a decrease in intracellular cyclic AMP.[12]

Growth hormone not only stimulates lipolysis but also inhibits lipogenesis. Hypophysectomized rats injected with GH exhibit reduced incorporation of glucose into fat as well as depletion of depot fat.[35] Recently, it was found that GH increased incorporation of long-chain fatty acids into triglycerides in isolated fat tissue,[36] however, such an effect has not been reported in other tissues.

Stimulation of lipolysis by GH does not cause fatty liver, perhaps, because the hormone also enhances oxidation of fatty acids. In man, respiratory quotients of the whole body[37] and the forearm[38] are lowered after GH treatment and there is also increased ketogenesis. These changes reflect increased oxidation of fatty acids. Attempts to demonstrate an effect of GH on fatty acid oxidation *in vitro* using labeled substrate have been generally unsuccessful. These negative results may be explained by the suggestion that the concentration of FFA in the plasma is not the sole determinant of FFA oxidation[38] and that high levels of intracellular FFA, induced by growth hormone, may be the major supply for oxidation reactions. GH infusion into the brachial artery induced a prompt reduction in glucose uptake by forearm tissues and there was a concomitant increase in fatty acid oxidation.

Adrenocorticotropin (ACTH). One of the prominent extra-adrenal actions of ACTH is its fat-mobilizing activity. *In vitro*, it is highly potent in releasing FFA from adipose tissue.[39] Administration of ACTH to intact and adrenalectomized animals increases lipolysis, an effect which does not depend on stimulation of the adrenal cortex.[40] In consequence, plasma FFA increase after ACTH administration and there is an elevation of liver lipids. The fat-mobilizing effect of ACTH is mediated through cyclic AMP which activates a lipase in adipose tissue.

Thyroid Hormones. Thyroid hormones influence lipid metabolism mainly by modifying the rate of oxidation and mobilization of FFA from adipose tissue. Rich *et al.*[41] first observed elevated plasma FFA levels in hyperthyroid subjects and also showed that administration of triiodothyronine (T_3) to normal individuals produced a rise in plasma FFA levels. Adipose tissue from thyrotoxic rats incubated *in vitro* releases FFA into the medium at an accelerated rate and exhibits an exaggerated response to epinephrine-induced lipolysis. Conversely, lipolysis and the effectiveness of catecholamines in mobilizing FFA are impaired in thyroid-deficient animals.

Most data suggest that the thyroid effect on lipolysis is to facilitate the action of other hormones rather than to directly stimulate mobilization of lipids.[42] A smaller dose of epinephrine is required to induce a maximum increase of plasma FFA in thyrotoxic patients than in control subjects.[43] Hypophysectomy in monkeys abolished the FFA response to epinephrine, but this was partially restored following TSH injection and completely corrected by T_3 administration.[44] Other studies suggest that fat mobilization by ACTH, TSH, GH and glucagon is similarly facilitated by thyroid hormones. Enhancement of the action of lipolytic hormones by thyroid hormone may be due to the fact that fat mobilization depends upon formation of CAMP and that thyroid hormones increase the amount of CAMP that is formed when adenyl cyclase activity is stimulated by lipolytic hormones.

Biosynthesis of fatty acids is increased by thyroid hormones. *In vivo* conversion of ^{14}C-acetate into fatty acids was greater in the liver of thyrotoxic rats than in that of normal animals. Conversely, fatty acid synthesis is reduced in thiouracil-fed rats. Lipid synthesis is decreased in hypothyroid individuals but is restored to normal by thyroid hormones. There are some investigators who claim that fat synthesis is decreased by thyroid hormones, however, there is little support for this finding.

Thyroid hormone enhancement of fat catabolism outweighs its influence on fat synthesis and is responsible for the changes in fat tissue which occur in thyroid disease. In thyrotoxicosis, there is loss of weight and the fat content of the body is below normal. Furthermore, many hyperthyroid patients lose weight because their energy expenditure is greater than the caloric intake hence there is mobilization of depot fat and increased oxidation of FFA. In hypothyroidism, plasma levels of FFA are depressed and there is diminished lipolysis in response to fasting or after administration of epinephrine or growth hormone.

BIBLIOGRAPHY

Protein Metabolism

1. Clark: J. Biol. Chem., *200*, 69, 1953.
2. Goodlad and Munro: J. Biochem., *73*, 343, 1959.
3. Munro: In *Mammalian Protein Metabolism*, Munro, ed. New York, Academic Press, Vol. I, Chap. 10, 1964.
4. Munro and Thomson: Metabolism, *2*, 354, 1953.
5. Kochakian, Tillotson and Austin: Endocrinology, *60*, 144, 1957.
6. Blanpin and Aschkenasy: Compt. Rend. Soc. Biol., *153*, 997, 1959.
7. Roche, Dumazert, Emond, and Roger: Compt. Rend. Soc. Biol., *136*, 326, 1942.
8. Manchester: In *Diabetes Mellitus*, Ellenberg and Rifkin, ed., New York, McGraw-Hill Book Co., 1970.
9. Lotspeich: J. Biol. Chem., *179*, 175, 1949.
10. Pozefsky, Felig, Soeldner and Cahill: Trans. Ass. Amer. Physicians, *81*, 258, 1968.
11. Wool and Krahl: Nature, *183*, 1399, 1959.
12. Wool: Amer. J. Physiol., *199*, 719, 1960.
13a. Herrera and Renold: Biochim. Biophys. Acta, *44*, 165, 1960.
13b. Mayne and Barry: J. Biochem., *99*, 688, 1966.
13c. Davidson and Goodner: Diabetes, *15*, 835, 1966.
13d. Mayne and Barry: Biochim. Biophys. Acta, *138*, 195, 1967.
14a. Korner: J. Endocr., *20*, 256, 1960.
14b. Robinson: Proc. Soc. Exptl. Biol. Med., *106*, 115, 1961.
15. Manchester: In *Mammalian Protein Metabolism*, Munro, ed., New York, Academic Press, Vol. IV, Chap. 33, 1970.
16. Leathem: In *Mammalian Protein Metabolism*, Munro, ed., New York, Academic Press, Vol. I, Chap. 9, 1964.
17a. Korner: Progr. Biophys., *17*, 61, 1967.
17b. Hjalmarson and Ahren: Acta Endocr. (Kobenhavn), *54*, 645, 1967.
18. Korner: J. Biochem., *81*, 292, 1961.

19a.Long, Katzin, and Fry: Endocrinology, 26, 309, 1940.
19b.Engel: Recent Progr. in Hormone Research, 6, 277, 1951.
20. Friedberg and Greenberg: J. Biol. Chem., 168, 405, 1948.
21. Munro: In Mammalian Protein Metabolism, Munro, ed., New York, Academic Press, Vol. IV, Chap. 34, 1970.
22. Bondy, Ingle and Meeks: Endocrinology, 55, 355, 1954.
23. Manchester, Randle, and Young: J. Endocr., 18, 395, 1959.
24. Noall, Riggs, Walker, and Christensen: Science, 126, 1002, 1957.
25. Weber, Srivastava, and Singhal: J. Biol. Chem., 240, 750, 1965.
26. Bass, Chambers, and Richtarik: Life Sci., 4, 266, 1963.
27. Clark: J. Biol. Chem., 200, 69, 1953.
28. Feigelson and Greengard: J. Biol. Chem., 237, 3714, 1962.
29. Kenney: In Mammalian Protein Metabolism, Munro, ed., New York, Academic Press, Vol. IV, Chap. 31, 1970.
30. Segal and Kim: Proc. Nat. Sci. USA, 50, 912, 1963.
31. Kreisberg, Owen and Siegal: Med. Clin. North America, 54, 1473, 1970.
32. Foley, London, and Prenton: J. Clin. Endocr. Metab., 26, 781, 1966.
33. Wellers and Leblane: C. R. Soc. Biol. (Paris), 160, 1785, 1966.
34. Tata: Progr. Nucl, Acid. Res., 5, 191, 1966.
35. Young: In Mammalian Protein Metabolism, Munro, ed., New York, Academic Press, Vol. IV, Chap. 40, 1970.
36. Breuer and Florini: Biochemistry, 4, 1544, 1965.
37a.Liao, Lin, and Barton: J. Biol. Chem., 241, 3869, 1966.
37b.Liao, Barton, and Lin: Proc. Nat. Acad. Sci. USA, 55, 1593, 1966.
37c.Liao and Lin: Proc. Nat. Acad. Sci. USA, 57, 379, 1967.

Carbohydrate Metabolism

1. Levine, Goldstein, Klein and Huddlestun: J. Biol. Chem., 179, 985, 1949.
2. Levine and Goldstein: Recent Progr. Hormone Res., 11, 343, 1955.
3. Park, Morgan, Henderson, et al.: Recent Progr. Hormone Res., 17, 493, 1961.
4. Levine: In Diabetes Mellitus, Ellenberg and Rifkin, ed., New York, McGraw-Hill Book Co., 1970.
5. Cuatrecasas: Proc. Nat. Acad. Sci. USA, 63, 450, 1969.
6. Villar-Palasi and Larner: Ann. Rev. Biochem., 39, 639, 1970.
7. Sharma, Menjeshwar and Weinhouse: J. Biol. Chem., 238, 1342, 1963.
8. Sokal and Ezdinli: J. Clin. Invest., 46, 778, 1967.

9. Bishop and Larner: J. Biol. Chem., 242, 1354, 1967.
10. Eisenstein and Strack: Endocrinology, 83, 1337, 1968.
11. Unger, Agiular-Parada, Muller, and Eisentraut: J. Clin. Invest., 49, 837, 1970.
12. Bitensky, Russell and Robertson: Biochem. Biophys. Res. Commun., 31, 706, 1968.
13. Exton and Park: Adv. in Enzyme Regulation, 6, 391, 1968.
14. ———: Pharmacol. Rev., 18, 181, 1966.
15. Fain: J. Biol. Chem., 239, 958, 1964.
16. Murad and Freedland: Proc. Soc. Exp. Biol. Med., 124, 1176, 1967.
17. Randle, Garland, Hales, and Newsholme: Lancet, 1, 785, 1963.
18. Boshell and Chaudalia: In Diabetes Mellitus, Ellenberg and Rifkin, ed., Chapter 4, New York, McGraw-Hill Book Co., 1970.

Fat Metabolism

1. Renold, Crofford, Stauffacher, and Jeanrenaud: Diabetologia, 1, 4, 1965.
2. Winegrad and Renold: J. Biol. Chem., 233, 273, 1958.
3. Vaughen: J. Biol. Chem., 236, 2196, 1961.
4. Schnatz and Williams: Diabetes, 12, 174, 1963.
5. Richard, Ruderman, and Herrera: Biochim. Biophys. Acta, 152, 632, 1968.
6. Basso and Havel: Clin. Res., 15, 127, 1967.
7. Mayes and Felts: Nature, 215, 716, 1967.
8. Ball and Jungas: Recent Progr. Hormone Res., 20, 183, 1964.
9. Gordon and Cherkes: Proc. Soc. Exptl. Biol. Med., 97, 150, 1958.
10. Jungas and Ball: Biochemistry, 2, 383, 1963.
11. Williams: In Textbook of Endocrinology, Williams, Ed., Philadelphia, W. B. Saunders Co., chapter 9, 1968.
12. Butcher, Baired, and Sutherland: J. Biol. Chem., 243, 1705, 1968.
13. Love, Carr, and Ashmore: J. Pharmacol. Exptl. Therap., 140, 287, 1963.
14. Jungas: Proc. Natl. Acad. Sci. U.S.A., 56, 757, 1966.
15. Levine: New Eng. J. Med., 283, 175, 1970.
16. Eymer, Schwartz, and Weinges: Klin. Wochenschr., 39, 631, 1961.
17. Williamson: In Adv. Enzyme Regulation, Vol. 5. London, Pergamon Press Ltd., 1965.
18. Sokal, Aydin, and Kraus: Am. J. Physiol., 211, 1334, 1966.
19. Weinges: Klin. Wochenschr., 39, 293, 1961.
20. Robison, Butcher, and Sutherland: In Cyclic AMP. New York, Academic Press, 1970.
21. Steinberg: Pharmacol. Rev., 18, 217, 1966.
22. Havel: In Lipid Pharmacology, Paoletti, Ed., Medicinal Chemistry, vol. 2, New York, Academic Press, 1964.
23. Winegrad: Vitamins and Hormones, 20, 141, 1964.
24. Rizack: J. Biol. Chem., 239, 392, 1962.

25. Carlson, Butcher, and Micheli: Acta Med. Scand., *187*, 529, 1970.

26. Brodie, Maikel, and Stern: *In* Adipose Tissue, Renold and Cahill, Eds., *Handbook of Physiology*, V. Baltimore, Williams & Wilkins Co., 1965.

27. Froberg and Oro: Acta Med. Scand., *176*, 65, 1964.

28. Gurin and Brady: Recent Prog. Hormone Res., *8*, 571, 1953.

29. Jeanrenaud and Renold: J. Biol. Chem., *235*, 2217, 1960.

30. Hays and Hill: Biochim. Biophys. Acta, *98*, 646, 1965.

31. Fain, Kovacev, and Scow: J. Biol. Chem., *240*, 3522, 1965.

32. Klausner and Heimberg: Am. J. Physiol., *212*, 1236, 1967.

33. Dreiling, Bierman, Debons, *et al.*: Metabolism, *11*, 572, 1962.

34. Raben: New Engl. J. Med., *266*, 82, 1962.

35. Goodman: Endocrinology, *72*, 95, 1963.

36. ———: Ann. N.Y. Acad. Sci., *148*, 419, 1968.

37. Brown and Bennett: J. Clin. Invest., *38*, 993, 1959.

38. Zierler: In *Clinical Endocrinology*, II, Astwood and Cassidy, Eds., New York, Grune & Stratton, 1968.

39. Hollenberg, Raben, and Astwood: Endocrinology, *68*, 589, 1968.

40. Li, Fonss-Bech, Greschwind, *et al.*: J. Expt. Med., *105*, 335, 1957.

41. Rich, Bierman, and Schwartz: J. Clin. Invest., *38*, 275, 1959.

42. Hoch: Postgrad. Med. J., *44*, 347, 1968.

43. Harlan, Laszio, Bogdonoff, and Ester: J. Clin. Endocr., *23*, 33, 1963.

44. Goodman and Knobil: Proc. Soc. Expt. Biol. Med., *100*, 195, 1959.

Chapter

14

Physiology of Hunger and Satiety; Regulation of Food Intake

JEAN MAYER

In the course of the past two decades, considerable progress has been made in our understanding of the mechanism of regulation of food intake, of appetite, and of satiety. At the same time, realization of the vast reaches of our ignorance, and of the fact that many of the often repeated "common sense" generalizations in the area of hunger, satiety and their abnormalities are but clichés which mask our ignorance, has grown correspondingly. After a long period of quiescence—from the pre-World War I period to the post-World War II era—research is now proceeding actively along several lines of attack: study of central mechanisms, particularly those based on mid-brain structures; study of gastrointestinal factors; interconnection of metabolic factors—particularly the metabolism of the adipose tissue—with neural and behavioral events; extensive examination of the various types of errors, inborn or acquired, which may lead to obesity or to anorexia, and relevance of these to the normal physiology of regulation of food intake; study of the influence of environmental factors—both ecological and psychological—on food intake. In addition to the new interest in the application of modern operant conditioning techniques to problems of food intake, there is a renewal of interest in the analysis of human sensations of hunger, appetite and satiety, which had lagged since the mid-nineteenth century. On such broad research activity rests the hope that progress will accelerate in this important and long-neglected field.

DEFINITIONS

The words appetite, hunger, satiety, regulation of food intake, limitation of food intake, obesity, overweight, anorexia have all been used in a variety of senses and this semantic confusion has in turn often created apparent contradictions where basic agreement in fact prevailed. Words such as hunger, appetite and satiety represent sensations and, as such, tend to take on highly subjective colorations. Studies in progress in my laboratory reveal great differences in the sensations of mild and extreme hunger in man as well as in the reasons that subjects state caused them to stop eating. Nevertheless, we shall attempt to give a series of working definitions of the terms which will be used in this chapter.

Appetite. The complex of sensations, up to a point pleasant, or at least not unpleasant, by which the organism is aware of desire for and anticipation of ingestion of palatable food. Specific appetites relate to desire for specific foods or nutrients.

Hunger. The complex of unpleasant sensations felt after prolonged deprivation (during the "hunger state") which will impel an animal or a man to seek, work or fight for immediate relief by ingestion of food (thus exhibiting "hunger behavior"). The passage from appetite to hunger is dependent on duration of deprivation, rate of energy expenditure, etc.

Satiety. The cessation of the urge to eat.

Regulation of Food Intake. The servomechanism or mechanisms whereby the body adjusts ingestion of food to requirement for homeostasis and for growth.

Limitation of Food Intake. The complex of sensations and factors which impels the organism to stop eating even though food is still available, whether energy requirements for maintenance and growth have or have not been covered.

Obesity. Excessive accumulation of body fat.

Overweight. Weight in excess of normal range.

Anorexia. Pathological absence of appetite or of hunger behavior in the presence of manifest energy needs.

CHARACTERISTICS OF THE REGULATION OF FOOD INTAKE

Regulation of Caloric Intake. Leaving aside temporarily the conscious aspects, such as sensations of hunger, appetite and satiety, let us examine the manner in which homeostasis is maintained and the expected pattern of growth achieved. The problem can be reformulated into the fourfold question: (1) Is there a regulation (or are there regulations)? (2) What is regulated? (3) How well is it regulated? (4) How is it regulated? In short, what are the mechanisms in terms of structure and function? That order will be followed in reviewing the available evidence.

Is there a regulation? Gasnier and A. Mayer[1] first showed that this question is best answered not by considering the food intake, but by observing the constancy, within a given environment, of total body weight, water content, reserves other than water, nitrogen balance and fat content. Their data on large numbers of animals carefully followed for long periods gave conclusive evidence that a regulation does exist.

What is regulated? Gasnier and A. Mayer further showed that three types of regulations could be defined:

Biometric Regulation. This is not, properly speaking, a mechanism but is a result of the very structure of the animal: it sets limits both upwards and downwards to energy exchange, the upper limit being the "summit" metabolism, the lower the basal metabolism. The limits change with the physiologic state.

Adaptation of Intake to Output: short-term (day-by-day) regulation of energy intake. This is perhaps the most important mechanism. A number of studies in different animals have shown the high correlation between output—modified by cold, exercise, etc.—and energy intake, as well as the sensitivity of intake of volume of food to changes in the caloric density of the diet.

Correction of the Errors in the Short-Term Regulation by Successive Compensations: long-term regulation of reserves. If energy balance was achieved exactly each day, intake and output would be equal, and in a plot of one against the other, all points would fall on the line bisecting the axes of coordinates. Actually, in such a plot, the points fall on a band spread on both sides of this line. The day-by-day regulation is thus not sufficient to ensure constancy of body weight and reserves. Gasnier and A. Mayer showed, however, that the distribution of the points was not random but lent itself to the following conclusions. On a given day, the farther away from the modal change the extra reserves deviated, the greater the chances that during the next 24 hours (*a*) if the change is in the same direction, it will be small, or (*b*) if the change is in the opposite direction, it will be large enough to approach or pass the mode. There is thus a long-term mechanism which, in effect, under constant environmental and physiologic conditions tends to maintain the constancy of body weight.

How well do these regulations function? Four parameters have been defined to describe how well both the short-term and the long-term regulations function: precision, reliability, sensitivity and rapidity.[1,2] For the short-term regulation, for example, the precision is inversely proportional to the difference between energy intake and energy output; the reliability is inversely proportional to the variability of the intake-to-output ratio; the sensitivity is inversely proportional to the dependence of the precision on the magnitude of intake; the rapidity is inversely proportional to the lag in adjustment of intake to output. The variation of such parameters as temperature, exercise, caloric dilution, state of hydration, changes in the nature of the diet, etc., characterizes the extent to which regulatory mechanisms are able to respond to such challenges. For example, in adapted animals, as the temperature falls both energy output and energy intake increase; the reliability of the short-term regulation adjusting intake to output increases, its precision remaining the same.[1,2] As regards the long-term regulation, body reserves increase, the precision and reliability of the regulation increase, but the sensitivity and rapidity decrease, with increasing metabolic intensity. The picture of the effect of enforced exercise on food intake is equally striking: the precision of the regulation is good within a wide range of activity. Below this range (in the "sedentary" range), and above it (in the "exhaustion" range) the precision deteriorates (Fig 14–1).

How do the regulations work? The answer to the question: what are the mechanisms of these regulations? is still tentative. We shall review briefly the anatomical support of

these regulations and the possible modes of integration of these mechanisms. It should be unnecessary to note again that, when one speaks of mechanisms of regulation, the interval of time considered is all-important. Short-term studies demonstrate the influence of a multiplicity of factors on appetite and emphasize instability. Experiments of longer duration—no less than one day and preferably longer periods—emphasize stability. It is essentially with the mechanisms underlying this stability that we are concerned.

It should be equally unnecessary to point out at the outset that *all* investigators whose hypotheses are about to be reviewed have repeatedly acknowledged the weakness of any general theory of appetite founded on response to only one stimulus, and none of them —least of all me—have attempted to enact such systems. The problem has been to identify the mechanism by which the metabolic state of the organism competes with such variable influences as taste, emotions. habitis, etc., to permit long-time homeostasis,

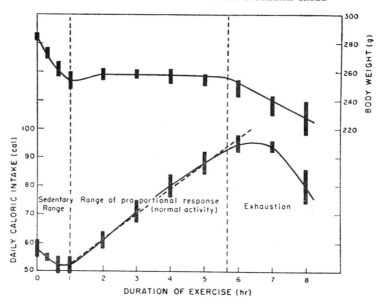

VOLUNTARY CALORIC INTAKE AND BODY WEIGHT
AS FUNCTIONS OF EXERCISE IN NORMAL RATS

Fig. 14-1. This figure illustrates the fact that the precision of the regulation of food intake as a function of exercise is good within the middle range of energy expenditure, in particular, normal activity, and poor both in the range of excessively low activity (sedentary range) and excessively high activity (exhaustion range). Within the range of normal activity, the reliability and sensitivity are constant, and the rapidity increases with energy expenditure.[2]

REGULATION OF CALORIC INTAKE AND WEIGHT: MORPHOLOGIC ASPECTS AND POSSIBLE MECHANISMS

Anatomic Basis. *Gastrointestinal Tract.* Haller was the first to suggest (in his *Elementa physiologica*, in 1777) that hunger was a gastric sensation. In his chapter, *"Famis causa proxima"*—the immediate cause of hunger— he stated that hunger sensations were due to the excitation of stomach nerves. For over a century and a half this theory was the most generally accepted. It was only in 1911 that it was tested experimentally by Cannon and Washburn[3] who showed that hunger sensations appeared simultaneously with contractions of the stomach. The hunger contractions were further investigated by Carlson[4] who found that during starvation the tonus of the empty stomach and the frequency and intensity of its contractions became progressively more pronounced, at least until the fourth day. The desire for food decreased. These gastric hunger contractions are relatively powerful; they occur in series of from twenty to seventy and last usually between half an hour and an hour and a half; they alternate with periods of quiescence. The contractions are seen in newborn babies before any food has been consumed. Their presence is general in land vertebrates, whether homeotherms or poikilotherms.

Hunger contractions are present even when there is some food in the stomach. The only time when the fundus does not exhibit them is immediately after a large meal. They occur after isolation from the brain and spinal cord, though at longer intervals and with less vigor. They are inhibited by a variety of stimuli: by the tasting or chewing of a palatable food, or even of an inert substance like paraffin wax (unless the contractions have become tetanic in nature), by stimulation of the gastric mucosa by ice cold water, acid, alcohol, smoking, by tightening of the belt, by vigorous muscular exercise, by sudden application of cold, by emotions such as fear or rage, by epinephrine, by glucagon or by intravenous glucose given under conditions such that normal utilization takes place. Inhibition of gastric contractions can be brought about also by irrigation of the duodenum by glucose. That this inhibition persists when the stomach is denervated or in auto-transplanted denervated gastric pouches has led to the postulation of secretion of a chalone by the duodenum or the liver. Interesting modifications of gastric tone take place in disease: duodenal ulcer and diabetes cause an increase, pulmonary tuberculosis and vitamin B_1, a decrease.

Carlson considered that the vagi were the main, if not the only, afferent pathways for the gastric hunger impulses and that the "primary hunger center" must therefore be the "sensory nuclei of the vagi" in the medulla (fasciculus solitarius). The existence of pressure- or tension-sensitive receptors in the stomach wall has been demonstrated.

The possible relation of intestinal phenomena to hunger has attracted some attention. The forward movement of food in the small intestine has been studied by a number of authors, in particular by Quigley.[5] The character of the peristaltic movement has been shown to be dependent on the composition of the chyme. The small intestine, like the stomach, obtains its supply of extrinsic nerve fibers from two sources: a bulbar autonomic (parasympathetic) supply by way of the vagi and a thoracic autonomic (sympathetic) supply by way of the splanchnic nerves and the superior mesenteric ganglia. Stimulation of the vagi causes contraction or increased tonus in the musculature of the intestine; stimulation of the splanchnic nerves generally inhibits its tonus. Psychological states and stimulation of portions of the cerebral cortex may produce contractions or relaxation of the walls of the small and large intestines. Epinephrine, like splanchnic stimulation, inhibits intestinal movements; oxygen, organic acids and bile increase them. The sensory fibers from the intestine are carried by the vagus and the splanchnic nerves.

Central Nervous System. Autopsies of patients with hypothalamic obesity suggested a role for the hypothalamus in the control of food intake. Experimental work by investigators on both sides of the Atlantic eliminated the pituitary from consideration as the prime suspect in the development of adiposity. The work of Hetherington and Ranson[6] and

Brobeck and co-workers[7] demonstrated that bilateral involvement of the ventromedial nuclei causes hyperphagia in the rat. It has since been shown that, in that species, unilateral destruction of the ventromedial nucleus may cause very slow development of obesity.[2] Hypothalamic obesity has been produced in the mouse by Mayer and his associates;[8] in that species, bilateral involvement of the ventromedial area is necessary for even the slightest degree of hyperphagia to appear. Obesity follows superficial lesions of the base of the anterior hypothalamus in the monkey, and lesions caudal to the paraventricular nuclei in the dog. Conversely, Anand and Brobeck[9] found that, in rats, bilateral destruction of more lateral parts of the hypothalamus is followed by complete cessation of eating (Fig. 14–2). Teitelbaum and Stellar[10] have confirmed this finding, though noting that this inhibition may be temporary, with resumption of eating dependent on the nature and consistency of the food presented. Morrison and Mayer,[11] noting that lesions in the lateral hypothalamus or subthalamus at the same rostrocaudal level as the ventromedial nucleus cause both aphagia and adipsia, tried to see whether these two responses were separate consequences of the lesions. They found that the patterns of food or water exchange cannot be reproduced by deprivation of sham-operated rats of either food or water. Daily water intubation facilitated the "escape"

from inhibition of eating and drinking. Localization of "aphagic" and "adipsic" lesions did not completely coincide and their histologic location suggested that the median forebrain bundle was as important as the lateral area proper in the control of water and food intake.[12] Morgane[13,14] in a careful anatomical analysis of this phenomenon has concluded that lesions causing aphagia may interfere with at least two systems of fibers, of which the more important is lateral to the median forebrain bundle; only destruction of this system (and of the median area of the pallidum) causes an irreversible aphagia. Other areas have also been shown to interfere with the regulation of food intake; bilateral damage to the ventromedial portion of the thalamus, of the rostral mesencephalic nuclei, of the temporal area of the amygdalum or the hippocampus causes hyperphagia. Destruction of the frontal area of the amygdalum or the hippocampus decreases food intake. Separation of the frontal lobes from their thalamic connections in rats, frontal lobotomy in man, and selective decortication in various types of animals also lead to hyperphagia.

Stimulation of various areas of the central nervous system has also proved rewarding. Larsson,[15] for example, studied the results of electrical stimulation of the hypothalamus and the medulla and of intrahypothalamic injections in sheep and goats. He found that stimulation of the hypothalamus, just caudal

REGULATION OF ENERGY EXCHANGE

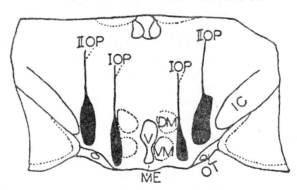

Fig. 14-2. Transverse section through tuberal region of hypothalamus. Medial lesions (I OP) induced hyperphagia and obesity, while lateral lesions (II OP) abolished feeding. ME, median eminence; OT, optic tract; IC, internal capsule; DM, dorsomedial nucleus; VM, ventromedial nucleus; V, third ventricle. (From Anand and Brobeck, Yale J. Biol. Med., *24*, 123, 1951.)

to the optic chiasma backwards throughout the hypothalamus, lateral to the sagittal level through the columna fornix descendens and the mammillothalamic tract resulted in hyperphagia. The most pronounced effect was obtained by stimulation of the region of the lateral hypothalamic nucleus, anterior to the columna fornix descendens or at the same transverse level as this tract. Rumination was seen on electrical stimulation of the same structures as gave hyperphagia. Mastication, licking and swallowing could be elicited as single effects without the simultaneous occurrence of hyperphagia. These results were taken by Larsson to suggest that it is an oversimplification to speak of a mammillothalamic or an anterolateral hypothalamic "feeding center." Although electrical stimulation of both these areas, particularly the latter, causes hyperphagia, the fact that extramasticatory and licking movements as well as hyperphagia are obtained diffusely in other areas supports the conclusion that centers directing feeding behavior and centers having to do with motivation to eat rest on centers which are in part different.

Finally, before leaving the anatomic description of central nervous areas involved in the regulation of food intake, it might be noted that some experiments performed by Sudsaneh and me,[16] described below, suggest that the ventromedial area of the hypothalamus exercises some measure of control over gastric contractions.

Use of Behavioral Techniques to Define the Role of Central Neural Structures Involved in the Regulation of Food Intake. The use of the behavioral techniques developed by B. F. Skinner and his associates has made it possible to better define the role of central neural structures in the regulation of food intake. It is also opening a trail which may some day give a more precise metabolic and neurologic basis to the concepts of hunger, satiety, appetite and specific appetites. An early experiment was that by Anliker and me, which compared the feeding behavior of normal animals with that of animals with various types of hyperphagia.[17] This clearly demonstrated that, as previously suggested by Brobeck[7] and by Miller, Bailey and Stevenson,[18] the ventro-

medial area appears to act as a "satiety" brake inhibiting constantly activated lateral "feeding" areas. (Similar techniques have permitted Rozin and Mayer[19] to study the characteristics of the regulation of food intake in the fish.)

Again on the basis of results obtained by behavioral techniques, Teitelbaum[20,21] has suggested that qualitative effects on taste were necessary concomitants of the destruction of the ventromedial area or of lateral hypothalamic lesions. Animals with ventromedial hypothalamic lesions cease to be hyperphagic if presented with diets the consistency or taste of which they do not like. Under such conditions, they may eat less than normal animals. The significance of this interesting observation is difficult, however, to evaluate at present. Lesions performed with the stereotaxic instruments are notoriously complex and it may well be that Teitelbaum was studying the effect of the destruction of a number of anatomically contiguous centers; the fact that animals can maintain their weight when feeding themselves through a gastric fistula suggests that taste (if not exaggeratedly aversive) is not an essential component in the regulation of food intake, although it obviously is one of the factors influencing food intake at a given time.

Another important behavioral technique which has contributed to our knowledge of central nervous areas involved in the regulation of food intake is that of Olds, who combined lever pressing for food in the rat with auto-excitation of a number of central areas.[22] The auto-excitation of certain areas (corresponding roughly to parasympathetic nuclei) acts as an additional reward and leads the animal to a tremendous increase in the rate of lever pressing. The auto-excitation of other areas (corresponding roughly to the areas in which Hess has obtained stimulation of the sympathetic system) acts as a negative reinforcement and decreases rates of lever pressing. The combination of Olds' auto-excitation technique with the use of an electric grid permitting the examination of the circumstances under which the drive to eat is particularly intense has allowed Morgane[23] to explore the role of the ventromedial area, the pallidum, the median forebrain bundle, and the lateral areas. His results seem to indicate that the lateral area should be subdivided into at least two subareas, an extreme lateral one—excitation of which leads to extreme rates of lever pressing for food, to considerable hyperphagia, and to the crossing of the electrified grid to obtain food, even when the animal is fed—and the properly lateral area, excitation of which leads to some hyperphagia, even in fed animals, but not to the crossing of the grid. These experiments, together with those on the effect of lateral lesions, do suggest the presence in the lateral hypothalamus of two systems of fibers, one having to do with purely quantitative aspects of the regulation of food intake (and presumably subject to ventromedial "satiety" inhibition) and one having to do with more qualitative aspects of appetite, the relation of which to the ventromedial area is still obscure.

PHYSIOLOGIC MECHANISMS OF REGULATION

Gastric Contractions as a Basis or a Component of Hunger and of Short-Term Regulation of Food Intake. The views of Carlson[4] on the relation between gastric pangs, hunger and the regulation of food intake are summarized in his well-known book *The Control of Hunger in Health and Disease*. They constitute the oldest attempt to account experimentally for these phenomena. For Carlson, the consciousness of gastric sensations carried by the vagi is the kernel to the problem. Hunger is defined by him as "a more or less uncomfortable feeling of tension and pain referred to the region of the stomach." While he considers that an explanation of hunger pangs is an explanation of hunger, he does recognize that "many apparently normal persons experience in hunger, besides the gnawing pressure-pain sensation in the stomach, a feeling of weakness, 'emptiness,' headache and sometimes nausea," but calls these states or symptoms "accessory hunger phenomena" because "they are not always present in hunger and their relative preponderance depends on the length of starvation and on some individual peculiarity in the person. It must be admitted, however, that in some individuals these accessory

phenomena appear to overshadow, if not entirely to suppress, the pressure-pain sensations from the stomach." In turn, Carlson, struck by the fact that insulin hypoglycemia leads to gastric contractions and hunger feelings, postulated that blood glucose levels were involved in the occurrence of hunger.

The theory received wide, if temporary, acceptance. Although the existence of hunger pangs has been abundantly confirmed, accumulating facts led observers to doubt whether gastric movements provided a sufficient basis for Carlson's generalizations. For example, Adolph[24] showed, by diluting the ration of animals with inert material, that differences in the bulk of the diet—in spite of their effect on the stomach—had only a transient influence on food intake. Complete bilateral vagotomy, which abolishes the motor response to insulin hypoglycemia, does not prevent or even impair the augmentation of food intake produced by insulin administration. The existence of patients in whom bilateral vagotomy has been performed for the treatment of gastric ulcers enabled Grossman and Stein[25] to extend these findings to human subjects; they found that the sensations of hunger continued to occur after complete vagotomy. The sensations included feelings of emptiness and weakness. In those persons in whom epigastric pangs of distress associated with individual gastric sensations were a part of the sensation-complex of hunger, vagotomy —by abolishing the contractions—eliminated that particular sensory component. Though the removal of this fraction of the sensory complex was recognized by the subject, it did not delay hunger or change the response to it. Vagotomy actually simply shifted the emphasis to the extragastric components, in particular the feelings of weakness and emptiness associated with the desire for food. Incidentally, the observation of Grossman and Stein appeared to disprove not only the essential nature of gastric contractions as a basis of hunger and regulation of food intake (the two concepts are not separated by Carlson) but Carlson's suggested mode of perception of these contractions as well. In two patients who had undergone sympathectomy, persisting gastric contractions were no longer associated with a feeling of distress.

Grossman and Stein concluded that the splanchnic nerves are the afferent pathways for the distress associated with gastric hunger contractions and that no such pathway exists in the vagus nerves.

With the decrease of the significance of hunger pangs, interest in their causation died down and stayed dormant for several decades. Scott[26] and his associates could find no correlation between blood sugar levels and the onset and prevalence of hunger contractions. Experimental work on the testing of the glucostatic hypothesis (see below) has revived interest in both hunger contractions and their control by showing the negative correlation between gastric hunger contractions and glucose utilization, by demonstrating the striking effect of glucagon in inhibiting gastric contractions and, finally, by indicating that gastric hunger contractions may be in part under the control of the ventromedial hypothalamic area.

It is legitimate to conclude from these studies, and from more recent ones conducted in my own laboratory on the nature and timing of hunger sensations in men, women and children, that hunger pangs are an important component of the sensory complex identified subjectively as hunger. At the same time, in spite of the metabolic and neural concomitants of hunger contractions, available evidence makes it impossible to base a mechanism of regulation of food intake exclusively or even principally on their perception. It remains true, however, that any theory purporting to interpret the regulation of food intake which cannot account for the occurrence of hunger pangs is doomed at the outset.

Thermostatic Component in the Regulation or the Limitation of Food Intake. Brobeck,[27] struck by the fact that the hypothalamus appears able to deal with a number of different stimuli which affect feeding behavior and to make suitable adjustments of food intake, hypothesized that a number of such stimuli may operate through their effect on the heat balance of the body. He accordingly advanced a thermostatic hypothesis, which postulated that "animals eat to keep warm and stop eating to prevent hyperthermia." The actual experimental evidence

for his view rested first of all on the observation that short-term exposure to high environmental temperature is followed by reduction of food intake. Kennedy,[28] however, has indicated that, under experimental conditions not dissimilar to those in which Brobeck's animals were placed, dehydration and pyrexial tissue breakdown may have played a major part in the weight loss following an acute exposure to heat. Acute exposure to cold also caused depression of food intake at first. Working with hypothalamic, hyperphagic rats, he demonstrated that in the long run—and as long as his animals stayed within the range of adaptation—they showed similar rates of weight gain at high and at low temperatures.

Another piece of evidence used in support of a thermostatic scheme is the fact that a change from a "high carbohydrate" to a "high fat" diet usually increases food intake and a change to a "high protein" diet usually decreases it. The specific dynamic action of protein is higher than that of carbohydrates which in turn is greater than that of fat. This was taken by Brobeck to indicate that modifications of intake follow perceptions of differences in specific dynamic action. It must be noted, however, that the specific dynamic action of a dietary mixture cannot be calculated by adding up the specific dynamic actions of its constituents if these were fed singly, but is usually lower and far less sensitive to changes in composition (within the usual range) than would be the case if the specific dynamic action were additive for the various nutrients. It has been repeatedly shown that in most strains, the effect on total caloric intake of changing from a high carbohydrate to a high fat diet is transient (though there are strains of animals which continue to eat more on a high fat diet, as do certain types of obese animals). Finally, there is no doubt that diets very high in protein do reduce the food intake of normal animals. The problem of the mechanism of this effect has been recently re-examined in my laboratory,[29] The fact that the effect is as marked, at a protein level of over 60 per cent, in animals in which the ventromedial hypothalamus has been lesioned shows that the effect is not mediated through the hypothalamic "satiety" centers. Above the 60 per cent level, and as the proportion of protein in the diet is further increased, food intake decreases in such a way that the protein intake remains constant, giving an appearance of a regulation based on protein intake. Inasmuch, however, as protein levels appear to have little or no effect in the 8 to 60 per cent range (which encompasses the range of protein levels normally encountered by rats living on natural foods rather than on semi-synthetic laboratory diets), it seems doubtful that this interpretation is the correct one. It appears more likely that one is dealing here with a "safety valve" effect, which indeed could be based on an abnormally high specific dynamic action (or excessive blood amino acids, or other mechanisms), which limits food intake when more than a given amount of protein is ingested but which does not come into play at lower levels. This safety mechanism would have to be situated elsewhere than at the ventromedial (satiety) centers. (Incidentally, it is possible that below a certain minimum intake of protein some other mechanism also comes into play to decrease hunger. In man, Dole and his co-workers[30] have obtained spontaneous reduction on diets excessively low in protein.)

Perhaps the most cogent experimental argument in favor of the existence of a thermostatic influence on feeding is the observation of Andersson and Larsson[31] that refrigeration of the preoptic area causes feeding in a fed goat. Cessation of feeding is observed in this animal, even when fasted for a prolonged period, when the preoptic area is warmed. The effect of cooling and warming on drinking behavior is the opposite of that on eating. While the effects demonstrated by Andersson and Larsson are clear-cut, the fact that the differences of temperature used in the experiment are enormous (of the order of $10°$ C in the vicinity of the thermode, of 1 to $1.5°$ C at a distance of 6 mm) casts some doubt as to the applicability of the results under physiologic conditions. Results recently obtained in several laboratories, mine in particular, indicate, incidentally, that the temperature of the ventromedial area remains remarkably constant in a variety of nutritional situations.

I feel that a thermostatic factor is an important component in the hunger satiety mechanism. I am inclined to believe that, while progressive exposure to cold may have a facilitatory effect on feeding (over and beyond its effect on energy requirements) and exposure to heat, particularly if sudden, a clearly inhibitory effect on feeding, variation in heat balance is probably not the agency through which metabolic requirements influence food intake so as to insure caloric homeostasis. On the other hand, it appears that an elevation of body temperature may exert a safety valve effect (similar to that demonstrated for very high protein diets) which overrides any other factor which might promote feeding so as to prevent any further heat load on an already overloaded organism.

Souleirac's Theory of Regulation of Carbohydrate Appetite by Intestinal Absorption. Souleirac limited himself to the study of appetite for carbohydrate in rodents. However, his numerous publications later collected in book form deserve a somewhat detailed analysis. His work[32] has the original merit of being directed towards the quantitative account of a qualitative appetite, and thus provides facts which may eventually be used to integrate taste and calorie intake. Souleirac was struck by the observation that phloridzin, which, according to Carlson, increases gastric contractions, inhibited appetite for carbohydrate. Thyroidectomized and adrenalectomized animals, both of which present hypoglycemic tendencies, also show diminished appetite for carbohydrate. The observation led to a search for possible correlations between carbohydrate appetite and physiological characteristics. Using a self-selection method, Souleirac systematically examined the quantitative and qualitative variations of uptake of different types of sugar after removal of the anterior pituitary, thyroid, and adrenal glands, alloxanization of the pancreas, and administration of the corresponding hormones: anterior and posterior pituitary extracts, thyroxin, "cortine" and deoxycorticosterone and insulin. He concurrently studied the modifications of taste threshold for carbohydrates and the effect of he endocrine disturbances just listed on the ntestinal absorption of carbohydrates. Similar studies were made after administration of epinephrine, ergotamine, pilocarpine, acetylcholine and atropine, after spinal section in the cerebral region and hypothalamic lesions, or after administration of glucose, riboflavin and phosphate. The effects of cold and physical exercise also were examined. Estimations of blood glucose and of serum amylase were made after these procedures. Souleirac found that there was no correlation between either absolute blood sugar level or the level of serum amylase and carbohydrate consumption. On the other hand, he found that all hormones with an effect on carbohydrate metabolism modified the taste threshold for glucose, though the interpretation of the modifications was difficult. By contrast, the correlation between the taste for carbohydrates and the intestinal absorption of carbohydrates was clear-cut. Any condition which increased intestinal absorption increased consumption and, conversely, if carbohydrate absorption was decreased, carbohydrate intake was decreased. For instance, injections of glucose depressed absorption of glucose and glucose intake; phloridzin and thyroidectomy decreased glucose absorption and intake; insulin and alloxan diabetes increased glucose absorption and intake. The only exception was provided by atropine, which slightly decreased the proportional absorption of glucose from the intestine but considerably increased the total. Souleirac explains the effect of atropine by the intense thirst it produces.

Although the facts invoked by Souleirac are clear enough as far as they go, it seems regrettable that no data are ever given on the caloric intake of the experimental animals, but only on the amount of carbohydrate solution ingested. The omission is all the more regrettable because the solid food available, cereals and greens, constituted a high carbohydrate diet. One would like to know also what the fluid (water) consumption in the different experimental situations was. Examination of the available information raises the question, which is not discussed by Souleirac, of how the organism detects the fact that carbohydrate is being absorbed. Souleirac

observed that spinal section at the level of the sixth to seventh cervical vertebrae did not eliminate the response of the carbohydrate intake to endocrine stimulation, but then it would not interrupt splanchnic sensory connections. The increased intake after atropine treatment could conceivably lend itself to an interpretation based on the effect of the drug on the vagus. The fact that vagotomy and sympathectomy, which would seem to eliminate afferent impulses from the intestine to the central nervous system, while eliminating hunger pangs, do not eliminate feelings of emptiness, weakness and desire for food[25] makes it unlikely that the regulation of food intake is based exclusively, or even primarily, on awareness of intestinal absorption. A humoral or hormonal intermediary could, of course, operate independently of intermediary nervous pathways, but there is no indication of the existence of such a link with the higher centers.

Souleirac suggests that the effect of the hypothalamus on the regulation of food intake is mediated through intestinal absorption; excitation of the hypothalamus would bring about a diminution of carbohydrate absorption and consumption; the action of the hypothalamus would be antagonistic to that of the pituitary and the balance between these organs would determine carbohydrate intake. While, in Souleirac's experiments, consumption of sugar solution increased after hypothalamic lesions, it is difficult to appreciate the significance of his finding, as it cannot be compared with the increases in total food and water consumption which follow the operation. The incidental finding that unilateral lesions lead to increased carbohydrate consumption is of interest in the light of the fact that slow development of obesity follows the production of unilateral hypothalamic lesions in the rat.[2]

Thus, the facts presented by Souleirac, although offering an undeniable challenge, do not appear to support the mechanism he wants to base them on. His observation that any modification of carbohydrate metabolism can affect appetite, and even taste, is in agreement with the postulation of the glucostatic theory. It appears doubtful, however, whether, strong though the appetite for carbohydrate (or protein or salt) may be, hunger and the regulation of food intake are simply summations of selective hungers and partial regulations. Such selective appetites do exist and can be extremely compelling; the "salt wars" are bloody illustrations of their strength. Yet, compelling though such appetites are, they do not appear to overrule the general regulation. Men and animals will, it is true, eat after satiety has apparently been obtained if the supplement offered is particularly appetizing or contains a nutrient of which they have been deprived. Yet, no mammal will increase its food consumption from, say, a low-protein diet simply to satisfy a need for protein or a specific amino acid.

Glucostatic Component of the Regulation of Food Intake. The glucostatic mechanism in the regulation of food intake, proposed by Mayer and his co-workers in the early fifties,[2] postulated that, in the ventromedial (satiety) hypothalamic centers (and possibly in other central and peripheral areas as well), there existed glucoreceptors sensitive to blood glucose in the measure that they utilize it. This concept was based on the facts that the central nervous system is dependent for its function on the availability of glucose; that carbohydrates are preferentially oxidized, and are not stored to any appreciable amount, so that their depletion is rapid, and that, in the interval between meals, there is an incomparably greater proportionate drop of carbohydrate reserves than of reserves of proteins and fat; only intake of food will replenish fully these depleted stores. Furthermore, carbohydrate metabolism is not only regulated by a complex edifice of endocrine interrelationships; it is, in turn, a regulator of fat oxidation and fat synthesis, of protein mobilization and breakdown, and of protein synthesis; thus, a mechanism of regulation of food intake based on glucose utilization could be—as it should be—successfully integrated with energy metabolism and its components. Such a theory also permitted successful interpretation of the known effects of cold, exercise, diabetes mellitus, hyper- and hypothyroidism, and other metabolic changes, provided the additional postulate was made that carbohydrate metabolism in the ventromedial area differed from that in the brain

in general. In particular, it was postulated that the ventromedial area was highly glucoreceptive and that, unlike the rest of the brain, would show varying rates of utilization. Such a theory could also account for such facts as the self-perpetuating effect of hyperphagia, which of itself causes a more rapid utilization of glucose.

Early experimental work designed to test the theory has often been misinterpreted and, apparently not infrequently, continues to be misinterpreted. Because of the (then) insuperable difficulty in measuring glucose utilization in the ventromedial area, and the postulate that, in general, ventromedial utilization must parallel peripheral utilization, an attempt was made by Mayer and Van Itallie to correlate hunger feelings (and later, by Stunkard, gastric contractions) with diminished peripheral glucose utilization in an easily accessible area, i.e., the forearm. Utilization was measured by capillary-venous (or arteriovenous) differences (or "Δ-glucose"); in patients at rest, variations of blood flow were not taken into effect. It was found that, in general, there was a satisfactory degree of correlation between small Δ-glucose and the appearance of subjective feelings of hunger and of gastric contractions. (That the correlation is far from perfect, even when carotid-jugular vein determinations are made, is emphasized in recent work.) It was also shown, in particular by Stunkard and Wolff,[33] that, whenever glucose utilization is proceeding satisfactorily, a slow intravenous glucose infusion in hungry individuals eliminates both the feeling of hunger and gastric contractions. In diabetics, and in hunger diabetes, glucose infusion does not affect hunger to a similar degree. While other authors at times have not observed the correlation between cessation of hunger and rises in glucose utilization,[34] they may have been operating under some of the conditions described by Van Itallie[35] when peripheral glucose arteriovenous differences are not reliable indices of over-all glucose utilization by the body, much less by the satiety mechanisms: such conditions include changes in circulation dynamics because of increase in blood flow, rapid rises in blood glucose, certain effects of insulin, and the presence of overriding dom-nant conditioning. Again the peripheral arteriovenous differences, although still associated in the thinking of many workers with the foundation of the glucostatic theory, have never really held any direct significance in it and were used in this early work "merely to obtain more reliable information about the changes which take place in carbohydrate supply than is available from arterial or venous glucose alone."[35]

It is interesting to note that Van Itallie and Hashim[36] have shown the reciprocal relation of blood nonesterified fatty acid levels and arteriovenous glucose differences. While these authors point out that it is unlikely that nonesterified fatty acid levels *per se* act directly as a signal to the food regulatory centers, their work provides yet another indirect way to evaluate patterns of metabolic utilization and their possible correlation with the hunger-satiety balance.

Major recent developments have entirely altered the status of our knowledge in this field by developing means of assessing, much more directly, hypothalamic events in the regulation of food intake, rather than having to rely on mere statistical correlations. These include the effect of glucagon on hunger feelings and gastric contractions and the role of the ventromedial area in the regulation of gastric contractions, the elucidation of the mode of action of goldthioglucose, the demonstration of the special characteristics of the metabolism of the ventromedial hypothalamic area, and the determination of the electrical activity of the ventromedial hypothalamic area under the influence of variations of blood metabolites, glucose in particular.

Action of Glucagon. Hypothalamic Glucostatic Control of Gastric Hunger Contractions. Stunkard, Van Itallie and Reiss[37] made the interesting observation that the injection of 2 mg of glucagon reproducibly eliminates gastric contractions (and hunger sensations) in human subjects. Their results demonstrated that the elimination of gastric contractions lasts as long as glucose utilization proceeds actively and ceases when glucose utilization is reduced, even though the absolute level of blood glucose be still well above the fasting level.

Stunkard also had the opportunity to observe a patient who had lost practically all of his brain cortex in an accident and was incapable of feeding himself.[38] After one week of fasting, he exhibited almost continuous gastric contractions. A variety of treatments, including the infusion of amino acids and induction of pyrexia (by rolling the patient in an electric blanket), did not inhibit gastric contractions. The only treatment (with the exception of food) which proved effective in inhibiting gastric contractions was the administration of glucagon.

Mayer and his co-workers found that in rats, too, intravenous injections of glucagon inhibit gastric hunger contractions. The dose found to be 100 per cent effective in a large series of animals was 75 μg. The inhibition starts between 45 and 60 seconds after the administration of glucagon. By the time inhibition takes place, the glucose in the blood has already risen considerably from the control fasting values and inorganic phosphorus has decreased, indicating active utilization. Blood glucose continues to increase as inorganic phosphorus returns to the fasted level and gastric hunger contractions appear.[16]

Mayer and Sudsaneh[16] found that rats in which the ventromedial hypothalamic area has been destroyed show no significant difference in their pattern of fasting contractions from that seen in normal animals. The inhibitory response to epinephrine and to norepinephrine is normal. On the other hand, the intravenous administration of 75 μg of glucagon almost invariably fails to produce complete inhibition of hunger contractions in animals with lesions of the ventromedial nuclei, whether the animals are allowed to become and remain obese, or whether they are reduced to their preoperative weight after demonstrating this hyperphagia. Response of these animals to prolonged exposure to cold is delayed, on the average, by 100 per cent. The failure of the animals to respond to glucagon and the delay in response to prolonged exposure to cold are obviously not caused by refractoriness of gastric contractions as such. The finding may be interpreted as indicating that the ventromedial area does exercise a definite measure of control over gastric hunger contractions and does so in response to an increase in its glucose utilization. An anatomical basis for such a mechanism may be provided by the existence of the bundles of Schutz which seem to originate in the general area of the ventromedial hypothalamus and go down to the roots of the vagus.

Mode of Action of Goldthioglucose. In 1949, Brecher and Waxler[39] observed a syndrome of hyperphagia and obesity in mice after a single intraperitoneal or subcutaneous injection of goldthioglucose. The observation was confirmed by Marshall, Barrnett and Mayer[40] who showed that goldthioglucose caused extensive damage to the ventromedial area as well as, in varying degree, to the supraoptic nucleus, the ventral part of the lateral hypothalamic area, the arcuate nucleus, and the median eminence. Marshall and Mayer[41] showed that there was minimal impairment of functions other than the regulation of food intake, unlike that which is observed with stereotaxic lesions. Goldthioglucose-obese animals, unlike animals made obese by stereotaxic lesions, will not infrequently mate and rear their young. As in stereotaxic hypothalamic animals, goldthioglucose-treated animals show impairment of satiety mechanisms as well as impaired reaction of the regulation of food intake to cold, exercise, and caloric dilution. Mayer and Marshall[42] later showed that goldthiogalactose, goldthiosorbitol, goldthiomalate, goldthioglycerol, goldthiocaproate, goldthioglycoanilide, and goldthiosulfate did not produce the brain damage which follows goldthioglucose administration. Neither were hyperphagia and obesity seen following such treatments, even though toxicity of such compounds is similar to that of goldthioglucose. It was also shown that, in the rat, goldthioglucose caused lesions which were similar to those seen in the mouse. The fact that simultaneous administration of sodium thioglucose protects animals against hypothalamic damage is probably traceable to competitive inhibition. On the basis of these observations, Mayer suggested that the toxic gold moiety of accumulated goldthioglucose destroyed the ventromedial neurons specifically because of the affinity of these cells for the glucose component of the molecule, in accordance with the general proposal that

glucose is a cardinal activator of the satiety center.

Debons and co-workers,[43] using radioautographic and neutron-activating analytical techniques, confirmed and considerably extended these conclusions. The Brookhaven co-workers first determined the gold content of the rostral, middle, and caudal portions of brains for controls. They found that some gold accumulated in the brain of all gold-treated animals with, however, notable differences in the localization of the gold. Animals treated with goldthiomalate failed to show any hypothalamic localization of the gold. Animals which received goldthioglucose but failed to become obese had a lesser total gold content of the brain, and the amounts of gold localized in the medial sections were less than in the case of the animals which developed the hyperphagic syndrome. In goldthioglucose-treated animals, radioautographic localization of gold-activity was found consistently in four regions. The greatest concentration was in the hypothalamus, chiefly at the lateral angles and floor of the third ventricle. (Histologically, this region consisted of collapsed glial scar tissue and, in some instances, showed cystic changes.) There was also a second and discrete concentration of radioactivity in the midline, dorsal and cephalad to the optic chiasma and immediately dorsal to the anterior commissure; a third in the caudal portion of the septum and ventral-hypocampal commissure; and a fourth labeled area in the hindbrain in the midline at about the level of the vestibular nuclei in the floor of the fourth ventricle. The fact that goldthioglucose, but not goldthiomalate, administration leads to such localization, even though gold diffused throughout the brain in either case, was taken by the authors as a probability that the gold moiety is responsible for the focal accumulation of sufficient gold in the hypothalamus to produce a destructive lesion which can result in hyperphagia and obesity. Luse, Harris and Stohr,[44] in electronmicroscopy studies of the early lesion, noted that goldthioglucose brought about initial changes in the hypothalamic oligodendroglia cells followed by focal neuronal degeneration. Luse and Harris suggest that the oligondendroglia cells, within certain areas of the central nervous system, share a high degree of specificity to glucose.[45]

Debons and his colleagues[43] point out that, while it is true that the foci of gold accumulation in the hindbrain, in the hypocampal commissure, and above the optic chiasma are at sites where lesions have been reported by Perry and Liebelt,[46] this by no means proves the suggestion of these authors that such extrahypothalamic lesions indicate that gold-thioglucose passes through deficient areas in the blood-brain barriers and is not selectively accumulated at "gluco-receptor" sites. Indeed, they add, in view of the extreme chemical specificity demonstrated for the goldthioglucose molecule, consideration must be given to the possibility that the sites of extrahypothalamic gold accumulation may themselves be glucoreceptive areas.

Arees and Mayer[47] have subjected Perry and Liebelt's hypothesis, that a nonspecific weakness in the blood-brain barrier in the ventromedial areas is responsible for the gold-thioglucose effect, to critical experimental test. They purposely increased the permeability of the blood-brain barrier in the cortex by inducing a local (electrolytic) lesion. It has often been demonstrated that many substances, such as dyes, electrolytes, or more complex molecules, which do not enter an intact brain will readily enter at the site of any focal lesion. Their test demonstrated that such lesions do not increase brain permeability to goldthioglucose.

More important, they were able to demonstrate that a reasoning based on the existence of glucoreceptors permitted the discovery of important new facts. They showed that destruction of cells with special affinity for glucose and a special role in the regulation of food intake made it possible to locate and stain nerve fibers, whose function had hitherto only been postulated.

It is well known that destruction of neurons causes their axons to degenerate. This process, which is believed to occur over the course of several days, is referred to as secondary or wallerian degeneration. Degenerating axons, whether or not myelinated, are more argyrophilic than normal fibers. A number of silver techniques have been devised to take advantage of this characteristic and to stain fiber pathways. Arees and Mayer[47] used a modification of one of the recent techniques, that used by Heimer[48] in 1967, which stains both the degenerating fibers and their points of termination ("boutons terminaux"). They reasoned that tracing axons of neurons which were selectively destroyed by gold-thioglucose (either because the neurons are glucoreceptors or because they are in close topological and functional relationship to the glucoreceptors) would enable them to define fibers involved in the regulation of food intake. Indeed, they found that they could demonstrate the hitherto unseen (though universally postulated) fibers connecting the ventromedial area and the lateral area. The axons extended from the ventromedial area in a dorsolateral and slightly rostral direction and terminated in the medial half of the lateral area. Most fibers passed ventral to the fornix bundle, whereas those coming from the dorsal-most boundary of the lesion passed just dorsal to the bundle. Some isolated fibers appeared to traverse the fornix bundle directly. Termination degeneration was lightest in the rostral and caudal regions of the lateral hypothalamus and heaviest in its middle region. No terminal degeneration was observed in the lateral half of the lateral hypothalamus.[49] The last finding is perhaps related to behavioral evidence, particularly that already cited obtained by Morgane,[13] which suggests that this area has to do with the more qualitative aspects and is not subject to ventromedial inhibition.[23]

As mentioned previously, Sudsaneh and Mayer[16] have shown that destruction of the ventromedial area eliminates the inhibition of gastric hunger contractions brought about by administration of glucagon and the consequent hyperglycemia and increase in glucose utilization. The fact that gastric hunger contractions continued to be responsive to epinephrine and norepinephrine suggested that they are not refractory to local agents. They proposed[16] that the glucoreceptor system in the ventromedial area involves the dorsal longitudinal fasciculus (bundle of Schutz). The demonstration by Ridley and Brooks[50] that destruction of the ventromedial area also eliminates the gastric acid secretion, which normally follows hyperglycemia, was seen as perhaps involving the same structure.

Arees and Mayer[47] found that the lesions brought about in the ventromedial area by goldthioglucose do cause the degeneration of the bundle of Schutz. This descending pathway was shown to terminate in the central gray region of the mesencephalon at the level of the superior colliculus, indicating that the axons linking the ventromedial area to the nucleus of the vagus, like those linking it to the lateral area, are part of the glucoreceptor system.

Finally, it is interesting to note that the fact that mercury thioglucose can replace goldthioglucose in the production of ventromedial lesions[51] confirms the general character of the findings obtained with goldthioglucose.

Special Metabolic Characteristics of the Ventromedial Area. A number of recent experiments have emphasized the metabolic heterogeneity of the hypothalamus and the very special metabolic characteristics of the ventromedial area. Larsson,[52] seeking to test the glucostatic hypothesis, reasoned that the hunger state must be accompanied by changes in the concentration of compounds through which brain tissue, which cannot burn or store fat, can nonetheless achieve some energy storage in the form of phosphagens (creatine phosphate) and adenosine triphosphate. One would expect rates of incorporation of glucose and phosphorus to be particularly affected in the ventromedial area, if it was designed to be sensitive to the rate of utilization of glucose. These workers studied the incorporation of glucose labeled with ^{32}P and ^{14}C in three areas, one including the "feeding" and satiety areas and two situated directly above the optic chiasma, the upper one cutting across the columna fornicis. In hungry rats the sample including the feeding area showed a preferential uptake of ^{32}P, indicating an increase of physiological activity over that in the fed state. In the fed state, by contrast, activity of the two control regions was enhanced, whereas that of the feeding area was proportionally decreased. Experiments with ^{14}C-labeled glucose showed the same type of response. In hungry rats the region that included the feeding area had a greater uptake of glucose as compared with the control areas. Although these studies demonstrated that various parts of the hypothalamus differ in their metabolic reactions, interpretation was difficult because the experimental samples studied and compared with "control" areas included both the ventromedial and lateral areas, as well as other structures presumably not directly concerned with the regulation of food intake.

Chain, Larsson, and Pocchiari,[53] in a subsequent study, confirmed differences in the fate of radioactive glucose, particularly in the labeling of amino acids, in different parts of the rabbit brain. Andersson, Larsson, and Pocchiari[54] extended the findings and mapped the incorporation of ^{14}C-labeled alanine, aspartic acid, glutamic acid, gamma-aminobutyric acid, glutamine, and arginine in the hypothalamus of the goat, again demonstrating differences in uptake in various parts of the brain. Interpretation of the results, beyond the demonstration of heterogeneity of the hypothalamus, is again difficult. The fact that alloxan diabetes eliminates the sensitivity of the ventromedial area to goldthioglucose, indicating the insulin dependence of the area,[55] has already been mentioned.

Anand,[56] studying glucose and oxygen uptake of various parts of the hypothalamus in the monkey, arrived at more clear-cut results, because of the better anatomical definition of his sample. He found that, in the fed animals, there is a relative increase in oxygen and glucose uptake per unit of nucleic acid by the satiety (ventromedial) region as compared with that of the feeding center. In the starved animal, the brain's uptake of oxygen and glucose is less than that of the feeding region. In this experiment, the arteriovenous glucose difference was low in the starved animals and high in those that had been fed. Anand concluded that the results demonstrated an increase in activity of the satiety centers in the fed state, accompanied by an increase in the uptake of glucose, and presumably determined by the changes in availability of glucose. He stated:

". . . the medial regions are activated as a result of changes in the levels of the blood sugar produced by food intake, which subsequently produces satiety and abolition of further eating by inhibiting the lateral mechanisms. The electroencephalographic recordings from feeding and satiety centers under conditions of hyperglycemia lend further support to this hypothesis, as changes in the activity of satiety centers are more pronounced than changes in the activity of feeding centers."[56]

Perhaps the most direct and striking demonstration of the existence of hypothalamic glucoreceptors regulating food intake, and of their special metabolic character, was the finding by Glick and Mayer[57] that infusion of minute amounts of phlorhizin into the cerebral ventricles of rats (in the vicinity of the hypothalamus) causes dramatic hyperphagia. Phlorhizin is a drug that interferes with cellular transport of glucose in a variety of tissues (kidney, intestine, red cells, and, under certain conditions, skeletal muscle).[58] The amounts given were less than those necessary for system effect. The duration of the hyperphagia is a function of the dose. While these findings do not specifically indicate where the glucoreceptive cells are, they point out again the idiosyncrasies of hypothalamic glucoreceptors, inasmuch as other cells in the central nervous system tissue have not been shown to be affected by phlorhizin.

Electroencephalographic Determinations. Anand and his co-workers[59] have evaluated, in rats and monkeys, the role of changes in the blood levels of glucose in various hypothalamic areas. Electrodes were implanted in the lateral, ventromedial, and various control areas of the hypothalamus. Still other electrodes were implanted in the cortex. Connections were brought through the skin at the back of the neck. Four or five days after the operation, hyperglycemia was produced by the intravenous injection of concentrated glucose solution. The consequent rise in blood glucose caused an increase in the frequency of encephalographic waves from the ventromedial (satiety) area (from 6 or 7 per second to 9 or 10 per second). The glucose injection was followed by a drastic decrease in activity in the lateral (feeding) area, with reductions in potential of two-thirds or more being noted. Electric activity of control areas in other parts of the hypothalamus was not affected. Conversely, hypoglycemia

(produced by intravenous injection of insulin) caused a reduction in frequency of ventromedial waves (from 6 or 7 per second to 2 or 3). Activity in the feeding area was increased.

Changes in blood amino acid and blood lipid concentrations did not affect the electric activity of the satiety and feeding centers. An increase in glucose utilization after the consumption of a meal was similarly found to be associated with a doubling of the frequency of ventromedial pulsation and a decrease in the activity of the feeding centers.

Effect of Glucose on Activity of Single Neurons in the Hypothalamus. In an impressive series of experiments utilizing 109 mongrel dogs and 47 cats, the effect of glucose and insulin on the electric activity of single hypothalamic neurons was examined by Anand and his collaborators,[60] with striking results. The experiments were well controlled —for example, in osmolarity of solutions infused. Microelectrodes were placed in the required sites under vision by a micromanipulator. The femoral vessels were cannulated for blood sampling and infusions.

The response of single neurons in the feeding centers to glucose infusion showed a decrease in spike frequency. In the satiety centers the spike frequency was markedly increased. This increase in the spike frequency of the neurons of the satiety center and the decrease in the feeding centers occurred within five to fifteen minutes after glucose infusion. The change in spike frequency was sustained for a period lasting half an hour to an hour, with the maximum occurring about half an hour after infusion. A second infusion two hours after the first caused a lesser change in the spike frequency. Other hypothalamic areas did not respond to glucose infusion, nor did the satiety areas respond to saline infusions. The response of single satiety-center neurons to insulin infusion is a transitory increase followed by a prolonged decrease in spike frequency. The changes in spike frequency when glucose and insulin were perfused were much more closely correlated with arteriovenous differences than with glucose levels, suggesting to the Indian workers that the activity of the satiety centers is much more closely correlated to glucose utilization than to absolute blood glucose levels, and that their reaction to insulin makes their metabolism representative of that of extracerebral tissues.

The glucostatic mechanism appears to be one of the essential processes through which metabolic requirements influence the feeding mechanism and through which energetic homeostasis is maintained. There are, of course, many other factors that influence food intake at a given time. A thermostatic component, sensitive to elevations of body temperature, may act on a safety valve situated in another hypothalamic area to shut off feeding behavior.[61] Other safety valves may be similarly sensitive to protein imbalance,[62] to excessively high intakes of protein,[62] to gastric distention, and to dehydration. Metering of food intake by the mouth or the pharynx, taste, emotions, and habits may at a given moment also influence intake. Long-term factors, such as the state of the adipose tissue, also appear to regulate food intake. (It may well be, however, that, because of the relation of free fatty acid release to the size and metabolic state of fat cells, and because of the mutual interrelation of glucose and fatty acid availability, the particular factor is mediated through the glucostatic mechanism.)

Long-Term Regulation of Food Intake and Body Weight. While the likelihood of the existence of a long-term mechanism of regulation of intake and body weight, correcting the errors of the short-term mechanism, comes out very strongly from the experiments of Gasnier and A. Mayer, the mechanism of such a regulation (the existence of which has since been postulated by a number of authors, in particular G. C. Kennedy[63]) is still unclear. Experiments conducted in my laboratory indicate that the efficiency of food utilization by an animal which has once been obese and then reduced is greater than before obesity had taken place. This would suggest that, as postulated by Kennedy, adipose tissue does play a considerable role in long-term homeostasis and that perhaps the level of enzymatic activity within this tissue tends to be more self-perpetuating than that of the fat content. It is of course possible that the long-term mechanism works through short-term components: more rapid

uptake of nutrients, in particular glucose, could take place whenever the steric hindrance due to accumulated fat in the adipose tissue is relieved by fat loss: Quaade has pointed out some of the effects on heat load of the body caused by the insulation due to increased adipose tissue.[64]

Hunger and Satiety Sensations in Man. Until a 1965 study conducted by Mayer, Monello and Seltzer,[65] there had been a complete dearth of systematic information on the sensory aspects of hunger and satiety in man. While much remains to be found, this study provided 400 elements of information each on 800 persons, adults and adolescents, obese and nonobese. The study revealed the existence of a multiplicity of sensations recognized by various individuals as hunger signals, with significant differences being found between age groups, the sexes and individuals. There is also an element of variability in the timing and the sequence of hunger sensations. Changes in moods associated with changes in the state of nutrition and degrees of urge are also more complex and more variable than hitherto recognized.

A major finding of the study was that, while hunger is associated with sensations, which increase in number and intensity as deprivation progresses, satiety—the cessation of the urge to eat—is not necessarily associated with any specific sensation, nor does it coincide simply with the disappearance of hunger sensations. It is often associated, particularly in adults, with changes in mood. In growing youngsters and some adults, while sensations of gastric fullness frequently accompany satiety, this is by no means general, even in individuals in whom it is a frequent concomitant of satiety. The sensory picture is thus not inconsistent with the phenomenon of satiety being dependent on events occurring largely at the subconscious or unconscious level, such as the hypothalamic level. It is obvious, however, that the timing of satiety is too rapid to make it dependent on "metabolic" monitoring of the food ingested. A more likely physiologic explanation is the possible presence of subsidiary chemoreceptors in the gastrointestinal tract and, perhaps, a reflex secretion of glucagon with, as a result, an indirect effect on the ventromedial hypothalamus. (Incidentally, comparison between the hunger and satiety pictures in obese and nonobese individuals suggests that abnormalities of satiety may be more prevalent than abnormalities of hunger.)

Recent work by Schachter[66] suggests that obese individuals are responsive to "outside" cues, while normal-weight subjects respond to "inside" cues. In a society which is highly punitive towards the obese,[67] it seems possible that individuals, whose physiological regulatory systems are inadequate, are driven to meter the intake which they will allow themselves through "outside" cues. These may form a more or less logical system "built in" as a result of information (or misinformation) concerning the caloric value of food. The observations of Schachter can, therefore, be interpreted as demonstrating that many obese subjects have a physiologically deranged regulatory mechanism, compensated for by psychological methods, rather than proving a psychogenic etiology of their obesity.

Conclusion. The existence of a regulation of food intake—perhaps mediated by a long-term and a short-term mechanism—which ensures homeostasis is clear. In addition to metabolic influences, probably mediated through a glucostatic component acting on the ventromedial hypothalamic area, with a thermostatic component acting perhaps on another area (preoptic?) as a "safety valve," also acting on various areas are a number of factors—gastric contractions (probably in part regulated through the hypothalamus), gastric distension, metering by mouth and pharynx, water balance, extremes of environmental temperature (acting above and beyond their effect on energy balance), a host of psychologic factors (taste, habits and emotions) and social and cultural habits and pressures which at a given moment will influence the subject to increase or decrease intake. These various factors interact. For example, taste may be in part dependent on the physiologic state.[68] It seems to me, having studied a large number of forms of experimental and human hyperphagias and anorexias, that the wonder is not that there should be a great diversity of disturbances in the regulation of food intake, producing many different types of obesities and excessive thinness: the wonder is

that in most animals and men, with feeding behavior subject to so many influences, the mechanism of regulation of food intake works so extraordinarily well.

BIBLIOGRAPHY

1. Gasnier and Mayer: Ann. Physiol. Physiochem. Biol., *15*, 145, 157, 186, 195, 210, 1939.
2. Mayer: Nutr. Abstr. Rev., *25*, 597, 871, 1955.
3. Cannon and Washburn: Am. J. Physiol., *29*, 441, 1911–12.
4. Carlson: *The Control of Hunger in Health and Disease*. Chicago, University of Chicago Press, 1914.
5. Quigley: Ann. New York, Acad. Sci., *63*, 6, 1955.
6. Hetherington and Ranson: Am. J. Physiol., *136*, 609, 1942.
7. Brobeck: Physiol. Revs., *26*, 541, 1946.
8. Mayer, French, Zighera, and Barrnett: Am. J. Physiol., *182*, 75, 1955.
9. Anand and Brobeck: Yale J. Biol. Med., *24*, 123, 1951.
10. Teitelbaum and Stellar: Science, *120*, 894, 1954.
11. Morrison and Mayer: Am. J. Physiol., *191*, 248, 1957.
12. Morrison, Barrnett, and Mayer: Am. J. Physiol., *193*, 230, 1958.
13. Morgane: Am. J. Physiol., *201*, 420, 1961.
14. ———: J. Comp. Neurol., *117*, 1, 1961.
15. Larsson: Acta Physiol. Scand., *32*, suppl. 115, 1, 1954.
16. Mayer and Sudsaneh: Am. J. Physiol., *197*, 274, 1959.
17. Anliker and Mayer: Am. J. Clin. Nutr., *5*, 148, 1957.
18. Miller, Bailey, and Stevenson: Science, *112*, 256, 1950.
19. Rozin and Mayer: Am. J. Physiol., *201*, 968, 1961.
20. Teitelbaum and Epstein: Psychol. Revs., *69*, 74, 1962.
21. ———: Proc. *First Internat. Symposium on Olfaction and Taste*, Oxford, England, Pergamon Press, 1963, p. 347.
22. Olds: Science, *127*, 315, 1958.
23. Morgane: Science, *133*, 887, 1961.
24. Adolph: Am. J. Physiol., *151*, 110, 1947.
25. Grossman and Stein: J. Appl. Physiol., *1*, 263, 1948.
26. Scott, Scott, and Zuckhardt: Am. J. Physiol., *123*, 423, 1938.
27. Brobeck: Yale J. Biol. Med., *20*, 545, 1948.
28. Kennedy: Proc. Roy. Soc. (B), *137*, 535, 1950.
29. Krauss and Mayer: Nature, *200*, 123, 1963.
30. Dole, Schwartz, Thayson, Thorn, and Silver: Am. J. Clin. Nutr., *2*, 381, 1954.
31. Andersson and Larsson: Acta Physiol. Scand., *52*, 75, 1961.
32. Souleirac: Bull. Biol. France, Belgique, *81*, 274 432, 1947

33. Stunkard and Wolff: J. Clin. Invest., *35*, 954, 1956.
34. Bernstein and Grossman: J. Clin. Invest., *35*, 627, 1956.
35. Van Itallie: Ann. New York Acad. Sci., *63*, 89, 1955.
36. Van Itallie and Hashim: Am. J. Clin. Nutr., *8*, 587, 1960.
37. Stunkard, Van Itallie and Reiss: Proc. Soc. Exptl. Biol. Med., *89*, 258, 1955.
38. Stunkard: Am. J. Clin. Nutr., *5*, 203, 1957.
39. Brecher and Waxler: Proc. Soc. Exptl. Biol. & Med., *70*, 498, 1949.
40. Marshall, Barrnett, and Mayer: Proc. Soc. Exptl. Biol. & Med., *90*, 240, 1955.
41. Marshall and Mayer: Am. J. Physiol., *178*, 271, 1954.
42. Mayer and Marshall: Nature, *178*, 1399, 1956.
43. Debons, Silver, Cronkite, Johnson, Brecher, Tenzer, and Schwartz: Am. J. Physiol., *202*, 743, 1962.
44. Luse, Harris, and Stohr: Anat. Record, *139*, 250, 1961.
45. Luse and Harris: Arch. Neurol., *4*, 139, 1961.
46. Perry and Liebelt: Proc. Soc. Exptl. Biol. & Med., *106*, 55, 1961.
47. Mayer and Arees: Fed. Proc., *27*, 1345, 1968.
48. Heimer: Brain Res., *5*, 86, 1967.
49. Arees and Mayer: Science, *157*, 1574, 1967.
50. Ridley and Brooks: Amer. J. Physiol., *209*, 319, 1965.
51. Sandrew and Mayer: Fed. Proc., *31*, 397, 1972.
52. Larsson: Acta Physiol. Scand. *32* (Suppl. 115): 7, 1954.
53. Chain, Larsson and Pocchiari: Proc. Roy. Soc. Biol. (London) *152*, 283, 1960.
54. Andersson, Larsson and Pocchiari: Acta Physiol. Scand., *51*, 314, 1961.
55. Debons, Krimsky and Likuski: Amer. J. Physiol., *214*, 652, 1968.
56. Anand: Amer. J. Clin. Nutr., *8*, 529, 1960.
57. Glick and Mayer: Nature (London), *219*, 1374, 1968.
58. Lotspeich: Harvey Lect., *56*, 63, 1960–61.
59. Anand, Dua, and Singh: Electroenceph. Clin. Neurophysiol., *13*, 54, 1961.
60. Anand, Chhina, Sharma, Dua, and Singh: Amer. J. Physiol., *207*, 1146, 1964.
61. Brobeck: Yale J. Biol. Med., *20*, 545, 1948.
62. Krauss and Mayer: Amer. J. Physiol., *209*, 479, 1965.
63. Kennedy: Proc. Roy. Soc. (B), *14*, 578, 1952–53.
64. Quaade: Lancet, *2*, 429, 1963.
65. Mayer, Monello and Seltzer: Postgrad. Med., *37*(6), A97, 1965.
66. Schachter: Science, *161*, 751, 1968.
67. Monello and Mayer: Amer. J. Clin. Nutr., *13*, 35, 1963.
68. Titlebaum and Mayer: Experentia, *19*, 539, 1963.

Chapter

15

Nutrition in Relation to Acquired Immunity

A. E. AXELROD

Much attention has been directed toward the possibility of a relationship between nutritive state and resistance-susceptibility to infection. With this in mind, many experimentalists have sought for dietary factors that could influence the resistance or susceptibility of a host to infectious disease. Many of these studies have certainly been motivated by the hope that suitable manipulation of the diet might influence the incidence and course of the infection for the benefit of the host. Ultimately, these experimental investigations were designed to find application in the human resources against infectious disease. Unfortunately, these interrelationships have proved to be exceedingly complex, and definitive statements on the relationship of specific dietary components to resistance to infection are difficult to make. This controversial subject has been reviewed by Kolmer in a previous edition of this book.[1]

The preponderance of efforts in these endeavors has been directed toward a possible relationship between diet and "natural" or "innate" resistance.

The determinants of resistance to infectious disease are multiple in nature, and count among their members the classic antigen-antibody interaction. In many instances, this reaction may represent a most significant facet of the intricate mechanism involved in resistance to infection. In this chapter, we shall discuss only the interdependence between nutrition and antibody formation or actively acquired immunity.

STATUS PRIOR TO 1955

This subject has been discussed fully in two review papers appearing in 1955[1,2] and there is little need to recapitulate this material *in extenso*. A brief summation of this field as it existed in 1955 is, however, in order. From a morass of data accumulated by numerous investigators, there emerged the significant fact that individual nutrients could play an important role in the process of antibody formation. Dietary deficiencies of these nutrients frequently led to impaired antibody production in experimental animals. Generalizations at this point were particularly dangerous but it appeared that a severe protein deficiency as well as deficiencies of pyridoxine, pantothenic acid and pteroylglutamic acid produced the most consistent deleterious effects upon antibody formation. This is not to imply that the function of other dietary factors was completely dissociated from the phenomenon of antibody synthesis. On the contrary, the need for certain of these dietary components, particularly members of the vitamin B complex, could be demonstrated clearly on occasion. A review of the literature made it apparent that a distressing variability existed in the results of different investigators. In some cases, seemingly contradictory data were reported. It is very probable that many of these discrepancies could be attributed to (1) the type, dosage or route of administration of the antigen, (2) species of animal, (3) methods of quantitating the antibody response and (4) specificity, and, perhaps, degree of the deficiency state. This latter point was particularly evident in some of the earlier studies. It seemed obvious that more conclusive data, collected with vigorous control of these factors, were required before the results of different experimenters could be fairly compared. It was suggested that more positive information in this field would be forthcoming if the phenomenon of antibody formation was treated as an entity completely dissociated from that of resistance to infection. With this operational procedure, studies would be designed *primarily* to investigate antibody production, not merely to attempt correlations between antibody formation and resistance to infection as had frequently been the case. As will be emphasized later, such correlations are of obvious importance in a study of the relationship of nutrition to infectious disease. However, an exclusive devotion to this aspect of the problem would, in my opinion, only impede experimental progress toward the elucidation of the mechanistic role of the nutritive factors in antibody synthesis.

Thus, the data accumulated prior to 1955 definitely established the fact that antibody response, as measured by the content of circulating antibodies, was markedly diminished in a variety of nutritional deficiency states. Concurrently, attention was being directed toward the mode of action of these nutritional factors. The difficulties encountered were many and were largely attributable to our ignorance of the precise mechanisms involved in the process of antibody synthesis. Information was sought on the role of biologic factors involved in the mechanism of synthesis of a protein (antibody) when, in actual fact, knowledge of the pathways of protein biosynthesis was tenuous. As a further complication, antibody protein is one which must be fabricated through the stimulus of an agent foreign to the host. Some information in this field has been garnered and can be summarized briefly.

A state of inanition usually accompanies the deficiencies under consideration. It became extremely important, therefore, to determine whether the effects observed in the deficiency were actually due to the specific absence of the nutritional factor or to the non-specific effects of caloric restriction (inanition). The accumulated evidence argued strongly against any significant role of inanition *per se* and supported the viewpoint that the effects observed were due specifically to the nutritional factor in question. This conclusion was further strengthened by numerous observations showing little correlation between growth and antibody responses of experimental animals in various deficiency states. This latter observation has served as the basis for the suggestion that antibody response might be utilized as a more sensitive criterion of nutritional adequacy than the frequently employed growth response.

In attempting to arrive at the mode of action of nutritional factors, we must consider the possibility that the antibody-synthesizing cells, whatever they may be, suffer a severe derangement in the deficiency state. Such damage may be manifested either by structural changes demonstrable by histologic techniques or by disturbances in functional activity. Cells of the lymphoid series have been implicated as the sites of antibody synthesis. Although histologic studies in nutritional deficiencies have yielded discordant results, it appears that lesions of these cells do occur in pyridoxine-deficient animals. Thus, the deleterious effect of this deficiency upon antibody production may be referable to damage to the lymphoid cells. Experiments in our laboratory have indicated a disturbance in the functional activity of splenic cells from pantothenic acid-deficient rats immunized with diphtheria toxoid. Splenic cells from immunized pantothenic acid-deficient rats, in contrast to those from normal immunized rats, were found to be unable to fabricate antibody when cultured *in vitro* or when passively transferred to normal rats. Also the mean DNA content of isolated splenic nuclei from immunized pantothenic acid-deficient rats was found to be lower than that from comparable controls. These results may mean that the deficiency interfered with the acceleration of cellular division that normally accompanies antibody production in the spleen. Since cellular division is always preceded by an increase in DNA content, the participation of pantothenic acid in DNA synthesis becomes an intriguing possibility.

It must be recognized that the serum antibody level utilized as a measure of antibody response probably reflects an equilibrium between the rate of antibody synthesis and release from the sites of synthesis on the one hand, and the rate of destruction of circulating antibody on the other. A change in any one of these factors could obviously affect the content of circulating antibodies. Thus, it becomes important to evaluate the effects of a nutritional deficiency upon antibody *release* and *degradation* before any positive statements can be made regarding any direct relationship between nutritional factors and antibody synthesis. Such experiments have been conducted and suggest that the decreased level of circulating antibody in the vitamin deficiencies cannot be attributed to a faulty release mechanism or to excessive destruction of antibody. It seems more likely, though not definitely proven, that there is a disturbance in the process of antibody synthesis.

CURRENT STATUS

More recent studies conducted, in the main, since 1955 and not covered in the two reviews cited earlier[1,2] are in general agreement with previous observations demonstrating the inhibitory effects of nutritional deficiencies upon antibody production in experimental animals. Rats,[3-7] mice,[8] and guinea pigs[9] have served as experimental subjects in these studies and a variety of antigenic stimuli, *i.e.* vaccine from a strain of *C. kutscheri*,[3] vaccines of *S. typhi, B. melitensis* and heterologous erythrocytes,[4-7] diphtheria toxoid,[9] and swine influenza virus,[8] has been employed. Zucker *et al.*[3] have noted the inhibitory effects of pyridoxine and pantothenic acid deficiencies upon antibody production and the lack of such an effect in a partial thiamin deficiency. Giunchi *et al.* have also observed the deleterious result of a pantothenic acid deficiency.[4,5,6] A requirement for ascorbic acid in the development and maintenance of acquired immunity has been reported by Bersins,[9] while Underdahl and Young[8] could find no such need for

vitamins A, D or E. Wissler *et al.*[7] utilized the phenylalanine antagonist, B₃-thienyl alanine, to demonstrate the requirement of phenylalanine for antibody synthesis. Bianchi *et al.*[10,11] were unable to observe an effect of pyridoxine deficiency, induced by the pyridoxine antagonist, deoxypyridoxine, upon antibody production to typhoid vaccine in rats and rabbits. This result is in marked contrast to the consistent findings of other workers in this field demonstrating the inhibitory action of a dietary-induced pyridoxine deficiency in experimental animals. More specifically, it is not in agreement with the observations of Stoerk[12] and ourselves[13] who have also employed the same antagonist to develop this deficiency state. The failure of Bianchi *et al.* to present definitive data on the degree of their induced deficiency state makes it difficult to evaluate their discordant result.

Scrimshaw *et al.*[14] reviewed in 1959 the relationship between vitamins and antibody formation. Harmon *et al.*[15,16] have reported that specific deficiencies of vitamin A, pantothenic acid, pyridoxine, or riboflavin produced an impairment of antibody synthesis in swine to the antigenic stimuli of *Salmonella pullorum* antigens or human erythrocytes. Antibody-synthesizing capacity was restored following repletion of the deficient pigs with a control diet. Paired-feeding studies demonstrated that the deleterious effects of the deficiency states were not due to concomitant inanition. Leutskaja[60] reported that chickens deprived of vitamin A developed a lower antibody titer in serum to the antigen from the nematode *Ascaridia galli* than those given vitamin A. In mice, the development of anaphylactic sensitivity and the production of circulating antibodies to horse serum were depressed by pyridoxine deficiency.[17] The significant role of folic acid in antibody production has been well documented in studies demonstrating the inhibition of antibody response by treatment with the folic acid antagonists, methotrexate and aminopterin. In these studies, antibody production was investigated in rabbit splenic cells,[18] dogs,[19] guinea pigs,[20] and mice [21] with the antigenic stimuli of *Brucella suis*,[18] attenuated virus of distemper vaccine,[19] diphtheria toxoid,[20] ovalbumin,[20] and typhoid-paratyphoid A and B vaccine.[21]

Moore and Lawrence[69] in an investigation of the effect of histidine decarboxylase inhibitors upon antibody production have shown that the combination of semicarbazide plus a vitamin B_6-deficient diet significantly inhibited antibody formation to salmonella flagellar antigen in rats. Under their experimental conditions, insignificant inhibition resulted from the feeding of vitamin B_6-deficient diet alone. Evidence for the development of a pronounced vitamin B_6 deficiency was not presented. Inhibition of splenic antibody (19S)-forming cells was observed in mice treated with semicarbazide plus a vitamin B_6-deficient diet or the α-hydrazino analogue of histidine alone or in combination with a vitamin B_6-deficient diet after immunization with sheep erythrocytes. Semicarbazide plus a vitamin B_6-deficient diet also markedly diminished production of plaque-forming cells producing 7S antibody. A deficiency of pyridoxine decreased antibody response to a synthetic peptide and sheep erythrocytes in the rat.[70] Deoxypyridoxine further decreased antibody response in the vitamin B_6-deficient rats and this effect was partially reversed by glycine or serine, serine being more effective. Impaired antibody production has been observed in chicks fed diets partially deficient in vitamin A, pantothenic acid or riboflavin (S. pullorum antigen),[71] in rats partially deficient in riboflavin (L. icterohaemorrhagiae as antigen)[72] and in scorbutic guinea pigs (sheep erythrocytes as antigen).[73] In the latter study, the inhibitory effect of scurvy occurred mainly in the early stages of antibody formation. We[73a] have failed to demonstrate any effect of severe scurvy in guinea pigs upon primary or secondary circulating antibody formation to diphtheria toxoid. Ströder et al.,[74] utilizing tetanus toxoid, diphtheria toxoid, influenza virus and sheep erythrocytes as antigens, studied circulating antibody production during and after development of rickets in rats. Impairment in antibody production was noted only in the case of tetanus toxoid when this antigen was injected into rats with developed rickets. Woodruff[75] has shown that inanition per se adversely influences antibody

response of adult mice to infection with Coxsackie virus B_3. This finding differs from the more common observation that inanition is without effect upon antibody synthesis.

Interest in the influence of variations in dietary amino acids and proteins upon the immune response continues. Deficiencies of tryptophan[70,84] and phenylalanine[70] decreased antibody response in rats while deficiencies of tryptophan and nicotinic acid did not significantly influence immunological response in young swine.[76] Pretreatment of Swiss mice with the amino acid analogue, cycloleucine, prevented antibody response to sheep erythrocytes by reducing the number of antibody-forming cells in the splenic pulp.[77] Effects of varying levels of methionine,[70,78,84] valine[78] and lysine[79,84] upon antibody response in the rat have been reported. As might be expected, the dietary balance of amino acids can play a significant role in determination of the immune response. Gill and Gershoff[80] have studied the effects of methionine deficiency or excess and the effects of one of its antagonists, ethionine, on the primary, early secondary and late secondary antibody response in Cebus albipron monkeys. The primary antibody response to a synthetic polypeptide was resistant to methionine deficiency, methionine excess and ethionine administration. The early secondary response was depressed both by ethionine and by excess methionine; it was resistant to methionine deficiency alone. The late secondary response was unaffected by methionine deficiency plus ethionine or by previous administration of a methionine excess diet; however, previous treatment with a methionine excess diet plus ethionine caused an enhanced antibody response. Kenney and co-workers[81–83] have investigated the effects of protein depletion and repletion upon antibody response in rats. The depression of antibody titers in protein deficiency could be attributed largely to the reduction of antibody-forming cells in spleen.

A comprehensive review of the relation between nutritive factors and antibody formation has been presented by Scrimshaw et al.[85]

The studies discussed thus far have dealt with the relationship of various deficiency states to antibody production in experimental animals. A series of observations has, however, concerned itself with the effects of large dosages of various vitamins administered to animals maintained on *normal* diets during the periods of active immunization. This experimental design tends to express the pharmacologic action of the vitamins rather than their more commonly recognized functions as nutritional factors. Solarino,[22] in reviewing the work of his school has reported the stimulatory action of pantothenic acid, riboflavin, *p*-aminobenzoic acid, nicotinic acid and vitamin E upon antibody production in rabbits to vaccines of *Vibrio cholerae*, and *S. typhi* and to heterologous erythrocytes. Flavonoids were without effect. This author stresses the possible harmful effects of higher dosages of certain of these vitamins upon antibody synthesis. In comparable experiments with rabbits, Segagni[23] noted that the administration of vitamin E led to an earlier and more extensive formation of antibodies following stimulation with typhoid vaccine, O-streptolysin or staphylococcus toxoid. This stimulatory effect was, however, only temporary. Richou,[24] on the other hand, failed to observe any effects of pantothenic acid administration to rabbits immunized with staphylococcus toxoid and negative results with folic acid, pantothenic acid, and pyridoxine were obtained by Lamanna and Taviani[25] in rats vaccinated with *S. typhi*. Butturini and Casa[26] concluded that ascorbic acid and vitamin E actually block the formation of antistreptolysin in guinea pigs.

More recently, Tashmukhamedov[86] has reported that injections of vitamin B_{12} substantially improved immunogenesis in rabbits immunized with tetanus toxoid and Bliznakov *et al.*[87] have noted that treatment of mice with coenzyme Q_{10} stimulated the immune response to sheep erythrocytes.

Studies in the human have failed to demonstrate any effect of malnutrition upon the isohemagglutinin content[27] or antibody formation to diphtheria toxoid.[28] An investigation by workers in South Africa[29] suggested that the capacity for antibody formation against typhoid vaccine in patients with kwashiorkor was equal to that of control subjects. However, interpretation of these experiments is difficult, since all patients were responding well to treatment with high-protein diets during the experimental period of antibody production. Antibody responses to tetanus and typhoid vaccines were diminished in one human subject consuming a low-protein diet composed of skim milk solids.[30] This effect was not observed in another subject who ate the same quantity of protein in the form of egg yolk. A pyridoxine deficiency induced by deoxypyridoxine did not affect antibody response to typhoid vaccine or the A and B blood group substances.[31] Hodges and co-workers have studied the immunologic responses of men deficient in pantothenic acid,[32] pyridoxine,[33] or both pantothenic acid and pyridoxine.[34] Pantothenic acid deficiency depressed the antibody response to tetanus antigen but not that to typhoid antigens. Of interest was their observation that antibody formation was not impaired in subjects receiving the pantothenic acid-deficient diet supplemented with the antagonist, omega-methyl-pantothenic acid. The authors suggest that the antagonist may have acted as an active vitamin in the process of antibody formation. Only a slight impairment of antibody production against tetanus and typhoid vaccines was noted in pyridoxine deficiency. However, a combined deficiency of pyridoxine and pantothenic acid, induced by feeding a deficient diet plus the antagonists, deoxypyridoxine and omega-methyl-pantothenic acid, markedly depressed the antibody responses to tetanus and typhoid antigens. Vitamin supplementation and re-immunization restored normal antibody production. Immunization with polio antigens was not affected in this combined deficiency state.

Najjar *et al.*[88] determined serum levels of IgM, IgA and IgG in infants with marasmic malnutrition. The levels of these three immunoglobulins were significantly higher than those of well-nourished infants 3 to 6 months of age. In older marasmic infants, the levels of IgM in those between 7 and 12 months and of IgA in those between 13 and 30 months were significantly higher than the corresponding levels in the well-nourished infants. In children with kwashiorkor, Reddy and Srikantia[89] reported that significantly higher titers to TAB vaccine were observed when nutritional rehabilitation was achieved with 50 gm of protein daily as compared to 30 gm of protein. Impairment of antibody response to yellow fever vaccine was noted in children with kwashiorkor.[90,91] The antibody response to polio and the clinical response to smallpox vaccines appeared to be normal in the malnourished children.[91] Scrimshaw et al.[85] have offered a critical evaluation of the relationship in human populations between antibody formation and protein deficiency.

Studies on the relationship between nutritional state and antibody formation have been conducted in our laboratory over an extended period of time. Early work with diphtheria toxoid had demonstrated a requirement for a number of vitamins, particularly of the B complex, in antibody synthesis in the rat. In a continuation of these studies, we have found that deficiencies of the amino acids, tryptophan and methionine, markedly inhibit antibody response. Deficiencies in vitamin E (conducted in collaboration with Dr. S. Ames of The Distillation Products, Inc.) and choline were without effect. The absence of any deleterious action of a choline deficiency is of some interest, since this deficiency state produced a marked weight loss as well as an extreme hemorrhagic condition of the kidney. A similar lack of correlation between antibody response and severity of the symptomatology of deficient animals has been noted frequently. Marked decreases in the avidity of serum antibody were observed in rats with pyridoxine and pantothenic acid deficiencies. Thus, in these deficiency states there was a qualitative difference in the type of antibody formed as well as a diminution in the total quantity of antibodies produced. This qualitative change is manifested by a lowered ability of the antibody to combine with the antigen and most likely results from the synthesis of altered antibody molecules. The effect of a pyridoxine deficiency upon circulating antibody formation has been studied in the guinea pig.[35] Pyridoxine deficiency was produced in very young guinea pigs by feeding a highly purified diet lacking pyridoxine. The deficiency state was produced in more mature animals by administering the pyridoxine antagonist, deoxypyridoxine, to

guinea pigs receiving the pyridoxine-deficient diet. Pyridoxine deficiency produced by either of these procedures depressed both circulating antibody formation and the degree of the early, Arthus-type skin hypersensitivity reaction to diphtheria toxoid. The latter reaction is associated with circulating antibodies.

Further studies were designed to investigate the role of nutritional factors in the various phases of the anamnestic response to diphtheria toxoid in the rat.[13] Deficiencies of pantothenic acid, biotin, pyridoxine and tryptophan produced marked inhibition of the secondary (booster) as well as of the primary response to this antigen, the inhibition of the booster response being most pronounced. Intensive nutritional therapy given *only* during the secondary phase failed to elicit antibody formation. In no case was an anamnestic effect seen in these supplemented animals, despite their immediate and marked growth response to the nutritional therapy. Repeated injections of diphtheria toxoid were unable to overcome the inhibitory effect of a pyridoxine deficiency induced by dietary means or by the administration of the pyridoxine antagonist, deoxypyridoxine. Thus, it seems clear that adequate nutrition during the primary phase is essential for the attainment of a satisfactory booster response. Subsequent experiments demonstrated that a pyridoxine deficiency induced by the administration of deoxypyridoxine during the secondary phase could significantly inhibit the secondary response. This inhibition was apparent three days after the booster injection. It should be stressed that these animals received an adequate diet during the primary phase and were therefore permitted to initiate the events, template or adaptive enzyme formation, which under normal circumstances would be triggered by the secondary stimulus to accelerate the processes of antibody synthesis. A pyridoxine deficiency in the secondary phase inhibited this normal sequence. These results can most likely be ascribed to the deleterious effects of an acute pyridoxine deficiency upon the lymphoid apparatus. Thus, the successful attainment of a satisfactory anamnestic response to diphtheria toxoid in the albino rat requires a state of adequate nutriture during *both* the primary and secondary phases of this process. Control experiments demonstrated again that inanition was not a factor in these studies. It was further noted that the high content of circulating antibody produced by anamnesis in normal animals was not affected by a subsequent acute deficiency of pyridoxine.

Our studies described thus far utilized only particulate antigens. In order to obtain further information regarding the antigenic specificity of these deficiency effects, it was considered advisable to repeat these experiments with a nonparticulate antigen. Influenza virus was chosen since it represents a nonparticulate antigen of clinical interest whose corresponding serum antibody can be readily determined by a specific neutralization procedure. Antibody formation to this virus was markedly diminished in pantothenic acid- and pyridoxine-deficient rats.[36] Of considerable interest was the observation that antibody synthesis was not impaired in rats with severe thiamin deficiency. Inanition was without effect. These results parallel our previous observations with other antigens and further emphasize the general nature of this phenomenon as well as the specificity of action of the vitamins as regards antibody production.

It is conceivable that the impairment of antibody production in the vitamin-deficient animals may be traced to a disturbance in some phase of antigen metabolism. It, therefore, seemed appropriate to investigate antigen metabolism in these deficiency states (Pruzansky and Axelrod, unpublished observations). A heterologous serum protein, bovine gamma globulin, was utilized as a model to investigate the metabolic fate of an antigen. ^{131}I-labeled bovine gamma globulin was injected intravenously into riboflavin-, pyridoxine-, and pantothenic acid-deficient rats and into control rats pair-fed with the riboflavin-deficient group. Since the rates of removal of bovine gamma globulin from the blood were essentially the same in the various groups, it was felt that the mechanism involved in the removal of a foreign protein (and, presumably also of an antigen) from the blood is not impaired in these vitamin deficiencies. In agreement with our studies

in pantothenic acid deficiency described earlier in this paper, we have shown (Axelrod and Seaborn, unpublished observations) that splenic cells from pyridoxine-deficient rats treated with diphtheria toxoid, in contrast to those removed from normal immunized rats, were unable to produce antibody when passively transferred to normal non-immunized rats. These experiments have been interpreted to indicate that pyridoxine deficiency results in a loss of the functional activity of antibody-producing cells. Utilizing the procedure of Jerne *el al.*[61] for the estimation of individual antibody-synthesizing cells, we have shown recently that the number of antibody-producing splenic cells following antigenic stimulus is markedly diminished in pyridoxine deficiency.[92] This decreased cellular immune response was independent of the inanition associated with the deficiency and was restored to normal by the administration of pyridoxine shortly before immunization. Accumulation of antigen by rat spleen did not appear to be deranged in pyridoxine deficiency. Similar observations were made in pantothenic acid-deficient rats (Lederer and Axelrod, unpublished observations).

In contrast to the requirement for a high level of circulating antibodies in combating certain infections, it may be desirable in some disease states to inhibit the antibody response to various antigens. This is the case for hypersensitivity (allergic) reactions where the presence of certain "antibodies" is necessary for the manifestation of the disease. The inhibition of the undesirable "antibody" response by the induction of a vitamin deficiency state suggests itself. A specific vitamin deficiency can be produced either by limiting the dietary intake of the vitamin or by utilizing a specific vitamin antagonist. In our own laboratory, we have been able to lessen the severity of the early (Arthus-type) hypersensitivity reaction to diphtheria toxoid in the guinea pig by the administration of deoxypyridoxine.[35]

We have found that pyridoxine-deficient guinea pigs inoculated with *Mycobacterium tuberculosis*, BCG, exhibited depressed delayed-hypersensitivity skin reactions to the allergen, purified protein derivative (PPD).[37]

Deoxypyridoxine treatment of previously sensitized animals also depressed skin reactivity. However, *in vitro* tests and passive transfer experiments demonstrated that cells of the pyridoxine-deficient animals were sensitive to PPD. Thus, the sensitization mechanism had not been inhibited by the deficiency at the cellular level even though ability to respond to the allergen was affected. One can speculate that pyridoxine or its coenzyme is an essential component in the sequence of reactions between sensitized cell and antigen. Later studies[38] indicated that a pyridoxine deficiency affects in parallel manner both systemic and skin reactivity to PPD. These results render unlikely the possibility that the decreased skin reactivity to PPD of pyridoxine-deficient guinea pigs results from skin abnormalities produced by the lack of pyridoxine. Since similar results were obtained with killed BCG as an immunizing agent, it would appear that impairment of growth of BCG in pyridoxine-deficient animals is not a dominant factor in the production of depressed reactivity. Animals immunized with BCG during a state of pyridoxine deficiency rapidly acquired reactivity when supplied with pyridoxine. Neither skin nor systemic reactivity was affected in inanition controls or ascorbic acid-deficient animals. Anaphylactic sensitivity to bovine serum albumin was not depressed in pyridoxine-deficient guinea pigs. The differential effect of pyridoxine deficiency upon endotoxin and PPD reactivity in the guinea pig permitted the conclusion that differences in basic mechanisms must be involved.[39]

It is becoming increasingly evident that host nutrition is a factor of crucial significance in the development of hypersensitivity phenomena. The inhibitory effect of a pyridoxine deficiency has already been cited.[35,37,38] Mueller *et al.*[40] have demonstrated that ascorbic acid deprivation in the guinea pig can abolish tuberculin sensitivity as measured by the PPD skin reaction. Supplementation with ascorbic acid restored sensitivity. In a later paper,[41] evidence was presented that ascorbic acid deficiency interferes with the actual induction of delayed hypersensitivity rather than with the skin reactivity. Results of passive transfer experiments and studies of

the *in vitro* mitotic response of lymphocytes suggest, however, that delayed tubercular hypersensitivity is not qualitatively lost at the cellular level in scorbutic guinea pigs.[62,63] Perhaps the scorbutic state affects the tuberculin skin response at a more "peripheral" level, possibly in the inflammatory response. The tuberculin reaction could also be inhibited by administration of the folic acid antagonist, amethopterin.[42] Passive transfer experiments with lymph node cells suggested that amethopterin did not inhibit tuberculin sensitization of cells but probably suppressed multiplication of cells altered by contact with tuberculin.[43] This antagonist was also capable of suppressing the development of delayed skin hypersensitivity and the specific febrile response to ovalbumin and diphtheria toxoid.[20]

Studies on the effects of 6-mercaptopurine and methotrexate on passive delayed hypersensitivity reactions indicated that, in the guinea pig, the suppression of delayed cutaneous hypersensitivity reactions by these compounds was due primarily to an immunosuppressive and not to an anti-inflammatory reaction.[93]

Experimental allergic encephalomyelitis (EAE) has been regarded as a specific manifestation of hypersensitivity which may have an autoimmune basis. It is, therefore, of considerable interest to note that the course of development of this disease is amenable to nutritional manipulation. In 1957, Schneider *et al.*[44] reported that susceptibility of homozygous BSVS mice to acute disseminated encephalomyelitis was nutritionally dependent, folic acid and vitamin B_{12} being the most effective nutritional factors studied. Supplementation of a highly purified diet with these vitamins restored in great measure the susceptibility of the mice to this disease. Biotin was less effective. This study was followed by the observations that EAE was suppressed in scorbutic guinea pigs[40] and in guinea pigs treated with amethopterin.[45] The protective effect of amethopterin was reversed by folinic acid.

Studies in the human have indicated that tuberculin sensitivity is impaired in malnourished children.[94,95] Passive transfer of delayed hypersensitivity to tuberculin was achieved in children with protein-calorie malnutrition by injection of material from lymphocytes of a tuberculin-positive donor.[96] These results suggested that there was no impairment of the delayed hypersensitivity reaction in malnourished children. Patients with Hodgkin's disease who showed evidence of a deficiency of pyridoxal phosphate were anergic.[97]

Our studies on skin homotransplantation afford another illustration of the possible usefulness of an induced vitamin deficiency state in preventing or diminishing the extent of a hypersensitivity reaction. It is generally agreed that the failure of an homologous transplant is due to an acquired immune response, perhaps of the delayed hypersensitivity type, in the recipient to the antigens of the donor tissue. The subsequent antigen-antibody interaction is assumed to effect the rejection of the donor tissue. On this basis, a successful transplant would be established if the immune response of the host could be blocked. The soundness of this hypothesis has been verified.[46,47] A high proportion of successful skin homotransplants can be achieved in pyridoxine-deficient rats of certain strains. The deficiency state was induced by the omission of pyridoxine from the diet or by the administration of the pyridoxine antagonist, deoxypyridoxine. Partial tolerance to skin grafts in normal rats was achieved by utilizing a state of immunological inertness induced by pyridoxine deficiency.[48] In these experiments, microsomal ribonucleic acid extracts derived from splenic cells of a normal rat, which later served as the skin donor, were administered to a pyridoxine-deficient rat of another strain. Skin homografting was performed after the ribonucleic acid-treated recipient had received intensive pyridoxine therapy. Later experiments[49] indicated that the biological effects of these extracts could be ascribed to their ribonucleic acid content. The ribonucleic acid effect was manifested only when administered during a state of pyridoxine deficiency. Tolerance of CBA/J mice to skin grafts from C3H/HeJ mice has been achieved by injection of C3H/HeJ splenic cells into pyridoxine-deficient CBA/J recipients.[64] Skin grafting was performed subsequent to pyridoxine therapy. Similar experiments conducted in our laboratory with mice of C57 B1/6J strain have indicated that the dose of splenic cells required for induction of tolerance in C57 B1/6J females to C57 B1/6J male skin isografts can be reduced if the cells are administered to recipient females in a state of pyridoxine deficiency.[98] In this sex-linked histocompatibility system, a male skin isograft transplanted to a female behaves like a homograft and is rejected. The ability of a pyridoxine deficiency to prolong viability of grafts has since been demonstrated in mice with skin[17,65] and ovarian[50] grafts and in dogs with skin grafts.[51] Administration of semicarbazide to rats receiving a pyridoxine-deficient diet improved survival of skin homografts.[99,100] Pyridoxine deficiency alone[99,100] or deoxypyridoxine plus a pyridoxine-deficient diet[100] had little effect. Smellie and Moore[101] have presented results which suggest that semicarbazide plus a pyridoxine-deficient diet may cause significant prolongation of canine renal homo transplants. Treatment with amethopterin has been reported to enhance survival of skin,[52] lung,[53] marrow[54,55] and tumor[56] grafts. The inactivity of this antagonist has been noted in skin[57] and renal[58] homografts.

Mechanism of Action of Pyridoxine. The precise role of pyridoxine in the sequence of events leading to its various effects upon immune phenomena has not yet been elucidated. Since antibodies are proteins, we considered the possibility that the inhibitory effect of this deficiency upon antibody synthesis could be a reflection of the requirement for this vitamin in the general process of protein biosynthesis. Our experiments to this end showed that pyridoxine deficiency in the rat produced a consistent decrease in incorporation of L-valine-l-^{14}C into proteins of liver, spleen, and serum.[66] Incorporation into proteins of subcellular fractions, *i.e.* nuclear, mitochondrial, microsomal, and soluble fractions, was affected in similar manner by this deficiency state. Incorporation by deficient animals ranged from 50 to 75 per cent of that of controls. Simple inanition was without effect and the diminished rate of incorporation was restored by administering pyridoxine 24 hours before injection of labeled valine. Utilizing a cell-free system capable of incorporating amino acids, we have since demonstrated that ribosomes isolated from liver or spleen of pyridoxine-deficient rats exhibited a decreased capacity for incorporating DL-leucine-l-^{14}C when compared to ribosomes isolated from corresponding tissues of normal rats.[67]

The relation of pyridoxine to protein biosynthesis and the known profound effects of a pyridoxine deficiency upon cellular growth suggest a role for this vitamin in metabolism of nucleic acids. At the enzymatic level, it has been established that pyridoxal phosphate is involved in the production of "active formaldehyde" via conversion of serine to glycine and that this C_1 unit participates in biosynthesis of purine bases and of thymidylic acid from deoxyuridine-5'-phosphate. Our results indicate that pyridoxine-deficient rats possess fewer cells and less DNA per milligram of splenic tissue. Studies on incorporation of labeled precursors of nucleic acids provide evidence for a decreased biosynthesis of DNA and RNA in pyridoxine deficiency.[68]

Our next series of experiments dealt with effects of a pyridoxine deficiency upon polysomes and messenger RNA, components which play a fundamental role in protein biosynthesis.[67] These experiments clearly indicate that a pyridoxine-deficient rat possesses fewer polysomes per unit of liver or spleen tissue than a corresponding control. Accordingly, the decreased incorporation of amino acids into protein by ribosomes isolated from liver and spleen of pyridoxine-deficient rats may be attributed to the decreased level of polysomes in these animals. These results suggest a decreased biosynthesis of RNA, particularly messenger RNA, in pyridoxine deficiency. This suggestion was investigated by determining incorporation of orotic-6-^{14}C acid into RNA associated with ribosomes. A decrease in RNA and, particularly, messenger RNA synthesis in pyridoxine deficiency was shown.

Apparently pyridoxine deficiency impairs nucleic acid synthesis with subsequent deleterious effects upon cell multiplication and protein biosynthesis. The adverse effects of pyridoxine deficiency upon immune responses can be explained on this basis. It is known that administration of an antigen stimulates an intensive multiplication of host cells in certain organs concerned with immune responses, e.g., spleen, lymph nodes. Although the mechanism of antigenic activity in this proliferation process is not clear at present, there is no doubt that requirements for DNA are increased at this step of the immune response. Since pyridoxine is required for DNA synthesis, its relative absence would represent a decisive deterrent to antibody synthesis. Furthermore, an accelerated production of specific mRNA would be expected to accompany synthesis of antibody by immunologically competent cells. Accordingly, a lack of pyridoxine would be manifested by a decreased rate of mRNA synthesis and, ultimately, by inhibition of the immune response. Thus, the deleterious effects of pyridoxine deficiency upon development of an immune response could be visualized at the sites of cellular proliferation as well as synthetic capacities of the cell.

Mechanism of Action of Pantothenic Acid. Previous investigations have demonstrated an impairment of antibody response to a variety of antigenic stimuli in pantothenic acid-deficient rats. The molecular basis of this impaired response is not clearly defined. Since antibodies represent a class of proteins, efforts have been directed toward elucidation of the role of pantothenic acid in protein synthesis.[102] We demonstrated a decreased incorporation of intravenously injected labeled amino acids into serum albumin in this deficiency state, thus implicating pantothenic acid as a significant factor in the metabolism of protein other than circulating antibodies. However, we could find no evidence for the malfunctioning of the enzymatic processes involved in protein synthesis. Thus, hepatic polysomal profiles and *in vitro* incorporation of labeled amino acids by a polyribosomal system were not affected in the pantothenic acid-deficient rats. Similarly, the synthesis of nascent polypeptides remained normal in pantothenic acid-deficient rats receiving an intravenous pulse of radioactive amino acids. Since our data indicated that the decreased rate of incorporation of amino acids *in vivo* in pantothenic acid-deficient rats was not due to a decreased synthesis of protein in liver, we explored the possibility that the defect in this deficiency may be the inability to secrete newly synthesized proteins into the extracellular compartment. Our preliminary data support this hypothesis and indicate that the intracellular transport of newly synthesized proteins is impaired in liver cells from pantothenic acid-deficient rats.

SUMMARY

The detrimental effects of specific dietary deficiencies upon the development of acquired immunity in experimental animals have been amply documented. In particular, the requirements for amino acids and certain members of the vitamin B complex are recognized. These requirements are certainly influenced by various factors such as the type of antigen and host species. In some deficiency states, the type as well as the total amount of antibody protein can be affected. The anamnestic (booster) response seems to be particularly sensitive to the absence of required nutrients. The roles of ascorbic acid and the fat-soluble vitamins, A, D and E, in antibody synthesis are inconsistent and require further clarification. The nutritional requirements for carbohydrates, lipids and minerals have not been investigated.

In man the present situation in regard to a relationship of nutritional state to acquired immunity remains indeterminate. Conflicting data in this area may be attributable, in part, to variations in response to different antigenic stimuli and to the difficulties inherent in the control and evaluation of nutritional status in man. Further clarification must await studies utilizing well-defined, specific deficiencies in human subjects. The experiments of Wayne and associates[31] and Hodges et al.[30,32-34] represent a beginning in this direction. Considerable attention has been devoted to the possible effects of protein-calorie deficiency and general malnourishment upon the immune response.[85] In this connection, the lack of an effect of general inanition upon the immune response in experimental animals should be noted.

The pharmacologic action of certain vitamins in stimulating antibody production in normal experimental animals requires confirmation in man.

The significance of the animal experimenta-

tion must also be evaluated critically. Generally speaking, these experiments have employed a severe deficiency state of the particular nutritional factor in question and have undoubtedly yielded much useful information. However, serious consideration must be given to the possible occurrence of nonspecific secondary effects in these severely debilitated animals. In agreement with the view expressed by Horwitt,[59] I visualize the need for controlled studies in experimental animals only *partially* deprived of specific nutrients. Such studies would bear a closer relationship to the degree of nutritional depletion commonly encountered in the human. This approach is utilized in the experiments of Panda and Combs[71] and Muranyi et al.[72]

It must be reemphasized that an antibody response may represent only one facet of a complex mechanism determining resistance to infection. In many instances, no correlation exists between the ability to fabricate antibodies and the degree of resistance to an infectious agent. Such a circumstance has been nicely illustrated by Zucker et al.[3] It is obvious, then, that a decreased immune response resulting from a nutritional deficiency will be of significance in the phenomenon of resistance to infection *only* in instances where resistance can be explained in terms of recognized immunological reactions.

Numerous experiments have demonstrated the influence of nutritional state upon hypersensitivity reactions. Such effects are in accord with the role of nutritional factors in antibody production and lend encouragement to the hope that undesirable states of hypersensitivity may become amenable to inhibition by nutritional means or by the application of antimetabolites. The beneficial effects of vitamin deficiencies upon experimental allergic encephalomyelitis and various homografts may be cited in this connection.

BIBLIOGRAPHY

1. Kolmer: Chapter 18 in *Modern Nutrition in Health and Disease*, Wohl and Goodhart, Philadelphia, Lea & Febiger, 1955, pp. 498–509.
2. Axelrod and Pruzansky: Vitamins and Hormones, *13*, 1, 1955.
3. Zucker, Zucker and Seronde, Jr.: J. Nutrition, *59*, 299, 1956.

4. Giunchi, Scuro, Sorice and Fidanza: Riv. Ist. Sieroterap. Ital., *28*, 281, 1953.
5. Giunchi, Fidanza, Scuro and Sorice: Int. Zeit. Vitaminforsch., *25*, 1, 1953.
6. ————: Exp. Med. and Surg., *12*, 430, 1954.
7. Wissler, Frazier, Soules, Barker and Bristow: Arch. Path., *62*, 62, 1956.
8. Underdahl and Young: Virology, *2*, 415, 1956.
9. Bersins: Zhur. Microbiol. Epidemiol. i Immunobiol., *9*, 18, 1955.
10. Bianchi and Cortesi: Acta Vitaminol., *8*, 269, 1954.
11. ————: Acta Vitaminol., *9*, 219, 1955.
12. Stoerk: Ann. N.Y. Acad. Sci., *52*, 1302, 1950.
13. Axelrod: Am. J. Clin. Nutr., *6*, 119, 1958.
14. Scrimshaw, Taylor and Gordon: Am. J. Med. Sci., *237*, 367, 1959.
15. Harmon, Miller, Hoefer, Ullrey and Luecke: J. Nutrition, *79*, 263, 1963.
16. ————: J. Nutrition, *79*, 269, 1963.
17. Hargis, Wyman and Malkiel: Inter. Arch. Allergy, *16*, 276, 1960.
18. Sterzl: Nature, *189*, 1022, 1961.
19. Thomas, Baker and Ferrebee: J. Immunol., *90*, 324, 1963.
20. Friedman, Buckler and Baron: J. Exp. Med., *114*, 173, 1961.
21. Berenbaum: Biochem. Pharmacol., *11*, 29, 1962.
22. Solarino: Int. Zeit. Vitaminforsch., *27*, 373, 1957.
23. Segagni: Minerva Pediatrica, *7*, 985, 1074, 1124, 1955.
24. Richou: C. Rend. Acad. Sci., *243*, 111, 1956.
25. Lamanna and Taviani: Acta Vitaminol., *9*, 57, 1955.
26. Butturini and Casa: Acta Vitaminol., *9*, 65, 1955.
27. Kahn, Stein and Zoutendyk: Am. J. Clin. Nutr., *5*, 70, 1957.
28. Havens, Jr., Bock and Siegel: Am. J. Med. Sci., *228*, 251, 1954.
29. Pretorius and de Villiers: Am. J. Clin. Nutr., *10*, 379, 1962.
30. Hodges, Bean, Ohlson and Bleiler: Am. J. Clin. Nutr., *10*, 500, 1962.
31. Wayne, Will, Friedman, Becker and Vilter: Arch. Int. Med., *101*, 143, 1958.
32. Hodges, Bean, Ohlson and Bleiler: Am. J. Clin. Nutr., *11*, 85, 1962.
33. ————: Am. J. Clin. Nutr., *11*, 180, 1962.
34. ————: Am. J. Clin. Nutr., *11*, 187, 1962.
35. Axelrod, Hopper and Long: J. Nutrition, *74*, 58, 1961.
36. Axelrod and Hopper: J. Nutrition, *72*, 325, 1960.
37. Axelrod, Trakatellis, Bloch and Stinebring: J. Nutrition, *79*, 161, 1963.
38. Trakatellis, Stinebring and Axelrod: J. Immunol., *91*, 39, 1963.
39. Stinebring, Trakatellis and Axelrod: J. Immunol., *91*, 46, 1963.
40. Mueller, Kies, Alvord, Jr. and Shaw: J. Exp. Med., *115*, 329, 1962.
41. Mueller and Kies: Nature, *195*, 813, 1962.
42. Friedman, Buckler and Baron: Fed. Proc., *20*, 258, 1961.
43. Friedman and Buckler: Fed. Proc., *22*, 501, 1963.
44. Schneider, Lee and Olitsky: J. Exp. Med., *105*, 319, 1957.
45. Brandriss: Science, *140*, 186, 1963.
46. Axelrod, Fisher, Fisher, Lee and Walsh: Science, *127*, 1833, 1958.
47. Fisher, Axelrod, Fisher, Lee and Calvanese: Surgery, *44*, 149, 1958.
48. Axelrod and Lowe: Proc. Soc. Exp. Biol. Med., *108*, 549, 1961.
49. Lowe and Axelrod: Transplantation, *3*, 82, 1964.
50. Parkes: Nature, *184*, 699, 1959.
51. Humphries, Jr., Harms and Moretz: J. Am. Med. Assoc., *178*, 490, 1961.
52. Berenbaum: Nature, *198*, 606, 1963.
53. Blumenstock, Collins, Thomas and Ferrebee: Surgery, *51*, 541, 1962.
54. Thomas, Collins, Herman, Jr. and Ferrebee: Blood, *19*, 217, 1962.
55. Uphoff: Proc. Soc. Exp. Biol. Med., *99*, 651, 1958.
56. ————: Transpl. Bull., *28*, 110, 1961.
57. Brooke: Transpl. Bull., *26*, 453, 1960.
58. Zukoski, Lee and Hume: J. Surg. Res., *2*, 44, 1962.
59. Horwitt: Ann. N.Y. Acad. Sci., *63*, 165, 1955.
60. Leutskaja: Dokl. Akad. Nauk SSSR, *159*, 938, 1964.
61. Jerne, Nordin and Henry: in *Cell Bound Antibodies*, Ed. Amos and Koprowski, Philadelphia, Wistar Institute Press, pg. 109, 1963.
62. Zweiman, Schoenwetter and Hildreth: J. Immunol., *96*, 296, 1966.
63. Zweiman, Besdine and Hildreth: J. Immunol., *96*, 672, 1966.
64. Axelrod and Trakatellis: Proc. Soc. Exp. Biol. Med., *116*, 206, 1964.
65. Herr and Coursin: J. Nutrition, *88*, 273, 1966.
66. Trakatellis and Axelrod: J. Nutrition, *82*, 483, 1964.
67. Montjar, Axelrod and Trakatellis: J. Nutrition, *85*, 45, 1965.
68. Trakatellis and Axelrod: Biochem. J., *95*, 344, 1965.
69. Moore and Lawrence, Jr.: Transplantation, *8*, 224, 1969.
70. Gershoff, Gill, Simonian and Steinberg: J. Nutrition, *95*, 184, 1968.
71. Panda and Combs: Proc. Soc. Exp. Biol. Med., *113*, 530, 1963.
72. Muranyi, Bertok, and Kemenes: Zeit. f. Immunitats und Allergie-forsch. *127*, 1, 1964.
73. Ravic-Scerbo and Lucjuk: Nutr. Abstr. and Rev., *38*, 2560, 1968.
73a. Kumar and Axelrod: J. Nutrition, *98*, 41, 1969.
74. Ströder, Lange, Emmerling and Finger: Zeit, Kinderheilk., *107*, 165, 1969.
75. Woodruff: J. Infect. Dis., *121*, 164, 1970.

76. Harmon, Becker, Jensen and Baker: J. Animal Science, *31*, 339, 1970.
77. Frisch: Biochem. Pharmacol., *18*, 256, 1969.
78. Bhargava, Hanson and Sunde: J. Nutrition: *100*, 241, 1970.
79. Gerzymisch and Hock: Arch. Exp. Veterinaermed., *22*, 25, 1968.
80. Gill and Gershoff: J. Immunol., *99*, 883, 1967.
81. Kenney, Arnrich, Mar and Roderuck: J. Nutrition, *85*, 213, 1965.
82. Kenney, Roderuck, Arnrich and Piedad: J. Nutrition, *95*, 173, 1968.
83. Piedad-Pascual, Arnrich and Kenney: J. Nutrition, *100*, 389, 1970.
84. Kenney, Magee and Piedad-Pascual: J. Nutrition, *100*, 1063, 1970.
85. Scrimshaw, Taylor and Gordon: in *Interactions of Nutrition and Infection*, Geneva, World Health Organization, Monograph Series, No. 57, pg. 148, 1968.
86. Tashmukhamedov: Federation Proceedings, *25*, No. 1, Part II, T143, 1966.
87. Bliznakov, Casey and Premuzic: Experientia, *26*, 953, 1970.
88. Najjar, Stephan and Asfour: Arch. Dis. Child., *44*, 120, 1969.
89. Reddy and Srikantia: Ind. J. Med. Res., *52*, 1154, 1964.
90. Brown and Katz: Trop. Geogr. Med., *18*, 125, 1966.
91. ———: E. Afr. Med. J., *42*, 221, 1965.
92. Kumar and Axelrod: J. Nutrition, *96*, 53, 1968.
93. Borel, Fauconnet and Miescher: Int. Arch. Allergy, *33*, 583, 1968.
94. Harland and Brown: E. Afr. Med. J., *42*, 233, 1965.
95. Lloyd: Brit. Med. J., *3*, 529, 1968.
96. Brown and Katz: J. Pediatrics, *70*, 126, 1967.
97. Chabner, DeVita, Livingston and Oliverio: New Eng. J. Med., *282*, 838, 1970.
98. Trakatellis and Axelrod: Proc. Soc. Exp. Biol. Med., *132*, 46, 1969.
99. Moore: Nature, *215*, 871, 1967.
100. Moore: J. Cardiovasc. Surg. *9*, 63, 1968.
101. Smellie and Moore: Surg. Gyn. Obstet., *128*, 81, 1969.
102. Roy and Axelrod: Proc. Soc. Exp. Biol. Med., *138*, 804, 1971.

Chapter

16

Nutrition and Cell Growth

MYRON WINICK

AND

JO ANNE BRASEL

During the past few years newer techniques in biology have made it possible to study cellular growth of organs in a quantitative manner. In 1962 Enesco and LeBlond serially measured DNA content of a number of rat organs.[1] Since DNA content per diploid cell is a constant for any particular species,[2] these investigators were able to calculate the number of cells in the various organs of the rat at any particular time, simply by dividing the total DNA content analyzed by 6.2 picograms (the DNA content of all diploid rat cells). Once the number of cells is determined then the weight per cell, total protein content per cell, or total lipid content per cell can be determined by either weighing the organ or ascertaining the total protein or lipid content of the organ and dividing by the number of cells. This can be expressed as a weight/DNA, protein/DNA, or lipid/DNA ratio.

Thus by simple biochemical techniques it has become possible to follow growth by monitoring the contribution made by increase in cell number and the contribution attributable to increase in cell size. It should be recognized that total DNA content, while accurately reflecting cell number in no way differentiates one cell type from another. In addition, although the ratios as outlined above give an overall average for these materials per cell, no single cell may actually contain this quantity of material. Individual cells, especially when differing in type, might vary widely in their composition of either proteins or lipids.

Within these limitations, however, this "chemical" approach to cellular growth has allowed certain generalizations to be made which have given rise to an overall picture of growth on a cellular level.

Careful examination of all non-regenerating organs by these methods reveals three distinct phases of growth. The first is characterized by a proportional increase in weight, protein and DNA content; the number of cells is increasing whereas the ratios or the size of the individual cells is not changing. Simple hyperplasia is occurring. This phase ends as the rate of net DNA synthesis begins to slow while weight and protein content continue to increase giving rise to a transitional phase of hyperplasia and concomitant hypertrophy which lasts until net DNA synthesis stops. After this point, all growth is by hypertrophy. Finally when weight stabilizes and net protein synthesis stops, growth is finished.[3]

These data allow us to view the overall growth of any organ as a continuous accretion of protoplasm made up of water, proteins and in some cases lipids. The ultimate packaging of this protoplasm into individual cells depends on the rate of DNA synthesis. At present the mechanisms controlling the period during which DNA may be synthesized by an organ and the mechanisms governing the rate of synthesis during that period are largely unknown.

Brain. In whole rat brain DNA synthesis and hence cell division stops at about 20 days of age. Total protein continues to increase until about 99 days of age when the brain reaches its final size. However, more detailed examination reveals that different regions have their own pattern of cellular growth.[4] In cerebrum, DNA synthesis continues until about 21 days postnatally. After this the cells continue to accumulate protein and lipid. Total cerebral lipid content is achieved somewhat later and total protein content around 99 days of age. In cerebellum, DNA synthesis stops at 17 days postnatally. Net protein synthesis actually becomes negative for a short period after this and the size of the individual cerebellar cells decreases. This decrease in cell size probably reflects the maturation of larger more primitive cells into smaller more mature cells. In brain stem, total cell number is increased to 14 days of age. Thereafter there is an enormous increase in the protein/DNA ratio. This increase probably not only reflects an increase in the size of the brain stem cells but also in growth, myelination and enlargement of neuronal processes from other brain regions into the brain stem. Hippocampus is an area which demonstrates a type of cellular growth somewhat unique to central nervous system. There is a discrete rise in DNA content between the 14th and 17th day of life. The increase corresponds to a migration of neurones from under the lateral ventricle into the hippocampus which occurs on the 15th day after birth in the rat.[5]

The ultimate cellular makeup of the various regions depends then on the rate of cell division within the particular region, the time that cell division stops, the type of cells dividing and whether or not cells are migrating to or from the region.

In human brain the sequence of events is not as clearly defined as in rat brain. Studies initially indicated that DNA synthesis was linear prenatally, began to slow down shortly after birth and reached a maximum around 8 to 12 months of age.[6] More recent studies have tended to modify these results somewhat and would extend the time beyond the first year of life.[7] Moreover, Dobbing and Sands[8] have recently shown that two peaks of DNA synthesis may occur normally in human brain. The first peak is reached at about 26 weeks of gestation and the second around birth. They have interpreted these results as corresponding to the peak rate of neuronal division and the peak rate of glial division respectively.

There are still very few data on the cellular growth of various regions of human brain. What data are available would indicate that the rate of cell division postnatally is about the same in cerebrum and cerebellum and stops at about the same time in both areas, that is, between 12 and 15 months of age.[9] The number of cases studied, however, is too small to attempt too precise a statement.

In brain stem, DNA synthesis continues at a slow but rather steady rate until at least 1 year of age. The exact cell types involved and the migratory patterns of the cells in the developing human brain are not as clearly worked out as in the rat brain. For obvious reasons, radioautography cannot be done. What is known then is the result of careful histological and histochemical examination of brains of fetuses of various ages. In a series of elegant studies Duckett and Pearse[10] have shown that during fetal life the brain not only increases linearly in weight but undergoes a series of biochemical changes. Glycolysis is present during the 2nd month of fetal life; oxidative mechanisms appear during the 3rd month; and activity and localization of a number of enzymes reach a mature pattern during the 7th month of fetal life.

In addition there is evidence that the presence of acetylcholinesterase indicates tissue excitability.[11] The activity of this enzyme is localized in neurons of the anterior horn of the spinal cord as early as the 10th week of embryonic life according to Duckett and Pearse.[12] This correlates well with the time that movement of the lower limb can be elicited by proper stimulation.[13]

Two specific cell types, the Cajal-Retzius cells[14] and the monamine oxidase cells[15] are present only in fetal life disappearing before birth. Their function is unknown. Serial analysis of lipids in human brains would indicate that the lipid/DNA ratio rises shortly after birth until at least 2 years of age. This is reflected in a rise in both the cholesterol/DNA and phospholipid/DNA ratios.[16] Thus postnatal lipid synthesis is occurring at a more rapid rate than DNA synthesis. This is undoubtedly related to the rapid myelination which is occurring during this period of life.

Although the descriptive work in human brain would suggest that cellular growth is governed by the same principles as those governing cellular growth in rat brain, more data are needed to complete the picture. Indirect measurements have been used to follow normal growth of human brain. The most common of these is cranial circumference. Some correlations have been made between increase in cranial circumference and cellular growth of the brain. Approximate formulas have been worked out relating head circumference to brain weight, protein and DNA content during the first year of life.[17]

In summary, normal cellular growth of mammalian brain is made up of an early proliferative phase in which cell division predominates and the quantity of protein and lipid per cell remains relatively constant. The rate of proliferation of cells appears to be separated into two peaks: one probably neuronal and the other glial. At the same time, cells migrate from certain regions of the brain to other regions. In human brain, there is evidence that certain cell types appear and disappear during this early phase of growth.

Later growth is characterized by a slowing and finally a cessation of cell division in spite of a constant rate of net protein synthesis, except in cerebellum, and an increasing rate of myelin synthesis. Finally myelination is completed and net protein synthesis stops. The mechanisms controlling the rate of cell division and the migratory patterns of cells are just beginning to be investigated.

Muscle. There has been a number of studies of cellular growth in skeletal muscle of rats. Enesco and Puddy[18] determined that 35 per cent of the nuclei in samples of 4 different limb muscles lay outside the muscle fibers in male Sherman rats at 16, 36, and 86 days of age. Since the percentage of nuclei outside the fiber did not change over the age span studied, an increase in DNA content, even if uncorrected for nonfiber nuclei, will proportionately reflect growth in muscle cell nuclei. This study, using combined histometric and chemical techniques, shows clearly that the number of individual muscle fibers does not increase postnatally but, contrary to earlier concepts, the number of nuclei within the fiber, as well as fiber size, shows significant increments. Note, however, that this study was carried out in normal animals, and the constant percentage of fiber to nonfiber nuclei may not hold true in abnormally growing animals. The DNA content of various striated muscles rises to fixed levels by 90 to 95 days of age, while increase in weight, myofibrillar proteins and sacroplasmic proteins continues until 140 days of age.[19] Thus it appears that hyperplasia of muscle fiber nuclei continues until some 90 days postnatally and hypertrophy of muscle fibers continues to approximately 140 days in the rat.

Cheek et al.[20–22] have also measured total muscle mass and total muscle nuclear number in the Sprague-Dawley rat. Using an ingenious technique, they measured DNA concentration in a sample of skeletal muscle and assessed the total muscle mass from determinations of total noncollagen protein or potassium in pulverized, defatted, dried carcass, or from determination of total muscle intracellular water or calcium content of bone. Total muscle nuclear number then equals [(DNA concentration in mg/gm) times (Muscle mass in gm)] divided by (DNA content per nucleus). The validity of these methods depends upon the muscle samples being representative of muscle throughout the body and upon the accuracy of noncollagen protein or potassium or intracellular water as reflections of total muscle mass or of calcium content as a reflection of bone mass. These investigators point out that the four different methods give similar results for grams of muscle in normal rats at different ages, and that these values are, in turn, similar to values using creatinine excretion[23] to determine muscle mass and to values obtained by dissection techniques.[23] The literature on the constancy of DNA from one muscle to another is contradictory. Although Cheek et al.[24] report agreement for DNA concentration in several muscles of normal male Sprague-Dawley rats, and in five muscles studied in young Macaca mulatta monkeys, Enesco and Puddy[18] find agreement only in certain muscles in male Sherman rats. In addition, there are differences noted with age. In hypophysecto-mized rats,[25] DNA content of various muscles may differ. These data suggest that DNA concentration may vary between different muscle groups even in the normally growing animal and, therefore, that calculation of total muscle nuclear population from the DNA content of a single sample may not provide entirely accurate values although trends with growth, disease or therapy might well be assessed in this way. However, to our knowledge, no studies of the constancy of DNA in various muscle groups with malnutrition or overnutrition have been reported. In the animal these possible pitfalls in methodology can be avoided by removing *in toto* one or more specific muscles or muscle groups and by measuring directly the weight, DNA, and protein content when studying either normal or abnormal growth.

Using the noncollagen protein method, Cheek *et al.*[23] have measured total muscle mass in normal male and female Sprague-Dawley rats from 3 to 14 weeks of age. In the male, muscle mass increases linearly during this period from approximately 15 to 144 gm. The female begins with the same amount of 15 gm at 3 weeks, but the rate of growth is less rapid, especially after 8 weeks of age. The adult female at 14 weeks achieves a muscle mass of 90 gm. These sex differences are erased if muscle mass is compared to total body weight rather than age.[23] For example, at a body weight of 200 gm, both sexes have a muscle mass of approximately 70 gm. This study does not document the time of cessation of growth in total muscle mass.

Using indirect methods, Cheek *et al.*[20,24] have also assessed growth in muscle "cell mass" during normal growth. Maximum muscle cell mass is reached in normal male Sprague-Dawley rats by 14 weeks, which is slightly earlier than the age noted for the quadriceps muscle by Gordon *et al.*[19] using total muscle analysis. Normal female rats[20] show values similar to males at 3 weeks; thereafter, until 13 weeks, individual "cell mass" is greater in the female; after 13 weeks, the male values exceed the female ones. This catch-up by the male occurs between 8 and 13 weeks, *i.e.*, after cessation of DNA replication.

Using a single muscle sample for DNA content determinations,[20] total muscle nuclear population in normal male Sprague-Dawley rats is achieved by 8 weeks of age with a spurt in DNA accumulation during puberty (6 to 8 weeks). In the female after 3 weeks of age the number of nuclei increases much more slowly than in the male. In addition, there is little acceleration during puberty, resulting in final nuclear numbers of approximately two-thirds of the male value at 14 weeks. The discrepancy between the figure of 90 to 95 days, cited earlier, and this value of 8 weeks or 56 days for the age of cessation of DNA growth in rat skeletal muscle may relate to the problems of extrapolation from a single specimen to total muscle DNA content.

Methods for assessing muscle cell growth in the human must be adapted to biopsy sampling for the biochemical measurements of DNA and protein. All of the reservations we have noted about the reliability of a single sample for the assessment of DNA content of the entire skeletal musculature pertain to human studies as well as to rat data. However, such biopsy data are the only ones available for the human.

Creatinine excretion has been used to measure total muscle mass. Graystone[23] ably reviews the early studies supporting the high correlation between the fat-free body mass and urinary creatinine levels. Under the conditions of a low-creatinine, low-hydroxyproline diet for 3 days prior to and including 3 consecutive days of urine collections, (muscle mass in Kgm) equals [(mean urinary creatinine excretion in gm/day) times (20)]. The derivation of this factor of 20 is well documented in Graystone's paper. Linear relationships with high coefficients of correlation are obtained in normal children with no apparent sex difference when creatinine excretion in mg per day is plotted against body weight. When height is used as a baseline, normal males and females have similar amounts of muscle per unit height until a height of 137.5 cm is reached. Thereafter, growth in muscle mass in boys accelerates rapidly, achieving values at early adolescence of $1\frac{1}{2}$ to 2 times the values per unit height noted in normal females. Sex differences, especially in later childhood, occur when creatinine excretion is compared to either chronological age or bone age. Graystone[23] has also determined the mathematical relationships between creatinine excretion and total body water, extracellular volume, total body chloride, total body potassium, and intracellular water. This remarkable investigation documents normal growth in muscle mass in childhood and describes its relationships to the other major body compartments. It provides valuable baseline information for the study of abnormal growth. However, if muscle mass calculations are to be made from creatinine excretion values in abnormal growth states, such as malnutrition, it will be very important to determine if Graystone's factor of 20 holds for the abnormal state as well.

Using a single muscle biopsy and 24-hour creatinine excretion, Cheek[26] calculated total muscle nuclear population from the equation: [(DNA content per gm of muscle) divided by (DNA content per diploid nucleus)] times (total muscle mass in gm). He determined that muscle nuclear number in male infants increases linearly with age, length, total body water, and basal oxygen consumption. No data are available for males between $1\frac{1}{2}$ and 5 years of age. From 5 to $10\frac{1}{2}$ years the mathematical relationship between muscle nuclear number and age is again linear; however, the slope of the line is less; i.e., the rate of DNA replication in muscle tissue is less rapid in the older boys. At the age of $10\frac{1}{2}$ years, the rate of DNA replication in muscle tissue again accelerates. From 5 to 16 years, growth in muscle nuclear number is linear with total body water and basal oxygen consumption. Estimates of the number of muscle nuclei in males at various ages are shown below.

Age	Nuclear Number
2 months	0.22×10^{12}
1.5 years	0.34×10^{12}
5 years	0.90×10^{12}
10 years	1.22×10^{12}
16 years	3.10×10^{12}

These results represent an over 14-fold increase in nuclear number from 2 months to 16 years of age.

In normal females from 6 to 17 years, growth in muscle nuclear number is linear with age but in contrast to males there is no acceleration in the rate of DNA replication during adolescence. Muscle nuclear number is also linear with height, total body water, and basal oxygen consumption. There are sex differences with age and height, but not with total body water or basal oxygen consumption.

Using the protein/DNA ratio, Cheek[26] has followed growth in "cell mass" in normal children. When this ratio is related to an indicator of lean body mass such as total body water, a definite sex difference is noted. During the mid-childhood years, females have a larger "cell mass" than males. "Cell mass" reaches stable, presumably adult, levels at a total body water value of 20.3 liters, which is equivalent to the age of $10\frac{1}{2}$ years in the normally growing female. The end point for "cell mass" in males is not defined. However, "cell mass" continues to increase in males to at least 16 years of age. By $14\frac{1}{2}$ years of age (total body water of 30 liters) male values equal female values and thereafter exceed them.

Although these extensive studies of Cheek and his co-workers depend upon assumptions of constancy of DNA content and constancy of ratios of fiber to nonfiber nuclei in all skeletal muscle and at all ages from birth to adolescence, their importance to our understanding of cellular growth in human muscle cannot be overstated. The validity of the assumptions remains to be substantiated and the numerical results may change with further studies. However, the trends described in cell growth with maturation and development cannot be expected to change significantly and therein lies their import. This group has used the only techniques currently available for the study of human muscle growth and has provided a wealth of data that can be altered or changed only with the advance of technology.

Placenta. Since placenta is readily available for study, abnormalities in fetal growth that are paralleled in the placenta could more easily be investigated using this tissue. With this in mind, placental growth has been examined in the normal rat and human and under certain abnormal conditions known to affect the growth of the fetus.

Using radioautography, Jollie has demonstrated that labeled mitotic figures do not appear in the trophoblastic layer of rat placenta after the 18th day of gestation.[27] Our own studies demonstrate that although weight, protein, and RNA rise linearly until the 20th day, DNA fails to increase after the 17th day owing to a cessation of DNA synthesis.[28] Thus three phases of cellular growth may be described in rat placenta just as in the other organs of the rat. From 10 days until about 16 days of gestation DNA synthesis and net protein synthesis are proportional, cell number increases, whereas cell size is unchanged. This is the period of pure hyperplasia. From 16 to 18 days, as a consequence of a slowing in the rate of DNA synthesis with protein synthesis continuing at the same rate, hyperplasia and hypertrophy are occurring together. Finally, around 18 days, cell division stops altogether. Weight and protein still continue their linear rise. The ratios rapidly increase. Hypertrophy is occurring alone.

Maturational changes occur throughout gestation. Therefore, growth by cell division is not necessary for certain of these maturational changes to occur. During the final period of hypertrophy certain electron microscopic changes take place in the rat placenta. There is a reduction of the "placental barrier" with the appearance of endothelial and trophoblastic fenestrations. Increased micropinocytotic activity, irregularities at the inner plasma membrane, and the appearance of large vacuoles can all be seen in the so-called element III. There is also approximation of inner and outer membranes at points of constriction and formation of pedicle-like foot processes.[27]

Concomitant with these morphologic changes, profound functional changes also take place. There is a change in the selectivity of transportable materials and an increase in the transport rate of certain materials. Also glycogen, which had previously been deposited in copious amounts, rapidly becomes depleted.[29]

Although the exact timing of events is not as clear as with the rat, available data indicate that the human placenta grows in a qualitatively similar manner. Placenta is the only human tissue in which cellular growth has been studied throughout its entire life span. Therefore, it is not known whether the sequence to be described is characteristic for other human tissues. However, studies cited in the previous section would indicate that human brain grows in a qualitatively similar manner.

At least until the fetus reaches 3,500 gm, fetal weight gain is accompanied by a linear increase in the weight of the placenta. In addition both total protein and RNA increase linearly to term. DNA, however, ceases to increase after the placenta reaches about 300 gm. This corresponds to a fetal weight of about 2,400 gm or a gestational age of 34 to 36 weeks.[30] Thus, as was previously demonstrated in the rat, cell division ceases before term. In the human this appears to be about the 35th week of gestation.

Although the cellular events are similar during the growth of human and rat placenta, there is one quantitative difference. The RNA/DNA ratio is twice as high in the rat. The reason for this difference is unknown, but it may be due to increased connective tissue within the human placenta. Fibroblasts contain relatively little RNA. Possibly the trophoblasts contain equal quantities of RNA in both species.

In summary, the normal cellular growth of placenta proceeds through an orderly sequence of changes as gestation progresses. Therefore, the time at which a stimulus is exerted may be as important as the nature of the stimulus itself. The same stimulus acting early might interfere with cell division, whereas later it cannot. Conversely, the nature of the cellular effects produced might give a clue to the time an unknown stimulus was most active. In any event, the DNA, RNA, and protein content of the placenta can be examined under conditions known to affect both fetal and placental growth. The similarity in the growth pattern between rat and human placenta also suggests the possibility of using the rat as an experimental model.

EFFECTS OF MALNUTRITION
ON CELLULAR GROWTH

Brain. The most common method employed in altering the nutritional status of neonatal rats is to vary the number of pups nursing from a single mother. The normal rat litter consists of from 8 to 12 pups and therefore a nursing group of 10 animals has arbitrarily been considered as normal. Malnutrition is imposed by increasing the size of the nursing group to 18 animals and overnutrition by decreasing the size to three animals.

More recently, other methods of undernutrition have been employed. Protein restriction in the lactating mother reduces the quantity of milk produced without altering its composition. Allowing the animals to nurse for only a single 8-hour period per day also reduces the quantity of milk consumed. All of these methods produce a total caloric restriction as well as a restriction in individual nutrients, the most notable of which is protein. Thus far, all three methods have produced comparable results on brain growth and we will, therefore, examine them together.

In order to produce qualitative changes in the milk without changing the quantity produced, the nursing animal must be artificially fed. There are two procedures which have been employed, repeated tube feeding and gastrostomy with continuous infusion of liquid. Both are time consuming, extremely tedious and technically quite difficult. At present no data on cellular growth of the brain are available which use these feeding techniques although Miller has extensively used the former to study protein synthesis in developing liver.[31]

Employing the "large and small litter" technique, McCance and Widdowson[32] demonstrated a number of years ago that growth rate of the nursing pups was inversely proportional to the number of animals in the group. Moreover, they demonstrated the weight of the brain was reduced in the undernourished animals and increased in the overnourished animals. Perhaps the most important finding in these experiments was that no matter what the state of nutrition after weaning,

the undernourished animals never attained normal size and their brains never recovered normal weight. Other experiments with neonatal pigs confirmed these results.[33] Profound growth retardation in the pigs was produced in the neonatal period and complete recovery in either body size or brain size could not be obtained even when maximum nutritional rehabilitation was attempted.

Previous studies had indicated that undernutrition later during the growing period of the rat would retard growth but that nutritional rehabilitation could restore normal body weight and brain weight.[34] The determining factor in recoverability appeared to be the time at which malnutrition occurred. The earlier the undernutrition, the less likely was recovery after discontinuing the stimulus. Thus there is something different about early growth than later growth which allows the older animal to recover from malnutrition.

The studies of normal cellular growth outlined above suggest a possible explanation. Early organ growth is mainly due to cell division and an increase in the number of cells. Later organ growth is due to hypertrophy with already present individual cells becoming larger. When the original McCance and Widdowson experiments were repeated and compared with animals undernourished at two later times during the growing period, it became clear that if malnutrition were imposed during the proliferative phase of growth, the rate of cell division was slowed and the ultimate number of cells reduced.[35] Moreover this change was permanent and could not be reversed once the normal time for cell division had passed. In contrast, undernutrition imposed during the period when cells are normally enlarging will curtail this enlargment but, on subsequent rehabilitation, the cells will resume their normal size. These experiments demonstrated that total brain cell number could be permanently reduced by undernourishing the rat during the first 21 days of his life and that no matter what is attempted thereafter this reduction in cell number would persist.

If the reduction in brain size in the animals reared in litters of 18 was due to a reduced cell number, how about those reared in litters of 3? When these experiments were performed,[36] it became clear that these over-nourished animals had an increased number of brain cells when compared to brains of animals nursed in normal-sized litters. Thus the number of cells attained by the developing rat brain depends, in part, on the nutrition of the animals during the period of time when brain cells actively are undergoing proliferation. Subsequent experiments have demonstrated that the rate of cell division can actually be manipulated in either direction by changing the state of nutrition during the proliferative phase.[37] Thus undernutrition for the first 9 days of life produced a deficit in brain cell number which can be entirely overcome by overnourishing the animal for the next 12 days. It should be noted here that, as pointed out earlier, we cannot differentiate one cell type from another with these methods. It is therefore possible that the deficit is made up by proliferation of a different cell type than was inhibited during the earlier restriction.

Malnutrition during the first 21 days of life also inhibits lipid synthesis in whole rat brain. The rate of cholesterol and phospholipid synthesis is reduced and the total brain quantity of these materials lowered.[38] This reduction is proportional to the reduction in DNA or cell number and, hence, the ratios of these lipids to DNA or the amount of these lipids per cell is unchanged. If the malnutrition continues beyond the proliferative phase of growth, the continued inhibition of lipid synthesis will result in a reduced lipid content per cell. Enzymes involved in lipid synthesis such as galactocerebroside sulfokinase are also reduced in activity by malnutrition during the first 10 days of life.[39]

Regional patterns of cellular growth are also modified by malnutrition during the nursing period.[40] Cerebellum, where the rate of cell division is most rapid, is affected earliest (by 8 days of life) and most markedly. Cerebrum, where cell division is occurring at a slower rate, is affected later (at 14 days of life) and less markedly. The effects produced include a reduced rate of cell division in both areas, as well as a reduction in overall protein synthesis and in the synthesis of various lipids. In addition to these effects on areas of rapid cell division, the increase in DNA content

which normally appears in hippocampus between the 14th and 17th day is delayed and perhaps even partially prevented. It would appear from these data that those regions in which the rate of cell division is highest are affected earliest and most markedly and that cell migration is also curtailed. Whether this is actually an interference with migratory patterns or an inhibition of cell division at the source below the lateral ventricle is not fully known. But data to be discussed shortly strongly suggest that the latter accounts for at least some of the reduced cell number in hippocampus. Regional patterns of lipid synthesis and the effects of malnutrition on these patterns have not been clearly established. What data are available, however,[41] suggest that areas where myelination is most rapid are most vulnerable to the effects of early malnutrition.

In all of the discussion to this point, individual cell types have not been considered. At present, three types of studies have been conducted on malnourished animal brains during rapid growth. The first is careful histologic examination, employing a variety of special stains, the second is histochemical examination in an attempt to differentiate effects on patterns of specific enzyme development and the third is radioautographic studies to determine the effect of undernutrition on the division of particular cell types. Unfortunately the same species have not been employed in all of these studies which makes cross comparisons difficult.

Histologic changes have been observed on the central nervous systems of rats,[42] pigs and dogs[43] reared after weaning on protein deficient diets. Both neurones and glia in spinal cord and medulla degenerate. These changes persist even after intensive rehabilitation with a protein-rich diet lasting for as long as 3 months. The changes could be made more severe either by beginning the restriction at an earlier age or by extending the duration of the deficient diet. In pigs it has also been demonstrated that severe undernutrition early in life produces histologic changes in the cortex itself. Neurones in the gray matter are reduced in number and appear swollen. More recently histochemical changes have been described in the brains of rats submitted to early malnutrition.[44] The appearance of a variety of enzymes, demonstrable by special staining techniques, is delayed and the ultimate quantity obtained is reduced. Thus early malnutrition produces specific histologic and histochemical changes within the cells of the central nervous system. Again, the earlier the malnutrition, the more severe the damage and the more likely it is to persist.

Radioautographic studies indicate that in neonatal rats malnourished for the first 10 days of life only glial cell division is inhibited in cerebrum since neuronal cell division ceases prior to birth. In cerebellum, the rate of cell division of external granular cells, internal granular cells and molecular cells is reduced.

In addition the rate of cell division in neurones under both the third and lateral ventricle is decreased.[15] This reduction in neurones under the lateral ventricle explains, at least in part, the reduced DNA content in hippocampus 5 days later since these are the cells which are destined to migrate into the hippocampus.

The effect of malnutrition on the human brain has only been studied to a limited extent.[9,16] The data indicate that in marasmic infants who died of malnutrition during the first year of life, wet weight, dry weight, total RNA, total cholesterol, total phospholipid and total DNA content are proportionally reduced. Thus the rate of DNA synthesis is slowed and cell division curtailed resulting in a reduced number of cells. Since the reduction in the other elements was proportional to the reduction in DNA content, the ratios are unchanged and, hence, the size of cells or the lipid content per cell is not altered. Again it is to be emphasized that these are "average" cells we are describing and it is quite possible that certain cells, i.e. those with lipid being actively deposited, are being affected differently than those in which this is not occurring. If the malnutrition persists beyond about 8 months of age not only are the number of cells reduced, but also the size of individual cells are reduced. In addition the lipid per cell is also reduced. Thus in human brain there is a similar type of response to malnutrition. During proliferative growth

cell division is curtailed, during hypertrophic growth the normal enlargement in cells is prevented.

It is obviously not possible to collect recovery data in infants, but indirect data suggest that the situation might also be similar to the situation in animals. Since head circumference was correlated with these cellular parameters and was reduced in proportion to the reduction in the number of cells in these infants, their head circumferences were appropriate for their brain sizes and cell number and reduced for their ages. In similar children recovering from this type of severe marasmus, this reduced head circumference persisted even after maximum rehabilitation until they were at least 5 years old. Regional effects of malnutrition in the human have been studied and the data indicate reduction in cell number will occur in cerebrum, cerebellum and brain stem in children who died of marasmus during the first year of life.[9] Thus available data indicate that the effects of malnutrition on human brain are qualitatively quite similar to the effects on rat brain. However, the quantitative events have still not been worked out.

Muscle. During hyperplastic growth in the rat, protein-calorie malnutrition results in a retardation in the rate of DNA synthesis in gastrocnemius muscle.[45] There is little change in the protein/DNA ratio, and the number of nuclei remain reduced even after adequate refeeding. Malnutrition in the more mature postpubertal animal[45] results in a reduced protein/DNA ratio only, and this change is reversed with refeeding.

In muscle of young rats fed a diet low in both calories and protein, Hill et al.[46] have found a reduction in both DNA content and protein/DNA ratio. By contrast, when the animals were restricted in calories but were fed adequate protein, less reduction in either muscle growth or muscle nuclear number was noted. In these animals the protein/DNA ratios were either normal or slightly increased. These authors postulate that reducing caloric intake will affect DNA replication primarily, while reduction of both caloric and protein intake has more serious effects on intracellular protein synthesis as well.

In laboratory studies of malnutrition, one

can usually produce a specific type of malnutrition. In clinical studies, however, patients rarely exhibit pure marasmus or pure kwashiorkor, but present a picture of mixed protein-calorie malnutrition. In the literature on muscle growth in human malnutrition, the age of onset, duration of malnutrition, severity of malnutrition, and type of dietary deficiency are variable, and hence it is difficult to generalize regarding effects on cellular growth of muscle. It seems clear, however, that whether estimated from cadaver analysis,[47] biopsy specimen,[48] limb measurements,[49] or creatinine excretion,[49–51] muscle growth is more severely and disproportionately reduced than the reduction in total body weight alone would indicate. Loss of total body potassium[51] and muscle tissue protein[47,48] can often be severe. Concomitantly, there is an increase in total body water when compared to body weight which is primarily due to expansion of the extracellular fluid compartment.

In a study of 9 male Peruvian infants from 5 to 30 months of age suffering from severe malnutrition,[50] gluteal muscle samples were analyzed for DNA and protein content and creatinine excretion was used to assess muscle mass. The most striking change was a reduction of the protein/DNA ratio, indicating a loss of "cell mass." There was only a slight reduction in muscle nuclear number when compared to infants of a similar height. These data conflict with data cited elsewhere in this chapter which have demonstrated decreased DNA content in other tissues with severe infantile malnutrition. There are several possible explanations for this discrepancy. First, the calculation of nuclear number depends on the DNA concentration of the biopsy specimen, which may not reflect DNA content in muscles throughout the body. Second, the calculation depends on the assumption that the factor for conversion of creatinine excretion to muscle mass is the same in normal and malnourished children. This has not been entirely substantiated; indeed Alleyne's work[51] suggests that the factor of 20 may be in error for malnourished children. Finally, DNA replication and cell division are time-related phenomena and are logically better compared with controls of the same chronological age rather than the same height as was done in this study. Since these Peruvian children were retarded in growth, one might expect reductions in nuclear number if the comparisons were made against an age baseline. Until further studies substantiate the validity of the factor of 20 for creatinine excretion conversion or until the DNA content of an entire muscle is measured, we must conclude that the extent of the effects of infantile malnutrition on muscle nuclear number has not yet been precisely delineated.

Placenta and Fetus. During intrauterine life all organs of the fetus are in the hyperplastic phase of growth. At no other time should the organism be more susceptible to nutritional stresses. And yet only recently has any information about fetal malnutrition been forthcoming. This is true probably for two reasons, one operational and the other philosophical. The first was the relative inaccessibility of the fetus for experimental manipulation. The second has been the generally accepted view of the fetus as the perfect parasite, extracting its needs from its mother. Recently, as researchers have ventured to study the uterus, this widely accepted viewpoint is being challenged. Fetal malnutrition may result from reduced maternal circulation, inadequate nutrients within the maternal circulation, or faulty placental transport of specific nutrients. The first two situations are now being extensively investigated in experimental animals.

The supply of blood to a single fetus in an animal delivering a litter of fetuses may be reduced spontaneously. It is not uncommon to see a "runt" in a litter of dogs or cats, and it is common knowledge that these animals will survive only with special care and that they will never reach the same final size as their littermates even if this special care is given. Occasionally the same situation occurs in a litter of pigs. Recently Widdowson has studied the cellular changes which take place in the organs of these spontaneously occurring "runt" pigs. Her findings indicate that cell division has been curtailed in heart, kidney, brain and skeletal muscle, the only organs so far studied. Cell size was also reduced in all organs studied when compared to littermate controls.[53]

In the rat, blood supply can be artificially reduced by clamping the uterine artery supplying one uterine horn. Using this technique, Wigglesworth[54] has compared the growth of the fetuses in the ligated horn to that of the fetuses in the unligated horn. Growth rate was reduced in proportion to the distance of the particular fetus from the ligated artery. Those at the uterine end closest to the ligation generally died. As one progressed farther away from the ligated uterine artery and closer to the intact ovarian artery, growth rate increased. More recently the cellular growth of various fetal organs including placenta has been studied in surviving animals within the ligated horn. Ligation on the 13th day of gestation will affect the rate of cell division in placenta and all fetal organs except the brain. Ligation on the 17th day will curtail cell division in the fetal organs again sparing brain, but in placenta cell size will be reduced with cell number remaining normal.[55] Thus in currently available animal studies in which blood supply has been either artificially or spontaneously curtailed, the rate of cell division in fetal organs excluding brain has been retarded. Placenta, moreover, responds in a manner that might have been predicted from the earlier studies involving early postnatal malnutrition. Ligation during the period of hyperplasia results in reduced cell number, whereas ligation during hypertrophy results in reduced cell size. Therefore, by determining the final effect on placental growth at delivery, it may be possible to pinpoint the time at which a stimulus producing such a result must have been active. As we shall see, this possibility may have relevance in the human, where placenta is the only tissue readily available for study. Another abnormality was defined in placentas from the ligated horns, elevation of total organ RNA content and hence an elevation of the RNA/DNA ratio or RNA per cell.[55] Such elevations in tissue RNA/DNA have been described in several tissues under a variety of circumstances. Clamping the aorta results in an increased RNA/DNA ratio in the left ventricle.[56] Repeated nerve stimulation results in an elevation of the RNA/DNA ratio in the innervated muscle,[57] injection of estrogen results in an

increased RNA/DNA ratio in the uterus, and removal of one kidney will result in an increased RNA/DNA ratio in the contralateral kidney.[58] The exact significance of this change is unknown, but it has been described under conditions requiring increased protein synthesis. This increase in placental RNA/DNA ratio may therefore represent an abortive attempt by placental cells to increase their rate of protein synthesis secondary to the stress of vascular insufficiency.

Maternal protein restriction in rats will also retard both placental and fetal growth. In placenta, cell number (DNA content) was reduced by 13 days after conception, cell size (protein/DNA ratio) remained normal, and the RNA/DNA ratio was markedly elevated. Retardation in fetal growth first became apparent at 15 days, followed by a progressive decrease in cell number in all the organs studied. By term there were only about 85 per cent of the number of brain cells in control animals.[55] These data agree with previous data of Zamenhof[59] which showed a similar reduction in total brain cell number in term fetuses whose mothers were exposed to a slightly different type of nutritional deprivation. Thus the cellular changes produced by severe prenatal food restriction are reflected in the placenta even earlier than in the fetus, but retardation of cell division in all fetal organs including brain can be clearly demonstrated.

By employing radioautography after injecting the mother with tritiated thymidine, cell division can be assessed in various discrete brain regions. Differential regional sensitivity can be demonstrated in this way by the 16th day of gestation in the brains of fetuses of protein-restricted mothers. The cerebral white and gray matter are mildly affected. The area adjacent to the third ventricle and the subiculum are moderately affected, whereas the cerebellum and the area directly adjacent to the lateral ventricle are markedly affected.[60,61] These data again demonstrate that the magnitude of the effect produced on cell division is directly related to the actual rate of cell division at the time the stimulus is applied. Moreover they demonstrate that the maternal-placental barrier in the rat is not effective in protecting the fetal brain from discrete cellular effects caused by maternal food restriction.

The subsequent course of these animals born of protein-restricted mothers can be examined. Lee and Chow have reported that even if these animals are raised normally on foster mothers they demonstrate a permanent impairment in their ability to utilize nitrogen.[62] Data from our own laboratory demonstrate that if these animals are nursed on normal foster mothers in normal-sized litters, they will remain with a deficit in total brain cell number at weaning. Thus we can again see early programming of the ultimate number of brain cells. This program, moreover, is written *in utero* in response to maternal nutrition.

These same newborn pups of protein-restricted mothers may be subjected to postnatal nutritional manipulation. If they are raised in litters of three on normal foster mothers until weaning, the deficit in total number of brain cells may be almost entirely reversed.[60] Although quantitatively the number of cells approaches normal, qualitatively the deficit at birth might very well be made up by an increase in cell number in different areas from those most affected *in utero*. Thus although it may appear that optimally nourishing pups after exposing them to prenatal undernutrition will reverse the cellular effects, this may not actually be so in specific brain areas.

Perhaps the most analogous situation to the situation in humans is exposing these pups, malnourished *in utero*, to subsequent postnatal deprivation. One can raise these animals on foster mothers in groups of 18. Animals so reared show a marked reduction in brain cell number by weaning. This effect is much more pronounced than the effect of either prenatal or postnatal undernutrition alone.[63,64] Animals subjected to prenatal malnutrition alone, as previously described, show a 15 per cent reduction in total brain cell number at birth. Animals subjected only to postnatal malnutrition show a similar 15 to 20 per cent reduction in brain cell number at weaning. In contrast, the "doubly deprived" animals demonstrate a 60 per cent reduction in total brain cell number by weaning. These data demonstrate

that malnutrition applied constantly throughout the entire period of brain cell proliferation will result in a profound reduction in brain cell number, greater than the sum of effects produced during various parts of the proliferative phase. It would appear that the duration of malnutrition as well as the severity during this early critical period is extremely important in determining the ultimate cellular makeup of the brain.

Recent experiments by Widdowson[53] in the guinea pig demonstrate that caloric restriction during gestation markedly reduces birth weight of the offspring and curtails the rate of cell division in the brain. In the skeletal muscle not only is there a reduction in cell number, but the actual number of muscle fibers is reduced, and each muscle fiber has an increased number of nuclei. These animals when fed normally after birth fail to recover normal height or weight.[53]

The animal data, then, clearly demonstrate that undernutrition due to either reduced blood supply or reduced availability of nutrients will curtail placental and fetal growth, retard the rate of cell division in various fetal organs, and result in an animal whose organs contain fewer cells. Evidence also indicates that animals born after developing in this type of intrauterine environment will carry these cellular deficits for the rest of their lives. However the two types of "malnutrition" produce very different effects on brain. In the vascular insufficiency model brain is spared whereas in the maternal malnutrition model brain is markedly affected. Human placenta goes through the same three phases of growth as those described for the organs of the rat. Cell division ceases at about 34 to 36 weeks of gestation, whereas weight and protein increase until nearly term.[30]

Placentas from infants with "intrauterine growth failure" show fewer cells and an increased RNA/DNA ratio when compared to controls.[65] Fifty per cent of placentas from an indigent population in Chile showed similar findings.[63] Placentas from a malnourished population in Guatemala had fewer cells than normal.[66] In a single case of anorexia nervosa in which a severely emaciated mother carried to term and gave birth to a 2500-gm infant, the placenta contained less than 50 per cent of the expected number of cells.[63] Thus both vascular insufficiency and maternal malnutrition will curtail cell division in human placenta. The cellular makeup of the placenta in both of these situations strongly suggests that both stimuli have been active for some time prior to the 34th to 36th week of gestation.

The effects of these stimuli on the cellular growth of the fetus are more difficult to assess. Indirect evidence suggests that cell division in the human fetus may be retarded by maternal undernutrition. Fetal growth is retarded and birth weight reduced.[67] If one examines available data on infants who died after exposure to severe postnatal malnutrition, three separate patterns emerge. Breast-fed infants malnourished during the second year have a reduced protein/DNA ratio but a normal brain DNA content. Full-term infants who subsequently died of severe food deprivation during the first year of life had a 15 to 20 per cent reduction in total brain cell number. Infants weighing 2000 gm or less at birth who subsequently died of severe undernutrition during the first year of life showed a 60 per cent reduction in total brain cell number.[63] It is possible that these children were deprived *in utero* and represent a clinical counterpart of the "doubly deprived" animal. It is also possible that these were true premature infants and that the premature is much more susceptible to postnatal malnutrition than the full-term infant.

Other Tissues. The normal cellular growth patterns for most of the organs of the rat have been worked out. In general, weight and protein continue to increase until about 100 days of age. By contrast, DNA reaches a maximum before this in all organs. The time at which it does so varies with the particular organ. In brain and lung DNA reaches a maximum at about 21 days of life; in liver, spleen and kidney at about 40 days of age; in submaxillary gland at about 45 days of age; and in heart at about 65 days of age. Malnutrition during the period of hyperplastic growth results in a reduced number of cells in all of these organs.

In the human, cellular growth patterns have been studied in 16 organs during normal fetal development. The data indicate that total cell number, as measured by total organ DNA content, increases in all organs from 13 weeks of gestation until term. Cell size, as measured either by weight/DNA or protein/DNA ratios, remains unchanged throughout gestation in heart, kidney, spleen, thyroid, thymus, esophagus, stomach, large and small intestines, and tongue. In brain, lungs, liver, adrenal gland, and diaphragm, cell size increases slowly from the beginning of the 7th month of gestation until term.

More limited data during the first year of life demonstrate that cell number continues to increase rapidly in heart, liver, kidney and spleen. Heart cell size begins to increase after 3 months of age, whereas in kidney, liver, and spleen cell size does not change during the first year.

Children who died of marasmus during the first 2 years of life showed marked reductions in cell number in all organs studied. As described in a previous section, brain cell size was also reduced when the malnutrition extended into the second year. In contrast, cell size in the other organs was not significantly reduced even if the malnutrition persisted beyond the first year.

BIBLIOGRAPHY

1. Enesco and LeBlond: J. Embryol. Exp. Morph., *10*, 530, 1962.
2. Boivin, Vendrely, and Vendrely: Compt. Rend. Acad. Sc., *226*, 1061, 1948.
3. Winick and Noble: Develop. Biol., *12*, 451, 1965.
4. Fish and Winick: Pediat. Res., *3*, 407, 1969.
5. Altman and Das: J. Comp. Neurol., *126*, 337, 1966.
6. Winick: Pediat. Res., *2*, 352, 1968.
7. Dobbing: Reported at Symposium of The American Pediatric Society, Atlantic City, May 1970.
8. Dobbing and Sands: Nature, *226*, 639, 1970.
9. Winick, Rosso, and Waterlow: Exp. Neurol., *26*, 393, 1970.
10. Duckett and Pearse: Proc. Fifth Internat. Cong. Neuropath. Cong. Ser., 100, p. 738. Amsterdam, Excerpta Medica Foundation, 1966.
11. Nachmansohn: *In* Barron, ed. *Modern Trends in Physiology and Biochemistry*, New York, Academic Press, p. 38, 1952.
12. Duckett and Pearse: Anat. Rec., *163*, 59, 1969.
13. Auguslinsson: *In* Sumner and Myrbäck, eds. *The Enzymes*, Vol. 1, New York, Academic Press, p. 443, 1950.
14. Duckett and Pearse: J. Anat., *102*, 183, 1968.
15. ———: Rev. Can. Biol., *26*, 173, 1967.

16. Rosso, Hormazbel, and Winick: Am. J. Clin. Nutr., 23, 1275, 1970.
17. Winick and Rosso: Malnutrition and central nervous development. Proc. NICHD Conf. on Neurophysiological Methods of Assessment. Palo Alto, Calif., June, 1969. U.S.G.P.O. 1973 (in press).
18. Enesco and Puddy: Am. J. Anat., 114, 235, 1964.
19. Gordon, Kowalski, and Fritts: Am. J. Physiol., 210, 1033, 1966.
20. Cheek, Brasel, and Graystone: In Cheek, ed.: Human Growth, Philadelphia, Lea & Febiger, chapter 22, 1968.
21. Cheek, Powell, and Scott: Bull. Johns Hopkins Hosp., 116, 378, 1965.
22. Graystone and Cheek: Pediat. Res., 3, 66, 1969.
23. Graystone: In Cheek, ed.: Human Growth, Philadelphia, Lea & Febiger, chapter 12, 1968.
24. Cheek, Holt, Hill, and Talbert: Skeletal muscle cell mass and growth: The concept of the DNA unit. Pediat. Res., 5, 312, 1971.
25. Beach and Kostyo: Endocrinology, 82, 882, 1968.
26. Cheek: In Cheek, ed.: Human Growth, Philadelphia, Lea & Febiger, chapter 24, 1968.
27. Jollie: Am. J. Anat., 114, 161, 1964.
28. Winick and Noble: Nature, 212, 34, 1966.
29. Correy: Am. J. Physiol., 112, 263, 1935.
30. Winick, Coscia and Noble: Pediatrics, 39, 248, 1967.
31. Miller: Fed. Proc., 29, 1497, 1970.
32. McCance and Widdowson: Proc. Roy. Soc. Lond., 156, 326, 1962.
33. Widdowson and McCance: Proc. Roy. Soc. Lond., 152, 88, 1960.
34. Jackson and Steward: J. Exper. Zool., 30, 97, 1920.
35. Winick and Noble: J. Nutr., 89, 300, 1966.
36. ———: J. Nutr., 91, 179, 1967.
37. Winick, Fish and Rosso: J. Nutr., 95, 623, 1968.
38. Davison and Dobbing: Brit. Med. Bull., 22, 40, 1966.
39. Chase, Dorsey, and McKhann: Pediatrics, 40, 551, 1967.
40. Fish and Winick: Pediat. Res., 3, 407, 1969.
41. Culley and Lineberger: J. Nutr., 96, 375, 1968.
42. Platt: Proc. Roy. Soc., London, 156, 337, 1962.
43. Platt, Heard and Steward: In Munro and Alison, ed.: Mammalian Protein Metabolism, vol. II, New York, Academic Press, chapter 21, 1964.
44. Zeman and Stanbrough: J. Nutr., 99, 274, 1969.
45. Winick: Pediat. Clin. N. Amer., 17, 69, 1970.
46. Hill, Holt, Parra, and Cheek: Johns Hopkins Med. J., 127, 146, 1970.
47. Waterlow: West Indian Med. J., 5, 167, 1956.
48. Hagerman and Villee: Physiol. Rev., 40, 313, 1960.
49. Standard, Wills, and Waterlow: Am. J. Clin. Nutr., 7, 271, 1959.
50. Cheek, Hill, Cordano, and Graham: Pediat. Res., 4, 135, 1970.
51. Alleyne: Clin. Sci., 34, 199, 1968.
52. Graham, Cordano, Blizzard, and Cheek: Pediat. Res., 3, 579, 1969.
53. Widdowson: Malnutrition during pregnancy and early neonatal life. Presented at the Symposium on Fetal Malnutrition, New York City, January, 1970.
54. Wigglesworth: J. Path. and Bact., 88, 1, 1964.
55. Winick: In Adamson, ed.: Diagnosis and Treatment of Fetal Disorders, New York, Springer-Verlag, 1968.
56. Gluck, Tainer, Stern, et al.: Science, 144, 1244, 1964.
57. Logan, Mannell, and Rossiter: J. Biochem., 51, 482, 1952.
58. Karp, Brasel, and Winick: Am. J. Dis. Child., 121, 186, 1971.
59. Zamenhof, Van Marthens, and Margolis: Science, 160, 3823, 1968.
60. Winick: Am. J. Obs. Gyn., 109, 166, 1971.
61. Winick and Velasco: Proc. Intern. Congr. Nutr., 8th, Prague, 1969. Excerpta Medica Ser. #213, 1970.
62. Lee and Chow: J. Nutr., 87, 439, 1965.
63. Winick: Fed. Proc., 29, 1510, 1970.
64. Winick, Fish and Rosso: J. Nutr., 95, 623, 1968.
65. Winick: J. Pediat., 71, 390, 1967.
66. Dayton, Filer and Canos: Fed. Proc., 28, 488, 1969.
67. Smith: J. Pediat., 30, 229, 1947.

PART IV

Malnutrition

Chapter

17

Vitamin Analyses in Medicine

Herman Baker

AND

Oscar Frank

INTRODUCTION

When some diseases were first recognized as deficiencies of one or another vitamin, the vitamins were assayed mainly by their effect upon growth and health of one or another laboratory animal. In man, vitamin deficiencies underlie numerous diseases; conversely, numerous diseases induce vitamin deficiencies. Hypovitaminosis may reflect decreased dietary intake, absorption defects, decreased hepatic avidity, storage, and conversion to active metabolic forms, excess utilization, destruction or excretion. Increased vitamin demands are evident in liver disease,[1-3] pregnancy, hyperthyroidism, growth, neoplasia, anemia, and tissue repair. Some antimetabolites interfere with normal vitamin metabolism. Their structural similarity to cell components enables them to compete for vitamin-dependent sites in metabolism; in this manner they can cripple or distort metabolism. Some antimetabolites may substitute for the vitamin in a coenzyme, thereby producing a faulty enzyme which blocks or modifies a specific biosynthetic pathway.[4]

Vitamins are organic substances required in minute quantities whose effects are based not on caloric values but exclusively on their catalytic activity. Elucidation of their structure, then practical biosynthesis are exciting chapters in organic chemistry. Their identification as prosthetic groups of enzymes fulfilled the revolution in biochemistry begun by Sir Frederick Gowland Hopkins.

The recognition of vitamin structure permits their determination by the tools of analytical chemistry, but, while such methods are widely used in industrial production, the minute quantities in body fluids and tissues limit the purely chemical approach to a few vitamins. Microchemical methods, based on the most sensitive colorimetric and, in particular, fluorometric techniques, are in use for determination of thiamine, riboflavin, ascorbic acid, and some of the fat-soluble vitamins. Vitamin D, on the other hand, is determined by animal assay or, indirectly, by use of alkaline phosphatase. Its metabolism in man is being studied with the use of ^{14}C or ^{3}H vitamin D.[7]

Since vitamins, especially the water-soluble ones, enter into the coenzymes for fundamental cellular mechanisms, they are required by invertebrates and by unicellular organisms, such as bacteria, and most algae. One way to analyze circulating vitamins is to measure enzyme function. Since many enzymes have vitamin-containing coenzymes, prolonged vitamin deficit diminishes coenzyme synthesis. Apoenzyme deficiency also diminishes enzyme activity, independent of vitamin concentration.[8] The analysis of circulating enzyme activity as a measure of vitamin status is not accurate in the presence of apoenzyme deficits; this was shown in liver disease.[8,9] For example, vitamin B_6 (as pyridoxal phosphate) is a coenzyme for a large number of reactions involving amino acids. This is because pyridoxal phosphate is a general "claw"

523

which the body uses to grasp the amino acid molecule. If one suffers from a B_6 deficiency, any enzyme requiring pyridoxal phosphate as a coenzyme is supposedly affected and, as B_6 deficiency increases, the degree of inhibition of the appropriate enzymes also increases. However, all B_6-dependent enzymes are not affected *equally* because there is an equilibrium between enzyme⇌apoenzyme + coenzyme and the affinities of the different apoenzymes for the coenzyme vary. In a moderate degree of deficiency, where some coenzyme is present but the amount is limited, those enzymes in which apoenzyme and coenzyme have a high affinity will be least affected, while those with a low affinity may be almost completely inactivated: the available supply of coenzyme will be preferentially distributed and, as a deficiency increases, reactions are eliminated in turn, but not all together. In general, reactions most essential to life tend to be the last eliminated.[9a] Therefore, the choice of enzymes as a measure of vitamin status does not permit a safety time-factor in which to reverse the vitamin depletion before untoward clinical signs appear. The measure of the circulating vitamins *per se* permits one to detect vitamin deficiency before biochemical and clinical signs appear: the decrease in circulating vitamin titer is the earliest warning signal of impending biochemical and clinical vitamin deficiency. For example, the plasma ascorbate level fell to zero after 41 days of ascorbate depletion, whereas clinical signs of scurvy did not appear for 134 days.[9b] In a study on folate, the first sign of impending biochemical and clinical folate deficiency was a depressed serum folate level: it took approximately 14 to 18 weeks for the biochemical lesion to appear and 20 weeks for the clinical symptoms to appear—depressed folate levels were apparent after 3 weeks. It therefore seems that there is still ample storage of vitamin-containing enzymes to maintain biochemical functions (enzymes), but the earliest sign of enzymatic malfunction remains the depressed circulating vitamin level.

Before the introduction of microbiological assays for B_{12} in human serum, deficiency could be diagnosed only by signs of hematological stimulation upon administration of liver extracts or B_{12} preparations. A similar problem was presented by folic acid.[10] Because folic acid is metabolically related to vitamin B_{12}, microbiologic assays had to be devised for differential diagnosis. This has been solved not only for the B_{12}-folic acid duo, but also for thiamin, biotin, pantothenic acid, riboflavin, nicotinic acid, folinic acid, and vitamin B_6.[1] These additions to the diagnostic armory have proved their value for assaying these vitamins in biologic fluids and tissues.

Use of protozoa to assay biologically active materials is not so well known, because of historical reasons, as the use of bacteria or fungi. Protozoan assays have several advantages over other biological, physical, or chemical assays.[1] These include unusually high sensitivity and specificity, especially for vitamins and organic nutrients, fewer restrictions on size or physical state of the molecule to be assayed, and marked sensitivity to many pharmacologically interesting compounds. Because of their ability to obtain exogenous metabolites by phagocytosis and pinocytosis, as well as by diffusion, osmosis and active transport, particle-ingesting protozoa may be used to assay soluble vitamins and vitamins in particulate form, including small molecules like nicotinic acid and the bulky ones like B_{12}. Protozoan assays are easy to do, require minimal space and inexpensive materials, and environmental conditions can be easily controlled.

Except for the *Lactobacillus casei* method for detecting folate activity, bacteriologic assays for vitamins have not been successful for assay in biologic fluids and tissues:[1,11] they proved to be either insensitive or non-specific. Introduction of protozoan-based techniques for estimating vitamins in biologic fluids and tissues met the practical needs,[1] since they have a sensitivity and specificity for vitamins much like man's.[1,12] By conjoint use of adequate chemical methods for β-carotene, vitamins A, C, and E, one can gauge vitamin imbalances in many metabolic and nutritional diseases.[2]

The development of protozoal techniques for such purposes introduces a new chapter in vitaminology. As nutritional biochemistry deepens into insights of intracellular happenings, the need arises for detecting essential metabolites as components of enzymes or of complex cofactors for enzymes with tools mimicking metazoan metabolic patterns. Microbial assays, which depend on sensitive and specific growth responses, point to a rather uniform characteristic of life: maintenance and growth depend on vitamins. Vitamins function as parts of enzymes. If the enzyme mediates electron transfer, one finds nicotinic acid or riboflavin; carboxylation or decarboxylation, thiamin or biotin; one-carbon transfer, folic acid and B_{12}; two-carbon transfer, pantothenic acid; three-carbon transfer or synthesis of a single carbon group, B_{12}; and nitrogen transfer, vitamin B_6. On a micro scale, protozoa respond to a great variety of vitamins in most of their molecular forms with a comprehensiveness matching chick or rat assays.[12] The criticism that protozoa generally grow more slowly than bacteria and that radioactive tracers like $^{60}CoB_{12}$ are faster analytical tools are of minor importance: more valid comparisons are with the growth rate of the chick or rat. One keeps in mind the economy of the protozoan assay and freedom from radioactivity hazards.

For a while, many investigators needed convincing about the applicability of protozoa for, not only assaying vitamins, but also for detecting drug toxicity: the excellent reproducibility, sensitivity, and metabolic similarity to man and metazoa have made certain protozoa favorable reagents for such use.[1] For example, *Ochromonas malhamensis* has a B_{12} requirement seemingly identical with man's;[1] this is now the official method in Britain for measuring vitamin B_{12} and has replaced *Lactobacillus leichmannii*, chicks, and rats for practical purposes. It is in routine use for monitoring the industrial production of B_{12}. We have given elsewhere much of the biochemical applications of microbiological assays,[1,13] so we shall keep theory brief while showing how microbial vitamin assays serve as an increasingly valuable clinical tool for investigating nutritional status, notably vitamin interrelationships.

We shall also discuss briefly the value of accurately charting vitamin involvement in metabolic processes for evaluating malnutri-

tion, keeping in mind that body vitamins are commonly determined by assessment of biologic fluids and tissues. Laboratory tests assume a correlation between the amount of nutrient in tissues, blood or urine and bodily function. Their usefulness, therefore, depends in a large measure on establishing such a relationship and finding the range in which changes in concentration can be interpreted. In all instances, however, the usefulness of various tests designed for nutritional investigation rests with an appreciation of the distinction between those techniques which reflect only the supply of nutrients to the body and those which indicate abnormal metabolism brought about by the nutritional deficiency.[1] In selecting an appropriate method for studying a nutritional problem, it is necessary to have clearly in mind the objectives of the investigation. These objectives fall into three categories, namely: clinical diagnosis, fundamental research, and nutritional survey work.[1,14]

In this section, we shall describe application of methods for the analysis of vitamins in biologic fluids and tissues: methods for vitamin analyses in pharmaceutical preparations and foodstuffs have been treated extensively by others.[15]

Many laboratories use variations of the assays referred to here and elsewhere.[1] More significance should be attached to the usefulness of *differentials* permitted by a specific assay, rather than to the absolute values: absolute values may deviate with varied methods. It is important to establish a normal range of a method, so that laboratory-to-laboratory variations in obtaining absolute values do not alter the conclusions, *e.g.,* ability to identify vitamin imbalance.

The development of protozoal assay techniques[1] for nutritional surveys brings a new realism to analytical survey procedures. Inadequacies in methodology hampered previous studies of this sort: some methods were not sensitive nor specific enough, making indirect methods necessary. In many instances, the fluid analyzed—urine—did not yield data correlating well with vitamin status owing to large variations in these 24-hour samples. Data thus gathered permitted only rough estimates of nutritional status. With these specific and sensitive protozoal techniques, blood and plasma values could now serve as an index of vitamin status. Earlier we had seen no gross circulating diurnal variations in vitamin titers, as frequently seen in urine specimens, except when dietary intakes were designed to cause gross vitamin overload. Once blood, serum, plasma or tissue is collected, the specimens can be stored frozen and shipped for assay; the vitamin titers do not significantly vary in specimens so handled.[1,52]

The easier quantitative determinations of vitamins in body fluids and tissues permitted by protozoal techniques should elucidate the significance of vitamins not merely in classical nutritional deficiencies but in the wider field of metabolic disturbances generally. Overt vitamin deficiencies are produced by malabsorption, by inhibitors of vitamin function, and sometimes strikingly by drugs and other toxic substances. Vitamin deficiencies may appear whenever an individual's metabolism is so deranged as to require enhanced quantities of a vitamin to cure or to counteract certain symptoms; B_6-dependent infants are a good example.

As with other constituents of blood or serum, deviation of vitamin titers from the normal range can mean different things: reduced intake or absorption, increased utilization, increased demand, increased excretion; all decrease titers; their opposites increase. In our studies we were able to recognize subtle nutritional deficiency states lacking overt signs, i.e., subclinical nutritional deficiencies.[52,225] Subclinical malnutrition, as the very phrase implies, is not obvious— but it exists; it is a warning signal for approaching biochemical and clinical lesions. It remains to learn how malnutrition due to subclinical deficiencies contributes to ill-health on aging.

A vitamin is often the etiological focus of a disease, e.g., vitamin B_{12} and folic acid in macrocytic anemias. Because of the obvious importance for diagnosis and therapy, determination of the "nucleogenic" vitamins B_{12} and folic acid is a necessity in the routine of clinical hematology. Where connections between vitamins and a disease are less clear, a wide field remains for discovery of correlations between physiologic or pathologic events and vitamin and enzyme content of body fluids and tissues.

A glance at vitamins in clinical practice reveals a wide panorama with attractive opportunities in hepatic conditions, renal dialysis technique, oxalosis and calculus disease, in obscure but widely spread neurological diseases, and in many dermatological disorders. Astute clinical observations, combined with knowledge of vitamin metabolism, could make vitamin analysis a powerful tool.

The potential importance of an apparently wide variation in individual human nutritional needs has become evident not only in our studies but also others. Because the concept of extreme human variability tends to destroy the orderliness of science, this subject has been overlooked. Many diseases have their roots in faulty nutrition, but once the extreme variability of human need is recognized, medical scientists may have a better understanding of a host of diseases of unknown etiology. In any event, once the analytical facility for vitaminology is set up, one can turn it into a valuable tool for diagnosing a variety of metabolic imbalances.[1,2]

VITAMIN A AND β-CAROTENE

The chemistry, metabolism and new researches in vitamin A have recently been treated in great detail.[16,17] A ready reference for many of the analytical procedures adopted for vitamin A has also been published.[18]

Many macro- and microphysiochemical methods[1,15] can be used for determining vitamin A and carotenes in a wide variety of materials: the choice depends on the materials to be assayed. Bioassays and thin-layer chromatography[15,20] have been widely used for assaying vitamin A and carotenes, but these methods have little value in estimating the vitamin in small samples of biologic fluids and tissues. The most widely used system for such purposes depends on a series of color reactions to demonstrate the presence of vitamin A or carotenes. The best-known method is based on the Carr-Price reaction[19]—a reaction between the carotenes or vitamin A and $SbCl_3$ in chloroform: this reaction yields a blue color in the presence of extracts of carotene and vitamin A-containing substances. Maximum blue color is reached after 5 seconds and, as the blueness then drops quite rapidly, the measurement must be carried out during this short interval: the reaction is, therefore, carried out directly in the spectrophotometer. Measurement of maximum light absorption can be carried out with any spectrophotometer or similar optical apparatus. With this method, the constants for carotene and vitamin A are usually uniform from one instrument to another.

In serum, the fractionation or concentration of vitamin A and carotenoids is unnecessary.[21] A combined determination is made by means of the blue color with $SbCl_3$ at various wavelengths. Human serum contains vitamin A, carotenoids, and small amounts of free carotene. Since carotenoids also react with $SbCl_3$ with a blue color, corrections become necessary when determining vitamin A.[1]

Most procedures customarily employ serum or plasma. Care must be taken not to use hemolyzed samples, since it has been shown[22,23] that hemolysis of blood gives very high values for vitamin A, but not for carotene.[24] This method[1] is useful for determining vitamin A in lyophilized tissues.[1,16] A new colorimetric procedure for macro- and microanalysis of serum vitamin A has been recently introduced.[25] This method is based on the blue color produced by trifluoroacetic acid with vitamin A.

Samples for assay may be stored frozen without loss of vitamin activity. Use of conical glass-stoppered centrifuge tubes minimizes evaporation and also ensures good packing of the centrifuged, precipitated protein.

The determination of vitamin A is restricted largely to blood studies, since this vitamin is not normally present in sufficient amounts to be measured in the urine of most animals. Injury to the kidneys or the action of certain drugs may cause its excretion in the urine.[18] In the blood there are found both vitamin A and β-carotene. Tests of vitamin A absorption in terms of "tolerance curves" have been employed in examining the nutritional state of individuals, especially in cases of celiac disease. As a measure of the storage of this vitamin, the assay of the vitamin A content of liver biopsy material has been used in certain select cases. Normal values for carotene range between 40 to 150 μg per 100 ml of serum and for vitamin A 25 to 70 μg per 100 ml of serum. In a study of vitamin A levels in infants and children,[26] the average fasting level under 6 months of age was found to be 24 μg; 32 μg in the group 6 months to 1 year, and 38 μg in children over 1 year. The serum carotene level is rather high toward term in pregnancy.[27] In cord blood it is about 25 per cent of that in the maternal blood.[28] The serum vitamin A level is about 25 per cent lower toward term in pregnancy.[27,28] In cord blood it is about 50 per cent of that in maternal blood.[28]

Infants and young children[1] have only a limited capacity for converting carotene into vitamin A. Conversion of carotene is also limited in diseases of the intestine, liver, kidney and in diabetes. In hypothyroidism conversion is almost completely blocked.[1] How vitamin A is derived from carotene is still receiving intensive research: opinions vary as to mechanisms.

A significant seasonal variation has been reported for carotene but not for vitamin A.[29] It was noted in a study of nutrient intake and serum levels that the serum level of carotene reflected the nutrient intake of carotene, but that the serum level of vitamin A did not reflect the nutrient intake of vitamin A.[30] There appears to be no significant difference between fasting and random sampling of blood on the vitamin A level, provided that no form of vitamin A concentrate has been ingested.

Following a single oral dose of vitamin A in oil or in aqueous dispersion, the level of vitamin A in the blood rises to a maximum in about 3 hours for the latter and 5 hours for the former menstruum, and in both cases returns to normal in approximately 24 hours.[26] The magnitude of the response to the test dose is greater with vitamin A dispersed in aqueous media; however, in normal subjects, total absorption is essentially the same.

The relationship between serum levels and liver stores has been examined using the fluorescence microscopy method.[31] Good correlation between liver stores and serum levels of this vitamin was found. Blood levels of vitamin A and carotene have been called an expression of liver function.

It is believed that the vitamin A alcohol level of the blood is a better index of hepatic storage and vitamin A nutrition than is the total vitamin A level.[32] The latter is influenced by a postprandial rise, whereas the alcohol level is not. In the fasting state, 80 per cent of the vitamin A circulates in the blood as the alcohol form. The elevation of blood vitamin A in the postprandial state is due largely to an increase in the ester form. The ester variety disappears in about 24 hours after the ingestion of the vitamin. The separation of the ester and alcohol form is carried out best by the chromatographic absorption method.[18]

VITAMIN D

Vitamin D deficiency can be defined biochemically as a disease in which the calcification process cannot keep pace with the synthesis of the organic matrix of bone.[33] The current methodology and metabolism involving studies of vitamin D have been reviewed in excellent treatises.[34,35] In determining the state of nutrition with vitamin D, one has to rely on such indirect methods as blood levels of calcium, inorganic phosphate, and alkaline phosphatase. No satisfactory chemical methods are available to measure either the concentration of this vitamin, its provitamin, or a metabolic product.

In rickets there is generally a decreased blood level of inorganic phosphorus and an associated rise in alkaline phosphatase activity. Alteration of serum calcium is not so consistent, but there is generally a low level. These changes are, however, not specific for vitamin D deficiency. In uncomplicated cases of hyperactivity of the parathyroid, there is generally an elevated serum calcium associated with a decreased level of serum phosphate. The alkaline phosphatase is increased above normal in various conditions other than rickets, such as hyperparathyroidism, Paget's disease, osteomalacia, and metastatic carcinoma.

One of the difficulties with chemical methods is in separating interfering substances such as cholesterol and retinol which have similar chemical and physical properties with vitamin D;[35] a further complication is the small amounts of vitamin D which occur in biologic fluids and tissues. Thus, any reagent to be used for vitamin D detection must be extremely sensitive and specific for vitamin D. Since there is no such reagent, work has centered around the separation of vitamin D from cholesterol and retinol by a variety of chromatographic and photometric procedures,[36-38] as well as by thin-layer chromatography:[39] they all suffer from a variety of limitations.

The use of alkaline phosphatase as a means of evaluating the state of vitamin D nutrition[40] has become popular, especially in survey studies. This method requires only 5 to 20 lambda of serum. The reagent, sodium p-nitrophenyl phosphate, is a colorless compound but, with the splitting off of the phosphate group, the chromogenic salt of p-nitrophenol is liberated. This product of the phosphatase reaction on the reagent serves directly as a measure of enzymatic activity. One p-nitrophenyl phosphate unit is equivalent to 1.8 Bodansky units: one King-Armstrong unit is equivalent to 7.3 units of p-nitrophenyl phosphate. The normal level of serum alkaline phosphatase is given as 1.5 to 4.0 Bodansky units for the adult and 5 to 14 units for the child.

Most of the procedures for the determination of inorganic phosphorus in blood or serum use protein-free serum or blood extracts.[41] The extract is treated with molybdate in acid solution, forming phosphomolybdate. This is reduced by excess molybdate to give a blue color. Normal serum inorganic phosphorus levels range between 3 to 4.5 mg per cent for adults and 4 to 6 mg per cent for children. Serum calcium has also been used. An empirical rule for determining if a child is rachitic is to calculate the product of the serum phosphorus and serum calcium. If it is below 30, rickets is present or will develop, but not if it is above 40.

A bioassay for vitamin D in sera of animals and humans has also been used.[42] Thomas *et al.*[43] assayed the sera of 18 normal subjects and found them to contain between 0.7 and 3.1 I.U. of antirachitic activity per ml. The predominant antirachitic activity was associated with the alpha globulins of serum.

In adults, the body's needs for vitamin D are usually met by its own synthesis. Liver oils are rich in vitamin D: tuna fish, 7,000 to 50,000 I.U. per gm; cod fish, 60 to 300 I.U. per gm. The mammalian liver contains little vitamin D.[43a] Recent reports[43b] indicate that the active circulating form of vitamin D_3 is 25-hydroxy-cholecalciferol; this form is activated by the liver. Another, more potent, form is believed to be 1,25-dihydroxy-cholecalciferol. This form is synthesized by the kidney from 25-hydroxy-cholecalciferol and returned to the circulation to activate bone formation.

VITAMIN E (TOTAL TOCOPHEROLS)

There are many methods for determining vitamin E:[1,15,44–47] all are either biological or chemical. The former measures bio-potency of tocopherols without quantitating the tocopherols and takes longer to complete.

The standard biological method is the rat antisterility assay in which female rats are depleted of vitamin E and mated with normal males. The material to be tested is administered in divided doses for some days after conception: the standard is given the same way. The rats are autopsied after 20 days of pregnancy and the numbers of living fetuses, dead fetuses, and resorption sites recorded.[46] The chemical methods are not all suitable for determining vitamin E in all types of samples, e.g., in biologic fluids and tissues. Determination of tocopherol in animal tissues can be carried out by means of column[47] or thin-layer chromatography,[48] but these are not suitable for large-scale nutrition studies involving biologic fluids. Another method involves the oxidation of tocopherol to tocopherolquinone, but this is not practical because of the interference of carotene and the rigid controls necessary for precise results. Another oxidimetric color reaction employs the Emmerie-Engel reaction.[49] This is based on the reduction of ferric ions to ferrous ions, which

form a red color with a,a'-dipyridyl. Reading the reaction at 520 mμ in a suitable instrument yields the results. This method has advantages over other techniques: it is rapid, reproducible, and well suited to determine tocopherols in micro amounts.[44] All the tocopherols give maximum color in the short time before measurements are made. The procedure measures total tocopherols in serum, plasma, or tissues.[44] Tocopherols and carotenoids are extracted into xylene and the optical density of the extract is read at 460 mμ to measure carotenoids. This reading is subtracted from that at 520 mμ.[1] The maximum peak of absorption for tocopherols is at 520 mμ and is developed 1.5 minutes after adding reagents.[1] Some workers use direct measurement for vitamin E in blood at 295 mμ, but this is not recommended:[1] the low extinction value of tocopherol and interfering substances make it impractical. Serum or plasma may be stored frozen for 1 month without loss of tocopherol activity. When measuring vitamin E in tissue, it is important to know how results are affected by interfering substances, e.g., steroids in liver tissue.[1] Extraction by column chromatography and determination of vitamin E by gas-liquid chromatography aid in standardizing the technique when tissue vitamin E analysis is undertaken.

A procedure to determine 1 to 20 μg of α-tocopherol, extracted from 0.5 to 1.5 gm of animal tissue, by means of chromatographic techniques and the Emmerie-Engel reaction has been described.[1] This is an accurate and reproducible method for the determination of tocopherol in macro- and microquantities of plasma.[1,50] Many workers have found it useful in population and experimental studies of plasma tocopherol.[1,51,52]

In rats with experimentally induced vitamin E deficiency the erythrocytes are abnormally susceptible to hemolysis by H_2O_2.[53] In man[54] it has been shown that, in a variety of clinical conditions, the degree of hemolysis by this test is inversely related to the serum tocopherol concentration. Normal adults usually have serum tocopherol levels greater than 0.5 mg per 100 ml and it has been shown that, at and above this level, relatively little hemolysis ($<$ 20 per cent) occurs.[55,56]

VITAMIN K

There are several methods for vitamin K determination in pharmaceutical preparations and extracts from biological materials. The Irreverre-Sullivan reaction is particularly useful for testing the fractions from column chromatography.[57,58] The K vitamin may be differentiated from other quinones by spectrography or by a color test;[58] biological methods use chicks which are better suited for animal assays than laboratory mammals.

Vitamin K is required to maintain normal plasma levels of the protein prothrombin (factor II) and of the three other clotting factors: VII, IX and X.[59] Thus the prominent sign of vitamin K deficiency is an increase in the time required for the blood to clot. The clinical manifestation is hemorrhage.

In general, prothrombin is measured by its ability to form thrombin which reacts with fibrinogen to form a clot. Actually, in most cases, prothrombin activity, not its concentration, is measured. An excellent discussion of the various methods used has been detailed.[59,60] For clinical purposes, the plasma prothrombin time of Quick, with various modifications, has been used widely.[60] This test is carried out by drawing fresh blood and placing it in a tube containing a measured amount of thromboplastin. A clot normally should form in 25 to 40 seconds. In general, if the prothrombin clotting time is not greater than 20 to 25 per cent above normal, bleeding does not occur on the basis of prothrombin deficiency.

In view of the number of variable factors other than prothrombin content that influence the prothrombin time, plus the variety of methods used in determining it,[60] it is not surprising that it is difficult to define a prothrombin concentration below which hemorrhage will occur. Many believe that a prothrombin concentration between 5 to 10 per cent of normal is a safe range.

THIAMINE

The many methods proposed for the analysis of thiamine can be classified into animal, microbiological, chemical, or physical: each has certain advantages and disadvantages.[1]

Chemical, microbiological, and erythrocyte transketolase methods are the most frequently used for measuring thiamine in biologic fluids and tissues.

The chemical assay for thiamine depends upon the alkaline oxidation of thiamine by ferricyanide into thiochrome, which exhibits an intense blue fluorescence in ultraviolet light and can, therefore, be measured fluorometrically: the details of this reaction have been reviewed.[61] As with all fluorometric determinations, selection of appropriate purification procedures and blanks is most important. A purification method using synthetic zeolite Decalso has been modified for nutrition surveys.[62]

The assay of blood for thiamine by the thiochrome method presents problems,[63,64] since hematin catalyzes the destruction of thiochrome in alkaline solutions.[65] This seems to have been circumvented by removal of the hematin by precipitation with trichloroacetic acid. The retention of thiamine in proteins precipitated with trichloroacetic acid and incomplete hemolysis of red cells may limit the usefulness of this procedure:[66,67] also, the supernatants from trichloroacetic acid precipitates show a marked increase in fluorescence upon storage, which necessitates their analysis for thiamine immediately after preparation.[68] A macro[69] and micro[70] procedure for thiamine in blood, employing the thiochrome method, has been reported and reviewed in detail.[65] Urine contains free thiamine so that it can be diluted and assayed directly by the thiochrome method, without prior treatment. A method for tissue thiamine has been described which permits the differentiation between thiamine and thiamine disulfide content by the thiochrome procedure.[71]

The main drawback of the thiochrome procedure is interference by fluorescing of non-thiamine substances: this is seen especially with urine. Its adequacy in detecting thiamine deficiency has been questioned by nutritional survey teams.[72] The measurement of red blood cell transketolase activity has been proposed for thiamine assay.[73,74] Transketolase is a thiamine-dependent enzyme. It catalyzes transfer of a 2-carbon fragment from a ketose to the aldehydic carbon of the aldose. The method involves incubation of hemolyzed washed red blood cells in a buffered medium with an excess of ribose-5-phosphate, both in the presence and absence of excess thiamine pyrophosphate. Disappearance of ribose-5-phosphate[73] by condensation with a 2-carbon intermediate to yield sedoheptulose-7-phosphate[74] is the indicator of thiamine activity.

Microorganisms which require thiamine fall into five categories. They may require (a) intact thiamine, (b) the pyrimidine moiety, (c) the thiazole moiety, (d) either the pyrimidine or the thiazole moiety, and (e) both moieties. Man and other animals utilize only intact thiamine. Hence, the assay organism must respond only to the intact vitamin for use in assessing thiamine status. Compared with chemical methods, microbiologic assay methods for thiamine are more sensitive, more specific, require less equipment and material for assay—important considerations when many biologic samples are to be analyzed.

Microbiological methods based on lactobacilli and yeast[65,75,76] suffer from poor reproducibility, partly because non-chemically defined media are used; also, lactobacilli are often stimulated nonspecifically by substances in biologic materials,[77,78] since these stimulants are inadequately supplied in published basal media. The phytoflagellate *Ochromonas danica* requires intact thiamine.[1] It does not respond to the thiazole or pyrimidine moieties as do the yeasts,[79,80] nor can it combine the thiazole and pyrimidine moieties.[80] It is a photosynthetic micro-animal with a mammalian-like requirement for not only thiamine but also biotin.[1] It can assay 100 pg/ml of thiamine in biologic fluids and tissues. It also uses aseptically added thiamine pyrophosphate (cocarboxylase). Its metazoan-like permeability, as inferred from its sensitivity to a wide variety of antimetabolites, coupled with counteraction of these growth inhibitors by appropriate metabolites, makes it also a versatile instrument for mode-of-toxicity drug studies.[81,82] The medium supports heavy, rapid growth and is not appreciably stimulated by natural fluids such as blood. The method, based on *O. danica*

has been successful for assaying biologic fluids and tissues: others have confirmed it.[83]

Lactate and pyruvate blood levels are of little value, especially in mild thiamine deficiency and severe liver disease.[84,85] Transketolase values are of little diagnostic usefulness during severe liver disease: levels are low and never recover, even after thiamine treatment.[85,86] This prompted reports that a transketolase apoenzyme deficiency exists in severe liver disease.[85,86] Transketolase level is useful only in frank, long-standing thiamine deficiency,[84] when transketolase levels are invariably low but increase after thiamine treatment.

We have seen thiamine-normal individuals who show no increase in transketolase activity when thiamine pyrophosphate (TPP) is added to the red cell hemolysate.[86,87] In contrast, in thiamine deficiency the introduction of TPP into the hemolysate increased the transketolase activity, indicating a thiamine deficiency. We have also seen some thiamine-deficient individuals who, when treated with thiamine, do not show any increases in their deficient transketolase levels. Only upon the introduction of exogenous TPP into the hemolysate does transketolase activity increase, indicating a phosphorylating defect of administered thiamine *in vivo*. We have observed another group which, when treated with thiamine, still have deficient transketolase activity, despite added *in vitro* TPP. Most of the members of the latter group had liver disease. In some instances the transketolase level returned to normal when positive nitrogen balance was restored. This group thus seemed to have an apotransketolase deficiency; *i.e.*, an inability to form or couple the protein moiety of the enzyme to the coenzyme.[87]

A better approach for determining thiamine status is an assay for the intact vitamin, an assay which is sensitive and specific, and which permits the earliest evaluation of total thiamine status and not of one of the many thiamine-dependent enzymes which depend on sufficient apoenzyme as well as coenzyme. Also, these enzymes may or may not be important in assaying thiamine nutriture (see Introduction for discussion of enzyme assays). Blood thiamine, as measured with *O. danica*, seems to be a more sensitive indicator of thiamine deficiency. This is especially true in severe liver disease.[1,2,88]

A method for measuring tissue saturation with thiamine involves the determination of half-disappearance of intravenously administered thiamine. The faster the thiamine disappearance, the more depleted are the tissue stores.[88]

Thiamine excretion tests have been carried out either in the fasting state or for varying periods of time following oral or parenteral administration of this vitamin: microbial methods,[1–3,65,88] automated thiochrome methods[89] and ^{35}S thiamine HCl[90] have been used. With the thiochrome method there is present in urine an interfering fluorescent substance called F_2.[91] This material has been identified as N-methyl-nicotinamide.[92] There is now reason to believe that there are other extraneous substances in urine that also contribute to this fluorescence.[86] One of the most troublesome problems in the determination of urinary thiamine has been how to obtain a satisfactory blank.

A colorimetric method[93] uses p-amino-acetophenone, which couples with thiamine to produce an insoluble purple-red compound. Such substances as uric acid and ascorbic acid interfere with the development of the color. The removal of these interfering substances is difficult. The method also is not sensitive for material with a low content of thiamine.

The load test method has also been used, but there is considerable disagreement as to what level of excretion indicates a deficiency state. A variety of forms of thiamine are present in urine. For example, it may be present as thiamine, thiochrome, cocarboxylase and as various degradation products, such as thiazole and pyrimidine moieties.[94] A method for determining the metabolites of thiamine in urine has been designed.[95] This method is based on the fact that bakers' yeast can synthesize thiamine from equal molar concentrations of pyrimidine and thiazole.

In our experience[1,96] and those of others,[97] it was found that an oral dose of thiamine made little change in the amount of thiamine in blood, whereas there was the expected increase in urinary excretion. When compar-

ing oral absorption of thiamine[1,3] we have consistently found that thiamine propyl disulfide is better absorbed than thiamine hydrochloride. Circulatory and urinary thiamine levels are increased approximately tenfold with thiamine propyl disulfide. In contrast, thiamine hydrochloride will produce only slight increases in circulating levels and approximately threefold increase in urinary levels.

The amount of cocarboxylase in whole blood varies directly with the amount of total thiamine, as determined by biologic methods, and also with the degree of tissue saturation.[98] The decarboxylation of pyruvic acid requires the coenzyme cocarboxylase (thiamine pyrophosphate), and a deficiency of thiamine results in an elevation of blood pyruvic acid. The elevation of blood pyruvic levels, however, is not a specific indicator of thiamine lack, since other pathologic conditions are associated with an increase in the amount of this substance in blood. Except in severe thiamine deficiencies, the determination of fasting pyruvic levels in blood is not a reliable indicator of thiamine deficiency.[99]

Since both lactic and pyruvic acid are normally formed during carbohydrate metabolism, it was thought that the determination of the level and ratio of pyruvic and lactic acid in blood might be a reliable aid in evaluating thiamine nutrition. A test based on the fact that the rate of breakdown of pyruvic acid is directly related to the metabolic load of glucose and lactic acid was proposed.[100] Accordingly, the simultaneous determination of these three constituents under proper conditions was used to provide information regarding thiamine nutrition. The validity of such a test depends on pyruvate and lactate levels; these are not reliable in the case of thiamine evaluations.[84,99]

In conclusion, our experience shows that the protozoan method utilizing *Ochromonas danica* is best suited for determining metabolically active thiamine in man and animals.[1]

Urinary load tests are of little value in grading the severity of a deficiency, not only of thiamine, but of most vitamins. There has been considerable variation reported in the results from individuals supposedly under similar conditions.[99] These divergencies may be explained in part by: (a) differences in absorption from gastrointestinal tract, (b) various renal threshold levels, (c) differences in the rate and volume of urine excreted, (d) inadequate emptying of the bladder, (e) varying amounts of the test dose administered, and (f) different degrees of tissue breakdown as the result of the deficiency state. All these factors must be considered when urinary excretion studies are used to evaluate the nutrient state. Since we know so little about the renal threshold and metabolism of these nutrients, estimations upon urine, with or without test doses, are not valuable for assessing nutriture.[101]

BIOTIN

There are no chemical methods for biotin assay[102] but a variety of biotin-requiring microorganisms are available: *Saccharomyces cerevisiae*,[103] *Lactobacillus casei*,[104] *Lactobacillus arabinosus* (now *L. plantarum* ATCC #8014),[105] *Micrococcus sodonensis*,[106] *Neurospora crassa*,[107] and *Rhizobium trifolii*.[108] None has been applied satisfactorily for assaying biotin in biologic fluids. *Lactobacillus casei* is not specific because it requires certain unidentified factors which affect the validity of biotin assays, particularly if the sample is low in biotin and relatively potent in unknown factors. *S. cerevisiae*, since biotin is strongly but variably spared by aspartic acid, oleic acid, and pimelic acid, is thus not specific in its biotin requirement[109] despite its development as an ultra micro assay for biotin.[110] Because the flagellate *Ochromonas danica* has a specific and sensitive biotin requirement[111] like man and animals, it has been utilized as a reagent for biotin in blood, serum, urine, brain, and liver tissue:[1] it has also been used in nutrition surveys for biotin.[1,2,52,84] The other method widely used utilizes *Lactobacillus plantarum*:[105] unlike *O. danica* it has its drawback as to specificity.

Pimelic acid, aspartic acid, Tween 80, alone or in combination, do not stimulate growth of *O. danica*:[111] these compounds spare biotin as an essential medium for some yeasts and lactobacilli.[112] Desthiobiotin, the sulfur-free analog of biotin, competitively inhibits the growth of *O. danica*.[111] Because *O. danica* is phagotrophic, it presumably ingests and digests low-molecular forms of biotin, e.g., biocytin: other organisms cannot use biocytin.[113]

RIBOFLAVIN

As with most vitamins, the first assays developed for riboflavin depended on the biological response of animals.[114]

Until recently none of the laboratory procedures available has been entirely satisfactory for measuring riboflavin in biologic fluids and tissues.[115] Microbial and chemical methods have been used for riboflavin assay.[65,116] But, because of interfering substances and technical difficulties, these techniques have not been used widely for biological fluids and tissues. Such difficulties have restricted riboflavin estimation to urinary excretion, in terms of μg per gm of creatinine, with inconsistent results.

The fluorometric method has been widely applied.[117] It has been used to measure free riboflavin, riboflavin 5-phosphate (FMN) and flavin adenine dinucleotide (FAD) in natural products as well as biologic fluids.[65,118] The most widely used assays are microbial and the most specific of these uses *Tetrahymena pyriformis*, a protozoan ciliate, for assaying riboflavin in biologic fluids and tissues. This method gives excellent correlation with the more cumbersome fluorometric assays.[1,119] *Tetrahymena pyriformis* responds equally on a molar basis to riboflavin, FMN and FAD. The growth curve for riboflavin is superimposable on those for FMN and FAD when molarities are taken into account. Therefore *T. pyriformis* permits estimation of total riboflavin.

The riboflavin requirement for *T. pyriformis* is specific, sensitive, rapid, and reproducible enough for assay of large numbers of biologic fluids and tissues.[1,52,84] Traces of fatty acids result in too high riboflavin values when *other* assay organisms[116,120,121] are used—an obvious drawback when dealing with fatty acid and lipid-rich fluids and tissues. In assay of fluids and tissues for riboflavin by the *Lactobacillus casei* method,[120] growth stimulation and drift in blood and tissues were noted.[119] Tween 80 (polyoxyethylene sorbitan monooleate) lessened but did not eliminate drift. Presumably, traces of other fatty acids and other compounds in the fluids and tissues were stimulating *L. casei*, thus yielding falsely high riboflavin values. Obviously, removal of traces of fats from 1-ml aliquots of biologic fluids would entail great losses of sample material and time, especially if many samples were to be assayed. The *Lactobacillus* medium gave high blanks.[119]

Since *T. pyriformis* in riboflavin-limited media is not stimulated by fats in blood and tissues or by ingredients in the medium, use of *T. pyriformis* obviates the drawbacks listed for lactobacilli.[1,78] The *T. pyriformis* method[119] has proved readily adaptable to routine or large-scale assays,[1,2,52,106] not only because it is sensitive and specific for riboflavin, but also because it is simple, inexpensive and requires few precautions.

The fluorometric procedure is too slow and poorly suited for large-scale studies because of the involved preliminary procedures before determinations can be made.[118] Special precautions must be taken: tissues have to be finely ground at 0 to 4° C, centrifugation must be at 4° C and, until neutralized, the samples must be kept as cold as possible to prevent hydrolysis of flavin adenine dinucleotide. Other sample aliquots must then be kept at room temperature in the dark for 2 days to complete hydrolysis of FAD to FMN: then, after incubation and neutralization, care must be taken to protect the samples from light, since both riboflavin and FMN are more sensitive to destruction by light in the concentrated salt solution needed for the final fluorometric determination. Caution must be taken to dilute the samples properly to prevent interferences from other substances present. The calculations are laborious. Considering the lengthy preliminary procedures and the extra precaution necessary for fluorometric analysis, with only a slight gain in sensitivity, e.g., 0.1 ng per ml with the fluorometric analysis versus 0.5 ng per ml with the *T. pyriformis* assay (values practically meaningless in analysis of biologic fluids and tissues), the *T. pyriformis* method has fewer pitfalls and permits more assays per unit effort.

In a preliminary survey of riboflavin disappearance in 32 randomly selected subjects, after intravenous administration of 5 mg flavin mononucleotide, the half-time clearance for riboflavin in 27 subjects with riboflavin levels above 100 ng/ml was slower than in 5 subjects with levels below 80 ng/ml.[119] Clearance of intravenously administered riboflavin may be useful as a rapid measure of tissue avidity for riboflavin: the more depleted the riboflavin tissue pool, the quicker the clearance of administered riboflavin from the circulation.

Different methods have been developed for the determination of riboflavin in urine based on either the use of microbiologic[1,120] or fluorometric procedures.[118] The latter methods involve measuring the fluorescence produced by the flavin in urine when subjected to light of prescribed wavelengths. The quantity of riboflavin in urine can also be assayed by measuring the rate of acid produced by *Lactobacillus casei*. The high levels of urea cause lowering of the titrimetric microbiologic results with *L. casei*.[99]

Extensive investigations have been carried out in the hopes of correlating urinary riboflavin excretion with nutritional status. Some of the various methods employed have determined the amount of urinary riboflavin excreted in, for example, 1 hour while fasting, during 24 hours and after the administration of load tests.[99] There is no consistent agreement among workers in the interpretation of their results.[122] It has been demonstrated that not only is the excretion of riboflavin affected by the dietary intake, but that excretion is proportional to the volume of urine excreted and inversely related to the level of protein intake.[123]

The value of load tests in appraising riboflavin nutrition has not been settled. It is unlikely that urinary excretion is an accurate estimation of riboflavin nutriture, since changes in tissue saturation are expected with different levels of intake.[124]

There is a wide variation for serum riboflavin values. The total riboflavin content of red blood cells[125] or whole blood[119] is considered to be a reasonable, sensitive and practical index of riboflavin nutritional status.

An enzymatic approach utilizing NADPH$_2$-

dependent glutathione reductase from red cells has been proposed for measurement of riboflavin status in man.[125a,b] The enzyme has FAD as a cofactor and is sensitive to riboflavin nutritional status (see Introduction for critique on enzyme assays), however, the specificity in combined deficiencies (e.g. B_6) has been questioned.[125c] There seems to be no abnormal metabolite in the urine of ribo-flavin-deficient subjects which could serve as a marker for a riboflavin-deficient state.

NIACIN (NICOTINIC ACID)

Recognition that many bacteria require niacin for growth has resulted in the develop-ment of microbial assay methods for niacin and closely related niacin-active compounds. Many methods are not specific,[117] causing drifts in organism growth, due to an incom-plete medium or stimulatory substances in the unknown sample. The use of *Tetra-hymena pyriformis* has obviated these objec-tions. The protozoan is sensitive and specific for niacin and niacinamide.[1,126] Microbial assay methods are particularly well adapted to the simultaneous assay of many samples. The microbial method used by many investi-gators employs *Lactobacillus plantarum* ATCC #8014.[126,127] *L. plantarum* responds to niacin, niacinamide and nicotinuric acid:[117] nico-tinuric acid is not biologically active. Hence *T. pyriformis* has a higher degree of specificity.

There are several chemical methods for niacin determination.[128,129] Most are based on the use of organic reagents which yield colored niacin derivatives that can be quan-titated photometrically: most are plagued by extraction difficulties as well as by a lack of specificity for niacin. The two principal metabolites of niacin and niacinamide ex-creted in urine of man are N^1-methylnico-tinamide (MN) and the 6-pyridone of MN. MN reacts with ketones in alkaline solutions to produce a green fluorescent compound. An excess of acid converts this compound to another more stable substance with a blue fluorescence that may be measured with a fluorophotometer. The pyridone does not interfere with MN determinations. The original method[130] and modifications[127] have been used. This method measures non-

metabolic catabolites of niacin. Most niacin in blood and tissues is found as NAD, NADH_2, NADP, and NADPH_2. Chemical methods used for niacin determinations in blood[131] and tissues[132] depend on the highly fluorescent products formed with both pyri-dine nucleotides after proper extraction.

An enzymatic-fluorometric method for the determination of pyridine nucleotides in tissue has been developed which is based on the observation that a neutralized alkaline extract of tissues contains NADH_2 and NADPH_2 plus smaller amounts of NAD and NADP which arise from auto-oxidation. The auto-oxidation was compensated by adding simul-taneously alcohol dehydrogenase and acetal-dehyde, to completely oxidize the NADH_2 to NAD and glucose-6-phosphate, and glucose-6-phosphate dehydrogenase to reduce all of the NADP to NADPH_2. The NAD and NADPH_2 are measured fluorometrically.[133,134] This method has been extremely useful for study-ing alcoholism:[135] the NAD:NADH ratio permits an indirect measure of alcohol de-hydrogenase activity as well as a measure of alcohol oxidation *in vivo*.[135]

The number of products of niacin metab-olism that appear in the urine are many and they vary from species to species. The end products of niacin metabolism in man are MN and its pyridone. In addition to these and other derivatives, a number of inter-mediates on the tryptophan-niacin pathway are excreted: therefore, MN excretion is par-ticularly susceptible to the influences of non-nutritional factors. Since both MN and the pryidone depend on methylation for their formation, a lower excretion might be ex-pected no matter what the niacin intake is, if insufficient methyl groups are available.[136] Workers disagree on what percentage of niacin is excreted as MN.[99] They also have diverging views regarding the significance of 24-hour urinary excretion studies. One group contends that the determination of MN for a 24-hour period is of little help in evalu-ating niacin nutrition. Another group feels that there is reasonably good correlation be-tween the excretion of this compound and dietary and clinical findings.[99] The different findings in different studies undoubtedly are due in part to the variety of methods used, as well as to inter- and intra-individual variations. Differences among persons in methylating ability may also partly account for variance. At present, the excretion levels of MN in the urine during fasting and after administration of load test doses of niacin are the only chemical procedures available for appraising niacin nutrition.

There is an acute need for more accurate methods for estimating body niacin. Assay with *T. pyriformis* can fill this void. Use of *T. pyriformis* permits a wider assay range and more comprehensive responses than does the the use of *Lactobacillus plantarum*. In our hands the range of *L. plantarum* was 3 to 30 ng/ml, as compared with 1 to 300 ng/ml for *T. pyriformis*. Some naturally occurring niacin derivatives were tested with *T. pyriformis*:[126] only niacin and niacinamide permitted full growth. Nicotinmethylamide and ethylamide showed some activity, but compounds having other modifications of the carboxyl groups did not elicit growth. Trigonelline (the betaine of nicotinic acid), which has no animal activity, proved inert for *T. pyriformis*. The organism's requirement seems to parallel that of higher animals. MN and its 6-keto derivatives, some of the principal excretion products in man, are not active for *T. pyriformis*.

The cellular components of whole blood contribute the greatest niacin activity. Such results are to be expected since red blood cells contain much NAD and NADP activity.[137-139] The chief excretory products of nicotinic acid in human urine include nicotinuric acid (nicotinoylglycine) and N^1-methylnicotinamide (MN). *Tetrahymena pyriformis* does not respond to either compound, whereas *L. plantarum* does,[140] another point of specificity favoring *T. pyriformis*, if one assumes that clinical status is reflected by niacin activity rather than by niacin plus its catabolic derivatives. Highly pigmented urines do not interfere with this assay as they do for the MN determination.[130]

The biosynthesis and metabolism of nicotinic acid in disease have received little attention; metabolic studies deal mainly with normal animals and man.[1,226,227] After a tryptophan load dose, the main catabolites in the urine are nicotinuric acid, MN, nicotina-mide, quinolinic acid, kynurenine, 6-pyridone, anthranilic acid, and 3-hydroxyanthranilic acid.

VITAMIN B_6

Vitamin B_6 can be determined microbiologically, enzymatically or chemically.[15,141,142] Some chemical analyses are done by measuring the fluorescence of the cyanohydrin of pyridoxal.[143] Chromatographic methods have also been used.[15,144] Microbiological determinations can be carried out with *Escherichia coli* mutants, *Saccharomyces carlsbergensis* 4228, *Streptococcus faecalis*, and *Lactobacillus casei*.[142,145] No assay has been used successfully for the detection of vitamin B_6 in biological fluids nor has any been correlated with the clinical signs of B_6 deficiency. Indirect methods for determining B_6 status in biological fluids include the transaminase method, the xanthurenic acid-kynurenine method, and a method utilizing circulating leukocytes. The transaminase system is based on the dependence on pyridoxal-5-phosphate of the alanine (SGPT) and aspartic (SGOT) transaminases in the serum. B_6 deficiency results in decreased plasma alanine and aspartic transaminases: the alanine enzyme appears to be more sensitive.[146] Two other enzymatic methods have been developed for the estimation of pyridoxal phosphate in biologic materials. One is based on tyrosine decarboxylase and the liberation of CO_2.[147] The other depends on the tryptophanase-catalyzed breakdown of tryptophan to indole, pyruvic acid, and ammonia.[148]

It seems probable that, using the enzyme methods, only free pyridoxal phosphate or that loosely bound to protein is measured. Thus, any pyridoxal phosphate bound with holoenzymes would not be measured.[99] A disturbance of B_6 metabolism, through derangement of tryptophan metabolism, gives rise to excretion of excess xanthurenic acid in the urine and some workers have used xanthurenic excretion as an index of B_6 status in man. There is disagreement about the validity and specificity of the xanthurenic acid titer as an index of B_6 deficiency:[149] e.g., high xanthurenic acid levels in human urine have been found, unrelated to pathologic or clinical changes due to B_6 deficiency:[150] riboflavin deficiency also produces high urine levels of tryptophan catabolites:[9a] nongravid women[151] and women in the last trimester of pregnancy[152] have been reported to excrete tryptophan catabolites equivalent to 2 to 3 times the tryptophan intake even though the absorption of vitamin B_6 was normal. Marked increases in xanthurenic acid excretion occur in toxemias of pregnancy[153] although xanthurenic acid itself is not toxic.[149] Elderly subjects were found to excrete about twice as much xanthurenic acid as young subjects in a 24-hour period after tryptophan loading, a defect abolished by vitamin B_6 therapy.[154] The tryptophan load test is not a real test of absolute B_6 deficiency. An intake of 10 gm DL-tryptophan upsets the amino acid balance and causes a severe stress that does not exist under normal conditions.[155]

The leukocyte method estimates pyridoxal phosphate in isolated leukocytes: it is based on a coenzyme-catalyzed tyrosine decarboxylase system from S. faecalis.[156] A comparison of pyridoxal phosphate content of circulating leukocytes in nonpregnant women, women at term, and umbilical cord blood showed higher values in nonpregnant controls: cord blood showed the highest values.[157] Enough data are not yet on hand to evaluate this method.

4-Pyridoxic acid has frequently been used as an indicator of B_6 status.[142,160] It is the principal excretion product from B_6 ingestion in man.[149,158] However, it has been reported that, in subjects on a normal diet, pyridoxic acid excretion accounted for only about half the intake of vitamin B_6.[159] This method is, therefore, not a totally reliable indicator of B_6 status.

The increased urinary excretion of oxalate in B_6-deficient rats and man[161] suggests the possible use of urinary oxalate as a criterion of B_6 adequacy.

Tetrahymena pyriformis has been used to assay for vitamin B_6.[1,162] Its vitamin requirements cannot be bypassed; e.g., its vitamin B_6 requirement cannot be satisfied or even spared by amino acids, including D-alanine, effective for such bacteria as Streptococcus faecalis and Lactobacillus casei.[142,163] Response to D-alanine also makes Saccharomyces carlsbergensis unreliable for assaying B_6 in

blood.[163] Because T. pyriformis has a lesser response to pyridoxol (pyridoxine), it has been criticized as being less valuable for assaying B_6 in plants where pyridoxal predominates. This does not detract from its use for assaying B_6 in biological fluids and tissues where pyridoxal and pyridoxamine predominate.

Measurement of vitamin B_6 activity using enzyme systems involves knowledge of two variables: (a) concentration of coenzyme pyridoxal phosphate, and (b) concentration of apoenzyme. Normal enzyme activity would indicate adequate concentration of both components, but decreased activity could mean a decrease in either or both. Since T. pyriformis has a mammalian-like requirement for vitamin B_6, it permits a direct measure of all metabolically active vitamin B_6 in man, rather than merely a determination of the function of individual enzymes which may not give a true reflection of the vitamin B_6 status.

With Tetrahymena pyriformis the B_6 distribution in blood was studied.[162] In 15 normal subjects, the plasma to red cell ratio ranged between 1.5 and 4.6 The mean B_6 for whole blood is 37 ± 6, for red cells 20 ± 3, and plasma 59 ± 13 ng per ml. Tetrahymena pyriformis, like man and animals, does not utilize B_6 in the presence of B_6 antagonists;[162] it is inhibited by D-, L-, and DL-penicillamine and isonicotinic acid hydrazide: penicillamine is the more potent B_6 antagonist.

PANTOTHENIC ACID

Chemical and animal methods for pantothenate assay are unsuited for biologic materials.[164,165] Saccharomyces carlsbergensis, Lactobacillus plantarum,[1,166] Lactobacillus casei, Acetobacter suboxydans,[15] and Tetrahymena pyriformis[1,166] have been used. S. carlsbergensis lacks specificity: this yeast produces its own pantothenate.[165] L. casei was replaced by L. plantarum because L. casei needs a complex medium for growth and is stimulated by fatty material in biologic materials, when assaying for pantothenate.[166] Pantothenyl alcohol is inactive for A. suboxydans but pantoic acid is very active,[15] so that the alcohol must be hydrolyzed to pantoic acid before using this assay. *T. pyriformis* is used[166] when non-specific contamination from natural products becomes a drawback.[13] Pantothenol and pantoyl lactose (with or without the addition of D-alanine) and coenzyme A are inactive for *Tetrahymena*[167] and *L. plantarum*; neither of which is stimulated by fats.[1]

There is no free pantothenate in blood. It is all bound. The vitamin can be released by an alkaline phosphatase and an enzyme from avian liver.[165] This liberates pantothenate from coenzyme A in a variety of foods and tissues. Treatment with Diastase gives more reliable results as compared with autolysis, acid hydrolysis, treatment with Mylase P, or combination of Diastase and papain or liver enzyme and alkaline phosphatase.[166] Diastase is free from pantothenate contamination. The other enzymes contain enough pantothenate to make results unreliable. In urine, the vitamin is unbound: results show no increase with enzyme hydrolysis. Pantothenic acid shows the same concentration in blood and cerebrospinal fluid.[1]

L. plantarum and *T. pyriformis* are reliable reagents for pantothenate in tissues and biologic fluids.[165,166,168] Results with both organisms are similar.[1,166]

VITAMIN C (ASCORBIC ACID)

Vitamin C is the only water-soluble vitamin for which there is no microbial assay. Biological assays generally have been replaced by chemical methods. Biological tests are only used now to ensure that it is ascorbic acid that is being measured.

Methods for determining ascorbic acid are many.[169,170] The methods of choice for determination of ascorbic acid status in humans involve plasma or serum ascorbic acid concentration[1] and white blood cell-blood platelet ascorbate concentration, which is more closely related to tissue stores.[1] Two types of procedures are used. One is based upon the oxidation of ascorbic acid by 2,6-dichlorophenolindophenol and the other is based upon the color formed by treating with 85 per cent H_2SO_4 the derivative produced by coupling oxidized ascorbic acid with 2,4-dinitrophenylhydrazine.[170] Titra-

tion and colorimetric techniques using 2,6-dichlorophenolindophenol suffer from interference from pigments and extraneous reducing substances in biologic fluids.[99] A modified method, using a combination of the two procedures,[171,172] has been devised and has served well in large-scale nutrition surveys and clinical situations.[2,52]

Samples for total ascorbate assay are best stored frozen, after precipitation of protein and separation of the acid extract containing the ascorbate. Ascorbate remains stable for 2 months when treated in this way. Samples not so treated should be processed within 2 weeks of freezer storage. Some solutions used in the procedure are labile and are best made fresh if the test is done infrequently.

Polarography and spectrophotometry have been used to measure ascorbate. Polarography offers no advantages over the chemical methods. Spectrophotometric methods are not adequate because of the weak absorption of ascorbate and prevalence of interfering substances.[169] Enzymatic and chromatographic assays have been used,[169] however, they have limited use in biologic materials. The most satisfactory chemical assays are based on reduction of 2,6-dichlorophenolindophenol or the formation of a colored dinitrophenylhydrazine derivative.[170] Dichlorophenolindophenol is blue in neutral and pink in acid solutions. In acid extracts ascorbic acid reduces dichlorophenolindophenol, at pH 1 to 4, to the colorless leuco form. Thiosulfate, ferrous, cuprous, stannous salts, and heated sugar solutions (reductones) interfere with this method because they also reduce indophenol.

The dinitrophenylhydrazine methods are very sensitive and specific for ascorbate.[170] The reaction depends upon the coupling of 2,4-dinitrophenylhydrazine to the keto groups of carbon 2 and 3 of diketogulonic acid to form a *bis*-2,4-dinitrophenylhydrazone—an osazone. In strong acid the osazone rearranges to a stable reddish-brown product which can be measured photometrically. Ascorbic acid must first be oxidized to dehydroascorbate for this reaction to occur. In the modified method,[1] 2,6-dichlorophenolindophenol is used as the *oxidizer*. We found dichlorophenolindophenol to be superior to

Norit or copper:[1] copper ions caused precipitate to form in the extracts. The use of dichlorophenolindophenol simplifies the method, especially for large-scale studies. The strong acid medium permits the dehydroascorbate to be hydrolyzed to diketogulonic acid so that hydrazone formation can take place.[173] Other reductones react slowly with dinitrophenylhydrazine and their osazones are unstable in high acid concentrations. Addition of thiourea as a reducer adds specificity by avoiding interference from non-ascorbate chromogens.[1]

A 3-hour incubation of the acidic extracts at 37° C works well. Five per cent metaphosphoric acid has been used to extract ascorbic acid, precipitate protein, inactivate the enzymes which oxidize ascorbate acid, and produce the required acidic milieu for the analysis.[170] We have found 5 per cent trichloroacetic acid (TCA) equally effective.[1] Once ascorbate is extracted with TCA, it can be stored frozen before assay. We have obtained excellent recoveries of ascorbate (96 to 102 per cent) and no gross errors due to the formation of chromogenic materials with sugars or glucuronic acid.

In adults, plasma ascorbate levels of 0.4 to 1.4 mg per cent reflect a daily ascorbate intake of 70 mg or more; less than 0.2 mg per cent indicate less than a 25-mg daily intake of ascorbate. In children, a plasma concentration of approximately 1.0 mg per cent indicates an ascorbate intake of about 1.5 mg per kg body weight, whereas ascorbate intake of 0.2 mg per kg will give serum ascorbate levels of 0 to 0.1 mg per cent.

When tissues are saturated with vitamin C, the plasma ascorbate levels lie between 0.8 to 1.5 mg per cent: the whole blood levels are between 1.0 to 1.5 mg per cent, and the buffy coat ascorbate levels are between 25 to 35 mg per cent.

A wide variety of load test methods for the analysis of ascorbic acid nutrition has been proposed. In general, individuals with low intakes of ascorbic acid excrete less of a given dose than do those on an adequate or saturating intake. The load test provides a fairly good index of tissue depletion and parallels moderately well the fasting plasma levels. However, the load test does not distinguish between varying degrees of deficiency states. The sensitivity of load tests may be increased if larger doses are administered.[99]

The known products of ascorbic acid catabolism do not offer great possibilities for assessment of ascorbic acid status, partly because ascorbic acid is basically a carbohydrate and many of its known metabolic products can arise from other sources. The products of ingested ascorbate excreted in urine are primarily oxalate, 2,3-diketogulonic acid, ascorbic acid and dehydroascorbic acid.[174] On an individual basis, all patients with scurvy will have serum ascorbate levels of zero, but not all persons with zero ascorbic acid levels will have scurvy.[1] Increased amounts of ascorbate are excreted in urine with increasing intake.[228]

Complete elimination of vitamin C from the diet, as seen by us in 5 patients on a complete restriction of food and vitamins, resulted in a serum ascorbate of zero within 35 to 40 days; the whole blood levels reached zero in about 80 to 90 days, and the white cell levels reached zero in 100 to 120 days. When the white cell level reached zero, clinical scurvy became manifest. White cell ascorbate seems best to reflect tissue stores, while plasma levels reflect intake within the preceding weeks.[1]

VITAMIN B_{12}

Most studies agree that protozoan methods are the most sensitive and specific way to measure metabolically and clinically active forms of B_{12} in biologic fluids and tissues or in B_{12}-containing products.[1,2,12] These methods employ the protozoans *Euglena gracilis* or *Ochromonas malhamensis*.[1] Such methods can be used to follow B_{12} metabolism *in vitro* or *in vivo*.[1,2,175]

Assay of vitamin B_{12} by physiochemical means is difficult because B_{12} occurs in exceptionally low concentrations in nature. Such assays are usually carried out on relatively concentrated solutions of the vitamin, *e.g.*, pharmaceutical preparations and B_{12} feed concentrates, and then only when the B_{12} is freed from interfering impurities.[15]

The availability of ^{57}Co, ^{58}Co, ^{60}Co-vitamin B_{12} has permitted the wide application of tracer techniques for detecting B_{12}.[176] They are more expensive and less adaptable to routine use than the microbiological ones with discrepancies between results.[177–179] Since the Schilling test is biological, the factors influencing reproducibility are multiple and not all apparent.[180] Radioactivity techniques require close cooperation between patient and analyst throughout. The Schilling test, for example, requires that the patient fast for 12 hours and drink no water for 4 hours before the test. After the radioactive oral dose, the patient must wait 90 to 120 minutes for the intramuscular dose of non-labeled vitamin B_{12} and the urine must be carefully collected for 24 hours after the load doses.[1] In the B_{12} absorption feces test, the feces must be diligently collected by the patient for 1 to 7 days after a radioactive load dose.[1] In the hepatic-uptake test,[181] the radioactivity after an oral dose is measured with a surface scintillation counter over the liver after the radioactivity has disappeared from the intestine, either spontaneously or after purgation. Indeed, in these tracer tests, the patience of patient and tester is critical.

The measurement of serum vitamin B_{12} level by radioisotope dilution with albumin-coated charcoal has been introduced[182] and has been adapted to intrinsic-factor assay.[183] This method is based on the adsorption of free B_{12} by albumin-coated charcoal. Residual B_{12} is then determined directly by radioactivity counts with the use of labeled B_{12}. Charcoal absorption of B_{12} has been used for the isotopic determination of B_{12}-binding capacity and concentration in biologic fluids.[184] Another method uses zinc sulfate instead of charcoal.[185] Validity of the charcoal assay of bound B_{12} or B_{12}-binding capacity of body fluids is questionable, especially when dealing with gastric materials.[181]

Biochemical tests for B_{12} have been introduced. Some workers have found an increased urinary excretion of aminoimidazolecarboxamide (AIC) in patients with untreated pernicious anemia;[186] however, this test is not specific for B_{12} deficiency, since high AIC is also excreted during folate deficiency[187] and other unrelated stress situations.[188] Proper propionic metabolism depends on the B_{12}-coenzyme for conversion of malonyl CoA to succinyl CoA. In severe B_{12} deficiency propionic acid excretion rises and falls after B_{12} treatment. Folate deficiency does not affect this pattern.[188] Such results indicate that methylmalonyl CoA isomerase is lowered in B_{12} deficiency, hence methylmalonic acid (MMA) excretion should increase during this vitamin deficiency. This reasoning has been substantiated: MMA excretion is indeed high during a B_{12} deficiency.[189] There seems to be no correlation between urinary titer of MMA and degree of hematological or neurological abnormalities. In some patients, MMA excretion continued even after the hematologic abnormalities and serum vitamin B_{12} returned to normal.[190] Other workers have used preloading with saline or valine as a means of increasing MMA excretion during B_{12} deficiency:[191] preloading with propionic acid does not seem suitable.[190] Unfortunately the MMA excretion method is complex and not very accurate.[192]

Lactobacillus lactis was the first microorganism used to identify the then unknown vitamin B_{12} in the refined liver extracts used for treating pernicious anemia.[1] *L. lactis* Dorner (ATCC 8000), *L. leichmannii*, and *Escherichia coli* mutants have also been used to assay for vitamin B_{12}.[193,194] When the lactic acid bacteria are used, deoxyribosides replace B_{12} in the assay and can invalidate results.[12] Methionine will do the same when the *E. coli* mutant or thermophiles are used for B_{12} assay.[12] Bacterial assays thus lack specificity.[1,12]

Although B_{12} can be assayed biologically with mice, rats, chicks, and radio cobalt, the protozoan method of assay is preferred because of its economy, sensitivity—detects 1 pg B_{12}/ml—and relative freedom from stimulation in biologic fluids and tissues. Neither deoxyribosides nor methionine can replace the B_{12} requirement.[1,12] *Euglena gracilis* is not as specific for B_{12} as *O. malhamensis*.[1,12] Serum and blood from normal subjects have a growth-promoting effect on *Euglena* above that seen with *Ochromonas*.[193] The reason for such stimulation is obscure, since no known pseudoforms of B_{12} have yet been found in biologic fluids. That the *O. malhamensis* method is superior for assay of B_{12} in natural materials was made clear by the agreement of *Ochromonas* and chick assays.[1,12] When *Ochromonas*, *Euglena*, *L. leichmannii*, and *E. coli* assays for B_{12} in blood, serum, and urine were compared, *Ochromonas* was the most dependable.[195] Serum or whole blood can be assayed, which simplifies the procedure.[1]

The specific vitamin B_{12} requirement of *O. malhamensis* still remains undisputed: it is exactly like man's and is unlike *Euglena's*.[1,12] B_{12} was the only vitamin to overcome the antagonistic action of various thyroactive compounds on the growth of *O. malhamensis*.[196] These findings suggested that *O. malhamensis*, like animals, could be used as an indicator of thyroactive substances and thyroid antagonists in man.[1] Because of its simplicity and specificity, we routinely use *O. malhamensis* for assaying B_{12}.[1]

FOLATES

Chick assays were probably the first determinations of what is now called folic acid (pteroylglutamic acid, PGA). Like all animal assays they were costly and time-consuming. Chemical methods are not useful for unfractionated biological materials.[1] They are applicable mainly to pharmaceutical preparations, particularly those having folic acid as sole active constituent. Chromatographic methods are valuable for differentiating folates in biologic fluids, when coupled with appropriate microbial assay systems.[197]

Indirect methods for determining folate status have been proposed.[197–199] One depends on estimating the formiminoglutamic acid (FIGLU) arising from histidine catabolism. FIGLU is normally converted into glutamic acid by donating its formimino group to tetrahydrofolate (THF). In severe folate deficiency no acceptor THF is available, hence large amounts of FIGLU are excreted. Urocanic acid, the precursor of FIGLU, is also excreted in folate deficiency. Many methods are available for estimating FIGLU[192,199] and urocanic acid.[192,197,199] Both tests are nonspecific for folate deficiency:[192,199] abnormal urinary excretion of histidine catabolites is found in patients with vitamin B_{12} deficiency as well as in folic-deficient patients.[192,199] Indeed many pregnant women with folate megaloblastic anemias, as proven by treatment, excreted *normal* amounts of FIGLU.[200] Folic acid abolishes the excretion of abnormal histidine catabolites, but so does vitamin B_{12}, methionine or glycine.[192,199,201] Increased excretion of histidine catabolites is, therefore, not a specific index of folate deficiency. Alanine interferes with the FIGLU determination[202] and makes determinations unreliable.

Another indirect test proposed to detect folate deficiency is one which measures excretion of 4(5)-amino-5(4)-imidazolecarboxamide (AIC). AIC, as the ribotide, is formylated *in vivo* to yield formamidoimidazole carboxamide ribotide, an intermediate in purine synthesis. The formyl group is donated by N^{10}-formyl-THF. In folate deficiency, this conversion should be crippled because N^{10}-formyl-THF is lacking: the substrate AIC accumulates.[192] However, AIC is increased in B_{12} as well as folate deficiency.[203,204] This test,[205] like that for FIGLU, does not distinguish between folate and B_{12} deficiency.[192,199]

Recently tritiated folic acid became available, making possible a non-microbiological method for studying folic metabolism. It obviated inhibition of microbial folate assay organisms by folic antagonists. This technique has been used to monitor uptake, metabolism, and excretory products of folic acid.[192,199,206] The ³H-labeled compounds excreted after intravenous ³H-folate were N^{10}-formyl folate, *p*-amino-benzoylglutamate, and PGA. The N^5-methyl-THF that was also excreted was not labeled but was displaced from the liver and did not arise from the administered labeled folic acid.[199,207]

Nearly all microbiologic assays for folate activity have used *Streptococcus faecalis*, *Lactobacillus casei*, and *Pediococcus cerevisiae*.[1,199] Earlier it appeared that these organisms did not lend themselves to detecting folic acid deficiency in man; *e.g.*, in one study using *S. faecalis* there was no detectable activity in the fasting serum of humans:[208] our own studies confirm this.[209] Administration of a loading dose of folic acid with subsequent assay by *S. faecalis* has been used as a workable means of detecting folic acid deficiency, but this technique has drawbacks.[210] Because of the multiplicity of folic acid factors reported in whole blood, the microbiologic assay for folic acid in *whole blood*, not serum, is regarded as valueless.[1] Our results show that almost no administered folic acid is taken up by the red cell *per se*, despite the high plasma folate level.[138,139] We therefore chose serum, not whole blood, for assaying the folate status of man.[1,11] Red blood cells contain a multiplicity of materials which stimulate growth of folate requirers. They also contain many forms of folylpolyglutamates which are not detectable unless properly deglutamylated to free folate.[211] Anticoagulants also affect folic acid activity.[212] Serum apparently is low in these folic bypassing substances, but may be rich in some PGA polyglutamates or N^5-methyltetrahydrofolic acid, which are available to *L. casei* only.[213,214] *Streptococcus faecalis* is inferior to *L. casei* in its utilization of N^5-methyl-THF[1,193,199] and the PGA polyglutamates.[1,11,199] In short, ability to utilize PGA polyglutamates may underlie the superiority of *L. casei* over *S. faecalis*.[1,11,199,215,216]

In 1945 an *L. casei* method for detecting folic acid was described[217] but was virtually unused for biologic fluids until 1959. Our experience with *L. casei* then showed that serum *L. casei* activity correlated with the clinical picture, even though we did not know then to which folate in serum the bacterium was actually responding.[11,212,218] The clinical worth and specificity of this *L. casei* method[11] has been confirmed.[199,218,219,220]

Since this *L. casei* method was introduced, minor modifications have been advocated.[199,219,221–223] They do not materially affect the end result.

The *L. casei* serum folate method has been extremely useful as a tool in studying folate metabolism. Combined with *S. faecalis* and *P. cerevisiae*, these assays yield a picture of total folates, one comprising oxidized and reduced mono- and polyglutamates.[1]

An oral folic acid tolerance test based on *L. casei* has been developed and applied to investigation of intestinal absorption of folates in normal subjects, patients with folate deficiency anemia, and patients with folate malabsorption associated with sprue.[224] The sensitivity of this test eliminates the need for priming doses of folic acid and urinary collections, as needed for other tests,[199] and permits a direct assessment of folate absorption in various clinical conditions.

Detection of folic acid activity in biologic fluids and tissues is of the utmost importance: it pinpoints the cause of the megaloblastic anemias, *e.g.*, it distinguishes between vitamin B_{12} and folate deficiencies. Because morphology of the abnormal red cell does not help diagnose the specific vitamin deficiency, one must rely on assay methods for the differential diagnosis. The *L. casei* method,[1] unlike the FIGLU method, defines specifically the folate status[1,2] in man, and has been useful in studying many aspects of folate metabolism. This method for detecting folate activity in biologic fluids and tissues has proven to be the most reliable for such purposes.[1,2,52,106,199]

BIBLIOGRAPHY

1. Baker and Frank: In *Clinical Vitaminology: Methods and Interpretation*, New York, Interscience Publishers, 1968.
2. ———: World Review Nutrition, *9*, 124, New York, Karger, 1968.
3. Leevy and Baker: Med. Clin. N. Amer., *54*, 467, 1970.
4. Karnofsky and Young: Fed. Proc., *26*, 1139, 1967.
5. Buckle: Proc. Roy. Soc. Med., *60*, 48, 1967.
6. Krehl and Hodges: Amer. J. Clin. Nutrition, *17*, 191, 1965.
7. Avioli: *The Fat Soluble Vitamins*, DeLuca and Suttie (Eds.) Madison, Wisconsin, University Wisconsin Press, p. 159, 1970.
8. Fennelly, Frank, Baker, and Leevy: Amer. J. Clin. Nutrition, *20*, 946, 1967.
9. Banyl: Amer. J. Clin. Nutrition, *23*, 52, 1970.
9a. Dalgleish: In *The Scientific Basis of Medicine Annual Reviews*, London, Athlone Press, p. 127, 1961.
9b. Crandon, Lund, and Dill: New Eng. J. Med., *223*, 353, 1940.
10. Kahn: Med. Clin. N. America, *54*, 631, 1970.
11. Baker, Herbert, Frank, Pasher, Hutner, Wasserman, and Sobotka: Clin. Chem., *5*, 275, 1959.
12. Ford and Hutner: Vitamins & Hormones, *13*, 101, 1955.
13. Hutner, Cury, and Baker: Anal. Chem., *30*, 849, 1958.
14. Pearson: In *The Vitamins*, vol. 7, György, Pearson (Eds.), New York, Academic Press, p. 1, 1967.
15. Strobecker and Henning: In *Vitamin Assay Tested Methods*, Germany, Verlag Chemie, Weinheim/Bergstr., p. 33, 1965.

16. Schwieter and Isler: Vitamins A and Carotene In *The Vitamins*, Vol. I, 2nd ed., Sebrell, Jr., and Harris (Eds.), New York, Academic Press, p. 5, 1967.

17. Roberts and DeLuca: In *The Fat Soluble Vitamins*, DeLuca and Suttie (Eds.), Madison, Wisconsin, University Wisconsin Press, p. 227, 1969.

18. Roels and Makadevan: Vitamin A In *The Vitamins*, Vol. III, 2nd ed. Gyorgy and Pearson (Eds.), New York, Academic Press, p. 139, 1967.

19. Carr and Price: Biochem. J., *20*, 497, 1926.

20. Bolliger: In *Thin-Layer Chromatography*, Stahl, (Ed.), New York, Academic Press, p. 220, 1965.

21. Inhoffer and Pommer: Vitamin A and Carotenes: Determination In *The Vitamins*, Vol. I, Sebrell, Jr., and Harris (Eds.), New York, Academic Press, p. 87, 1954.

22. Sobel and Snow: J. Biol. Chem., *171*, 617, 1947.

23. Bieri and Schultze: Arch. Biochem. Biophys., *34*, 273, 1954.

24. Utley, Brodovsky, and Pearson: J. Nutrition, *66*, 205, 1958.

25. Neeld, Jr. and Pearson: J. Nutrition, *79*, 454, 1963.

26. Kagen: Nutrition Symposium Series, *7*, 31, 1953.

27. Hummel: J. Bio. Chem., *180*, 1225, 1949.

28. Nordmann, Arnaud, and Nordmann: Clin. Chim. Acta, *12*, 304, 1965.

29. Raiha: Pediatrics, *32*, 1025, 1963.

30. Merrow, Krause, Browe, Newhall, and Pierce: J. Nutrition, *46*, 445, 1952.

31. Popper: Physiol. Rev., *24*, 205, 1944.

32. Popper, Steigmann, Dublin, Dymewicz, and Hesser: Proc. Soc. Exper. Biol. & Med., *68*, 676, 1948.

33. DeLuca, Weller, Blunt, and Neville: Arch. Biochem. Biophys., *124*, 122, 1968.

34. DeLuca, and Suttie (Eds.): Vitamin D In *The Fat-Soluble Vitamins*, New York, Academic Press, p. 1, 1969.

35. Kodicek, and Lawson: Vitamin D In *The Vitamins*, György, and Pearson (Eds.), New York, Academic Press, p. 211, 1967.

36. Theivagt and Campbell: Anal. Chem., *31*, 1375, 1959.

37. Strobecker and Pies: Arch. Pharm. Ber. Dtsch. Pharmaz Ges., *294*, 800, 1961.

38. Osadca and DeRitter: Feedstuffs, *35*, 26, 1963.

39. Heaysman and Sawyer: Analyst, *89*, 529, 1964.

40. Bessey, Lowry, and Brock: J. Biol. Chem., *164*, 321, 1946.

41. György (Ed.): In *Inorganic Phosphate in Whole Blood and Serum*, New York, Academic Press, 1951.

42. Warkany, Guest, and Grabill: J. Lab. Clin. Med., *27*, 557, 1942.

43. Thomas, Morgan, Connor, Haddock, Bills, and Howard: J. Clin. Invest., *38*, 1078, 1959.

43a. Dam and Sondergaard: Fat Soluble Vitamins. In *Nutrition*, vol. 2, Beaton and McHenry, Eds. New York, Academic Press, p. 2, 1964.

43b. Norman: Amer. J. Clin. Nutrition, *24*, 1346, 1971.

44. Quaife, Scrimshaw, and Lowry: J. Biol. Chem., *180*, 1229, 1949.

45. Freed: Vitamin E in *Methods of Vitamin Assay*, New York, Interscience Publishers, p. 363, 1966.

46. Bunnell: Vitamin E. Assay by Chemical Methods In *The Vitamins*, Vol. 6, New York, Academic Press, p. 261, 1967.

47. Bieri, Pollard, Prange, and Dam: Acta Chem Scand., *15*, 783, 1961.

48. Bollinger: In *Dunnschicht-Chromatographic*, Stahl (Ed.), Berlin, Springer, p. 217, 1962.

49. Emmerie and Engel: Recueil Trav. Chim. Pays-Bas, *60*, 104, 1941.

50. Haskin and Schuttringer: Amer. J. Clin. Nutrition, *19*, 137, 1966.

51. Bieri, Teets, Belavady, and Andrews: Proc. Soc. Exptl. Biol. Med., *117*, 131, 1964.

52. Baker, Frank, Feingold, Christakis, and Ziffer: Amer. J. Clin. Nutrition, *20*, 850, 1967.

53. György and Rose: Ann. N. Y. Acad. Sci., *52*, 231, 1949.

54. Gordon and Nitowsky: Amer. J. Clin. Nutrition, *4*, 391, 1956.

55. MacKenzie: Pediatrics, *13*, 346, 1954.

56. Binder and Spiro: Amer. J. Clin. Nutrition, *20*, 594, 1967.

57. Irreverre and Sullivan: Science, *94*, 497, 1941.

58. Dam and Sondergaard: The Determination of Vitamin K In *The Vitamins*, Vol. 6, György, and Pearson (Eds.), New York, Academic Press, p. 245, 1967.

59. Suttie: In *The Fat Soluble Vitamins*, DeLuca, and Suttie (Eds.), Madison, Wisconsin, Univ. Wisconsin Press, p. 447, 1969.

60. Page and Culver (Eds.) Hemorrhagic Diseases In *Syllabus of Laboratory Examinations in Clinical Diagnosis*. Cambridge, Massachusetts, Harvard University Press, p. 186, 1962.

61. Maier and Metzler: J. Amer. Chem. Soc., *79*, 4386, 1957.

62. Manual for Nutrition Surveys, International Committee on Nutrition for National Defense, U.S. Government Printing Office, Washington, D.C., p. 136, 1963.

63. Burch, Bessey, Love, and Lowry: J. Biol. Chem., *198*, 477, 1952.

64. Pence, Miller, Dutcher, and Thorp: J. Biol. Chem., *158*, 647, 1945.

65. Pearson: In *The Vitamins*, Vol. 7, György, and Pearson (Eds.), New York, Academic Press, p. 53, 1967.

66. Baker, Pasher, Frank, Hutner, Aaronson, and Sobotka: Clin. Chem., *5*, 13, 1959.

67. Mickelson and Yamamoto: In *Methods of Biochemical Analysis*, Vol. 6, Glick, (Ed.), New York, Academic Press, p. 191, 1958.

68. Dube, Johnson, Yu, and Storvich: J. Nutrition, *48*, 307, 1952.

69. Rindi and Perri: Intern. Z. Vitaminforsch, *32*, 398, 1962.

70. Burch: In *Methods in Enzymology*, Vol. 3, Colowick, and Kaplan, (Eds.), New York, Academic Press, p. 946, 1957.

71. Bonvicino and Hennessy: Intern. Z. Vitamin-forsch, *30*, 89, 1959.

72. Interdepartmental Committee on Nutrition for National Defense, Nutrition Survey. The Kingdom of Thailand. Department of Defense, Washington, D. C., Feb., 1962.

73. Brin: Ann. N. Y. Acad. Science, *98*, 528, 1962.

74. Dreyfus: New Eng. J. Med., *267*, 596, 1962.

75. Edwards, Kaufman, and Storvich: Amer. J. Clin. Nutrition, *5*, 51, 1957.

76. Banhidi: Acta Physiol. Scand., *50*, 1, 1960.

77. Drebil, Evans, and Neven, Jr.: J. Bacteriol., *74*, 818, 1957.

78. Hutner, Cury, and Baker: Analytical Chem., *30*, 849, 1958.

79. Krampitz and Woolley: J. Biol. Chem., *152*, 9, 1944.

80. Baker, Frank, Fennelly, and Leevy: Amer. J. Clin. Nutrition, *14*, 197, 1964.

81. Frank, Baker, Ziffer, Aaronson, Hutner, and Leevy: Science, *139*, 110, 1963.

82. Hutner, Provasoli, and Baker: Microchem. J., *1*, 95, 1961.

83. Myint and Houser: Clin. Chem., *11*, 617, 1965.

84. Fennelly, Frank, Baker, and Leevy: Brit. Med. J., *2*, 1290, 1964.

85. ———: Proc. Soc. Exp. Biol. Med., *116*, 875, 1964.

86. Cole, Turner, Frank, Baker, and Leevy: Amer. J. Clin. Nutrition, *22*, 44, 1969.

87. Baker: Amer. J. Clin. Nutrition, *20*, 543, 1967.

88. Leevy, Baker, ten Hove, Frank, and Cherrick: Amer. J. Clin. Nutrition, *16*, 339, 1965.

89. Pelletier and Medere: Federation Proc., *30*, 522, 1971.

90. Thomson, Baker, and Leevy: J. Lab. Clin. Med., *76*, 34, 1970.

91. Najjar and Wood: Proc. Soc. Exp. Biol. Med., *44*, 386, 1940.

92. Mickelson, Condiff, and Keys: J. Biol. Chem., *160*, 361, 1945.

93. Alexander and Levi: J. Biol. Chem., *146*, 399, 1942.

94. Pearson: Amer. J. Clin. Nutrition, *20*, 514, 1967.

95. Ziporin, Nunes, Powell, Waring, and Sauber-lich: J. Nutrition, *85*, 287, 1965.

96. Sorrell, Frank, Aquino, Thomson, Howard, and Baker: Amer. J. Clin. Nutrition, *25*, 125, 1972.

97. Burch, Bessey, Love, and Lowry: J. Biol. Chem., *198*, 477, 1952.

98. Goodhart and Sinclair: J. Biol. Chem., *132*, 11, 1940.

99. Krause: In *Modern Nutrition in Health and Disease*, 4th Ed., Wohl and Goodhart (Eds.), Philadelphia, Lea & Febiger, p. 531, 1968.

100. Horwitt and Kreisler: J. Nutrition, *37*, 411, 1949.

101. Sinclair: New Eng. J. Med., *245*, 39, 1951.

102. György and Langer, Jr.: In *The Vitamins*, Vol. 2, Sebrell, Jr. and Harris (Eds.), New York, Academic Press, p. 280, 1968.

103. Hertz: Proc. Soc. Exp. Biol. Med., *52*, 15, 1943.

104. Schull and Peterson: J. Biol. Chem., *151*, 201, 1943.

105. Wright and Skeggs: Proc. Soc. Exp. Biol. Med., *56*, 95, 1944.

106. Aaronson: J. Bacteriol., *69*, 67, 1955.

107. Hodson: J. Biol. Chem., *157*, 383, 1945.

108. West and Woglom: Cancer Res., *2*, 324, 1942.

109. The Association of Vitamin Chemists, Inc.: Biotin In *Methods of Vitamin Assay*, Freed (Ed.), New York, Interscience, p. 245, 1966.

110. Glick and Ferguson: Proc. Soc. Exp. Biol. Med., *109*, 811, 1962.

111. Baker, Frank, Matovitch, Pasher, Aaronson, Hutner, and Sobotka: Anal. Biochem., *3*, 31, 1962.

112. Terroine: Vitamins and Hormones, *18*, 1, 1960.

113. Wright, Cresson, Skeggs, Peck, Wolf, Wood, Valiant, and Folkers: Science, *114*, 635, 1951.

114. Bliss and György: In *The Vitamins*, Vol. 7, György and Pearson (Eds.), New York, Academic Press, p. 134, 1967.

115. Goldsmith: In *Nutrition*, Vol. 2, Beaton and McHenry (Eds.), New York, Academic Press, p. 109, 1964.

116. Barton-Wright: In *Microbiological Assay of the Vitamin B-Complex and Amino Acids*, London, Pitman, p. 35, 1952.

117. Freed: In *Methods of Vitamin Assay*, 3rd Ed., New York, Interscience, p. 150, 1966.

118. Burch: In *Methods in Enzymology*, Vol. 3, Colowick and Kaplan (Eds.), New York, Academic Press, p. 960, 1957.

119. Baker, Frank, Feingold, Gellene, Leevy, and Hutner: Amer. J. Clin. Nutrition, *19*, 17, 1966.

120. Snell: In *The Vitamins*, Vol. 3, Sebrell and Harris (Eds.), New York, Academic Press, p. 372, 1954.

121. Horwitt: In *Modern Nutrition in Health and Disease*, Wohl and Goodhart (Eds.), Philadelphia, Lea & Febiger, p. 335, 1960.

122. Rivlin: New Eng. J. Med., *283*: 463, 1970.

123. Sarett, Klein, and Perlzweig: J. Nutrition, *24*, 295, 1942.

124. Mickelson: In *Present Knowledge of Nutrition*, New York, The Nutrition Foundation, Inc., p. 61, 1967.

125. Bessey, Horwitt, and Love: J. Nutrition, *58*, 367, 1956.

125a. Glatzle, Korner, Christeller and Wiss: Internat. J. Vit. Res., *40*, 166, 1970.

125b. Tillotson and Baker: Amer. J. Clin. Nutrition, *25*, 425, 1972.

125c. Sharada and Bamji: Internat. J. Vit. Res., *42*, 43, 1972.

126. Baker, Frank, Pasher, Hutner, and Sobotka: Clin. Chem., *6*, 572, 1960.

127. Goldsmith and Miller: In *The Vitamins*, Vol. 7, György and Pearson (Eds.), New York, Academic Press, p. 139, 1967.

128. Friedemann and Frazier: Arch. Biochem., *26*, 361, 1950.

129. Official Methods of Analysis, Association of Official Agricultural Chemists, Washington, D.C., p. 660, 1960.

130. Huff and Perlzweig: J. Biol. Chem., *167*, 157, 1947.
131. Levitas, Robinson, Rosen, Huff, and Perlzweig: J. Biol. Chem., *167*, 169, 1947.
132. Fergelson, Williams, Jr., and Elvehjem: J. Biol. Chem., *185*, 741, 1950.
133. Lowry, Roberts, and Kapphahn: J. Biol. Chem., *224*, 1047, 1957.
134. Lindall and Lazarow: Metabolism, *13*, 259, 1964.
135. Lieber: In *The Biological Basis of Medicine*, Vol. 5, Bittar and Bittar (Eds.), New York, Academic Press, p. 318, 1969.
136. Ellinjer and Coulson: Biochem. J., *38*, 265, 1944.
137. Hoagland, Ward, and Shank: J. Biol. Chem., *241*, 2367, 1966.
138. Baker, Frank, Thomson, and Feingold: Amer. J. Clin. Nutrition, *22*, 1469, 1969.
139. Sorrell, Frank, Aquino, Thomson, and Baker: Amer. J. Clin. Nutrition, *24*, 924, 1971.
140. Leder and Handler: J. Biol. Chem., *189*, 889, 1951.
141. Storvich, Benson, Edwards, and Woodring: In *Methods of Biochemical Analysis*, Vol. 12, Glick (Ed.), New York, Interscience, p. 183, 1964.
142. Sauberlich: In *The Vitamins*, Vol. 7, György and Pearson (Eds.), New York, Academic Press, p. 169, 1967.
143. Toepfer, Polansky, and Hewston: Anal. Biochem., *2*, 463, 1961.
144. Korytnyk, Fricke, and Paul: Anal. Biochem., *17*, 66, 1966.
145. Storvich and Peters: Vitamins and Hormones, *22*, 833, 1964.
146. Cinnamon and Beaton: Amer. J. Clin. Nutrition, *23*, 696, 1970.
147. Umbreit, Bellamy, and Gunsalus: Arch. Biochem., *7*, 185, 1945.
148. Wada, Morisue, Sakamoto, and Ichibara: J. Vitaminol. (Japan), *3*, 183, 1957.
149. Leitch and Hepburn: Nutrition Abst. Rev., *31*, 389, 1961.
150. Gassman, Knapp, and Gartner: Klin Wochschr., *37*, 189, 1959.
151. Marquez and Reynolds: J. Amer. Dietet. Assoc., *31*, 1116, 1955.
152. Turner and Reynolds: J. Amer. Dietet. Assoc., *31*, 1119, 1955.
153. Wachstein and Gudartis: J. Lab. Clin. Med., *42*, 98, 1953.
154. Ranke, Tauber, Hornick, Ranke, Goodhart, and Chow: J. Gerontol., *15*, 41, 1960.
155. György: Vitamins and Hormones, *22*, 885, 1964.
156. Boxer, Pruss, and Goodhart: J. Nutrition, *63*, 623, 1957.
157. Wachstein, Moore, and Graffeo: Proc. Soc. Exp. Biol. Med., *96*, 326, 1957.
158. Holtz and Palm: Pharmacol. Rev., *16*, 113, 1964.
159. Reddy, Reynolds, and Price: J. Biol. Chem., *233*, 691, 1958.
160. Huff and Perlzweig: J. Biol. Chem., *155*, 345, 1944.
161. Gershoff: Vitamins and Hormones, *22*, 581, 1964.
162. Baker, Frank, Ning, Gellene, Hutner, and Leevy: Amer. J. Clin. Nutrition, *18*, 123, 1966.
163. Haskell and Wallnofer: Anal. Biochem., *19*, 659, 1967.
164. Hubbard, Hintz, Libby, and Sutor, Jr.: J. Assoc. Office Agr. Chemists, *48*, 1217, 1965.
165. Bird and Thompson: In *The Vitamins*, Vol. 7, György, and Pearson (Eds.), New York, Academic Press, p. 209, 1967.
166. Baker, Frank, Pasher, Dinnerstein, and Sobotka: Clin. Chem., *6*, 36, 1960.
167. Dewey and Kidder: Proc. Soc. Exp. Biol. Med., *87*, 198, 1954.
168. Malgras, Meyer, and Pax: Ann. Inst. Pasteur, *93*, 792, 1957.
169. Knox and Groswami: Advan. Clin. Chem., *4*, 121, 1961.
170. Roe: In *The Vitamins*, Vol. 7, György and Pearson (Eds.), New York, Academic Press, p. 27, 1967.
171. Roe: In *Methods of Biochemical Analysis*, Vol. 1, Glick (Ed.), New York, Interscience, p. 134, 1954.
172. Schwartz and Williams, Jr.: Proc. Soc. Exp. Biol. Med., *88*, 136, 1955.
173. Penny and Zilva: Biochem. J., *37*, 403, 1943.
174. Baker, Hodges, Hood, Sauberlich, and March: Amer. J. Clin. Nutrition, *22*, 549, 1969.
175. Baker and Frank: In *The Vitamins*, Vol. 7, György, and Pearson (Eds.), New York, Academic Press, p. 293, 1967.
176. Rosenthal: In *The Vitamins*, Vol. 2, Sebrell, Jr., and Harris (Eds.) New York, Academic Press, p. 151, 1968.
177. Reizenstein: Blood, *27*, 744, 1966.
178. Woodliff and Armstrong: Med. J. Austral., *1*, 1023, 1966.
179. Mahmud, Ripley, and Doscherholmen: J.A.M.A., *216*, 1167, 1971.
180. Lawar, Jr., McCracken, Miller, and Goldsmith: Amer. J. Clin. Nutrition, *16*, 402, 1965.
181. Glass: Physiol Rev., *43*, 529, 1963.
182. Lau, Gottlieb, Wasserman and Herbert: Blood, *26*, 202, 1965.
183. Gottlieb, Lau, Wasserman and Herbert: Blood, *25*, 6, 1965.
184. Grossowicz, Sulitzeam, and Merzbach: Proc. Soc. Exp. Biol. Med., *109*, 604, 1962.
185. Hift: So. Afr. J. Med. Sci., *29*, 84, 1964.
186. Luhby and Cooperman: Lancet, *2*, 138, 1962.
187. Herbert, Streiff, Sullivan, and McGeer: Lancet, *2*, 45, 1964.
188. Coward and Smith: Clin. Chem. Acta, *12*, 206, 1965.
189. Barness, Young, Mellman, Kahn, and Williams: New Eng. J. Med., *268*, 144, 1963.
190. Kahn, Williams, Barness, Young, Shafer, Vivacqua, and Beaupre: J. Lab. Clin. Med., *66*, 75, 1965.

191. Gompertz, Jones, and Knowles: Lancet, *1*, 424, 1967.
192. Johns and Bertino: Clin. Pharmacol. Therapeutics, *6*, 372, 1965.
193. Baker and Sobotka: Advances Clin. Chem., *5*, 215, 1962.
194. Skeggs: In *The Vitamins*, Vol. 7, György, and Pearson (Eds.), New York, Academic Press, p. 278, 1967.
195. Baker, Frank, Pasher, and Sobotka: Clin. Chem., *6*, 578, 1960.
196. Baker, Frank, Pasher, Ziffer, Hutner, and Sobotka: Proc. Soc. Exp. Biol. Med., *107*, 965, 1961.
197. Blakley: In *The Biochemistry of Folic Acid and Related Pteridines*, New York, Wiley Interscience Div., p. 32, 1969.
198. Ellegaard and Esmann: Lancet, *1*, 308, 1970.
199. Chanarin: In *The Megaloblastic Anaemias*. Philadelphia, F. A. Davis Co., 1969.
200. Chanarin: Proc. Roy. Soc. Med., *57*, 384, 1964.
201. Eichhorn and Rutenberg: Lancet, *2*, 906, 1965.
202. Cooperman, Luhby, and Singer: Proc. Soc. Exp. Biol. Med., *131*, 434, 1969.
203. McGeer, Sen, and Grant: Canad. J. Biochem., *43*, 1367, 1965.
204. Herbert, Streiff, Sullivan, and McGeer: Lancet, *2*, 45, 1964.
205. Luhby and Cooperman: Lancet, *2*, 1381, 1962.
206. Cherrick, Baker, Frank, and Leevy: J. Lab. Clin. Med., *66*, 446, 1965.
207. McClean and Chanarin: Blood, *27*, 386, 1966.
208. Chanarin, Anderson, and Mollin: Brit. J. Haematol., *4*, 156, 1958.
209. Baker, Frank, Gellene, and Leevy: Proc. Soc. Exp. Biol. Med., *117*, 492, 1964.
210. Gerdwood: Brit. Med. Bull., *15*, 14, 1959.
211. Bird, McGlohon, and Vaitkus: Canad. J. Microbiol., *15*, 465, 1969.
212. Hutner, Nathan, and Baker: Vitamins and Hormones, *17*, 1, 1959.
213. Larrabee, Rosenthal, Cathou, and Buchanan: J. Amer. Chem. Soc., *83*, 4094, 1961.
214. Herbert, Larrabee, and Buchanan: J. Clin. Invest., *41*, 1134, 1962.
215. Baker, Frank, Feingold, Ziffer, Gellene, Leevy, and Sobotka: Amer. J. Clin. Nutrition, *17*, 88, 1965.
216. Jeejeebboy, Pathare, and Noronba: Blood, *26*, 354, 1965.
217. Teply and Elvehjem: J. Biol. Chem., *157*, 303, 1945.
218. Herbert, Baker, Frank, Pasher, Sobotka, and Wasserman: Blood, *15*, 228, 1960.
219. Herbert: J. Clin. Invest., *40*, 81, 1961.
220. Herbert: Trans. Assoc. Amer. Physicians, *75*, 307, 1962.
221. Waters and Mollin: J. Clin. Pathol., *14*, 335, 1961.
222. Hansen: In *On the Diagnosis of Folic Acid Deficiency*, Goteborg, Sweden, Orstadius Baktryckeri AB, 1964.
223. Herbert: J. Clin. Pathol., *19*, 12, 1966.
224. Baker, Frank, Sobotka, Ho, Cohen, Janowitz, Ziffer, and Leevy: J.A.M.A., *187*, 159, 1964.
225. Baker, Frank, and Hutner: Science, *169*, 313, 1969.
226. Okuda: J. Biochem. (Japan), *48*, 13, 1960.
227. Reddi and Kodicek: Biochem. J., *53*, 286, 1953.
228. King: J.A.M.A., *142*, 563, 1950.

Chapter

18

Radiologic Findings in Nutritional Disturbances

ROBIN C. WATSON,

HERMAN GROSSMAN,

AND

MORTON A. MEYERS

The roentgenographic findings in nutritional disorders are somewhat varied: they may be distinctive, as in scurvy or rickets, but they are often non-specific, as in osteoporosis and osteomalacia, and the diagnosis may depend upon secondary manifestations.[1-3] Also, it must be pointed out that any radiographic abnormality occurs only in the face of prolonged deficiency or excessive intake. In all probability the most striking changes are seen in this day and age as a result of malabsorption rather than deficient intake. However, particularly in underdeveloped areas, the latter is still a dominant factor. Generally, the earliest and most specific findings are seen in the child and adolescent, rather than in the adult, although with gastrointestinal abnormalities this probably is reversed.

OSTEOPOROSIS

Over the years there has been a considerable blurring of the meaning of "osteoporosis," which has become a vague, all-embracing word.[4,5]

In the normal subject there is a balance detween osteogenesis and osteolysis and an abequate degree of bone mineralization. Osteoporosis represents a breakdown in this mechanism: there is a defect in osteogenesis while osteolysis proceeds at the normal rate and the process of bone mineralization is unimpaired. The result is that there is an overall loss of bone mass with respect to the volume of bone present, and the bone elements, therefore, become sparse and brittle.

Radiographically there is thinning of the cortical bone with an overall loss of bone density, and the distance between the normally mineralized longitudinal, but thin, trabeculae becomes increased (hence the term "porotic"), while there is a concomitant loss of transverse trabeculae.[6] These changes are usually first apparent in the spine; however, in advanced cases, the process may be seen to involve all bones. Fractures due to the brittle quality of the bone are common and deformities may result. Most often seen are crush fractures of the spine with collapse of the vertebral endplates and anterior wedging of the bodies, resulting in increased lordotic curves. Pseudofractures are not seen in this condition.

Osteoporosis may be seen in relation to:
1. Senile and post-menopausal patients.
2. Malnutrition.
3. Hypovitaminosis C.
4. Endocrine disorders, such as Cushing's disease, acromegaly, hypothyroidism and hyperthyroidism.
5. The congenital defect of osteogenesis imperfecta.
6. Idiopathic.

Difficulty in interpretation results from the fact that there must be extensive loss of the mass of bone before this becomes radiographically apparent. Furthermore, the

547

findings are non-specific and there is no way of differentiating, say, postmenopausal osteoporosis from that found in multiple myeloma.

Osteoporosis is, perhaps, most often seen in elderly patients, usually of reduced circumstances, in whom there is an associated dietary insufficiency, including vitamin C. Although there are perhaps fewer of these individuals than in the past, they exist in both rural and urban areas.

SCURVY

Abnormalities in the skeleton in infantile scurvy have been studied by Park.[7] There is a disturbance of endochondral bone growth, with subperiosteal hemorrhagic manifestations occurring without associated trauma. The bone changes occur quite symmetrically throughout the skeleton and are more widely distributed than are gross subperiosteal or intramedullary hemorrhages. Like the changes in rickets, those of scurvy are most marked where growth in length is normally most rapid; at the sternal end of the middle ribs, the lower end of the femur, the upper end of the humerus, both ends of the tibia and fibula, the lower end of the radius and ulna, in approximately the order given.

The columns of cartilage cells in the pro-liferative cartilage in infantile scurvy tend to be irregular rather than linear. Whether this change represents a purely scorbutic process or whether it depends in part on an associated or antecedent rickets is not entirely certain. Scurvy interferes with the mechanism for removal of calcified cartilage matrix; it suppresses the formation of new trabeculae and, wherever there is bone already formed, resorption proceeds. These changes, morphologically important in themselves, affect the structure of bone also from a functional point of view by diminishing its capacity to withstand mechanical stress.

Roentgenographic changes are often diagnostic or suggestive. The costochondral junctions of the ribs are wide (Fig. 18–1A and B). The abrupt bony swelling culminates in a ridge where bone and cartilage meet. The sternochondral plate may be displaced posteriorly by atmospheric pressure where the cartilage has been pushed backward at the line of its separation from the bony shaft.

In the early stages, the changes in the bone are nonspecific, presenting poorly discernible trabeculae and thin cortices. As the disease progresses a thick white line at the metaphysis (Figs. 18–2 and 3) develops. Spurs develop at the cartilage-shaft junction and sub-epiphyseal atrophy casts a transverse line or

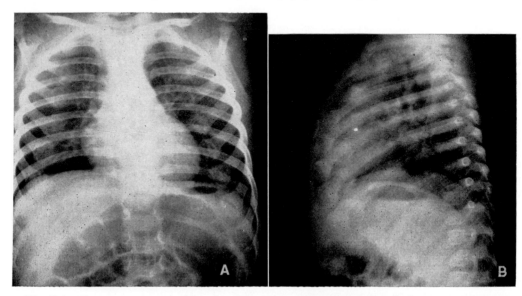

Fig. 18-1. Twenty-seven-month-old male with scurvy. Frontal and lateral chest roentgenograms demonstrate bony swelling at the costochondral junctions of the ribs.

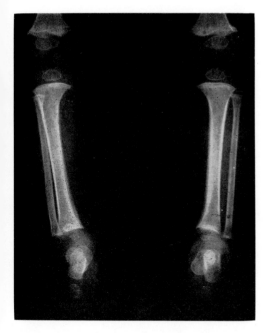

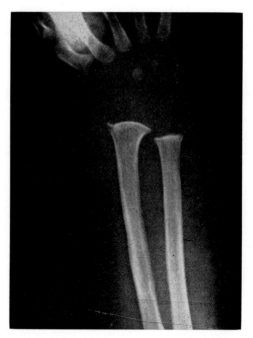

Fig. 18-2. Ten-month-old male with scurvy demonstrating a thick white line at the metaphyses of the long bones of the knees. Linear breaks are present in the bones proximal and parallel to the white lines of the distal femurs. Spurs are present and best seen at the ends of the femurs and medial aspect of the right tibia. The ossification centers have central rarefaction with heavy ring shadows on the margins. Periosteal new bone is along the medial aspects of the tibias.

Fig. 18-3. Eight-month-old female with scurvy showing dense white lines and rarefaction at the distal ends of the radius and ulna. The "corner sign" of scurvy, noted at the distal, lateral aspect of the radius is due to a defect at the angle between the provisional zone of calcification and the cortex.

band of diminished density[8] (Fig. 18–2). This zone of rarefaction is a linear break in the bone proximal and parallel to the white line. Peripheral metaphyseal clefts, the so-called "corner sign," are characteristic of scurvy[7] (Fig. 18–3). Ossification centers have central rarefaction with heavy ring shadows (Fig. 18–2) on the margins. Epiphyseal separation may occur along the line of destruction, with linear displacement or compression of the epiphysis against the shaft. Subperiosteal hemorrhages often appear on the larger long bones[8,9] (Fig. 18–4A and B). During healing the elevated periosteum becomes calcified (Fig. 18–4B), creating a heavy shell of subperiosteal bone. This shell of bone gradually shrinks and forms a new cortex. Subperichondrial hemorrhages over the epiphysis are said not to occur in scurvy.

OSTEOMALACIA

In most countries osteomalacia is now considered to be the adult form of rickets. It represents an abnormality of the mineralizing process while both osteogenesis and osteolysis proceed at a normal rate.[10] The result of the mineral deficiency is that the bone becomes soft and pliable. Whereas in osteoporosis the thin and brittle bones fracture easily, in osteomalacia there is more likely to be bending of the bony structures. The bone mass is still of normal volume, but there is a loss of bone density.[11]

Most often osteomalacia is related to malabsorption as a result of a variety of conditions, such as sprue, steatorrhea, pancreatic insufficiency, Crohn's disease, gastric or small bowel resections, fistulas or chronic ulerative colitis. Radiographically the bone density is decreased; however, this may be hard to recognize. The trabeculae are poorly defined and coarse, with widening of the inter-

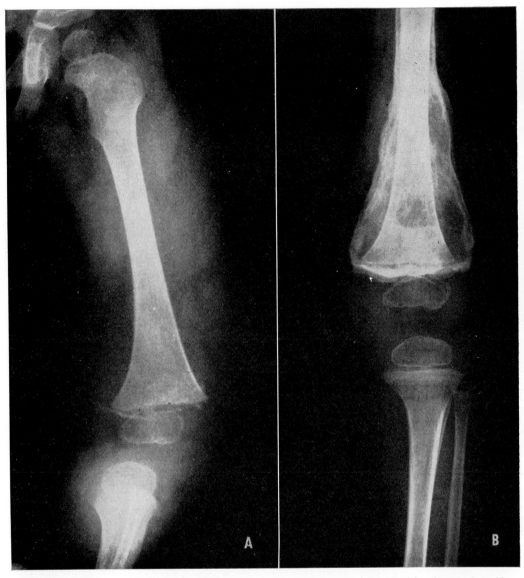

Fig. 18-4. Twelve-month-old male with healing scurvy. *A.* Fracture of the provisional zone of calcification of the distal femur with early calcification. Displacement of the soft tissues is due to hematoma which has not begun to calcify. *B.* Extensive calcification of elevated periosteum after 2 weeks of vitamin C therapy.

trabecular spaces. The most striking feature is that, in areas of stress, pseudofractures appear as thin radiolucent lines extending across the cortex at right angles to the long axis of the bone.[12] These fractures are most often symmetrical and bilateral. With treatment, the margins of these fractures become sclerotic, but angulation often occurs at the site. One theory is that the fractures are related to pulsating periosteal blood vessels; however, this seems unlikely. In partially treated or untreated cases, these zones of lucency remain for considerable periods of time. The bones most commonly affected are the first or lower ribs, the pubic rami, the transverse processes of the lumbar vertebra, lateral scapular borders, tibiae and fibulae, and the shafts of the femoral necks. In chronic and untreated cases, gross skeletal deformities may result.

RICKETS

Rickets, a disease of infancy and childhood, is a metabolic disorder of bone characterized by formation of normal collagen, matrix and osteoid with a disturbance in calcium and phosphorous metabolism, which prevents the normal deposition of calcium salts in the growing parts of the skeleton. The skeleton becomes weak, is unable to withstand the stress and strain to which it is ordinarily subjected and yields and deforms. For the development of ordinary rickets, a deficiency must exist both in the short ultraviolet radiations of the sun and in the vitamin D present in certain foods. Osteomalacia is merely deficiency rickets occurring after endochondral growth has come to an end.

The roentgenograms give the most accurate information regarding rickets. The costochondral junctions, the most actively growing bones, are not accessible for clear radiographic study early in the course of rickets. The lower end of the femur is too thick and the junction of the epiphysis with the diaphysis is too uneven for slight changes to show distinctly. The lower ends of the radius and ulna are most useful for the study of rickets by x-ray pictures because of their small size and convenient location. Significant changes are often visible in the ulna when the radius appears to be normal.

The changes at the cartilage-shaft junction are characterized by total or partial lack of calcification of the terminal segment of the shaft. This "invisible" provisional zone of calcification is seen only in rickets (Fig. 18–5A). Cupping, spreading, cortical spurs, and fraying at the ends of bones are also seen in rickets, but not one of these changes itself is characteristic of rickets, since it may be seen in other conditions, such as congenital syphilis or scurvy.

Cupping may not be evident until treatment is begun, because of the lack of lime salts in the organic tissue which forms the cup (Fig. 18–5B and C). Cupping may be seen in scurvy, to a slight degree, in the ulnae of young, especially premature, infants whose bones are growing rapidly.

Cortical spurs are linear shadows which extend as prolongations of the shadows of the cortex along the sides of the proliferative cartilage[13] (Fig. 18–5B). They are not always in the direct line of the cortex, but are external to it, since they lie in the perichondrial-periosteal layer which envelops the cortex. Such shadows may be found on one or both sides; they may be straight and in line of the cortex or they may arch outward. The shape and direction of the spurs are determined by the configuration of the proliferative cartilage. In the x-ray film it can often be seen that the spurs lie external to the cortex, overlapping and seeming to splint the cartilage-shaft junction. This represents a new cortical layer forming outside the old. Spur formation also occurs in congenital syphilis.

Fraying consists of thread-like calcified shadows extending from the end of the shaft into the transparent cartilage[14] (Fig. 18–5B). These frayed densities are neither straight nor parallel but extend in various directions, exactly as would be expected from the disorder in the underlying pathological condition.

In severe rickets the shaft of the bone shows a diffuse rarefaction caused by the loss of lime. The cortex may be thin and, in places, invisible. Strands of osteoid may extend from the poorly defined cortex to the almost invisible periosteum, which contains enough lime salts to cast hair-like shadows sticking out from the sides of the bones (Fig. 18–5A). Other changes in the shaft which may be visible are complete or partial fracture, callous formation, curvature of the shaft, with great thickening on the concave side, or displacement of the epiphysis on the diaphysis.

Healing rickets is first observed in the provisional zone of calcification. A transverse linear recalcified density develops in the ricketic metaphysis beyond the visible end of the shaft and at a level the epiphyseal plate would have reached in the absence of rickets (Fig. 18–5B). As healing continues, the new provisional zone of calcification thickens. The metaphyseal spongiosa also recalcifies and fuses with that of the provisional zone of calcification. The cortex heals more slowly and is less conspicuous roentgenographically.

However, when layers of osteoid have been deposited under the periosteum, recalcification of this osteoid discloses a diffuse layer or cortex, which may be of uniform density or lamellated (Fig. 18–5C).

Complete healing can be achieved in deficiency rickets. Distortion and sclerosis in the bone remain visible in the same level of the shaft for years and cortical thickening on the concave surfaces of curvature deformities may also remain. Most bowing and angulation deformities result from displacement of the epiphyseal cartilage. Angulation deformities may also be secondary to pathologic fractures.

The Separation of Scurvy and the Incidence of Scurvy in Association With Rickets. Scurvy may be distinguished from rickets by the tenderness and pain present with scurvy, which exceeds anything found in rickets. The various hemorrhagic phenomena seen with scurvy do not occur in rickets. Difficulty may be encountered in distinguishing the enlargement of the costochondral junctions found in scurvy from that found in rickets and differentiation may be impossible.

Vitamin D and C deficiency occurs commonly together, since it is necessary to give both vitamins as accessories to the diet. If one

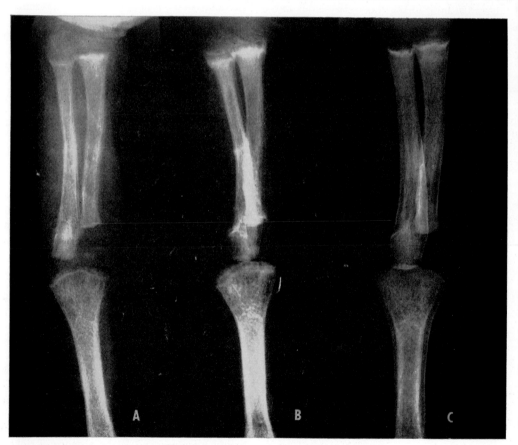

Fig. 18-5. A ten-month-old male during various stages of rickets.

   A. Non-calcified provisional zone. Fraying of the distal humerus. Strands of calcified osteoid projecting out from the sides of the bone.

   B. Cupping, spread metaphysis, fraying and cortical spurs. Transverse linear recalcified density develops in ricketic metaphysis. A fracture in the midshaft of the radius. Greenstick fractures are common in the long bones.

   C. Metaphyseal spongiosa recalcifies and fuses with that of the provisional zone of calcification. Diffuse layer of recalcified cortex.

is not given, it often happens that the other is omitted also. The association is thus due to chance, not to any interrelationship between the two vitamins in a chemical sense. However, a deficiency in one vitamin may prevent deficiency in the other from expressing itself by characteristic symptoms and signs. If vitamin D deficiency is sufficiently severe and prolonged, the lattice of calcified matrix framework, which is so characteristic a feature of scurvy, cannot form at all or forms imperfectly. In scurvy it is the collapse of the brittle lattice framework that is responsible for the fractures and the development of subperiosteal hemorrhage, and probably the pain and tenderness. Thus, as a result of suppressing the development of the lattice, vitamin D deficiency may prevent or modify important symptoms of scurvy, typical roentgenographic signs, and characteristic histology.

IRON DEFICIENCY ANEMIA

Roentgenographic changes in the skeleton in association with congenital hemolytic anemia result from increased proliferation of hematopoietic tissue in the bone marrow.

In 1936 Sheldon[15] first described a child with changes in the skull in association with iron deficiency anemia. In the 1960's many other reports[16-20] described changes in the skull in children with iron deficiency anemia. Lanzkowsky[21] recently reported several children with iron deficiency anemia who had changes in the metacarpals, as well as in the skull.

The degree of change in the roentgenograms of the skull and metacarpals is variable with iron deficiency anemia. Children with marked changes are similar to those seen with severe congenital hemolytic anemias. The diploic space of the skull is widened in a non-uniform manner. The occipital squamosa is usually not wide, due to normally deficient marrow in this portion of the skull. The trabeculae may be perpendicular to the inner table presenting a radial pattern which may have a "hair-on-end" appearance (Fig. 18-6A and B).

Involvement of the long bones has been only described in a few patients.[21,22] The metacarpals show widening due to expansion of the medullary space, prominent trabeculae, and thinning of the cortices (Fig. 18-7).

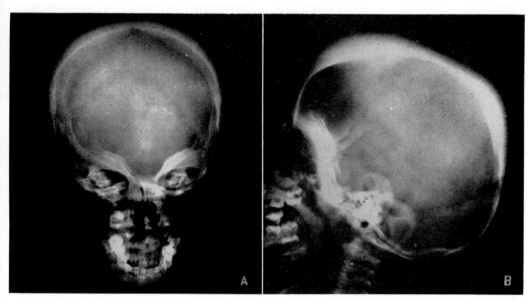

Fig. 18-6A and B. Frontal and lateral views of the skull in a young child with iron deficiency anemia demonstrating non-uniform widening of the diploic space with a "hair-on-end" appearance. (Courtesy of Dr. Philip Lanzkowsky.)

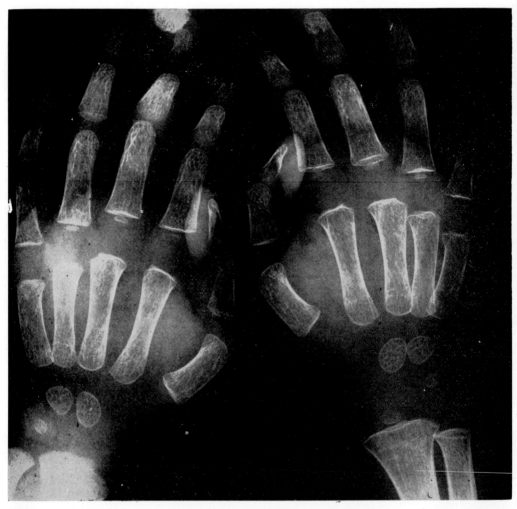

Fig. 18-7. The hands of a child with iron deficiency anemia demonstrating widening of the metacarpals, prominent trabeculae of the bones of the hands and thin cortices. (Courtesy of Dr. Philip Lanzkowsky.)

HYPERVITAMINOSIS A

Early roentgenographic findings of chronic vitamin A poisoning may be limited to widened sutures in the skull and a bulging anterior fontanelle (Fig. 18-8A and B). The long bones (Figs. 18–9A and 10) may be normal at this stage of the disease. The 2-year-old patient represented in Figures 18–8 to 10 was seen for anorexia and vomiting. Because her fontanelle was full, a skull x-ray film was taken and demonstrated sutural diastasis. The dense line at the metaphyses of all long bones suggested lead poisoning. The "history of a poor eater" raised the possibility of pica, but careful questioning revealed that "extra" cod liver oil had been given, 100,000 units of vitamin A and 15,000 units of vitamin D, 1 to 3 times a day intermittently during the previous 6 months. Serum vitamin A level was elevated. The dense line was considered to be due to excess vitamin D. Two weeks after the diagnosis and the cessation of vitamin A, cortical hyperostosis was present on the ulnae (Fig. 18-9B), and the fibulae. The bone changes are usually symmetrical. Three week after admission to hospital the serum vitamin A became normal but the hyperostosis continued.

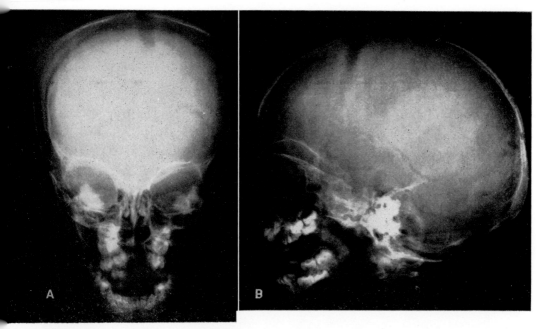

Fig. 18-8A and B. Skull in frontal and lateral projections of a 2-year-old female with hypervitaminosis A showing wide sagittal and coronal sutures.

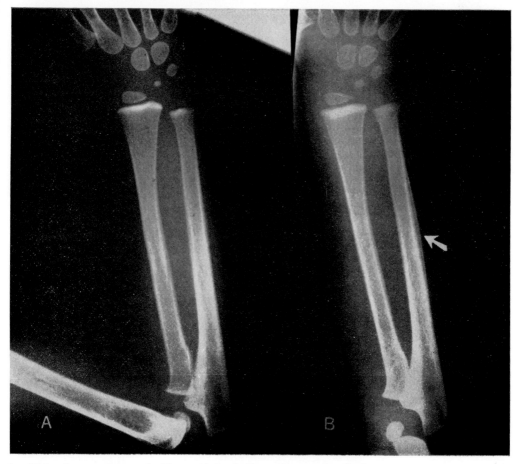

Fig. 18-9. Same patient as in Figure 18–8. *A.* Dense line at the distal end of radius and ulna. No subperiosteal new bone. *B.* Three weeks later periosteal new bone seen on the lateral aspect of the ulna.

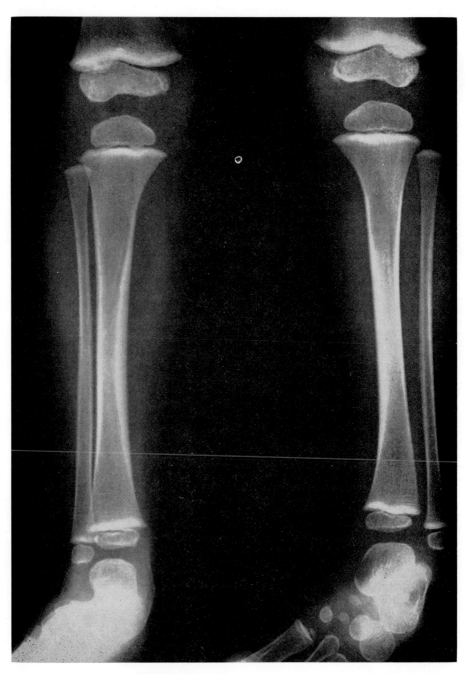

Fig. 18-10. Same patient as in Figure 18-8. Initial roentgenograms of the metaphyses at the knees and ankles demonstrate dense lines. No periosteal new bone is present.

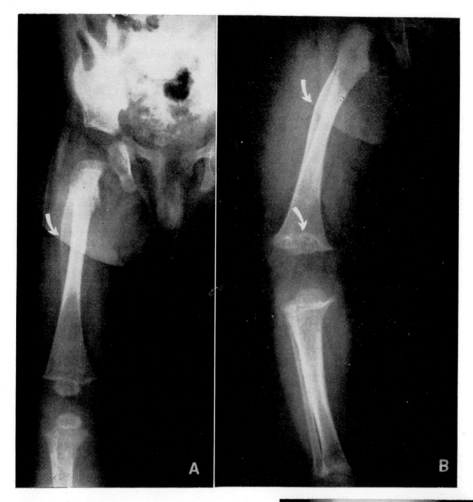

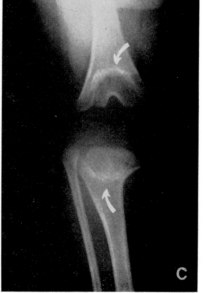

Fig. 18-11. Frontal view of the right lower extremity of an 18-month-old child who had received 50,000 to 250,000 units of vitamin A since 3 months of age.

A. Cortical hyperostosis of the femur.

B. The cortical thickening is more dense and there is metaphyseal cupping of the femur and tibia 4 months after initial diagnosis. The distal end of the tibia is not affected.

C. Nine months after the initial x rays the cartilage plates are narrow and the epiphyseal ossification center and their respective shafts are fusing in the central segments of their cartilage plates. The ossification centers are buried into the metaphyseal cups. The joint spaces are increased. The defects were bilateral and symmetrical. (A, B and C courtesy of Dr. A. Geffin.)

When soft tissue swellings are noted in association with clinical symptoms of vitamin A toxicity, e.g., anorexia, pruritus, alopecia, desquamation of the skin, cortical thickening of long bones is present (Fig. 18–11A). Although vitamin A then is eliminated from the diet, the changes in the bones continue. The subperiosteal new bone continues to thicken (Fig. 18–11B). These cortical thickenings usually stop short of the ends of the shafts. In some patients there is metaphyseal cupping, splaying of the affected end of the shaft, hypertrophy of the contiguous epiphyseal ossification center and premature fusion of this center with the shaft (Fig. 18–11B and C). Premature fusion of the center with its shafts is most often seen at the distal ends of the femurs and results in arrested growth, with permanent shortening of the affected bones. Although these changes at the metaphyses and epiphyses were demonstrated in experimental animals,[23,24] it was not until Pease[25] reported 7 patients in 1962 that this complication of vitamin poisoning was universally accepted. Cortical hyper-

ostosis of ribs (Fig. 18–12) also occurs with vitamin A poisoning.

Caffey[26] reviewed the many diseases which cause cupping of the metaphyses. He believes that the basic defect is a reduced growth in the arterial segment of the epiphyseal plate. The "walls" of the cup are dependent on the periosteal and metaphyseal arteries, not on the epiphyseal arteries and, therefore, the peripheral zones of the bones continue to grow. Caffey suggests that, in vitamin A poisoning, spontaneous immobilization occurs, due to exquisite pain and hyperesthesia. Immobilization causes slowing and stagnation of the blood, which leads to thrombosis of the arteries of the epiphyseal plate.

HYPERVITAMINOSIS D

In the presence of an excess of vitamin D an increased mobilization of mineral occurs with secondary hypercalcemia and phosphatemia.[27] Calcific deposits occur in the renal tubules with secondary renal failure, and

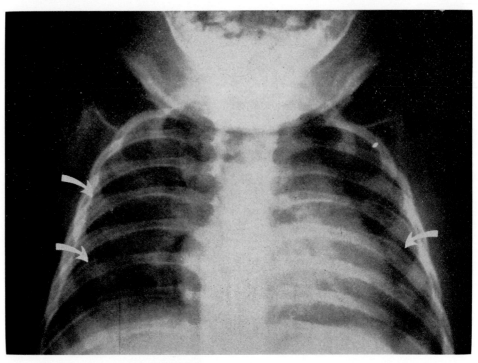

Fig. 18-12. Same patient as in Figure 18-11. Chest roentgenogram shows cortical hyperostosis of many ribs due to vitamin A poisoning.

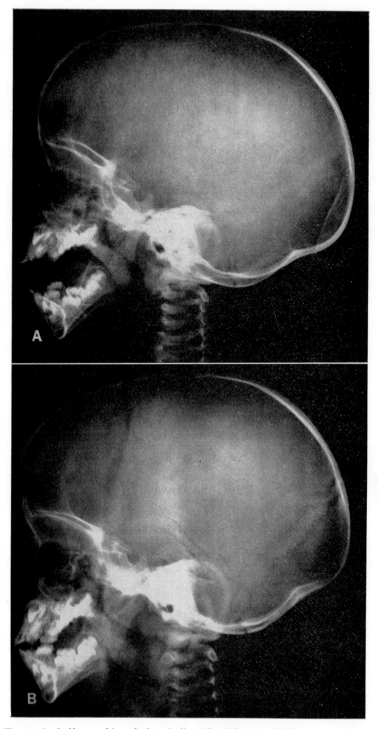

Fig. 18-13. Two-and-a-half-year-old male hospitalized for failure to thrive.

A. Lateral skull roentgenogram at time of admission is normal.

B. Two months later when the child had gained weight and was well, the lateral skull roentgenogram demonstrates wide coronal and lamboid sutures.

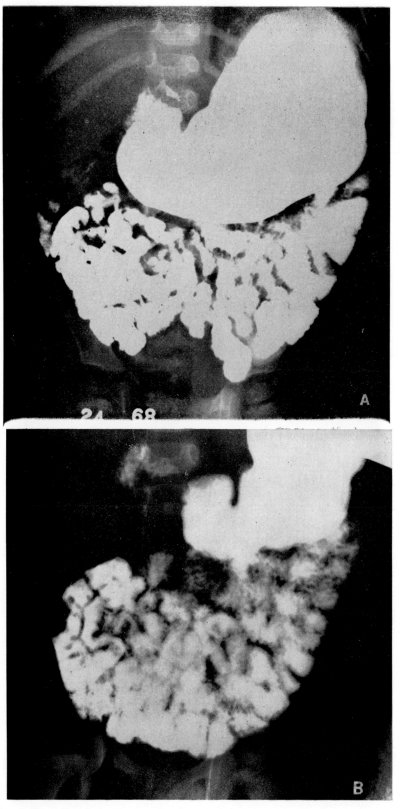

Fig. 18-14. *A.* Gastrointestinal series 2 weeks after admission demonstrates a large stomach and separated loops of small intestine with thickened valvulae conniventes. *B.* Four weeks after the original study when the patient was well, a repeat intestinal series shows the small intestine to be normal.

sometimes death results. In the growing child the zone of provisional calcification becomes relatively dense in comparison to the adjacent metaphyseal region. In addition, extensive periarticular and vessel calcification may be present with, in some cases, premature vascular calcification.[28,29] When the calcium intake is correspondingly high thickening of the bony cortex may result so that, instead of decreased density, the bones may, in fact, be more dense. Distinguishing between this entity, hypercalcemia and hypovitaminosis D can be difficult radiographically.

SUTURAL DIASTASIS FOLLOWING RAPID WEIGHT GAIN

Sutural diastasis has been considered a sign of acute raised intracranial pressure in children, especially under the age of 10 years. Capitanio and Kirkpatrick[30] described 3 children with nutritional deprivation who developed increased head circumference and cranial sutures following the correction of malnutrition. In 1970, two other reports[31,32] added 9 more children with these changes related to nutrition. The increased head circumference and separation of the cranial sutures (Fig. 18–13A and B) are due to cellular growth of the brain, when nutrition is improved in previously malnourished young children.[33] Although the sutural diastasis simulates increased intracranial pressure, there are no abnormal neurologic signs or symptoms. No increased intracranial pressure has been noted, and, in the one patient who had a pneumoencephalogram, the lateral ventricles were normal.

Distention of the stomach may be apparent on abdominal x rays in nutritional deprivation. One patient had a small bowel study done as part of the work-up for "failure to thrive." Thickened valvulae conniventes and separation of loops, noted (Fig. 18–14A) on an early examination, were normal (Fig. 18–14B) on a repeat examination 1 month later. The pathogenesis of the gastrointestinal changes is not known, but it was thought that these findings were due to edema, although the serum albumin was normal.

MILK-ALKALI SYNDROME

With excessive ingestion of milk and alkali, usually related to peptic ulcer disease, insoluble calcium and phosphate precipitates may occur.[34] This can result in a renal tubular deposition of calcium, with visible demonstration of nephrocalcinosis. To a certain extent the condition can be relieved by limiting the intake of calcium. Soft tissue calcification, usually periarticular in nature, is also a feature of this syndrome; however, the most common finding is that of calculi within the upper urinary tracts.[35]

FLUOROSIS

When fluorine is used to excess, probably above levels of 4-million parts per million in water, or in the treatment of osteoporosis, multiple myeloma or Paget's disease, certain side effects may be demonstrated.[36] Arguments persist as to the exact mechanism by which fluorine exerts its effects but, in all probability, it acts by decreasing the solubility of bone salts, thus impairing the process of osteolysis. Radiographically there are seen to be thickening and coarsening of the trabeculae and similar changes in the cortex. The overall result is one of increased density of the bony structure, although the underlying abnormality is sometimes difficult to visualize. Similar changes, of course, are seen in cases of myelosclerosis and myelofibrosis.

LEAD AND BISMUTH

Both these heavy metals have an affinity for bone and act by replacing calcium. In these days the effects of bismuth are rarely seen as it is seldom used for the treatment of syphilis in the growing child, except when the mother has been treated during pregnancy. However, cases of lead poisoning still present themselves where eating of lead paint has been the causative factor. In the growing child deposition of heavy metals is principally seen in the region of the metaphyses of long bones, particularly where there is accelerated growth, i.e. the knee, ankle, and wrist. Intoxication makes itself evident by the visualization of zones of increased density in this

region. Confirmation may be obtained by
the visualization of heavy metal content in the
GI tract, together with widening of the skull
sutures, indicating increased intracranial pressure.

GASTROINTESTINAL DISTURBANCES

In the last several years, there have been
exciting advances in the radiologic diagnosis
of gastrointestinal abnormalities that may
lead to nutritional disturbances. While the
clinical presentation is often non-specific,
gastrointestinal contrast studies may be crucial
in making the correct initial diagnosis, in
outlining the site and extent of disease or in
indicating the likely underlying entities requiring further investigation. In many of
these conditions roentgen interpretation relies upon subtle but characteristic findings.
It must be emphasized that x-ray abnormali-

ties may reflect pathologic anatomic changes
or physiologic disturbances.

MALABSORPTION SYNDROME

Sprue. This group of diseases includes
celiac diseases of children, nontropical sprue
(gluten-induced enteropathy, idiopathic
steatorrhea) and tropical sprue. Characteristic radiologic changes in the small intestine
are present in almost all patients during the
active phase of the disease.[37,38] The *sine qua
non* of this deficiency state include:

1. dilatation of small bowel loops, either
diffusely or more marked in the mid and
distal jejunum, and

2. hypersecretion, shown by dilution of
the barium suspension often with striking
flocculation and segmentation (Fig. 18–15A
and B). Frazier *et al.*[39] have shown that the
classic "deficiency pattern" of segmentation
within the small bowel is not necessarily

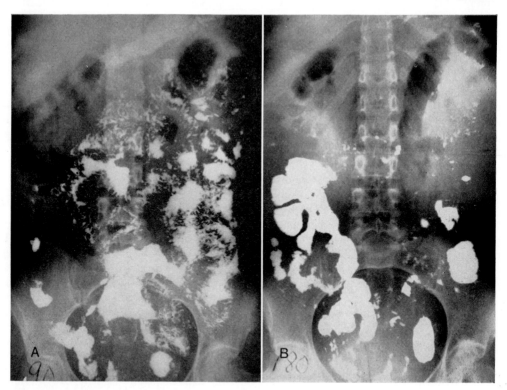

Fig. 18-15. Non-tropical sprue.
A. At 90 minutes, there is conspicuous fragmentation and flocculation of the barium suspension. Disordered motor activity is apparent.
B. At 180 minutes, segmentation of the contrast within ileal loops occurs, further reflecting hypersecretion.

associated with disordered motor function of the intestinal wall, but is dependent upon the quality of the contents of the intestinal lumen. The loops are flaccid and contract poorly, so that the transit time through the small bowel may be delayed. Little intrinsic change occurs in the mucosal folds. Their appearance is dependent upon the amount of secretions and peristaltic disorder. Short nonobstructive intussusceptions may transiently occur.[40]

The peculiar relationship of sprue and lymphosarcoma of the bowel[41] must be kept in mind. Not only may lymphoma present with sprue-like malabsorption,[42] but it has been shown that the incidence of lymphoma complicating well-documented chronic cases of adult celiac disease is about 7 per cent.[43] Roentgen study may be helpful in the distinction.[38]

Malabsorption and a sprue-like radiologic pattern may result from vascular insufficiency of the small bowel.[44,45] This must be suspected clinically if malabsorption appears in middle or later life, particularly if accompanied by abdominal angina or manifestations of atherosclerotic occlusive disease elsewhere. Abdominal aortography and selective arteriography may be crucial in establishing the diagnosis. Revascularization procedures have been shown to reverse the steatorrhea.[45]

Whipple's Disease (Intestinal Lipodystrophy). While the multisystem involvement of this disease is shown by the major clinical manifestations of diarrhea, steatorrhea, arthralgias, increased skin pigmentation, lymphadenopathy and serous effusions, it is the intestinal symptoms which are usually predominant by the time the diagnosis is established.

Small intestinal series demonstrate definite thickening of the mucosal folds in the jejunum and duodenum and only occasionally in the ileum (Fig. 18–16). The coarsened folds are frequently wild and redundant in outline and may present slightly nodular contours. No significant hypersecretion nor dilatation is shown; any flocculation or segmentation is minimal. There is normal peristaltic activity and transit time from stomach to cecum is within normal limits.[46,47]

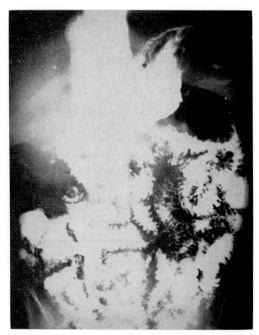

Fig. 18-16. Whipple's disease. Markedly prominent valvulae conniventes without hypersecretion or dilatation.

The diagnosis can be established by intestinal mucosal or lymph node biopsy. The small bowel villi are swollen and the lamina propria is infiltrated with macrophages containing PAS-positive bodies. These have been shown to be bacteria.[48] Improvement in the radiologic picture may parallel the clinical remission on long-term antibiotic therapy.[47]

Scleroderma (Diffuse Systemic Sclerosis). The hallmarks of sclerodermatous involvement of the alimentary tract are dilatation and a marked diminution in peristaltic activity. These reflect the underlying pathologic changes of collagen replacement of the muscular layers. Bacterial overgrowth in the intestinal lumen is now recognized as a major cause for steatorrhea in patients with scleroderma.

The esophagus is most commonly involved and presents hypomotility and some dilatation. Poor drainage results, and characteristic roentgen findings include failure of the esophagus to empty on prone films and stasis even in the erect position, with air-fluid levels (Fig. 18–17A).

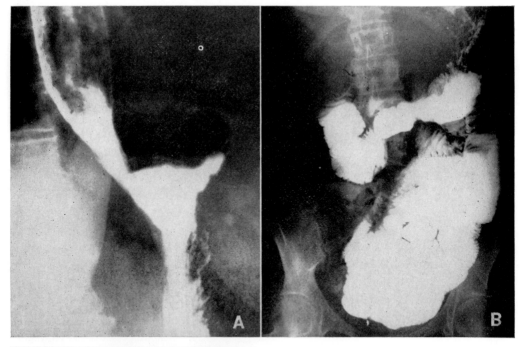

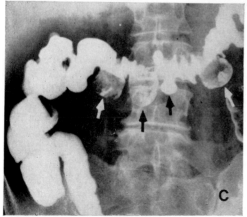

Fig. 18-17. Scleroderma.
A. Despite a non-obstructed lumen, differential fluid levels persist in the esophagus and stomach in the upright position.
B. Diffuse involvement of the small bowel results in gross dilatation, most evident in the descending duodenum and jejunum.
C. Asymmetric involvement of the colon is shown by large wide-mouthed pseudosacculatious (arrows).

In the intestines, large flaccid loops are seen without hypersecretion. The dilatation may appear most striking in the descending duodenum (Fig. 18–17B). Transit time is often markedly prolonged. Colonic dilatation and hypotonicity may also be present, with characteristic secondary pseudosacculations projecting from the antimesenteric border of the transverse colon (Fig. 18–17C).

Amyloidosis. The presence of malabsorption in some patients with amyloidosis has been well established.[49] In a report from the Mayo Clinic, Herskovic et al.[50] reviewed 103 patients with amyloidosis and were able to find 6 with documented steatorrhea. With known gastrointestinal involvement, the incidence of malabsorption may approach 50 per cent.[51] Radiologically, markedly diminished motility, conspicuous valvulae conniventes and, rarely, tumor-like deposits, scattered throughout the intestinal tract, may be present.[51]

Disaccharidase Deficiency. This is probably the most common abnormality of the small bowel in man, the only known mammal in whom lactase activity in the small intestine is maintained after weaning. Diarrhea, cramps and flatulence after milk ingestion clinically indicate the disorder, which can be easily confirmed roentgenologically.[52,53] When 50 gm of lactose are added to the usual barium mixture, characteristic changes occur in the small bowel series. These include dilution of the barium, particularly noticeable in the ileum and colon, and dilatation of the small bowel (Fig. 18–18). These effects are secondary to the ingress of water into the bowel lumen in response to the osmotic forces of the disaccharide. Rapid intestinal motility accompanies the dilatation.

Intestinal lactase deficiency occurs as an isolated phenomenon and is also common in a variety of intestinal disorders. This radiologic technique is the most valuable screening aid for it. The addition of lactose to the barium sulfate mixture does not interfere with the examination of the small bowel in patients without disaccharidase deficiency. When a lactase deficiency is discovered, a conventional small bowel examination with barium alone is indicated to identify any morphologic abnormality.[53]

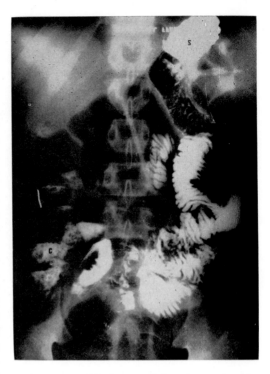

Fig. 18-19. Massive small bowel resection for volvulus following gastrojejunostomy. Few small bowel loops, primarily jejunal as shown by their mucosal pattern, remain between the stomach pouch (S) and the cecum (C).

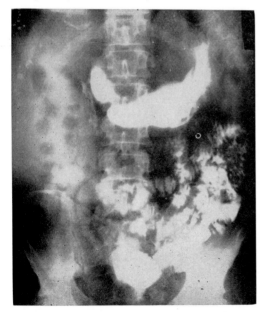

Fig. 18-18. Lactase deficiency. A barium-lactose mixture results in progressive dilution and hypermotility.

Small Bowel Resection. The severity of malabsorption after small bowel resection generally depends on the extent and site of resection, presence of the ileocecal valve and the condition of the remaining small bowel and other digestive organs.[54] These parameters of the "short-gut syndrmoe" can be evaluated by roentgen study (Fig. 18-19). On occasion, the exact extent of resection performed in the past is not known when malabsorption becomes a serious problem of management. Since the normal length of small intestine is variable, more important than knowledge of the length of bowel *removed* is an accurate appraisal of the length of the *remaining* functioning loops.

This is best accomplished by measurements derived from roentgen study after the passage of an opaque tube. This obviates the inaccuracy inherent in measuring the continuity of superimposed barium-filled loops.

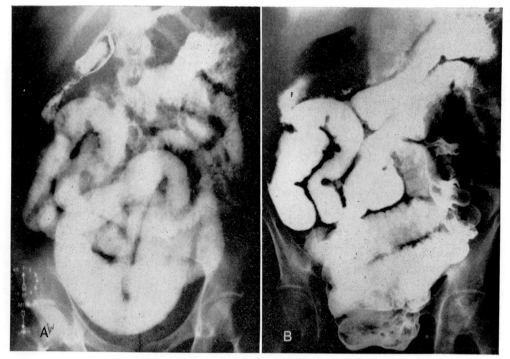

Fig. 18-20. Enteric fistula producing malabsorption following ileotransversostomy.
A. Dilatation and hypersecretion of small bowel loops. While there is no flocculation or segmentation, these changes constitute a sprue-like pattern.
B. During another examination, the fistula (F) between the distal ileum and descending duodenum is demonstrated.

Enteric fistulas (Fig. 18-20A and B) and inadvertent gastroileostomy[55] result in a similar condition by by-passing the absorptive mechanisms of the small bowel.

Diverticula, Blind Loops and Strictures. Common to all these conditions, which may result in malabsorption, is stasis of intestinal contents and bacterial overgrowth. Normally, the small bowel flora consists of predominantly gram-positive and anaerobic organisms. The ileocecal valve serves to separate two distinct groups of organisms: above, mainly streptococci, lactobacilli and fungi; below, coliforms, bacteroides, and anaerobic lactobacilli.[56] In a variety of disease states, an overgrowth of bacteria especially the anaerobic bacteroides, lactobacilli and clostridia may occur and cause steatorrhea by deconjugating and/or dehydroxylating primary bile salts in the intestinal lumen.[57]

Diverticulosis of the small bowel is readily recognized as multiple outpouchings without gross intrinsic contractility from the mesenteric borders of the loops. Blind loops may be a complication of (side-to-side) intestinal anastomoses, an obstructed postoperative loop, as in the afferent-loop syndrome following a Billroth II gastrojejunostomy (Fig. 18–21), or multiple strictures of the intestine, as in the stenotic phase of regional enteritis,[38] or post-radiation changes (Fig. 18–22). In radiation enteritis, lymphatic dilatation, bowel thickening and avascularity may also contribute to the malabsorption.[58]

Parasitic Diseases. The enteritis caused by infestation with Giardia lamblia[59] or Strongyloides stercoralis[60] is reflected by roentgen alterations, which may first draw the attention of the clinician to the diagnosis.

Dysgammaglobulinemia. Hypogammaglobulinemia may underlie a clinical pattern of repeated infections and chronic or intermittent diarrhea and mild steatorrhea. In 1966, Hermans and his co-workers[61] noted

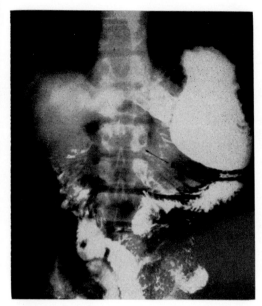

Fig. 18-21. Afferent loop syndrome. The massively distended, obstructed afferent loop (*A*) following a Billroth II gastrojejunostomy constitutes a blind loop leading to malabsorption.

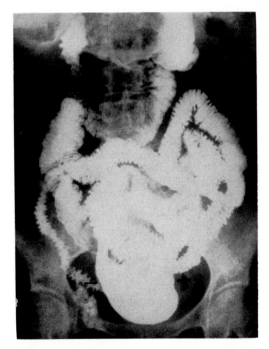

Fig. 18-22. Blind loop secondary to radiation effects. Stasis within a fixed, distended loop as a consequence of multiple strictures

the association of nodular lymphoid hyperplasia of the small intestine, with or without giardiasis, in cases of dysgammaglobulinemia with a disproportionate deficiency of the IgA and IgM components. These nodular hyperplastic lymphoid follicles in the lamina propria can be recognized as tiny, 1- to 3-mm filling defects, primarily in the duodenum and jejunum[62] (Fig. 18–23A and B). Their recognition may be an important clue in directing the clinician to evaluation of the gamma globulins and to intestinal biopsy for information necessary in management.

Uncommon Constitutional Disorders. In recent years, a number of uncommon systemic diseases in which malabsorption may be a significant complication of the syndrome have been recognized. Radiologic abnormalities in the gastrointestinal tract have been noted or are a conspicuous feature in the Canada-Cronkhite syndrome,[63] mastocytosis,[64] Degos' disease,[65] a-beta-lipoproteinemia (Bassen-Kornzweig syndrome),[66] and Waldenstrom's macroglobulinemia.[67]

PROTEIN-LOSING ENTEROPATHY

A major development during the past few years has been the recognition that excessive gastrointestinal protein loss is a major cause of hypoproteinemia seen in association with a wide variety of disorders. Loss of protein secondary to exudation through an inflamed or ulcerated mucosa (as in regional enteritis or ulcerative colitis) or secondary to obstructed outflow of the gastrointestinal lymphatics (as in lymphoma or Whipple's disease) is well known. In an excellent review, Waldmann[68] has compiled over 40 such gastrointestinal disorders and emphasizes that, in many of these patients with clearly defined gastrointestinal tract diseases, hypoproteinemia and edema may be the only clinical manifestations.

Giant Hypertrophy of the Gastric Mucosa (Menetrier's Disease). Massively enlarged gastric rugae may be the site of loss of plasma proteins, particularly albumin, into the lumen.[69] They characteristically are more prominent along the greater curvature and usually do not extend to involve the gastric antrum. The hypertrophied folds

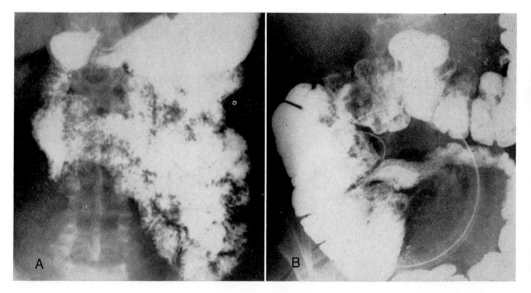

Fig. 18-23. Nodular lymphoid hyperplasia of the small intestine associated with hypogammaglobulinemia. Two different cases illustrate multiple punctate to nodular submucosal filling defects in the jejunum (A) and terminal ileum (B).

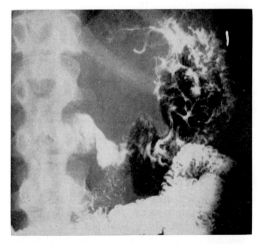

Fig. 18-24. Menetrier's disease. Markedly enlarged gastric folds, particularly prominent in the upper two-thirds of the stomach.

maintain pliability and are not nodular or ulcerated (Fig. 18–24).

Intestinal Lymphangiectasia. This recently recognized syndrome reflects a generalized disorder of the development of lymphatic channels. First defined by Waldmann in 1961, it is characterized by excessive loss of serum protein into the intestine with massive edema (often asymmetric), chylous effusions, hypoalbuminemia and hypogammaglobulinemia. The dilated lymphatic vessels invariably present in the intestinal wall may leak protein through an intact epithelium or may rupture and discharge their contents into the lumen of the gut. Isotopic studies are helpful in documenting the serum protein loss into the intestine.

The condition is being recognized with increased frequency and roentgen study plays an important role in its diagnosis. The characteristic appearance in the small bowel series consists of enlargement of the valvulae conniventes of both jejunum and ileum, increased secretions and minimal or absent dilatation of the bowel (Fig. 18–25A and B). The fold enlargement may assume a "cobblestone" pattern. Punctate filling defects occasionally seen may represent the enormously enlarged villi secondary to dilated submucosal lymphatics.[70]

Hypoalbuminemia, itself, below a level of 2.5 gm per cent due to other causes (*e.g.*, nephrosis or hepatic cirrhosis) may result in edema of the bowel with diffusely thickened intestinal folds,[71] but usually does not exhibit increased intraluminal secretions.

Lymphangiographic findings support the concept that this disease is a systemic lymphatic dysplasia.[70,72] In the lower extremities, either hypoplasia of lymph vessels or dilated, varicose lymphatics are present. In the abdomen, hypoplasia of lymph nodes or moderate contrast reflux into mesenteric lymphatics, associated with possible obstruction of the cisterna chyli and enlarged lymph nodes, have been demonstrated.

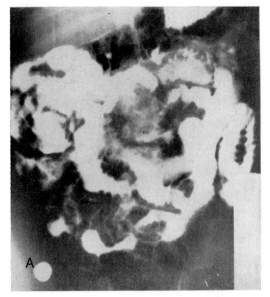

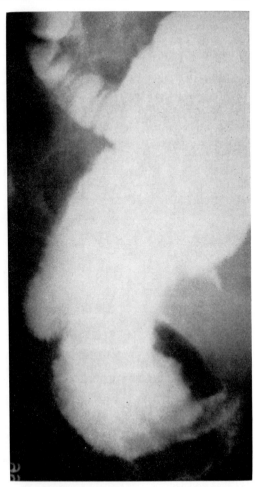

Fig. 18-25A and B. Intestinal lymphangiectasia. Three-year-old child with severe protein-losing enteropathy.

A. Prominent mucosal folds within mildly dilated small bowel loops containing increased secretions.

Fig. 18-26. Villous adenoma of rectum. Large circumferential mucosal mass with diffusely irregular contours.

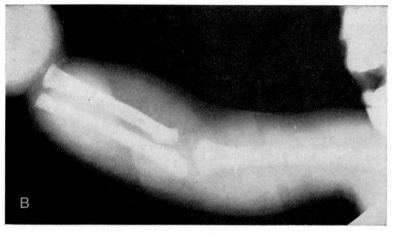

B. Edematous involvement of right upper extremity.

Villous Adenoma of the Colon. Among the neoplasms of the gastrointestinal tract which may produce excess secretion of mucus to result in severe protein loss, villous adenoma of the colon is one of the most prominent. It is commonest in the rectum, where, because of its usual soft consistency, it may be easily missed on digital palpation. On barium enema examination, it is revealed by its characteristically irregular polypoid or flame-shaped contours as the contrast agent fills in the interstices between its frond-like projections (Fig. 18–26).

BIBLIOGRAPHY

1. Gould: Am. J. Med. Sci., *223*, 569, 1952.
2. Barnett and Nordin: Brit. J. Radiol., *34*, 683, 1961.
3. Shapiro: Clin. Radiol. (Lond)., *13*, 238, 1962.
4. Harrison, Fraser and Mullan: Lancet, *1*, 1015, 1961.
5. Park: Pediatrics, *33*, 815, 1964 (supplement).
6. Steinbach: Radiol. Clin. N.A., *2*, 191, 1964.
7. Park, Guild, Jackson and Bond: Arch. Dis. Child., *10*, 265, 1935.
8. McLean and McIntosh: Am. J. Dis. Child., *36*, 875, 1928.
9. Kato: Radiology, *18*, 1096, 1932.
10. Albright, Burnett, Parson, Reifenstein and Roos: Medicine, *25*, 399, 1946.
11. Lasser: *Dynamic Factors in Roentgen Diagnosis*. Baltimore, The Williams & Wilkins Co., 1967.
12. Milkman: Am. J. Roent., *32*, 622, 1934.
13. Park: Harvey Lecture, *34*, 157, 1938–39.
14. Park and Jackson: J. Pediat., *13*, 748, 1938.
15. Sheldon: Proc. Roy. Soc. Med., *29*, 743, 1936.
16. Shahidi and Diamond: New Eng. J. Med., *262*, 137, 1960.
17. Britton, Canby and Kohler: Pediatrics, *25*, 621, 1960.
18. Moseley: J. Mount Sinai Hosp. (New York), *29*, 109, 1962.
19. Burko, Mellins and Watson: Amer. J. Roentgen. Rad. Ther., *86*, 447, 1961.
20. Ryan: Med. J. Australia, *1*, 844, 1962.
21. Lanzkowsky: Amer. J. Dis. Child., *116*, 16, 1968.
22. Holt and Hodges: *Year Book of Radiology*, 1958–1959 series, Chicago, The Year Book Medical Publishers, Inc. 1958, p. 51.
23. Wolbach: J. Bone and Joint Surg., *45*, 171, 1947.
24. Maddock, Wolbach, and Maddock: J. Nutr., *39*, 117, 1949.
25. Pease: J.A.M.A., *182*, 980, 1962.
26. Caffey: Am. J. Roent., *108*, 451, 1970.
27. Christiansen, Liebman and Sosman: Amer. J. Roent., *65*, 27, 1951.
28. Bauer and Freyberg: J.A.M.A., *130*, 1208, 1946.
29. Danowski, Winkler and Peters: Ann. Intern. Med., *23*, 22, 1945.
30. Capitanio and Kirkpatrick: Radiology, *92*, 53, 1969.
31. Sondheimer, Grossman and Winchester: Arch. Neurol., *23*, 314, 1970.
32. DeLevie and Nogrady: J. Pediat., *76*, 523, 1970.
33. Wincik and Rosso: J. Pediat., *74*, 774, 1969.
34. Wenger, Kersner and Palmer: Amer. J. Med., *24*, 161, 1958.
35. Burnett, Commons, Albright and Howard: New Eng. J. Med., *240*, 787, 1949.
36. Leone, Stevenson, Hilbish and Sosman: Amer. J. Roentgen., *74*, 874, 1955.
37. Laws, Booth, Shawdon and Steward: Brit. Med. J., *1*, 1311, 1963.
38. Marshak and Lindner: Seminars in Roentgenology, *1*, 138, 1966.
39. Frazier, French and Thompson: Brit. J. Radiol., *22*, 123, 1949.
40. Ruoff, Linder and Marshak: Am. J. Roentgen., *104*, 525, 1968.
41. Sherlock, Winawer, Goldstein and Bragg: *Progress in Gastroenterology*, Vol. II: New York, Grune & Stratton, 367–391, 1970.
42. Sleisenger, Almy and Barr: Amer. J. Med., *15*, 66, 1953.
43. Harris, Cooke, Thompson and Waterhouse: Amer. J. Med., *42*, 899, 1967.
44. Shaw and Mayard: New Eng. J. Med., *258*, 874, 1958.
45. Watt, Watson and Haase: Brit. Med. J., *3*, 199, 1967.
46. Clemett and Marshak: Radiol. Clin. N. A., *7*, 105, 1969.
47. Rice, Roufail and Reeves: Radiology, *88*, 295, 1967.
48. Trier, Phelps, Edelman and Rubin: Gastroenterology, *48*, 684, 1965.
49. Gilat and Spiro: Am. J. Dig. Dis., *13*, 619, 1968.
50. Herskovic, Bartholomew and Green: Arch. Intern. Med., *114*, 629, 1964.
51. Legge, Carlson and Wollaeger: Am. J. Roentgen., *110*, 406, 1970.
52. Laws and Neale: Lancet, *2*, 139, 1966.
53. Preger and Amberg: Am. J. Roentgen., *101*, 287, 1967.
54. Winawer, Broitman, Wolochowo, Osborne and Zamcheck: New Eng. J. Med., *274*, 72, 1966.
55. Katz and Karp: Am. J. Roentgen., *99*, 162, 1967.
56. Gorbach, Plaut, Nahas, Weinstein, Spanknebel and Levitan: Gastroenterology, *53*, 856, 1967.
57. Rosenberg, Hardison and Bull: New Eng. J. Med., *276*, 1391, 1967.
58. Tankel, Clark and Lee: Gut, *6*, 560, 1965.
59. Marshak, Ruoff and Lindner: Am. J. Roentgen., *104*, 557, 1968.
60. Louisy and Barton: Radiology, *98*, 535, 1971.
61. Hermans, Huizenga, Hoffman, Brown and Markowitz: Am. J. Med., *40*, 78, 1966.
62. Hodgson, Hoffman and Huizenga: Radiology, *88*, 883, 1967.
63. Orimo, Fujita, Yoshikawa, Takamoto, Matsuo and Nakao: Am. J. Med., *47*, 445, 1969.

64. Clemett, Fishbone, Levine, James and Janower: Am. J. Roentgen., *103*, 405, 1968.
65. Strole, Clark and Isselbacher: New Eng. J. Med., *276*, 195, 1967.
66. Stacy and Loop: Amer. J. Roentgen., *92*, 1072, 1964.
67. Khilnani, Keller and Cuttner: Rad. Clinics N. A., *7*, 43, 1969.
68. Waldmann: Gastroenterology, *50*, 422, 1966.
69. Reese, Hodgson and Dockerty: Am. J. Roentgen., *88*, 619, 1962.
70. Shimkin, Waldmann and Krugman: Am. J. Roentgen., *110*, 827, 1970.
71. Marshak, Khilnani, Eliasoph and Wolf: Am. J. Roentgen., *101*, 379, 1967.
72. Bookstein, French, and Pollard: Am. J. Digest Dis., *10*, 573, 1965.

Chapter

19

Clinical Evaluation of Nutrition Status

Harold H. Sandstead

AND

W. N. Pearson*

INTRODUCTION

Health has been defined as a "state of complete physical, mental and social well-being and not merely the absence of disease or infirmity."[1] Because "optimal" nutrition is necessary for "optimal" health, much attention has been directed toward its definition and measurement. For any given individual, many aspects of his nutritional status can be determined rather precisely if sufficient diagnostic acumen and equipment are available. Nutritional evaluation of large population groups requires utilization of the same basic methods. However, because time, personnel and facilities are frequently limiting, the observations obtained are often less complete, and in some instances, are less precise. The information necessary to provide a nutritional profile of a population has been summarized by a WHO expert committee[2] (Table 19-1). A complete discussion of all of the facets listed in the table is not possible in this chapter. Instead, aspects of the dietary, clinical, and biochemical procedures which have been found to be of value in nutritional evaluations will be discussed. A more detailed consideration of the nutritional biochemical measurements used in the evaluation of individuals may be found in Chapter 17. Other aspects of surveys are discussed in certain of the reviews cited in the bibliography.

* Died November 28, 1968.

PRE-SURVEY DATA COLLECTION

Prior to beginning a survey, certain data should be collected so that a general impression may be gained of the level of nutriture that is likely to be encountered in the population. From information concerning agricultural production, and the methods of food processing, storage and marketing, rough estimates can be made of the per capita intake of major foodstuffs. Socio-economic and cultural data are of use in the characterization of the distribution of food within families and the overall population as determined by income and customs.

Anthropometric information such as birth weights and lengths, and the heights and weights of older children, which are in part influenced by nutrition, can sometimes be obtained from public health statistics. The incidence of infectious diseases such as tuberculosis, measles, and dysentery, as well as parasitic diseases such as malaria, hookworm and schistosomiasis, may also be available from public health records. This latter information is of value because of the relationship of malnutrition to these diseases in developing countries. A disease which illustrates this interrelationship is measles. In Western Europe and the United States, measles is of little consequence as far as childhood mortality is concerned. However, in many underdeveloped countries, because it often exacerbates underlying protein-calorie malnutrition, it is a major contributor to

Table 19-1. Information Needed for Assessment of Nutritional Status

Sources of Information	Nature of Information Obtained	Nutritional Implications
(1) Agricultural data Food balance sheets	Gross estimates of agricultural production Agricultural methods Soil fertility Predominance of cash crops Overproduction of staples Food imports and exports	Approximate availability of food supplies to a population
(2) Socio-economic data Information on marketing, distribution and storage	Purchasing power Distribution and storage of foodstuffs	Unequal distribution of available foods between the socio-economic groups in the community and within the family
(3) Food consumption patterns Cultural-anthropological data	Lack of knowledge, erroneous beliefs and prejudices, indifference	
(4) Dietary surveys	Food consumption	Low, excessive or unbalanced nutrient intake
(5) Special studies on foods	Biological value of diets Presence of interfering factors Effects of food processing (*e.g.*, goitrogens)	Special problems related to nutrient utilization
(6) Vital and health statistics	Morbidity and mortality data	Extent of risk to community Identification of high-risk groups
(7) Anthropometric studies	Physical development	Effect of nutrition on physical development
(8) Clinical nutritional surveys	Physical signs	Deviation from health due to malnutrition
(9) Biochemical studies	Levels of nutrients, metabolites and other components of body tissues and fluids	Nutrient supplies in the body Impairment of biochemical function
(10) Additional medical information	Prevalent disease patterns, including infections and infestations	Interrelationships of state of nutrition and disease

infantile mortality.[3] A second example is the well known relationship between hookworm infestation and iron deficiency anemia.

Data obtained in the pre-survey evaluation should be interpreted with caution. Unfortunately, even in the most sophisticated countries, the reliability of public health, socio-economic and production information is sometimes suspect. Birth weights, for ex- ample, may be available from the cities but not from the rural areas. There may be much "folklore" but little reliable data regarding the incidence of certain diseases. Sometimes a disease is rampant but unrecognized in rural areas, while recognized but almost non-existent in the urban communities. Agricultural production figures may be in error for various reasons. Because of these potential pitfalls, pre-survey information should be used only as a rough guide with the understanding that it may be drastically modified after the actual survey is finished.

POPULATION SAMPLING

It is obvious that under most circumstances, only small populations can be examined in their entirety and that no population is sufficiently homogeneous to allow the use of a sample of one subject. Therefore, it is necessary to obtain an appropriate sample, which, when examined, will provide information from which valid inferences can be made concerning the entire population. Publications are available that treat this subject fully.[4-6] A summary of their content follows.

The Interdepartmental Committee on Nutrition for National Defense, which became the Nutrition Program of the Center for Disease Control, Health Services and Mental Health Administration, used a number of sampling approaches in its thirty-three surveys of foreign populations and the ten states surveyed in the U.S. National Nutrition Survey. In some instances, well-developed census and vital statistics data were available and were used in planning, while in others, the data were incomplete or unavailable. In these latter surveys, the sample was evolved by an "educated guess" based on general information concerning conditions in the country.

The survey of the West Indies[7] represents an example of a foreign survey in which it was possible to select the sample with the assistance of an expert and cooperative office of statistics. During the 1960 census, the islands had been divided into "enumeration districts." For the survey, these districts were grouped geographically and 8 of the 40 areas deliberately selected for study while, from the 32 remaining districts, 14 were randomly selected. Within each enumeration district, 15 dwelling units were randomly selected and the residents asked to participate in the survey. A roughly similar plan was followed in the U.S. National Nutrition Survey.[8]

Rarely can samples be selected so ex-quisitely. Often the country or region being surveyed has extremely varied topography which makes movement from place to place difficult. Such was the case in Ecuador.[9] In that country, credible census data made it possible to select geographic regions for study which contained populations with differing types of food production and consumption. Within each geographic region, reasonably accessible villages were randomly selected for study. In the two major cities (Quito and Quayaquil) the samples were taken on the basis of economic and occupational considerations.

When it is necessary to conduct a survey in limited time, biased sampling may be used. When this is done, those segments of the population that are thought to be in the greatest risk of malnutrition are examined. This usually includes pre-school children and pregnant and lactating women. Because malnutrition is most often associated with poverty, the lower socio-economic groups are studied. If individuals in this social class are found nutritionally adequate, groups higher on the socio-economic scale may usually be presumed to be nutritionally sound.

Accessibility of the high risk age groups for examination is often poor. Therefore, special efforts and preparations are necessary to accomplish their examination. Community leaders, teachers, nurses, social workers and physicians are frequently helpful in persuading mothers to come to Maternal and Child Health Clinics where they and their children can be examined. Examination of school children is usually more easily accomplished because school officials can usually assist in arranging for their examination.

CLINICAL APPRAISAL

The clinical appraisal of nutritional status includes four major aspects:

1. Historical evaluation of the dietary and medical experience.

2. Anthropometric measurement of growth, development and fatness.

3. Physical examination for signs consistent with deficiencies.

4. Biochemical assessment.

HISTORICAL EVALUATION

Surveys of the dietary intakes of populations have often been carried out independent of other clinical measurements of nutrition. Obviously, when carried out alone, they are of limited usefulness. Information obtained concerning the dietary habits of a population or of an individual is complementary to other aspects of the evaluation. The dietary data, when considered in terms of the overall survey results, are particularly valuable for the planning of remedial measures which may be necessary.

The usual aim of a dietary survey is to determine the foods and the quantity eaten by members of the target population, as well as the factors which influence their availability and consumption. The approaches used to gain this information usually include aspects of the following:[10] The homemaker or the person consuming the food may be asked to estimate (prospectively and retrospectively) the amounts and kinds of food eaten. Quantitation may be achieved either by actual measurement (weight or volume) of the food, or by estimation, using visual or descriptive comparisons of quantity. A diary may be utilized in prospective studies. The information gained may or may not be related to meals and eating patterns. Usual, unusual and new foods may all be included or only the usual, and their frequency may be recorded. The time interval covered may be as short as 1 to 3 days, 7 days, or occasionally longer. The distribution of food within the family or group, as well as economic condition of the group or individual, may be included.

Obviously the gathering of this information may be difficult and the techniques are not foolproof. The difficulties encountered in obtaining and interpreting dietary information have been exhaustively considered.[10-15] Problems include the duration of the survey, the reliability of the participants, the method of expression of the data, the reliability of available tables of food composition and the appropriateness of having food analysis performed. The following discussion will briefly consider these problems.

It is the consensus of experienced investigators that a 1-day dietary study of children or of adults does not give an accurate picture of the customary food intake.[16-24] More reliable "average" nutrient intake data may be obtained if the number of days studied is expanded to 7.[20] Observation periods longer than 7 days are unnecessary and difficult. Unfortunately, field conditions often preclude the study of individuals for longer than 1 to 3 days. Hence, 1-day records have frequently been used with full recognition of their limitations.[25-26] One- to 3-day records were utilized in the international surveys of the ICNND[27-28] with reasonably satisfactory results. Although the observations of Flores[13] may tend to refute the accuracy of the findings, short term surveys will probably continue to be used in under-industrialized regions where diets are monotonous. In this setting, the data are thought to be more representative of the intake than in the more economically advanced countries. If logistics allow, a 3-day record is obviously more desirable.

The gathering of accurate dietary information, which includes socio-cultural data, is one of the most demanding aspects of a nutrition survey. This is in part because of the intimate nature of food habits. The uncooperative, un-comprehending or dishonest informant is the bane of the interviewer. It has been shown that, when subjects keep their own food records, reliability may suffer.[29] This was true for housewives across the socioeconomic and intellectual scale.[30] To improve the reliability of dietary information, cross check methods have been devised. The same questions are asked in different ways at different times in the interview.[31] While this procedure will ferret out unreliable subjects, it is time consuming and, therefore, is utilized primarily in nutrition clinics or in studies where time is less important than is usually the case in the field. To circumvent some of the need for cross checking, socioeconomic information may be used to evaluate the history by inference. The combined problems of reliability and accuracy make it apparent that the quality of data obtained is dependent upon the skill, personality and sensitivity of the interviewer.

The reduction of food intake data to nutrient content (calories, protein, vitamins, etc.) has been traditional in the analysis of dietary survey data. This has usually been accomplished by the use of published food composition tables.[32-34] The composition of exotic foods or dishes, if known, has been obtained from food tables extant in the country or area of survey. For example, the INCAP-ICNND Food Composition Tables,[35] published in Spanish and English, have been particularly useful in Latin America. Most tables present analyses in terms of the edible portion of the food, so that food preparation and cooking losses are corrected. Estimates of the losses of vitamins in large-scale cooking may be obtained from data compiled by the U.S. National Research Council.[36] The nutrient losses from various vegetables and other foods prepared on a small scale, as in the home, may be obtained from a publication by Teply and Derse.[37]

Food composition tables have a number of serious limitations.[12,38,39] Perhaps their greatest flaw is that they present the total amount of a nutrient present, without consideration of its availability. Some nutrients, such as carotene and iron, are not well absorbed when present in certain foods. This is because some foods contain constituents that decrease the availability of certain nutrients.[3] Unfortunately, knowledge in this area is incomplete and appropriate correction of food tables to account for availability has not been possible.

In spite of their limitations, tables of food composition have been found to provide data amazingly close to the analyzed values for certain nutrients in various foods.[15,28,40,41] Chemically analyzed protein and calorie contents of the diets of approximately 300 individuals were found usually to be within 10 per cent of the calculated value. On the other hand, calculated values for fat tended to be considerably greater than the analyzed content.[12] Thus, food composition tables provide respectable estimation of certain nutrients under most circumstances.

From a clinical point of view, the detailed calculation of nutrient intake is not what is needed when one is confronted with an individual patient. Qualitative information concerning the adequacy of the diet is more to the point. This type of information can be obtained by reducing historical information to an assessment of the intake of the food groups, and appraising the cooking habits and economic status of the household. The frequency of intake of specific groups of food is particularly important. From this type of information, a qualitative estimate can be made as to whether the subject in question has had adequate intake of the essential nutrients. The unwieldy, time consuming calculation of the intake of individual nutrients can be avoided and clinically useful information rapidly obtained. The use of computers may be helpful in the refinement of the information.

After the food intake of a family or population has been measured and calculated into nutrients, the results must be expressed. Three methods have been used. These are the per capita intake, the "man value" and the "nutrition unit."

Per capita intake is useful for comparison of the availability of foodstuffs at time X vs time Y. It is easily calculated and provides important information in regard to the population as a whole. However, it may obscure the fact that a significant portion of the population is eating poorly due to factors such as economic status, and age. For example, while 80 per cent of a population may be eating well, the remaining 20 per cent may be malnourished, or older children and young adults may be well nourished, while infants and the elderly are malnourished.

The so-called "man values" were developed because of the limitations of per capita intake. In this procedure, family members are assigned fractional "man values" depending on age and sex. For example, in a family of four, the husband might be assigned 1.0, the wife 0.8, and the children 0.4 and 0.3 respectively. Thus the "man value" size of the family would be 2.5 and the daily consumption of the entire family would be divided by 2.5 rather than 4.0 to express intake in "man values." Nutrient intakes for each individual can also be calculated separately. However, because the intake of a single member of the household, such as the father, may markedly influence the apparent intakes of the remainder of the family, this system may be inequitable at times.[11]

To compensate for the shortcomings of the "man value" procedure, the "nutrition unit" concept has been developed. For example, the U.S.D.A. has used 3,000 calories as the basic unit and has expressed individual requirements as multiples or fractions of this unit.[42]

The results of dietary surveys may be interpreted in terms of international or national guidelines developed by agencies in various countries. This subject has been extensively reviewed by Young,[43] while the U.S. National Research Council has summarized the standards of eleven countries.[44] The recommended allowances for the U.S. and Canada are discussed in Chapter 9, p. 403 of this text. The recommended dietary allowances suggested by the Food and Nutrition Board of the National Research Council of the United States[44] are customarily used in this country, while those of the British Medical Association[45] are used in the United Kingdom. The ICNND has developed a guide for the interpretation of nutrient intake data obtained on surveys[4] (Table 19–2). The ICNND standards for calorie intakes are those of the U.S. National Research Council,[44] which were adopted from those proposed by F.A.O.[46] It should be pointed out that the ICNND guidelines apply only to a standard adult male.

The medical history should pertain to those aspects of health which may influence the individual's response to his nutritional experience. Information of obvious interest includes the history of infections, accidents, operations, and allergies. A general system review is most appropriate, as is the pregnancy history. In surveys of large populations, the depth to which the medical history can be explored will be limited by the pressures of time. In the case of the individual patient, however, a detailed history should be obtained as it is often helpful and necessary in the assessment of a given clinical problem.

ANTHROPOMETRIC EVALUATION

The assessment of growth and development in relation to age and sex is of particular importance in the nutritional appraisal of infants, children and adolescents. Retardation of growth and development is one of the nonspecific hallmarks of nutritional deprivation. Clinically, a variety of deficiency syndromes have been implicated. Although numerous anthropometric measures have been recommended, height (or length), weight, and skinfold thicknesses are generally the most informative.[47] In children, head, chest and arm circumference measurements are also useful,[48] while in adolescents, the degree of genital and secondary sexual development is an index of nutritional experience.[49,50] The non-specificity of these measurements must be kept in mind when findings are interpreted. Clearly, other varieties of ill health may also cause severe degrees of retardation, as may the combined effects of undernutrition and recurrent infection or parasitic disease.

Table 19-2. Suggested Guide to Interpretation of Nutrient Intake Data for Physically Active Young Adult Males*

Nutrient	Deficient	Low	Acceptable	High
Niacin (mg/day)	<5	5–9	10–14	≥15
Riboflavin (mg/day)	<0.7	0.7–1.1	1.2–1.4	≥1.5
Thiamine (mg/1000 calories)	<0.2	0.2–0.29	0.3–0.4	≥0.5
Ascorbic acid (mg/day)	<10	10–29	30–49	≥50
Vitamin A (IU/day)	<2000	2000–3499	3500–4999	≥5000
Calcium (gm/day)	<0.3	0.30–0.39	0.4–0.7	≥0.8
Iron (mg/day)	<6.0	6–8	9–11	≥12
Protein (gm/kg body weight)	<0.5	0.5–0.9	1.0–1.4	≥1.5

* Twenty-five years of age, 170 cm in height, weighing 65 kg.

If possible, it is desirable that height-weight observations on children from less developed areas of the world be compared with measurements obtained on well-nourished children from the same ethnic and geo-graphic background, as well as to standards from more affluent societies. Unfortunately, few standards for ethnic groups in the less developed countries are available. Standards for American children have been compiled

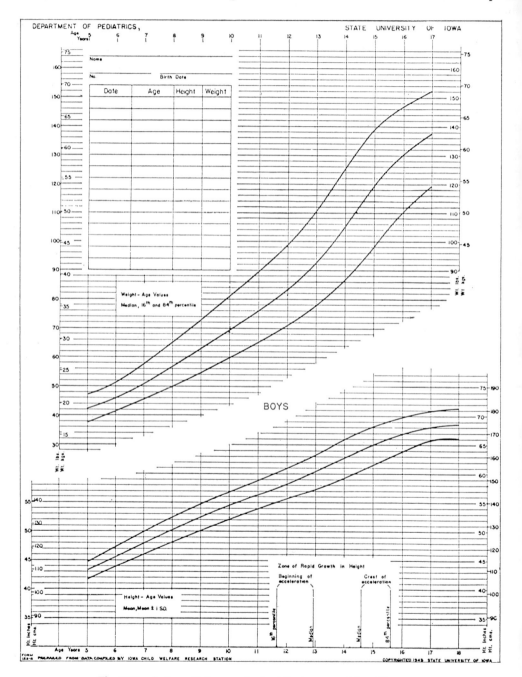

Fig. 19-1. Jackson-Kelly growth chart for boys, aged 5 to 18 years.

by several investigators. Those by Jackson and Kelly,[51] the so-called "Iowa Growth Charts," are based on data collected between 1920 and 1940 from 13,500 height and 11,000 weight observations of 1500 boys and 1500 girls in the State University of Iowa Well-Infant Laboratory and Pre-School Laboratory, as well as elementary and high schools in Iowa City. An example of their growth chart for boys 5 to 18 years of age is shown in Figure 19-1. Though Garn[52] considers these norms a generation obsolete, they are widely known and are acceptable for most purposes. Whether they should be used as normal standards for children world-wide, may be open to debate. As a practical matter, though, they or other American or English standards are usually the ones used on surveys and in clinics as a comparative index.

Growth charts are particularly useful for the determination of the growth pattern of an individual child over time. By plotting the child's growth, it can be ascertained how he relates to the normal, as well as whether events have occurred which have caused growth to slow. Unfortunately, in surveys of populations, longitudinal observations of individuals are almost never possible. The charts are then used to describe the population in terms of the norm. The factors which contributed to the population's position on the chart may in part be defined by the historical, physical and biochemical findings of the survey. These include socio-economic and dietary factors as well as infectious diseases and genetic characteristics. The last, while fundamental to growth potential, is probably the least important factor in the pathogenesis of the short stature of economically deprived populations. Secular trends in size of populations previously considered "short," as well as the height of their upper classes, support this concept. Factors such as maternal and childhood nutrition and infectious diseases appear to have far greater influences than has been accepted in the past.[53] Present knowledge indicates that the ultimate height and development of man is the result of many factors which influence the growth process from the time of conception to maturity.

The weight and height standards most frequently used for adults are the Medical Actuarial Tables of 1912.[54] Although new height-weight tables have since been published[55] in which "desirable weights" for men and women are given according to type of "body frame," the method for objective determinations of the "body frame" was not described. To permit such a judgment, Garn[52,56] has proposed the lateral bony chest measurement (by x ray) as a stature reference.

The collection of height and weight data requires a careful technician and accurate, good quality instruments. Ideally, the subjects to be weighed should be nude. This is often impractical. As a compromise, they should be dressed in similar amounts of clothing and an estimate made of the weight of the clothing. Nude weight then can be derived. Standing height should be taken with the head in a standard position. This may be accomplished by use of a bar projecting vertical to the measuring rod. The bar should be attached to the measuring rod in such a way that it can be positioned lateral to the subject's face in a position where the external auditory meatus and lateral angle of the orbit can be "lined up" adjacent to the bar, thus putting them on a line horizontal to the floor. The apex of the skull can then be measured with a second bar which projects vertically from the measuring rod. The measuring rod obviously must be vertical to the floor or a flat platform. Length of infants should be measured by placing the infant in a caliper box.

Fatness is an indirect indicator of the previous calorie intake. Fatness can be derived from measurements of body specific gravity, the lean body mass (by ^{40}K whole body counting), the fat free body (by deuterium oxide or T_2O), as well as by soft tissue roentgenograms or caliper measurement of the skin fold. The latter technique is suitable for surveys and, although it has been maligned,[57] if carried out properly, it will provide data which correlate reasonably well with the other techniques, such as the soft tissue roentgenogram.[58,59] Garn's[52] experience concerning the utility of various body sites for fat-fold measurements is summarized in Table 19-3. The lower thoracic site is the best location for measurement of all individuals including the obese; however, for the practical reason of accessi-

Table 19-3. Utility of Various Body Sites for Fat-Fold Measurements

Site	Comments
Deltoid-triceps	Difficult to avoid underlying muscle. Impractical in obese individuals.
Subscapular	Practical but hard to locate and replicate beyond 3 to 4 cm of fat.
Lower Thoracic	Practical up to 5 to 6 cm of fat.
Iliac	Impractical in fatter individuals.
Abdominal	Practical but difficult to replicate in very thin individuals.

bility, the subscapular and the deltoid-triceps sites are usually used, even though obesity increases the error. The method of triceps and subscapular skinfold measurement may be found in the manual of the ICNND.[4]

The combined measurements of skinfold and arm circumference have been used in the evaluation of calorie and protein reserves of children.[60,62] This measurement appears to be a reasonably good index of muscle mass and indirectly, therefore, of protein intake. While fatness does not correlate well with linear growth and hence adequate nutriture, muscularity does.[62] This measurement should, therefore, be an integral part of the evaluation of children.

PHYSICAL EXAMINATION

The physical examination is probably the least sensitive portion of the clinical evaluation for the detection of nutritional deficiencies. This does not detract from its value, however, because in surveys, if individuals are found to have physical abnormalities consistent with nutrient deficiencies, it is likely that large numbers of individuals in the population have "sub-clinical" deficiencies which may be detected by laboratory means. In the past, classical deficiency diseases were not rare in what are now the developed countries of the world. Fortunately, this is no longer true. Today, in these countries, the physician often finds physical abnormalities which are entirely non-specific in

etiology, but which, experience has shown, may be associated with nutrient deficiency. These lesions tax the observational abilities of the examiner, i.e., they are best recognized by an "experienced hand." In the less developed countries, classical deficiency diseases, such as kwashiorkor, pellagra, beri-beri, rickets and scurvy, are not so rare. The abnormalities they produce are easily recognized. At the same time, the frequency of non-pathognomonic abnormalities often found in the malnourished is also greater. Physicians working in this setting are often acutely aware of malnutrition and, therefore, possibly are more likely to recognize illnesses related to severe undernutrition than physicians from the developed countries. Ironically, they may miss instances of marginal nutritional status because their criteria of normality tend to become altered by their patient population.

The parts of the body which most commonly exhibit abnormalities consistent with malnutrition include the integument, eyes, mouth, skeleton and nervous system. Almost all of the abnormalities which occur are non-specific. Trauma, exposure to the elements, and allergies may produce physical abnormalities which closely resemble the adverse effects of deficiencies. It seems possible that deficiency disease may in some instances increase susceptibility to trauma.

A vexing problem encountered in clinical surveys is that of examiner bias. Different examiners often grade the same lesion differently. The more non-specific and subtle the abnormality, the more divergent are the opinions. For example, judgments of degree of leanness have been found to relate to the examiner's own body build, in the case of women subjects to the contours of his wife.[63] Standardization of observers must be carried out at regular intervals throughout the survey.[57] This can be done by the use of slides which illustrate lesions consistent with nutritional deficiency and by duplication and comparison of findings between observers.

Certain of the clinical signs which may be associated with nutrient deficiency are listed in Table 19–4. In addition to the following discussion, they have been considered by others.[4,64]

Table 19-4. Some Clinical Signs of Probable Nutritional Significance

Area of Examination	Clinical Sign
Hair	Lack of luster
	Easy pluckability
Skin	Follicular hyperkeratosis
	Petechiae, purpura
	Pellagrous dermatitis
	Scrotal and vulval dermatitis
Face	Nasolabial seborrhea
Eyes	Xerosis of conjunctivae
	Keratomalacia
	Corneal vascularization
	Circumcorneal injection
	Blepharitis
	Photophobia
	Bitot's spots
Lips	Cheilosis
	Bilateral Angular Fissures
	Bilateral Angular Scars
Tongue	Edema
	Glossitis
	Magenta Tongue
Gums	Swollen Interdental Papillae
	Bleeding
Teeth	Mottled enamel
Glands	Thyroid enlargement
	Parotid enlargement
Skeleton	Enlarged wrist epiphysis
	Bossing of the skull
	Beading of the ribs
	Bowed legs
Neurological	Absent vibratory sense in the feet
	Hyporeflexia
	Decreased position sense
	Tender calf muscles
Extremities	Dependent edema

CUTANEOUS MANIFESTATIONS OF DIETARY DEFICIENCY

Healthy skin results from adequate nutrition, protection from trauma, and cleanliness. Poorly nourished skin appears to be less resistant to exogenous insults. Perhaps for this reason, persons suffering from poor nutrition are found to have abnormalities of the integument which do not fit any clear descriptive category. Although the skin lesions mentioned in this section have traditionally been thought of as due to deficiency of a single nutrient, the fact that single nutrient deficiencies almost never occur outside of the experimental laboratory suggests that they are probably due to mixed deficiencies, one nutrient perhaps being predominant.

An apparent association between follicular hyperkeratosis and vitamin A deficiency was first reported by Frazier and Hu.[65] Their patients had rough, dry skin with hyperkeratotic plugs in hair follicles. Current evidence suggests that the relationship of vitamin A lack to this lesion is tenuous. An early study that indicated they might not be related was done in Britain during World War II.[66] Recent nutrition surveys have supported this concept.[67] Using supplements other than vitamin A, such as essential fatty acids and the vitamin B complex, others have found that deficiencies of these nutrients may, in some way, contribute to its occurrence.[68-70] It appears from these observations that the finding of vitamin A deficiency in individuals with this lesion was coincidental.

The principal form of seborrheic dermatitis associated with nutrient deficiency is the so-called "naso-labial seborrhea." It is found when secretion by sebaceous glands of the face have been excessive. This lesion can be produced in man by riboflavin[71,72] and pyridoxine deprivation.[73,74] Defective metabolism of essential fatty acids has been proposed as an explanation.[75] Of interest is the fact that, in several surveys, the incidence of this lesion has not been found to correlate with the historical intake of riboflavin.[67]

The classic cutaneous lesions of pellagra occur symmetrically on areas of the body, such as the back of the hands, the face and neck, that are exposed to sunlight and on surfaces subjected to recurrent trauma, such as the elbows. They are hyperpigmented and desquamating. Sometimes, if severe, they are erythematous and resemble a second or third degree burn. Therapeutically, they respond to niacin and/or tryptophan. According to some investigators they may be partially responsive to riboflavin.[76] A rash which may be confused with that of pellagra is the rash observed in infants with severe protein calorie malnutrition (kwashiorkor). This rash typically occurs on the legs, perineum and trunk, in areas not necessarily exposed to sunlight. Of interest is the fact that this cracked, peeling, hyperpigmented, crazy pavement like rash is not found in all cases. A finding which suggests that other deficiencies occurring in association with protein deficiency may contribute to its occurrence.

The cutaneous manifestations of ascorbic acid deficiency (scurvy) include perifollicular hemorrhages, petechiae and ecchymosis. Perifollicular hyperkeratosis and curious corkscrew like abnormalities of the hair of the extremities and trunk may be seen. Ecchymoses typically occur on weight bearing surfaces, such as the back of the arms, the buttocks and in and around joints.[77-81]

OCULAR LESIONS OF DIETARY DEFICIENCY

The eye is a sensitive target of certain nutritional deprivations. Its vulnerability to vitamin A lack is dramatically illustrated by the fact that A deficiency is one of the major causes of blindness in the world. The numerous lesions of the eye which may occur as a consequence of nutritional deficiencies have been reviewed by McLaren.[82]

The Bitot spot originally described by Hubbenet[83] and later named after Bitot[84] is a rare lesion composed of foamy, greyish white mucoid secretions and epithelial debris. It typically occurs on the exposed portion af the lateral bulbar conjunctiva. Until recently, it was thought pathognomonic of vitamin A deficiency. It is now apparent that there is no correlation between its presence and the vitamin A status of adults determined biochemically.[85] It seems likely that the Bitot spot is caused by abnormalities in the secretions and the conjunctival epithelium of the eye which occur because of poor nutriture in other dietary factors. When found, the nutritional status of the patient should receive further investigation.[86]

When A deficiency is severe, the epithelium of the conjunctiva becomes keratinized. As a result, it takes on a dull, wrinkled appearance in place of its usual bright, moist luster. This change, xerosis, may also affect the cornea, although drastic corneal changes leading to blindness may precipitously occur before conjunctival changes are seen.[87]

Liquefactive necrosis of the cornea (keratomalacia) may follow xerophthalmia. Bacteria may then invade the eye. The iris may prolapse and the lens and other ocular contents may be extruded.[88] The rapidity with which these events take place, makes ocular changes consistent with A deficiency, a medical emergency.

Corneal vascularization from in-growth of capillaries from the limbic plexus was described in riboflavin deficient patients by Sydenstricker et al.[89] On the basis of their studies, it was thought diagnostic of the deficiency until studies were carried out in riboflavin deficient volunteers.[90,91] As in the case of the Bitot spot, it appears that this non-specific lesion may sometimes reflect a generally poor nutriture. It is not possible at present to define what deficiencies contribute to its occurrence. Currently, its presence should be considered an indication for a more extensive nutritional evaluation.

Fissuring and sogginess of the outer canthi (blepharitis) may sometimes be found in nutritionally deprived individuals. According to Vilter et al.,[74] in some it reflects deficiency of pyridoxine and/or other B vitamins.

ORAL LESIONS OF NUTRIENT DEFICIENCIES

The lips, tongue and membranes of the mouth mirror the adverse effects of nutrient deficiencies on the entire gastrointestinal tract. Though non-specific and non-diagnostic, the effects are easily recognized. Therefore, examination of the mouth is an important part of the clinical nutritional evaluation.

Edema, accompanied by flaking, crusting and cracking of the epithelium of the lips (cheilosis) is often found in riboflavin deficiency, but may also be a consequence of exposure to the elements or constant mouth breathing. The relationship of the riboflavin status to the response of the lips to these other factors is unknown. Experimentally, this lesion has been produced in man by riboflavin deprivation,[71,92-94] and by feeding the riboflavin antagonist galactoflavin.[95] In contrast, urinary riboflavin excretions have not been found to correlate well with the presence of this lesion in nutrition surveys.[67] The apparent nutritional non-specificity of this lesion is attested to by its also being observed in patients with niacin[96] or iron deficiency.[64]

Angular stomatitis or fissuring at the angles of the mouth also occurs in riboflavin deficiency.[71,91] It has also been reported in patients with iron or pyridoxine deficiency.[64] Other causes of this lesion include herpes stomatitis and ill-fitting dentures. When caused by nutrient deficiency, the lesions are almost always bilateral, a finding less constant when non-nutritional factors are the cause. Deep fissures often leave scars which may be seen at the time of examination.

The tongue is particularly sensitive to nutritional disease. Atrophy of its filliform papillae, hypertrophy of its fungiform papillae, erythema, pain, loss of taste and fissure formation may be produced by a variety of deficiencies, occurring alone or in concert. The nutrients in question include, iron, zinc, folic acid, vitamin B_{12}, pyridoxine, niacin and riboflavin.[97-99] In addition, riboflavin deficiency may sometimes result in the tongue taking on a magenta hue.[71] The fact that nutritional disease in man almost always results in deficiency of several nutrients at one time, makes it difficult to implicate a specific nutrient as the cause of clinical abnormalities of the tongue in any given instance. Appreciation of the significance of these tongue lesions should prompt the clinician to investigate the status of individuals in which they are found in more depth. Non-nutritional abnormalities also occur on the surface of the tongue. One long thought due to a deficiency, but now no longer thought related to nutrition, is geographic atrophy of the tongue papillae.

The gingiva is frequently found abnormal in surveys of groups without ready access to dental care. The most frequently found lesions reflect chronic infection of the gum margin and include hypertrophy of the gum as well as inflammation and atrophy. The margin of the gum may be tender and may bleed easily. Rarely, hemorrhages and swelling of the papillae are found. Abnormalities of these types are usually thought to be due to poor hygiene and do not necessarily relate to nutritional status. The changes of scurvy are those of marginal bleeding, hemorrhagic interdental papillae and, occasionally putrefaction of the gum.[100] With putrefaction, the bone may be destroyed and the teeth may fall out. Similar loss of teeth may occur in patients with periodontal disease due to poor hygiene. In the latter instance, the role of nutrition in the loss of the teeth is a subject of debate. The observations of Krook et al.[101] suggest that a low calcium to phosphate ratio may be a factor. The reader is referred to Chapter 27 for a more complete discussion of the nutritional factors which have been implicated.

Teeth reflect the effect of nutritional events which occurred at the time the teeth were formed. For example, excessive ingestion of fluoride may lead to chalky white mottling and brownish discoloration of enamel. Characteristically, these individuals have a lower incidence of caries compared to those not exposed to fluoride.[102,103] Constituents of the diet such as carbohydrate and phosphate, as well as the consistency of the diet influence the occurrence of caries. This aspect of dental health is discussed in Chapter 27. The examining physician should be as alert as the dentist to the abnormalities which may be observed in the teeth, as skilled dental examiners are not always available to perform this critical portion of the examination.

LESIONS OF GLANDS ASSOCIATED WITH NUTRIENT DEFICIENCY

Enlargement of the parotid gland has been observed fairly frequently in certain populations in association with malnutrition.[104] It also has been described in patients with diabetes mellitus.[105] The specific cause of the enlargement is unknown. Protein and/or B vitamin deficiencies have been associated with the lesion in some populations.[104] Gross enlargement is easily recognized, because the lateral facial contour obscures the lobules of the ear. When not so evident, enlargement may be detected by palpation. It is usually firm, non-tender and easily outlined.

Nutritional causes of thyroid enlargement include iodine deficiency,[106] large excesses in iodine intake[107] and the presence of goitrogenic substances in water or the diet.[108,109] Palpation of the thyroid with the head slightly extended will reveal whether the gland is enlarged. Empirically, it has been suggested that a thyroid which is palpably 4 to 5 times enlarged, is a grade I goiter. Glands of this size are usually readily visible when the head is thrown back. If the gland is easily visible with the head in its normal position, it is classified as grade II. Palpation is not needed for diagnosis. A grade III goiter is very large and can be recognized from a considerable distance.[110]

NEUROLOGICAL, SKELETAL AND EXTREMITY ABNORMALITIES IN NUTRITIONAL DISEASE

Abnormalities in neurologic function may result from a variety of deficiencies, the best known of which are vitamin B_{12} and thiamine. Pyridoxine, pantothenic acid, niacin, and riboflavin have also been implicated according to some authorities.[111,112] In this country, neurologic abnormalities associated with malnutrition are most frequently found in chronic alcoholics, individuals who have had surgery on the gastrointestinal tract, and who have subsequently developed a malabsorption syndrome, and in people with pernicious anemia. Although examination of these individuals most often reveals abnormalities in peripheral nerve function, careful examination not uncommonly will reveal abnormalities in central function as well. On surveys, neurologic assessment is usually limited to the lower extremities. Deep tendon reflexes, vibratory sense, response to firm palpation of the calf muscle and gait are the parameters tested. A more detailed evaluation is appropriate when an individual patient is evaluated. Descriptions of the neurological syndromes associated with nutritional deficiencies may be found in reviews[111,112] and most neurologic texts.

Rickets and osteomalacia are the major unequivocal nutritional diseases of the skeleton (Chapter 20, p. 572). In most instances, inadequate exposure to sunlight and/or an inadequate dietary intake of vitamin D is the cause. The disease may be observed in otherwise well-nourished children or, as is often the case in developing countries, with other deficiencies.[113] In rare instances, malabsorption syndrome or an inborn error of metabolism are implicated in its occurrence. Bowing of the legs, bossing of the skull, enlargement of the epiphysis at the wrist, and enlargement of the costochondral junctions of the chest are the classic findings in children, while deformities of the pelvis and other weight bearing bones are found in adults. These abnormalities are readily recognized on physical examination and by x ray. The etiology of osteoporosis is less clear than that of rickets and osteomalacia. Some authorities have contended that it is due to calcium deficiency.[114,115] Resolution of this problem is in any case beyond the scope of this chapter.

Recognition of osteomalacia may be difficult without roentgenograms[116,117] for bone density. Unfortunately, these are often unavailable on surveys. X-ray films are also useful in the assessment of bone development in children. Standard x-ray pictures of the wrist were obtained for this purpose on many of the surveys of the ICNND and the National Nutrition Survey.[7,8]

The musculature of individuals, and presumably their protein status, can be assessed by measurement of the diameter of the biceps muscle.[61] This measurement, in addition to examination of the scapula for winging, has become a standard part of the examination of children for assessment of musculature.[7,8]

Edema of the legs, in the absence of underlying diseases such as congestive failure, varicose veins or nephrotic syndrome, is often an indicator of severe protein deprivation. This sign, which should alert the physician to this possibility, is routinely examined for in all nutritional evaluations.

LABORATORY ASSESSMENT OF NUTRITIONAL STATUS

The contribution of biochemistry to the assessment of nutritional status is shown in

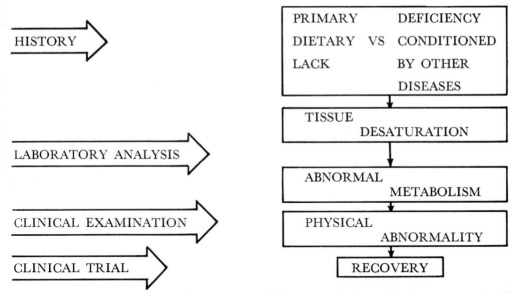

Fig. 19-2. Evolution of Nutritional Disease and Methods of Study.

Figure 19–2. Generalization beyond this is unwise as each nutrient has its own characteristic metabolic fate and therefore must be considered separately. Some of the laboratory measurements that have proven most useful in determination of nutritional status will be summarized here with interpretive guidelines. A more extensive exposition of the biochemical methods used in nutritional evaluation is presented in Chapter 17, p. 523. The selection of laboratory procedures for the nutritional evaluation of a population or of an individual depends on the purpose of the evaluation, as well as the availability of laboratory facilities and the time limitations on the study.

Samples of blood or urine are the usual materials obtained for laboratory assessment. Their collection, handling and storage is critical to the attainment of reliable data. The activity of the subjects may influence the data. It is therefore desirable that the subjects are sampled under similar conditions. Under most circumstances, the subjects should have fasted for 12 hours and sampling should be done the morning after between 8 and 10 A.M. In addition, their physical activity should have been similar. Obviously certain of these aspects of activity can be only irregularly controlled on most surveys.

Collection of timed urine specimens may prove difficult on surveys. The collection of "casual samples," and the relating of their content of vitamins or metabolites to the creatinine excretion has been shown satisfactory for survey purposes.[118–123] Because young children excrete less creatinine than adults, and larger amounts of certain vitamins per gram of creatinine, interpretive standards have been developed to take this into account.[123] The need for this is illustrated by the following: 7- to 9-year-old girls fed 2 mg of riboflavin daily excrete 55 per cent of their intake or 1900 μg/gm creatinine. In contrast, women 20 to 25 years of age will excrete 25 per cent of the same intake, or 35 μg/mg creatinine.[124] Specimen collection and handling, as well as the expression of data have been reviewed in more detail elsewhere.[123,125]

Calorie Status. Currently available biochemical tests are of little use in the appraisal of energy intake. Fortunately, anthropometric measurements such as height, weight, and skinfold thickness permit a reasonable approximation of this facet of nutritional status.

Protein Status. The procedures available for the assessment of protein nutriture are best characterized as "inadequate."

Though serum albumin and total protein are reduced in severe protein deficiency,[126,127] they are insensitive indices and their use as an index of the protein status of individuals and/or populations provides objective information for only the most severely deficient. Neither measurement has been useful in the evaluation of marginal to mild degrees of protein deprivation. Of the two measurements, the total serum protein is the least sensitive and, is therefore, of dubious value as a measure of body protein stores.[128,129] Indeed, populations consuming inadequate amounts of dietary protein may show elevated rather than depressed total plasma protein concentrations because of increases in the globulin fraction which often occur in response to parasitic infection or chronic disease.[130] Some have suggested that carefully determined plasma albumin levels relate well to protein status.[131-133] Others suggest the measurement is insensitive.[134,135] In the opinion of the author, the latter view, that plasma albumin concentrations become abnormal only after protein deprivation has been severe, is correct.[136]

Blood amino acid concentrations have been suggested as potentially useful in population studies.[137-139] It appears, however, that they are readily altered by the recent dietary intakes of protein and may, therefore, give a false impression of protein availability.[136]

Excretion of products of protein metabolism have also been proposed as indices of protein nutriture. The relationship of creatinine excretion to height appears useful,[140-141] as does the ratio of urinary nitrogen to creatinine. Nitrogen/creatinine ratios have been shown to be greater in countries where large amounts of protein are consumed than in countries where intake of protein is lower.[142,143] The sulfate/creatinine ratio has also been proposed as a measure of the qualitative and quantitative aspects of dietary protein intake.[144] Excretion of hydroxyproline, an index of collagen formation, is thought to reflect active growth.[145,146] Therefore, the urinary content of this amino acid related to creatinine (millimols/millimol) has been suggested as an indirect index of the protein status of children.[147]

The analysis of anagen hair roots for volume, protein or DNA appears to be a sensitive, quantitative measurement of protein-calorie nutriture. According to Bollet,[148] these parameters of hair growth become abnormal before serum albumin and transferrin levels decrease in protein malnourished individuals. If further study substantiates these observations, this index of assessment of protein status may prove to be the most sensitive yet available.

Iron. Iron deficiency anemia is probably the most common anemia in the world. It is therefore one of the more frequently observed abnormalities found on any nutrition survey. Most commonly, severe deficiency is related to some conditioning factor, such as parasitism, geophagia or abnormal bleeding. Infrequently, dietary deficiency alone will result in severe anemia. An associated deficiency of some other hematemic agent such as folic acid is not uncommon. The anemia which occurs may also be modified by non-nutritional factors, such as chronic infection or altitude. Because the pathogenesis of the anemia may therefore be complex, utilization of the hemoglobin level alone as an index of iron nutriture, is probably unwise. The mean corpuscular hemoglobin concentration (MCHC) value, which may be calculated from the hemoglobin and hematocrit, can be utilized with more confidence.

If facilities allow, more specific measurement of iron status, such as the serum iron concentration and transferrin saturation,[149,150] should be utilized in the assessment. The major difficulty encountered in their use on surveys is the fact that there is a diurnal variation in their concentrations in blood.[151] Specimens should, therefore, be obtained in the morning. The most sensitive clinical index of iron stores is the histochemical examination of the bone marrow for hemosiderin.[152] Obviously this method is not adaptable to surveys. Interpretative standards are presented in Table 19-5.

Vitamin A. Because liver stores of the vitamin are large, the serum level usually does not reflect the recent intake. In spite of this, consistently low serum levels in a population are considered good evidence for an inadequate level of vitamin A nutriture.

The serum carotene level relates more closely to intake and absorption than does the level of vitamin A. Carotene usually ranges from 75 to 150 μg/100 ml in individuals consuming reasonable amounts of carotenoid containing foods. Because little carotene is normally stored in the body, the serum level decreases rapidly when it is unavailable. Low levels may be found in blood within 2 months of withdrawal.[66] Thus the serum concentration is a relatively sensitive index of the dietary intake and/or the absorption of carotene. Serum carotene and vitamin A concentrations do not always correlate.[48] This is due

Table 19-5. Suggested Guide to Interpretation of Blood Data
(National Nutrition Survey)

	Deficient	Low	Acceptable
Hemoglobin (gm/100 ml):			
Men	<12.0	12.0–13.9	≥14.0
Female*	<10.0	10.0–11.9	≥12.0
Children (2–5 yrs)	<10.0	10.0–10.9	≥11.0
Children (6–12 yrs)	<10.0	10.0–11.4	≥11.5
Hemoglobin Concentration (MCHC): (gm/100 ml RBC)			
For all ages and sex		30	≥30
Serum Iron (μg/100 ml)			
Men		<60	≥60
Women*		<40	≥40
Children (2–5 yrs)		<40	≥40
Children (6–12 yrs)		<50	≥50
Transferrin Saturation (%)			
Men		<20	≥20
Women*		<15	≥15
Children (2–5 yrs)		<20	≥20
Children (6–12 yrs)		<20	≥20
Red Cell Folacin (mμg/ml)			
All ages	<140	140–159	≥160–650
Serum Folacin (mμg/ml)			
All ages	< 3.0	3.0–5.9	≥ 6.0
Serum Albumin (gm/100 ml)			
Adults	< 2.8	2.8–3.4	≥ 3.5
Children (1–5 yrs)		<3.0	≥ 3.0
Children (6–17 yrs)		<3.5	≥ 3.5
Serum Ascorbic Acid (mg/100 ml)			
All ages	< 0.1	0.1–0.19	≥ 0.2
Plasma Carotene (μg/100 ml)			
Adult*		<40	≥40
Children (1–17 yrs)		<40	≥40
Plasma Vitamin A (μg/100 ml)			
All ages	<10	10–19	≥20

* Non-pregnant, non-lactating

to the fact that vegetables contain non beta-carotene carotenoids which are detected in the chemical assay for carotene.[153] The interpretive guide recommended by the ICNND and used in the U.S. National Nutrition Survey of 1967–1970 is shown in Table 19–5.

Ascorbic Acid. The average plasma ascorbic acid concentration of a population is a rough index of its ascorbic acid intake. While the white blood cell-platelet ascorbic acid concentration is a superior measure of tissue stores,[68,154] it is technically difficult and is therefore impractical for mass application. The relationship of the dietary intake to the plasma ascorbic acid value is also reasonably good when applied to individuals (Table 19–6). This interpretive guide is probably valid over the entire age spectrum, if the intake is calculated on the basis of body weight. Data available on children suggest that an intake of approximately 1.5 mg of ascorbic acid/kg. of body weight or less will result in a serum concentration in the vicinity of 0.1 mg/100 ml. The ICNND and National Nutrition Survey guidelines for the interpretation of serum ascorbic acid levels are shown in Table 19–5.

Thiamine. Thiamine status can be assessed directly by measurement of the urinary excretion of the vitamin per 24 hours or per gram of urinary creatinine, and indirectly by assay of the erythrocyte transketolase activity. An interpretive guide for the urinary excretion of thiamine is shown in Table 19–7. Using this guide, a good correlation has been found between the average thiamine/creatinine ratios of adult populations and their average thiamine intake/1000 calories, as ascertained by dietary survey.[124]

Table 19-7. Suggested Guide for Thiamine Excretion† (National Nutrition Survey)

Age Group	Deficient	Low	Acceptable
1–3	<120	120–175	≥176
4–6	<85	85–120	≥121
7–9	<70	70–180	≥181
10–12	<60	60–180	≥181
13–15	<50	50–150	≥151
Adult*	<27	27–65	≥66

† Values are micrograms per gram of creatinine
* Non-pregnant, non-lactating

The erythrocyte transketolase activity also correlates well with thiamine status.[155,156] This enzyme functions in the hexose monophosphate shunt, in which pentose and TPNH are generated by the degradation of hexose. Thiamine pyrophosphate is essential in this sequence; therefore, erythrocytes from thiamine deficient individuals show a reduced rate of metabolism of ribose 5-phosphate. This assay has not received extensive use in surveys. It is expected that it will in the future, in part because of the refinements developed by Warnock,[157] which have increased its sensitivity and reliability.

Riboflavin. The urinary excretion of riboflavin is the current index of choice for the assessment of the riboflavin intake.[94] The relationship between intake and excretion of riboflavin is more direct than it is for thiamine. This is because riboflavin itself is its own principal urinary metabolite. In contrast, there are more than 20 urinary metabolites of thiamine. Thiamine itself rarely represents more than one-half of the total quantity excreted. An interpretive guide for riboflavin excretion is shown in Table 19–8.[123]

Riboflavin status may also be assessed by measurement of the erythrocyte content of the vitamin.[158–159] Although this technique appears to be quite sensitive and a practical index of status, it has not received wide application in individual patients or in the field.

Niacin. The biochemical evaluation of niacin status is complicated by the fact that tryptophan is its precursor. Approximately

Table 19-6. Ascorbic Acid Intake vs. Serum Ascorbic Acid Level

Intake/Day (mg)	Serum Ascorbic Acid (mg/100 ml)
<10	<0.1
10–29	<0.2
30–70	0.2–0.5
≥70	0.6–1.4

Table 19-8. Suggested Guide for Riboflavin Excretion† (National Nutrition Survey)

Age Group	Deficient	Low	Acceptable
1–3	< 150	150–499	≥ 500
4–6	< 100	100–299	≥ 300
7–9	< 85	85–269	≥ 270
10–15	< 70	70–199	≥ 200
Adult*	< 27	27–79	≥ 80

† Values are in micrograms per gram of creatinine
* Non-pregnant, non-lactating

1 mg of niacin may be derived from 60 mg of tryptophan.[160] The major metabolic products of niacin in man are N^1methylnicotinamide and its pyridone. These products are derived from both dietary niacin and tryptophan. The use of urinary N^1methylnicotinamide per gram of creatinine as an index of niacin status has proven less than satisfactory. As an alternative, the ratio of pyridone to N^1methylnicotinamide excretion has been proposed.[161]

Folic Acid. Assessment of the folate nurture of large populations is unwieldy as the method for assay of the vitamin is microbiological.[168] In spite of this problem, the experience of the National Nutrition Survey indicates that measurement of serum and/or erythrocyte concentrations of folic acid is a valuable component of the laboratory assessment. The guidelines for folate status used in the National Nutrition Survey are presented in Table 19–5.

Other Nutrients. Space does not allow consideration of the laboratory assessment of other nutrients such as iodine, zinc, other trace elements, pyridoxine, tocopherol, cyanocobalamin, vitamin D, and other vitamins. Some are considered in the ICNND manual[4] or in Chapter 17, p. 523. Deficiencies of certain of these nutrients account for specific clinical syndromes. With the exception of iodine, however, their satisfactory laboratory assessment in large populations has not been reported. Difficulties in methodology are in part responsible. Lack of apparent clinical importance of others has also been a factor. It is expected that, with increased understanding of their metabolic functions in man, and with improvements in methodology, the assessment of their concentrations in the blood and urine of population groups will be recognized as needed additional information for the assurance of adequate nutritional health of the public.

Interpretation of Laboratory Results. Some have found it perplexing that there is often a poor correlation between biochemical and clinical findings on surveys. This is, of course, to be expected because of the nonspecific nature of many clinical lesions and the wide spectrum of nutritional disease. In the usual course of events, laboratory abnormalities become evident sometime before physical effects are seen. Figure 19–2 illustrates this disparity. Plough and Bridgeforth[67] have considered this subject in detail. They express the opinion, as have others, that the laboratory and dietary intake data are more apt to show a more positive relationship than are laboratory and physical findings. The clinician should, therefore, not be discouraged when his clinical examination of a patient is non-diagnostic. The history and the laboratory assure him of a reasonable degree of diagnostic accuracy and sensitivity.

BIBLIOGRAPHY

1. W.H.O. International Health Conference, New York, 1946.
2. W.H.O. Technical Report Series No. 258, W.H.O., Geneva, 1963.
3. Scrimshaw: In *Mammalian Protein Metabolism*, edited by Munro and Allison, Vol. 2, New York, Academic Press, 1964.
4. Interdepartmental Committee on Nutrition for National Defense: *Manual for Nutrition Surveys*, 2nd Ed., Washington, D.C. 1963.
5. Doll (ed.): *Methods of Geographical Pathology*. London, Blackwell Scientific Publication Ltd., 1959.
6. Perez, Scrimshaw and Munoz: Bull. W.H.O., *18*, 217, 1958.
7. Interdepartmental Committee for Nutrition in National Defense: *West Indies Nutrition Survey*, Bethesda, Md., N.I.H., 1962.
8. *National Nutrition Survey Guidelines and Procedures*, Nutrition Program Center for Disease Control, HSMHA, Rockville, Md., 1970.
9. Interdepartmental Committee for Nutrition in National Defense: *Ecuador Nutrition Survey*, Bethesda, Md., N.I.H., 1960.
10. Young and Trulson: Am. J. Publ. Hlth., *50*, 803, 1960.

11. Leitch and Aitken: Nutrition Abstr. and Rev., *19*, 507, 1950.
12. Whiting and Leverton: Am. J. Pub. Hlth., *50*, 815, 1960.
13. Flores: Am. J. Clin. Nutrition, *11*, 344, 1962.
14. Stefanik and Trulson: Am. J. Clin. Nutrition, *11*, 335, 1962.
15. Eagles, Whiting and Olson: Am. J. Clin. Nutrition, *19*, 1, 1966.
16. Young, Chalmers, Church, Clayton, Gates, Hagan, Steele, Tucker, Wertz, and Foster: Univ. Mass. Agr. Exp. Sta. Bulletin 469, Amherst, Mass., 1952.
17. Roberts and Waite: J. Home Ec., *17*, 80, 1925.
18. Waite and Roberts: J. Am. Diet. Assoc., *8*, 323, 1932.
19. Koehne: J. Am. Diet. Assoc., *11*, 105, 1935.
20. Trulson: Assessment of Methods of Dietary Intake, Ph.D. Thesis, Harvard University, 1951.
21. McHenry, Ferguson and Gurland: Canad. J. Pub. Hlth,, *36*, 355, 1945.
22. Yudkin: Brit. J. Nutr., *5*, 117, 1951.
23. Young, Franklin, Foster and Steele: J. Am. Diet. Assoc., *29*, 459, 1953.
24. Chappell: Brit. J. Nutrition, *9*, 323, 1955.
25. Anderson and Sandstead: J. Am. Diet. Assoc., *23*, 101, 1947.
26. Eads and Meredith: Public Health Rpts., *63*, 777, 1948.
27. Schaefer: In *Nutrition, A Comprehensive Treatise*, edited by Beaton and McHenry, Vol. 3, New York, Academic Press, 1966.
28. Combs and Wolfe: U.S.P.H.S. Repts., *75*, 707, 1960.
29. Leitch: Proc. Nutr. Soc., *14*, 86, 1951.
30. Morrison, Russell and Stevensen: Brit. J. Nutr., *3*, V, 1949.
31. Burke: J. Am. Diet. Assoc., *23*, 1041, 1947.
32. Watt and Merrill: Composition of Foods— Raw Processed, Prepared. Agricultural Handbook No. 8, Washington, D.C. 1950.
33. Nutritive Value of Foods, Home and Garden Bulletin No. 72, U.S.D.A., Washington, D.C., 1960.
34. *Food Values of Portions Commonly Used* (10th ed), Church and Church, Philadelphia, J. B. Lippincott Co., 1966.
35. INCAP-ICNND, Food Composition Tables for use in Latin America ICNND, Bethesda, Md., N.I.H., 1961.
36. Committee on Food Composition Tables of Vitamin Retention in Large Scale Cooking, N.A.S.-N.R.C., Washington, D.C. 1946.
37. Teply and Derse: J.A.D.A., *34*, 836, 1958.
38. Mayer: Postgrad. Med., *28*, 295, 1960.
39. Harris: Fed. Proc., *22*, 138, 1963.
40. Valassi and Reynolds: Am. J. Clin. Nutrition, *18*, 203, 1966.
41. Miller and Payne: J. Nutrition, *74*, 413, 1961.
42. Stiebling, Monroe, Coons, Phipard and Clark: U.S.D.A. Misc. Publication No. 405, 1941.
43. Young: In *Nutrition, A Comprehensive Treatise*, edited by Beaton and McHenry, Vol. 2, New York, Academic Press, 1964.
44. Recommended Dietary Allowances Publication 1694, N.A.S.-N.R.C., Washington, D.C., 1968.
45. Report of the Committee on Nutrition, British Medical Association, London, 1950.
46. Food Agr. Org. U.N.-F.A.O. Nutrition Studies 15, Calorie Requirements, 1957.
47. Brozek *et al.*: Human Biology, *28*, 111, 1956.
48. Sandstead, Carter, House, McConnell, Horton and VanderZwaag: Am. J. Dis. Child., *121*, 455, 1971.
49. Gómez-Leal, Castillo, Sanchez-Medel, González-Pineda and Gomez-Mont: Rev. Invest. Clin. Organo Hosp Enfermedades Nutr. Mex, *10*, 247, 1968.
50. Prasad and Oberleas: Ann. Int. Med., *73*, 631, 1970.
51. Jackson and Kelly: J. Pediatrics, *27*, 215, 1945.
52. Garn: Am. J. Clin. Nutrition, *11*, 418, 1962.
53. Guzman: In *Malnutrition, Learning and Behavior*, edited by Scrimshaw and Gordon, Cambridge, Mass, MIT Press, 1968.
54. Medical Actuarial Mortality Investigation, New York, *1*, 38, 1912.
55. Halpern, Glenn and Goodhart: J.A.M.A., *173*, 1576, 1960.
56. Garn: Ann. N.Y. Acad. Sci., *110*, 429, 1963.
57. Bridgforth: Am. J. Clin. Nutrition, *11*, 433, 1962.
58. Garn and Gorman: Human Biology, *28*, 407, 1956.
59. Garn: Science, *124*, 178, 1956.
60. Jellife: World Health Organ. Monograph Ser. No. 53, 1966.
61. Jellife and Jellife: J. Trop. Pediat., *15*, 177, 1969.
62. Frisancho and Garn: Am. J. Clin. Nutr., *24*, 541, 1971.
63. McGanity and Darby: In *Methods for Evaluation and Nutritional Adequacy and Status*, edited by Spector, Peterson and Friedemann. Department of the Army, Office of the Quartermaster General, Washington, D.C., 1954.
64. Jolliffe, Ed.: *Clinical Nutrition*, 2nd ed., New York, Paul B. Hoeber, Inc., p. 334, 1960.
65. Frazier and Hu: Arch. Int. Med., *48*, 507, 1931.
66. Hume and Krebs: Medical Rsch. Council Special Rpt. Series 264, London, 1946.
67. Plough and Bridgforth: U.S.P.H.S. Rpts., *75*, 699, 1960.
68. Srikantia and Belavady: Ind. J. Med. Res., *49*, 109, 1961.
69. Clarke and Okoro: J. Trop. Med. Hyg., *65*, 27, 1962.
70. McLaren: Am. J. Clin. Nutrition, *18*, 467, 1966.
71. Sebrell and Butler: U.S.P.H.S. Rpts., *54*, 2121, 1939.
72. Horwitt, Hills, Harvey, Liebert and Steinberg: J. Nutrition, *39*, 357, 1949.
73. Mueller and Vilter: J. Clin. Invest., *29*, 193, 1950.
74. Vilter, Mueller, Glazer, Jarrold, Abraham, Thompson and Hawkins: J. Lab. & Clin. Med., *42*, 335, 1953.

75. Mueller and Iacono: Am. J. Clin. Nutrition, *12*, 358, 1963.
76. Prinsloo *et al.*: Proc. Nutr. Soc. S. Africa, *3*, 66, 1963.
77. Crandon, Lund and Dill: New Eng. J. Med., *223*, 353, 1940.
78. Ralli and Sherry: Medicine, *20*, 251, 1941.
79. Vilter, Woolford and Spies: J. Lab. & Clin. Med., *31*, 609, 1946.
80. Cutforth: Lancet, *1*, 454, 1958.
81. Chazan and Mistilis: Am. J. Med., *34*, 350, 1963.
82. McLaren: *Malnutrition and the Eye*, New York, Academic Press, 1963.
83. Hubbenet: Ann. Oculist (Paris), *2*, 263, 1860.
84. Bitot: Gaz. Hebd. Sci. Med. Bordeaux, *10*, 284, 1863.
85. Darby, McGanity, McLaren, Paton, Alemu and Medhen: U.S.P.H.S. Rpts., *75*, 738, 1960.
86. McLaren: Brit. Med. J., *1*, 926, 1963.
87. McLaren: E. African Med. J., *37*, 321, 1960.
88. Sydenstricker, Sebrell, Cleckley and Kruse: J.A.M.A., *114*, 2437, 1940.
89. Boechrer, Stanford and Ryan: Am. J. Med. Sci., *205*, 544, 1943.
90. Hills, Liebert, Steinberg and Horwitt: Arch. Int. Med., *87*, 682, 1951.
91. Sebrell and Butler: U.S.P.H. Rpt., *53*, 2282, 1939.
92. Jolliffe, Fein and Rosenblum: New Eng. J. Med., *221*, 921, 1939.
93. Horwitt: Bull. U.S. Nat. Rsch. Council, Washington, D.C., *116*, 1948.
94. Horwitt, Harvey, Hills and Liebert: J. Nutrition, *41*, 247, 1950.
95. Lane, Alfrey, Mengel, Doherty and Doherty: J. Clin. Invest., *43*, 357, 1964.
96. Goldsmith: Am. J. Clin. Nutr., *6*, 479, 1958.
97. Dreizen: Arch Envir. Hlth, *5*, 66, 1962.
98. Follis: *Deficiency Disease*, Springfield, Charles C Thomas, 1958.
99. Henkin, Schechter, Hoy *et al.*: J.A.M.A., *217*, 434, 1971.
100. Lind: *Treatise on Scurvy*, 2nd ed., London, Millar, 1757.
101. Henrickson, Krook, Bergman *et al.*: Svensk Tandlak T, *62*, 329, 1969.
102. Dean, Arnold and Elvove: Pub. Health Rept., *57*, 1155, 1942.
103. Russell, Littleton, Leatherwood, Sydow and Greene: U.S.P.H.S. Rpt., *75*, 717, 1960.
104. Sandstead, Koehn and Sessions: Am. J. Clin. Nutr., *3*, 198, 1955.
105. Davidson, Leibel and Berris: Ann. Int. Med., *70*, 31, 1969.
106. Follis: Am. J. Trop. Med. Hyg., *13*, 137, 1964.
107. Suzuki *et al.*: Acta Endocrinologica, *50*, 161, 1965.
108. Jirousek and Reisenaur: Endocrinologia Experimentalis, *1*, 271, 1964.
109. Gaitan, Island and Liddle: Trans. Assoc. Amer. Physicians, *82*, 141, 1969.
110. Perez, Scrimshaw and Munoz: *In Endemic*

111. Victor and Adams: Am. J. Clin. Nutr., *9*, 379, 1961.
112. Hornabrook: Am. J. Clin. Nutr., *9*, 398, 1961.
113. Aboul-Dahab and Zaki: Am. J. Clin. Nutr., *13*, 98, 1963.
114. Walker, A. P.: Am. J. Clin. Nutr., *16*, 327, 1965.
115. Anon: Lancet, *1*, 180, 1970.
116. Exton-Smith, Millard, Payne, Wheeler: Lancet, *2*, 1153, 1969.
117. ———: Lancet, *2*, 1154, 1969.
118. Aykroyd, Sebrell, Jolliffe, Shank, Lowry, Tisdall, Moore, Wilder and Zamecnik: Canad. Med. Assoc. J., *60*, 329, 1949.
119. Plough and Consolazio: J. Nutrition, *69*, 365, 1959.
120. Hegsted, Gershoff, Trulson and Jolly: J. Nutrit., *60*, 581, 1956.
121. Louhi, Yu, Hawthorne and Storvick: J. Nutrit., *48*, 297, 1952.
122. Clarke, Cosgrove and Morse: Am. J. Clin. Nutrition, *19*, 335, 1966.
123. Pearson: Am. J. Clin. Nutr., *11*, 462, 1962.
124. ———: Am. J. Clin. Nutrition, *20*, 514, 1967.
125. ———: In *Nutrition, A Comprehensive Treatise*, edited by Beaton and McHenry, Vol. 3., New York, Academic Press, 1966.
126. Dean and Schwartz: Brit. J. Nutrition, *7*, 131, 1953.
127. Waterlow: Fed. Proc., *18*, 1143, 1959.
128. Keys, Taylor, Mickelsen and Henschel: Science, *103*, 669, 1946.
129. Youmans, Patton, Sutton, Kern and Steinkamp: Am. J. Pub. Health, *33*, 955, 1943.
130. Arroyave, Scrimshaw, Pineda and Guzman: Am. J. Trop. Med. & Hygiene, *9*, 81, 1960.
131. Schendel, Hansen and Brock: S. African Med. J., *34*, 791, 1960.
132. Bronte-Stewart, Antonis, Rose-Innes and Moodie: Am. J. Clin. Nutrition, *9*, 596, 1961.
133. Brock: Fed. Proc., *20*, 61, 1961.
134. Keys *et al.*: *Biology of Human Starvation*, Vol. I., Rochester, Univ. Minnesota Press, 1950.
135. Bakker, Blick and Luyken: Doc. Med. Geograph. Trop., *9*, 1, 1957.
136. Sandstead: In *Amino Acid Fortification of Protein Foods*, edited by Scrimshaw and Gordon, MIT Press, Cambridge, Mass., 1971.
137. Whitehead: Nature, *204*, 387, 1964.
138. Whitehead and Dean: Am. J. Clin. Nutrition, *14*, 320, 1964.
139. ———: Am. J. Clin. Nutrition, *14*, 313, 1961.
140. Arroyave and Wilson: Am. J. Clin. Nutrition, *9*, 170, 1961.
141. Vitori and Alvarado: Pediatrics, *46*, 696, 1970.
142. Interdepartmental Committee for Nutrition in National Defense, *Uruguay Nutrition Survey*, Besthesda, Md., N.I.H., 1963.
143. Interdepartmental Committee for Nutrition in National Defense, *Paraguay Nutrition Survey*, Bethesda, Md., N.I.H., 1967.

Goiter, W.H.O. Monograph Series No. 44, Geneva, 1960.

144. Evaluation of Protein Quality, Publication No. 1100, N.A.S.-N.R.C., Washington, D.C., 1963.

145. Smiley and Ziff: Physiological Reviews, *44*, 30, 1964.

146. Jones, Bergman, Kittner and Pigman: Proc. Soc. Exp. Biol. & Med., *115*, 85, 1964.

147. Howells and Whitehead: J. Med. Lab. Tech., *24*, 98, 1967.

148. Bollet and Owens: Nature, *228*, 465, 1970.

149. Beutler: New Eng. J. Med., *256*, 692, 1957.

150. Beutler, Robson and Buttenwieser: Ann. Int. Med., *48*, 60, 1960.

151. Bothwell and Finch: *Iron Metabolism*, Boston, Little, Brown, 1962, p. 153.

152. Rath and Finch: J. Lab. & Clin. Med., *33*, 81, 1948.

153. Roels: In *The Vitamines*, 2nd ed., edited by Sebrell and Harris, New York, Academic Press, 1967.

154. British Med. Council Sp. Rept. No. 280, London, 1953.

155. Brin: Ann. N.Y. Acad. Sci., *98*, 528, 1962.

156. Brin, Dibble, Peel, McMullen, Bourquin, and Chen: Am. J. Clin. Nutrition, *17*, 240, 1965.

157. Warnock: J. Nutr., *100*, 1057, 1970.

158. Burch, Bessey and Lowry: J. Biol. Chem., *175*, 457, 1948.

159. Bessey, Horwitt and Love: J. Nutrit., *58*, 367, 1956.

160. Horwitt, Harvey and Rothwell, Cutler and Haffron: J. Nutrit., *60*, Suppl. 1, 1956.

161. DeLange and Joubert: Am. J. Clin. Nutrition, *15*, 169, 1964.

162. Luhby and Cooperman: In *Advances in Metabolic Disease*, edited by Levine and Luft, New York, Academic Press, 1964.

Chapter

20

Clinical Manifestations of Certain Vitamin Deficiencies

Harold H. Sandstead

INTRODUCTION

The classical deficiency diseases of beriberi, pellagra, scurvy and rickets occur infrequently in the North America of today. Such has not always been the case. Prior to the discovery of the vitamins and the subsequent elucidation of their roles in human nutrition, these diseases were more prevalent. In fact, their near disappearance from the scene of American medicine is largely the result of the striking advances in communication, education, food technology and public health which began with World War II and have accelerated in pace ever since. The modern student is thus often unaware of the impact these diseases have had and, in fact, still have on large segments of the world's population. It is the intent of this chapter to briefly review the history of these diseases and their clinical features. Details of their biochemistry are considered elsewhere in conjunction with discussions of the metabolism and requirements for specific vitamins.

Today, in North America and Northern Europe, these diseases, when they occur, usually are associated with social or medical pathologic conditions of some variety. In contrast to other regions, they seldom occur primarily. In addition, they almost never are due to a single deficiency, except under experimental conditions. Thus, they are, in fact, mixed deficiency syndromes whose "major" manifestations reflect derangements induced by lack of the most limiting nutrient, and whose "minor" manifestations are induced by the associated deficiencies.

Examples of social pathologic conditions often associated with these diseases include alcoholism, social isolation, food faddism, ignorance and neglect of individuals unable to care for themselves, such as small children or the elderly. Medical causes that may contribute to their occurrence include intestinal malabsorption syndrome, senility, psychosis and iatrogenic factors. In the technologically less advanced parts of the world, social factors, such as customs, taboos, poverty, lack of education, poor agricultural practices and poor systems of food delivery and storage, play a much greater role in their genesis.

It is evident, therefore, that, when they occur, these syndromes are the consequence of a variety of factors which ultimately result in the patient not having access to, not eating, or not utilizing a diet adequate in all nutrients. The complexity of their pathogenesis, therefore, must be kept in mind when one is confronted with a patient with clinical manifestations consistent with one of them. Only by determining the root cause can their recurrence be avoided. In addition, an understanding of underlying causes will make it possible for the physician and public health worker to prevent their occurrence in the first place.

BERIBERI

Beriberi is an ancient disease that has been endemic in the Orient for over 4000 years. Although it generally occurs in populations whose staple is polished rice, it has been observed in individuals subsisting on unenriched white flour.

Clarification of the cause of beriberi began toward the end of the last century with the studies of Takaki, Director General of the Japanese Naval Medical Service. He conducted a clinical trial in which he added meat, milk and barley to the polished rice diet of sailors to see if he could prevent the occurrence of beriberi during a long voyage. His success lead to improvement of the diet of the navy and near disappearance of the disease among Japanese sailors. Antedating the concept of vitamins by roughly 25 years, he attributed the prevention to the increased dietary protein.[1]

Unaware of Takaki's observations, a Dutch physician, Eijkman, working in Java during the 1890's, discovered that feeding polished rice to fowl produced a fatal polyneuritis. Influenced by the discoveries of Pasteur and Koch, he at first thought the disease infectious. Later he attributed it to a toxic effect of the starch in the polished rice, which could be overcome by a substance in the husk.

Eijkman's successor, Grijns, extended the studies on the "factor" and enunciated the concept that beriberi was due to a deficiency of a heat labile substance present in the husks of grain.[1] Clinical studies were inconclusive until 1910, when Frazer and Stanton clearly affirmed that "beriberi is a disorder of metabolism" due to a lack of a substance extractable from rice that is essential for nerve tissue. Soon after this, Vedder, a U.S. Army physician, enlisted the help of Williams, a chemist, to help in the search for the unknown factor. Many years later, Williams and his associates isolated and subsequently synthesized thiamine. The German chemist, Casimir Funk, also searched for the factor. His studies led him intuitively to propose in 1912 that the missing factor was a "vital amine" and to coin the word vitamine. The vitamin concept was thus born.[1]

Clinically, beriberi, like many other diseases, presents a spectrum of manifestations. Their presence seems in part to be determined by the chronicity of the deficiency, its severity and stress factors which may acutely increase the rate of metabolism of the patient.[2] Thus, individuals subsisting on a diet of 0.2 to 0.3 mg of thiamine per 1000 calories, which is slightly less than the thiamine requirement, may become gradually depleted and develop peripheral neuropathy. Their extremities of maximal use are most affected. They experience paresthesia, hyperesthesia, anesthesia, formication and weakness. Initially, their deep tendon reflexes are increased: later they may be absent. Their muscles are often tender and may atrophy. Foot and wrist drop occur. Fatigue, decreased attention span and impaired capacity to work are striking. This type of beriberi is so called "dry" or "atrophic beriberi."

If the patient has been subsisting on something less than 0.2 mg of thiamine/1000 calories, deficiency will be more severe and he will develop so called "subacute" or "wet beriberi." In addition to neurological manifestations, cardiovascular signs and symptoms will be more apparent. Dependent edema may be seen. The heart is often enlarged, with the right side being particularly prominent and the pulmonary second sound accentuated. With the slightest effort, tachycardia occurs. The patient complains of palpitation as well as dull precordial and epigastric pain. The venous pressure is often increased while the circulation time may be shortened or normal, due to arteriovenous shunting. Digestive disturbances with anorexia and constipation commonly occur. Anorexia may be quite striking. As the disease advances, the neurological manifestations become increasingly evident.

Fulminant cardiac failure may be precipitated in the above types of patients by physiologic stress, even if the individual has shown little previous evidence of thiamine deficiency. This type of cardiac failure has been given the colorful name of "Shoshin beriberi" after the region in China where it was studied. Patients so afflicted rapidly succumb with cardiac failure, which seems to be primarily rightsided. Systolic hypotension, venous distension and peripheral cyanosis are prominent. Pulmonary congestion is reported to occur late in the illness and the patients are said to expire in extreme agony and fully conscious.[2]

In the western world, where thiamine deficiency heart disease is most often associated with alcoholism, the cardiac features of the illness are similar to those observed in oriental beriberi.[3] Such patients typically have been drinking to the exclusion of eating for some weeks, thus depleting their body stores of thiamine. (Such depletion can be produced experimentally in man in roughly 12 to 14 days.) Almost always they are also deficient in other B vitamins and/or protein. In addition to cardiac failure, they often present a variety of neurological abnormalities attributable to thiamine deficiency, such as peripheral neuropathy, myelopathy, cerebellar signs and Wernicke's encephalopathy or its residual effects.[4]

It is generally held that the cardiac failure of thiamine deficiency is of the high output variety. However, it should not surprise the clinician to find an occasional patient with low output failure responsive to thiamine. Biochemically and physiologically, such a phenomenon is quite understandable, as the cardiac metabolism of pyruvate is grossly compromised by thiamine lack.[5] Further evidences of myocardial injury in thiamine deficiency are non-specific electrocardiographic abnormalities. In thiamine deficient experimental animals similar physiologic derangements have been produced, both with and without microscopic pathology.[6,7] The essential factors influencing the incidence of morphologic injury are the severity and the acuteness of the deficiency.

The superimposition of the toxic effects of alcohol on the myocardium may cause some confusion in diagnosis; therefore, it is essential that the patient's response to therapy with thiamine be the principal criterion used. Patients with heart failure due to thiamine deficiency do not respond to digitalis or diuretics. In contrast, therapy with thiamine (5 to 10 mg 3 times daily) is followed by a rapid disappearance of tachycardia, ventricular gallop and other evidences of congestive failure. Unfortunately the response of the neurologic lesions may be slow, in contrast to the heart. Their poor response reflects the limited regenerative capacity of nervous tissue.

The most acute type of thiamine deficiency, Wernicke's encephalopathy,[4] is rare in the Orient. It occurs primarily in alcoholics and in patients with pernicious vomiting, such as may occur in pregnancy or following surgery on the upper gastrointestinal tract. Acute administration of glucose to such severely deprived patients may precipitate the encephalopathy. Manifestations range from mild confusion to coma. Ophthalmoplegia with sixth nerve weakness and lateral and/or vertical nystagmus are seen. Cerebellar ataxia is often evident. If untreated, death is common. If the patient survives, damage to the cerebral cortex may result in a psychosis (Korsakoff's). Retentive memory and cognitive function are severely impaired. Confabulation is a common characteristic of such patients.

Because of the high mortality, morbidity and sequelae of Wernicke's encephalopathy, it is imperative that thiamine be included in the therapeutic regimen of all patients admitted to hospitals for the various illnesses associated with alcoholism. In addition, thiamine, as well as the other vitamins, should be given to those who are unable to eat for any extended period. Thus iatrogenic disease, due to thiamine deprivation or other vitamin deficiencies, may be avoided.

Though infantile beriberi is rarely if ever seen in the Occident, it still occurs in the Orient, in regions where enrichment of rice with thiamine has not been instituted. In these places, beriberi is still an important cause of infant death. Nursing babies whose mothers subsist largely on polished rice and who show evidence of thiamine deficiency are particularly at risk. Typically, the infants become ill between the 1st and 4th month of life.[8]

The clinical onset of infantile beriberi may be sudden. It may present as acute cardiac failure in a previously healthy appearing child. In others, the signs may be primarily neurological, with aphonia (silent crying) or features suggestive of meningitis. In some infants, the signs may come and go. In others, death is prompt. Recovery is often rapid and dramatic following administration of thiamine.[9]

The diagnosis of thiamine deficiency can be made more rapidly and objectively today than in the past. Advantage is taken of the role of thiamine pyrophosphate in the transketolase reaction of the pentose shunt. (See chapters 5 and 19A.) The activity of the enzyme in erythrocytes is determined with and without added thiamine pyrophosphate. If the baseline activity is low and addition of thiamine pyrophosphate causes a striking increase, this is interpreted as metabolic evidence consistent with thiamine deficiency.[10,11]

Thiamine status may also be assessed by measurement of the urinary excretion of the vitamin. This has been a useful technique for assessing the thiamine status of populations. For technical reasons, it generally has not been utilized for evaluation of individuals. Further discussion of the biochemical assessment of thiamine status is present in chapter 19A.

PELLAGRA

Pellagra is a mixed deficiency disease, the major manifestations of which are primarily due to a deficiency of niacin or its precursor tryptophan. Classically it occurs seasonally, is often chronic and tends to recur. Historically, it appears to be a relatively new disease, in that it was not recognized by European physicians or in the Middle East until after the introduction of corn (maize). It seems probable, however, that populations subsisting on *Sorghum vulgare* have suffered from the disease from antiquity. This supposition is based on Sandwith's description of pellagra in non-corn eating Egyptians from upper Egypt, and on his report that physicians who had been working in India recognized the disease when shown photographs of his Egyptian experience.[12] The fact that pellagra continues to occur today among Indians who live on *Sorghum vulgare* (Joware)[13] is also supportive. Whether pellagra occurred in the pre-Columbian New World is unknown.

The association of pellagra with maize was reported in the mid 18th century by Casal and Frapollie.[14] Casal noted its seasonal occurrence, the relation of the dermatitis to sunlight and described the good therapeutic effect of milk.[15]

The first clear enunciation of the relationship between a poorly balanced diet and pellagra was by Cerri in 1795.[15] His observations were generally disregarded for 120 years until Goldberger reported his classic studies in the early 1900's. The dilemma and confusion of scientists prior to Goldberger is well presented in Roberts' text, *Pellagra*, which appeared in 1913.[12] At that time, pellagra had reached epidemic proportions in the southeastern United States and affected an estimated 10,000 persons nationally.

The careful epidemiologic and experimental studies of Goldberger disproved the infection and toxin hypotheses and established that the disease was caused by a lack of some nutrient or nutrients in the corn on which the populace subsisted. He favored a deficiency of cystine and/or tryptophan.[15,16] Despite Goldberger's observations and the subsequent efforts of others, pellagra continued to be a serious public health problem throughout the south until after 1938 when Elvehjem et al.[17] isolated niacinamide from liver and demonstrated that it would cure black tongue in dogs. Of interest is the fact that Funk[18] had isolated niacin in 1912 and had suggested that it might be lacking from the diet of pellagrins. Other major factors in the eradication of pellagra were the social and economic changes which occurred throughout the country as a result of World War II.[16] Since that time, in the United States and Northern Europe, it has become a disease of the alcoholic, the elderly recluse and others with bizarre eating habits. It may also rarely occur in patients with malabsorption syndromes, thyrotoxicosis, diabetes mellitus, neoplasia and serotonin producing tumors (carcinoid).

The multiple deficiency aspects of pellagra emerged when it became possible to treat pellagrins specifically with niacin. Examples of other nutrients which the pellagrin may lack include protein, riboflavin, pyridoxine, thiamine, folic acid, vitamin A, iron and zinc. The presence of these associated deficiencies contributes to some of the clinical findings noted below.

The clinical features of classical endemic pellagra were graphically described and related to the gross and microscopic pathology by Roberts in 1913.[12] More recently, Follis[19] reviewed the pathologic condition. While the disease adversely affects all systems of the body, the most striking symptoms and signs involve the integument, nervous system and gastrointestinal tract. Generally the patients are apathetic, anorexic, have neurasthenia, complain of intermittent pain in their extremities and body. They appear pale and may have severe weight loss. If the disease has been chronic, the skin over exposed surfaces and pressure points may be thickened, hyperkeratotic and hyperpigmented without evidence of inflammation, while moist areas, such as the vulva and scrotum, may be macerated and erythematous. When deficiency is severe, the rash may resemble a severe burn and may be secondarily infected. Areas classically involved are the backs of the hands, the elbows, the neck (Casal's necklace), and the anterior chest.

Neurological manifestations may be a prominent feature. Peripheral neuropathy, myelopathy and encephalopathy may all occur. In less severe disease, peripheral nerve abnormalities may predominate. Both sensory and motor modalities may be affected. With increased chronicity and, presumably, more severe deficiency, myelopathy, which may progress to full blown combined cord degeneration, may occur.[12,19] Involvement of the brain may result in mania and, shortly before death, in seizures and coma. Prior to the availability of specific therapy, the psychiatric aspects of pellagra accounted for a high percentage of admissions to mental institutions in endemic areas.

The gastrointestinal tract is affected from mouth to anus. The mouth shows a number of non-specific lesions which emphasize the multiple deficiency aspects of the disease. These include cheilosis, angular fissures, atrophy of the epithelium of the tongue with associated pain and inflammation. Hypertrophy of the fungiform papillae may also occur, as may gastric achlorhydria. The small intestinal mucosa is atrophic and may be inflamed. Non-specific colitis with bleeding may occur, while the rectum and anus are inflamed and painful. Malabsorption of fat and other nutrients occurs in association with the diarrhea.

Clinically less striking aspects include anemia, which may be macrocytic and responsive to folic acid, or hypochromic and microcytic and responsive to iron.[15] In some patients the anemia is mixed. The reproductive system may also be involved, resulting in amenorrhea and an apparent increased incidence of abortion.[12]

The biochemical pathogenesis of pellagra has been a fertile field for research. After the relationship between tryptophan and niacin became known (60 mg tryptophan is equivalent to 1 mg of niacin),[15] it was evident that Goldberger had been partially correct in his supposition that the quality of the dietary protein consumed is an important factor in the genesis of the disease.[16] In addition, it has been shown that, while the niacin in corn and other cereals, such as wheat, rice and barley, is present in amounts sufficient to prevent pellagra, it is firmly bound to indigestible constituents in the grain and is, therefore, poorly available to man and other monogastric animals. The alkaline treatment of corn, which is commonly done in Latin America, improves this availability. Such treatment coupled with the consumption of coffee, which may contain significant amounts of niacin, depending on the roast, presumably explains the rarity of pellagra among the corn eating peasants of the region.[15] A third factor in pathogenesis may be the amino acid pattern of certain grains. Studies by Gopalan et al.[20] suggest that the high leucine content of *Sorghum vulgare* induces an amino acid imbalance which apparently may produce pellagra in man and black tongue in dogs. It is thus evident that the biochemical etiology of pellagra is complex and that several characteristics of the food consumed interact to produce the disease.

The diagnosis of pellagra is usually straightforward in patients with the rash. If, however, their skin has not been exposed to sunlight or to minor trauma, the rash may be minimal or absent. Then, with only neurological and/or gastrointestinal manifestations evident, the diagnosis may be obscure. A careful dietary history will usually resolve the issue. In general, an intake of less than 9.0 mg of niacin daily, or less than 4.4 mg/1000 calories, including that formed from tryptophan, is inadequate. If facilities allow, the measurement of the 24-hour urinary excretion of N^1-methyl nicotinamide and pyridine in patients fed a diet containing 10 mg of niacin and 1000 mg of tryptophan is also informative. Patients with pellagra excrete less than 3.0 mg on this regimen, while well-nourished individuals excrete more than 7.0 mg.[15] Unfortunately, a more rapid laboratory method for niacin assessment, analogous to the erythrocyte transketolase assay for thiamine status, is not available.

Treatment of patients with pellagra should, in addition to nutrients, include attention to the various distressing manifestations noted above. Nutrient therapy includes 300 to 500 mg of niacinamide daily in divided doses plus administration of the other nutrients often deficient in such patients. The diet, at least initially, should be soft so as to be more easily eaten while the patient is acutely ill.

SCURVY

Scurvy is perhaps the oldest well described deficiency disease, in that it is referred to in the Ebers Papyrus and by Hippocrates.[21] Its occurrence among soldiers and explorers doubtless influenced the course of history, because those so afflicted were unable to carry out their intentions. Thus, it contributed to the failure of certain crusades,[22] frustrated long sea voyages and land explorations and, through its occurrence in the French navy, may have contributed to Nelson's triumph over Napoleon.[23] The first clearcut formulation of the cause of scurvy is attributed to Bachstrom, who, in 1734, noted that those who abstained from fresh vegetables and fruits developed the disease. He is said to have been the first physician to discard the "humor concept" in favor of the hypothesis that lack of a specific type of food could result in disease.[21] It should be noted, however, that Lancaster, a British sea captain had demonstrated the preventive value of lemon juice 134 years earlier[21] and that the French explorer, Cartier, had learned 200 years previously of the curative value of a decoction of pine needles and bark.[22] Contemporary with Bachstrom, James Lind, a British naval physician, conducted a controlled therapeutic experiment on scorbutic sailors which conclusively demonstrated the preventive and curative value of citrus fruit. He published

his findings and recommendations in 1753. Forty-two years later, the Admiralty followed his advice:[22] a decision which, as noted above, may have changed the course of history. Scurvy among infants became a severe clinical problem in the late 19th century, when pasteurization and the boiling of infant formulas became the vogue. It continued to be not uncommon in this age group until the evolution of modern pediatric feeding practices. This was in spite of the fact that Waugh and King[24] had isolated and crystalized vitamin C from lemons in 1932, and had shown it to be identical with the "hexuronic acid" of Szent-Györgyi.[25] The following year Reichstein et al.[26] accomplished its synthesis.

Today scurvy is rare where modern medicine is practiced and nutrition education has had an impact. When it occurs, it is usually the result of neglect of individuals who, because of psychiatric difficulty, age, alcoholism or ignorance, are unable or unwilling to care for themselves. In infants, it is found, except in a rare instance, only among the artificially fed: its occurrence reflects a lack of understanding on the part of mothers of the nutritional needs of children.

The clinical manifestations of scurvy appear to reflect the role of the vitamin in the metabolism of mesenchymal cells, which form connective tissue, osteoid and dentine.[27] Osteoblastic activity is retarded, new wounds do not heal and old wounds open up. In addition, it appears from animal studies that scurvy may impair the production of vasohumoral agents by the kidney.[28] Such a phenomenon would allow an abnormal distribution of blood flow in capillary beds, resulting in engorgement and subsequent extravasation. In addition, because of impaired collagen formation, the supporting matrix for the capillary bed may be inadequate.

Under usual circumstances, the onset of clinical scurvy in adults is delayed for 4 to 5 months from the time dietary vitamin C is restricted. The severity of the restriction and the previous body stores of the individual dictate the time of onset. Plasma concentrations of ascorbic acid, on the other hand, reflect the recent intake of the vitamin and fall to low levels in 3 to 4 weeks. A decline in white blood cell-platelet vitamin C occurs more slowly, reaching low levels after 20 to 24 weeks. The decrease in white blood cell-platelet ascorbic acid is believed to reflect tissue saturation, as signs of clinical scurvy appear roughly 2 weeks after the white blood cell-platelet concentration of the vitamin has become negligible.[29]

In infants, scurvy occurs most commonly between the 5th and 24th month of age. The peak incidence is between 8 and 11 months. The time of onset reflects the body stores at birth, the duration of nursing, which provides adequate ascorbic acid, the rate of growth and its duration and the vitamin C content of the food.

Early symptoms in adults include anorexia, weakness, neurasthenia and aching in the joints and muscles. The first specific clinical sign is an increased prominence of the hair follicles, on the thighs and buttocks. This is due to keratin plugging of their lumens. Hairs within the follicles become coiled and fragmented and have a characteristic cork-screw appearance after they erupt. Peri-follicular hemorrhages, which ultimately result in the deposition of brown hemoglobin pigment, occur. With time, the purpuric lesions coalesce and form ecchymoses which spread from the lower extremities to the rest of the body, particularly those areas exposed to trauma. Hemorrhage may also occur in muscles, in and around joints, in gastrointestinal mucosa, in the kidneys and into the pericardium. The gingiva at the base of teeth become hemorrhagic and finally necrotic. This abnormality first appears at the base of the molars. The interdental papillae become swollen and bluish red in color and may become secondarily infected. With time, the teeth fall out. A curious finding is the hemorrhage which may occur in old scars, premonitory of their subsequent dehiscence. Death may occur suddenly, once the clinical signs have become extensive and severe.

In infants, the clinical features are somewhat different from those of adults. The onset is usually insidious. Failure to thrive may be an early clue. A common presentation is for the infant to be irritable, to have tender extremities and pseudo paralysis. Purpuric lesions, which may be overlooked, are also present. If teeth are erupting, hemorrhage of the adjacent gum may be seen. A striking finding is the apprehension of the infant when it is handled. Other hemorrhagic manifestations which occur include epistaxis, retrobulbar hemorrhage, hematuria and bloody diarrhea.

X-ray examination of the extremities often reveals a ground glass appearance of the bones with a thinning of the cortex. A radiolucent area may surround the epiphyseal plate. The center of ossification may be displaced. Following initiation of treatment, calcification of the periosteum will outline the sub-periosteal hemorrhage. The radiolucency noted above initially affects the shaft, giving rise to the "corner sign" of Park. This is seen at the lateral margin of the junction between the metaphysis and epiphysis. The absence of calcification in this region is starkly apparent and constitutes an early roentgenographic sign of the disease.[29] Radiographic examination of the chest shows findings analogous to the extremities. The external appearance and palpation of the costochondral junctions are characteristic. Posterior subluxation of the sternum results in the sharp end of the ribs being palpable, while the displaced cartilages are related to the ends of the ribs in a manner analogous to a bayonet attached to a rifle.

Anemia occurs in both adult and infantile scurvy. While in experimental subhuman primates it is clear that ascorbic acid has a sparing effect on the folic acid requirement, and will prevent the occurrence of megaloblastic anemia,[30,31] this relationship is more obscure in man.[32,33] This is probably related to the fact that single nutrient deficiencies are rare in man. Thus, the anemia associated with human scurvy may have components of iron, folic acid and ascorbic acid deficiencies simultaneously, in addition to reflecting the effects of infections which may be present.

The prevention and treatment of scurvy is straightforward; therefore, the disease should occur only on rare occasions in modern society. Ten mg of ascorbic acid daily will prevent the disease in infants and adults. Several times this amount is provided by a diet containing a mixture of fresh fruits and vegetables. Animal sources which contain significant amounts of ascorbic acid are liver and raw milk. Because the vitamin is readily destroyed by heat, oxygen and storage, the content of ascorbic acid in processed foods is significantly decreased. To correct for this loss, ascorbic acid is often added to processed foods normally considered important sources of the vitamin.

RICKETS AND OSTEOMALACIA

Rickets and osteomalacia comprise a disease of the skeleton characterized by decreased deposition of calcium in osteoid. This failure of calcification results in a decreased structural rigidity of bone. Skeletal deformities, which are the clinical hallmarks of the disease, are the consequence of the soft bones.

One of the earliest "modern" descriptions of rickets is the medical thesis prepared by Whistler in 1645.[34] He describes the softness of the bones, their contorted shapes, the rachitic rosary and other chest deformities. He also alludes to the poor muscular development, delayed tooth eruption and poor nutritional status of the children. A more comprehensive description, De Rachitide, was published by Glisson in 1650. From these texts it may be inferred that rickets was a serious and common affliction of children in the Northern Europe of that day.

The relationship of the deformities to decreased bone mineral was documented in 1842 by Marchand.[35] Sixteen years later a clear description of the morphologic pathology was provided by Müller.[35] By the turn of the century, the failure of rachitic children to absorb calcium and phosphorus was appreciated. Experimental animal studies reported in 1921 documented the predictive value of the product of the serum calcium and phosphorus concentrations in the diagnosis of the disease.[36] The same year Park and Howland described the curative effects of vitamin D.[37]

Since these early days, it has become evident that rickets and osteomalacia may be caused by a variety of etiologies other than lack of exposure to ultraviolet light or dietary inadequacy of vitamin D. Certain of these causes are inborn errors of metabolism, others are related to disorders of gastrointestinal function or to substances toxic to the kidney or gastrointestinal tract. Today, these "metabolic" causes are more commonly implicated than is dietary deficiency. The near elimination of dietary rickets in advanced countries may be credited to a general appreciation of the causes of the disease, its prevention and cure, and the implementation of vitamin D enrichment. Dietary rickets is still found in countries where children are customarily shielded from the sun, vitamin D enrichment of food is not practiced and fish oils or vitamin preparations containing vitamin D are not given. The same is true of osteomalacia in women, who because of custom, continue to wear heavy veils.

Classically, dietary rickets was a disease of temperate countries. Long winters, with little ultraviolet light, due to the angle of the sun, cloud cover, and smog over industrial centers, resulted in a high incidence of the disease. From 1901 to 1908, in Dresden, 94 per cent of 287 autopsied children under 2 years of age were rachitic.[38] A similar study on material obtained in Baltimore from 1926 to 1942 showed that greater than 50 per cent of the children had been affected. When grouped by age according to month, severe rickets was found in 12 to 43 per cent.[35] Today the disease is rare in Baltimore.

Rapid growth increases the susceptibility of premature infants and babies to rickets.[39] One of the earliest signs is craniotabes. The normal remodeling of bone results in removal of hydroxyapatite. Failure to calcify new osteoid results in a softening of the skull and delayed closure of the fontanelles. The habitual position of the child molds the skull with resultant flattening of the chronically dependent surface, usually the occiput. Thickening (bossing) of the skull over the frontal and parietal eminences also occurs. This may be particularly impressive in infants with anemia, giving the skull the appearance of a "hot cross bun."

The shafts of the extremities are also soft. In response to the influence of gravity and position, they may become severely misshapen. Epiphyseal growth and the failure of calcification result in knobby deformities at the ends of the long bones. Displacement of the epiphysis may occur. Thus, posterior tilting of the lower tibeal epiphysis by the weight of the foot results in initiation of the classical saber shin deformity, and displacement of the distal radial and ulnar epiphysis by the weight of the infant on his pronated hand results in a conspicuous bulging at the wrist.[39]

Dentition typically is delayed: teeth may erupt out of order. While the enamel of deciduous teeth is unaffected, permanent teeth formed during the rachitic interval may be severely injured. Their enamel is thin, pitted and sometimes absent.

Enlargement of the costochondral junctions, the so-called "rachitic rosary," is an early sign of rickets. Occasionally, posterior displacement of the sternum occurs in response to force exerted by the diaphragm and intercostal muscles, thus forming a trough. In other instances, the sternum may move anteriorly, forming a "pigeon breast." With softening, the inferior ribs may bend inward, forming a "Harrison's Groove." If the ribs become very soft, the bellow function of the chest may he severely compromised. Later in life, rachitic deformities of the chest may limit pulmonary function.

Just as the chest and extremities are twisted, so is the spine. Early in life a dorsolumbar kyphosis occurs. Later, after the child begins to walk, the kyphosis may disappear and severe lordosis develop. The deformity of the back and twisting of the tibia and femur grossly alter the gait, so that the patient may waddle in a manner similar to that seen with congenital dislocation of the hips.

The musculature of the rachitic child is often hypotonic. "Pot belly" is common. Motor development may be retarded. Other nutrient deficiencies may be present, but are inconsistent. The presence of scurvy, because of its effect on the metabolism of osteoblasts, retards the development of rickets.[35]

X-ray abnormalities occur both in the epiphysis and shaft. The junction of the epiphysis and metaphysis typically shows a concave cupping of the metaphysis, with spreading of the junction. The inner margin of the cup is often fringed and stippled. Stippling reflects the incomplete deposition of calcium and phosphorus that occurs in early rickets.

X-ray abnormalities in the shaft reflect the normal remodeling of bone and subsequent failure of calcification. Osteoid is not radioopaque; therefore, the trabeculae appear coarse and the cortex is thin. In extreme instances, the bone is nearly translucent.

When vitamin D is given, calcium is deposited in the provisional zone of cartilaginous calcification. Thus an opaque line (Müller's line), separate from the rest of the metaphysis, appears on the x-ray film

Osteomalacia is metabolically identical to rickets, except that it occurs in adults. Because longitudinal growth has stopped, only the shafts of the long bones and flat bones, such as the pelvis, are affected. The remodeling process results in softening, distortion and an increased susceptibility to fracture. Some of the most distressing signs of the disease are the pelvic deformities which occur in women as a consequence of multiple pregnancies and lactation, low dietary calcium and nonexposure to ultraviolet irradiation. Even today, osteomalacia of this etiology is said to be endemic in Northern India, Japan and Northern China.[40]

X-ray findings in osteomalacia reflect resorption of bone and failure to calcify osteoid. Gross asymmetrical deformity of the pelvis with narrowing of the outlet is typical. Minute ribbonlike fracture of long bones also occur.

The pathogenesis of dietary rickets and osteomalacia seems to be roughly as follows.[39] Deficiency of vitamin D, either of dietary origin or due to lack of ultraviolet irradiation results in decreased absorption of dietary calcium and phosphorus. As a result, hydroxyapatite formation is decreased and plasma levels of calcium tend to decline. In response to the lowering of plasma calcium, the parathyroid glands release parathormone. Bone resorption and phosphate excretion are accelerated through the influence of the hormone. Thus the plasma concentration of ionized calcium is maintained. In bone, calcification of cartilage and new osteoid is inhibited and bones become soft. Flat bones and the shafts of long bones become distorted in both children and adults. In children, the cartilaginous growth sites on the ends of bones over grow, resulting in knobby deformities.

From this simple scheme, the expected serum concentrations of calcium, phosphorus and alkaline phosphatase which occur in rickets and osteomalacia can be predicted. In infants and children, serum calcium may be normal or low: phosphorus is low and alkaline phosphatase is quite elevated. In adults, serum calcium is usually normal to low-normal. Serum phosphorus is low and alkaline phosphatase is increased. Because the methods of analysis and expression of results differ in various laboratories, numerical values have not been given.

Rickets and osteomalacia due to other causes are morphologically and clinically similar to the dietary disease. When related to intestinal malabsorption, not only is vitamin D absorption decreased, but calcium malabsorption may be so severe as to be little affected by endogenous vitamin D derived from ultraviolet irradiation.

As a consequence of abnormalities in renal tubular phosphate reabsorption, severe depletion in the anion may occur. Serum levels may be so low as to impair the formation of hydroxyapatite. This phenomenon appears to account for the vitamin D resistant rickets associated with certain renal tubular diseases. On the other hand, renal tubular acidosis promotes calciuria, thus decreasing the amount of calcium available for bone. This form of rickets is also vitamin D resistant, as is the rickets of idiopathic primary calciuria.

The prevention and treatment of dietary rickets is straightforward. Enrichment of milk with 400 international units of vitamin D per quart has been shown to be a very effective preventive measure. This level of intake has been suggested as the recommended daily allowance for children. Treatment requires the administration of both vitamin D and calcium. Three thousand to 5000 IU of vitamin D and 1 to 2 pints of milk daily is usually sufficient. In instances of vitamin D resistance, considerably larger amounts are required (up to 500,000 IU daily). In patients with malabsorption syndrome and osteomalacia, severe restriction of dietary fat to less than 30 gm daily may be required to correct the malabsorption of calcium. Prevention of excessive losses of calcium in the feces will often allow restoration of bone, if several grams of calcium are given daily. Modest amounts of vitamin D ($\pm$ 5000 IU) will also facilitate the process. If it is not possible to decrease the dietary fat, large doses of vitamin D (50,000 to 100,000 IU) may have a salutary effect.

Details of the biochemistry of vitamin D and its active metabolites are presented in chapter 5B, as is additional information concerning dietary sources and human requirements of the vitamin.

BIBLIOGRAPHY

1. Williams. *Toward the Conquest of Beri Beri*, Cambridge, Harvard University Press, 1961.
2. Platt: Fed. Proc. *17*, 8, 1958.
3. Blankenhorn: Circulation *11*, 288, 1955.
4. Victor and Adams: Am. J. Clin. Nutr. *91*, 379, 1961.
5. Olson: Fed. Proc. *17*, 24, 1958.
6. Hundley: Fed. Proc. *17*, 27, 1958.
7. Follis: Fed. Proc. *17*, 23, 1958.
8. Burgen: Fed. Proc. *17*, 39, 1958.
9. Ramalingaswami: Fed. Proc. *17*, 44, 1958.
10. Brin, Dibble, Peel, McMullen, Brouquin and Chen: Am. J. Clin. Nutr. *17*, 240, 1965.
11. Warnock: J. Nutr. *100*, 1057, 1970.
12. Roberts: *Pellagra*, C. V. Mosby, St. Louis, 1913.
13. Gopalan and Srikantia: Lancet *1*, 954, 1960.
14. Majors: *Classic Description of Disease*, 3rd ed. Springfield, Charles C Thomas, 1945, p. 607.
15. Goldsmith: in *Nutrition a Comprehensive Treatise II*. Ed. Beaton and McHenry, New York, Academic Press, 1964, p. 109.
16. Sydenstricker: Am. J. Clin. Nutr. *6*, 409, 1958.
17. Elvehjem, Madden, Strong and Wooley: J. Biol. Chem. *123*, 137, 1938.
18. Funk: *The Vitamins*, Baltimore, The Williams & Wilkins Co., 1922.
19. Follis: *Deficiency Disease*, Springfield, Charles C Thomas, 1958, p. 316.
20. Gopalan, Belvady and Krishmanurthi: Lancet *2*, 956, 1969.
21. Friedman and Jolliffe: in *Clinical Nutrition*, 2nd ed. by Joliffe, New York, Hoeber Medical Division, Harper & Row, 1962, p. 656.
22. Majors: *Classic Description of Disease*, 3rd ed. Springfield, Charles C Thomas, 1945, p. 585.
23. Davidson: in *Textbook of Medicine*, ed. Beeson and McDermott, 11th ed. Philadelphia, W. B. Saunders Co., 1963, p. 1218.
24. Waugh and King: J. Biol. Chem. *97*, 325, 1932.
25. Szent-Györgyi: Biochem. J. *22*, 1387, 1928.
26. Reichstein, Grussner and Oppenhauer: Helv. Chem. Acta *16*, 1019, 1933.

27. Follis: *Deficiency Disease*, Springfield, Charles C Thomas, 1958, p. 175.
28. Akers and Lee: Proc. Soc. Exp. Biol. Med. *82*, 195, 1953.
29. Woodruff: in *Nutrition a Comprehensive Treatise II*, ed. by Beaton and McHenry, New York, Academic Press, 1964, p. 265.
30. May, Nelson, Lowe and Salmon: Am. J. Dis. Child. 80, 191, 1950.
31. Woodruff, Dutra, Misra and Darby: Fed. Proc. *17*, 498, 1958.
32. Zuelzer, Hutoff and Apt.: Am. J. Dis. Child. *77*, 128, 1949.
33. Vilter, Woolford and Spies: J. Lab. Clin. Med. *31*, 609, 1946.

34. Majors: *Classic Description of Disease*, 3rd ed: Springfield, Charles C Thomas, 1945, p. 594.
35. Follis: *Deficiency Disease*, Springfield, Charles C Thomas, 1958, p. 361.
36. Howland and Kramer: Am. J. Dis. Child. *22*, 105, 1921.
37. Park and Howland: Bull. Johns Hopkins Hosp. *32*, 341, 1921.
38. Schmorl: cited by Follis: *Deficiency Disease*, Springfield, Charles C Thomas, 1958, p. 380.
39. Park: in *Clinical Nutrition*, 2nd ed. by Jolliffe, New York, Hoeber Medical Division, Harper & Row, 1962, p. 506.
40. Snapper: in *Clinical Nutrition*, 2nd ed. by Joliffe, New York, Hoeber Medical Division, Harper & Row, 1962, p. 261.

Chapter

21

Protein-Calorie Malnutrition *

Fernando E. Viteri

AND

Guillermo Arroyave

INTRODUCTION

The body needs to ingest food in adequate amounts to obtain energy, as well as protein and the other essential nutrients to maintain normal metabolic functions at any age and physiological state. While in the case of children these amounts have to account for maintenance and growth, in adults the needs in general are for maintenance purposes only. In the adult woman, pregnancy and lactation represent periods of growth and, consequently, of increased nutritional requirements.

Large segments of the world's population live under conditions where the availability and intake of food are in deficit in relation to their needs.[1] This is the case in many developing areas where food consumption is deficient both in quantity and quality. Insufficient food intake leads to chronic caloric deficiency, and ingestion of foods with insufficient protein concentration induces protein deficiency in vulnerable groups. This is particularly true when the protein is of poor quality, as is the case with most vegetable proteins. The problem with the latter is that

* Scientific articles published on this subject are much more numerous than those cited in the present Chapter. However, because of limited space, the reader is often referred to some comprehensive reviews on the subject. Publications cited at the beginning or at the end of paragraphs or sections are general references for the topic dealt with. Through these, as well as through the more recent specific articles cited, many other important references may be easily located by those interested in a deeper approach to the subject.

the bulk of the food often imposes a limit to its intake. Also, amino acid deficiencies further limit the utilization of such protein sources, so that small children cannot satisfy their naturally elevated nitrogen and specific amino acid requirements.

These dietary factors, associated with many other health problems to be described later, lead to primary chronic protein-calorie malnutrition (PCM). In conditions conducive to primary PCM, the intakes of other essential nutrients, such as vitamins and minerals, are also generally low; however, serious manifestations of their specific clinical deficiencies are less common than one would expect. This is due to the fact that, when the calorie and protein intake is the limiting factor, the requirements for other nutrients diminish. Nevertheless, in PCM, vitamin or mineral deficiencies may become overt.

Primary PCM should be differentiated from secondary PCM, which is the consequence of a primary disease that leads either to inadequate food intake or utilization or to increased nutritional requirements. Examples of secondary PCM are psychological disorders, obstructive gastrointestinal lesions, primary malabsorptive problems, diseases inducing cachexia of metabolic, infectious or neoplastic origin, as well as endocrine disorders.

This chapter deals only with primary PCM, that is, the situation where energy and protein intake are apparently the most limiting factors in malnutrition.

604

EPIDEMIOLOGIC AND ETIOLOGIC CONSIDERATIONS

All of the developing areas of the world have several common characteristics, among which are low weight of newborn babies, high disease prevalence, small physical size of their inhabitants, elevated mortality rates, particularly during infancy and early childhood (Table 21–1), and, as a consequence, short life expectancy. The main reasons for these characteristics are two: undernutrition and poor environmental health. These situations lead to decreased productivity and increased waste of human and economic capital, including food. This perpetuates and often aggravates underdevelopment, thus worsening nutrition and health and, therefore, establishing a vicious cycle. This general picture, associated with a large concentration of still unproductive young people, provides the background for underdevelopment.

Table 21-1. Mortality Rates of Children 0-4 Years of Age*

Age	Guatemala (1965)	%	U.S.A. (1967)	%	Ratio Guatemala/U.S.A.
A. Infant mortality (deaths/1000 live births)					
0–28 days	35.9	39.1	16.6	73.8	2.2
1–11 months	55.9	60.9	5.9	26.2	9.5
1 year	91.8	100.0	22.5	100.0	4.1
B. Mortality in children between 1 and 4 years of age (deaths/1000 children of the corresponding age)					
1 year	50.0		1.4		35.7
2 years	35.2		0.9		39.1
3 years	24.9		0.7		35.6
4 years	15.6		0.6		26.0
1–4 years	30.3		0.9		33.7

* Compounded from data published by the Pan American Health Organization: *Las Condiciones de Salud en las Américas 1965–1968*. Washington, D.C., Organización Panamericana de la Salud, septiembre, 1970 (Publicación Científica No. 207), and INCAP.[3]

Table 21-2. Children Below 5 Years of Age in Central America, 1965-1967, Presenting Growth Retardation which, by the Gómez* Classification, Could Be Catalogued as Malnourished†

Country	Total population below 5 years of age	1st, 2nd, and 3rd degree malnourished No. of cases	%	Malnourished 1st degree No. of cases	%	2nd degree No. of cases	%	3rd degree No. of cases	%
Costa Rica	294,300	153,200	52.0	117,900	40.0	31,300	10.6	4,000	1.4
El Salvador	554,400	380,000	68.5	244,600	44.1	116,900	21.1	18,500	3.3
Guatemala	833,400	611,660	73.4	380,100	45.6	197,700	23.7	33,860	4.1
Honduras	346,900	221,300	63.7	143,000	41.2	71,200	20.5	7,100	2.0
Nicaragua	287,500	148,800	51.8	112,300	39.1	32,400	11.3	4,100	1.4
Panama	207,900	104,947	50.4	84,625	40.7	18,990	9.1	1,332	0.6
Total	2,524,400	1,619,907	64.2	1,082,525	42.9	468,490	18.6	68,892	2.7

* Gómez, F., *et al.*[2]

† Numbers are extrapolations from a statistically representative sample.

The magnitude of the problem varies from area to area. As an example, we can cite the figures obtained from a survey of the Central American region, where—by projecting to the total population of the area the prevalence obtained from a statistically representative sample—of all of the 2.5 million children below 5 years of age, 1.6 million could be categorized, on the basis of their body weight, as suffering or as having had undernutrition. Nearly one-third of them had been or were moderately or severely malnourished (second and third degree undernutrition) at the time of the survey.[3] These findings are presented in Table 21-2.

Adult undernutrition is more difficult to recognize, but is also prevalent in developing areas. In Guatemala, for instance, over 8 per cent of all medical admissions to the wards of government hospitals, are due to primary PCM.

From the epidemiologic point of view, PCM can be conceived as the consequence of the interaction of the environment on the host through an agent which, in this case, is the deficient availability of calories and protein at the cell level. The environment, host and agent factors are interwoven.

Environment. This can be considered at two levels:[4] (a) macroenvironment, at a regional or national level, and (b) micro-environment, at the family and individual level.

In the developing areas, the macroenvironment is that of poverty, not only in the strict economic sense, but also in the more important concept of poverty of human resources. Both are the cause and the consequence of lack of education, unsatisfactory health of the population, poor communications, low productivity, unfavorable economic balance and inadequate utilization of natural resources; all of these factors lead to inadequate food production, conservation, distribution, and consumption.

On the other hand, the microenvironment constituted by the family, which is the biological unit in terms of nutrition, receives the impact of the macroenvironment and further limits the availability of nutrients to the host. The factors operating at this level are meager purchasing power, faulty concepts of food utilization that conduce to poor food consumption practices and inadequate distribution of available nutrients among the members of the family. The latter is particularly evident in the case of small children and when disease strikes a member of the family, whose food is very often drastically restricted.

Host and Agent. Maternal malnutrition and infectious episodes during pregnancy are frequently the cause of prematurity and small, born-at-term infants. These children, already at a nutritional disadvantage, are the victims of poor feeding practices, especially in those regions where breast-feeding is being replaced early in life by artificial formulas in the face of prevailing inadequate education, hygiene and economic resources. All of these factors must be favorable for artificial lactation to be adequate.

This inadequate feeding takes place at a time when nutritional requirements are high per unit of body weight. The consequence is the increasing number of infants who suffer from early protein-calorie malnutrition, particularly in the urban areas. The most common type of severe malnutrition at this age is that of non-edematous PCM due to a predominant caloric deficiency.[5]

Even when properly breast-fed, complementary feeding practices for the child are poor, and thus induce some degree of PCM late in infancy. When weaning occurs, most children are fed diets that provide insufficient amounts of calories and proteins. Others receive only starchy gruels or high-carbohydrate low-protein diluted cereal drinks, which accentuate protein deficiency. Table 21-3 presents the median nutrient intake of rural Central American children, expressed as per cent of the recommended allowances for each age group. It is important to realize that, in the developing areas, children are smaller in size than those of the same age in the developed areas; consequently, their actual requirements are somewhat reduced because of their smaller size. Nonetheless, a decreased food intake for age, even when it could be fairly satisfactory for size, perpetuates undernutrition. If at this time the child is forced-fed diets which are high in calories but low in protein, he becomes acutely protein-deficient, in spite of being fat. This

Table 21-3. Median Nutrient Intake as Per Cent of Recommended Allowances of Nutrients Consumed by Preschool Age Children in the Rural Area of Guatemala, 1965 *†

	Age groups (years)			
Nutrients	1 (38)‡	2 (43)	3 (34)	4–5 (14)
Calories	63	66	80	48
Proteins	79	74	108	67
Calcium	72	69	101	72
Iron	56	71	103	66
Vitamin A	24	30	25	20
Thiamin	100	92	128	68
Riboflavin	50	46	50	31
Niacin	42	50	68	39
Vitamin C	40	60	56	20

* Over 90% of preschool age children consumed less calories and over 60% consumed less protein than the recommended allowances. The calories and protein consumption was lower than recommended in 80% and 40% of the families, respectively.
† Modified from: Flores, M., Menchú, M. T., Lara, M. Y., and Guzmán, M.: Arch. Latinoamer. Nutr., 20, 41, 1970.
‡ Figures in parentheses represent the number of children.

severe protein deficiency gives rise to edematous PCM of the "sugar baby" type.[6] More often, infants become the victims of mild-to-moderate repeated infections[7] and, by the time they are weaned, develop a common diarrhea syndrome known as "weanling diarrhea."[8] After weaning, children are fed the usual family foods, with little or no milk or other animal products, and, at this time or later, may also suffer from acute severe infections. As a consequence, their nutritional condition rapidly deteriorates. These children, who prior to weaning were growing at a slower rate and very often were somewhat underweight for their height, become frankly undernourished. Those who follow this path develop also the edematous type of PCM, but at the same time are somewhat emaciated. They suffer from a predominant pro-tein deficiency, superimposed on various degrees of caloric deficit.

The majority of children, however, do not develop a severe degree of PCM and, through a series of adaptive mechanisms, remain in a state of mild-to-moderate protein-calorie malnutrition. This condition is characterized only by growth retardation and by periods wherein they have a mild weight for height deficit, with or without traces of edema. Children who survive the critical weaning and preschool age periods continue to grow at a slower rate and, by this time, their calorie and protein requirements per unit of body mass are rapidly decreasing. Their daily diet continues to be low in both calories and protein but they usually can procure more food and often have already had most of the common childhood infectious diseases. Thus, these children can progress into adulthood without further serious risks of becoming severely undernourished. However, if a severe infection or diarrhea supervenes, they can still develop severe PCM, regardless of their age. Among the common childhood infections, measles and whooping cough are well known to precipitate severe protein-calorie malnutrition. In children and adults, repeated acute diarrheal episodes and massive parasitic infestations by hookworm, *Trichuris trichiura*, *Strongyloides*, malaria and *Schistosoma* plus other stresses, such as acute food shortage and severe physical or psychological stresses, can well induce severe PCM.

PHYSIOPATHOLOGY AND ADAPTIVE RESPONSES IN CALORIE DEFICIENCY AND IN PROTEIN DEFICIENCY

Through a series of physiological mechanisms, the body tends to maintain a dynamic equilibrium. These mechanisms are constantly in operation in a variety of aspects. A typical example is the tendency towards caloric equilibrium: after the ingestion of a meal, energy is stored mostly in the form of high energy phosphates, fat and glycogen. These are drawn upon to obtain energy during the daily regular and relatively short periods of fasting, as well as during periods of increased energy expenditure.

With longer periods of calorie and/or

protein restriction, the body progressively adapts itself in order to maintain as adequate a functional status as the limited supply of nutrients allows. Consequently, in the process leading to PCM, the body is dynamically adapting to it and continues to do so throughout, until the individual is "maximally adapted." This adaptation results in a decreased nutrient demand and in the attainment of nutritional equilibrium compatible with a lower level of cellular nutrient availability. If, at this point, the supply of nutrients becomes persistently lower than that to which the body can adapt, death supervenes. However, although in most instances the nutrient supply is low, it is not so inadequate as to cause death and the individual is thus able to live in a state adapted to the diminished intake. In this process, most functions are altered and have the following characteristics: (a) They are more susceptible to being overwhelmed by an overloading mechanism, whether physiological or pathological, because of diminished functional reserves. This overload brings about uncompensation or failure of adaptation, and consequently poses a threat to the

life of the host. In other words, the adapted PCM individual is a labile, functionally fragile subject. (b) Due to their dynamic nature, the degree of functional alteration generally correlates with the degree of protein depletion. Nevertheless, this correlation is influenced by the rate at which depletion occurs, or at which repletion takes place during nutritional rehabilitation.[9]

The adaptive metabolic processes in both calorie and protein malnutrition occur by hormonal interaction, by servomechanisms at the cellular level, and by yet poorly understood generalized body reactions. Briefly, calorie deficit induces the hormonal adaptations described in Table 21–4, which lead to increased fat mobilization from adipose tissue. Moreover, during the initial phases of deficiency, the individual shows decreased physical activity, and a lower basal energy expenditure per unit of lean body mass. The body composition is progressively altered by decreasing adiposity at a fast rate and lean body mass at a slower rate. Muscle catabolism produces an increased efflux of amino acid, primarily as alanine. As the caloric deficit becomes severe, basal energy expendi-

Table 21–4. Schematic Hormonal Adaptive Mechanisms from the Nutritional Standpoint

Hormone	Stimulus	Result	Hormonal activities in	
			Calorie deprivation	Protein deprivation
Insulin	↑ Glucose ↑ amino acids	↑ Protein synthesis (muscle) ↑ Growth ↑ Lipogenesis	Decreased	Decreased
Growth hormone	↓ Glucose ↑ amino acids	↑ Protein synthesis (body) ↑ Growth ↑ Lipolysis ↓ Urea synthesis	Increased	Variable, generally increased
Glucocorticoids	↓ Glucose ↓ amino acids	↑ Protein catabolism (muscle) ↑ Protein turnover (viscera) ↑ Neoglucogenesis ↑ Lipolysis	Increased	Generally decreased
Thyroid hormones	↑ Energy metabolism	Energy homeostasis ↑ Protein turnover	Decreased	Decreased

ture may be normal or even increased per unit of lean body mass, which then decreases at a faster rate.[9–11]

Without concomitant severe calorie restrictions, protein deficit induces the hormonal changes described in Table 21–4, as well as cellular adaptation mechanisms not directly hormonally mediated, but induced by the poor availability of amino acids. The latter involve decreased protein synthesis at the ribosomal level. The results from both mechanisms of adaptation are an internal shift in protein metabolism which consists of increased muscle protein catabolism and, as a consequence, a relatively increased amino acid availability at the visceral level. The composition of the free amino acid pool is altered. There is a decrease in the synthesis and catabolism of total body proteins, the latter predominating over the former. The end result is a longer half-life of some proteins, such as albumin, and a generally decreased protein turnover. In addition, the internal body distribution of protein changes. This is the case with albumin, which diminishes more in the extravascular than in the intravascular space. Urea synthesis decreases and amino acids are more efficiently recycled. Simple nitrogen-containing compounds, such as urea, apparently are more efficiently utilized as sources of non-essential nitrogen. In terms of body composition, there occurs a progressive reduction in lean body mass, due primarily to muscle and probably also to skin protein loss. Visceral protein is initially reduced ("labile protein") but then becomes stable or may even regain some of its total mass. Adiposity should remain essentially constant. As the body protein turnover and total body protein mass decrease, basal oxygen consumption also decreases.[9,12]

These adaptations, which lead to the sparing of body protein, are easily upset by forced calorie intake, primarily in the form of carbohydrates. Hormonal adaptation mechanisms are "fooled" and, as a consequence, internal protein shifts are impaired, thus inducing visceral amino acid depletion and a breakdown of adaptation. Infections leading to disease also upset adaptation by producing fever (increased calorie waste), which is accompanied by large nitrogen losses and shifts toward amino acid utilization for energy purposes. Amino acid utilization is also diverted for increased synthesis and for the turnover of special proteins, such as gamma-globulins (antibodies).[13,14]

When the adaptive mechanisms are maintained, the impact of PCM is diminished, and the length of time that an individual takes to go from mild to severe protein-calorie malnutrition is prolonged. As mentioned before, the individual has to sacrifice certain functions and some of his nutrient reserves and, for this reason, he becomes more susceptible to injuries which a well-nourished individual can well withstand with little repercussion. Among the nutrient reserves, total body K content is reduced[15,16] so that the malnourished subject is more liable to be depleted of this cation under conditions that promote increased potassium losses. His total circulating hemoglobin is reduced *pari passu* to decreased body oxygen demands; red cell production diminishes; and hemodilution takes place.[9,10,17] From the hemodynamic point of view, cardiac work decreases[18] and central circulation predominates over the peripheral circulation. Cardiovascular reflexes are altered, conducing to postural hypotension and diminished venous return. Hemodynamic compensation in severe PCM occurs mostly from tachycardia, rather than increased stroke volume. The renal plasma flow, glomerular filtration rate and tubular function decrease. As a consequence, in the severe cases, the renal concentrating ability and acidification mechanisms are impaired.[19] Before this occurs, chronic sodium retention and increased serum and urine antidiuretic activities lead to relatively increased total and extracellular body water.[20] Intracellular water is reduced in absolute terms because of losses in lean body mass, but intracellular overhydration may be present.[15,21] Physical strength is diminished, further inducing a reduction in the physical working capacity.[22,23]

Other alterations take place which have been found not to correlate directly with the degree of protein deficit, but which are always present in advanced protein deficiency. Among these, impaired intestinal absorption, moderately decreased capacity to transport protein-bound substances in blood, reduced gonadal function, and lowered local resistance to infection can be mentioned. Impaired intestinal absorption of lipids and disaccharides and a decreased rate of glucose absorption occur in severe protein deficiency; the greater the protein deficit, the greater the functional impairment. A decrease in gastric, pancreatic and bile production is also observed, with normal to low enzyme and conjugated bile acid concentrations. These alterations further impair the absorptive functions. Protein-deficient individuals are diarrhea-prone due to these alterations and possible also due to irregular intestinal motility and gastrointestinal bacterial overgrowth. Diarrhea *per se* aggravates the malabsorption.[24–28]

Finally, a generalized decrease in nervous system function is clearly apparent in severe PCM.[29,30] The etiology of these alterations has not been as yet elucidated. Several explanations have been proposed, among others, decreased brain potassium content and catecholamine production; reduced number of cells in the central nervous system when malnutrition occurs before 6 to 8 months of age, and small cell size when it occurs at a latter age.[31,32]

Decompensation from severe calorie deficiency occurs from inability to maintain internal energy supply, and results in hypoglycemia, hypothermia, impaired circulatory and renal functions, acidosis, coma and death. In the case of decompensation from protein deficiency, visceral functional failure also results from unavailability of amino acids. At the same time, an accelerated tissue breakdown takes place. The resulting alterations are mainly liver failure to synthesize certain proteins, such as albumin, several clotting factors, and transport proteins leading to fatty liver; increased free circulating cortisol, hemorrhagic diathesis, and jaundice in extreme cases; various degrees of renal failure with acidosis, as well as water and sodium retention; frankly decreased cardiac work, and tissue anoxia with pulmonary congestion. All of these factors lead to the development of clinical edema and, in extreme cases, skin lesions with hemorrhagic phenomena. In addition, there is fluid leakage into the gastrointestinal tract, increased susceptibility to pulmonary infections, water and electrolyte disturbances with hypokalemia and hypomagnesemia, frank central nervous system depression, and death.[33–35]

DIAGNOSTIC CHARACTERISTICS OF PROTEIN-CALORIE MALNUTRITION

The clinical and biochemical picture of PCM varies according to its severity and to the characteristics of the host, the environment and the agent.

Chronic Mild-to-Moderate PCM.[36] *Clinical.* It is obvious that the severe syndromes of edematous and non-edematous PCM, recognized as "kwashiorkor" and "marasmus," respectively, represent the critical end of a spectrum of varying degrees of deficiency.

However, before these severe stages are reached, children survive with insufficient calories, protein or both, a situation which does not allow them to grow and develop at the rate to be expected from their genetic potential. A long-standing restriction would be clearly manifested by a retardation in height and weight gain (Figs. 21–1 and 21–2). This reduced size may be a life-saving device to allow the children to survive on the restricted food available to them.

Under these chronic conditions, it is generally observed that body mass, although markedly retarded for the chronological age of the child, is adequate for its height. However, these children may be chronically affected by temporary periods of weight for height deficits. As judged by body composition studies, bone maturation and biochemical measurements, it is known that the malnourished child is not a small version of his well-nourished counterpart of equivalent chronological age. He shows an immaturity of biological development compatible with his retarded physical size. This includes deficits in lean body mass and adiposity, with relative overhydration affecting primarily the extracellular space. Without knowing the actual age of the subject, it is often difficult or even impossible to determine the presence or extent of malnutrition in these children.

Other characteristics of such cases, which are more difficult to attribute exclusively to

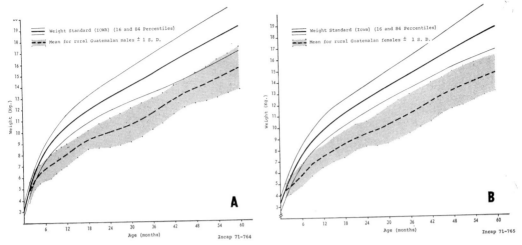

Fig. 21-1. Weight of rural Guatemalan male and female children below 5 years of age, in relation to that of U.S.A. children. Number of Guatemalan children in the sample: 431 males and 436 females.[3]

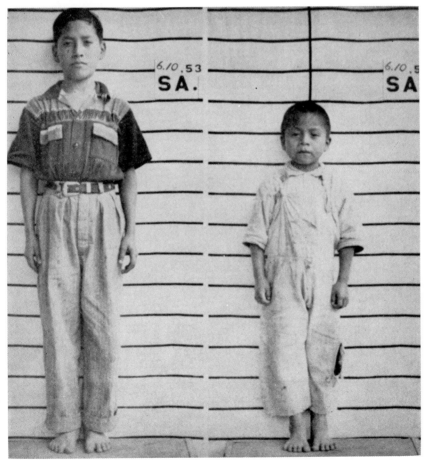

Fig. 21-2. Appearance of two 10-year-old children in the rural Central American region. The one at the left has always been well-nourished. The one at the right has been mild-to-moderately malnourished.

nutrition, are reduced physical activity, mental apathy, frequent episodes of ill-defined sickness, anorexia and diarrhea, and a higher fatality rate from common infectious diseases.

Recent studies have shown that there exists an association between retarded physical growth and development and some tests of psychomotor and mental development.[37] The isolated effect of malnutrition as a cause of this phenomenon is strongly suggested by present data derived from animal experimental work. Direct proof does not exist as yet in humans, although studies are now under way from which an answer to this question is expected. Nevertheless, it is beyond doubt that the responsible factor is the complex of social deprivation, of which nutrition is one of the most important components.[38]

Chronic PCM in adults generally results in marked leanness (Fig. 21–3), which, in severe cases, can reach a state resembling cachexia. Because their protein requirements per unit of body mass are much smaller than in children, the main manifestations are of primary calorie deficiency. Thus, physical activity and capacity for prolonged physical work are reduced, perhaps as a mechanism to keep themselves in caloric equilibrium on their low food intakes. Changes in body composition similar to those described for children can also be observed.[22,23]

Biochemical. Because of the characteristically low protein intake, subjects have a low excretion of urea N per unit of creatinine,[39] and a somewhat abnormal plasma free-amino acid pattern with a decrease of the branched essential amino acids.[40,41] It has been reported also that they excrete a lower amount of hydroxyproline in the urine, in good agreement with their slow growth rate.[42] Slight decreases in transferrin and albumin serum levels have been reported in these cases.[43,44] If lean body mass is reduced for height, this is manifested by a decreased creatinine/height index.[45]

Severe Protein-Calorie Malnutrition.
Clinical. Non-edematous PCM. Severe calorie deficiency is clinically recognized in children by the syndrome identified as *"marasmus"* in most parts of the world, or non-edematous severe PCM (Fig. 21–4). Its main charac-

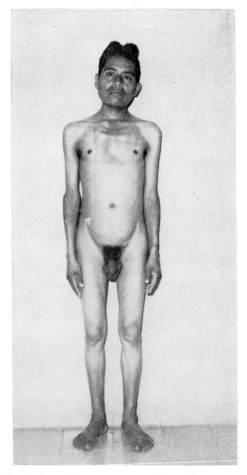

Fig. 21-3. Mild-to-moderate malnourished 36-year-old man.

teristics are: a child frankly small for his age who looks emaciated and, in extreme conditions, reduced to "skin and bones" because of an essentially total absence of adipose tissue. His skin is usually dry and "baggy," wrinkles easily and has lost its turgor. The hair is sparse, thin and dry, and can be pulled out easily; it loses its normal sheen and acquires a dull brown or reddish yellow color, giving it a lifeless appearance. The face resembles that of a monkey, with sunken cheeks in extreme cases, because of the disappearance of the Bichat fat-pad. The child is weak, looks hypotonic, and his pulse, blood pressure and temperature may be low. He is very sensitive to cold temperature, cries easily and is often found retracted from his

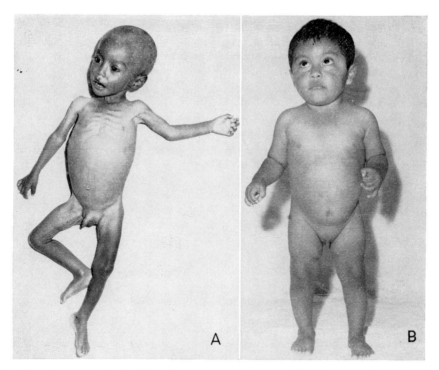

Fig. 21-4. Twenty-one-month-old child with severe non-edematous PCM (marasmus) on admission to the hospital and 4 months later, when fully recovered.

environment, sucking one or more fingers. Soon after therapy is initiated the child becomes alert and interested in his environment. His viscera are small and lymph nodes are easily felt. In adults, extreme emaciation is characteristic of calorie deficit (Fig. 21-5).

Common complicating features are eye lesions, due to hypovitaminosis A, and skin infections. The classical cases suffer from constipation and are ravenously hungry, but diarrhea, anorexia and vomiting, with dehydration, are not rare: dehydration, acidosis and electrolyte imbalances may, in fact, cause death. Postmortem examination shows only generalized atrophy, without fatty liver. Clinically, and post mortem, the child has no edema, although his total body water is increased for his size.[11,15]

Edematous PCM. The child with acute severe protein deficiency of the *"sugar baby"* type (Fig. 21-6) is usually almost normal in height for age: his body fat is normal or increased, but flabby, and he is clinically

edematous. The edema may be located only in the lower segments of the body, due to action of gravity, but generally his face is swollen, his cheeks look heavy and his eyelids are swollen shut. He is pale and the skin shines in the edematous areas. In other parts of his body the skin may be dry, atrophic or have large asymmetrical confluent areas of hyperpigmentation and hyperkeratosis. A peeling type of desquamation occurs in these areas, leaving underneath a fine, atrophic pinkish skin. Hair is atrophic, dry, depigmented and has a reddish tint, falls off easily and breaks upon rolling it between the fingers. Often, zones of alopecia are noted. The nails are brittle and have horizontal grooves. The general appearance is that of a hypotonic, miserable-looking child. He is apathetic and irritable at the same time. In the severest cases his apathy is profound. Anorexia is almost universal. Hepatomegaly is frequent, as are a swollen stomach and intestinal loops. Diarrhea is almost always present. Frequent complications are eye

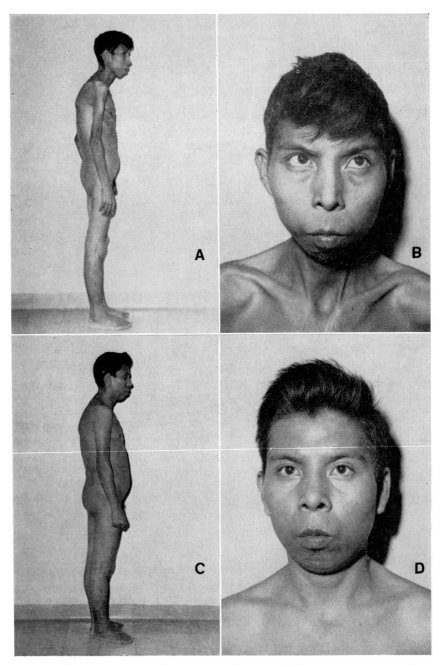

Fig. 21-5. Twenty-nine-year-old man with severe non-edematous PCM on admission to the hospital and 3 months later, when fully recovered.

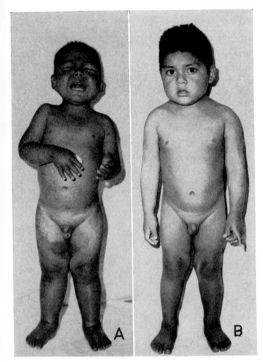

Fig. 21-6. Thirty-six-month-old child with severe edematous PCM and preservations of adiposity (kwashiorkor) on admission to the hospital and 4 months later, when fully recovered.

tion, both in children and adults, fall between these two extremes of pure caloric and pure protein deficiency. In these cases, a moderate-to-severe protein deficit may be superimposed on a severe degree of calorie deficiency, and vice versa, a moderate-to-severe degree of calorie deficit may be superimposed on a severe degree of protein deficiency (Fig. 21-7). These subjects, suffering from severe PCM with edema, together with pure protein deficiency, have been termed "kwashiorkor" cases. Clinical edema constitutes the main characteristic for its diagnosis. The mixed PCM cases have also been identified with a variety of terms, among which are "pluricarential syndrome," in Central America, "undernutrition," in other Latin American regions, and "protein malnutrition" in certain African and Asian countries.[1,35,36] In adults, a predominant protein deficiency can also conduce to edematous PCM (Fig. 21-8).

lesions due to vitamin A deficiency, cheilitis and cheilosis, as well as other manifestations of deficiencies of the vitamin B complex. Upper respiratory infections and dehydration, even in the presence of edema, are common and often lead to death. Intestinal motility is irregular, and these children often become dehydrated before they pass a huge liquid stool. As the child begins to recover he loses his edema and remains fat and flabby. This appearance often misleads the clinician who may consider him recovered because his weight may be normal. In fact, he is still severely protein deficient in terms of lean body mass.

Pulmonary edema with bronchopneumonia, septicemia, gastroenteritis and water and electrolyte imbalances are the most commonly found causes of death. At autopsy, generalized edema, visceral and muscle atrophy and severe fatty liver are found. Red bone marrow is centripetally retracted.

The majority of cases of severe malnutri-

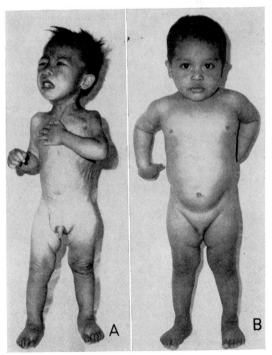

Fig. 21-7. Twenty-five-month-old child with severe edematous PCM superimposed on chronic caloric deficit. Besides being edematous, he appears wasted (marasmus-kwashiorkor). Pictures were taken on admission to the hospital and 4 months later, when fully recovered.

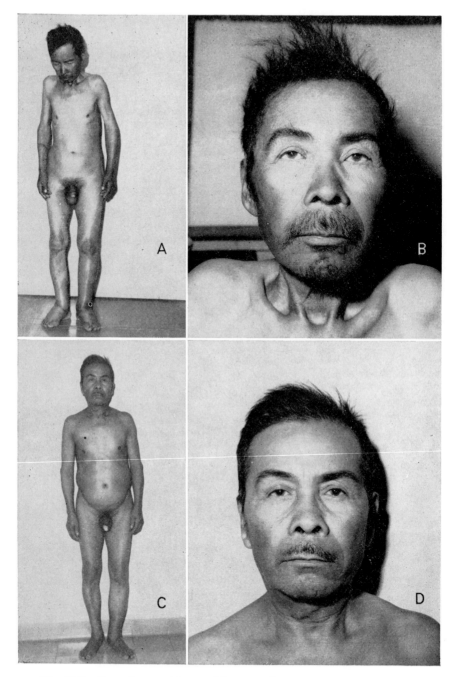

Fig. 21-8. Forty-six-year-old man with severe edematous PCM on admission to the hospital and 3 months later, when fully recovered.

Biochemical. In severe protein-calorie malnutrition several biochemical alterations can be observed. Many of these are distinguishing between the *edematous* and the *non-edematous* types.

Proteins and Nitrogenous Compounds. The child who has reached the severe stage of edematous PCM has been submitted to a severe negative balance of body proteins.[46] Consequently, his total body nitrogen is markedly reduced. Different organs share this protein loss to different extents.[47,48] The liver rapidly loses a fraction of proteins, while the loss of muscle protein is progressive and, because of its large mass, accounts for the major part of the protein loss. Kidney, brain and endocrine organs seem to retain their protein more efficiently. However, the importance of these different losses in terms of organ function cannot be derived from their relative magnitude. A low ratio of protein to DNA has been shown in muscle, liver, and brain, illustrating intracellular protein loss.[32,49] In the non-edematous PCM these changes are moderate, becoming severe only in the most advanced stages.

The concentration of several protein fractions in the body fluids is low. The blood plasma has been studied more at depth. Although present in both types of PCM, edematous and non-edematous, the changes to be described are more pronounced in the first type. In the second one, they may be totally absent. The concentration of total proteins is reduced, and the magnitude of the reduction is explained mainly by a decreased albumin concentration. The concentration of beta-globulins is also decreased. On the other hand, the gamma-globulin fraction concentration is either normal or increased; therefore, their per cent contribution to the total plasma proteins is always high.[35] Some plasma proteins with very specific functions may also be decreased. Among them, those associated with the transport of other nutrients and hormones are particularly important, such as transferrin,[43,50] ceruloplasmin,[50] retinol-binding protein (RBP),[51] alpha- and beta-lipoproteins,[52] as well as thyroxin[53] and cortisol-binding proteins.[54] Impaired blood transport may attain significance in the development of secondary metabolic abnormalities,

as has been shown in the case of lipids and vitamin A.[55] The blood concentration of urea nitrogen is found to be low, as is also its excretion in the urine. This reflects the low catabolic rate of body proteins and decreased urea synthesis, which are characteristic of primary protein deficiency.[12] When calories are the most limiting factor, urea production is increased, because body protein catabolism is elevated, as has been demonstrated in some non-edematous cases suffering mainly from marasmus.[56]

The excretion of urinary creatinine is decreased,[57,58] a consequence of the decrease in muscle tissue and lean body mass.[59]

The plasma free-amino acid pattern is abnormal in edematous PCM. A lowered concentration of valine, leucine, and isoleucine is a characteristic, as is also a very low tyrosine concentration.[60,61] The ratio of the branched essential to non-essential amino acids is low. Another finding, which is very characteristic, is a low tyrosine-phenylalanine ratio, due to a deficiency in phenylalanine hydroxylase.[62] In non-edematous PCM, plasma amino acid alterations may be absent.[40]

Hemoglobin concentration is variable, but often it is around 10 gm/100 ml because of hemodilution. Generally, the cells are normochromic and normocytic. Hypochromia can be present, if there exists a severe iron deficiency from other causes. Mild to overt megaloblastosis can occur because of folate deficiency.[63] The great majority of subjects are not anemic but physiologically adapted to the decreased oxygen demands.[10,17] Leukocytosis can occur, if infection is present: leukopenia and thrombocytopenia generally indicate the presence of gram-negative septicemia.

Although it has been observed that urinary amino acid excretion is abnormal, no consistent pattern seems to be evident. The abnormal metabolites, ethanolamine and beta-amino isobutyric acid, have been detected, suggesting a defect in transmethylation.[64] Excretion of urocanic acid has been shown to be abnormal after a histidine load.[65]

Carbohydrates. Usually blood glucose is normal. However, there is an increased tendency to hypoglycemia upon fasting.

This is compatible with the finding that liver and muscle glycogen stores are normal or low.[66] Some alterations revealed by clinical laboratory studies suggest abnormal metabolic handling of glucose. Furthermore, glucose tolerance tests give a diabetic type of curve, and insulin secretion is low.[67,68] Impaired glucose utilization, glycogenolysis and glycolysis have also been demonstrated. In addition, there are isolated pieces of evidence of impaired enzymatic steps along the glucose oxidation, the Krebs cycle and the galactose to glucose conversion paths.[66,69,70]

Lipids. Steatorrhea is a characteristic of edematous PCM, even when the diet is practically devoid of fat.[71] Lipid absorption has been found reduced.[72] Low levels of many serum lipid fractions, neutral fat, cholesterol, particularly its esters, vitamins A and E, and phospholipids have been demonstrated. These findings suggest that the changes in specific plasma proteins and physical chemical structure of the lipid-protein complexes account for impaired blood transport.[55,73,74] In fact, there is direct evidence for decreased lipoproteins as well as for RBP, the specific vitamin A-binding protein.[51] A great part of the fatty liver may well be the consequence of inability to mobilize fat.[74]

Vitamins.[75] Signs of water-soluble vitamin deficiencies vary with the local dietary patterns, but, even when intakes are low, serum concentrations of thiamin, riboflavin, vitamin C, niacin metabolites and folates may well be within the normal range, and overt clinical signs of deficiency of these factors are rarely seen. Vitamin B_{12} serum levels are often found to be high. All of the above findings suggest that, although the supply of these vitamins may be low, tissue demands are also decreased.

In the edematous type of PCM (kwashiorkor), serum levels of vitamins A and E are consistently lower than normal. In the case of vitamin A, poor vitamin intake and defective absorption and transport explain these alterations. This explanation may well apply also to vitamin E. All levels rise rapidly with therapy.

Water and Electrolytes.[34,76,77] Hypo-osmolarity is a common finding. Serum sodium levels are from normal to low. Potassium and magnesium serum levels are not decreased, except when excessive losses of the cations occur due to diarrhea and vomiting. In such cases, hypokalemia is accompanied by a loss of potassium from specific tissues such as muscle and brain.[78] This results in a decreased cellular potassium-to-nitrogen ratio. Mild acidosis is also common, on account of a decrease in the renal acidification mechanisms. Total serum calcium is somewhat low, primarily due to the protein-bound fraction.

Enzymes. The activity of several serum enzymes such as amylase, pseudocholinesterase and alkaline phosphatase is reduced. Their drop is consistent and quite parallel to that of albumin, so that they may be normal in non-edematous PCM.[35,79] Serum transaminases are elevated and reflect increased tissue transaminase activity and leakage from the cells.[80] Around 15 hepatic enzymes have been studied,[81,82] including dehydrogenases, oxidases and esterases; of these, 4 are clearly decreased in the edematous type of PCM: xanthine oxidase, glycolic acid oxidase, d-amino acid oxidase and cholinesterase. It has been pointed out that these enzymes are not involved in fundamental physiological functions and seem to be of relatively little importance. On the other hand, cytochrome C reductase, a key enzyme in electron transport, is well preserved.

More complex systems, which depend on the integrity of the mitochondria, have been studied. Oxidative phosphorylation is somewhat reduced, and phosphate uptake into phosphatides is about half the value seen in recovered children.[46]

Enzymatic changes in liver and PMN leukocytes have been studied comparatively.[83] It has been found that not only are changes in both tissues very similar, but that they are characteristically different in the edematous and non-edematous types. In summary, these changes are: increased activity of fumarase and aconitase, and decreased activity of isocitric dehydrogenase, glutamic dehydrogenase and aldolase in the edematous malnourished child. The reverse is true in the non-edematous patients. Muscle creatine phosphokinase activity has been found to be consistently low in children with the edematous type, while, in those suffering from the marasmic type, low or normal values can be observed.[84]

It is impossible to separate the effects of protein deficiency *per se* on enzymes from changes in activity which may reflect changes in functional pattern in response to adaptation. In general, the latter interpretation seems more plausible. Furthermore, the measurements done *in vitro* with reconstructed systems tell nothing about subcellular structure changes, which may alter linking of enzymes with their substrates and co-factors. These could well involve alterations in membrane structure at the cellular and subcellular level.

TREATMENT

Chronic Mild-to-Moderate Protein-Calorie Malnutrition. Children suffering from chronic protein-calorie malnutrition are, as mentioned before, smaller in height and lighter in weight than their counterparts of equivalent chronological age. Because these children are not only physically retarded but also proportionally immature, their protein and calorie intake should be calculated on the basis of their height, that is, as if the child were well-fed but younger, of an age for which his height would correspond to the 50th percentile. This means a higher calorie and protein intake per kg of body weight than that of children of the same chronological age. These intakes, therefore, will promote a retention of energy and protein to permit catch-up in growth and development. Of course, they should contain the appropriate concentrations of all the other essential nutrients. Even more, when marked deficiencies of other nutrients are also prevalent, administration of specific supplements is called for.

Severe Protein-Calorie Malnutrition. The severe, uncompensated forms of PCM require medical guidance during the initial phases of treatment.[85,86] In these cases, even when hospitalized, mortality is high, ranging from 11 to 50 per cent, depending on the centers where they are treated and on certain characteristics of the patients. Table 21–5 lists those characteristics which carry a poor prognosis.

The treatment of severe PCM may be divided into two phases:

(*a*) That oriented towards saving the patient's life by bringing him back to his adapted stage, and

(*b*) The rehabilitation or "consolidation of cure" phase. At this stage, body protein and energy repletion for the patient's height should be achieved.

The main objectives of the initial treatment are: therapy of infection and correction of water and electrolyte imbalances, as well as of other factors which lead to decompensation. It is during this phase that a cautious handling of the nutrition aspect is essential. This demands patience, and the personnel must be conscious of the fact that the most common causes of death are one or more complications and not malnutrition *per se*. Drastic therapeutic nutritional measures, such as high protein or calorie load from the start, may precipitate death by posing an "iatrogenic" overload on enzymatic and various physiologic functions which have reached "maximal adaptation" in several weeks or even months in the process of progressive malnutrition.

Table 21-5. Characteristics of Severely Protein-Calorie Malnourished Children Which Carry a Poor Prognosis

1. Stupor or coma.
2. Age less than 6 months.
3. Weight-for-height deficit greater than 40%.
4. Severe, protracted diarrhea.
5. Infection, primarily bronchopneumonia or measles.
6. Hemorrhagic tendency. Purpura is usually associated with septicemia.
7. Severe eye lesions.
8. Extensive exudative or exfoliative dermal lesions.
9. Extensive and deep decubitus ulcers.
10. Dehydration and electrolyte disturbances, particularly hyponatremia, hypokalemia, and probably hypomagnesemia.
11. Clinical jaundice or increased serum bilirubin and/or frankly elevated serum glutamic-oxalacetic and glutamic-pyruvic transaminases.
12. Hypoglycemia and/or hypothermia.
13. Total serum proteins below 3 gm/100 ml.

Maintenance of adequate urinary output is of primary importance. This is preferably accomplished by oral therapy, keeping in mind the fact that the severely PCM individual is hypo-osmolar. Therefore, solutions of around 280 mOs/liter are preferred. These should provide from 6 to 8 mEq/kg/day of K and, if needed, the potassium concentration can be raised to 10 mEq/kg/day so as to replace actual K losses which are usually 40 mEq/liter from diarrhea or vomiting. Sodium intake should replace losses (about 35 mEq/liter from diarrhea, and 12 mEq/liter from emesis), but, otherwise, it should be low (1 mEq/kg/day) because PCM patients have an excess of body sodium. An excess of sodium and osmolar overloads can easily induce cardiac failure. Magnesium should also be administered, particularly when diarrhea and vomiting occur. Usually 1 cc of Mg $SO_4.7H_2O$, 50 per cent solution, I.M. every 12 to 24 hours is adequate. This therapy is important if tetany, oculogyric crises, tremor and bizarre neurologic signs occur in the initial phases of realimentation. Unless severe, acidosis should not be treated. Usually, renal function will handle acid-base balance efficiently.

If needed, intravenous therapy can and should be used, following the general outline described for oral rehydration, except that K therapy should not exceed 6 mEq/kg/day; osmolarity should be kept at around 280 mOs/liter, and sodium must be kept low. Administration of plasma or other "protein-rich" fluids is contraindicated.

Shock, due to severe dehydration or gram-negative septicemia, should be treated as if the individual were not malnourished. In some of these cases blood transfusions are indicated, but hemoglobin concentrations should be brought only to about 10 gm/100 ml which is commonly the hemoglobin level these children achieve from adaptation. Transfusions of packed red cells are indicated only when severe anemia is present and cardiorespiratory failure is imminent. Again, hemoglobin concentration should be brought only to around 10 gm/100 ml.

Infection should be treated vigorously and, if possible, with the help of a laboratory, so that the infective organisms can be isolated and their sensitivity to antibacterial agents determined.

A free airway with adequate lung ventilation is essential. When pneumonia is present, tracheostomy should be undertaken, because it often happens that these subjects are weak and cannot clear their airways satisfactorily.

When severe hepatic failure occurs, it should be treated accordingly, as is done when cardiac failure supervenes. Diarrhea is treated mainly by diet. No anti-cholinergic drugs are used. Another general rule that must be followed is to guard the PCM patient from exposure to cold and hypothermia, as well as from hypoglycemia. During this initial phase of therapy a diet based on high-quality protein, such as milk-casein mixtures (to reduce lactose loads), casein alone, egg or fish protein, is recommended. In children this should provide, during 3 to 4 days, around 1 gm/kg/day of protein and 80 to 100 calories/kg/day, 20 per cent of the calories derived from vegetable fat. From then on, and based on the same ingredients, dietary therapy should be progressively increased to reach, in a 4- to 6-day period, from 3 to 4 gm of protein and from 120 to 180 calories/kg/day, 20 to 30 per cent from a fat source. In adults, calorie intakes at the start may be 50 calories/kg/day to reach, later on, 80 to 100 calories/kg/day.

Vitamins, including folate, should be administered from the beginning, to meet recommended allowances. On admission, the routine administration of a single high dose (20,000 mcg) of water-dispersible vitamin A is recommended to avoid acute eye lesions due to vitamin A deficiency when high calorie and protein diets are initiated. This is followed by a daily dose of 1500 mcg P.O.

The diet should also provide from 4 to 5 mEq/kg/day of K, 1 mEq/kg/day of Na, and adequate amounts of magnesium, calcium and phosphorus. Iron, in amounts from 16 to 32 mg, as $FeSO_4$, is routinely administered by mouth as soon as increased protein-calorie intakes are begun, in order to supply the excess requirements of this mineral produced by the rapid increase in total circulating hemoglobin.

With this initial regimen, the severely malnourished subjects begin a smooth recovery: they start to lose edema and to gain in body mass; their general state shows the first signs of improvement and anorexia is replaced by a frankly increased appetite. Then the patient may begin to eat a more varied diet; serum and urine values also start a trend towards normal and the hematological status initiates recovery. All of these changes are accompanied by a clear rise in nitrogen and energy retention. Except for sodium, mineral retention also increases. Rapid changes in weight should be avoided, particularly a rapid loss of edema. Usually, within 2 to 3 weeks of therapy, serum composition returns to normal limits, and consolidation of cure begins.

This second phase of therapy is accomplished only by dietary means. The patients should by then be receiving a complete mixed diet providing the protein and calorie levels reached in the later phase of the initiation of therapy. Progressive physical activity should be encouraged. Complete calorie and protein repletion generally is accomplished in a 6-

to 12-week period, depending on the deficits at the start of treatment. Calorie repletion is judged by weight-for-height, and is considered achieved when this index is 0.90 or more. Generally, in non-edematous PCM, normalization of weight-for-height is reached later than normalization of the creatinine/height index. In edematous PCM the opposite occurs. These changes are illustrated in Figures 21–9 and 10.

PREVENTION

Two are the aspects from which prevention can be approached: (1) measures to decrease the risk of individuals reaching severe PCM, and (2) improvement of the general nutritional status of the population, so that even chronic mild-to-moderate PCM cases become rare.

The first aspect of prevention is amenable to some direct actions. These include: (a) fostering of maternal lactation and adequate supplementation practices during infancy; (b) food supplementation programs of vulnerable groups, such as pregnant and lactat-

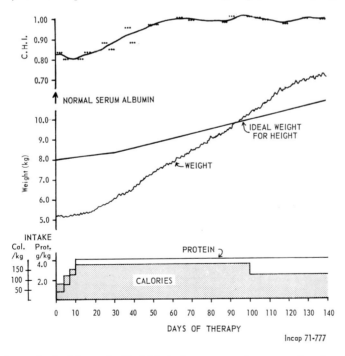

Incap 71-777

Fig. 21-9. Clinical record of a 16-month-old child during recovery from non-edematous PCM. His lean body mass (CHI) reached normal levels before his weight-for-height was normal.

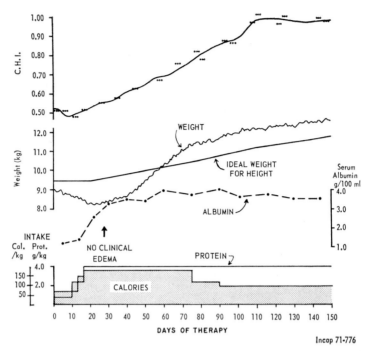

Fig. 21-10. Clinical record of a 20-month-old child during recovery from edematous PCM. His lean body mass (CHI) reached normal levels after his weight-for-height was normal.

ing women, children up to school age and above, if possible, and physically hard-working men; (c) improvement of sanitary conditions, and (d) specific nutrition education. For this last objective, nutrition education and recuperation centers[87] have been instituted in several countries. Their main objective is to educate the parents of chronic mild-to-moderate PCM children by having them participate actively in the nutrition rehabilitation of their own children. These centers must be (a) located in the community and adapted to the local environment; (b) supported by each community; (c) children must be rehabilitated by the proper feeding of locally available foods, and (d) the mothers must rotate in the care of the children, so as to have direct experience of the benefits that adequate nutrition brings to their children. Experience is accumulating on the effects of these specific preventive measures, indicating that they appear to fulfill their goals.

Improvement of the general nutritional status of the population, so that malnutrition is eradicated, requires a complex approach.

This is inseparable from the acceleration of socioeconomic development; the actions to bring this about are beyond the scope of this chapter.

BIBLIOGRAPHY

1. Scrimshaw and Béhar: Fed. Proc. *18* (Suppl. 3), 82, 1959.
2. Gómez, Ramos Galván, Frenk, Cravioto-Muñoz, Chávez and Vásquez: J. Trop. Pediat. *2*, 77, 1956.
3. *Evaluación Nutricional de la Población de Centro América y Panamá. Guatemala.* Instituto de Nutrición de Centro América y Panamá (INCAP); Oficina de Investigaciones Internacionales de los Institutos Nacionales de Salud (EEUU); Ministerio de Salud Pública y Asistencia Social. Guatemala, Instituto de Nutrición de Centro América y Panamá. 1969, 136 pp. plus 5 appendices.
4. Viteri, Béhar and Alvarado: Rev. Col. Med. (Guatemala) *21*, 137, 1970.
5. Soriano: Rev. Chilena Pediat. *39*, 475, 1968.
6. Waterlow: *Fatty Liver Disease in Infants in the British West Indies.* London, Her Majesty's Stationary Office, 1948 (Medical Research Council Special Report Series No. 263), 84 pp. plus 12 plates.

7. Mata, Urrutia and Gordon: Trop. Geogr. Med. *19*, 247, 1967.
8. Gordon, Chitkara and Wyon: Am. J. Med. Sci. *245*, 345, 1963.
9. Viteri and Alvarado: Rev. Col. Med. (Guatemala) *21*, 175, 1970.
10. Viteri and Pineda: In *Famine. A Symposium Dealing with Nutrition and Relief Operations in Times of Disaster.* Edited by Blix, Hofvander and Vahlquist. Almquist and Wiksells, Boktryckeri Aktiebolag, Uppsala, Sweden, 1971.
11. Kerpel-Fronius, Varga and Kun: Ann. Pediat. (Switzerland) *183*, 1, 1954.
12. Waterlow, Alleyne, Chan, Garrow, Hay, James, Picou and Stephen: Arch. Latinoamer. Nutr. *16*, 175, 1966.
13. Beisel, Sawyer, Ryll and Crozier: Ann. Intern. Med. *67*, 744, 1967.
14. Cohen and Hansen: Clin. Sci. *23*, 351, 1962.
15. Frenk, Metcoff, Gómez, Ramos-Galván, Cravioto and Antonowicz: Pediatrics *20*, 105, 1957.
16. Alleyne: Clin. Sci. *34*, 199, 1968.
17. Viteri, Alvarado, Luthringer and Wood: Vitamins Hormones *26*, 573, 1968.
18. Alleyne: Clin. Sci. *30*, 553, 1966.
19. Gordillo, Soto, Metcoff, López and García Antillón: Pediatrics *20*, 303, 1957.
20. Srikantia: In *Calorie Deficiencies and Protein Deficiencies.* Edited by McCance and Widdowson. London, J. & A. Churchill Ltd., 1968, p. 2033.
21. Brinkman, Bowie, Fansriss-Hen and Hansen: Pediatrics *36*, 94, 1965.
22. Keys, Brozek, Henschel, Mickelsen and Taylor: *The Biology of Human Starvation.* Vol. II. Minneapolis. University of Minnesota Press, 1950. p. 1002.
23. Viteri: In *Amino Acid Fortification of Protein Foods.* Report of an International Conference held at the Massachusetts Institute of Technology, September 16 to 18, 1969. Edited by Scrimshaw and Altschul. Cambridge, Mass., The MIT Press, 1971, p. 350.
24. Viteri, Flores and Béhar: In *VIIth International Congress of Nutrition. Abstracts of Papers. Hamburg, 3-10 VIII, 1966.* Hamburg, Germany, Pergamos-Druck, 1966, p. 4.
25. Bowie, Barbezat and Hansen: Am. J. Clin. Nutr. *20*, 89, 1967.
26. Barbezat and Hansen: Pediatrics *42*, 77, 1968.
27. Schneider and Viteri: Am. J. Clin. Nutr., *25*, 1092, 1972.
28. Mata, Jiménez, Cordón, Schneider, Viteri, Rosales and Prera: Am. J. Clin. Nutr., *25*, 1118, 1972.
29. Barrera Moncada: *La Edad Pre-Escolar.* Mérida, Venezuela, Talleres Gráficos Universitarios, 1964, 541 pp.
30. Geber and Dean: Courrier (Paris) *6*, 3, 1956.
31. Hoeldtke and Wurtman: Fed. Proc. *30*, 459, 1971.
32. Winick and Rosso: Pediatría (Chile) *12*, 159, 1969.
33. Wayburne: In *Calorie Deficiencies and Protein Deficiencies.* Edited by McCance and Widdowson. London, J. & A. Churchill Ltd., 1968, p. 7.
34. Garrow, Smith and Ward: *Electrolyte Metabolism in Severe Infantile Malnutrition.* London, Pergamon Press, 1968, 168 pp.
35. Trowell, Davies and Dean: *Kwashiorkor.* London, Edward Arnold Ltd., 1954, 308 pp.
36. Viteri, Béhar, Arroyave and Scrimshaw: In: *Mammalian Protein Metabolism.* Edited by Munro and Allison. Vol. II (Chapter 22). New York, Academic Press, 1964, p. 523.
37. Cravioto, DeLicardie and Birch: Pediatrics *38* (Suppl., Part II), 319, 1966.
38. Canosa: In: *Malnutrition, Learning, and Behavior.* Edited by Scrimshaw and Gordon. Proceedings of an International Conference co-sponsored by the Nutrition Foundation Inc. and the Massachusetts Institute of Technology, held at Cambridge, Mass., March 1-3, 1967. Cambridge, Mass., The M.I.T. Press, 1968, p. 389.
39. Arroyave: In: *Mild-Moderate Forms of Protein-Calorie Malnutrition.* Edited by Blix. Symposia of the Swedish Nutrition Foundation I. Båstad, August 29-31, 1962. Uppsala, Almqvist and Wilksells, 1963, p. 32.
40. Whitehead: In: *Calorie Deficiencies and Protein Deficiencies.* Edited by McCance and Widdowson. London, J. & A. Churchill Ltd., 1968, p. 109.
41. Arroyave: In: *Protein Calorie Malnutrition.* Edited by von Muralt. Berlin, Springer-Verlag, 1969, p. 48.
42. Whitehead: Lancet, *2*, 567, 1965.
43. McFarlane, Ogbeide, Reddy, Adcok, Adeshina, Gurney, Cooke, Taylor and Mordie: Lancet *1*, 392, 1969.
44. Hansen: In: *Calorie Deficiencies and Protein Deficiencies.* Edited by McCance and Widdowson. London. J. & A. Churchill Ltd., 1968, p. 33.
45. Viteri and Alvarado: Pediatrics *46*, 696, 1970.
46. Waterlow, Cravioto and Stephen: Adv. Prot. Chem. *15*, 131, 1960.
47. Garrow, Fletcher and Halliday: J. Clin. Invest. *44*, 417, 1965.
48. Halliday: Clin. Sci. *33*, 365, 1967.
49. Mendes and Waterlow: Brit. J. Nutr. *12*, 74, 1958.
50. Lahey, Béhar, Viteri and Scrimshaw: Pediatrics *22*, 72, 1958.
51. Goodman, Arroyave and Viteri: in preparation.
52. Cravioto: Bol. Med. Hosp. Infantil (Mexico) *15*, 805, 1958.
53. Beas, Mönckeberg and Horwitz (with Figueroa): Pediatrics *38*, 1003, 1966.
54. Alleyne and Young: Clin. Sci. *33*, 189, 1967.
55. Arroyave, Wilson, Méndez, Béhar and Scrimshaw: Am. J. Clin. Nutr. *9*, 180, 1961.
56. Reddy, Belavady and Srikantia: Indian J. Med. Res. *51*, 952, 1963.
57. Standard, Wills and Waterlow: Am. J. Clin. Nutr. *7*, 271, 1959.
58. Arroyave, Wilson, Béhar and Scrimshaw: Am. J. Clin. Nutr. *9*, 176, 1961.

21

59. Alleyne, Viteri and Alvarado: Am. J. Clin. Nutr. *23*, 875, 1970.
60. Holt, Snyderman, Norton, Roitman and Finch: Lancet *2*, 1343, 1963.
61. Arroyave, Wilson, Funes and Béhar: Am. J. Clin. Nutr. *11*, 517, 1962.
62. Cravioto: Am. J. Clin. Nutr. *11*, 484, 1962.
63. Adams and Scragg: J. Pediat. *60*, 580, 1962.
64. Edozien and Phillips: Nature *191*, 47, 1961.
65. Whitehead and Arnstein: Nature *190*, 1105, 1961.
66. Alleyne and Scullard: Clin. Sci. *37*, 631, 1969.
67. James and Coore: Am. J. Clin. Nutr. *23*, 386, 1970.
68. Becker, Pimstone, Hansen, Buchanan-Lee and MacHutchon: S. African Med. J. *43*, 1154, 1969.
69. Gillman, Gillman, Scragg, Savage, Gilbert, Trout and Levy: S. African J. Med. Sci. *26*, 31, 1961.
70. Metcoff, Frenk, Yoshida, Torres-Pinedo, Kaiser and Hansen: Medicine (Baltimore) *45*, 365, 1966.
71. Van der Sar: Documenta Neerlandica et Indonesica de Morbis Tropicis (Amsterdam) *3*, 25, 1951.
72. Jayasekera, De Mel and Collumbine: Ceylon J. Med. Sci. (D) *8*, 1, 1951.
73. Schwartz and Dean: J. Trop. Pediat. *3*, 23, 1957.
74. Flores, Sierralta and Mönckeberg: J. Nutrition *100*, 375, 1970.
75. Béhar, Arroyave, Tejada, Viteri and Scrimshaw: Rev. Col. Med. (Guatemala) *7*, 221, 1956.
76. Metcoff, Frenk, Gordillo, Gómez, Ramos Galván, Cravioto, Janeway and Gamble: Pediatrics *20*, 317, 1957.
77. Caddell and Goddard: New Eng. J. Med. *276*, 533, 1967.
78. Garrow: Lancet *2*, 643, 1967.
79. Arroyave, Feldman and Scrimshaw: Am. J. Clin. Nutr. *6*, 164, 1958.
80. McLean: Clin. Sci. *30*, 129, 1966.
81. Waterlow: Fed. Proc. *18*, 1143, 1959.
82. Burch, Arroyave, Schwartz, Padilla, Béhar, Viteri, and Scrimshaw: J. Clin. Invest. *36*, 1579, 1957.
83. Pineda: In: *Calorie Deficiencies and Protein Deficiencies*. Edited by McCance and Widdowson. London, J. & A. Churchill Ltd., 1968, p. 75.
84. Contreras, Pineda, Viteri and Arroyave: Fed. Proc. *30*, 231, 1971.
85. Garrow, Picou and Waterlow: West Indian Med. J. *11*, 217, 1962.
86. Alvarado, Viteri and Béhar: Rev. Col. Méd. (Guatemala) *21*, 231, 1970.
87. Bengoa: J. Trop. Pediat. *10*, 63, 1964.

Chapter

22

Obesity

JEAN MAYER

DEFINITION OF OBESITY

Obesity is a pathological condition characterized by an accumulation of fat much in excess of that necessary for optimal body function. As such, it is distinct from "overweight" which is defined as body weight much in excess of average. Both these definitions contain an element of imprecision, both from the physiological and the anatomical viewpoint. For example, populations which expect to be subjected at regular intervals to scarcity of food may consider a certain measure of obesity as desirable, indeed as necessary for survival. Such considerations, however, no longer apply to the United States, where longevity is greatest when obesity is least. The definition of overweight given above makes no mention of body type. Yet a professional football player may be muscular and lean at a weight for his height which is clearly excessive when seen on a physically inactive executive. At the risk of being trite, let us emphasize at the outset of this chapter the importance of careful physical examination of the patient: if a man, woman or child looks fat when undressed, he or she most likely is too fat. Visual observation by an experienced observer is a more reliable method than the automatic application of height-weight tables, at least, when the degree of overweight is not extreme. Obviously, however, we need quantitative data on both obesity and overweight if we are to carefully follow individual patients and relate weight and fat content to disease in population groups.[1]

DIAGNOSIS AND ESTIMATION OF OBESITY

A number of methods have been developed for the estimation of body fat (See Chapter 1). The execution of some of these methods is too complex for the practicing physician or nutritionist. We shall, therefore, concentrate, in this chapter, on the two basic methods, determination of weight and its relation to height, age and body type and skin-fold determinations.

Height-Weight Tables. The appearance of the naked patient is the usual basis for the diagnosis of obesity by the experienced clinician and, as a qualitative guide, is usually reliable. When a quantitative estimate is desired, the patient's weight is usually compared with the "standard" weight for his height as given by one of several tables. For children and adolescents, the standard is usually an average weight for height, age and sex. The variety of tables available includes the Baldwin-Wood, Bayer and Bayley, Stuart, Hathaway, Falkner, etc. Some of these tables show percentiles as well as medians. (See Chapter 1 for discussion of Height-Weight tables and Appendix for table of desirable weights for adults.) The Wetzel grid defines channels expressing percentiles of weight for height, independent of age.

Limitations of Tables. It is obvious that if overweight (weight in excess of average) is very marked, obesity (excessive fatness) is present. For moderate degrees of overweight, however, obesity is by no means clear. College football linemen are generally overweight: they are generally not obese. Conversely some extremely sedentary persons can be obese without being markedly overweight. Without a more direct measurement of adiposity, the diagnosis of obesity cannot be certain.

The standards derived from the "Build and Blood Pressure Study, 1959"[2] have additional weaknesses. First, there is some question as to how representative the insurance data are for the general population of the United States. Seltzer has shown that average weights in Metropolitan Life tables are 9 to 10 pounds less for men and 3 to 4 pounds less for women than the average values obtained in the National Health Examination Survey of the United States Public Health Service on a stratified, noninstitutionalized random sample of men and women from all classes and areas of the country from 1960 through 1962.[3] Secondly, the Metropolitan Life Insurance Company tables give no definitions of frames, so that the user is unable to characterize his frame in the same way as the authors of the tables.

Recent epidemiologic data have shown that properly defined variations in body structure are important not only in terms of defining obesity, but also possibly in terms of longevity. Analysis of the data of the "Build and Blood Pressure Study, 1959" tends to suggest this. In general, for each broad height category, mortality increased as weight increased. These data have been interpreted to mean that increased overweight is responsible for increased mortality. However, since persons who have the lowest weight for height (referred to by the life insurance companies' actuarians as underweights) and who must be for the most part dominant ectomorphs (rather than emaciated mesomorphs and endomorphs) have the highest longevity, it appears that this body type is associated with a longer-than average life expectancy. The significant association of obesity with bones and muscles larger than average, which Seltzer and Mayer[4] have demonstrated in females, suggests that, at least among females, there may be an association between increased mortality and body type, irrespective of adiposity. Gertler and White[5] and Spain, Bradess and Greenblatt[6] also have suggested the association of certain body types with specific diseases. The ultimate answer to the question of the relation of obesity to mortality may lie in treating each type of body build separately and in correlating the extent of adiposity of each category of body build with mortality and disease manifestations.

While one cannot quarrel with the general concept that excessive weight gain after growth has ceased is bad for the patient, it appears questionable to base the diagnosis of obesity and the prescription of an ideal weight for a given patient on height-weight tables, even those as seemingly sophisticated as the ones derived from the "Build and Blood Pressure Study, 1959." A knowledge of the patient's actual fatness is preferable not only from the viewpoint of diagnosing obesity, but also because it emphasizes that component of body weight which can, in fact, be modified.

MEASUREMENT OF SKIN-FOLD THICKNESS

Measurement of skin-fold thickness appears to be the simplest and most practical available method of determining the extent of obesity. These measurements, obtained by using a suitable caliper on selected sites, have been shown by comparison with results of other methods to give a good indication not only of subcutaneous fat (about 50 per cent of the total fat) but also of total body fat. The technique is simple and the caliper relatively inexpensive.[*] With proper directions and a minimum of demonstration by an experienced person, the physician can obtain reproducible measurements with the skin-fold caliper.

Standardization of skin-fold calipers has become a necessary requirement for universal comparability of fatfold measurements and conversion to total body fat. The accepted national recommendation is a caliper so designed as to exert a pressure on the caliper face of 10 gm per square millimeter and with a contact surface of 20 to 40 mm.[7][†]

* Calipers usually range in price from $65 to $75.
† Skin-fold calipers meeting these requirements include the Lange Skin-fold Caliper, manufactured by the Cambridge Scientific Industries, Inc., Cambridge, Maryland, and the Harpenden Skinfold Caliper, manufactured by British Indicators, Ltd., St. Albans, Hertfordshire, England.

The skin-fold measurement to be obtained is the (doubled) thickness of the pinched "folded" skin plus the attached subcutaneous adipose tissue. The person making the measurement pinches up a full fold of skin and subcutaneous tissue with the thumb and forefinger of his left hand at a distance about 1 cm from the site at which the calipers are to be placed, pulling the fold away from the underlying muscle. The fold is pinched up firmly and held while the measurement is being taken. The calipers are applied to the fold about 1 cm below the fingers, so that the pressure on the fold at the point measured is exerted by the faces of the caliper and not by the fingers. The handle of the caliper is released to permit the full force of the caliper arm pressure, and the dial is read to the nearest 0.5 mm. Caliper application should be made at least twice for stable readings. If the folds are extremely thick, dial readings should be made 3 seconds after applying the caliper pressure.

Sites Measured for Skin-fold Thickness. Various workers have used a number of sites, including the triceps, subscapular, abdominal, hip, pectoral and calf areas. For the general population, the Committee on Nutritional Anthropometry of the National Research Council has recommended the triceps and the subscapular skin-folds as good indexes of an individual's over-all fatness.[8]

Triceps Skin-fold. The triceps skin-fold is located at the back of the right upper arm midway between the acromion and olecranon processes. The midpoint can be marked with the aid of a steel tape. The arm should hang freely during the skin-fold measurement. Because of the gradation of subcutaneous fat thickness from shoulder to elbow, location of the midpoint is somewhat critical.

Subscapular Skin-fold. The subscapular skin-fold is located just below the angle of the right scapula (shoulder and arm relaxed). The fold is picked up in a line slightly inclined in the natural cleavage of the skin. Because the subcutaneous fat is fairly uniform in this region, precision of location is less critical.

The work of Seltzer, Goldman and Mayer,[9] among others, indicates that for obese individuals the triceps skin-fold, which is the easiest to measure, is also the most representative of

body fatness. No special advantage is gained in utilizing any other skin-fold in addition to the triceps skin-fold.

CRITERION FOR OBESITY

Extensive data on the distribution of triceps skin-fold values, such as those obtained by Young and Blondin[10] and Novak,[11] allow determination of the normal variation of such skin-folds in our population (at least for Caucasian subjects). The next step, setting up a cutoff point for obesity, is obviously arbitrary. Because of its association with certain body types, the distribution of fatness within the general population may not be strictly monomodal; it does, however, represent a continuum, and any cutoff point would be a practical rather than a theoretically based selection. Furthermore, while this selection may represent a common fat content, it may not represent a common risk, because the significance of a given body fat content may differ with body type. Finally, it must be noted that the relation of skin-fold thickness to body fat content is virtually independent of height.[12] This permits giving a single value for each sex and age as a cutoff point.

Based on these concentrations, Seltzer and Mayer have recommended that in the American population the qualification of obesity be reserved for those individuals less than 30 years old in whom the triceps skin-fold is greater by more than one standard deviation than the mean.[7]* Furthermore, the standard established for subjects 30 years old should be applied to men and women in the 30 to 50 year age group. Table 22–1 shows the details of this definition in numerical terms.

The very definition of standard deviation signifies that 16 per cent of the present American population less than 30 years of age are obese. Experience with obesity in children, adolescents and young adults indicates that

* The triceps skin-fold frequency distribution is typically skewed to the right. To normalize the distribution, the logarithmic mean rather than the arithmetic mean is determined before establishing the cutoff point. This prevents very obese members of the population from unduly influencing the determination of the mean.

Table 22-1. Obesity Standards for Caucasian Americans[1]

(minimum triceps skin-fold thickness in millimeters indicating obesity)[2]

Age (years)	Skin-fold measurements	
	Males	Females
5	12	14
6	12	15
7	13	16
8	14	17
9	15	18
10	16	20
11	17	21
12	18	22
13	18	23
14	17	23
15	16	24
16	15	25
17	14	26
18	15	27
19	15	27
20	16	28
21	17	28
22	18	28
23	18	28
24	19	28
25	20	29
26	20	29
27	21	29
28	22	29
29	23	29
30–50	23	30

[1] Adapted from Seltzer, C. C., and Mayer, J. A simple criterion of obesity. *Postgrad Med.* 38: A 101–107, 1965.
[2] Figures represent the logarithmic means of the frequency distributions plus one standard deviation.

experienced workers in the field, whatever the basis for their criteria, recognize at least a similar proportion as obese.* For example, for 16-year-old girls the median skin-fold thickness is 16 mm, corresponding to about 23 per cent of the body as fat. The suggested criterion for obesity is 25 mm, corresponding to 39 per cent of the body as fat. For persons

* This does not mean that a physician may not consider some patients whose skin-folds are slightly below our cutoff points to be too fat for their body builds. Our criteria define frank obesity.

more than 30 years old the proportion of obesity as defined by the criterion proposed here increases far above 16 per cent, in accordance with the general observation that middle-age obesity is more prevalent than obesity in the population at the younger ages.

PREVALENCE OF OBESITY

Childhood and Adolescence. We have no satisfactory national statistics for the prevalence and incidence of obesity in the general population. However, a number of reports point to a steady increase in prevalence both in children and adults. For example, a 1952–53 study showed more than 10 per cent of the boys and girls examined in the public schools of Newton-Brookline, Massachusetts, to be obese by the definition chosen—that is, they were in Channel A-4 or above on the Wetzel Grid.[13] Actually, a more specific definition of obesity, which should be based on body fat, would have shown that a number of boys and girls in Channel 3 had as great a proportion of body fat as those in Channel 4 and were, therefore, obese. In general, more children tended to be stocky than slender and more girls than boys ranged from stocky to obese. The obese children in high school with records from the first grade fell mainly into three groups. One half of the obese girls and nearly one half of the obese boys showed persistent obesity throughout their school years. About one third of the boys and girls became obese in the 6th to 8th grades. There also were those who showed year-to-year variation, especially in the junior high groups.

A survey of the school in the late sixties showed an increase in prevalence of obesity by over 20 per cent. Similar studies show increases in the same order for urban children. Children living in the country, particularly in areas where the climate is conducive to outdoors activity throughout the entire year, tend to be leaner.

Adults. Selective Service data show that the weight of draftees for any given height and age has increased during the past 50 years. A comparison of army inductees from World War I, World War II and 1957–58 reveals that in each period they were taller and heavier than their predecessors. Height increased a total of 1.2 inches, and weight increased 18 pounds.[14]

Insurance Data. Most of the weight data for the adult population is from life insurance studies and therefore does not represent a cross section of the population. Life insurance data deal with "overweight," defined in terms of the weight status in relation to average weight for a given age, height, and sex. They relate to presumably healthy persons in better than average economic circumstances, engaged in safe occupations, free of serious defects and selected for insurance after medical examination.

The 1959 Build and Blood Pressure Study of the Society of Actuaries produced new tables of average weight based on 5 million insured persons.[2] These new figures are more nearly representative of the general population than the previously used 1912 life insurance tables, because the new data include overweight persons rated as substandard risks because of weight only. Nevertheless, the figures do not represent a general population based on a nationwide probability sample.

These new tables of average weight indicate that men tend to weigh 1 to 5 pounds more than shown in the earlier tables, and women 2 to 6 pounds less. The increase in average weight is greatest for short men at most ages, with the greater differences occurring after age 45 for tall men and men of medium height. The decrease in average weight reflected on the new tables is greatest for younger women, with the differences from the previous years becoming less with advancing age. Average weight increases with age, increasing rapidly in men who are in their 20's and early 30's and most rapidly in women in their mid-30's and 40's.

The prevalence of weight deviation from desirable or best weight for ages 20 to 69 is shown in the following Metropolitan Life Insurance Co. data[15,16] (Table 22-2).

The table shows a considerable increase of overweight with advancing years. The greatest increase occurs from the 20's to the 30's. However, the percentage of overweight men remains fairly constant after the 30's while it continues to rise among women. The proportion of persons 20 per cent above

Table 22-2. Percentage of Persons Deviating from Best Weight[1]

Age (years)	Men		Women	
	10–19% above best weight	20% or more above best weight	10–19% above best weight	20% or more above best weight
20–29	19	12	11	12
30–39	28	25	16	25
40–49	28	32	19	40
50–59	29	34	21	46
60–69	28	29	23	45

[1] Adapted from Metropolitan Life Insurance Co., New York. Frequency of overweight and underweight, *Statistical Bulletin 41*:4, Jan. 1960.

best weight is the same for men and women in the 20's and 30's: Both are respectively 12 and 25 per cent overweight. Although the proportion continues to rise with advancing age, only about one third of the older men are overweight as compared with nearly one half of the older women. One is tempted to conclude that, contrary to some published articles, men may be doing a better job at keeping weight down with advancing years than women.

Recent data on height, weight, and selected body dimensions have been published by the National Center for Health Statistics, Public Health Service.[14] The height and weight data are presented as averages for age and sex and also selected percentiles by age, and sex. The data are descriptive of the adult, civilian, non-institutional population of the United States. They are not evaluated in terms of underweight, overweight, or desirable weight. Neither are they analyzed for association with morbidity or mortality. However, it is interesting to note that these 1960–62 averages show the population to weigh more than does the 1959 Build and Blood Pressure Study. A maximum average weight for men occurs between ages 35 to 54 and a maximum average for women between ages 55 to 64. Women, according to these recent data, thus appear to achieve maximum weights about two decades later than do men, and have a greater relative gain with age. Within each age group, the average weight for both men and women tends to increase with increasing height.

Data from the Manhattan Mental Health Study suggest that there is less overweight among the high socioeconomic class, particularly among the women in that class.[17] There is less correlation between overweight and class among the men, however, but even there the prevalence of overweight increases as socioeconomic status decreases except, perhaps, for the lowest group, constituted of laborers.

ETIOLOGY

As recently as 15 years ago, obesity was dealt with clinically as an almost exclusively psychological problem. The rationale was simple: Obesity is due to overeating. Overeating is due either to lack of self-control—that is, gluttony—or to more serious abnormalities of personality.

Fortunately, the intervening years have seen knowledge progress on a wide front. Oversimplifications are no longer tenable to those who are concerned with the problem and its prevention and management. Advances in scientific knowledge have not re-

sulted in any "magic bullet" based on diagnosis of specific neurophysiological or biochemical disturbances. However, the progress witnessed does open avenues for exploration and affords a more comprehensive understanding of the complexities involved.

Obesity, the result of a positive caloric balance, can be the outcome of a number of disturbances (Table 22–3). The variations in causes and subsequent manifestations indicate that not all obesity can be considered the same. For this reason, some investigators have come to use the plural term "obesities" rather than "obesity."

Obesity can be classified according to etiology, or underlying causes, or it can be classified according to pathogenesis—changes in the mechanisms involved in the development of obesity, such as the impairment of a physiological or biochemical process. Both classifications are intimately involved in the regulation of food intake.[1]

GENETIC FACTORS IN HUMAN OBESITY

In laboratory animals the role of genetic factors is clear-cut. The hereditary obese hyperglycemia syndrome of mice is an example of metabolic obesity. Other examples of hereditary obesity are: the yellow obesity, a dominant syndrome seen in mice hetero-

Table 22-3. Types of Human Obesity

Genetic: A multiplicity of genes have been studied by Newman, von Verschuer. Bauer, Gurney, Rony, Angel, and others; in congenital adpiose macrosomia; in monstrous infantile obesity; associated with Laurence-Moon-Biedl syndrome; associated with hyperostosis frontalis interna; associated with von Gierke's disease; in familial hypoglycemosis (congenital lack of alpha cells)

Of hypothalamic origin: In dystrophia adiposogenitalis, with discrete or diffuse hypothalamic injury; occasionally with panhypopituitarism and narcolepsy; Kleine-Levin syndrome

Of other central nervous system origin: After frontal lobotomy; in association with cortical lesions, in particular bilateral frontal lesions

Of endocrine origin: With insulin-producing adenoma of islands of Langerhans, with diffuse hyperplasia of islets and in association with diabetes; with chromophobe adenoma of pituitary gland without hypothalamic injury; in Cushing's syndrome (hyperglycocorticoidism); from treatment with cortisone or ACTH; in Bongiovanni-Eisenmenger syndrome; in disorders of reproductive system; gynandrism and gynism; aspermatogenic gynecomastia without aleydigism; male hypogonadism (sometimes with bulimia); postpubertal castration; menopause; ovarian disorder; paradoxical (Gilbert-Dreyfus) disorder

Otherwise induced: By immobilization in adults and children; by psychic disturbances; by social and cultural pressure

zygous for this gene[18]; the New Zealand obesity, a recessive syndrome of obesity and diabetes that differs in many ways from the obese hyperglycemia syndrome (to cite one difference, the affected animals will mate),[19] and a genetically controlled spontaneous degeneration of the ventromedial area of the hypothalamus.[20] Other examples of genetic obesity in various types of laboratory and farm animals have been discussed in previous papers.[21,22]

Familial Occurrence in Man. The demonstration of the hereditary nature of familial obesity in man is much more difficult. That obesity does "run in families" is well established. In a series of over 1000 obese patients in Vienna, Bauer[23] found that one or both parents were obese in 73 per cent of cases. This figure is close to that of 69 per cent found by Rony[24] for a series of 250 patients in Chicago. In his studies in Philadelphia, Angel[25] reported that half the offspring of obese-average parents were obese, as were two-thirds of the offspring of obese-obese matings. Eighty per cent of the obese children had at least one fat parent: the parents of 25 per cent of the obese children were both obese. Gurney,[26] in a previous survey of a similar population, had found that only 9 per cent of the children of average weight parents were overweight. Fellows,[27] studying the overweight fraction of a life insurance sample, observed that 58 per cent of the mothers and 43 per cent of the fathers were or had been overweight. Dunlop and Lyon,[28] studying a group of obese subjects in Edinburgh, reported that 69 per cent had at least one overweight parent (in 39 per cent, mothers only; in 12 per cent, fathers only; and in 18 per cent, both parents overweight).

Ellis and Tallerman[29] stated that 30 of 50 very obese children studied (60 per cent) had a parent of sibling similarly affected; 13 (26 per cent) had grossly overweight mothers, 6 (12 per cent) grossly overweight fathers, and in 3 cases (6 per cent) both parents were grossly overweight. Iversen,[30] following 40 obese children, found that in 78 per cent (31 cases) one or both parents were obese. In only 10 per cent (4 cases) was there no obesity in parents or siblings. Our own studies in Boston[3] also show a high degree of correlation between overweight in parents and in children.

Ethnic Differences. Interpretation of these data is difficult since cultural background interacts with genetics to determine the incidence of overweight. Angel[25] reported that the sizable obese group he studied showed a relative excess of first- and second-generation Americans: 42.7 per cent had American-born parents (more than half "old Americans"): 8.7 per cent were American-born with one foreign parent and one American-born parent: an unusual 35 per cent were American-born of foreign-born parents and 13.6 per cent were foreign-born. On the other hand, although it has been claimed on the basis of small samples that children of southern European[25] and Jewish[29] stock have an unusually high incidence of obesity, studies in Boston did not confirm this. Fry[31] did not find any significant association between ethnic (white) origin and severity of obesity. Johnson et al.[3] did not observe any significant difference between the incidence of obesity in two well-to-do suburbs of Boston: Brookline (mostly Jewish) and Newton (mixed background). The fact that in the southern United States overweight is more prevalent in Negro males than in Negro females,[32] may be the result of a socioeconomic situation in which Negro men are still frequently employed in jobs entailing physical labor, while Negro women no longer are, but are not yet subjected to social pressure for weight control. On the other hand, this difference between the white and the Negro population may be determined, at least in part, by genetic factors.

Several factors emphasize the significance of two tools—the study of twins and the study of sex ratios—that are applicable to problems such as that of genetic factors in human obesity. These are the possible interaction of environmental and genetic factors; the mixed genetic background of most human groups, particularly in Europe and North America; the fact that human genetics deals with generations with life expectancies similar to those of the geneticists; and the fact that some of the most useful tools of genetics (for example, parent-offspring and brother-sister mating) are not applicable to human studies.

Evidence from Studies of Twins. Siemens' Zwillings-Pathologie, the study of diseases in twins,[33] provides much more cogent evidence of the importance of genetic factors in the etiology of at least some forms of obesity than do simple demonstrations of familial association. The method is, briefly, as follows: Assuming that it is possible to diagnose with accuracy identical (monozygous) and fraternal (heterozygous) twins, it is then reasonable to say that pathological and other characteristics are hereditary which, if they occur at all, are always or nearly always present in both members of identical twin-pairs, but rarely or never appear in both members of fraternal twin-pairs. (This statement does not imply the reverse—that is, that characteristics found in members of both types of pairs are not hereditary.) The twin method has been applied by Newman, Freeman, and Holzinger[34] to measurable characteristics such as height, weight, and intelligence quotient. In this case, comparison of the variability of the quantity measured in identical twins and in fraternal twins permits a preliminary assessment of the role of heredity and environmental factors. (A comparison of variability among siblings and persons of the same age and sex obviously leads to a far less clear-cut distinction between environmental and hereditary causation.)

The study of Newman et al. bore on a large number of subjects, identical and fraternal twins and siblings of like sex. Variability of weight was included among the many physical and mental characteristics compared.[34] The correlation between identical twins for weight was found to be extremely high (0.973), exceeded only (and barely) by that for standing height (0.981), higher than right-finger and left-finger ridges (0.919 and 0.931), and intelligence characteristics (Binet, 0.910, Woodward-Mathews, 0.562). The ratio of standard errors of weight estimate for fraternal twins to identical twins is 2.2 (22.96 pounds for fraternal-twin weights as compared to 10.33 pounds for identical-twin weights), of the same order as height or head length and superior to all such ratios for mental traits. When twins and siblings are paired (the siblings being taken at comparable age), the mean pair difference in

weight of siblings is 10.4 pounds (with 32.5 per cent differing by more than 12 pounds), that of fraternal twins is 10.0 pounds (with 34.5 per cent differing by more than 12 pounds), and that of identical twins is 4.1 pounds, with only 2 per cent differing by more than 12 pounds.

Verschuer,[35] studying 57 pairs of identical twins from 3 to 51 years of age, found weight somewhat more variable than other physical characteristics, but still very constant from twin to twin. The average variation amounted to only 2.58 per cent. A separate calculation for identical twins reared and living in identical environments and for those reared and living in dissimilar environments showed the average percentage variation in body weight to be 1.39 per cent for the first group and 3.6 per cent for the second group. These results tend to demonstrate that, whereas environmental factors have a role in the control of body weight, genetic factors are of paramount importance.

Suggestive of the importance of genetic factors in the etiology of human obesity is the finding[25,26] that segregation can be shown to take place in the transmission of obesity. If the various types of mating—stout-stout, stout-nonstout, and nonstout-nonstout—are considered, the variability of weight of the offspring is relatively small for the first type (most of the offspring—73 per cent in this study—stout), least for the third type (almost none of the offspring—9 per cent in this study—stout), and largest for the matings of stout-nonstout (offspring almost evenly divided between obese—41 per cent—and nonobese—59 per cent). This is interpreted by Gurney as showing that stout persons carry gametes for slenderness, whereas slender ones rarely carry gametes for stoutness.

Evidence from Sex Ratios of Children. Perhaps the most striking indication of genetic determination in human obesity is the demonstration by Angel[3] that the sex ratios of children in the various types of matings (as characterized by weight) are statistically different from those for the population as a whole.

Evidence from the Study of Adopted Children. Finally, a recent study by Withers[36] attempts to differentiate genotype from phenotype in yet another way. He studied the possible correlation of overweight in adopted children and in their adoptive parents, and compared it to the correlation observed between weights of natural children and their biological parents in a South London suburb. The weight picture in natural children was found to be correlated to the weights of the biological parents; that in the adopted children showed no correlation. The evidence that genetic factors dictate predisposition to overweight—and to a significant extent its occurrence—in a society where food is abundant and hard physical labor unnecessary is, I believe, convincing, although the data that would permit the elucidation of the mechanism of hereditary transmission are still missing.

Somatotype, Obesity, and Genetics. Seltzer and Mayer,[4] studying the somatotypes of obese adolescent girls, showed that they differed from the nonobese population in features other than differences in amount of fatty tissue. Obesity did not occur in all varieties of physical types; it occurred more often in some physical types than in others. The obese adolescent girls appeared to be more endomorphic, somewhat more mesomorphic, and considerably less ectomorphic than the nonobese girls of comparable age drawn from the general population. The obese series was somatotypically more homogeneous and invariable than the general population, as manifested by the absence of subjects low in endomorphy and high or even moderate in ectomorphy. In nonanthropological language, the obese group was remarkable for large skeleton and muscle mass, which seemed to be present in spite of the extreme inactivity of these obese adolescent girls,[37] and by the absence of narrow, elongated extremities (very few girls with long, tapered fingers are obese). In adults the problem is more complex, since in that population group one must deal with physical types that are prone to a relatively sudden blossoming into middle-age obesity. Their results[38] show that, in that age group as well, the obese are not, as far as body build is concerned, identical to the nonobese in body components other than fat, but are once

again more endomorphic, more mesomorphic, and considerably less ectomorphic.

If there is a close correlation between obesity and body types in adolescents, this obviously argues further for the genetic determination of obesity, in that the hereditary character of the determination of body build has been repeatedly demonstrated. For example, Withers[36] has attempted to determine, in the working class population of a South London suburb, as well as in the samples from a boys' and a girls' school in a London borough (which he also reports on in his study of overweight in adopted children), the extent and manner in which endomorphy, mesmorphy, and ectomorphy were transmitted from parents to children. Several findings stood out when the results obtained in both studies were collated: The father definitely contributed mesomorphy to his sons, and the mother contributed her endomorphy to her sons. The father may also have transmitted his mesomorphy or ectomorphy to his daughters, and the mother her endomorphy or ectomorphy to her daughters, though the size of the population studied was too small to establish these correlations definitely.

Traumatic Factors. Experimental obesity has been produced in animals by both physiological and psychic trauma. For example, obesity may be produced by creating hormonal imbalances in animals. Likewise, animals can be punished until they overeat: soon they learn to overeat and, with removal of punishment, continue to overeat for a while.

Again, identification of an exact human counterpart type of obesity is elusive. However, studies of obese persons make it clearly evident that overeating is frequently associated with emotional trauma. The onset of obesity in a number of subjects can be identified with some particular stress period.[1] In some instances, this is self-limiting with disappearance of the stress, but in others the overeating and obese condition remain.

Human obesity resulting from physiological trauma is less clearly defined.

Environmental Factors. Such factors as culture, activity, and diet all exert at least a permissive effect in the development of obesity.[1,21,22] The nature of the diet, which in the present-day United States of America tends to be a concentrated source of calories, and the lack of opportunity to exercise in our cities are important elements in the etiology of obesity. This is particularly true if heredity or certain responses to stress predispose an individual to obesity.

The possible role of a particular type of diet in the etiology of obesity is frequently expressed as an important factor. A recent study of body fat, diet, and physical activity reveals little correlation between caloric intake and degree of body fatness. It reveals no correlation between degree of body fatness and the frequency of eating, nor any between the degree of body fatness and the consumption of one half of the total daily calories at one meal.[39]

The one general difference in this country between the food habits of people who are or are not obese is that the obese tend to "overeat" in the evening.[39]

Pathogenesis. An alternate classification of obesities relates to the actual mechanism involved within the individual.[22] Two categories of classification have been suggested, regulatory obesity and metabolic obesity.

Regulatory Obesity. In regulatory obesity the primary impairment is in the central mechanism regulating food intake.[1,22] Metabolism of the extracerebral tissue is normal except to the extent that it is modified by hyperphagia or by extreme adiposity. Experimental examples are the hypothalamic obesities induced in animals by surgical intervention or by gold thioglucose, or the obesities due to thalamic or frontal lesions, or the obesities resulting from forcing or conditioning an animal to overeat. In human subjects, this regulatory type of obesity might be likened to that resulting from immobilization or from extreme sedentariness.

A decreased tendency to move about is a common finding in studies of obese adults and obese children. A number of recent studies have demonstrated the extreme inactivity of the majority of obese children.

A study of incidence and prevalence of obesity in two suburban school systems showed that excessive weight gain among obese children generally occurred in the winter. This suggested that inactivity might be a major factor in the development of obesity.[13] A more detailed study comparing the food intake and activity schedules of 28 obese girls and 28 nonobese girls showed that the obese girls ate less but exercised strikingly less than the nonobese.[40] Similar studies with similar results have been conducted on other groups.[41] A new technique developed for time/motion studies in industry and involving the analysis of sample 3-second motion pictures (30,000 were taken and analyzed) has demonstrated unequivocally that obese girls not only devote less time to exercise than nonobese girls, but that they also expend far less energy during scheduled exercise periods.[37] Conversely, a number of experiments have demonstrated that increased exercise in obese children does not generally increase their food intake and is, therefore, an effective weight control measure.[42]

An explanation for this widespread inactivity among obese children is under investigation. There is convincing evidence that to a large degree inactivity antedates the development of obesity in an individual. Physiological causes may be involved. In most obese youngsters, psychological traumas consequent to the obesity seem to operate to make the inactivity self-perpetuating. Obese children, and obese girls in particular, show many of the characteristics of minority groups—obsessive concern with their condition, passivity, withdrawal, and expectation of rejection. These result in unhappiness, social isolation—and growing inactivity.

Metabolic Obesity. In contrast to regulatory obesity, where the excessive food intake is due to an error in the central mechanism, metabolic obesity is that type where the overeating results from an abnormality in the metabolism of fats and carbohydrates.[1,22] A number of experimental examples of metabolic obesity have been studied in great detail in this writer's laboratory.

In animals with metabolic obesity, one may observe an increase in lipogenesis over that seen in normal animals. This type of obese animal will make more fat even though it may not "overeat"—in fact, even in the presence of fasting.

Table 22-4. Principal Causes of Death Among Men and Women Rated for Overweight.
Attained Ages 25-74 Years

Ratio of Actual to Expected Deaths According to Estimates of
Contemporaneous Mortality Experience on Standard Risks
Metropolitan Life Insurance Company, Ordinary Department
Issues of 1925 to 1934, Traced to Policy Anniversary, 1950

	Men		Women	
Cause of Death	Deaths	Per Cent Actual of Expected Deaths	Deaths	Per Cent Actual of Expected Deaths
Principal cardiovascular-renal diseases	1,867	149	1,103	177
Organic heart disease, diseases of the coronary arteries and angina pectoris	1,377	142	697	175
Organic heart disease	748	*	515	*
Coronary disease and angina pectoris	629	*	182	*
Cerebral hemorrhage	247	159	226	162
Chronic nephritis	243	191	180	212
Cancer, all forms	385	97	476	100
Stomach	62	85	34	86
Liver and gallbladder	33	168	46	211
Peritoneum, intestines and rectum	103	115	93	104
Pancreas	19	93	21	149
Respiratory organs	39	78†	—	—
Breast	—	—	81	69
Genital organs	—	—	132	107
Uterus	—	—	103	121
Leukemia and Hodgkin's disease	26	100	23	110
Diabetes	205	383	235	372
Tuberculosis, all forms	24	21	20	35
Pneumonia, all forms	98	102	78	129
Cirrhosis of the liver	96	249	32	147
Appendicitis	76	223	41	195
Hernia and intestinal obstruction	39	154†	31	141†
Biliary calculi and other gall bladder diseases	32	152†	30	188†
Biliary calculi	19	206	50	284
Ulcer of stomach and duodenum	30	67	—	—
Puerperal conditions	—	—	43	162
Suicide	63	78	23	73
Accidents, total	177	111	74	135
Auto	76	131	27	120
Falls	32	131	—	—

* Satisfactory basis for comparison not available.
† Based on mortality rates on Standard risks for 1935–39.
NOTE: Percentages which have been underlined indicate statistically significant deviations from experience on Standard risks.

Examples of decreased fat mobilization or oxidation have also been described in the metabolic type of obesity. While it is likely that similar examples exist in man, these have not yet been documented.

RISKS OF OBESITY

The increase in mortality in the obese is well known and is summarized in Table 22–4. The effects of obesity on established disease are also important and are discussed in the next section under "indications for weight reduction."

TREATMENT OF OBESITY IN ADULTS

Medical History and Basic Data. It is essential that, in the medical history, particular attention be given to the age of onset of obesity and its past course: the psychologic aspects and prognosis are quite different in persons who become obese in their adult years and in persons who were obese as children and as adolescents. Persons who were obese as youngsters are much more likely to be obsessively concerned with self-image and to view their obesity as a badge of shame rather than as a medical problem which can be attacked by rather simple means; they are more likely to have failed repeatedly to control their weight in the past, they are more likely to be victims of as yet little understood physiologic or psychologic abnormalities.[43] While the classic "endocrine" abnormalities are rare, the possibility of hypothyroidism, hyperadrenocorticism and, in the male, hypogonadism should be ruled out. The possible occurrence of abnormal fluid retention also should be ruled out. Dietary habits should be investigated thoroughly, together with the familial psychologic and economic background. Patterns of hunger and satiety should be understood and their modification, when the patient is on a reducing diet, followed,[44] as they form the basis of decisions on the division of the calories allotted in the reducing diets among the proper number of meals and snacks, and of decisions on the eventual use of anorexigenic agents, their dosage, and timing of administration. The actual time spent in activities not involving

sitting or lying down, and some idea of the vigor with which these activities are pursued, should be known: these elements, together with the sex of the patient and his or her size and age, form the basis of the estimate of the daily caloric requirements for energy balance. An oral glucose tolerance curve is a useful element of information. (The presence of a marked secondary hypoglycemia may be an indication to attempt a low carbohydrate diet.) Serum iron data, as well as hemoglobin, etc., may be useful as possible indications of a tendency toward iron deficiency, a condition which seems much more prevalent among obese subjects than among the general population.

As regards psychologic data, it is important, before searching for possible psychogenic factors, to evaluate as carefully as possible the psychologic effects of obesity on the patient. The psychologic impact on the patient of newly discovered pathologic conditions (*e.g.*, diabetes, hypertension) ought also to be appraised in terms of their possible effect on motivation.

Indications for Weight Reduction. Outside of some (rare) situations involving either somatic or psychiatric problems, weight reduction is desirable in all obese individuals. The attitude that, in the absence of any clear reason for reducing the patient, he or she should be left alone is a counsel of laziness. Should one wait for hypertension or diabetes or immobilization consequent to the superimposition of excess weight on arthritis to do something about the problem? Furthermore, the patient's general fitness is visibly improved; his employability is increased in both government and industry; and, in a society which, for better or for worse, puts a great deal of emphasis on appearance, his social acceptability—and, in some cases, his happiness—is improved.

In some serious conditions indications for weight reduction are particularly pressing:

1. *Respiratory Difficulties.* The work of breathing is increased, if considerable additional weight is carried on the chest wall. Excessive adipose tissue also increases the complexity of the problem of keeping the whole body oxygenated. Obese people consequently have diminished exercise tolerance

and may show great difficulty in normal breathing, particularly in the presence of any—even mild—respiratory infection. At the extreme, very marked obesity may lead to the Pickwickian syndrome where, through decreased ventilation, accumulation of carbon dioxide in blood leads to lethargy and somnolence. Lowered oxygenation of arterial blood may also lead to reactive polycythemia, which may compound the possibility of thrombosis and abnormal blood clotting. Cardiac enlargement and congestive heart failure may also result from pulmonary difficulties due to extreme obesity. The removal of obesity is esssential to the treatment of the Pickwickian syndrome.[45] It can aid greatly the treatment of congestive heart failure.

2. *Hypertension.* While it is true that in some early reports the correlation between obesity and hypertension was exaggerated by the use of pressure cuffs of ordinary size, which excessively compressed the tissues in the upper arm, even when a cuff of proper size is used a significant association between obesity and hypertension is seen. In general, it can be said that hypertension is more prevalent among obese than among nonobese persons and that obese hypertensives show a greater morbidity and mortality rate and, in particular, a greater risk of coronary heart disease than nonobese hypertensives (or than obese nonhypertensives).[46,47]

The results of weight reduction on hypertension are by no means universally present but, when there is a change, it tends to be favorable, with the drop in blood pressure a function of the drop in body weight. Recent experience shows that, in large groups of hypertensives, at least half—and in some instances as many as 75 per cent—of the patients experience significant decreases in blood pressure (20 mm Hg systolic or 15 mm Hg diastolic) if they lose at least 15 pounds. While certain authors have claimed that the most important effect of weight reduction regimens is the curtailment in sodium chloride which accompanies the caloric restriction, it appears that this is only one of the variables involved. There is no doubt that, whatever the mechanisms involved, hypertension in an obese patient is a compelling indication for weight reduction. The favorable effect of

weight reduction on the survival of post-coronary patients is well documented.[47,48] While improvement in angina pectoris is always difficult to measure, there is little doubt that weight reduction is also a favorable factor in this condition.

3. *Endocrine and Metabolic Disturbances.* Hirsutism and menstrual irregularities, much more frequent among obese women than among nonobese, can often be mitigated after sufficient weight loss. There are somewhat conflicting reports on the association of obesity with high cholesterol levels, triglycerides and fatty acids.[1] It is probable that such conflicts are due to a lack of differentiation of the phase of obesity (active weight gain, static obesity) and to our inability at present to differentiate among various forms of obesity. It can be stated in general that, while abnormal plasma lipid levels frequently fail to respond to weight reduction, any response which takes place, particularly in blood cholesterol level, tends to be favorable; *i.e.,* the abnormally high lipid level is decreased temporarily or permanently.

There is a high prevalence among obese subjects of impaired glucose tolerance and, in many cases, of hyperglycemia. This type of maturity-onset "diabetes," which often responds dramatically to weight reduction, may be less likely to lead to vascular degeneration than juvenile, "nonobese" types of diabetes,[49] nevertheless, avoiding the need for insulin, preventing skin and other infections related to hyperglycemia, and avoiding the risk of acidosis provide strong indications for immediate institution of weight reduction in such patients. After suitable weight reduction, insulin can very frequently be replaced by oral hypoglycemic agents. In many cases, the need for pharmacologic agents to control blood sugar may be eliminated altogether. For example, in a large series of obese diabetics, glucose levels returned to normal in nearly 75 per cent of those achieving the desired weight reduction. Glucose tolerances were improved in about half of the remainder.

4. *Other Pathologic Conditions.* Serious difficulties in reproduction associated with obesity can often be diminished or eliminated by weight reduction. The risk of toxemia and

delivery problems can be decreased if the woman's weight is controlled preferably by reduction before the beginning of pregnancy (See Chapter 23 for discussion of obesity and pregnancy). Infertility in obese men may be the result of excessively high temperature of the scrotum, if it is surrounded by folds of adipose tissue.

While there is a significant association between obesity and gallbladder disease, there is as yet no documented evidence that, once the disease is present, it is ameliorated by weight reduction.

Certain skin problems may similarly be mitigated or eliminated by weight reduction. Obesity, because it restricts normal heat loss by the body, tends to promote excessive perspiration. Contact or friction between moist skin areas in adjacent folds often leads to rashes, inflammation and furuncles, While obesity, *per se*, probably does not cause varicose veins, weight reduction considerably lessens the risk of ulcers and other skin complications in women who have varicose veins.

A number of bone and joint diseases are greatly benefited by weight reduction, which decreases the pressure on the damaged structure and facilitates mobility. Rupture of intravertebral disks, osteoarthritis and intermittent claudication are examples in point.

In spite of steady advances in anesthesiologic and surgical techniques, obese patients still have an increased risk in operations and, if possible, should be reduced before elective procedures.

Finally, especially in adolescents but also in many obese adults, particularly in women, the adverse psychologic effects of obesity— "losing one's looks," anxiety about its effects on marital relationships, etc.—may, by themselves, constitute a pressing medical indication for weight reduction.

Contraindications to Weight Reduction. Certain diseases, in particular tuberculosis, gout and diverticulitis, are often quoted as examples of conditions in which weight reduction is contraindicated. Actually, weight reduction, if needed, can be accomplished safely in these diseases if done very gradually with a sensible dietary regimen. Weight reduction is contraindicated in Addison's disease, regional ileitis and ulcerative colitis:

it is, however, rarely associated with these diseases.

Cases in which rapid weight loss was associated with profound depression or acute psychosis have received wide attention and have frequently been cited as illustrating the dangers attendant on weight reduction. While such cases are indeed documented, the following points must be made: (1) The occurrence of depression or psychosis during weight reduction is very rare: (2) the patients had manifestly unstable personalities before the reduction therapy: (3) treatment was usually aimed at a rapid rate of weight loss and was based on a drastic curtailment of food intake, rather than aimed at a slow rate of weight loss with the combination of increased exercise and a moderate diet to create the caloric deficit necessary for weight loss. Previous instances of successful weight loss, even though the lower weight was not maintained, can be taken as a sign that the patient can probably tolerate a course of weight reduction. Certainly, in the enormous majority of cases, the physician need not fear such drastic psychologic complications of treatment, although regular checks of the patient's outlook and a careful examination of the degree of hunger and fatigue experienced by the patient with proper remedial measures, if both appear excessive, are essential parts of the sound therapy of obesity.

Methods of Weight Reduction. It cannot be emphasized enough that the various methods which we are about to examine are not alternative methods. Diet and exercise are complementary measures in establishing the caloric deficit. The manipulation of the dietary schedule and the use of artificial sweeteners, formula diets and anorexigenic agents are all directed at making the limitation in caloric intake more acceptable. Salt restriction may help to provide a more even rate of weight reduction, by avoiding excessive fluid retention. Psychologic support is always an essential element of any long-term therapy.

Dietary Regimen. A proper diet must provide all necessary nutrients, other than calories, in sufficient amounts, be palatable, easily available from the viewpoints of economics and convenience and be limited in calories, so as to permit the desired caloric deficit. Ideally, the diet must be such as to help in the reeducation of the patient, so that, by increasing somewhat the size of the portions, it will provide a proper maintenance diet when the desired weight has been obtained.

The determination of the desired deficit is based on the fact that a pound of fatty tissue is the caloric equivalent of approximately 3500 calories. This means that a daily deficit of 500 calories will lead, over a long enough period, to an average rate loss of 1 pound a week; a deficit of 1000 calories to an average rate of loss of 2 pounds a week. This rate of 2 pounds a week is, incidentally, as much as should be lost by a patient not under close, frequent medical supervision: if patients are very obese and are followed very carefully, both metabolically and psychologically, greater rates of weight loss can be obtained safely, at least at the beginning of the reduction regimen, but indications for such a rapid rate must be pressing (*e.g.*, impending surgery).

It is generally true that, in ambulatory, busy patients, a caloric intake of less than 1500 calories for men and 1000 for women is poorly tolerated over long periods. An increased rate of energy expenditure through stepped up physical activity makes it possible to obtain a caloric deficit of 500 or 1000 calories per day without having to cut food intake below these (low) limits.

Once the rate of weight loss has been decided (*e.g.*, 2 pounds per week, tantamount to a deficit of 1000 calories per day), a guess is made as to the requirements to maintain the patient, given his or her size and pattern of activity. Let us assume that the best guess is of the order of 2200 calories. Adding an hour of walking to the usual activity pattern will bring it to 2500 calories: the diet should be geared then to provide 1500 calories, with the intake adjusted as the results of the trial become available over, say, a 2-week period.

Determining the caloric content of the diet is but one aspect of dietary prescription. Knowledge of the patient's familial and economic status, his usual eating pattern, his tastes and the capabilities of the person who does the marketing and cooking are necessary before the choice of foods to be included in the diet can be made (always remembering that the more varied a diet, the greater the chances that it will be nutritionally adequate, thus eliminating the need for nutritional supplements, such as vitamin pills).

Education of the patient as regards the caloric content of the various foods in various-sized portions is essential not only to the success of the weight reduction program, but also of the subsequent maintenance program. Models are a necessary tool in demonstrating the size of portions. Such expressions as an "average" potato or an "average" serving of lean meat are understood to mean widely different sizes by various individuals.

The distribution of the food in a number of meals and snacks is a matter for individual prescription and experimentation: a "good" reducing diet is one on which the patient does not become too hungry. Knowing the normal pattern of hunger and satiety of the patient, a guess can be made as to the number of meals and snacks which will prevent the development of excessive hunger. If this does develop once caloric restriction is instituted, further fragmentation of the daily food allowance may help to mitigate the problem. If this is still unsuccessful, a clear indication for the use of anorexigenic agents exists.

There is at present no evidence available to support the idea that some of the more extreme diets recently popularized have any advantage over a calorically restricted, balanced, "normal" diet. A low protein, low fat, "rice" type diet was popular a few years ago. It was followed by a very low protein diet, dubbed the "Rockefeller" diet by its promoters. The very high protein, moderate carbohydrate diet has been recommended by a number of groups in part on the basis of a misconception of the order of magnitude of the specific dynamic action of proteins in a mixed diet. The high fat, low carbohydrate (or carbohydrate-free) diet reappears every now and then under a variety of names, most recently the "DuPont" or "Pennington" or "Mayo" diet. With alcohol added, it has become the "drinking man's diet." Again, advocates of these diets who are sincere are apparently misguided on a number of counts. While it is true that a high fat diet depresses fat synthesis, it by no means prevents fat deposition when fat is copiously available in the diet. Fat does have "satiety" value, but so do other foods. A carbohydrate-free, high fat diet does cause an immediate weight loss (over and above the steady decrease due to caloric deficit), but this is due to partial de-hydration and is of no lasting significance in a program designed to reduce adiposity, not simply to decrease weight, *per se*, over the short term. A diet high in fat, where calories and alcohol can be consumed *ad libitum*, not only tends to make your patients fat (and inebriated) but also may be highly atherogenic.

A balanced diet, containing no less than 12 to 14 per cent of protein, no more than 30 per cent of fat (with saturated fats cut down), and the rest carbohydrates (with sucrose cut down to a very low level), pro-vided by foods of sufficient variety is in-finitely preferable to the fad diets mentioned (and their congeners, the grapefruit diet, the banana diet, the hard boiled egg diet, etc.).

Formula diets have become very popular in the past 10 or so years. Whether purchased in liquid form or as powders to be suspended in water, their main advantage is that they provide strictly established amounts of food (3 times 300 calories or 4 times 225 calories per day, in general) and thus provide a sim-ple, rigid regimen which does not need to be based on any knowledge of foods and food values. While this is often an advantage at the beginning of the reducing period (2 to 4 weeks), it should not retard the dietary education which, sooner or later, is absolutely necessary to carry the patient over a pro-longed weight reduction period and through the maintenance, lifelong phase. The enor-mous majority of patients do not, in fact, stay exclusively on such formula diets, and, as the formula diet is supplemented by other foods, its intrinsic value is lost. Formula diets may, nevertheless, be found useful during main-tenance, as the exclusive replacement of one meal a day.

Bulk-producing agents (such as methyl-cellulose) have not been shown to have any special merit. Apples, celery, raw carrots or salads are more palatable, more likely to be-come parts of a lifelong dietary pattern and,

thus, are superior on all counts to artificial bulk-producing agents. Work done in our laboratory suggests that bulky foods may be particularly valuable as satiety adjuncts, not so much because of their stomach-filling role as because they slow down the course of the meal and provide time for satiety phenomena to supervene. Artificial bulk-producing agents do not make a similar contribution to satiety.

The use of artificial sweeteners can be a useful adjunct to reducing diets. Certainly there is little to say for the extensive consump-tion of sucrose, an "empty" source of calories which, in large amounts, may excessively stimulate insulin production. A small amount of sucrose (*e.g.*, one sourball once or twice a day at the end of a meal as "dessert," or as a snack, if a meal is excessively delayed) is useful with some patients, but the use of sugar in the numerous cups of tea and coffee often consumed by reducing patients and the use of sugar-containing soft drinks should be strictly eliminated. If reducing patients have to drink a number of cups of black coffee a day (a questionable practice for some patients on other grounds) and if the coffee has to be sweetened, the use of saccharine and other artificial sweeteners should be encouraged.

Strict restriction of salt is a therapeutic procedure which should be prescribed only if the clinical picture warrants it. On the other hand, cutting down on the salt intake de-creases the tendency to excessive fluid reten-tion seen in many reducing obese subjects, particularly middle-aged and older women and sedentary individuals. It may also have some effectiveness in the prevention of hyper-tension. Salt restriction is a much sounder and safer way to prevent excessive water re-tention during weight reduction than the use of diuretics which, if prolonged, may cause renal damage. It is unfortunate that certain "reducing" pills containing diuretics (ammonium chloride) are still available for over-the-counter sale. Patients ought to be warned against such preparations.

Anorexigenic Agents. The current anorexi-genic agents are sympathomimetic amines, amphetamines and related compounds. It is generally agreed that they act chiefly by stimulating the ventromedial (satiety) hypo-thalamic centers, but they may have other accessory actions, including some stimulation of spontaneous activity and of free fatty acid release by the adipose tissue. The dosages used vary from patient to patient (from 5 to 20 mg per day for the amphetamines). They are most usefully employed after the hunger-satiety pattern on the desired reducing diet has been determined and whatever adjustment can be made by shifting snacks has been effected, so that the physician knows that the critical periods of extreme hunger are in fact covered. There is little point in giving a small or moderate dose early in the morning, so that the effect has worn off by the end of the afternoon, if one is dealing with a patient who is hungry, eats and overeats only in the evening. A frequently successful practice is to give a long-acting amphetamine preparation in the morning with a booster in the late afternoon.

In general, the effective duration of amphetamine treatment is considered to be of the order of a month to 6 weeks, although recent results suggest that some patients continue to respond for much longer periods: amphetamines are most useful at the onset of treatment and with patients who have become obese relatively recently. Unfortunately, in many, if not most patients, some side effects are observed; dry mouth, restlessness, irritability, insomnia and sometimes constipation. Cardiac patients are not good candidates for amphetamine therapy because of the adrenergic effects of such agents on the heart (increase in heart rate, potentiation of cardiac arrhythmias); in cases of moderate hypertension, the favorable effect of steady weight loss on blood pressure often outweighs the slight risk of increase due to the amphetamine. The superiority of modifications of the amphetamines (such as phenmetrazine, phentermine, chlorphentermine and benzphetamine) both in terms of effectiveness and avoidance of side effects is not yet convincing to this observer. Supplementation of amphetamine therapy with sedatives or tranquilizers can be useful in certain cases.

It cannot be emphasized enough that the use of such agents by a physician does not in any way decrease the importance of dietary prescription and dietary instruction, as previously described. It goes without saying that patients should also be warned against increasing the dose of the prescribed agent on their own or supplementing it with over-the-counter medications (most of which are worthless and some of which are dangerous).

Exercise. The value of exercise in the prevention of obesity and the treatment of moderately obese persons in otherwise good health is well established.[1,50] Its value in the prevention of heart disease is also well established.[1,51,52] Let it be recalled simply that exercise is the great variable in energy expenditure. Caloric equivalent of exercise of various types has been given. The caloric expenditure due to exercise is proportional to the duration of exercise; it is also proportional to the weight of the subject, so that an obese person will use up proportionately more calories to perform the same task than a thin subject. The caloric expenditure increases rapidly with the intensity with which the exercise is performed. Exercise does not increase voluntary food intake in inactive subjects until it has reached a certain critical duration and intensity, depending on the individual.

While obviously a very obese subject, even one in good cardiovascular state, should not be put suddenly to exercise: it is a good idea to start him to walk every day and to increase the duration and eventually the intensity of the exercise as his weight reduction progresses. An understanding of the schedule and of the mode of life of the patient is necessary if exercise is going to be built into his daily life. Advantage of every opportunity for walking, stair climbing, etc., can be taken, so as to restore mobility in patients used to the constant use of automobiles and elevators.

The physician must remind the patient that the insulation provided by the excessive adiposity will restrict his rate of heat loss on hot days, so that particular caution must be exercised in the summer to interrupt the exercise with sufficient rest periods and keep hydrated (preferably with water!).

Thyroid Preparation. There is still too much thyroid hormone prescribed to obese patients (usually in the form of desiccated thyroid preparation) without any clear indication that the patient is in a hypothyroid state. Such medication is based on the misconception that most obese patients are hypo-metabolic, an old idea originating from relating basal oxygen consumption to body weight. At present, sophisticated methods (I uptake, PBI determinations, etc.) should be used before a diagnosis of hypothyroidism is arrived at and acted on. The administration of thyroid hormone is in part self-defeating anyway, as it depresses endogenous thyroid secretion, the depression being very slow to reverse. If higher doses are given, tachycardia, palpitation, nervousness and insomnia appear, creating an unpleasant and a potentially dangerous situation.

Triiodothyronine has been advocated by some as a useful aid to dietary restriction. It enhances *in vitro* the lipolytic effect of epinephrine and is said not to depress thyroid action to the extent shown by thyroid preparations, and not to cause thyrotoxicosis. The evidence to support the claim of usefulness in reducing treatment is not sufficient to recommend its general use.

Other Methods. A number of "heroic" measures have recently been advocated. I have been unimpressed with total fasting as a therapeutic measure (as distinct from a research procedure). Published reports, including reports of accidents during total fasting, do not impel me to look at this method favorably, although there may be situations, such as impending surgery, where the risk of total fasting for a hospitalized patient, under close laboratory and psychologic supervision, may be less than that of continued extreme obesity. If surgery is contemplated, it is important that the patient have a week of moderate feeding at the end of the fasting period and immediately before the operation. Patients ought to be strongly warned against self-administered total fasting, because of dangers to themselves (as well as to others, if they drive a car!).

Surgical procedures, which permit temporary bypass of part of the small intestine, have been used in "intractable" obesity. In patients in whom adequate follow-ups are available, the experience has been miserable. Not only did the patients exhibit serious difficulties while the shunt lasted (including some cases of uncontrollable hypocalcemia),

but the weight was generally recovered rapidly after the shunt was discontinued.

Psychologic Support. The physician should be concerned with certain psychologic aspects of the therapy of obesity. In order of increasing diagnostic and therapeutic difficulty, these are:

1. The psychology of weight reduction. He should ease the discomforts attending the continued sensations associated with a prolonged period of caloric deficit, such as mitigating hunger and fatigue by appropriate measures and counseling, and fixing realistic short-term and long-term targets, arriving at the latter by his clinical judgment, based on the actual body structure of the patient and his mode of life and capabilities.

2. The psychology of being obese. Particularly in patients who were obese in adolescence, when the body image appears to be developed, there is a galaxy of psychologic traits, which appear to be due to the obesity-obessive concern with self-image, such as passivity, expectation of rejection, and progressive withdrawal, which must be coped with, if the patient is to be a happy, well-adjusted person. Many of these psychologic effects of obesity may tend to make the obesity self-perpetuating.

3. Psychologic factors leading to obesity. These are the least known and thus are particularly difficult to deal with adequately. Anxieties and stresses which burden an obese patient may be instrumental, if the patient is otherwise predisposed to obesity by genetics and by constitution, in causing overeating and immobilization and, hence, weight accumulation. The development of new interests can be useful, particularly in middle-aged women with little to do outside of the home, too much time on their hands, and a tendency to view their interpersonal relationships in terms of sitting down together at meals.

TREATMENT OF OBESITY IN CHILDREN AND ADOLESCENTS

We have seen earlier that the concept of childhod obesity as "puppy fat" which, left to itself, will disappear does not correspond to the facts as we know them. Treatment of obesity in children and adolescents is desirable but must be conducted with the thought in mind that any drastic caloric reduction may be accompanied by cessation of growth and, therefore, be essentially self-defeating. The following additional considerations should be kept in mind.

(1) An obese child is not necessarily an otherwise well-fed child. There is evidence, for example, that a low serum iron, indicative of a tendency towards anemia, is of much more common occurrence among fat adolescents than among normal-weight young people of the same age.[53] Similar observations have been made concerning fat babies.

(2) Moderately obese children and adolescents are generally characterized by intakes not in excess of the average for their age, sex, and height, but by drastically reduced energy expenditure. In fact, many such moderately obese youngsters may be eating somewhat less than average, but are incredibly inactive. Under these conditions, to further reduce intake in an effort to cause weight loss (or at least fat loss) may compromise growth in length. Considerable measures of success have been achieved in weight reduction programs conducted in summer camps[54] and in a school[42] where a program of vigorous *daily* physical activity was instituted, with food habits improved by careful painstaking instruction, but without prescribed caloric restriction.

(3) In the case of extremely obese children, a degree of caloric restriction can usually be imposed without resultant impairment of growth. As with adults, instruction and prescription in diets must be conducted with food models or with real food portions, so that the concept of portion size is firmly understood. In general, small children are best indoctrinated with their mothers present. Older children and adolescents should be seen separately from their parents. If, as is often the case, one or both parents also have a weight problem, it is often more effective to make both dieting and exercise a family affair. The obese child, often a lonely, unhappy person isolated from his or her contemporaries by the early and massive discrimination against the obese characteristic of our society, should receive as much encourage-ment and companionship from his family as possible.

(4) It may be useful to restate that an estimation of fat, rather than weight, is particularly important during growth. Whereas, in adults, a weight gain means usually accumulation of fat, in growing youngsters it may mean true (protein) growth, growth and fat accumulation, fat accumulation alone, and even, in some cases (particularly during the puberty "growth spurt" of boys), growth with loss of fat. It is, therefore, essential to supplement the readings of the scale with careful examination of the patient and, preferably, with skin-fold measurements.

BIBLIOGRAPHY

1. Mayer: *Overweight: Causes, Cost and Control*, New York, Prentice-Hall, 1968.
2. Build and Blood Pressure Study, 1959. Soc. of Actuaries. Chicago, 1, 1959.
3. Seltzer and Mayer: J.A.M.A., *201*, 221, 1967.
4. Seltzer and Mayer: J.A.M.A., *189*, 677, 1964.
5. Gertler and White: *Coronary Disease in Young Adults*, Cambridge, Harvard University Press, 1954.
6. Spain, Bradess, and Greenblatt: Amer. J. Med. Sci., *229*, 294, 1955.
7. Seltzer and Mayer: Postgrad. Med., *38*, A101, 1965.
8. Committee on Nutritional Anthropometry, Food and Nutrition Board, National Res. Council (A. Keys, chairman). Recommendations concerning body measurements for the characterization of nutritional status. In *Body Measurements for Human Nutrition* (J. Brozek, ed.), Detroit, Wayne Univ. Press, 10, 1956.
9. Seltzer, Goldman, and Mayer: Pediatrics *36*, 212, 1965.
10. Young, Tensuan, Sault, and Holmes: J. Amer. Diet. Assoc. *42*, 409, 1963.
11. Novak: Ann. N.Y. Acad. Sci. *110*, 545, 1963.
12. Garn and Haskell: A.M.A. Dis. Child. *99*, 746, 1960.
13. Johnson, Burke, and Mayer: Amer. J. Clin. *4*, 231, 1956.
14. National Center for Health Statistics: Weight by Height and age of adults, U.S. 1960–62. Vital and Health Statistics. Public Health Serv. Pub. No. 1000–Series 11, No. 14, U.S. Gov't. Printing Office, May, 1966.
15. Friis-Hansen: Pediatrics *28*, 169, 1961.
16. Metropolitan Life Ins. Co., N.Y. Frequency of overweight and underweight. Statistical Bulletin, *41*, 4, 1960.
17. Moore, Stunkard and Srole: J.A.M.A. *81*, 962, 1962.
18. Carpenter and Mayer: Amer. J. Physiol. *193*, 499, 1958.

19. Bielschowsky and Bielschowsky: Austr. J. Exp. Biol. Med. Sci. *34*, 181, 1956.
20. Vidal and di Roberti: Medicina (Buenos Aires) *3*, 185, 1943.
21. Mayer: Physiol. Rev. *33*, 472, 1953.
22. Mayer: Nutr. Abstr. Rev. *25*, 597, 1955.
23. Bauer: *Constitution and Disease: Applied Constitutional Pathology*, 2nd ed., New York, Grune & Stratton, 1945.
24. Rony: *Obesity and Leanness*, Philadelphia, Lea & Febiger, 1940.
25. Angel: Amer. J. Phys. Anthrop. *7*, 433, 1949.
26. Gurney: Arch. Intern. Med. *57*, 557, 1936.
27. Fellows: Amer. J. Med. Sci. *181*, 301, 1931.
28. Dunlop and Murray Lyon: Edinburgh Med. J. *38*, 561, 1931.
29. Ellis and Tallerman: Lancet *2*, 615, 1934.
30. Iversen: Acta Paediat. Scand. *42*, 8, 1953.
31. Fry: Amer. J. Clin. Nutr. *1*, 453, 1953.
32. Hundley: *Weight Control*, Ames, Iowa State College Press, 1956.
33. Siemens: *Einfuhrung in die allgemeine und spezielle Vererbungspathologie des Menschen: Ein Lehrbuch fur Studierende und Arzte.* Berlin Springer, 1923.
34. Newman, Freeman, and Holzinger: *Twins: A Study of Heredity and Environment.* Chicago, University of Chicago Press, 1937.
35. von Verschuer: Die vererbungsbiologische Zwillingsforschung: Ihre biologischen Grundlagen: Studien an 102 eineiigen und 45 gleichgeschlechtlichen zweieiigen Zwillingsund an 2 Drillingspaaren. Ergebn. Inn. Med. Kinderheilk. *31*, 35, 1927.
36. Withers: Eugenics Rev. *56*, 81, 1964.
37. Bullen, Monello, Cohen, and Mayer: Amer. J. Clin. Nutr. *12*, 1, 1963.
38. Seltzer and Mayer: J. Amer. Diet. Assoc. *55*, 457, 1969.
39. Beaudoin and Mayer: Fed. Proc. *11*, 436, 1952.
40. Johnson, Burke, and Mayer: Amer. J. Clin. Nutr. *4*, 37, 1956.
41. Stefanik, Bullen, Heald, and Mayer: Res. Quart. *32*, 229, 1961.
42. Seltzer and Mayer: Amer. J. Publ. Health *60*, 679, 1970.
43. Monello and Mayer: Amer. J. Clin. Nutr. *13*, 35, 1963.
44. Monello and Mayer: Amer. J. Clin. Nutr. *20*, 253, 1967.
45. Walker: Arch. Int. Med. *93*, 951, 1954.
46. Bjerkedal: Acta Med. Scand. *159*, 13, (Fac. 1), 1957.
47. Mayer: Postgrad. Med. *46*, 195, 1969.
48. Marks: Diabetes *11*, 544, 1962.
49. Hundley: J. Amer. Diet. Assoc. *32*, 417, 1956.
50. Mayer: Ann. N.Y. Acad. Sci. *131*, 502, 1965.
51. Mayer: J. Amer. Diet. Assoc. *52*, 13, 1968.
52. Mayer: Med. Today *2*, 25, 1968.
53. Seltzer, Wenzel, and Mayer: Amer. J. Clin. Nutr. *13*, 343, 1963.
54. Bullen, Monello, Cohen, and Mayer: Amer. J. Clin. Nutr. *12*, 1, 1963.

PART V

Nutrition During "Physiologic" Stress

Chapter

23

Nutrition in Pregnancy

ROBERT W. HILLMAN

AND

ROBERT S. GOODHART

"Basic to an understanding of the role of nutrition in reproduction is the concept that pregnancy is a normal state, not a pathological one. Since pregnancy is normal, a pregnant woman's nutritional status and her diet should be thought of as contributions to normal processes leading to the birth of a healthy, full-term baby; they should not be thought of as means of forestalling or treating possible complications."[1]

Optimum development of the infant is necessarily a function of parental diet—an ongoing, long-term, as well as immediate, relationship. However much of the information relating to maternal and fetal nurtiture remains too controversial and too contradictory to permit clinical application.

The several reasons for this difficulty include both those common to all nutritional problems and some that are unique to the gravid state.[5,6]

1. The ethical, moral, and legal limitations of investigating the human subject are compounded by the need to consider the interests of the child (and of the father) as well as of the mother.

2. Animal studies, characterized by species and strain differences, cannot readily be extrapolated to human experience.[7-9]

3. Intra- as well as inter-individual variations preclude simple and valid conclusions from limited observations.[3]

4. Factors such as parental age, birth rank, and birth interval influence the outcome of pregnancy.[10,11]

5. The mother's preconception diet (and possibly that of *her* mother) is important.[11-13]

6. The ability of the organism to adapt to suboptimal intakes of dietary essentials complicates the problem of establishing optimum quantities and proportions of these substances. Metabolic mechanisms peculiar to pregnancy seem to sustain successful reproduction in the presence of nutritional adversity.[2,12]

7. Nutritional deprivation typically is most severe when a wide range of nonnutritional adversities concurrently disposes to maternal and fetal complications.[2,13,14] Clinical and epidemiologic studies have been comparatively unsuccessful in dissociating nutritional factors from other elements of the socioeconomic environment with which variations in perinatal experience are also closely identified. Psychologic factors, in particular, are being implicated in the causation of untoward effects.[15-20]

8. Assessment of the outcome of pregnancy obviously is a function of the criteria adopted. A wide range of indices—maternal and fetal, early developing and late appearing—represents not only a convenient battery of parameters for evaluating reproductive experience, but, unfortunately, also an equal number of opportunities for inconsistent and even incompatible interpretation.[14]

Notwithstanding these limitations and with due consideration for the bias inherent in predominantly positive reports, impressions of a generally favorable influence of good nutrition on the outcome of pregnancy probably are valid.

OBSERVATIONS ON OTHER SPECIES

The present, considerable support for the relationship of maternal nutrition to ante-, peri-, and postnatal events derives as much from observations on lower species as on man. Livestock breeding, in particular, has provided extensive opportunities for modifying pregnancy and lactation through alterations in diet. Studies of mammalian reproduction (*e.g.*, sheep, seals) under so-called natural conditions have provided valuable information concerning the role of major aliments and of trace elements, such as calcium, phosphorus, copper, and cobalt.[21] Laboratory animal studies, although possibly less applicable to human experience, have identified probable generic needs in reproduction for both protein components and specific micronutrients. The experimental production of congenital malformations by Warkany[8] and others[22-24] has emphasized the importance of timing, dose, and duration in the manipulation of essential elements. In some instances, an excess as well as a deficiency of a required substance (*e.g.*, a fat-soluble vitamin) evidently conduces to a wide variety of deleterious effects, ranging from neonatal death, through successively earlier gestational mishaps, to actual failure of conception. Malformations may be induced during either the organogenic or the pre-organogenic period. To a considerable degree, they appear to be specific for the nutrient as well as the species and strain involved. Although these experimental nutritional states are more extreme and more acute than those commonly experienced by pregnant women, concern seems appropriate for the possibility of nutritional as well as pharmaceutical[25] stress in the early stage of human gestation.

OBSERVATIONS ON MAN

Evidence for the role of nutrition in human pregnancy is derived from three categories of observation: (1) records of large population groups with varying socioeconomic and health status; (2) data for supervised hospital and clinic groups; and (3) controlled prospective studies of patients receiving prescribed diets and/or nutritional supplements. Much of this and other pertinent information have been reviewed by Garry and Wood,[26] Burke and Stuart,[27] Josey,[28] Stearns,[29] Hepner,[14] Dalderup,[30] and Seifrit.[31]

Population studies relating to maternal nutriture have originated principally in the United Kingdom, where, during World War II, overall improvement in diet was associated with improved perinatal experience, often despite otherwise unfavorable socioeconomic conditions.[32-34] Numerous and for the most part smaller and better controlled studies have supported this impression of benefits attributable to good maternal nutrition in that country.[13,35-37] Toverud in Norway,[38] Riquelme and Alvorado in Chile,[39] Dean in Germany,[40] Antonev in the Soviet Union,[41] Berry in Africa,[42] Hamlin in Australia,[43] Gopolan in India,[44] and Ebbs, Tisdall and Scott in Canada[45] have reached similar conclusions. In this country, Burke and Stuart[46] and their associates have provided major support for good dietary practices during pregnancy. Other observations, direct and indirect, have corroborated their findings.[47-52] Borquin and Benum[53] observed that women with better nutriture responded more favorably to treatment for recurrent abortion.

Although these reports largely affirm impressions of a favorable influence of good maternal nutriture, negative and/or equivocal observations also have been registered.[54-60] The wide range of laboratory findings that appears to be compatible with normal reproductive function has been emphasized by Macy[61] and by McGanity, Darby, Bridgforth and their colleagues at Vanderbilt University.[62] The Vanderbilt experience indicated no advantages to dietary intakes in excess of recommended allowances or to vitamin supplementation.

Except where maternal deprivation is much more extreme than that commonly encountered in this country, it is difficult to ascribe specific clinical benefits to dietary improvement during gestation.

Special laboratory investigations that may be expected to resolve problems of major clinical significance include studies of placental function. Reviews by Page,[63] Dancis,[64] Davies,[65] Villee,[66] and Sternberg[67] identify this organ with the active transport and synthesis of nutrients as well as of hormones. Additional evidence tends to affirm its role in regulating the fetal blood concentrations of these substances.[68-72]

The optimum nutriture for parenthood remains to be determined—as does the degree of deprivation below which adaptation cannot ensure successful reproduction. However, there are a few parameters of perinatal experience in respect to which present, limited evidence appears to support some dietary recommendations for the pregnant woman.

BIRTH WEIGHT

Unsatisfactory maternal nutriture is generally recognized as a factor in the causation of low infant birth weight—the most widely accepted index of prematurity.[10,13,62,73,96] Gravidas who are underweight at the time of conception and those who fail to gain weight adequately during the first and second trimesters seem especially disposed to have newborn in the lighter weight range and to incur premature separation of the placenta and an overall increase in morbidity and mortality. However, infant birth weight is correlated more closely with maternal weight and maternal height at conception than with maternal weight gain during pregnancy.[13,86] In a survey of primiparas exclusively, Thomson found that the birth weight of the infants rose as the caloric value of the mothers' diets increased and the incidence of low birth weight fell. However, when the data were statistically adjusted to control for the fact that the women with greater caloric intake were from the upper social classes and were taller, heavier, and healthier, Thomson found that maternal social class and stature were much more important than the diet in pregnancy.[97,98]

Large infants apparently are associated with adiposity. Baumgartner et al.[73] showed that neonates with birth weights 1 to 2 pounds above average (post mature) fared as poorly as infants of the same degree of underweight at birth. As indicated by the often adverse experience of the large infants born to dia-

betic mothers, big babies are not always the "best" babies.[100]

Although birth length and duration of gestation may constitute more valid indices, the relative simplicity of determining birth weight encourages its adoption as the principal criterion for routine estimation of infant maturity. And although birth weight does appear to be a function of birth length, these measurements are not consistently well correlated, and the critical component of body composition is only infrequently assessed. Thomson[13] has appropriately stressed the *quality* of babies, which is just as variable as size and "probably of more practical importance." The improved assessment of infant maturation in relation to maternal nutriture would seem to require better standardized criteria with suitable adjustments for ethnic, familial, and sex differences, if normal biologic variations are not to be mistaken for differences in nutritional state,[14,101,102] and if more valid concepts are to be formulated concerning the extent to which the maternal diet governs fetal well-being and chances for survival.

CONGENITAL DEFECTS

Although extremely severe malnutrition existing during the first year of life may very well be a definite contribution to a long-lasting retardation in mental development, the specter of millions of children doomed to mental retardation as a result of malnutrition *in utero* and/or during the first year of life cannot be supported by available factual knowledge.[103]

Arbeter et al.,[104] in studies of severely malnourished children and adults, found that phagocytosis is not defective in malnutrition except when there appears to be severe iron deficiency or when there appears to be increased iron utilization during recovery from malnutrition.

Experiments with animals[8,22-24] and the indictment of pharmaceutical agents[25,105,106] in the causation of congenital abnormalities have reinforced a disposition to implicate malnutrition, notably deficiency states, in the etiology of these aberrations.[3,8,107,108] Evidence that only a small proportion (less than

10 per cent) is directly attributable to genetic factors,[23,106,109] also has furthered the hope that improvements in maternal nutriture may reduce their incidence. However, in the small proportion of congenital malformations in which major environmental factors have been suspected, efforts to identify nutritional deficiencies have been largely unsuccessful. Epidemiologic studies, notably by Coffey and Jessop[110] and by Anderson, Baird, and Thomson[111] in the United Kingdom, have detected a greater frequency of anomalies among the offspring of the lower socio-economic groups. However, except for areas of endemic goiter, other studies[112] have not demonstrated an increased occurrence among the children of the presumably under-nourished. The principal evidence has been reviewed by Millen,[23] Ashley-Montagu,[89] and the Committee on Maternal Nutrition of the Food and Nutrition Board, National Research Council.[1]

The administration of folic acid antagonists to pregnant women with malignant disease has been followed by the birth of deformed infants.[113] Together with the increased frequency of malformations among infants of diabetic mothers, these observations provoke concern for the possible untoward effects of unidentified, dietary and/or endogenous anti-metabolites.

TOXEMIA

The term *toxemia* is a misnomer that is frequently applied to all hypertensive disorders of pregnancy.[114] It is interpreted here as applying to *preeclampsia*, which the Committee on Terminology of the American College of Obstetricians and Gynecologists has suggested be defined as hypertension with proteinuria and/or edema appearing after the twentieth week of pregnancy.[114] *Eclampsia* in most cases represents an end result of preeclampsia. A dramatic decrease in mortality from the acute toxemias of pregnancy occurred during the years from 1940 to 1961–1965. It dropped from 52.2 per 100,000 live births in 1940 to 6.2 in 1961–1965.[114] The reasons for this decline have not been defined.

Preeclampsia is primarily a disease of primigravidas and is more common among the very young primigravidas and those past 30. The diagnosis is suspect in a multipara unless she has some predisposing factor, such as antecedent hypertension, diabetes, or multiple pregnancy. The chance of a woman developing toxemia is increased many times in multiple pregnancies, the risk increasing again when twinning occurs in primigravidas. The only incontrovertible cause of preeclampsia is pregnancy: it does not occur in any other circumstance. The only certain cure is the termination of pregnancy.[114] "No convincing evidence has come to light that simply supplementing the diet of the pregnant woman affects the incidence of toxemia."[114]

An influence of maternal nutriture on the occurrence of toxemia is widely claimed.[13,30,50,54,62,74] However, because the precise nature of this relationship is yet to be established, dietary recommendations for the prevention and management of this major, maternal complication remain largely empirical, directed toward control of the most readily determinable but variably significant parameter, body weight.

The normal curve of weight gain is sigmoid, there being little gain during the first trimester, a rapid increase during the second, and some slowing in the rate of increase during the third. In one study of a large group of Scottish primigravidas a total weight gain of 12.5 kg (27.5 lb), with an average rate of gain of slightly less than 0.5 kg (1.1 lb) per week during the second half of pregnancy, was found to be associated with the lowest overall incidence of pre-eclampsia, prematurity (low birth weight), and perinatal mortality.[115] The products of conception account for only about one-half of the total weight gained; the expanded maternal blood volume plus enlargement of the reproductive organs for about 18 per cent: the remainder normally is fat plus 1 or 2 kg of "excess" body water at term.[115]

One of the characteristics of toxemia is edema, and water retention means added weight. In many cases, therefore, toxemia is associated with a gain in weight. But there is no evidence that excessive weight gain, whether in the form of fat or water, causes toxemia.[114,134,135] The rate of gain is important. After about the twentieth week of pregnancy, a sudden increase in weight is cause for suspecting that water is being retained.[114]

In general, toxemia occurs most commonly among patients who are overweight at conception and those who gain weight excessively during the second and third trimesters. A smaller, though often more serious, increment in toxemia is noted among women who are markedly underweight at conception and who fail to gain adequately during the antenatal period. Notwithstanding the apparently successful reproductive pattern of many underweight women who also may fail to show a weight increase during pregnancy, notably in Asiatic countries,[44,90,120] these gravidas appear to be the most vulnerable of the "high risk" patients in this part of the world. However, the pregnant woman who develops a sudden, excessive gain in weight, irrespective of previous pattern, remains the greatest hazard in terms of toxemia *per se*.

In addition to these abnormal weight patterns, extensive, albeit inconclusive, evidence has implicated more specific nutritional factors in the causation of toxemia.[117–124] In particular, variations in the intake and/or metabolism of protein, salt, and single vitamin components (*e.g.*, ascorbic acid, B_6) of the diet have been suspected on the basis of epidemiologic, clinical, and laboratory observations.

Although the apparently significant decrease in toxemia in parts of Europe during both World Wars has been variously attributed to a reduction in calories, in fat, and in protein, as well as to an increased intake of relatively unrefined carbohydrate products, the many non-nutritional as well as dietary factors operating during these periods of comparative privation preclude ascribing the improved perinatal experience to any one food component.[13,30] In this country, although reduced serum protein concentrations have not been consistently demonstrated, plasma electrophoretic studies have been consistent with the present consensus that a high rather than a low protein intake protects against the development of toxemia.[117,118,125–130]

Notwithstanding considerable laboratory evidence to suggest increased vitamin B_6 requirements during pregnancy,[124–131] especially in toxemic patients, dietary supplementation with pyridoxine, except for a possible reduction in the incidence of dental caries,[132] appears not to influence the frequency or course of toxemia, or of other maternal or fetal complications.[124–133] Nevertheless, a conditioned deficiency attributable to impaired phosphorylation may be present.[133]

Reports by McCartney *et al.*,[136] by Plentl and Gray,[137] and by Chesley[122] indicate that toxemia is associated with an excess of sodium in the fat-free tissue components; findings consistent in part with the view that retention of salt and water, while not a fundamental cause,[117–120] often is a major manifestation of this condition. Stearns[29] and Soichet[15] have emphasized the effects of emotional stress on maternal metabolism and the occurrence of toxemia. It also must be borne in mind that abnormal weight patterns may indicate other conditions apparently aggravated by, though not the direct result of, pregnancy, such as diabetes mellitus.[38] Nevertheless, a sudden gain in weight, especially after the twentieth week, should alert one to the potentiality of acute toxemia.

ANEMIA

Although rarely the most serious development, anemia probably is among the most prevalent systemic complications of the gravid state. The generic problem of standardizing diagnostic criteria and especially of distinguishing between physiologic and pathologic, maximal and optimal, usual and normal, and acceptable and desirable conditions probably is most apparent in a consideration of this "anemia of pregnancy." Notwithstanding substantial agreement on mechanisms and measurements, clinicians differ on the questions of significance and, particularly, of the practical management and prevention of a low hemoglobin concentration during different phases of the antepartum period.

Numerous observers have associated anemia in pregnancy with other complications, both fetal and maternal.[44,139–150] Although a causal relationship is suspected in some instances, the influence of a common denominator is more often implied. The several anemias of pregnancy are characterized by different morphologic and clinical attributes and by different, but commonly interdependent, etiologies. Although they should be distinguished from preexisting anemias of "specific" origin (*e.g.*, sickle cell anemia, thalassemia, mixed hemoglobinopathies),[15] most if not all of these more usual types also are not peculiar to pregnancy, but more probably are precipitated by and exaggerated during gestation. Moreover, they frequently coexist, with consequent hematologic confusion resolved only by extensive laboratory investigation and/or therapeutic trial.

Iron. Although factors in addition to iron deficiency evidently are operative in a significant proportion of cases, concern in this country is principally with the hypochromic normocytic (usually) anemia, which is encountered so commonly as to be considered, if not normal, certainly not remarkable. The principal problem is that of the so-called physiologic anemia of pregnancy.[134,152,153] Hemodilution undoubtedly occurs during normal pregnancy, followed by hemoconcentration in labor and the puerperium.[154–156] Estimates place the transitory and highly variable increase in circulating plasma at 20 to 40 per cent (higher in other extracellular spaces), and that of the circulating hemoglobin at about half that figure in a majority of untreated cases. However, abundant evidence suggests that, in most instances, a fall in hemoglobin can be appreciably limited by adequate and timely supplies of iron.[150, 153–168] On occasion, prematernal stores appear ample, as in many Bantu mothers who, despite a seemingly unsatisfactory state of general nutrition, may maintain normal hemoglobin readings throughout pregnancy.[169–171] However, the blood hemoglobin level, though probably of more practical value than red cell mass and serum iron content, is not a reliable index of marrow iron reserves, which may seem low in patients with ostensibly adequate hemoglobin concentrations, and even normal in patients with apparent anemia.

According to Pritchard,[172] ". . . if iron is readily available to the bone marrow, an average of about 0.5 g. of iron will be utilized in augmenting maternal erythropoiesis during pregnancy.

"The iron that is directed to the fetus and placenta, exclusive of the maternal hemoglobin in the placenta, amounts to about 0.2 to 0.3 g. Therefore, if iron is readily available, iron utilization induced by pregnancy with a single fetus amounts to about 0.8 g. and with multiple fetuses somewhat more. If prorated over the later half of pregnancy, when practically all of the placental transfer to the fetus takes place, the iron needed for pregnancy totals nearly 6 mg. per day. To this amount must be added the 0.5 to 1.0 mg. of iron that is lost through the gut, the urinary tract, and the skin and its appendages each day.

"This relatively large amount of iron might be obtained from the following sources:

"*Maternal iron stores:* The iron stores of women are seldom large enough to supply all the iron that is needed. When calculated from histochemical evaluation of marrow reticuloendothelial iron and measurements of iron stores by quantitative phlebotomy, the stores of healthy young American women average about 0.3 g.

"*Diet:* Food rarely provides sufficient iron to permit 6 to 7 mg. to be absorbed each day. Diets currently consumed by American women contain on the average about 6 mg. per 1000 calories. Pregnant women appear to ingest from dietary sources 13 or 14 mg. of iron per day, most of which is not absorbed.

"*Supplementation:* A simple ferrous salt during pregnancy will easily furnish sufficient iron to the mother and fetus."

The routine administration of iron throughout the prenatal period, even before the increased rate of absorption that characteristically prevails in the third trimester, has been questioned as being unnecessary and possibly as being contraindicated.[173,174] However, the difficulty if not the impossibility of distinguishing between normal and abnormal features of the maternal state and of estimating iron reserves at conception moves many observers to advocate iron supplements for all pregnant women. Ascorbic acid may enhance iron absorption, whereas large quantities of milk and, as practiced in some areas, ingestion of clay and cornstarch may interfere with this function.[175,176] The adverse influence of a possible complicating infection, notably occult involvement of the urinary tract, also must be borne in mind.[11, 153,177,178]

Folic Acid. Although macrocytic anemias of pregnancy are common in many countries (e.g., Asia and South America),[44,146,178,179] and have been credited with a significant frequency in the United Kingdom (Giles and Shuttleworth;[140] Chanarin et al.[180]) and even among some clinic populations in the United States, they do not constitute the major problem in this part of the world. However, folic acid metabolism appears altered in pregnancy, even in the absence of the megaloblastic anemia it commonly corrects.[166–178, 181–190] Compared with nonpregnant controls, pregnant women show an increased rate of clearance of intravenously administered folic acid, notably in the last trimester. Plasma clearance is especially rapid in instances of twin pregnancy and of megaloblastic anemia. A deficiency state is further suggested by impaired absorption of folic acid in pregnancy, most evident in anemic patients, and by an increased excretion of formiminoglutamic acid (FIGLU), which responds to folic acid administration. Folic acid is frequently recommended, not only in the less common megaloblastic, macrocytic anemia, but also as a routine adjunct to iron in the treatment and prevention of the more usual, hypochromic anemias.[148,187–189] Folic acid also appears beneficial in the hemolytic anemias associated with the hemoglobinopathies, and has been credited with prevention of other fetal and maternal complications.[148,187] Folate requirements have been estimated as "close to 300 μg per day."[19] Protein supplements may enhance folate effectiveness in instances of severe dietary limitation.

SPECIAL CONSIDERATIONS

Calcium. The perennial concern for calcium metabolism during pregnancy notwithstanding, the question of optimum intake seems far from being resolved.[192] Total fetal needs appear to be about 20 to 30 gm, an estimated 30 per cent of which usually is provided by or passes through maternal stores. Although a negative calcium balance appears almost inevitable during pregnancy and especially lactation, women with an average daily intake as low as 300 mg appear to deliver and to nurse successive, healthy children without clinical evidence of calcium depletion when vitamin D is in adequate supply.[192–197] Gravidas long accustomed to a low calcium intake (e.g., less than $\frac{1}{2}$ gm daily) appear to adjust satisfactorily to these levels, in part probably because of the decreased excretion and increased absorption of this mineral that reportedly ensures its more efficient utilization during pregnancy.[192–197] An adequate intake of magnesium and, particularly, avoidance of excessive phosphorus also appear conducive to positive calcium balance.[198]

NUTRITIONAL MANAGEMENT

Implicit in the nutritional management of the pregnant or lactating woman is the need to individualize each patient's regimen with due concern for the psychologic factors that, directly and indirectly, affect maternal metabolism.[15–20] The personal prescription should be based on the Recommended Dietary Allowances of the National Research Council (1968 Revision, Table A-1 in Appendix), which provide for general increases over levels advised for nonpregnant women, particularly in respect to protein, calcium, iron, and calories.

Although these recommendations should ensure a margin of safety in respect to all dietary essentials, nutritional adequacy at the time of conception cannot always be assumed,[11–13] and a corrective rather than merely a sustaining regimen may sometimes be required. Similarly, an overly rigid adherence to the recommendation for an increase in calories may lead to hyperalimentation in individuals with habitual and/or pregnancy-inspired substandard energy expenditure. Regular exercise should be advocated not only because it enhances overall metabolic function and general well-being, but because, by permitting a greater caloric intake, it also provides for a wider choice of protective foods.

DIET IN PREGNANCY

The caloric intake should be sufficient to maintain the calculated "ideal" body weight, with an additional 200 kcal per day during gestation. The minimum energy vehicle required to ensure meeting vitamin and mineral needs has been estimated at 2000 kcal daily. Protein needs should be met readily through an addition of 10 gm to the maintenance level of 1 gm per kg of ideal weight, provided that at least two-thirds of the total nitrogen component is of animal origin. Fat should contribute approximately 30 per cent of the total calories, assuming satisfactory tolerance. The carbohydrate component should consist predominantly of complex polysaccharides, although simple sugars may be indicated for the patient with hyperemesis. Meals should be individually balanced and consumed on a regular, consistent schedule even when small frequent feedings are advised for such conditions as nausea in the first trimester and abdominal fullness toward term.

The best index of nutritional needs is the condition of the patient, and, notwithstanding its limitations, body weight probably remains the most practical single parameter.[134] In the individual of normal weight and body composition, a total gain of 20 to 28 pounds during pregnancy is commensurate with the most favorable outcome of pregnancy. It also represents an acceptable objective above the ideal level for the initially substandard or overweight patient. A smaller-than-average gain, which appears compatible with a normal pregnancy experience in a majority of gravidas in some areas,[44,116] actually may prove advantageous to selected overweight subjects in this country. Carefully worked out dietary plans make it possible to minimize the weight gain of obese women without any statistical penalty. Obviously, such a restricted intake must be accompanied by a high protein, mineral, and vitamin dietary intake to be safe. Drastic weight reduction during pregnancy seems ill-advised and, obviously, should never be achieved at the expense of essential dietary constituents.

Patients with complicating conditions such as diabetes mellitus require special dietary regimens compatible with their optimum overall medical management. Gravida with prediabetes ("pregnancy diabetes") also may benefit from modified programs, although the sometimes advocated pattern of low carbohydrate intake and small doses of insulin appears to convey few benefits apart from a reduction in newborn weight. Weight gain should be regular and even, avoiding both the inadequate early increase identified with prematurity and the later, excessive—often sudden—increment associated with toxemia. A total gain of about 3 pounds over the first four months (1.5 pounds in the first ten weeks), with a subsequent average gain of 0.8 pound per week, seems a reasonable goal. Thomson noted an overall favorable experience among women who gained about 1 pound per week in the last trimester.[13]

Salt. Although benefits have been ascribed to a large salt intake[199] and some observers believe its limitation to be harmful,[117–121] many obstetricians favor some routine restriction of dietary sodium during pregnancy. However, until its metabolic role is better understood, salt probably should not be restricted for healthy women. The practice of routinely restricting sodium intake and at the same time prescribing diuretics is potentially dangerous. A daily intake of 2.5 to 5.0 gm (more in summer months) may be allowed in the absence of specific contraindications such as hypertensive cardiovascular and renal disease.

Vitamins. Although a number of vitamins, including biotin,[200] have been reported to be low in maternal tissue fluids during gestation, with the possible exception of folic acid there seems to be no empiric justification for routinely prescribing vitamin supplements for healthy pregnant women.

Iron. Iron supplements appear to be indicated for all pregnant women, especially those with a history of anemia, multiple births, or frequent pregnancies. A hemoglobin level below 11 gm per 100 ml in the first trimester, 10.5 per 100 ml in the second trimester, or 10 gm per 100 ml in the third trimester represents almost certain evidence of iron deficiency. Beyond the seeming advantages of a sustained, satisfactory hemoglobin concentration throughout pregnancy, this practice appears warranted by estimates of the usual blood loss during parturition (500 ml of blood; @200 mg of iron) and by the frequency and unpredictability of complicated delivery (*e.g.*, cesarean section; 1000 ml of blood; @400 mg of iron) and of ante-, intra-, and postpartum hemorrhage. Adequate reserves of iron, together with protein and other essential nutrients, conduce to rapid recovery and to the mother's ability to nurse and otherwise meet the needs of the newborn infant. Oral preparations providing 30 to 60 mg of iron daily during the last four or five months of pregnancy generally are sufficient to protect any existing iron stores. For the treatment of overt anemia and the replenishment of stores, 200 mg of elemental iron daily are adequate: this is equivalent to about three tablets daily of ferrous sulfate or ferrous fumarate, or six tablets daily of ferrous gluconate. The parenteral administration of iron (intramuscular preparations to 1000 mg in four or more doses; intravenous preparations in repeated or single doses)[201-203] frequently is attended by adverse reactions and consequently should be reserved for the occasional patient who is unresponsive to ingested iron or the patient with an extremely low hemoglobin level close to term.[204] A large intake of milk may interfere with iron absorption and contribute to anemia in women with marginal dietary representations of this element.

Other Hematopoietic Substances. Folic acid (200 to 400 μg daily) probably should be prescribed for most prenatal patients, particularly those in marginal economic groups. Gravida with refractory anemia and hemoglobinopathies, as well as those with a macrocytic or dimorphic pattern, may require larger doses (1 mg daily).

Calcium. Although calcium salts have been advocated in some instances (*e.g.*, leg cramps), supplementation generally is unnecessary. When indicated, the gluconate or lactate form seems preferable (0.5 to 1.0 gm, four times daily).

Adequate intakes of magnesium, copper, and potassium usually are assured through a balanced dietary regimen. Beyond concern for adequate iodine consumption under special circumstances, other mineral components rarely need to be considered in uncomplicated pregnancy.

DIET IN LACTATION

The nutritional management of lactation consists essentially of a selective, quantitative extension of those measures advised during pregnancy.[13,19,23,44] Although the quality of breast milk varies from person to person[203] and, in the same person, from day to day, this variability does not appear attributable to short-term modifications of the maternal diet.[13,205,206] An insufficiency of liquids, protein, or calories appears to affect the amount more than the composition of mammary secretion.[205] Severe, sustained malnutrition evidently results in a reduced energy, protein and fat content, as well as in a significantly smaller volume of breast milk.[206] Since the estimated caloric efficiency of milk production is at most 60 per cent, and that of protein is about 50 per cent, intakes of 1000 kcal and of 20 gm of protein per day above the allowances for nonpregnant women are recommended. The intake of calcium should be at least equal to that prescribed during pregnancy, and an adequate supply of vitamin D also must be assured.

BIBLIOGRAPHY

1. Maternal Nutrition and the Course of Pregnancy, Nat. Acad. Sci., Washington, D.C., 1968,
2a. Beaton: Fed. Proc., *20*, (Supp. 7), Pt. 3, 196, 1961.
2b. Beaton and Arroyane: Fed. Proc., *22*, Pt. 1, 608, 1963.
2c. Beaton, Arroyane and Flores: Amer. J. Clin. Nutr., *14*, 269, 1964.
3. Anon.: Nutr. Rev., *18*, 260, 1960.
4. Woollam: J. Col. Gen. Pract., *8*, (Supp. 2), 35, 1964.
5. Hillman: Missouri Med., *59*, 312, 1962.
6. Hillman: Med. Clin. N. Amer., *48*, 1141, 1964.
7. Vincent and Huzon: Bull. World Health Organ., *262*, 143, 1962.
8a. Warkany: J.A.M.A., *168*, 2020, 1958.
8b. Warkany: Borden Rev. Nutr. Res., *21*, 1, 1960.
9. Schaefer: Mod., Proc. Western Hemisphere Nutrition Congress, p. 43, A.M.A., 1965.
10. McKeown and Record: Brit. J. Prev. Soc. Med., *11*, 102, 1957.
11. McGanity: Proc. Western Hemisphere Nutrition Cong., p. 199, A.M.A., 1965.

12. Bagchi and Bose: Amer. J. Clin. Nutr., *10*, 586, 1962.
13a.Thomson: Brit. J. Nutr., *5*, 158, 1951.
13b.Thomson: Brit. J. Nutr., *12*, 410, 1958.
13c.Thomson: Brit. J. Nutr., *13*, 509, 1959.
13d.Thomson: Proc. Nutr. Soc., *16*, 45, 1957.
13e.Thomson and Billewicz: Brit. Med. J., *1*, 243, 1957.
13f.Thomson and Billewicz: Proc. Nutr. Soc., *22*, 55, 1963.
13g.Thomson and Hytten: Proc. Nutr. Soc., *19*, 5, 1960.
13h.Thomson and Hytten: Proc. Nutr. Soc., *20*, 76, 1961.
14. Hepner: J.A.M.A., *168*, 1774, 1958.
15. Soichet: Amer. J. Obstet. Gynec., *77*, 1065, 1959.
16. Wiehl, Berry and Tompkins: in Epidemiology of Mental Disorder. Am. Ass'n Advancement Science, Washington, 1959.
17. Blau, Slaff, Easton, Welkowitz, Springarn and Cohen: Psychosom. Med., *25*, 201, 1963.
18. McDonald, Gynther and Christakos: Psychosom. Med., *25*, 357, 1963.
19. Mayer: Postgrad. Med., *30*, 380, 1963.
20. Paffenberger and McCabe: Amer. J. Pub. Health, *56*, 400, 1966.
21a.Marston: Physiol. Rev., *32*, 66, 1952.
21b.Marston: Nutr. Rev., *15*, 8, 1957.
21c.Marston: Nutr. Rev., *17*, 270, 1959.
22. Hale: Texas Med. J., *33*, 228, 1937.
23a.Millen: *The Nutritional Basis of Reproduction*, Springfield, Charles C Thomas, 1962.
23b.Millen and Woollam: Proc. Nutr. Soc., *19*, 1, 1960.
24. Frazer: J. Chron. Dis., *10*, 97, 1959.
25. Adamsons and Joelsson: Amer. J. Obstet. Gynec., *96*, 437, 1966.
26. Garry and Wood: Nutr. Abst. Rev., *15*, 591, 1946.
27. Burke and Stuart: in *A.M.A. Handbook of Nutrition*, 2nd ed., Philadelphia, The Blakiston Co., 1951.
28. Josey: Amer. J. Clin. Nutr., *2*, 303, 1954.
29. Stearns: J.A.M.A., *168*, 1655, 1958.
30. Dalderup: Vitamins Hormones, *17*, 223, 1959.
31. Seifrit: J. Amer. Dist. Assn., *39*, 455, 1961.
32. Sutherland: Lancet, *2*, 953, 1946.
33. Baird: J. Obstet. Gynec. Brit. Emp., *52*, 217, 339, 1945.
34. Moncrieff: Acta Pediat., *36*, 167, 1948.
35. Balfour: Lancet, *1*, 208, 1944.
36. Cameron and Graham: Glasgow Med. J., *24*, 1, 1944.
37. The Peoples League of Health: J. Obstet. Gynec. Brit. Emp., *53*, 498, 1946.
38. Toverud: in *Nutrition in Relation to Health and Disease*, New York, Milbank Memorial Fund, 1950.
39. Riquelme and Alvorado: Acta Pediat. Espanola, *113*, 310, 1952.
40. Dean: Med. Res. Council Spec. Rep. Ser. No. 275, 1951.

41. Antonev: J. Pediat., *30*, 250, 1947.
42. Berry: Brit. Med. J., *2*, 819, 1955.
43. Hamlin: Lancet, *1*, 64, 1952.
44a.Gopolan: Bull. W.H.O., *26*, 2, 1962.
44b.Gopolan and Belanady: Fed. Proc., *20* Pt. 3, Supp. 7, 177, 1961.
45. Ebbs, Tisdall and Scott: Milbank Mem. Fund Quart., *20*, 35, 1942.
46a.Burke and Stuart: J.A.M.A., *137*, 119, 1948.
46b.Burke: Amer. J. Clin. Nutr. *2*, 425, 1954.
47. Jeans, Smith and Stearns: J. Amer. Diet. Assn., *31*, 576, 1955.
48. Ferguson and Hinson: J. Louisiana Med. Soc., *105*, 18, 1953.
49. Brantley: North Carolina Med. J., *18*, 1, 1957.
50. Block, Lipsett, Redner and Hirschl: J. Pediat., *41*, 300, 1952.
51. Crump: J. Nat. Med. Assn., *54*, 432, 1962.
52. Herrell, Woodyard and Gates: Metabolism, *5*, 555, 1956.
53. Borquin and Benum: Amer. J. Clin. Nutr., *5*, 63, 1954.
54a.Smith: J. Pediat., *30*, 229, 1947.
54b.Smith: Amer. J. Obstet. Gynec., *53*, 599, 1947.
55. Williams and Fralin: Amer. J. Obstet. Gynec., *43*, 1, 1942.
56. Speert, Graff and Graff: Amer. J. Obstet. Gynec., *62*, 1009, 1951.
57a.Dieckmann, Turner and Ruby: Amer. J. Obstet. Gynec., *50*, 701, 1945.
57b.Dieckmann: *The Toxemias of Pregnancy*, 2nd ed. St. Louis, C. V. Mosby Co., 1952.
58. Kyhos, Vaglio, Severinghaus, Nutley, Hagedorn and Knowlton: Amer. J. Digest. Dis., *16*, 436, 1949.
59. Petry: Obstet. Gynec., *7*, 219, 1956.
60. Scrimshaw: J. Amer. Diet Assn., *26*, 21, 1950.
61a.Macy, Mayer, Kelly, Mack, DiLoreto and Pratt: J. Nutr. (Supp. 1), *52*, 1, 1954.
61b.Macy: J.A.M.A., *168*, 2265, 1958.
62a.McGanity, Cannon, Bridgforth, Martin, Densin, Newbill, McClellan, Christies, Peterson and Darby: Amer. J. Obstet. Gynec., *67*, 491, 501, 539, 1954.
62b.McGanity, Bridgforth, Martin, Newbill and Darby: J. Amer. Diet. Assn., *31*, 582, 1955.
62c.Darby, Bridgforth, Martin and McGanity: Obstet. Gynec., *5*, 528, 1955.
62d.McGanity, Bridgforth and Darby: J.A.M.A: *168*, 2138, 1958.
63. Page: Amer. J. Obstet. Gynec., *75*, 705, 1957.
64. Dancis: Amer. J. Obstet. Gynec., *82*, 167, 1961.
65. Davies: *Survey of Research in Gestation and the Developmental Sciences*, Baltimore, The Williams & Wilkins Co., 1960.
66. Villee: *The Placenta and Fetal Membranes*, Baltimore, The Williams & Wilkins Co., 1960.
67. Sternberg: Amer. J. Obstet. Gynec., *84*, 1731, 1962.
68. Report of a WHO Scientific Group: WHO Tech. Rep. Series 280, Geneva, 1964.
69. Adamsons: in Symposium on the Placenta: Its Form and Functions. Birth Defects Original Article Series, Vol. 1, No. 1, 1965.

70. Wong and Latour: Amer. J. Obstet. Gynec., *94*, 942, 1966.
71. Stenger, Henry, Cestari, Eitzman and Prytowsky: Amer. J. Obstet. Gynec., *94*, 261, 1966.
72. Hensleigh and Krantz: Amer. J. Obstet. Gynec., *96*, 5, 1966.
73a. Baumgartner, Pessin, Wegman and Pakter: Pediatrics, *6*, 329, 1950.
73b. Baumgartner: Bull. WHO, *26*, 175, 1962.
74. Editorial: J.A.M.A., *167*, 470, 1958.
75. Williams: Brit. Med. J., *2*, 1338, 1957.
76. Widdowson: Amer J. Clin. Nutr., *3*, 391, 1955.
77. Beilley and Kurland: Amer. J. Obstet. Gynec., *50*, 202, 1951.
78. Douglas and Scadron: Med. Clin. N. Amer., *35*, 733, 1951.
79. Fisher and Fry: Obstet. Gynec, *11*, 92, 1958.
80. Abramowicz and Kass: New Eng. J. Med., *275*, 938, 1966.
81. Kerr: Amer. J. Obstet. Gynec., *45*, 950, 1943.
82. Stewart and Hewitt: J. Obstet. Gynec. Brit. Com., *67*, 812, 1960.
83. Fields and Davis: Obstet. Gynec., *19*, 423, 1962.
84. Emerson: Brit. Med. J., *2*, 516, 1962.
85. Lesinski: Bull. WHO, *26*, 183, 1962.
86. Kaltreider: *Effects of Height and Weight on Pregnancy and the Newborn*, Springfield, Charles C Thomas, 1963.
87. Clements: Fed. Proc. 20 Pt. 3, Supp. 7, 165, 1961.
88. Mitchell: *Comparative Nutrition of Man and Domestic Animals*, New York, Academic Press, 1962.
89. Ashley-Montagu: *Prenatal Influences*, Springfield, Charles C Thomas, 1962.
90. WHO Expert Committee on Nutrition, 6th Report, 245, 1962.
91. Vincent and Hugon: Bull. W.H.O., *262*, 143, 1962.
92. Anon.: Nutr. Rev., *16*, 6, 1958.
93. WHO Expert Committee on Maternal and Child Health, 3rd Report, WHO Tech. Rep. Ser., 217, 1961.
94. Barnes: in Papers and Discussion of the Second International Conference on Congenital Malformations, July 14–19, 1963.
95. Rossi: Connecticut Health Bulletin, *78*, 267, 1964.
96. Naeye: Arch. Path., *79*, 284, 1965.
97. Thomson: Brit. J. Nutr., *13*, 509, 1959.
98. Siegel and Morris: Maternal Nutrition and the Course of Pregnancy, p. 22, Nat. Acad. Sci., Washington, D.C., 1968.
99. Churchill, Neff and Caldwell: Obstet. Gynec., *28*, 425, 1966.
100. Naeye: Amer. J. Obstet. Gynec., *95*, 276, 1966.
101. Mellin: J.A.M.A., *180*, 11, 1962.
102. Moiyama: Canad. J. Pub. Health, *50*, 60, 1959.
103. Barnes: Fed. Proc., *30*, 1429, 1971.
104. Arbeter, Echeverri, Franco, Munson, Velez and Vitale: Fed. Proc., *30*, 1421, 1971.
105. McKay and Lucey: New Eng. J. Med., *270*, 1231, 1292, 1964.

106. Lucey: in Proceedings of Symposium on the Placenta, Its Form and Functions. Birth Defects Original Article Series Vol. 1, 1965.
107. WHO Expert Committee on Human Genetics, 2nd Report, WHO Tech. Rep. Ser. 282, 1964.
108. Hammond: Proc. Nutr. Soc., *19*, 1, 1960.
109. Lenz: *Medical Genetics*, Chicago, Chicago University Press, 1963.
110. Coffey and Jessup: Irish J. Med. Sc., *393*, 391, 1958.
111. Anderson, Baird and Thomson: Lancet, *1*, 1304, 1958.
112. Edwards: Brit. J. Soc. Prev. Med., *12*, 115, 1958.
113. Thiersch: In *Ciba Foundation Symposium on Congenital Malformations*, London, J. & A. Churchill Ltd., 1960.
114. Report of Working Group on Relation of Nutrition to the Toxemias of Pregnancy: Maternal Nutrition and the Course of Pregnancy, p. 163, Nat. Acad. Sci., Washington, D.C., 1968.
115. Hytten and Thomson: Ibid, p. 63.
116. Hauck: J. Obstet. Gynec., Brit. Com., *30*, 885, 1963.
117. Brewer: *Metabolic Toxemia of Late Pregnancy. A Disease of Malnutrition*, Springfield, Charles C Thomas, 1966.
118. Reboud, Groulade, Groslambert and Colomb: Amer. J. Obstet. Gynec., *86*, 820, 1963.
119. Nelson, Zuspan and Mulligan: Amer. J. Obstet. Gynec., *94*, 310, 1966.
120. Mengert and Tacchi: Amer. J. Obstet. Gynec., *81*, 601, 1961.
121. Pike: J. Amer. Diet. Assn., *44*, 176, 1964.
122. Chesley: Amer. J. Obstet. Gynec., *95*, 127, 1966.
123. Clemetson and Andersen: Obstet. Gynec., *24*, 774, 1964.
124. Klieger, Evrard and Pierce: Amer. J. Obstet. Gynec., *94*, 316, 1966.
125. Alfonso and De Alvarez: Amer. J. Obstet. Gynec., *86*, 815, 1963.
126. Robinson, London and Pierce: Amer. J. Obstet. Gynec., *96*, 226, 1966.
127. Leathem: *Reproductive Physiology and Protein Nutrition*, New Brunswick, Rutgers University Press, 1959.
128. Glowinski, *et al.*: Foreign Mail, J.A.M.A., *180*, 83, 1962.
129. Werch, Lewis and Ferguson: Obstet. Gynec., *11*, 676, 1958.
130. Smith, De Alvarez and Forsander: Amer. J. Obstet. Gynec., *77*, 326, 1959.
131. Wachstein: in *The Promotion of Maternal and Newborn Health*, New York, Milbank Memorial Fund, 1955.
132. Hillman, Cabaud and Schenone: Amer. J. Clin. Nutr., *10*, 512, 1962.
133. Hillman, Cabaud, Nilsson, Arpin and Tufano: Amer. J. Clin. Nutr., *12*, 427, 1963.
134. Haley and Woodbury: Surg. Gynec Obstet., *103*, 227, 1956.

135. Fish, Bartholomew, Colvin, Grimes, Lester and Golloway: Amer. J. Obstet. Gynec., 78, 743, 1959.
136. McCartney, Pottinger and Harrod: Amer. J. Obstet. Gynec., 77, 1039, 1959.
137. Plentl and Gray: Amer. J. Obstet. Gynec., 78, 742, 1959.
138. Stephens, Page and Hare: Diabetes, 12, 213, 1963.
139. Traylor and Torpin: Amer. J. Obstet. Gynec., 62, 898, 1951.
140. Giles and Shuttleworth: Lancet, 2, 1341, 1958.
141. McClean: Pediatrics, 7, 136, 1951.
142. Zilliacus and Putkinen: quoted by Josey in reference 28.
143. Sisson and Lund: Amer. J. Clin. Nutr., 6, 376, 1958.
144. Woodruff: J.A.M.A., 167, 715, 1958.
145. Raiha, Lind, Johanson, Kehlberg and Vara: Ann. Pediat. Fenniae, 2, 69, 1956.
146. Layrisse, Aguero, Blumenfield, Wallis, Dugarte and Ojeda: Blood, 15, 724, 1960.
147. Stapp: Obstet. Gynec., 27, 718, 1963.
148. Fraser and Watt: Amer. J. Obstet. Gynec., 89, 532, 1966.
149. Roszkowski, Wojcicka and Zaleska: Obstet. Gynec., 28, 820, 1966.
150. Barry: J. Irish Med. Assn., 53, 105, 1963.
151. Henrikse and Watson-Williams: Amer. J. Obstet. Gynec., 94, 739, 1966.
152. Rovinsky and Jaffin: Amer. J. Obstet. Gynec., 95, 787, 1966.
153a. Holly: Obstet. Gynec., 5, 563, 1955.
153b. Holly: Postgrad. Med., 26, 418, 1959.
153c. Holly: Amer. J. Obstet. Gynec., 80, 946, 1960.
153d. Holly: Amer. J. Obstet. Gynec., 93, 371, 1965.
154. Miller, Williams and MacArthur: Amer. J. Obstet. Gynec., 78, 303, 1959.
155a. Pritchard: Amer. J. Obstet. Gynec., 77, 74, 1959.
155b. Pritchard, Baldwin, Dickey and Wiggins: Amer. J. Obstet. Gynec., 84, 1271, 1962.
156. Tjan and Okey: Amer. J. Obstet. Gynec., 84, 1316, 1962.
157. Gohres, Albert and Dodek: Amer. J. Obstet. Gynec., 84, 764, 1962
158 Edgar and Rice: Lancet, 1, 599, 1956.
159. Gatenby: Proc. Nutr. Soc., 15, 115, 1956.
160. Fisher and Biggs: Brit. Med. J., 1, 385, 1955.
161. Benstead and Theobold: Brit. Med. J., 1, 407, 1952.
162. Kerr and Davidson: Lancet, 2, 483, 1958.
163. Morgan: Lancet, 1, 9, 1961.
164. Hood and Bond: Obstet. Gynec., 16, 82, 1960.
165. Berk and Novick: Amer. J. Obstet. Gynec., 83, 203, 1962.
166. Krishna Menon and Lakshmi: J. Obstet. Gynec., India, 12, 382, 1962.
167. Leading Article: Lancet, 1, 309, 1963.
168a. Lowenstein, Hsieh, Brunton, deLeeuow and Cooper: Postgrad. Med., 31, 72, 1962.
168b. Lowenstein, Brunton and Hsieh: Canad. Med. Assn. J., 94, 636, 1966.
169. Gerritsen and Walker: J. Clin. Invest., 33, 23, 1954.

170. Turchetti, Cornbrink, Krawitz and Metz: Amer. J. Clin. Nutr., 18, 249, 1966.
171. Partwardhan: Amer. J. Clin. Nutr., 19, 63, 1966.
172. Pritchard: Maternal Nutrition and the Course of Pregnancy, p. 74, Nat. Acad. Sci., Washington, D.C., 1968.
173. Lapan and Friedman: Amer. J. Obstet. Gynec., 76, 96, 1958.
174. Hytten and Duncan: Nutr. Abst. Rev., 26, 855, 1956.
175. Anon.: Nutr. Rev., 18, 35, 1960.
176. Edwards, McDonald, Mitchell, Jones, Mason and Trigg: J. Amer. Diet. Assn., 44, 109, 1964.
177. Giles and Brown: Brit. Med. J., 2, 10, 1962.
178. Scott: Brit. Med. J., 2, 354, 1963.
179a. Woodruff: Brit. Med. J., 1, 1297, 1955.
179b. Ojo: J. Trop. Med. Hyg., 68, 32, 1965.
180a. Chanarin, MacGibbon, O'Sullivan and Mollin: Lancet, 2, 634, 1959.
180b. Chanarin, Rothman and Watson-Williams: Lancet, 1, 1068, 1963.
181. Spies: Surg., Gynec., Obstet., 89, 76, 1946.
182. Scott: J. Obstet. Gynec. Brit. Emp., 61, 646, 1956.
183. Metz, Stevens and Brandt: Brit. Med. J., 2, 1440, 1962.
184. Dawson: J. Obstet. Gynec. Brit. Com., 69, 38, 1962.
185. Henderson: Obstet. Gynec., 24, 752, 1964.
186. Metz, Festenstein and Welch: Amer. J. Clin. Nutr., 16, 472, 1965.
187. Benjamin, Bassen and Meyer: Amer. J. Obstet. Gynec., 96, 310, 1966.
188. Alperin, Hutchinson and Levin: Arch. Int. Med., 117, 681, 1966.
189. Hansen and Rybo: Nord. Med. 76, 853, 1966.
190. Vitale: Nutr. Rev., 24, 289, 1966.
191. Willoughby and Jewell: Brit. Med. J., 2, 1568, 1966.
192. Kerr, Loken, Glendening, Gordon and Page: Amer. J. Obstet. Gynec., 83, 2, 1962.
193. Page and Page: Obstet. Gynec., 1, 94, 1953.
194. Comar: Ann. N.Y. Acad. Sci., 64, 279, 1956.
195. Nicolaysen, Egg-Larsen and Malm: Physiol. Rev., 33, 424, 1953.
196. Bronner: Science, 132, 472, 1960.
197. Goss: Obstet. Gynec., 20, 199, 1962.
198. Briscoe and Ragan: Amer. J. Clin. Nutr., 19, 296, 1966.
199. Robinson: Lancet, 1, 178, 1958.
200. Bhagavan: Internat. J. Vit. Res., 39, 235, 1969.
201. O'Sullivan, Higgins and Wilkinson: Lancet, 2, 483, 1955.
202. Scott and Govan: Brit. Med. J., 2, 1259, 1954.
203. McClanahan, Henderson and Gready: Obstet. Gynec., 12, 439, 1958.
204. Bhatt, Jashi and Shah: Amer. J. Obstet. Gynec., 94, 1098, 1966.
205. Kevany, J.: in Proc. Western Hemisphere Nutrition Congress 1965. p. 50, A.M.A. Chicago, 1966.
206. Anon.: Nutr. Rev., 24, 105, 1966.

Chapter

24

Nutrition in Infancy and Adolescence

SELMA E. SNYDERMAN

AND

L. EMMETT HOLT, JR.

GENERAL CONSIDERATIONS

The physician who is responsible for the diet of infants and children faces different problems in different countries and population groups. In underdeveloped countries and among the underprivileged ignorance of nutrition is profound and malnutrition is widespread; the problem is to provide adequate intakes of calories and specific nutrients. In well-developed countries, and particularly in the United States, the reverse is the case; the public has been made overconscious of nutrition—concerned about nutrients which are of no practical importance; the problems by and large are those of overnutrition and the task of the physician is to re-educate the public as to what is important and what is not. Our basic knowledge—and it is far from complete—will be considered under three headings: (1) the nutritional requirements of the normal child, (2) the extent to which a margin of safety beyond these levels is desirable to promote health, and (3) nutrition in pathologic conditions in which increments or decrements of particular nutrients are indicated.

PECULIARITIES OF NUTRITION IN EARLY LIFE

The phenomenon of growth involves more than an increase in size; it involves changes in function and in body composition which are reflected in nutritional requirements. These differences in requirements are seen particularly during the period of infancy, for it is then that growth is most rapid and that most of the chemical maturation is accomplished. In terms of body weight the infant needs more of all nutrients. Not only does he require the nutrients for growth but, in addition, because of his higher metabolic rate and more rapid turnover of nutrients, his requirements for maintenance are higher than those of the adult. His relatively large surface area involves relatively greater losses of heat and water through the skin. The development of the skeleton imposes special nutritive requirements. The absence of teeth requires that his food be finely subdivided. In contrast to these handicaps there are certain nutrients in regard to which he is in a favored position, having received during fetal life a surplus which is stored in the liver and which will tide him over the early months. Iron, copper and vitamin A are in this category.

Nutritional Requirements in Early Life. *Energy Requirements.* The caloric requirements of the newborn infant are 2 to 3 times as great as those of the adult in terms of body weight. Average figures for boys are given in Figure 24–1, which also indicates the distribution of calories needed during the period of growth. The basal heat production of the infant is high; this is due in part to his relatively greater body surface which favors loss of heat by conduction and convection, in part to his larger proportion of active metabolic tissue. It should be pointed out that what is commonly referred to as basal metabolism—

CALORIC REQUIREMENTS DURING CHILDHOOD

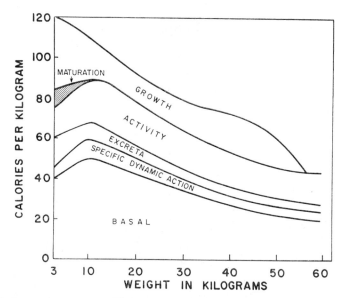

Fig. 24-1. Caloric requirements per kilogram throughout childhood. The ordinate under the upper curve shows the average requirement in calories per kilogram. The space between the curves indicates the allowance for the various factors which make up the total. Modified from Barnet's *Pediatrics* (courtesy of Appleton-Century-Crofts).

namely, metabolism under conditions of rest—is actually not basal in the growing child, for it represents the requirement for growth as well as for maintenance. Energy required for growth is greatest in the newborn period, decreasing rapidly during the first year and more gradually up to the time of puberty, when a spurt in growth occurs. A special requirement for chemical maturation quite apart from that demanded by increase in body size exists in infancy. The requirement for activity is surprisingly great, particularly in small infants; crying alone has been shown to double the metabolic rate.[1] The energy lost in the excreta is somewhat greater in early infancy than later; this, however, represents only a small fraction of the total energy requirement. There is considerable variation in the caloric requirements of individual infants, due chiefly to differences in activity. A placid infant may thrive on as little as 70 calories per kg. whereas one who cries a great deal may require 130 calories or even more.

Protein Requirements. Protein is required for maintenance (wear and tear) of tissues, for growth of new tissue and for maturation of tissues. At birth, roughly 2 per cent of the body consists of nitrogen as contrasted with a trifle over 3 per cent for the adult. Most of this change occurs during the first year. The zone of requirements for high quality protein at different ages is shown in the accompanying figure (Fig. 24–2). It would appear that breast milk, which commonly furnishes an intake ranging between 2.0 and 2.5 gm/kg, provides only a small margin of safety; however, its quality, constancy of composition and regularity of administration render this small margin adequate. Cow's milk was formerly regarded as considerably inferior to breast milk in biological value and for this reason higher protein intakes have been commonly given. Recent work, however, has shown that when cow's milk is processed in such a way as to avoid curd indigestion the protein is utilized virtually as efficiently as that of breast milk, and that intakes greater than 2.5 gm per kg are not necessary even in the early months of life.

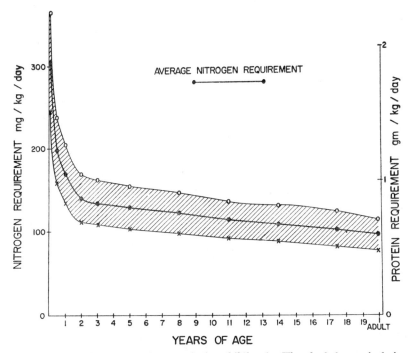

Fig. 24-2. The average nitrogen requirement during childhood. The shaded zone is designed to cover individual variations. The upper border of the zone represents a level of intake upon which virtually all individuals (95 per cent of the population) can be expected to thrive. The lower figure represents a figure below which a normal individual cannot be expected to thrive. (From Holt and Snyderman, Nutr. Abstr. & Rev., *35*, 1, 1965).

As infancy advances the curve of protein requirement falls off sharply, more sharply than the curve for caloric requirement. The reason for this is that activity is now the major function for which calories are required, and activity, unlike growth and maintenance, does not involve additional expenditure of nitrogen.[2] The widely used formula that 15 per cent of the total calories should consist of protein, a proportion which obtains in most American diets at all ages appears to provide well in excess of mimimal requirements in infancy and even more so as the child grows older. It should be borne in mind, however, that in the case of older children taking a mixed diet an allowance must be made for irregularities of intake and deficiencies of mastication. An increase of 25 per cent to cover this is not excessive. Beyond this, an allowance must finally be made for protein quality on diets in which a major portion of the protein is of vegetable origin. On mixed American and European diets increasing the

intake by the factor 1.2 should suffice, but as the quality of the protein declines, as may be the case in underdeveloped areas where the chief reliance is upon a single vegetable protein, the quantity may need to be doubled; it may not be practicable to do this because of the large quantity of food required. It is in such situations that manifestations of protein deficiency are commonly encountered.

Amino Acid Requirements. It has been generally accepted since the time of Mendel[3] that the limiting factors in protein diets are the essential amino acids from which it follows that adequacy of a diet could be obtained by providing a diet which met the minimum requirements of each essential amino acid. Much effort has been expended in determining individual requirements of the essential amino acids at different ages so that these figures could be applied in practical dietetics. It now appears that these figures are of limited usefulness, since they were determined under very special conditions and are not applicable to many other conditions. The amino acid requirements of adults[4-26] and older children[27-31] were determined under conditions of maximum sparing of the essential amino acids, generous caloric intakes and generous provision of "unessential" nitrogen (unessential amino acids and ammonium salts) to minimize the utilization of essential amino acids for energy or for the synthesis of unessential amino acids. The figures obtained no doubt represent close approximations to absolute minima but when applied to natural diets of high protein quality it appears that these minimum figures may have to be doubled or more than doubled before the protein needs of the organism are met.[32] The limiting factor in most human diets appears to be not an essential amino acid but nitrogen—essential or unessential.[33,34] As the quality of the protein diet deteriorates, the discrepancy between the adequacy of the diet and the minimal essential amino acid requirement values diminishes and, of course, when one comes to the seriously deficient proteins upon which Mendel's concept was based, the essential amino acids are indeed limiting.

The studies of essential amino acid requirements of infants[35-44] were not determined under conditions of maximum sparing of essential amino acids, the experimental diets employed being based on the pattern of human milk. The values obtained, though of greater practical value, may not represent absolute minimal requirements.

Amino Acid Patterns and Biologic Values. There is no doubt that the nutritional quality of a protein food or a protein diet is determined by its amino acid *pattern* and primarily by its pattern of essential amino acids. Supplementation of a diet with a single amino acid will often result in improved growth performance. In the past, this phenomenon has been attributed to an effect of the supplement upon the *content* of that particular amino acid in the diet—a deficiency was being met. However, with our growing knowledge of interrelationships between amino acids, particularly the competition of certain related amino acids for transport systems, it seems that the benefits of supplementation can be attributed to correction of an amino acid imbalance rather than to meeting a deficiency

in an absolute requirement—to an approach to a more ideal amino acid pattern.

A number of efforts to delineate an ideal amino acid pattern as a standard of reference have been made. In a recent consideration of the subject by a joint committee of FAO and WHO[32] the conclusion was reached that no artificial pattern was superior to that of whole egg or of human milk and that it was not possible to say that the pattern of one of these foods was superior to that of the other. Several scoring procedures have been devised to evaluate the nutritional quality of a diet from its amino acid pattern. Although of some value, these procedures, as we have pointed out elsewhere, are subject to considerable errors. As a guide to the quality of the protein of a diet it is necessary to evaluate that diet by criteria discussed elsewhere in this volume, notably the criteria based on nitrogen balance (biologic value and net protein utilization). It is preferable that such data be determined for the species under consideration and the time of life for which their application is desired. Although there is marked parallelism between protein quality as evaluated in the rat and man, there are notable exceptions. The rat, for example, makes a rather poor showing on human milk.

Fat Requirement. There is some evidence that humans, like other animals, require small quantities of polyunsaturated fatty acids. The long-continued use of a fat-free diet has been followed by undesirable consequences. Chwalibogowski[45] fed two infants on a fat-free diet for more than a year. Their clinical course and development did not appear in any way abnormal, although some evidence of rickets was obtained. Hansen and Wiese,[46] maintained a child with chylothorax on a fat-free diet for 2 years and observed increased frequency of skin infections and the development of eczema. More recently they studied a large group of infants[47] maintained on a fat-free diet in whom a scaly dermatitis developed; a number of infants also had loose stools and unsatisfactory weight gain. The addition of small amounts of polyunsaturated acids to the diet cured this.

The older pediatric literature contains many references to the deleterious action of volatile (short-chain) fatty acids, and their higher concentration in cow's milk was long blamed for some of the shortcomings of artificial feeding. It now appears, however, that the short-chain fats are digested as well as, if not better than, their long-chain analogs. Shorter chain fats and fats containing unsaturated linkages are somewhat more readily absorbed.[48,49] In feeding normal infants it appears desirable to include a certain amount of fat in the diet, but a strong case for feeding particular fats cannot be made, for the differences are small. In conditions of steatorrhea, however, the superior absorption of certain fats appears to have some practical advantage.

Carbohydrate Requirement. Although infants have been fed on carbohydrate-free diets for many months,[45] this is not a practical procedure. The development of ketosis is difficult to avoid. As a rule, roughly half of an infant's caloric requirement is supplied as carbohydrate.

Mineral Requirements. These are, for the most part, not accurately defined. With the exception of iron, the breast-fed infant appears to be adequately provided with minerals and it may be assumed that the quantities ingested are well above his minimal requirements. A 12-pound infant ingesting 800-ml breast milk per day would receive the following quantities of minerals:

exist. If the protein intake is adequate oxidation of the sulfur derived from the sulfur-amino acids will meet all the body's needs for sulfur.

The only important mineral deficiency likely to be encountered in feeding the normal infant is that of iron. This may be the most common nutritional deficiency of infancy, the exact prevalence depends on the criteria used for diagnosis. Both cow's milk and breast milk provide insufficient iron and, after the stores present at birth become depleted, iron deficiency develops unless a supplement is given. It is current practice to give supplementary iron in the formula or as a natural solid food such as reinforced cereal. A total iron intake of 1 mg/kg/day up to 15 mg total has been recommended.[49a] This fulfills the requirement as well as allowing for variations in absorption and in iron stores.

Under exceptional circumstances, when a milk-free diet must be used, fortification of the diet with calcium may be advisable. An intake of 200 to 300 mg per day appears to be adequate.

A factor complicating the exact determination of mineral requirements is the phenomenon of "supermineralization." When more mineral is given more is retained and the body may become, for a time at least, somewhat richer in mineral. This phenomenon is particularly striking in the case of calcium

		Intake			*Per cent of intake retained**
	mg/day	*mg/kg/day*	*mM/day*	*mM/kg/day*	
Na	120	21.6	5.2	0.95	40–55
K	420	75.7	10.8	1.96	20–30
Ca	250	45.0	6.2	1.13	15–20
Mg	30	5.4	1.2	0.22	20–30
Cl	330	59.2	8.4	1.53	20–30
P	200	36.0	6.4	1.16	15–20

* According to Swanson, Am. J. Dis. Child., *43*, 10, 1932.

Deficits of these minerals do not ordinarily arise from inadequate intake; they may, however, arise from pathologic processes in which there are abnormal losses of electrolytes from the gastrointestinal tract, kidney and, at times, the skin. A dietary requirement for oxidized sulfur does not appear to

and phosphorus and it appears that hyperalimentation of these elements may temporarily increase their storage in the bones. Whether this is beneficial or not is not established. Although claims have been made that a generous calcium intake prevents osteoporosis in later life, some observations made in animals[50,51] suggest that calcium more rapidly acquired during the growth period is more loosely held in adult life and may predispose to senile osteoporosis. Evidence that this holds for man is not available.

The requirements of children for the trace elements—copper, manganese, cobalt, zinc and selenium—are not known with accuracy. Iodine is discussed elsewhere (Chapter 8, Section A). The intake of fluorine has recently assumed considerable importance. An excess of this element leads to discoloration and mottling with increased brittleness of the dental enamel (fluorosis), whereas a deficiency predisposes to dental caries. The margin of safety between the two is a relatively small one. It has been estimated that if drinking water contains less than 1 ppm of fluorine, cariogenic effects may be expected. A concentration between 1.0 and 1.5 ppm is thought to be ideal.[52] Concentrations up to 2 ppm may lead to white mottling; beyond this level, brown mottling and fragility of the teeth may be encountered. Milk itself may contain as much as 2 ppm of fluorine but this does not lead to fluorosis since the fluorine exists in an insoluble form. The control of the fluorine content of drinking water has become a public health problem (see Chapter 27); it is a matter of particular importance during the period of dental development.

Vitamin Requirements. The requirements of infants for the vitamins which are established as dietary essentials are given in the following table:

Vitamin A	Not accurately known 1500 i.u. per day is definitely protective
Vitamin C	25–35 mg per day[53,54]
Vitamin D	400 I.U. per day[54]
Thiamin	0.20 mg per day[55]
Riboflavin	0.50 mg per day[56]
Pyridoxine	0.50 mg per day[57]

The requirement for nicotinic acid is a conditional one. If the intake of tryptophan is sufficient, it appears that the nicotinic acid required can be synthesized from this source. However, when the protein intake is marginal, nicotinic acid must be supplied as such. The requirement is commonly expressed in terms of niacin equivalents, 60 mg of tryptophan being equivalent to 1 mg niacin. Another B factor for which the requirement is conditional is choline. With a sufficient intake of methionine the needs of the body for additional choline appear to be insignificant, but, when the intake of methionine is limited, choline becomes a dietary factor of importance. The quantitative relationships between these conditionally required factors and their antecedents remain to be accurately defined.

It would appear that extremely small amounts of folic acid and B_{12} are needed by the human organism. These vitamins are synthesized in the large intestine, but it is questionable if they can be absorbed from the large gut in significant amounts. B_{12} requires no consideration in the infant's diet, nor does folic acid, provided the diet contains an adequate amount of vitamin C and provided antibiotics are not being given.

Other known B factors—pantothenic acid, biotin, and inositol—important as catalysts in metabolic reactions, are not yet established as normal dietary essentials. The same is true of lipoic acid.

In infant feeding ascorbic acid and vitamin D are the chief factors which merit concern. Milk provides limited amounts of these vitamins and in sterilization much of the ascorbic acid is destroyed, hence it is regarded as good practice to provide the daily requirement by means of a vitamin supplement or by orange or tomato juice. A number of proprietary feedings are now fortified with adequate amounts of C.

Since unfortified cow's milk and even breast milk cannot be relied on to furnish adequate vitamin D, this must be supplied independently or some fortified milk used.

Vitamin A deficiency is seen in infants only under exceptional circumstances, as when skimmed milk has been employed for feeding for a prolonged period.

On the basis of the peroxide reaction[58] it has been claimed that vitamin E deficiency exists in many premature infants and in certain forms of steatorrhea, notably cystic fibrosis of the pancreas.[59] As yet it has not been possible to establish beyond question clinical benefit from supplementation with vitamin E in these conditions. Instances of a macrocytic anemia with multinucleated erythroblasts in the bone marrow have been reported in patients with kwashiorkor,[60] who have responded to the administration of vitamin E and some of its congeners. A symptom complex consisting of edema, anemia, reticulocytosis and thrombocytosis, which is responsive to vitamin E therapy, has been described. It occurred in small premature infants fed a proprietary formula supplemented with iron and with a high content of polyunsaturated fatty acids. Presumably, the increased vitamin E requirement associated with this type of fat was further increased by oxidation by the iron in the gastrointestinal tract.[60a]

Vitamin K deficiency occurs in various clinical conditions associated either with malabsorption from the intestine, liver disease, or prolonged oral antibiotic therapy. In the newborn infant it is commonly recommended that a single dose, not to exceed 2 mg, be given after birth as prophylaxis for hemorrhagic disease of the newborn.

At one time pyridoxine deficiency was observed in infants fed a proprietary feeding which had been subjected to unusual thermal treatment.[57] This defect was soon corrected and with the recognition of this possible deficiency it appears unlikely that it will recur.

Water Requirement. The infant is peculiarly susceptible to lack of water. His obligatory water loss through the kidney and the skin is considerably greater than that of the adult, and in addition he is far more subject to pathological processes causing water loss, notably vomiting and diarrhea. Symptoms of dehydration appear rapidly and have serious consequences. For the healthy infant, in a temperate climate, the minimum water requirement is probably in the neighborhood of 75 ml per kg. A daily intake of 150 ml per kg ($2\frac{1}{4}$ ounces per pound) may be regarded as providing an adequate margin of safety,[61] but under subtropical or tropical conditions it may have to be increased to 175 ml per kg or even more.

INFANT FEEDING

Overnutrition in Childhood. The emphasis on nutrition in well-developed countries has all been directed to the prevention of dietary deficiencies, the objective being to meet nutritional requirements and to provide in addition a generous margin of safety. This margin of safety has a two-fold purpose —to compensate for the defects in our knowledge of requirements and to build up stores of specific nutrients that can be drawn upon to combat future situations of stress. The possibilities of overnutrition with specific nutrients have received relatively little attention. An approach to an optimal diet—or rather an optimal range of nutrient intakes—requires a critical consideration of the risks as well as the advantages of generous margins for safety.

Needs for specific nutrients must be established by surveys in which both physical status and dietary intake have been measured. Laboratory criteria of deficiency, when applied, must be based not on deviations from an average of a healthy population, but on correlations with clinical deviations from health. Generosity in a margin of safety should bear some relation to the risk of deficiency. Finally, the extent to which effective reserves can be stored by a generous diet must be critically examined. In the case of calories there is no question that reserves of flesh can be accumulated that are effective against future situations of caloric deficit. When it comes to specific nutrients, this does not necessarily follow. Much has been written about protein "reserves," but if reserves are to be defined as "a moiety retained by intakes above the minimal adequate that is effective against some form of stress," evidence of the reality of a protein reserve is difficult to find. Halac[62,63] and Holt *et al.*[64] were unable to demonstrate such a reserve in rats. Carbohydrate reserves in the form of glycogen are real but transitory. Fat reserves in the form of adipose tissue are synonymous with caloric reserves.

The situation as to reserves of minerals and vitamins is far from clear and needs much further study. That fat-soluble vitamins can be stored in body fat for long periods is clear enough, but in the case of the water-soluble vitamins the quantities stored effectively and their duration in the body are still largely unknown, and the same is true for the minerals. Even when it can be shown that the body contains more of a particular nutrient after a high intake, it does not follow that this constitutes a useful reserve. With deprivation it may be excreted faster and the end result may be no different.

The effects of overnutrition in the pediatric age group have received some attention. Obesity in the infant is said to predispose to obesity in the older child and adult, often causing psychological problems and in many instances being caused by them. A vicious cycle may thus develop, the remote results of which as far as health is concerned become apparent only in adult life.

Overnutrition with protein, apart from specific hypersensitivities to foods, may under certain circumstances cause difficulty. "Protein fever"[65] described in infants on high protein diets was actually dehydration fever, the result of an increased demand for water to excrete urea. A sudden shift from a low to a high protein intake may cause difficulty, possibly because hypertrophy of the liver, a needed response to a high protein intake, has not had time to develop. Temporary loss of appetite and failure to gain weight may occur.

The pediatric literature contains many references to fat intolerance attributed to an excess of fat in the diet, the presenting symptom being steatorrhea. At the present time, it is more generally believed that the loss of intestinal tolerance for fat is not induced by fat feeding but is merely demonstrated by giving fat. Steatorrhea *per se* is not an indication for reducing the fat intake. The fat lost in the stool does no harm in transit; it does not appear to "wash out" other nutrients. The real indications for reducing the fat intake are ketosis, lipemia and a fatty liver.

An excessive proportion of carbohydrate in the diet of infants and young children led to a syndrome described by German pediatricians as Mehlnährschaden, a picture which we now describe as kwashiorkor or pre-kwashiorkor and which we attribute to a deficiency of protein rather than to an excess of carbohydrate.

Acute toxic episodes occur occasionally as a result of ingesting a large quantity of some mineral. Occasionally, the use of an iron tonic in excess gives rise to hemosiderosis.

Hypervitaminosis is seen particularly with the fat-soluble vitamins which cannot be readily excreted in the urine. Hypervitaminosis A, though relatively uncommon, is seen from time to time as the result of the administration of a vitamin concentrate in spoonful rather than drop quantities. Hypervitaminosis D, common for a time in England and on the continent of Europe, is today less common now that attention has been called to it. Hemolytic disease of the newborn from excessive vitamin K administration is now rarely seen. The tolerance of the body for water-soluble vitamins is such that large excesses can be taken with apparent impunity.

Little is known about possible remote effects of overnutrition of specific nutrients in humans. One may suspect that untoward results such as have been observed in animals[67] may occur, but the evidence is not at hand.

Breast Feeding. Many good and some poor arguments are adduced in support of breast feeding and the subject is surrounded with a certain amount of emotionalism. For most mothers, successful nursing is a satisfying emotional experience and is to be encouraged from that point of view unless there are reasons to the contrary. From the point of view of the welfare of the child, the writers are not impressed with the views of certain psychiatrists that failure to nurse at the mother's breast will cause emotional deprivation and subsequent psychologic maladjustment. The advantage to the child is in the somatic field. The strongest argument for maternal nursing is that it is a relatively foolproof method. When artificial feeding is carried out under ideal conditions—by an intelligent and careful mother or nurse, under experienced medical guidance and with a milk supply that is beyond question—the risk is a negligible one, but under less ideal conditions the infant may suffer and the morbidity and mortality of the artificially fed infant may run far ahead of the breast fed. It is obvious that in some countries, in some areas and with some groups of people the encouragement of nursing is a matter of the greatest importance. A rare contraindication to the use of breast milk is the onset of hyperbilirubinemia due to the presence of pregnane-3 (alpha); 20 (beta)-dial. This steroid inhibits hepatic glucuronyl transferase activity in the newborn.[67a]

Breast Feeding vs. Breast Milk. How much of the over-all superior results with breast feeding are due to the safety of the method and how much to the superior nutritional qualities of breast milk is a much debated question. Adequate data on infants artificially fed on human milk obtained from a breast milk dairy would settle the matter, but such data are not available. In their absence, conclusions must he drawn from data where artificial feeding is carried out under ideal circumstances and from biochemical and nutritional studies of the two milks. As stated above, the results of ideal artificial feeding appear to be comparable to those of breast feeding. One can state with assurance that the important nutritional differences have been overcome. It is possible, however, that factors of minor importance remain to be discovered in which breast milk may possess some small advantage. One or two claims for such substances[68,69] have recently been made, but await confirmation.

Practical Considerations in Breast Feeding. If the mother is healthy and the child is receiving an adequate quantity of milk—something that can be determined by periodically weighing before and after nursing—it can be assumed that he will be adequately nourished. After the second month, a supplement of iron should be provided, usually in the form of solid food since human milk is deficient in iron and the hepatic stores, present at birth, have been exhausted. Vitamin supplements providing C and D are commonly given to breast-fed infants, not so much because of the risk of deficiency during this period, but because of the risk that at weaning these supplements may be overlooked, unless they have become habitual.

Details of the technique of breast feeding may be found in standard pediatric texts.

Artificial Feeding. Successful artificial feeding with cow's milk involves three problems: (1) meeting the nutritional requirements of the child, (2) avoiding certain mechanical difficulties of digestion caused by the curd of the milk and (3) avoiding pathogenic microorganisms. The bacteriologic problem is solved by heat treatment of the milk—pasteurization, boiling or autoclaving and by scrupulous care of the utensils, nipples and bottles, all of which are heat sterilized. Cleanliness on the part of the mother or nurse in preparing and giving the feeding is also essential.

The curd problem, too, is conveniently solved by heating the milk. This causes the lactalbumin to coagulate in fine particles; the subsequent coagulation of the casein in the infant's stomach occurs about these micellae and the resulting curd is friable and easily digestible rather than tough and resistant. The beneficial effect varies with the amount of heat applied. Pasteurization improves the digestibility of the curd, but does not overcome the difficulty as completely as does boiling or autoclaving. However, terminal sterilization by raising the milk to the boiling temperature in the feeding bottles is routine practice, so that even when fresh pasteurized milk is used the subsequent heat treatment takes care of the curd problem. The all-important consideration is the nutritive property of the feeding, a consideration of which demands some knowledge of the differences between cow's milk and breast milk.

Differences Between Breast Milk and Cow's Milk. As is shown in Table 24–1, cow's milk is richer in protein by reason of its higher content of casein; it is comparable in fat content although the content of polyunsaturated fatty acids is sometimes lower. It contains considerably less sugar (lactose). Its mineral content is higher, individual minerals being from 3 to 5 times as abundant as in breast milk. Most vitamins, too, are present in higher concentrations in cow's milk, exceptions being vitamins C and D, nicotinic acid and inositol.

Provided the bacteriologic problem and the mechanical problem of the curd are taken care of by the heat treatment, undiluted and unmodified cow's milk can be and is often used for infant feeding and with success. Such difficulties as are attributed to it are of a minor nature. It may require a few days for the infant to adapt to the higher protein intake, if a change to whole cow's milk is suddenly made. It has also been pointed out[70,71] that, because of the higher protein

Table 24-1.   Average Percentage Composition of Mature
Breast Milk and Cow's Milk*

Constituents	Breast milk Per cent		Cow's milk Per cent	
Water	87.6		87.2	
Total solids	12.4		12.8	
Protein	1.1		3.3	
Casein		0.4		2.7
Lactalbumin		0.4		0.4
Lactoglobulin		0.2		0.2
Fat	3.8		3.8	
Lactose	7.0		4.8	
Ash	0.21		0.71	
Sodium		.015		.058
Potassium		.055		.138
Calcium		.034		.126
Magnesium		.004		.013
Iron		.00021		.00015
Chlorine		.043		.100
Phosphorus		.016		.099
Sulfur		.014		.030
Vitamin content per 100 ml				
Vitamin A	53.00 μg		34.00 μg	
Carotenoids	27.00 μg		38.00 μg	
Thiamin	16.00 μg		42.00 μg	
Riboflavin	43.00 μg		157.00 μg	
Nicotinic acid	172.00 μg		85.00 μg	
Pyridoxine	11.00 μg		48.00 μg	
Pantothenic acid	196.00 μg		350.00 μg	
Folic acid	0.18 μg		0.23 μg	
Choline	9.00 mg		13.00 mg	
Inositol	39.00 mg		13.00 mg	
Biotin	0.40 μg		3.50 μg	
B$_{12}$	0.18 μg		0.56 μg	
Vitamin C	4.30 mg		1.80 mg	
Vitamin D	0.4–10.0 i.u.†		0.3–4.0 i.u.†	
Vitamin K	26 D.G. units‡		100 D.G. units‡	
Calories per ounce	22		21	
Calories per 100 ml	71		69	

* Taken largely from National Research Council Bulletin No. 254, 1953.
† International units
‡ Dam-Glavind units.

and mineral content of cow's milk, infants so fed have a greater obligatory water requirement for renal excretion; hence with the same fluid intake they have a slightly smaller margin of safety against dehydration. For these reasons, and also because of tradition based on experience before the curd problem was solved, the general practice has continued of diluting cow's milk to reduce its protein content, the caloric deficit being made up with a carbohydrate supplement.

In the United States evaporated milk has largely replaced fresh milk for infant feeding. It is estimated that about 80 per cent of American bottle babies are fed on evaporated milk or on some prepared milk feeding marketed in evaporated form. The constancy of the product, its sterility and the complete avoidance of curd indigestion have been responsible for its increasing popularity.

Modified Milks. Commonly used and convenient modifications of this type are the following:

Evaporated milk	3 oz
Water	7 oz
Cane sugar	½ oz
	10 oz

Whole milk	7 oz
(or reconstituted whole milk prepared from milk powder)	
Water	3 oz
Cane sugar (1 tbsp)	½ oz
	10 oz

These formulas, approximately isocaloric with breast milk, furnish 20 calories to the ounce. The percentage distribution of calories in breast milk, cow's milk and in a widely employed modification given above is as follows.

	P	F	C
Breast milk	8%	50%	42%
Cow's milk	20%	51%	29%
Common milk modification	15%	35%	50%

The range in percentage distribution of calories which can be used successfully in infant feeding is a wide one, there being no need to simulate closely the composition of breast milk, as was once thought necessary. By tradition more protein is commonly given to artificially fed infants, but, as pointed out above, the difference in biologic value between the proteins of breast milk and cow's milk is a negligible one. Experience with feedings providing only 10 per cent of the calories as protein has been altogether satisfactory.

Carbohydrates commonly used as supplements in artificial feeding are cane sugar, lactose and maltose-dextrin mixtures. There would seem to be little choice between them. Starch and cereals may also be used, although their absorption is slightly less complete.

The heat treatment used in destroying bacteria in milk and in rendering the curd more digestible also exerts some untoward effects on the nutritive properties of the milk, which may have to be repaired. Most important is the loss of vitamin C; much of this is lost during pasteurization and a further loss occurs during terminal sterilization; hence all artificially fed infants should be given a supplement of 25 mg ascorbic acid in some form. Boiling the milk destroys some thiamin, and autoclaving even more; this vitamin is, however, amply supplied in cow's milk and, unless autoclaving has been unduly prolonged (a half hour or more), the loss is not serious. Autoclaving milk also causes some destruction of pyridoxal, the chief form of vitamin B_6 present in milk. As ordinarily carried out in the processing of evaporated milk, the loss is not serious. At high temperatures several of the amino acids, notably lysine, may react with the lactose of the milk, forming compounds which render the amino acid unutilizable by the body, although still present by analysis. This so-called Maillard or "browning" reaction assumes significant proportions only when liquid milk has been subjected to autoclaving for half an hour or more. The possibility of thermal inactivation of a fraction of the protein is, however, a reason for using a protein intake slightly higher than that of breast milk. In the preparation of evaporated milk it has been estimated that about 11 per cent of the lysine has been inactivated.[72] Lysine is, however, present in cow's milk protein in a somewhat higher concentration than in breast milk protein and does not appear to be a limiting amino acid.[73]

A number of proprietary infant foods are available—some in powdered or evaporated form; others are dispensed in individual containers ready for direct feeding. Some of these are simple modifications of milk with added carbohydrate; others are "humanized milks" which imitate to a greater or lesser extent the caloric proportions, the mineral content or the fat of breast milk. They save trouble in preparing the formula and several of them are adequately reinforced with vitamins and iron. These foods are all satisfactory and convenient; the advantage of the humanized products is, however, questionable.

Practical Infant Feeding. Feedings for an entire day are usually prepared at one time, being put into the feeding bottles, which are then terminally sterilized by standing in boiling water for 10 minutes and are then refrigerated until used. The necessity of carrying out this procedure has been recently questioned. Under standard conditions prevailing in American cities (a pure municipal water supply and excellent milk hygiene) there would seem to be a minimal risk of contaminating a feeding with a pathogenic organism. Fischer[74] observed no untoward effects from omitting terminal sterilization in data obtained in Philadelphia under conditions of good pediatric care and Vaughan[75] showed that no differences could be obtained even in an underprivileged group in Georgia. Other pediatricians,[76] however, have viewed this innovation with alarm. Before feeding the infant the bottle is commonly warmed to the body temperature, although it has been shown that such warming is actually unnecessary.[77]

The technique of feeding is important. The rubber nipple (which must be sterilized before use) must have an opening wide enough to permit the milk to drop out of the bottle without shaking. Smaller nipples cause the baby to suck in much air and may lead to vomiting. It is also important to hold the bottle at such an angle that the nipple is always full of milk and to hold the baby vertical for a few moments after feeding to enable him to "burp" and bring up swallowed air. Regularity of feeding, though it need not be made a fetish, on the whole is to be preferred, as it is with breast feeding. Some latitude may, however, be given the child as to the quantity he takes at each feeding. As a rule his appetite is an excellent guide to follow.

In planning artificial feeding for a baby one should: (1) estimate the caloric requirements from the weight (roughly 100 calories per kg); (2) estimate the daily quantity of formula needed—from a knowledge of the calories furnished by the formula; (3) divide this into the number of feedings desired.

Most babies will require 6 feedings a day which may be given at four-hour interals around the clock. At the age of two months a night feeding can usually be omitted and only 5 feedings given. It is wise to check the calculation of the formula to make sure that an adequate protein allowance (2.5 gm per kg) and water allowance (150 per kg) are provided.

An initial artificial feeding is always in the nature of an experiment. An individual baby may need more or less than the calculated requirement. A steady weight gain and the appearance of health are the best indications of success. *Provided air swallowing and consequent distention of the stomach are avoided* one can usually rely on the baby's appetite as to the quantity of food needed. If he steadily refuses some of his bottle, he probably needs less and if he drinks it ravenously and cries before mealtime, he probably needs more.

The artificially fed infant should be given a supplement containing 25 mg ascorbic acid, and vitamin D in some form to insure an intake of 400 international units a day. A need for other vitamin supplements on an ordinary milk formula has not been established. Cereals and homogenized baby foods can be fed by spoon at any age, replacing a portion of the formula feeding, but there is no particular advantage in giving them to small infants. Their purpose is twofold—to provide iron and to educate the child to accept solid foods. Since the iron stored at birth takes care of the needs of the early weeks, a good case cannot be made for giving iron before the age of 2 months. Training to eat solid foods is likewise readily accomplished at the age of 3 or 4 months; it should not be delayed beyond the first half year. A great variety of canned meats, vegetables, fruits and soups is now available for infants. As these are introduced, calculation of calories becomes highly inaccurate and feeding by appetite becomes the rule. By the age of 7 or 8 months, it should be possible to reduce meals to 4 a day, the last one being milk alone, and by the age of a year, 3 meals a day should suffice. As teeth come in, the need for homogenized foods disappears.

Digestive Disturbances. A discussion of the causes, pathologic physiology and therapy of acute and chronic digestive disturbances is beyond the scope of this chapter. These disturbances provide some of the most difficult problems with which the physician has to deal. In the presence of vomiting, oral alimentation is out of the question and, in the case of diarrhea, its value is limited by the hyperperistalsis. Parenteral nutrition must be relied on to replete stores of water and electrolyte, to correct abnormalities of acid-base equilibrium and to supply needed calories.

In conditions of acute dehydration and shock, restoration of the circulation is the matter of first concern. An electrolyte solution, preferably with an excess of fixed base, should be given without delay, followed by a transfusion of whole blood or plasma to maintain plasma volume. The repair of extracellular fluid deficits requires the further administration of an electrolyte solution to which potassium may be added, when it is clear that the kidneys are functioning; Darrow's solution[78] is satisfactory for that purpose. One can only guess at the severity of the dehydration from clinical appearances and continue intensive treatment until the signs of dehydration—particularly lack of skin turgor—have disappeared. There are, however, limits to the rate at which intravenous fluid can be safely administered. A 5-kg infant should rarely be given more than 1500 ml by vein a day, given by continuous drip or by intermittent push infusions. This corresponds to a rate of about 1 ml per minute for a continuous drip. A more rapid rate, not exceeding 15 to 20 ml per minute may be employed with push infusions in which a fraction—not exceeding 250 ml—may be given at one time.

Parenteral Nutrition. This becomes important whenever the requirements of the body cannot be met by the oral route. To the extent that the organism cannot be nourished parenterally it must live on its own tissues. It is the general experience, particularly with infants, that most of the fatalities which occur in severe digestive disorders when these cannot be readily controlled are due to nutritional failure. The chief minerals of intracellular fluid, potassium, magnesium and phosphorus, must be given cautiously for only a limited rise in their concentrations in the plasma can be tolerated. Considerable experience has been obtained in recent years in the parenteral administration of potassium, largely as a result of the

pioneer work of Darrow. Much can be done to restore the diminished cell concentrations of this element, which occur in conditions of dehydration and in other pathologic states, by giving infusions with several times the concentration of potassium found in extracellular fluid. Provided the kidneys are functioning as much as 35 mEq per liter may safely be given. Potassium so given may at times serve to replete the cellular deficit of sodium from the cells. Unfortunately, the restoration of the K/Na balance in the cells is not a simple matter. Active metabolic processes are concerned in maintaining the differences in concentration inside and outside the cell; when these are deranged the cell may not be able to accept potassium[79] which is presented to it in the extracellular environment. Nevertheless, the provision of this element as is done in Darrow's solution[78] permits the cell to accept it when it can. Signs, symptoms and biochemical changes of magnesium depletion and its therapy are discussed in Chapter 6, Section B.

The recent introduction of total parenteral nutrition ("hyperalimentation") routines has made it possible to maintain even the smallest infant for prolonged periods of time on intravenous feeding. The insertion of a catheter into the superior vena cava and the use of a peristaltic pump to control the speed of delivery have allowed the use of hypertonic dextrose solutions which insure adequate caloric intake. In addition to protein hydrolysate solutions, electrolytes, and vitamins, periodic infusion of fresh blood or plasma is used to provide trace substances as well as unidentified factors. Normal growth and development, as well as adequate nitrogen retention, have been attained in these infants.[80-82] Nutritional and procedural aspects of this method of feeding are considered in Chapter 36.

It should be pointed out that the administration of plasma or whole blood, valuable though it may be in maintaining plasma volume, is of negligible importance from the point of view of providing nitrogen for nutritional purposes. The proteins so administered have slow turnover rates and it is only as they are degraded that the constituent amino acids become available. Amino acids given as such can, however, be rapidly used.

Oral Feeding in Digestive Disturbances. Vomiting presents an obvious barrier to oral alimentation, but the situation in the case of intestinal disturbances—acute and chronic diarrheas—is not so obvious and has provoked differences of opinion in regard to their management. Restriction of the oral intake has been the policy generally favored. In its support was the observation that it resulted in decreased stooling and stool losses; also the general philosophy that rest favored recovery of a disordered function.

The philosophy of rest, however, has not gone unchallenged. Coleman[83] and Dubois[84] some years ago questioned the value of resting the intestine in typhoid fever and their results have revolutionized the dietary treatment of that disease. Likewise in the pediatrics field Schick and Wagner[85] in studying chronic intestinal indigestion (celiac disease) concluded that the therapy of use was preferable to that of rest of the disordered function. Their work was supported by the subsequent observations of McCrae and Morris[86] in celiacs and by Black *et al.*[87] on sprue in adults, all of which pointed to the conclusion that, regardless of stooling, the administration of fat in steatorrhea improved fat absorption.

There has, however, been little direct evidence with which to answer the two leading questions involved: (1) what is the effect of feeding on absorption of the food itself and of other substances, and (2) how does oral feeding affect the duration of the digestive disorder? If feeding increases the net loss of caloric food or of water and electrolyte, or if it delays recovery, it is contraindicated, and if it does none of these things and favors absorption it would seem to be indicated. The studies of Chung[66] on infantile diarrhea, carried out at different levels of food intake, failed to reveal any "washing out" of minerals or other foodstuffs caused by food administration; the amount of each foodstuff absorbed—whether calorigenic foodstuff, mineral or water—was found to be roughly proportional to the intake. The administration of food increased stool volume and stooling, but in every instance, and for every food ingredient studied, either net absorption was increased or loss was decreased. A study designed to evaluate the effect of feeding on the duration of infantile diarrhea was made by Chung and Viscorova[88] who treated alternate cases: (*a*) by a conventional plan of initial starvation with a gradual resumption of food and (*b*) by offering full caloric feeding from the start. The duration of the disorder was found to be identical in the two groups, indicating that the duration of the disturbance is not influenced by the feeding. Similar observations have been made by others.

A series of studies of various forms of steatorrhea—celiac disease,[89] cystic fibrosis of the pancreas, biliary atresia[90] and steatorrhea of prematurity[91]—was carried out by the group at New York University with a view to determining the effect of varying fat intakes. Similar observations on the steatorrhea of kwashiorkor were made by Gomez *et al.* in Mexico.[92] Although the stool fat output increased with increasing fat intake, fat absorption was correspondingly increased and only clinical benefit was observed. The conclusion drawn from these studies was that intestinal intolerance in these states was not induced or indeed affected in any way by the administration of the poorly tolerated foodstuff. The increased stooling was interpreted as a *demonstration of existing intolerance* rather than as a relapse. These recent observations serve to support the views expressed in former years by Dubois,[84] Schick,[85] Park[93] and others, and would seem to point to a more liberal oral feeding policy than has generally prevailed. It is of course quite possible, particularly in the chronic disorders, to feed these patients satisfactorily without using the poorly tolerated foodstuff to any great extent. It is, however, not necessary to do so, nor should the conclusion be hastily drawn that relapses when they occur are due to breaches of a prescribed diet. In celiac disease in particular such untoward events occur quite irrespective of the diet employed. The idea of "food intoxication" once widely held is now largely abandoned. It is now believed that the manifestations of "food intoxication" accompanying a digestive upset are not caused by food but by dehydration associated with electrolyte losses and derangements of electrolyte metabolism.

The Allergic Infant. Food allergy presents a special problem in infant feeding. It may be observed even in the breast-fed infant. Hypersensitivity to the natural proteins of the mother's own milk has not been observed, but in rare instances[94] proteins ingested by the mother find their way unsplit into the milk in biological traces and, when the sensitivity of the infant is extreme, they produce symptoms. The mother herself may not be sensitive to the offending protein. Elimination of the particular food from the maternal diet is followed by the disappearance of the symptoms.

Hypersensitivity to one of the proteins of cow's milk—usually lactalbumin—is somewhat more frequently encountered and may be found in all degrees of severity. Idiosyncrasy of an extreme degree is rare, but very dramatic in its manifestations. A single drop of cow's milk may lead within a few minutes to urticaria, asthma, acute gastrointestinal symptoms, and shock of alarming proportions. Fatalities have been reported. In these circumstances the elimination of cow's milk from the diet must be scrupulously done. Goat's milk is often well tolerated by these infants, but at times there is sensitivity to this also and a milk-free diet must be given. Such extreme sensitivity is not permanent. By means of desensitization procedures in which small graded non-reactive doses are given, it appears that a complete tolerance can be established though this may require a year or more.

Lesser grades of food intolerance—sometimes to milk, eggs, wheat or other protein foods—are also recognized; the symptoms are usually gastrointestinal or cutaneous (usually urticaria) and they develop less promptly than in the extreme cases. Rubin[95] and others[96] have reported acute diarrheas due to milk allergy in the newborn period; usually the symptoms are less acute. Subjecting milk to autoclaving temperatures often denatures the lactalbumin to such an extent that it can be tolerated and a milk-free diet is not required. In older subjects the celiac syndrome has been related by several investigators to intestinal allergy to wheat gluten.[97]

Aside from the clearly demonstrable cases of allergy there is a wide zone in which respiratory, digestive and cutaneous manifestations are not so clearly related to allergy. It is our opinion that the diagnosis of food allergy is often uncritically made and food unnecessarily restricted. It should be appreciated that a positive skin test is not synonymous with clinical allergy; such tests are frequently encountered in normal subjects. Elimination tests—in the case of food allergy, elimination diets—are needed to establish the diagnosis. Only when the symptoms can repeatedly be made to disappear on removal of the dietary antigen and to recur when it is restored to the diet, *other factors remaining constant*, is one justified in assuming a causal relationship. In our experience, it is only in the exceptional case of digestive disturbance in early life that the diagnosis of allergy can be sustained by an environmental test. It is also a mistaken notion that a child's distaste for a particular food such as spinach indicates that he is allergic to it. An article of food to which a patient is hypersensitive is as a rule eaten with enthusiasm, even when—as in older subjects—its relation to forthcoming symptoms is known.

The construction of a complete elimination diet free from all antigenic protein has been solved by a preparation in which all nitrogen is supplied in the form of amino acids and non-antigenic polypeptides. The suspected food or foods can be added to this one at a time for diagnostic purposes. When cow's milk allergy is demonstrated there are now many milk-free feedings that are available; complete feedings based on meat or soybean protein may be employed as well as the protein hydrolysate.

Some allergic patients appear to be benefited by a reduction in the carbohydrate of the diet, for which fat is substituted. The underlying mechanism is not clearly understood, but appears to be related to a loss of fluid, chiefly extracellular, which occurs under these circumstances and which limits inflammatory reactions.

The Premature Infant. The premature infant presents peculiar nutritional problems. His caloric requirements are high, he absorbs certain foodstuffs—notably fats and fat-soluble vitamins—poorly. He is known to have a greater need for vitamin C than the mature infant and it seems not unlikely that other special nutritive requirements exist. He often regurgitates and aspirates his food with serious consequences. It is in the smallest premature infants that these difficulties are more often encountered. The small premature infant is born with negligible reserves of body fat and is poorly equipped to withstand caloric deprivation, yet it is often impossible to feed him maintenance diets for some days; one must proceed cautiously. If medical complications prevent early feeding, intravenous therapy should be used. The tendency of the premature infant to develop symptomatic hypoglycemia can be prevented by the use of intravenous glucose.

The basal energy requirement of the premature is as high and perhaps higher than that of the full-term infant and his growth rate is more rapid; the caloric loss in the excreta—largely unabsorbed fat—is also greater. These are, however, partly compensated for by the low activity of these infants, so that the total caloric requirement is only moderately elevated. Most of these infants will gain well on 125 calories per kg. some on less than this.

The composition of the premature infant's feeding has been a controversial matter. In years past, breast milk has been regarded as the ideal food and the results with it appeared to be satisfactory. The avidity with which these infants retain protein[98] however, suggested that the low protein content of breast milk might be suboptimal for these infants. The question is still unsettled. Higher protein intakes than that of breast milk will lead to increased nitrogen retention, but whether or not this is advantageous from the point of view of health is not established.

By and large premature infants absorb fat poorly although this steatorrhea is not apparent clinically. Tidwell and Holt[99] showed that it could be substantially reduced by substituting more unsaturated fats for butter in the feeding. Because of the limited absorption of fat, low fat feedings have frequently been advised.[100] However it now appears that unabsorbed fat in the intestine is completely innocuous. Morales et al.[91] have shown the interesting fact that the percentage of fat absorbed by the premature remains relatively constant regardless of the intake. They were able to increase the total fat absorbed by increasing the fat intake without untoward effects, thereby achieving a total fat absorption comparable to that of full-term infants. This also is true for the fat-soluble vitamins which, like fat, are poorly absorbed; the absorption defect is met by increasing the intake.

Premature infants have a peculiar need for vitamin C, particularly when relatively high protein feedings are given. Levine and Gordon[101] demonstrated that unless this vitamin was generously supplied a characteristic defect of aromatic amino acid metabolism appeared with the excretion of so-called tyrosyl compounds (hydroxyphenyllactic acid and hydroxyphenylpyruvic acid) in the urine. It has been subsequently demonstrated that ascorbic acid activates p-hydroxyphenylpyruvic acid hydroxylase activity, the enzyme necessary for the further degradation of these metabolites of tyrosine. A special requirement of the premature infant for vitamin E has been suggested. Both the anemia of prematurity[102] and a syndrome[103] consisting of edema, skin changes, elevated platelet count, and morphologic changes in the red blood cells have been attributed to deficiency of this vitamin.

In summary, the feeding of the premature infant should provide, as soon as this can be tolerated, a caloric intake of 125 calories per kg. This can be accomplished satisfactorily by cow's milk mixtures as well as by breast milk. The defect of fat absorption can be overcome in several ways: by giving more protein and carbohydrate, by giving more fat or a more readily absorbable fat. An increased requirement of fat-soluble vitamins is best established for vitamin D of which the intake should be no less than 2000 international units per day. Single dose therapy of 300,000 units has also proved safe and effective therapy lasting several months. A daily supplement of 100 mg ascorbic acid given for the early weeks is adequate to control tyrosyluria even on a relatively high protein intake. Peculiarities of the mineral requirements of the premature infant are not known to exist. Although the so-called anemia of prematurity[104] is a common event, this appears to differ in no sense from the physiologic anemia of the newborn and early infancy. Until recently it has been maintained that exogenous iron, though absorbed, was not readily utilized until the end of the second month of life. However, Gorten, Hepner and Workman[105] showed with labeled iron that even young prematures will utilize such iron for hemoglobin synthesis without difficulty.

The feeding of premature infants is rendered difficult by their imperfectly developed reflexes. Sucking and swallowing are often imperfectly performed by the small premature, who must in consequence be tube fed. A small rubber catheter introduced at mealtime was formerly in general use, but in recent years this has largely been replaced by a small polyethylene catheter[106] which can be left in place continuously. Regurgitation of food presents a greater danger of aspiration in the premature than in the mature infant, because the coughing reflex is often imperfectly developed. The use of a continuous oral drip or of small frequent feedings helps to reduce the volume of food in the stomach at any one time and thereby minimizes the risk of aspiration. Feeding by gastrostomy to avoid the risk of aspiration has been introduced recently.[107] Its recommendation as a routine procedure will have to await more extensive data. Total parenteral nutrition offers an alternative route of feeding when necessary.

Feeding Problems of Older Children. These are largely psychologic in origin. *Anorexia* is an exceedingly common condition which is said to occur in nearly 50 per cent of American homes. The difficulty usually arises from rigid ideas on the part of the parents or perhaps the grandparents as to what the child should eat and more particularly regarding the quantity he should eat, these being at variance with the child's appetite. Coaxing and forcing of food effectively destroy the appetite and a vicious cycle is started. In some instances this situation leads to psychogenic vomiting. Often the child learns to capitalize on the concern of the parents regarding his nutrition. He enjoys being the center of attention and may hold out for special privileges in return for eating. The therapy is simple, but sometimes difficult to carry out in a home where there are opinionated adults. It is to set before the child a well-balanced diet, sweets being withheld until protein foods are eaten. Comments on the desirability of eating are withheld and after a limited time—no longer than twenty minutes—the meal, if uneaten, is quietly removed, no food being offered until the next meal, when a similar procedure is followed. A few strong-willed children will resist until the third day, but most of them will become hungry and capitulate before this, often eating ravenously foods which before they were unwilling to touch.

Pica. The eating of dirt or of any inedible material, though uncommon, presents a serious problem. Its cause is not understood. The theory that the habit starts from an effort to compensate for some dietary deficiency is not established in man, although this has been observed in experimental animals. The habit which is seen more frequently in urban ghetto areas has been related to emotional deprivation.[107a] The danger from the ingestion of toxic substances is a serious one, the most frequent difficulty being from the ingestion of lead from paint or plaster. The habit may be difficult to break and requires careful supervision.

With a few notable exceptions, such as pica, certain acutely ill infants, certain mental defectives, and a few situations of bad conditioning, the appetite of the infant remains an excellent guide to his dietary needs, a far better one than is generally supposed. The observations of Clara Davis[108] in which a group of normal infants were allowed to select their own diet from 8 months of age onward for several years bear eloquent testimony to this fact. Marked irregularities in the intake of particular foods were observed—a single food often being ingested in large quantities for a time, but such dietary enthusiasms corrected themselves and over a long period the intake proved to be a balanced one, the health record of these children being impressive. It is unfortunate that sweets were not included in this classic study for there is evidence that a "sweet tooth," if uninhibited, also tends to correct itself in time.

Unsolved Problems of Infant Nutrition.
In spite of the notable advances in infant feeding made during the past half century, there are many nutritional problems contributing heavily to infant mortality and morbidity which remain unsolved. *Frank nutritional failure* is still responsible for most of the deaths in infantile diarrhea. Uncertainty still prevails as to the cause of many of these diarrheas. Undiscovered microbial agents—producing enteral or parenteral infection—for which no specific therapy is available are doubtless responsible for many of these; their discovery is important. A knowledge of the mechanism whereby an infection—enteral or parenteral—damages the assimilatory mechanisms of the intestine would be invaluable. A temporary deficiency of disaccharide-splitting enzymes appears to explain certain cases of poor carbohydrate assimilation. A knowledge of the steps involved in assimilatory mechanisms, of the enzymes and coenzymes concerned, might make it possible to restore function even if the damaging agent could not be eliminated. A perfect parenteral feeding would eliminate the immediate need of the digestive tract; our present materials have well-recognized imperfections. Good criteria for the adequacy of specific nutrients, especially protein, are needed. The long-range effects of overnutrition in infancy merit further study.

The largest infant mortality problem, that of the smallest premature infants, may well be due to nutritional failure. Obvious causes of death are not found at autopsy and the diagnosis of physiologic immaturity is used to cloak our ignorance. A more precise definition of immaturity in terms of defective tissue enzymes and coenzymes might lead the way to replacement of some of the latter at any rate. It is quite possible that the small premature infant needs a variety of accessory substances which the mature infant can manufacture for himself. Their discovery might permit these subjects to survive without difficulty.

Finally it is possible that many diverse diseases of known and unknown origin may exert baneful effects upon intermediate metabolism that are as yet unsuspected. Accessory cofactors—unessential for the normal individual but essential for the disease state—remain to be discovered.

NUTRITION IN ADOLESCENCE

The nutritional requirements of the adolescent are conditioned primarily by the *pubertal growth* spurt. During this period, which in an individual child may be much more striking than average figures indicate, there is an increase in the apparent basal metabolic requirement which, as pointed out, includes the growth requirement. There is also an increased demand for calories and for nitrogen. The increased caloric need is ordinarily reflected in the appetite. Unless additional food is provided at mealtime the individual makes it up by eating between meals. Exceptionally, the increase in appetite is inadequate and one observes a spindly individual who compensates for his or her increased caloric need by taking little exercise. Figures collected by Gephart[109] for the caloric consumption of boys at boarding school were surprisingly large—much of this being consumed outside the dining room.

The need for additional nitrogen at the pubertal growth spurt has been stressed particularly by Johnston.[110] The additional caloric need and nitrogen need are thought to be proportional. Both are correlated with physiologic events, menarche in girls and the adolescent growth spurt in boys.[110a] Failure to meet the additional requirement for protein at this time is believed to be an important cause of loss of resistance to infections, particularly tuberculosis. The loss of resistance at this time of life is seen particularly in the female whose growth spurt is more rapid, though less prolonged (Fig. 24–3). Factors other than nutrition may, however, have some influence on loss of resistance such as the hormonal changes occurring at this time. The practical consideration would seem to be the maintenance of an adequate protein intake with the first evidences of puberty. The maintenance of an adequate diet is often difficult in girls who often attempt to achieve artificial standards of slimness by ill-advised dietary restrictions.

An extreme form of malnutrition, *anorexia*

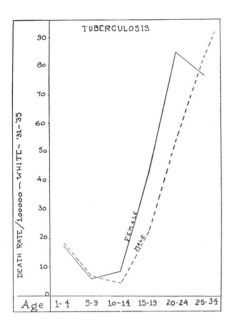

Fig. 24-3. Mortality rates in tuberculosis. Note the sharp rise in adolescence, the increase occurring first in the female, corresponding with the sex differences in pubertal phenomena. (J. A. Johnston, *Nutritional Studies in Adolescent Girls and Their Relation to Tuberculosis*, courtesy of Charles C Thomas.)

nervosa, is seen particularly in adolescence, although not confined to this time of life. The term implies that this is a neurosis and there is no question that this is the explanation of the majority of cases, in whom a psychologic disturbance is often very apparent. We are not, however, inclined to accept the view that all non-fatal cases exhibiting such extreme anorexia and malnutrition should be regarded as neuroses in contrast to Simmonds' disease, where the syndrome is brought about by total destruction of the pituitary. There is some evidence for the existence of transitory or incomplete pituitary lesions which may induce this picture. Such cases have been observed post partum (Sheehan's syndrome) and it may be that the endocrine changes at puberty induce similar changes. Such extreme forms of anorexia and malnutrition require expert psychotherapy, but forced feeding is at times necessary.

Obesity, although seen at all ages, may present a particular problem in the adolescent.

The adolescent girl has often been somewhat obese throughout childhood. In many, self-consciousness and vanity, coming with puberty, will correct the situation, but in others there develops an attitude of defeatism. There is withdrawal from social activities and sport and more indulgence in eating as a solace— a vicious cycle. The same factors operate at times in the male. The dietary management of obesity is discussed elsewhere in this volume (Chapter 22), but the psychologic factors seen particularly during the adolescent period must not be overlooked.

The problem of *simple goiter* or adolescent goiter is related to diet at this time of life. The classical work of Marine and his co-workers[111] served to relate this condition to a suboptimal intake of iodine. The demand for thyroid hormone is increased at the time of puberty and in the presence of an iodine shortage the gland responds by simple hypertrophy. The evidence cited by Marine *et al.* consisted of the demonstration of low iodine in the soil areas where adolescent goiter was more prevalent and of a reduction of goiter when the iodine intake was increased. Exception to this concept has been taken by Greenwald[112] who points to a number of discrepancies in the iodine content of the soil and the incidence of goiter, and particularly to variations in the incidence of goiter in the same locality from time to time. Goitrogenic substances in foods and drugs may perhaps play a role in the incidence of this disorder. The beneficial effect of iodine is, however, a fact beyond question, both prophylactically and therapeutically (Chapter 8, Section A). Endemic goiter is seen particularly in isolated communities, usually in mountainous regions some distance from the sea. The development of transportation invariably results in a sharp decrease in its incidence. Food with a higher iodine content begins to come in from other places and there is a greater tendency for the inhabitants themselves to travel.

NUTRITION IN PATHOLOGIC STATES

A number of pathologic conditions are seen in early life which present nutritional problems because of derangements of metabolism.

Some of these represent inborn errors and others are acquired.

1. Anomalies of Amino Acid Metabolism. A number of these respond to restriction of a specific amino acid or restriction of protein intake. Some respond to pharmacologic doses of vitamins. These and other inborn errors of metabolism are discussed in Chapter 39.

High protein diets may be useful in any condition associated with abnormal loss of protein from the body. One chronic situation where such loss from the bowel may not be readily appreciated is *cystic fibrosis of the pancreas*. In certain hypoglycemic states such as the Von Gierke type of glycogen storage disease, the blood sugar can be maintained by giving additional protein meals, a procedure which may help restore the normal growth of the child.

2. Anomalies of Carbohydrate Metabolism Correctable by Diet. Of particular importance in this group is *galactosemia*, a congenital condition involving a deficit in the enzyme system which converts galactose to glucose.

Analogous to the above condition is *hereditary fructose intolerance*, a rare familial condition presenting similar symptoms and caused by an enzymatic block in the conversion of fructose to glucose.[113]

An inherited deficiency of one of the sugar- or starch-splitting enzymes in the gastrointestinal tract may result in a diarrhea severe enough to interfere with growth. The specific defect can be demonstrated by following the blood sugar curve after loading with the appropriate carbohydrate. A complete remission can be obtained by omitting the proper carbohydrate from the diet. Specific inabilities to utilize lactose, maltose, sucrose and starch[114] have been reported.

3. Anomalies of Fat Metabolism. There are several disorders of fat metabolism which occur in children and which may be influenced by dietary therapy. The separation of idiopathic familial hyperlipemia into two forms is based on the response to diet: one responds to fat[115] and the other to carbohydrate restriction.[116] Low fat intake reduces the plasma lipid level and the number of attacks of acute abdominal pain to which individuals of the first group are subject. Carbohydrate-induced hyperlipemia occurs in children rarely. Familial hypercholesteremia occurs in the pediatric age group;[117] the response of atheromatous lesions to dietary therapy has not been significant.

The demonstration of a metabolic error in the catabolism of phytanic acid in Refsum's disease[118] makes dietary treatment of this rare neurologic disorder possible.[119] Since phytanic acid is of exogenous origin, restriction of foods containing this 20-carbon branched-chain fatty acid is indicated.

4. Anomalies of Vitamin Metabolism. Familial vitamin D resistant rickets[120] is an inherited metabolic disease associated with marked hypophosphatemia in the presence of relatively normal serum calcium and only slight to moderate elevation of the alkaline phosphatase. The clinical manifestations of rickets are quite variable. The fundamental defect is an impairment of the renal tubular reabsorption of phosphate as a result of an insensitivity to the action of vitamin D or one of its metabolites. Extremely large doses of vitamin D (50,000 to 500,000 units daily) are required. Since these amounts are close to the toxic range, and often beyond it, treatment should be carefully controlled by frequent serum calcium determinations as well as roentgenograms of the long bones.

The clinical features of vitamin B_6 dependency are limited to the central nervous system and include hyperirritability, convulsions with electroencephalographic changes and a significant elevation of the spinal fluid protein.[121] The disease appears to be an inborn error of metabolism of a brain enzyme dependent on vitamin B_6 the exact nature of which has not yet been elucidated. Symptoms may appear within a few hours or days after birth and are controlled specifically by the administration of large amounts of pyridoxine. Therapy must be continuous; symptoms have recurred promptly on withdrawal of the vitamin even after several years of continuous therapy.

Supplementation of the diet with vitamins A, D and E is required in the malabsorption syndromes with poor fat absorption. Steatorrheas are the only indication for vitamin E supplementation known at present.

5. **States Requiring Adjustment of the Mineral Intake.** Since there are a number of such states, space will be taken only to mention them. Situations in which additional sodium is required include Addison's disease, the salt-losing form of the adrenogenital syndrome, congenital tubular renal acidosis (Lightwood syndrome)[122] and hypotonic dehydration. Potassium supplementation is needed in the acute diarrheas, congenital alkalosis with diarrhea, congenital renal alkalosis, aldosteronism, periodic familial paralysis (hypokalemic type) and the treatment of diabetic coma. Sodium restriction is used in nephrotic and cardiac edema and potassium restriction is indicated in anuria. Calcium supplementation is necessary in the various forms of tetany. Restriction of calcium intake is indicated in idiopathic hypercalcemia (Lightwood[123] and Fanconi[124]) and in prolonged immobilization where bone decalcification may result in elevation of the serum calcium levels.

BIBLIOGRAPHY

1. Murlin, Conklin, and Marsh: Am. J. Dis. Child., 29, 1, 1925.
2. Protein Requirements. Nutritional Studies #16. Published by Food & Agr. Organization of United Nations. Rome, 1957.
3. Mendel: Harvey Lectures, 10, 101, 1914.
4. Rose, Johnson, and Haines: J. Biol. Chem., 182, 541, 1950.
5. Rose, Haines, Warner, and Johnson: J. Biol. Chem., 188, 49, 1951.
6. Rose, Haines, and Warner: J. Biol. Chem., 193, 605, 1951.
7. Rose, Warner, and Haines: J. Biol. Chem., 193, 613, 1951.
8. Rose, Haines, and Warner: J. Biol. Chem., 206, 421, 1954.
9. Rose, Lambert, and Coon: J. Biol. Chem., 211, 815, 1954.
10. Rose, Leach, Coon, and Lambert: J. Biol. Chem., 213, 913, 1955.
11. Rose, Borman, Coon, and Lambert: J. Biol. Chem., 214, 579, 1955.
12. Rose, Coon, Lockhart, and Lambert: J. Biol. Chem., 215, 101, 1955.
13. Rose, Eades, and Coon: J. Biol. Chem., 216, 225, 1955.
14. Leverton, Gram, Chaloupka, Brodousky, and Mitchell: J. Nutr., 58, 59, 1956.
15. Leverton, Gram, Brodousky, Chaloupka, Mitchell, and Johnson: J. Nutr., 58, 83, 1956.
16. Leverton, Johnson, Pazur, and Ellison: J. Nutr., 58, 219, 1956.
17. Leverton, Johnson, Ellison, Geschwender, and Schmidt: J. Nutr., 58, 341, 1956.
18. Leverton, Ellison, Johnson, Pazur, Schmidt, and Geschwender: J. Nutr., 58, 355, 1956.
19. Mertz, Baxter, Jackson, Roderick, and Weis: J. Nutr., 46, 313, 1952.
20. Swendseid, Williams, and Dunn: J. Nutr., 58, 495, 1956.
21. Swendseid and Dunn: J. Nutr., 58, 507, 1956.
22. Jones, Baumann, and Reynolds: J. Nutr., 60, 549, 1956.
23. Clark, Yess, Vermillion, Goodwin, and Mertz: J. Nutr., 79, 131, 1963.
24. Clark, Yang, Walton, and Mertz: J. Nutr., 71, 229, 1960.
25. Clark, Reitz, Vacharotayan, and Mertz: J. Nutr., 78, 173, 1962.
26. Clark, Mertz, Kwong, Howe, and DeLone: J. Nutr., 63, 71, 1957.
27. Nakagawa, Takahashi, and Suzuki: J. Nutr., 71, 176, 1960.
28. ———: J. Nutr., 73, 186, 1961.
29. ———: J. Nutr., 74, 401, 1961.
30. Nakagawa, Takahashi, Suzuki, and Kobayashi: J. Nutr., 77, 61, 1962.
31. ———: J. Nutr., 80, 305, 1963.
32. Joint FAO/WHO Expert Group on Protein Requirements, Geneva, 1963.
33. Snyderman, Holt, Dancis, Roitman, and Balis: J. Nutr., 78, 75, 1962.
34. Hundley, Sandstead, Sampson, and Whedon: Am. J. Clin. Nutr., 5, 316, 1957.
35. Pratt, Snyderman, Cheung, Norton, and Holt: J. Nutr., 56, 231, 1955.
36. Snyderman, Pratt, Cheung, Norton, and Holt: J. Nutr., 56, 253, 1955.
37. Snyderman, Norton, Fowler, and Holt: Am. J. Dis. Child., 97, 175, 1959.
38. Snyderman, Holt, Smellie, Boyer, and Westall: Am. J. Dis. Child., 97, 186, 1959.
39. Snyderman, Boyer, and Holt: Am. J. Dis. Child., 97, 192, 1959.
40. Snyderman, Roitman, Boyer, and Holt: Am. J. Dis. Child., 102, 157, 1961.
41. Snyderman, Boyer, Phansalkar, and Holt: Am. J. Dis. Child., 102, 163, 1961.
42. Snyderman, Boyer, Roitman, Holt, and Prose: Pediatrics, 31, 786, 1963.
43. Snyderman, Boyer, Norton, Roitman, and Holt: Am. J. Clin. Nutr., 15, 313, 1964.
44. ———: Am. J. Clin. Nutr., 15, 322, 1964.
45. Chwalibogowski: Acta Paediat., 22, 110, 1937.
46. Hansen and Wiese: Federation Proc., 5, 233, 1946.
47. Hansen et al.: Pediatrics, 31, 171, 1963.
48. Holt, Tidwell, et al.: J. Pediat., 6, 427, 1935.
49. Snyderman, Morales, and Holt: Arch. Dis. Child., 30, 83, 1955.
49a. Committee on Nutrition. Pediatrics, 43, 134, 1969.
50. Henry and Kon: Brit. J. Nutr., 7, 147, 1953.
51. Gershoff, Legg, and Hegsted: J. Nutr., 64, 303, 1958.

52. New York Academy of Medicine Committee on Public Health Relations: Report on Fluoridation of Water Supplies, Bull. New York Acad. Med., *28*, 275, 1952.
53. Hamil, Reynolds, Poole, and Macy: Am. J. Dis. Child., *56*, 561, 1938.
54. Recommended Dietary Allowances: National Research Council Food and Nutrition Board, Publ. 1694, Washington, D.C., 1968.
55. Holt, Nemir, Snyderman, *et al.*: J. Nutr., *37*, 53, 1949.
56. Snyderman, Ketron, Burch, *et al.*: J. Nutr., *39*, 219, 1949.
57. Report of the Tenth M. & R. Pediatric Research Conference: Vitamin B₆ in Human Nutrition, M. & R. Laboratories, Columbus, Ohio, 1953.
58. Gyorgy, Cogan, and Rose: Proc. Soc. Exp. Biol. Med., *81*, 536, 1952.
59. Nitowsky, Gordon, and Tildon: Bull. Johns Hopkins Hosp., *98*, 361, 1956.
60. Majaj, Dinning, Azzam, and Darby: Am. J. Clin. Nutr., *12*, 374, 1963.
60a.Ritchie, Fish, McMasters, and Grossman: New Eng. J. Med., *279*, 1185, 1968.
61. Pratt *et al.*: Pediatrics, *1*, 181, 1948.
62. Halac: Am. J. Clin. Nutr., *9*, 557, 1961.
63. Halac: Am. J. Clin. Nutr., *11*, 574, 1962.
64. Holt, Halac, and Kajdi: J.A.M.A., *181*, 699, 1962.
65. Hoag, Rivkin, Levine, and Wilson: Am. J. Dis. Child., *34*, 150, 1927.
66. Chung: J. Pediat., *33*, 1, 1953.
67. Ross: Federation Proc., *19*, 1190, 1959.
67a.Arias, Gartner, Seifter and Furman: J. Clin. Invest., *43*, 2037, 1964.
68. Gyorgy: Pediatrics, *11*, 98, 1953.
69. Mellander: Upssala Läkeref. Forhandl., *52*, 107, 1947.
70. Pratt and Snyderman: Pediatrics, *11*, 65, 1953.
71. Calcagno and Rubin: Pediatrics, *13*, 193, 1954.
72. Mauron: Arch. Biochem., *59*, 433, 1955.
73. Harper: J. Nutr., *67*, 109, 1959.
74. Fischer, C. C. and Whitman, M. P.: J. Pediat., *55*, 116, 1959.
75. Vaughan, V. C. *et al.*: J. Pediat., *61*, 547, 1962.
76. Report of Committee on Fetus and Newborn: Pediat., *28*, 675, 1961.
77. Holt, Davies and Hasselmeyer: J. Pediat., *61*, 566, 1962.
78. Darrow: J. Pediat., *28*, 515, 1946.
79. Kauhtio and Hallman: Acta Paediat., *39*, 328, 1950.
80. Wilmore and Dudrick: J.A.M.A., *203*, 140, 1968.
81. Filler, Erakles, Rebin and Das: New Engl. J. Med., *281*, 589, 1969.
82. Dudrick, Wilmore, Vars *et al.*: Ann. Surg., *169*, 974, 1969.
83. Coleman: J.A.M.A., *69*, 320, 1917.
84. Dubois: Arch. Int. Med., *10*, 177, 1912.
85. Schick and Wagner: Zeitschr. f. Kinderheilk., *35*, 263, 1923.
86. Macrae and Morris: Arch. Dis. Child., *6*, 75, 1931.

87. Black, Fourman, and Trinder: Lancet, *1*, 574, 1946.
88. Chung and Viscorova: J. Pediat., *33*, 14, 1948.
89. Chung, Morales, Snyderman, Lewis, and Holt: Pediatrics, *7*, 491, 1951.
90. Krahulik, Shoob, Morales, Snyderman, and Holt: J. Pediat., *41*, 774, 1952.
91. Morales *et al.*: Pediatrics, *6*, 86, 1950.
92. Gomez *et al.*: Lancet, *2*, 121, 1956.
93. Park: Proc. Connecticut State Med. Soc., 1924, p. 190.
94. Lyon: Am. J. Dis. Child., *36*, 1012, 1928.
95. Rubin: Am. J. Med. Sci., *200*, 385, 1940.
96. Rothman: Am. J. Dis. Child., *86*, 201, 1953.
97. Dicke, Weyers, and Van de Kamer: Acta Paediat., *42*, 34, 1953.
98. Rubner and Langstein: Arch. f. ges. Physiol., *39*, 39, 1918.
99. Tidwell, Holt, Farrow, and Neale: J. Pediat., *7*, 481, 1935.
100. Gordon and McNamara: Am. J. Dis. Child., *62*, 328, 1941.
101. Levine, Marples, and Gordon: J. Clin. Invest., *20*, 209, 1941.
102. Oski and Barness: Am. J. Dis. Child., *67*, 1045, 1965.
103. Hassan *et al.*: Am. J. Clin., *19*, 147, 1966.
104. Mackay: Arch. Dis. Child., *10*, 195, 1935.
105. Gorten, Hepner, and Workman: J. Pediat., *63*, 1063, 1963.
106. Kunz: H. J. Pediat., *41*, 84, 1952.
107. Steigman: Am. J. Dis. Child., *100*, 794, 1961.
107a.Millican and Laurie: In *The Child in His Family*, New York, John Wiley and Sons, Inc., 1970.
108. Davis: Am. J. Dis. Child., *36*, 651, 1928.
109. Gephart: Boston Med. Surg. J., *176*, 17, 1917.
110. Johnston: Ann. New York Acad. Sci., *69*, 881, 1958.
110a.Heald: *Adolescent Nutrition and Growth.* New York, Appleton-Century-Crofts, 1969.
111. Marine: Medicine, *3*, 453, 1924.
112. Greenwald: Transactions of the American Goiter Assn., *369*, 1950.
113. Levin, Oberholzer, Snodgrass, Stimler, and Wilmers: Arch. Dis. Child., *38*, 220, 1963.
114. Weijers and Van De Kamer: Acta Paediat., *52*, 329, 1963.
115. Holt, Aylward and Timbres: Bull. Johns Hopkins Hosp., *64*, 279, 1939.
116. Knittle and Ahrens: J. Clin. Invest., *43*, 485, 1967.
117. Rausen and Adlersberg: Pediatrics, *28*, 276, 1961.
118. Steinberg *et al.*: J. Clin. Invest., *46*, 313, 1967.
119. Eljjarn *et al.*: Lancet, *1*, 691, 1966.
120. Winters, Graham, Williams, McFalls, and Burnett: Medicine, *37*, 97, 1958.
121. Scriver: Pediatrics, *26*, 62, 1960.
122. Lightwood, Payne, and Black: Pediatrics, *12*, 628, 1953.
123. Lightwood: Arch. Dis. Child., *27*, 302, 1952.
124. Fanconi and Girardet: Helvet. Paediat. Acta, *7*, 314, 1952.

Chapter

25

Nutrition for the Aging and the Aged

Donald M. Watkin

GENERAL CONSIDERATIONS

Aging in man is a process beginning no later than conception and continuing until death. By the term "aging" is meant the progression of changes in biochemical processes which determine structural and functional alterations with age in the cells and noncellular tissue and hence in the whole organism. The aged are those persons in whom at least 65 per cent of the total changes associated with biologic aging have already occurred, assuming the life span (defined as the oldest age to which any member of a given species has survived) of man to be approximately 115 years.[1]

In man, aging is so modified by disease that its truly uncomplicated course is unknown. When an elderly man dies, he dies from disease or accident, although his demise may euphemistically be attributed to "old age." Prior to death the aged display interindividual variations in many measurable parameters which are far greater than those observed in younger populations. These greater variations are theoretically attributable to the lack of similarity among individuals in the temporal manifestation of aging patterns of the genome and in the lifetime accumulation of insults from environmental hazards, disease and trauma. They are reflected in the variety of values reported as minimum requirements for specific nutrients among the aged. Such reports only emphasize the fact that any nutritional recommendations directed at the aged as a class must be couched in terms so general as to be meaningless. Older individuals may or may not have special nutritional needs. If they do, these special needs spring from medical, psychological, social and economic factors as varied as the fingerprints of the aged themselves. Good nutrition for today's aged implies focusing attention on the specific needs of each individual.

For those experiencing the earlier stages of the aging process, good nutrition from conception through late maturity may mean the difference between continued active life and either death or a life plagued by disability. Since nutrition is an environmental factor over which man has relatively great control, man can use nutrition as one means of preventing complications of the aging process by disease. Although in general there is little evidence in man that nutrition can influence aging *per se*, certain animal studies (*v.i.*) suggest that nutrition may influence the aging of collagen, while others point to perinatal nutrition (*v.i.*) as a determinant of selected parameters of aging after maturity. Although present theory in molecular biology suggests that cell death, a major contributor to the aging process, may result from factors still beyond man's immediate control (*v.i.*), scientists, sociologists and economists are already anticipating the day when additional basic research and clinical investigation may provide the means by which man may forestall cell death, raise by several decades his average age at death and possibly even prolong his life span.[1a] For the present, good nutrition continues to play its most significant role during youth and middle age in the prevention of those diseases which ultimately manifest themselves as serious disabilities among the aged. In addition, it is well to remember that recent animal studies suggest that good nutrition is a perinatal environmental factor favorably influencing senescent processes after maturity.[1a]

Basically, ideal nutrition for an elderly person in good health differs insignificantly from that of younger individuals, assuming in both cases that caloric intake is proportional to energy expenditure.[1b] Organ systems and metabolic processes normally have sufficient reserve so that decrements in efficiency associated with physiologic aging require no compensatory adjustments in nutrient intake. Rarely, however, are elderly men and women unafflicted by disabilities. Often these are complicated further by socioeconomic problems.

Consider for a moment the plight of an elderly man who is edentulous and whose dentures are of an improper, painful fit. If barred by economic reasons from consulting a dentist, he may resort to the simple expedient of eating only those foods which can be consumed without teeth. Again his economic position and living arrangements may make it impossible for him to purchase and prepare well-balanced diets and dietary supplements of which many suitable for his dentition are now on the market. Instead he may revert to such standbys as bread, mashed potatoes and other easily swallowed, high-carbohydrate, low-protein foods.

Consider the case of an elderly woman crippled by arthritis living alone. Merely going to a store to buy food may be an insurmountable task. Even opening food containers, let alone preparing meats and vegetables, may be painful and disagreeable. As being alone and eating alone compounds her misery, she soon may revert to easily prepared foods which furnish calories but do little to supply the protein, minerals and vitamins needed for proper nutrition.

Consider the elderly patient with myocardial insufficiency whose diet should be low in salt; the elderly patient with hypercholesterolemia who had been advised to restrict his intake of saturated fats; the elderly diabetic who needs a carefully planned daily menu of six feedings; the elderly cancer patient whom surgery has left with a colostomy; or the elderly cirrhotic who has been told to eat a high-protein, sodium-restricted regimen.

Consider the 19-year-old whose cervical fracture sustained in an auto accident produced instant aging, telescoping 80 years into a few milliseconds.[1c] Plagued by paralysis; cachexia; neurogenic dysfunction of the bladder and bowel; bone dissolution leading to osteopenia, pathologic fractures and renal lithiasis; pulmonary insufficiency; cardiovascular instability; anemia; carbohydrate intolerance; upper gastrointestinal hemorrhage; pressure ulcers of the skin; severely restricted vocational opportunities; negligible pension rights; almost total dependency on others; plus the need for an indivdually tailored dietary regimen, he deserves to be numbered along with the nation's 8,000,000 aged living in poverty for whom solutions are only now beginning to surface. (*v.i.*)

Obviously, solutions exist on paper for all these individuals and for many more who have conditions amenable to nutritional therapy. However, their transformation into practice requires their being tailored to the individual, his environment, the social conditions under which he lives and his financial resources. These solutions can be found only in an interdisciplinary approach by physicians, nutritionists, social workers and, when necessary, hospital or visiting nurses. This approach should be emphasized in both theory and application during the education and training of all members of the interdisciplinary team. The food industry in particular, through the introduction of protective foods processed to provide long shelf life in any climate, packed in single-meal units in easy-to-open containers labeled in large letters and marketed on a sufficiently large scale to insure a truly low retail price, could help solve the practical problem of providing balanced diets for the great majority of the aged. The necessity for low retail prices to match the reduced earnings of the aged suggests the wisdom of marketing such products to appeal to the aging from youth through late maturity as well as to the aged themselves. Previous marketing experience indicates that food products labeled "for the aged" are not accepted by older people. This unwillingness of the aged to identify themselves with products obviously prepared for them does not prevent them from consuming large quantities of baby and junior foods whose purchase can always be explained as being for grandchildren. These purchases indicate a need, either real or conceived out of fear or ignorance, for inexpensive single service, easily opened foods requiring minimal effort in preparation and little mastication prior to deglutition.

Changing life styles among the nation's youth place many in the same socioeconomic position which has long characterized the needy aged. Early marriage, vocational inadequacies, entrenched seniority systems, high levels of unemployment and the dissolution of the institution of the extended family now confront youth with the same nutritional problems long faced by the needy aged.[1d]

Nutrition in the perinatal portion of the aging process has attracted long overdue attention for its influence on the physical and behavioral growth and development of children.[1e–j] Less well recognized and investigated is the influence of perinatal nutrition on senescent changes occurring in adult life. Animal studies[1k–s] in short-lived species have shown altered age-related patterns in various parameters correlated to the quality of perinatal nutrition. Similar prospective studies in man would require many decades, while retrospective studies, at least for the present, face methodologic obstacles of such magnitude that their credibility is seriously in doubt. Nonetheless, animal investigations and epidemiologic studies[1t–u] provide evidence supporting a high index of suspicion that perinatal nutrition may be a previously unsuspected environmental factor conditioning the aging process in adult life.

The requirements of the aging, aged 20 to 40, have received scant attention with the exception of those for pregnant and lactating women. Yet the two decades preceding age 40 represent the golden period during which nutrition may exert its maximum effect in the prevention of disease in adult life. In these two decades children experience release form parental authority; young men and women complete their educations and enter upon their respective careers; young men serve in the armed forces; married couples become

parents; and the exuberance of youth is mellowed by experiences, some traumatic and stressful, into the maturity of middle age. These events transpire in kaleidoscopic fashion providing little time for concern by the aging about the consequences of dietary indiscretion or nutritional neglect.

Preventive nutrition for the aging should begin, of course, before birth and continue through childhood and adolescence. Preschool and elementary school nutrition education programs are commonplace. Less common, however, are secondary school and college programs. Hence, at the very time when rebellious youths are gaining independence from parental control, nutrition education programs play an insignificant role. In universities, in business and among the professions, preventive nutrition is neglected entirely or hypocritically acknowledged but sidetracked in deference to matters of presumed higher priority. Even in the armed forces, where the means of indoctrinating troops with preventive nutrition is theoretically at hand, more attention is paid to food industry lobbyists, worried mothers, congressional complaints and the unthinking cravings of youth than to presently known knowledge on disease prevention by nutritional means. The lack of knowledge regarding preventive nutrition is no more evident than among many United States Peace Corps volunteers whose first realization of the interrelation of nutrition and health has come when they have encountered the cultural shock of malnutrition in developing countries. Lack of appropriate concern for preventive nutrition by government agencies has manifested itself not only in the defense establishment (v.s.) but even in the National Aeronautics and Space Agency where hardware considerations and astronaut whims have received higher priority. Other agencies are no less remiss.[2]

These examples highlight the urgent necessity of seizing every possible opportunity to teach young men and women, to indoctrinate them with and to habituate them to the virtues and the substance of preventive nutrition. When honest efforts fail, research must develop new approaches; however, with present opportunities unseized, firmer appli-

cation of known methods should take precedence over any wasteful scramble to develop
methodologic panaceas.

NEW POTENTIAL FOR NUTRITIONAL GERONTOLOGY

As agglomerates, nutrition and gerontology
share similar attributes. While rooted in
science, their contemporary images depict
desperate need; unrequited yearnings for
health, vitality and prowess; politically expedient maneuvers; consumer gullibility and
activism; administrative, legislative and juridi-
cal processes; flagrant commercialism; overt
quackery; and genuine dedication by persons
and institutions to the search for pragmatic
solutions for very real problems in both
spheres. The interrelations of nutrition and
aging, while scientifically intriguing, manifest
themselves in man only after the passage of
many decades. This creates a hind-sight
perspective which fails to provide surcease to
burdens or succor from distress occasioned by
long-term past indiscretions. Although scientists perceive the interrelationships most
trenchant in developmental aging, the elderly
are primarily concerned with how the interrelationships affect them and their lives at the
moment.

These differing viewpoints are irrecon-
cilable. The scientists, aware that cell death
(*v.i.*) is the irreversible process fundamental
to biologic aging, have thinly veiled contempt
for the elderly's often irrational quest for
nutritional panaceas. The aged, including
some once skeptical scientists, nonetheless
sustain themselves through confidence that
their dreams will be fulfilled. Hence they are
fair game for a broad spectrum of charlatans
motivated by profit, self-aggrandizement or
both.

While science and the hopes of today's
aged are presently incapable of integration
into a compatible aggregate, developments of
the past half-decade strongly suggest that
healthy overtures to the interrelations of
nutrition and aging are afoot. Happily, they
obviate the need for miracles and generate
advocacy of greater support for nutrition and
aging research among the millions of aged

who themselves may never benefit from new
discovery.

The low positions assigned nutrition and
gerontology in rank order of priorities have
severely limited resources apportioned to
amelioration of human needs in both fields.
These restricted resources have made impossible simultaneously meeting the exigencies of
those already old while protecting the future
interests of younger generations, including
the unborn and those yet to be conceived.

Recent developments are the harvest of
seed planted years ago in hostile environments by those whose vision included faith
in an eventual change in majority attitudes
toward the poor, the hungry and the old.
In the United States of America, the 1969
White House Conference on Food, Nutrition
and Health (WHCFNH) (in itself an under-
scoring by the new Administration of the
decisive role nutrition plays in national
ecology[2a]) stressed gerontology by incorporating into its own structure a Panel on Aging.
Community and state-wide preliminary conferences and special task force meetings, all
incorporating considerations of nutrition and
aging in their agenda, culminated in the
Washington WHCFNH in late November
and early December, 1969.

The final report of the Panel on Aging
comprised 11 recommendations each in turn
comprising varying numbers of specific components. These have been published.[2b]

The specific recommendations of the Panel
on Aging were assigned by the Subcommittee
on Nutrition of the Domestic Council to
various Federal Departments and Agencies
for evaluation and, where possible, implementation. The responses and reports on action
taken were compiled by the Subcommittee
on Nutrition and presented to a Follow-up
Conference of WHCFNH Staff and Panel and
Task Force Chairmen and Vice-Chairmen
at Williamsburg, Virginia, on February 5,
1971.[2c,2d]

The Panel on Aging in cooperation with
the Administration on Aging (AoA) of the
Department of Health, Education and Welfare (HEW) and HEW's Nutrition Program
conducted a 2-day Workshop in August,
1970, to examine means of implementing
recommendations I, IV, VI and VII.[2e] The

transcripts of the Workshop have been summarized.[2f] In February, 1971, the WHCFNH Follow-up Conference at Williamsburg reviewed the responses of various Federal Departments and Agencies and assessed actions in the intervening year.[2g] A highly structured system of preliminary conferences at municipal and state levels produced in the early months of 1971 grassroot expressions of opinion from the nation's elderly on six major issues dealing with nutrition which had been painstakingly constructed and phrased by the Technical Committee on Nutrition of the White House Conference on Aging (WHCoA) in a series of meetings in late 1970.[2h] Policy recommendations and suggestions for immediate action were prepared by all jurisdictions, assembled by the Technical Committee on Nutrition's Secretariat and offered for discussion, approval or revision at the national WHCoA in Washington.[2i]

Increasing public and professional interest and action plus the almost ninefold increase in funding for food stamps since the WHCFNH in 1969 have drastically changed the potential for adequate nutrition for the aged American.[2j–n]

Concern for nutrition among the aged and the aging has not been confined to the U.S.A. In the U.S.S.R., interest in the notorious longevity of certain Transcaucasian peoples has focused on their lifelong dietary practices.[2o] In other industrialized nations, well-subsidized projects provide adequate nutrition as part of national health and social security programs.[2p] While the aged in technically underdeveloped societies represent comparatively low percentages of total populations, their presence has not gone unnoticed by the public or by specialists in development planning.[2q] The difficult experiences of the technically advanced societies in coping with larger percentages of aged suggest strongly a need to plan ahead for the time when the enormous young populations of today's technically underdeveloped world will themselves be old. In these societies, great concern for nutrition during the pregnancy of mothers and the early lives of children has been manifest for years. As these concerns are translated into effective programs, their impact on aging throughout life may become more evident, and more non-genetically-elite[2r] may survive into advanced old age. The challenge for these societies is to plan well enough to leapfrog over the errors committed by presently developed societies into a more promising twenty-first century.

THE AGING PROCESS

The lack of evidence in adult man that nutrition can influence the aging process *per se* has been mentioned. This statement can be better understood if the nature of aging can be more clearly defined. Whether to regard aging as an indication of pathology or to look upon it as a normal process is to indulge in semantics. That aging occurs in man whether or not it is accompanied by disease is a *prima facie* assumption. Much of what is known of aging has come not from knowledge of man but from work in animals and even lower orders of life. Trends in molecular biology suggest the possibility that aging may be a phenomenon common to all living material, raising hopes that discoveries at the molecular level in any living matter may have direct bearing on the process in man.

Cell Loss. Aging has been attributed in large measure to either losses of cells by organ systems or the reduction in the cellular metabolism of tissues with age.[2s] Much convincing evidence exists to support the concept of cell loss with increasing age. Histologists can distinguish old from young tissues, especially those of heart, skeletal muscle, brain, cartilage and kidney which have no capacity for regeneration, by the reduction with age in the number of functioning parenchymal cells.[2t] Reduction in the volume of specific muscles in old rats has been interpreted as cell loss.[3] The number of non-glial cells per unit of cerebral cortex decreases with advancing age, the greatest slope being between 45 and 55.[3a] However, several brain stem structures show no reduction in cell number with age.[3b] In man, reductions in organ or organ system functions are commonly found in aging. These have been directly associated with demonstrable cell loss. For example, linear reductions in discrete renal functions[4,5] between age 30 and 90 indicate loss of functioning nephrons, a loss corroborated by quantitative counts in histologic sections.[6] Agewise decrements in body water unaccompanied by decrements in oxygen consumption per unit of body water[7] similarly suggest cell loss. Body composition studies[8,9,10,11] have revealed decreased fat-free as well as total body weight in advanced age. Studies of total body potassium measured either by K^{42} dilution techniques[12] or by estimation of K^{40} radiation in a whole body counter[13] have revealed agewise decrements suggesting cell loss.

Virtually all these data represent observations on age differences among groups of subjects representing different age categories. The data have, therefore, a built-in bias due to selective mortality, a bias which would be eliminated were it possible to assemble serial measurements on the same subject while that subject grows older.[13a] Longitudinal studies in man designed to overcome this bias have begun[13b,c] but so far have not been in operation long enough to provide meaningful data even in those parameters which can be measured. Hence, almost all information presently available is based on cross-sectional studies. Interpretations derived from such information therefore should be accepted with reservations introduced by the biasing effect of selective mortality.

Reduced Cellular Metabolism. While the bulk of evidence from cross-sectional studies supports the concept of cell loss with aging, the possibility remains that reduced organ or organ system performance may be due in part to reduced cellular metabolism with age. When enzyme activity in the heart, kidney and liver of young and old rats was measured and related to the deoxyribonucleic acid (DNA) content of tissues[14,15,16,17,18] no decrements in alkaline and acid phosphatase, succinoxidase, pyrophosphatase, pseudocholinesterase or D-amino acid oxidase were found. One enzyme, cathepsin, however, showed increased activity with aging. Other enzyme studies during protein deprivation and refeeding showed little evidence of decrements in protein synthesis in senescence.[19] In fact, these and other studies showing increased tryptophan peroxidase activity with age in rat liver[20] and increased ribonucleic acid (RNA) in the cells

of aged mice[21] have even suggested increased protein turnover with age.

Reductions of succinoxidase activity in whole tissue homogenates led to speculation that mitochondria (which contain essentially all succinoxidase activity) might lose enzyme activity with age. Studies of isolated liver and kidney mitochondria[17,22] failed to reveal decrements with age leading to the suggestion that impaired cellular enzyme activity may result from a loss of mitochondria from cells rather than changes in the enzyme activity of mitochondria themselves.

Studies in 193 men aged 21 to 95, mentioned briefly above,[7] showed no decrement in oxygen consumption with age per unit of body water, although body water per square meter of body surface decreased with age. These observations suggest that functioning cells are lost as man ages but that the oxygen uptake of functioning cells in old men is no different from that in young. This clinical evidence combined with the fact that even the maximum observed decrements in enzyme activity in animal tissues cannot account for the well-documented organ and organ system decrements in function, which may reach 60 per cent,[23] lead to the conclusion that cell death continues to be the major phenomenon on which to blame the functional impairment accompanying the aging process.

Biochemical Mechanisms Underlying Cell Death. Knowledge of possible biochemical mechanisms underlying cell death has increased with recent advances in understanding of the role of deoxyribonucleic acid (DNA) and ribonucleic acid (RNA) in protein synthesis. One hypothesis in explanation of cell death has been proposed by Wulff et al.[21] They compared the H^3 cytidine incorporation into RNA in young and old mice with data on RNA content of liver, dorsal root ganglia and Purkinje cells and observed that tracer uptake increased more, or decreased less, with age than RNA content. In other words, the ratio of tracer uptake to RNA content increased with age. In theory, these observations suggest that sites for RNA synthesis sustain damage with aging related to continual use. The damaged sites produce defective RNA which produces nonfunctioning enzymes. As substrate for protein synthesis accumulates, RNA synthesis undergoes derepression where this is possible (*e.g.*, in liver cells). Hence, increased production of RNA is required to maintain a functional level of enzymes in the presence of impaired RNA synthesis. Since defective RNA is less stable than normal RNA, the ratio of tracer uptake to RNA content increases.

The same authors have presented data from kidney, ventricular muscle and skeletal muscle to add to that described above.[21a] In addition, they concluded from data on the time course of labeling that RNA synthesis occurs in nuclei and that nuclear RNA subsequently moves to cytoplasm.

Wulff *et al.* have concluded that compensatory processes occur in an effort to maintain cell-sustaining enzyme activity, with senescence and death ensuing when the efficacy of this process falters.[21b]

In summary, the hypothesis of these investigators attributes aging to the accumulation of somatic mutations in DNA. This in turn yields defective RNA which is incapable of producing enzymes which can synthesize proteins from available amino acids. A cell will survive until functional enzymes fall below a critical level at which point cell death ensues.

The factors which may be responsible for errors in the synthesis of nucleic acids and proteins have been reviewed by Medvedev.[24] He includes random errors in RNA replication from DNA; radiation; microemission of heat and radiant energy; blocking of active groups; microdenaturation; incorporation of analogs and products of side reactions; and changes in ratio of substrates during the synthesis of RNA and proteins. These factors act on DNA and RNA in different ways. The synthesis of DNA is relatively unaffected. In addition, natural selection rapidly eliminates any negative characteristics arising from errors in DNA synthesis; likewise, it spares positive characteristics for future reproduction. Unlike DNA synthesis, RNA and protein synthesis are relatively unsheltered, a situation leading to damaged molecules which are retained and accumulated in cells.[24a,b] Since proteins are extremely specific for each function performed and since

they cannot replicate themselves exactly, changes in proteins form the molecular basis for cell death and eventually for death of the individual.

Medvedev suggests that aging is associated with a gradual weakening of the hereditary control of protein synthesis, *i.e.*, cellular RNA replication of DNA becomes less exact with the passage of time.[24,24a,24b] The process of aging could be altered therefore by eliminating the responsible factors mentioned above or by creating conditions unfavorable to the production and accumulation of damaged molecules. This might be done by eliminating or segregating the altered RNA templates so that only the correct RNA could function in protein synthesis. The rate of autoreproduction of correct RNA templates might be increased. Medvedev's suggestion[24] that tests be run on the immunization of young animals by proteins derived from the aged with a view toward the elimination of altered proteins by autoimmune reactions in the young, while theoretically possible, can be challenged by more recent considerations of immunological phenomena.[24c] Theoretically, the introduction of soluble RNA from young cells into old cells could increase production of perfect proteins. Favorable changes in memory among moderately impaired aged subjects after oral and intravenous injections of yeast RNA have been reported by Cameron *et al.*[24d–g] Reports of similar improvement after administration of magnesium pemoline,[24h] a drug which in theory stimulated RNA synthesis, have been tempered by disappointing results in the hands of the same and other investigators.[24i,j] By whatever method it is brought about, extension of the time period during which DNA effectively governs protein synthesis provides a major avenue of research into deceleration of the aging process.

More recently, Medvedev[24k,l] has postulated a process he calls "active aging." This implies a marked group of "aging" genes activated at a predetermined stage of life. These genes increase the rate of molecular reproduction, incorporate "noise" into the system and cause aging as a special case of random morphogenesis. This programmed aging would act in determining life span independently of previously mentioned mutagenic factors responsible for somatic mutations. Medvedev sees in "active aging" a theoretical mechanism for preventing the accumulation of mutations which, if allowed to continue indefinitely, could be evolutionarily lethal for a given species. In addition, Medvedev[24m] proposes not only that error-producing but also error-correcting systems exist, possibly in the form of specific repressors of the "aging" genes, or as error elimination and correction processes coded in definite genetic loci and possibly subject to maximal activation.

Another model theory of aging as a process has been presented by von Hahn.[24n,o] He observed that DNA from old animals was denatured at a higher temperature than DNA from young, suggesting stronger intramolecular bonding in old DNA. He also observed that residual histone is present in greater concentrations in old than in young DNA. He therefore suspects that histone may be the substance which represses structural genes, preventing the DNA helix from unwinding and, hence, from transcribing RNA, thereby preventing the formation of enzymes.

According to von Hahn, therefore, the aging of DNA appears to consist in large measure of the stabilization of the Watson-Crick double helix by firm binding of histone, as opposed to the temporary binding of histone to DNA which characterizes normal repression of RNA synthesis. Since local unwinding of the double helix is necessary for the transcription of genetic information, the observed effect of the firmer binding of histones could interfere with the transcribing mechanism, prevent the formation of RNA and enzymes and result in cell death.

Prevention of Faulty RNA Production. The hypotheses of Wulff, Medvedev and von Hahn emphasize the fact that aging need no longer be regarded as a mysterious, inexorable partner of life. Any process which can be described quantitatively ultimately will yield to measures directed at its control The prevention of faulty RNA production by control of environmental factors, nutrition being one factor directly under human control, offers one solution. Control of factors such as radiation and heat poses for man practical prob-

lems of great magnitude. However, control of substrate concentrations and ratios by appropriate nutrient intake, regulation of physical activity and possibly the administration of substances yet to be identified and tested are not only within man's reach but also feasible in terms of cost and management. More research is required to reveal the full impact of nutrition on the biochemistry of nucleic acid and protein synthesis. As knowledge unfolds, man can apply it to the prevention or deceleration of aging as he has applied knowledge of nutritional biochemistry to the prevention and treatment of deficiency and degenerative disease during the past century.

Maturation of Collagen as Index of Biologic Age. In those tissues which are in an essentially nondynamic state, molecular aging adds another dimension to the aging process. The above discussion of nucleic acid metabolism applies particularly to the labile proteins. Certain proteins, collagen and elastin for example, have such long half-lives as to preclude their being turned over at all.[25-27] Verzár[28] has studied the maturation of collagen as an objective index of "biological age" as distinguished from "calendar age" of men and animals. He observed that tendons from the tails of 30-month-old, senile rats showed greater contractility on heating to 65° C than tendons from the tails of 5-month-old, young rats. Verzár[28,28a] and Chvapil,[29] using heat- and sodium perchlorate-induced contraction of tendon, respectively, have also observed a prolonged relaxation time in old collagen as opposed to young. Chvapil[29] used this technique to quantify a specific example of the impact of nutrition on molecular aging. In animals whose lives had been prolonged by feeding them restricted diets, as first described by McKay,[30] he found tendons with biological age younger than the animals' calendar age. Holeckova, Chytil and Chvapil[31] also observed that fibers from the tail tendons of wild Norway rats showed a lower biological age than fibers from the tail tendons of domesticated animals of the same calendar age. Chvapil and Holeckova[32] later showed that intermittent feeding and fasting of domesticated Wistar rats led to an inhibition of the normally occurring agewise increase in stability of collagen in domesticated rats. Hence, altering the feeding pattern of the domesticated animals reduced the biologic age of their tail tendon fibers to that of their wild counterparts.

Molecular Aging of Collagen. The increased tension of biologically older collagen fiber has been attributed by Verzár,[28,28a] Bjorksten[33] and Piez[33a] to the increased number of hydrogen and ester bonds forming cross links between molecules within the fiber. The increased number of cross links in aging collagen are attributed by Verzár to the random contact between collagen molecules bathed in body fluids as they are shuttled about by Brownian movements. In a lifetime, during which collagen is neither renewed nor replaced, cross links between molecules would accumulate in increasing numbers. Confirmation of this hypothesis exists in the lower solubility of old collagen during thermally induced contraction at $65°$ C,[34] suggesting an increase in the number of cross links in older fibers. With aging, more ester (as opposed to hydrogen) bonds requiring hexose molecules for their formation have been postulated.[33,35] While these changes were once regarded as evidence of deterioration with advancing age, Verzár[28a] and Piez[33a] now suggest they represent a continuing and perhaps genetically programmed maturation process. Milch *et al.*[36,36a,b] have identified as aldehydes intermediary metabolites which stabilize the lattice structure of collagen against the adverse effects of pH or collagenase activity. Of the several carbohydrate metabolites studied, only those with aldehyde structure promote stability; others disrupt the collagen lattice structure. Among the aldehydes, glyceraldehyde, the major intermediary metabolite which is found in all known carbohydrate metabolic pathways, is the most potent stabilizer of collagen under conditions approximating those of extracellular body fluid. This research may lead to the means of preventing cross-link formation and thereby of slowing down the molecular aging of collagen.[28] The apparent reduction in cross-linkages in the tendons of rats whose lives have been prolonged by underfeeding or whose biological age was reduced by intermittent feeding and fasting suggests the role of nutrition in influencing the molecular aging process.

Since collagen constitutes 40 per cent of all protein in the body,[28] and since collagen is an important component of connective tissue on which all cells depend for contact with the external environment, molecular aging of collagen would seem to deserve a high priority in considerations of over-all aging in man. However, it is well to remember that ionizing radiation which shortens life and produces changes resembling aging[37] has been reported by Verzár[28] to have no effect on the biological age of rat tail tendon fibers. Although this negative effect has not been found by Baily,[38] the lack of agreement may be related to methodologic differences (irradiation in the wet *in vivo* or the dry state) or to the fact that Verzár measured a net effect of both scission and formation of cross-linkages within the collagen molecules.[39] In any event, the lack of a conclusive effect of radiation on collagen aging along with the impossibility of explaining cell death (except by invoking oxygen and nutrient transport failure) on the basis of collagen aging suggests that deterioration of RNA and labile protein synthesis with age remain the more significant problem at this time.

AGING AND SPECIFIC NUTRIENTS

Protein. The minimum daily requirement for protein has yet to be satisfactorily related to age in adult man. For reasons already mentioned, it is not surprising that various investigators using conventional nitrogen balance techniques have found increased,[40-43] decreased[44-46] and similar[47,48] minimum requirements for the aged when compared to the young. Nor is it surprising that adherents of the "allowance"[49] principle have seized upon this large intergroup variability to insist on a standard of protein intake for the elderly high enough to include even those who obviously deserve to be treated as special cases.

Among the evidence supporting a higher dietary protein allowance for the aged is the observation that serum albumin falls with aging while serum globulins show a compensatory rise.[50,51,52,53,54] In discussing their findings, most authors have generally blamed reduced protein synthesis by the liver for the lowered albumin content. Acheson and Jessop[54] found lower serum albumins among those with histories of low-protein intake and noted an agewise increase in γ-globulin which was reversed only in extreme old age. The success in increasing low albumin concentrations, encountered in a variety of conditions in all age groups, with diets containing ample quantities of high-quality protein has led to the inference that high-protein diets were desirable for the aged.

The varied results of nitrogen balance studies and the nonspecificity of serum albumin as an index of protein needs have led to additional methods of investigation seeking to portray more accurately the alterations in protein metabolism with advancing age.

Anabolic Hormones. The changes in nitrogen balance accompanying administration of anabolic hormones have been described by several investigators[55,56,57,58,59] whose work has suggested a superiority of male over female hormones in inducing nitrogen retention. Watkin *et al.*[60] studied nitrogen balances in eight elderly men on high- and low-protein diets before, during and after androgen administration. The androgen induced somewhat greater retention on the high- than on the low-protein diet, but the increment achieved by androgen administration on the low-protein regimen was less than the increment achieved by a high-protein diet alone. A variance analysis[61] performed on data from the four men fed high- and the four fed low-calorie diets during these studies showed no effect of the calorie difference but revealed a marked effect of the protein level. A modified "t" test analysis was performed to assess the role of dietary protein level on the response to androgen administration. This analysis revealed a significant effect of hormone therapy on nitrogen balance at both levels of protein intake. Of far greater significance, however, was the influence of the dietary protein level itself. The analysis revealed no significant hormone-protein interaction. From those studies, it was concluded that a high-protein diet is a far greater stimulus to nitrogen retention than either

added calories or an androgenic hormone. These studies confirmed the ability of aged men to retain nitrogen when fed diets containing adequate protein. The problems of side effects[62] as well as the cost and inconvenience of taking anabolic hormone preparations suggest the desirability of using increased dietary protein when greater protein anabolism is desired.

Changes in Protein Intake. Another approach has compared the metabolic responses of older and younger subjects to abrupt changes in protein intake. During investigations in four elderly and three middle-aged men, Watkin, Silverstone and Shock[63] studied whether old subjects retained their ability to adapt to sudden changes in dietary protein level. Diets were changed from medium- (7.0 gm nitrogen/day) to low- (4.3 gm nitrogen/day) to high- (13.3 gm nitrogen/day) protein content. After shifting from the medium- to the low-protein diet, the elderly men approximated a minimal level of nitrogen loss in 10 days and the middle-aged men in 14. When the dietary protein was raised from the low to the high level, the elderly retained more nitrogen than the middle-aged men, both during the first 5 days and for 30 days after the change. No statistically significant differences in cumulative nitrogen balances, however, were found after any shift in dietary protein level.

Similar observations were made by Couch *et al.*[64] in a 70-year-old man subjected to complete nitrogen withdrawal while he consumed a 2800-calorie diet containing all essential nutrients except amino acids. Well within the 12-day period of nitrogen deprivation, the subject reduced his urinary nitrogen to 2.5 gm/day, a level comparable to that observed in younger subjects.[65] When L-amino acids in the casein pattern were subsequently added to the basic regimen, he responded with strongly positive nitrogen balances.

These studies provide convincing evidence that the aged can adapt successfully to protein withdrawal. The positive nitrogen balances in both investigations following the addition either of more dietary protein or of L-amino acids indicate as well that protein synthesis in the aged increases rapidly when additional amino acid substrate is supplied in the diet.

Amino Acid Metabolism. The increased availability of pure amino acids and the development of chromatographic methods for the measurement of amino acids in biologic materials have made possible quantitative studies of amino acid metabolism in men of all ages. Those performed in the aged have added immeasurably to the information previously available[66,67] which had revealed deficiencies of methionine and lysine in diets self-selected by older individuals. In the first of a series of investigations, Tuttle *et al.*[68] studied five men aged 52 to 68 whose protein nitrogen intake was kept at 7.0 gm/day and whose calorie intake (30 to 40 calories/kg) was sufficient to maintain constant weight. After a 12-day control period, the subjects were given an L-amino acid mixture based on the composition of 18.75 gm of egg protein containing, in addition to the eight essentials, the L-forms of histidine, cystine and tyrosine. The test mixture was supplemented with glycine to bring the nitrogen intake up to that of natural food (7.0 gm/day). Although the mixture contained amounts of amino acids in excess of the quantities required for nitrogen equilibrium in young adults, all five older men went into negative nitrogen balance while receiving it. In addition, three subjects also went into negative nitrogen balance when fed egg protein in an amount duplicating the essential L-amino acid content of the amino acid mixture. These findings suggested that the minimum requirement of one or more of the essential amino acids is higher in older men or that the nonessential nitrogen source (glycine) may not be so well utilized by the aged as by the young for the synthesis of nonessential amino acids.

Minimum Requirement of Essential Amino Acids. Results of these investigations must be viewed in the light of others of slightly different design in which no increase in requirement for aged men was observed. Watts *et al.*,[69] using the nitrogen balance technique, measured the minimal amount of essential amino acids needed for nitrogen equilibrium in six Negro males ranging from 65 to 84 years of age. The authors also compared nitrogen balances in this aged group with those observed[70] in a group of 25-year-old men when both groups received the FAO reference and the milk patterns of essential amino acids. Positive balances at the 200, 280 and 360 mg tryptophan levels of the FAO pattern were in marked contrast to findings by Tuttle *et al.*[68] and, in the authors' opinion, cannot be simply explained by differences in experimental design. When compared to the minimum requirements for 25-year-old men described by Rose,[71] the minimum requirements of only two of the aged men while being fed the FAO patterns were slightly in excess of Rose's *minimum* for young men.

When these same aged men were fed essential amino acids in the milk pattern, Watts *et al.* observed methionine requirements ranging from 0.29 to 0.60 gm methionine as opposed to the 2.4 to 3.0 gm requirement reported by Tuttle *et al.*[72] All of the aged men were in nitrogen equilibrium on amino acid mixtures containing approximately half the methionine required for nitrogen equilibrium in 25-year-old men. The authors conclude that their studies indicate no higher requirement for men over 65 years of age than for men of 25.

Amount of Amino Acids in Relation to Total Nitrogen Content of Diet. Tuttle *et al.*[73] also studied the relation of the essential amino acid requirements of older men to the total nitrogen content of their diet. Previous studies[74] had indicated that men over 60 could maintain nitrogen equilibrium on 1.5 gm of essential nitrogen with amino acids proportioned in the egg pattern if the total nitrogen intake was 3.5 gm/day. The same men went into negative nitrogen balance when total nitrogen was raised to 7.5 gm/day. When the essential nitrogen component was raised to 3.0 gm, their nitrogen balance became positive. When the total nitrogen content was increased to 15 gm daily by the addition of glycine and diammonium citrate, their nitrogen balance again became negative.[73] The authors suggest that this dependence of essential amino acid requirement on total nitrogen intake may be characteristic of older men, since similar dependence has not been observed in younger men and women.[75] They also point out that these observations combined with those of food intake studies[66,67] showing self-selection of proteins low in biological value by the aged could justify an upward revision for dietary protein allowances for the elderly.

Source and Quantity of Nonessential Nitrogen. Other studies[76,77] in normal male and female subjects aged 20 to 24 fed limiting amounts of essential amino acids had revealed that the source as well as the quantity of nonessential nitrogen influenced nitrogen retention. Hence, Tuttle et al.[78] investigated the effect of the kind of dietary nonessential nitrogen fed on the dietary essential amino acid requirement in a group of six older men ranging in age from 50 to 70 years with an average age of 63. Nitrogen balance was measured while the subjects received three different levels (1.2, 1.8 and 2.4 gm amino acid nitrogen per day) of purified essential L-amino acids in whole egg pattern proportions supplemented by either glycine alone or by a mixture of nonessential L-amino acids in whole egg protein proportions in amounts needed to maintain total nitrogen intake at 7 gm daily. When the nonessential amino acid mixture replaced glycine as a source of supplemental nitrogen, greater nitrogen retention was observed in five out of the six subjects. Despite this increased retention, the requirement for nitrogen equilibrium still was greater than 1.2 gm of essential amino acid nitrogen daily in all but one subject. One additional subject achieved nitrogen equilibrium when the essential amino acid nitrogen intake was 1.8 gm daily. However, 2.4 gm daily were required to achieve nitrogen equilibrium in all subjects. These studies demonstrate clearly the great variability in amino acid requirement among the aged. They suggest that the nonessential amino acid as well as the essential amino acid composition of the diet may influence nitrogen retention. They also point toward the possibility of a failure of certain nonessential synthetic pathways with advancing age. Although they suggest an increased requirement for essential amino acids for the aged, the differences in experimental design between this study and that in younger men[79] leave room for some doubt and suggest the desirability of additional investigation.

Requirement for Specific Amino Acids. In studies of requirements for specific amino acids, Tuttle et al.,[72] Swendseid and Tuttle[80] and Tuttle et al.[81] have investigated the dietary requirement for methionine in six men aged 58 to 73 (average age 64) and for lysine in four men aged 53 to 64 (average age 59). The diets contained essential L-amino acids (except for cystine and methionine in the study of methionine requirement and for lysine in the study of lysine requirement) in the proportions of whole egg protein in amounts equivalent to 2.4 gm of essential amino acid nitrogen daily. They also contained 17 gm of nonessential L-amino acids proportioned in the whole egg protein pattern and enough additional glycine to bring the total dietary nitrogen up to 7 gm per day.

All of four men tested were in negative nitrogen balance on 2.1 gm or less of methionine daily. One of two subjects tested was in positive nitrogen balance on 2.4 gm methionine daily; one of three, on 2.7 gm daily; and all of three, on 3.0 gm daily. These estimates are well in excess of requirements ranging from 0.8 to 1.1 gm daily proposed by various investigators[82,83] for young men and women, and also in excess of the 0.29 to 0.60 gm daily noted by Watts et al. (v.s.). However, since the diets contained less than 50 mg cystine daily (all in the low-protein food present in the basal diet), the possibility exists that the increased requirement comes not from the need for sulfur-containing amino acids *per se* but rather from a decreased efficiency of conversion of methionine to cystine.

Two out of four subjects tested retained nitrogen on 1.4 gm lysine daily. The two subjects in negative balance on this amount (the two men in the group over 60) retained nitrogen when 2.8 gm lysine were fed daily. Even 1.4 gm lysine daily is well in excess of the 0.8 to 0.9 gm daily proposed as the requirement for the young by other investigators.[77,82]

The authors conclude that, under the experimental conditions imposed, elderly men require more than twice the amount of methionine and lysine needed for nitrogen equilibrium or retention in young adults.

Plasma Amino Acids. These authors have complemented previous studies by recent observations on the amino acid content of postabsorptive plasma of subjects fed diets containing various levels of dietary protein.[74,84,84a] In young men and in men over 60 who were in nitrogen equilibrium on a diet containing 45 gm of well-balanced protein (7.0 gm nitrogen), they observed relatively constant proportions of plasma amino acid concentrations and relatively constant essential/nonessential (E/N) ratios. When dietary protein was doubled, these proportions and ratios were essentially unchanged. However, when low-protein (3.5 gm nitrogen) diets were fed, the plasma essential amino acids except for lysine gradually fell until, after 60 days on the diet, they were reduced from zero day values by an average of 66 per cent. While the essentials fell, the plasma nonessentials rose so that the total amino acid concentration remained the same or actually increased. Hence, the plasma E/N ratios were reduced by as much as 55 per cent when the subjects consumed the low-protein diet for 60 days. The E/N ratios were much lower while subjects consumed the low-protein diet than were the ratios found in the same subjects on either self-selected diets or on the 7.0 gm nitrogen per day diet. On the 14.0 gm nitrogen diet, the E/N ratios reached maxima more rapidly than they attained the minima on the 3.5 gm nitrogen diet. In one subject who received for eight days a diet containing only 0.5 gm nitrogen per day, complemented by adequate calories, the E/N ratio at the end of the study was low and valine and threonine values were reduced while the alanine concentration was high. This suggested that removal of all protein from the diet results in virtually the same plasma amino acid pattern changes as does a diet containing 3.5 gm nitrogen.[84a]

Data presently available[74] which make direct comparisons between young and old subjects on the same diet are confined to one tabulation in which four college students were found to have total essential amino acid concentrations of 92 μ moles per 100 ml and an E/N ratio of 48, whereas five men over 60 were found to have total essential amino acid concentrations of 87 μ moles per 100 ml and an E/N ratio of 45. Both groups were consuming a 7 gm nitrogen diet.

Swendseid[74] tentatively regards the low E/N ratio as an indicator of inadequate protein nutritional status, provided disease states and dietary intake are given adequate consideration or are controlled.[84a] Since most of the increase in nonessential amino acids is confined to asparagine-glutamine and alanine, all actively involved in transamination,[85] Swendseid also raises the question as to whether the plasma concentrations of these amino acids would increase if metabolic processes were unable to supply adequate amounts of the keto acids necessary to synthesize these amino acids,[74,86] as might occur if a calorie deficit were combined with a low-protein diet. Some preliminary evidence[87,88] supporting this concept has been obtained in elderly, obese but otherwise healthy subjects undergoing starvation for 28 days. In contrast to the elderly men fed calorically adequate diets containing 3.5 gm of nitrogen, these men showed an approximately 30 per cent increase in branched-chain amino acids (valine, leucine, isoleucine) for 3 weeks, followed by a fall to normal or low values at the end of 4 weeks. The initial rise in the branched-chain acids was accompanied by a decrease in nonessential amino acids. The fate of the nonessentials during the fourth week in these preliminary studies was not reported.

Plasma Amino Acids During Starvation. In a report on prolonged starvation as a treatment for severe obesity, Drenick et al.[89] presented data on five subjects, aged 37, 38, 39, 52 and 71, whose plasma amino acids were measured at the beginning and at intervals during periods of starvation lasting from 22 to 90 days. These subjects showed initial high E/N ratios due to increased concentrations of branched-chain amino acids ranging from 19 to 29 per cent of total amino acids, compared with a range of 13 to 18 per cent in healthy, nonobese subjects. After 20 to 30 days of fasting, little change was observed. However, after 50 to 60 days, the branched-chain amino acids and the E/N ratios decreased. In one subject, the values fell in the normal range after 90 days of starvation.

No differences were apparent between the younger and the older subjects.

Swendseid notes two instances where protein undernutrition is not associated with low E/N ratios: the prolonged starvation of grossly obese subjects[89] and the administration for five-day periods of purified amino acid diets lacking in phenylalanine or lysine.[74] The complete absence of calories prevents the rise of nonessential amino acids. Caloric restriction (900 calories per day) superimposed on protein restriction (3.5 gm nitrogen per day),[84a] however, failed to prevent the rise in nonessential amino acids and the fall in E/N ratio. Abnormally high E/N ratios have been observed in gross obesity, in some diabetics and in healthy subjects on ketogenic diets.[86] All elevated ratios are caused by increases in branched-chain amino acids. Since these conditions have gluconeogenesis in common, a high E/N ratio may indicate increased gluconeogenesis.

Support for this thesis has been found in data from studies of the influence on plasma amino acid concentrations of variations in proportions of fat and carbohydrate fed young subjects on isonitrogenous diets containing 21.5 gm nitrogen per day.[89a] Urinary nitrogen excretion was greater on the high fat- than on the high-carbohydrate diet. On the high-fat diet, branched-chain amino acid concentrations were elevated, the alanine level decreased and the concentration of α-aminobutyric acid was increased. The lower alanine concentration suggests increased transamination of alanine to pyruvic acid, as would occur with increased gluconeogenesis. The high concentration of α-aminobutyric acid suggests an accumulation of this amino acid when threonine and methionine are more rapidly catabolized. Since studies with perfused rat and dog livers[89b,c] have shown liver, the chief site of amino acid catabolism, to be relatively ineffective in the oxidation of branched-chain amino acids, Swendseid et al. conclude that, in the presence of increased amino acid catabolism (as in gluconeogenesis), branched-chain plasma amino acid concentrations would rise.

Swendseid et al. have more recently studied[89d] in five groups of patients (college students receiving 14 gm dietary N per day; elderly men, 14 gm N per day; elderly men, 3.5 gm N per day; college students on a ketogenic diet; and grossly obese patients on ad libitum food intake) the effect on plasma amino acid concentrations over a 4-hour interval of the oral administration 12 hours postprandially of 175 gm of glucose dissolved in 200 ml of water. One additional group of college students and laboratory personnel was given only 200 ml of water 12 hours postprandially. Another similar group received 80 gm of corn oil homogenized with Tween 80 in water.

In the first three groups, glucose administration resulted in significant reductions of total essential amino acid concentrations below control values. No significant reductions of total nonessential amino acid concentrations were noted. However, alanine values were usually elevated. Students on the ketogenic diet and obese subjects showed decreases in essential (not significant) and nonessential (significant $p = < .05$) amino acid concentrations. The subjects receiving water and corn oil showed no changes in total essential or nonessential amino acid concentrations. Since the decreases of amino acid concentrations were well correlated with one another (cystine-H being the only exception), the authors developed proportionality patterns for the students and elderly men receiving high- and low-protein diets. Since glucose loading has been shown to increase protein synthesis,[89e,f] the study provided an opportunity to observe the amino acid pattern of a hypothetical protein being synthesized in old and young men and in old men on both high- and low-protein diets.

No quantitative or qualitative differences were observed between the subjects on high- and on low-protein diets. Nor were differences of statistical significance noted between college students and old men. The only suggestive differences between young and old were the consistently lower mean reductions (expressed as μ moles/100 ml) in plasma concentrations of essential amino acids of the elderly men on the high-protein diet when compared to the mean reductions of similarly fed college students. The authors conclude that the protein or proteins formed from amino acids removed from plasma following a glucose load have similar essential amino acid compositions in young subjects and in old subjects fed diets either adequate or restricted in protein.

In a study of the serum amino acid response in young men to isocaloric test meals, Yearick and Nadeau[89g] observed greater increases following high- (44 gm/day) than following moderate- (31 gm/day) protein meals but found no significant effects of the fat to carbohydrate ratios in the meals at either protein level.

Plasma Amino Acids on Diets Deficient in a Single Amino Acid. Swendseid *et al.*[87] and Swendseid[74] have also reported results of studies in which postabsorptive plasma amino acid concentrations were measured in subjects who for 7 days received diets deficient in single amino acids. When lysine, phenylalanine or tyrosine was lacking, total plasma amino acids tended to increase due to elevations in glycine, alanine and serine and also in some of the essential amino acids. The concentration of the amino acid lacking in the diet remained constant. The E/N ratio during the 7-day periods of these studies remained unchanged. In all subjects, nitrogen losses during the 7-day periods were in excess of 1 gm daily. When a diet deficient in valine was studied[89a] (because during low-protein diet studies valine had been reduced the most among essential amino acids in plasma), valine plasma concentrations fell rapidly; however, the threonine concentration rose and neither the E/N ratio nor the nonessential amino acid concentrations were changed. Hence, a marked difference was observed between negative nitrogen balances induced by omission of an essential amino acid and those induced by fasting or by a low-protein diet.

Plasma Amino Acids Following Test Doses of Branched-Chain Amino Acids. Swendseid *et al.*[89h] have studied the effect of 2-gm test doses of leucine, isoleucine and valine on concentrations of plasma amino acids in middle-aged and elderly obese and normal weight fasting subjects. In the succeeding four hours, leucine but not isoleucine or valine returned to fasting concentration. Leucine but not isoleucine or valine administration caused re-ductions in the plasma concentrations of the other branched-chain amino acids. No meaningful differences were observed in the responses of obese or normal weight subjects.

Protein Synthesis in Aging. Another investigative approach to the study of protein metabolism in aging has been taken by Sharp *et al.*[90] They fed N^{15} tagged yeast to four elderly female subjects (average age 66) and to one young male and one young female subject (both aged 24). During 5 days following the feeding of the tagged yeast, they observed retentions of absorbed N^{15} of 49.1 per cent in the elderly and 57.6 per cent in the young subjects. Based on the amount of N^{15} absorbed the amount of nitrogen (both fed and recycled) used for protein synthesis was 0.204 gm/kg/day in the elderly and 0.284 gm/kg/day in the young subjects. The mean N^{15} half-life was 61 days in the elderly and 86 days in the young. The turnover of N^{15} (protein, nitrogen) in the young was about one and one-half times that in the elderly. The authors concluded that the rate of protein synthesis is slowed by physiologic aging.

Another study of the rates of amino acid incorporation into protein was performed by Tschudy *et al.*[91] in a 54-year-old woman with lymphosarcoma during an inactive phase of her disease. The study of the rates of nitrogen incorporation into protein was designed to measure in quantitative terms the effect of variations in the protein calorie/total calorie ratio in the diet, and the differences between inactive and active phases of the disease. The incorporation rate was increased significantly only when both total calories and protein calories were simultaneously raised. This increased rate was associated with a more rapid metabolic pool turnover associated with the higher calorie intake but was unaccompanied by more nitrogen retention than when the patient was on an equally high-protein but lower-calorie diet. One year later, the patient was again studied,[92] this time with active neoplastic disease. She was unable to consume more than the low-calorie, low-protein regimen of the previous investigations. The rate of nitrogen incorporation into protein and the metabolic pool turnover rate were both increased to values equivalent to those observed on the high-calorie, high-protein diet of the earlier study. This investigation clearly indicates both that dietary intake must be carefully standardized among subjects and that disease must be excluded from all subjects if changes in rates of protein synthesis are to be correlated with aging *per se* and not with some extraneous factor.

In summary, the dietary protein needs of adult man have yet to be related satisfactorily to the aging process. The existence of great variation in protein requirement for nitrogen equilibrium among the aged is the only conclusive fact arising from many balance investigations. Agewise studies of serum proteins and of adaptations to protein withdrawal and to refeeding have led to no conclusions which could be related to aging *per se*. Studies using pure L-amino acids which have indicated greater requirements among the aged are counterbalanced by others of slightly different design in which indications of marked differences in amino acid requirement were not demonstrated. All these investigations show marked inter-individual variation among the aged. Differences based on age alone in the E/N ratios in plasma are so small as to lack significance. Turnover studies provide some evidence of slower protein synthesis but even this must be tempered by considerations of the sex and body composition of the elderly subjects studied and by the nature of the tagged protein fed. Obviously, a clear answer to the question of protein requirement must await more carefully controlled investigations in larger numbers of elderly and young subjects unimpaired by disease. Even more desirable would be longitudinal studies in the same subjects conducted at stated intervals over a span of many years.[13a]

Fat. Relating the aging process *per se* to quantitative or qualitative intake of dietary fat is complicated in man by the ubiquitous nature of the disease atherosclerosis. Since diagnosis of the presence, let alone quantification of the extent, of atherosclerosis is virtually impossible in man, short of autopsy or clinical indications of important vascular occlusions, experimental work in human subjects who are guaranteed free of atherosclerosis cannot be performed. The best compromise has been work in population groups known by experience to have low mortality rates attributable to and little autopsy evidence of atherosclerosis. Often these groups habitually consume diets low in total fat and/or diets containing fat, a high percentage of which is in the form of unsaturated oils.[93,94] However, since these same population groups often live under environmental circumstances which preclude optimum personal hygiene, public sanitation and preventive and curative medicine, they form a poor group in which to conduct studies relating dietary fat to aging *per se*.

Many carefully controlled clinical investigations[95-100] have left little doubt that substitution of unsaturated for saturated fats will depress serum cholesterol concentrations as well as those of other serum lipids which have been correlated in surveys of population groups with clinical evidences of atherosclerosis.[94,101,102] Consequently, it is customary to recommend that the aged who have statistically a great prevalence of atherosclerosis adhere to diets moderate in total fat, a high percentage of which should be in the form of unsaturated oil. Of greater importance are efforts directed at the prevention of atherosclerosis through the use of similar measures throughout youth and middle age. Despite strong circumstantial evidence in favor of restricting total fat and of substituting unsaturated for saturated fats, the Committee on Dietary Fat Levels of the Council on Foods and Nutrition of the American Medical Association[103] has cautioned that no direct causal relationship between dietary or serum lipids concentrations and atherosclerosis has been proved. The committee recommends that any manipulations with dietary fat be regarded as experimental procedures as far as the prevention and treatment of atherosclerosis is concerned.

The final report (1968) of the U.S. National Diet-Heart Study (1963–1965)[103a,b] on the feasibility of studying the effects of low-fat, low-cholesterol, high-polyunsaturated-fatty acid diets on serum cholesterol concentrations in both free-living and closed populations includes the recommendation that a 5-year, major definitive study of the effects of diet on the primary prevention of myocardial infarction be planned and put into operation as soon as possible. Such a study, if successfully completed, will provide data on which to base further recommendations on the use of diet control as a public health measure in the prevention of myocardial infarction and other manifestations of atherosclerosis. As observed in the final report,[103a] such data may have profound implications for major food processors in the United States and abroad. Properly designed, it could provide data relative to the impact of nutrition, if any, on the aging process *per se*.

At this point, it should be re-emphasized that prevention or treatment of atherosclerosis is not the prevention of aging. Atherosclerosis is a disease; aging is for the time being an inexorable biochemical process. It may at some future date be demonstrated that the biochemical changes associated with aging may be related to those leading to the disease atherosclerosis. The influence of quantitative and qualitative changes in dietary fat on plasma amino acid concentrations[89a,103c] suggests other relationships between dietary lipids and aging. For the present, however, it is well to remember that progress in understanding the aging process, progress which may well cause the aging process to submit to modification by man, is more likely to come from studies in basic chemistry, physics and mathematics[21,24,28,29,31,32,104] than from investigations primarily aimed at modifying a widespread chronic disease.

During the past half-decade, interest in the Fredrickson classification of serum lipid and lipoprotein patterns in persons with familial hyperlipoproteinemia has spread beyond academic centers to become a diagnostic reality in the evaluation of all age groups.[104a] The dietary management of each of the five types affords a means of protecting those affected from premature disability and death. The interrelationships of each of the types to aging as a biological process remain to be explored.

Carbohydrate. Carbohydrate once was called the "Cinderella of human nutrition,"[105] in large measure because it was a nutrient whose physiologic role in human nutrition

had been overlooked or given scant attention. As far as aging and its associated diseases were concerned, carbohydrate received far less attention by qualified investigators than either protein or fat. Studies applying various tolerance tests suggested[106,107,107a] that man's ability to metabolize carbohydrate is reduced with advancing age. On the other hand, it was reported that in diabetics greater carbohydrate tolerance was observed in patients fed a high-carbohydrate diet over periods of several weeks.[113] Concern was expressed by many authors at the "empty calories" found in the high-carbohydrate diets of certain categories of the aged.[108–110] Gustafsson et al.[111] presented strong evidence that consumption of large amounts of carbohydrate-containing foods, especially those which adhere for long periods on tooth surfaces, leads to a high caries rate in susceptible persons.

When carbohydrate is present as a high percentage of total calories in man's diet, lactescence appears in serum associated with a rise in the concentrations of S_f 20–400 β-lipoproteins.[103] This has been attributed to the accumulation of triglycerides synthesized endogenously from carbohydrate.[104a,112] Moreover, merely increasing the frequency of carbohydrate ingestion of a fixed amount daily from three times to six or more times clearly results in reduced insulin requirements in diabetics.[114,115] In studies with isocaloric, isonitrogenous diets, frequent carbohydrate ingestion has resulted in lower serum cholesterol concentrations and greater nitrogen retention than similar quantities ingested three times daily.[115] In a variety of ways, therefore, carbohydrate has long been a nutrient of great potential to those interested in the process of aging and its associated diseases.

The fact that carbohydrate is no longer the "Cinderella of human nutrition" is indicated by the plethora of studies dealing with its metabolism which have appeared in recent years. While the effects of carbohydrates on lipid metabolism in animals were observed previously,[115a] attention more recently has been stimulated by the papers of Yudkin[115b,c,d] and others [115e–k] indicting refined carbohydrates for hypertriglyceridemia and hypercholesterolemia and for an increased incidence of ischemic heart disease in man.[115d,l,m] The majority of studies have suggested that highly refined carbohydrates, particularly sucrose, when substituted isocalorically for complex carbohydrates such as starch, lead to an increase in the concentrations of serum cholesterol and serum triglycerides.[115i-o]

In regard to aging as a biologic process no meaningful studies of carbohydrate nutrition have been performed.

Minerals. *Calcium.* As is atherosclerosis, osteoporosis is often regarded as a manifestation of the aging process.[116,116a,116b] In its primary type, it is, however, a disease which much experimental and epidemiologic evidence relates to negative calcium balances, small in quantity but continued over long periods of time.[117,118,119,120,120a] This evidence is contradictory to the longstanding hypothesis of Reifenstein and Albright[55] that osteoporosis is associated with lack of adequate protein matrix. Therapy also has changed in that greater calcium intake, the ingestion of strontium[120b] and the use of sodium fluoride[120 c–h] have tended to supplant estrogen and androgen therapy. However, no single therapeutic regimen is clearly ascendant, leading many cautious investigators to acknowledge the pluralistic etiology of this disease.[116a,120i,j] Exton-Smith,[120k] in agreement with Garn et al.,[120l,m] has concluded that bone loss in old age cannot conclusively be related to calcium intake in adult life but that considerable evidence exists relating the amount of bone present in old age directly to the skeletal mass at maturity.

These investigations in osteoporosis have raised anew the question of the optimum calcium intake for man, and particularly for the elderly. Hegsted et al.[121] observed metabolic equilibrium for calcium among prisoners in Peru who were accustomed to low-calcium intakes with calcium intakes as low as 0.2 to 0.3 gm daily. Walter[122] also has observed adaptation to low-calcium diets. Malm,[123] working with elderly men, observed successful adaptation to diets containing from 0.9 down to 0.45 gm daily. In calcium balance studies in elderly men lasting for many months, he also observed cyclic alterations in calcium balance. These cyclic changes emphasize the caution which must be exercised in evaluating any parameter in the aged, especially when that parameter is measured only over a short period of time. Smith et al.[120i] have found higher serum calcium and phosphorus concentrations and greater antirachitic activity in the sera of Puerto Rican than in those of Michigan women, suggesting that sunlight exposure may be related to lower prevalence rates for osteoporosis in tropical climates. Calkins,[124] studying an aging male while in a metabolic research unit and later when the man worked on his own farm, found increased retentions of calcium, phosphorus and nitrogen during the second phase of the investigation. Hence, environment[120i] and activity[116a,b] are additional variables which must be standardized in comparing metabolic parameters in individuals or groups.

Higher calcium requirements for the aged than for the young have been reported.[125–127] On the other hand, no differences in requirements for old and young have been reported by others.[47,123] Calcium was not stored in one investigation[47] despite retention of large amounts of phosphorus and nitrogen. Similar findings were observed[60] in old men retaining large amounts of nitrogen and phosphorus at two dietary protein levels both with and without a potent synthetic androgen. By a re-evaluation of data collected from seven sources, Harrison[128] has inferred that there is little difference in the efficiency of calcium absorption among old men, young adults and older children, although his evaluation revealed a very high calcium absorption efficiency among infants.

Lutwak, Krook, Henrikson et al. have presented impressive evidence that bone resorption in human periodontal disease and in experimental models in animals can be prevented or reversed by adequate calcium intakes. They suggest that bone loss in general can be prevented at any age and under a variety of physiological states (e.g., posttraumatic immobilization) by the provision of calcium in at least the Recommended Daily Allowance if not higher in the dietary regimen.[128a,b,c,d]

On the whole, present evidence suggests that the calcium requirements of the aged in good health are at least equivalent to those of younger adults. In view of data on bone mineralization in old age,[129,130,131] not to mention data in osteoporosis (*v.s.*), long-term negative calcium balances, occasioned either by deficient intake in earlier adulthood or by some as yet undefined metabolic defect associated with aging, indicate a need in many aged persons for greater dietary intake of calcium. This in turn implies a need for greater consumption of milk, a product which is often unpopular among or too expensive for the aged. The problem of unpopularity may be resolved by education campaigns and the issue of cost, by the use of powdered skim milk. When milk or milk products are absolutely contraindicated, calcium gluconate or lactate may be needed to rectify a continued negative calcium balance. Attention to dietary calcium intake should be matched by encouragement of physical activity, the anabolic consequences of which have already been mentioned (*v.s.*).

Phosphorus. Dietary phosphorus has gained new significance as a result of some studies in rodents and primates[132] suggesting that increased dietary phosphorus may lead to greater protection against caries in childhood and adolescence. Animal studies suggest a similar role for phosphorus in improving bone structure. However, increasing the phosphorus content in the diets of the aged has yet to be undertaken experimentally and should be approached with considerable caution in view of the linear decrements in renal function associated with the aging process after age 30. Hyperphosphatemia is a common companion of azotemia in renal disease. Lives have been saved in acute situations or prolonged in chronic disease states by the prescription of such high-carbohydrate, low-protein, low-phosphorus diets as the rice diets.[46] When only conventional diets are available, phosphorus absorption may be prevented by the administration of two hourly, 30-ml doses of aluminum hydroxide gel, a procedure that will reduce urinary phosphorus concentration practically to zero and keep serum phosphorus concentrations in the normal range.[133,133a] The high-phosphorus diets associated with the ingestion of large amounts of meat and soft drinks by some segments of the population lower the calcium/phosphorus ratio in diets and may predispose those affected to osteopenia unless sufficient calcium is included in the diet to maintain a ratio of one or higher.[133b]

Fluorine, when consumed by children under five in drinking water with a concentration of one part per million (ppm), will protect teeth from dental caries during childhood and adolescence and preserve these instruments of mastication for use throughout adulthood and into old age.[134,135] Scientific data to support the contention of certain groups that fluoridation of drinking water in the recommended concentration is harmful have not been presented.

As mentioned in the discussion of calcium (*v.s.*), sodium fluoride in doses ranging from 50 to 150 mg/day[135a] has been under investigation as a treatment for osteoporosis. Both epidemiologic evidence[120h] and clinical investigation by balance study and bone density techniques[120e] have indicated a potential role for fluoride in prevention and treatment. Not all investigators have been enthusiasts,[120j,135b] the favorable effects being transitory or negligible in their hands. Toxic manifestations of sodium fluoride therapy such as anorexia, epigastric pain, ectopic calcification, optic neuritis and retinal damage[135a,b] serve as reminders that sodium fluoride therapy is still an experimental procedure. The potential hazards of the fluoride content of bones incorporated into whole fish flour is under investigation.

Iron in food or as a medication should be provided daily to individuals of all ages, with modifications in dosage to meet special requirements of childhood, pregnancy and lactation and disease. Aged males and postmenopausal females without blood loss due to disease may develop an iron deficiency on the basis of inadequate intake alone if the deficient diet is consumed over many years (see Chapter 6C). Parenteral iron is usually contraindicated by its inconvenience and expense, not to mention its potential carcinogenicity.[136]

Iodine is essential to the proper function of the thyroid gland throughout life. If iodinized salt is contraindicated as a source of iodine because of diets restricted in sodium, other iodine-containing medications should be administered to provide the appropriate amount of iodine daily.

Although *sodium* is an essential component of any diet, its restriction in therapeutic diets has caused it to become a household term to patients with congestive heart failure, hypertension, cirrhosis of the liver with ascites and other conditions associated with the retention of extracellular fluid. Among mature and elderly adults whose physicians prescribe low-sodium diets, two problems arise. First, it is difficult for a patient to secure meals low in sodium if he eats in restaurants or with others who practice no sodium restriction. Second, by lowering the palatability of diets, sodium restriction may lead to lowered food consumption and therefore to deficiencies in the intake of other essential nutrients.

The first problem is related to the general one of obtaining proper nutrition counseling and appropriate, low-cost foods as discussed in detail above. The second requires reeducation of the patient and, if necessary, the substitution of other sodium-free flavoring agents and condiments or of commercially available salt substitutes. Of paramount importance, however, is motivating the patient to adhere to his diet, and this is a task requiring great ingenuity on the part of his physician and of all others in the patient's immediate environment.

Hypernatremia is a serious and usually preventable problem seen not infrequently in patients whose medical condition requires feedings administered by tube.[137] If the tube feeding is high in protein and salt, the resulting load of urea and salt which must be excreted increases the obligatory renal water loss sufficiently to produce a negative water balance and hypernatremia. Hence, great care must be given to the water requirements of tube-fed patients, especially to those who are obtunded or comatose and unable to respond to the sensation of thirst. If hypernatremia occurs, the appropriate treatment is the administration of water, enough to add 4 per cent of the body weight in kg for each 10 mEq/liter increase in serum sodium above normal.[138]

Potassium is so widely distributed among natural foods that primary potassium deficiency is virtually unknown. Potassium is so effectively excreted that excessive potassium intake rarely causes difficulty in healthy man. In disease states, however, both hypo- and hyperkalemia may occur; for example, the former in association with complications of surgery and the latter in renal insufficiency. Hypokalemia can be corrected by parenterally administered solutions containing potassium salts and later by the oral administration of potassium-containing foods. Hyperkalemia can be treated by administration of pure carbohydrate and fat, either orally or parenterally, supplemented by appropriate vitamins. Such regimens reduce potassium intake and also minimize tissue breakdown, an endogenous source of potassium.[139] Hyperkalemia may be attacked more directly by the administration of sodium polystyrene sulfonate, a cation exchange resin prepared in the sodium phase with exchange capacity *in vivo* of approximately 1 mEq potassium per gm. This resin when given systematically over a period of a week may result in a loss of total body potassium of greater than 10 per cent, with associated deterioration of myocardial performance, delay in cellular glucose uptake and retention of water.[139a] In either the hypo- or the hyperkalemic state, monitoring serum potassium concentrations by flame photometry or electrocardiography is required for guidance in prescribing control measures.

Vitamins. Socioeconomic conditions and reduced physical activity among the aged may lead to sharp curtailment in intake of vitamin-containing natural foods. The high costs of protective foods and of dietary supplements available to the well-to-do may eliminate these as sources of vitamins for the less fortunate. Various diseases capable of inducing secondary deficiencies are more common among the aged. It is not surprising therefore that many authors have postulated and some have sought evidence for vitamin deficiency among the elderly.

Water-Soluble Vitamins. According to one group of investigators, B-complex vitamins and ascorbic acid supplements have resulted in improved "general vitality and vigor" among the aged studied.[140] According to others, administration of B-complex vitamins and ascorbic acid has resulted in improvement in symptoms previously attributed to nonspecific senility and cerebral atherosclerosis.[141,142] One psychiatrist, influenced by these reports, has blamed further dietary restrictions superimposed on an already borderline vitamin reserve for acute psychotic episodes in elderly adults.[143] Rafsky and Newman have reported greater ascorbic acid needs,[144] greater quantities of thiamine for "saturation"[145] and lower blood thiamin concentrations and lower urinary thiamin excretions[146] in the elderly fed diets qualitatively adequate for young adults. However, Horwitt et al.,[147] in a classic series of carefully controlled metabolic studies in institutionalized subjects, have failed to reveal differences in thiamin and riboflavin excretion between young and old. No correlation between age and urinary excretion has been found in studies during which test doses of various B-complex vitamins were administered.[148,149,150]

Vitamin B_{12} was found by Watkin et al.[151] to be retained in greater amounts by old than by young men when test doses were administered parenterally at four different dose levels. Various evidence led the authors away from the usual inference that these findings pointed to a dietary deficiency or a greater need for vitamin B_{12}. Old and young subjects alike had received good diets adequate in B_{12} for many months. Other studies had indicated no influence of previous diet on the excretion of parenterally administered vitamin B_{12}.[152] Agewise decrements in renal function could not be held responsible for the differences. Studies of the renal clearance of vitamin B_{12}[153] indicated that B_{12} excretion was proportional to plasma concentration and glomerular filtration rate at plasma concentrations over 1 mμg per ml. At lower plasma concentrations, no excretion occurred. Reports of increased plasma B_{12} concentrations in patients with chronic myelocytic leukemia[154] and in those with hepatic metastases[155] led to investigations indicating that B_{12} is bound in plasma of healthy and diseased persons to a substance in the glycoprotein portion of the α_1 globulin fraction of plasma proteins.[156–158] The same investigations indicated that the B_{12}-binding capacity of the substance in the glycoprotein was exceeded in normal men at concentrations over 1 mμg per ml. While explaining satisfactorily the findings of the renal clearance studies,[153] these observations cannot explain the agewise decrements in B_{12} excretion in tolerance tests[151] and agewise decrements in B_{12} plasma concentrations.[159,160,161] Hall and Finkler[161a–c] have identified two binding proteins, transcobalamin I (TC I) identical to that of Mendelsohn et al.[156] which carries endogenous B_{12} and transcobalamin II (TC II), a protein with the mobility of a β-globulin which functions as a carrier of recently administered B_{12}. In chronic myelocytic leukemia in relapse, the TC II binding capacity was markedly diminished, whereas that of TC I was greatly increased. In Addisonian pernicious anemia, TC II binding capacity was diminished or absent but that of TC I was unaltered. Still uninvestigated are the possibilities of age-related changes in the binding capacities of TC I, TC II or other as yet undescribed binding proteins. Extension of studies on B_{12} absorption, plasma transport, metabolism and excretion[162,163] to the field of gerontology may provide explanations and may also set patterns for better assessment of nutrition with respect to other vitamins in aging man.

Fat-Soluble Vitamins. Deficiencies in fat-soluble vitamins among adults in the United States are usually secondary to consumption of low-fat diets, to the interference with absorption caused by habitual ingestion of mineral oil as a laxative[164] or to diseases characterized by steatorrhea.[165,166] The aged who are clinically free from disease and who consume an adequate diet show few evidences of fat-soluble vitamin deficiencies.

There are no agewise decrements in plasma vitamin A and carotene concentrations.[167] Absorption of vitamin A by the intestine is unchanged by aging.[168] A significant decline in visual sensitivity revealed by light threshold has been observed in the aged.[169] However, no correlation between light threshold and serum vitamin A concentrations and no improvement in light threshold after administration of 100,000 I.U. vitamin A daily for as long as 76 days have been demonstrated.[170]

Diseases preventing absorption of vitamin D, calcium and phosphorus may lead to

senile osteomalacia. Immediate therapy
consists of administration of vitamin D, calcium and phosphorus, while the ultimate
objective is correction of the illness responsible for the secondary deficiency. An inverse relation of exposure to sunshine and the
prevalence of involutional osteoporosis has
been proposed by Smith *et al.* (*v.s.*).[120i]
Treatment of rheumatoid arthritis with
massive doses (150,000 to 500,000 I.U. daily)
of vitamin D has led to vitamin D intoxication.[171–173] Signs and symptoms have included metastatic calcification, hypercalcemia, azotemia, renal insufficiency, weakness, lassitude, anorexia, visual disturbances,
anemia, dermatitis and inflammation and
fatty deposits in the sclerae. These are
dramatic reminders that nutrients in pharmacologic doses are potentially as hazardous as
are drugs.

Except for individuals with bizarre eating
habits,[174] primary vitamin K deficiency is not
observed in adults. Man obtains the vitamin
not only in his food but also from synthesis by
the intestinal microflora. Hence, various
diseases and types of therapy which interfere
with fat absorption also interfere with absorption of vitamin K. In addition, sulfa drugs
and antibiotics if taken in amounts large
enough to substantially reduce the number of
intestinal microflora will reduce the amount
of vitamin K available for absorption. Any
condition reducing production or absorption
of vitamin K will reduce prothrombin synthesis for which the vitamin is essential. Hypoprothrombinemia in turn leads to poor
clotting, bleeding, purpura and inadequate
wound healing. When hypoprothrombinemia
continues despite parenteral administration
of vitamin K, severely impaired liver function
is suggested. The use of Dicumarol as an
anticoagulant following myocardial infarction
and in other diseases characterized by intravascular clotting has popularized the use of
vitamin K as an antidote in cases of Dicumarol overdosage.[175]

In experimental animals, vitamin E deficiency has produced disorders in reproduction
in females, sterility in males, abnormal red
blood cell susceptibility to destruction by
hydrogen peroxide, degenerative changes in
skeletal and cardiac muscle and encephalo-

malacia. Efforts to relate comparable conditions in humans to vitamin E deficiency
have not been supported by acceptable
data.[176a–c] Recently, however, more responsible investigations have substantiated
the relationship of vitamin E deficiency to
the increased susceptibility of red cells
from premature and full-term babies to
hemolysis by dilute solutions of hydrogen
peroxide,[176d,e] the shortening of erythrocyte
lifetime in adults[176f] and megaloblastic anemia
in infants.[176g] Patients with malabsorption
syndromes have manifested many classic
signs of vitamin E deficiency.[176c] The problem of evaluating lesser degrees of vitamin
E deficiency in man has been plagued by
methodological problems.[176c] Bunnell *et
al.*[176h] have estimated the α-tocopherol daily
intake in "average" American diets to range
from 2.6 to 15.4 mg, with an over-all average
of 7.4 mg daily. They suggest that this indicates the possibility of relatively low α-
tocopherol intakes in some portions of the
population. Among these could be aged
groups whose general dietary practice and
socioeconomic condition might exclude vegetable oils, the best source of vitamin E.

Horwitt[176i] has demonstrated in adults an
acceleration of α-tocopherol depletion by increasing the dietary intake of polyunsaturated
fatty acids. The rapid rise in polyunsaturated
oil consumption[176h] has raised the interesting
question of whether or not this may increase
the prevalence of vitamin E-deficiency disease
or at least increase vitamin E requirements.
To date, one excellent clinical study[176i] has
provided a negative answer. In consideration of the Horwitt findings (*v.s.*) and the
mean polyunsaturated oil intake (24 gm/
capita/day),[176k] the Food and Nutrition
Board's *Recommended Dietary Allowances*[49] suggests an adult tocopherol requirement of
from 10 to 30 mg per day. In mild criticism
of this recommendation, Herting concludes
his "Perspective on Vitamin E"[176c] stating:
"Faced with the knowledge that man requires
vitamin E, that the vitamin E content of
many foodstuffs is low, that a number of
observations suggest an incidence of suboptimal nutrition of vitamin E and that several presumably normal populations have
shown signs of vitamin E deficiency, it is

evident that every reasonable step should be taken to assure the normal requirement to healthy persons, and a generous amount to the ill, especially to those in whom the supply or absorption may be interrupted."

While Herting's argument is well documented, the caution of the Food and Nutrition Board reflects the diversity of reports in the clinical realm re man's need for vitamin E. It is encouraging to note that work even more recent than that mentioned above suggests a specific role for vitamin E in the processes of protein synthesis.[176l] As these investigations reveal the details of α-tocopherol function in human metabolism, a more secure place in human nutrition and perhaps in the biochemistry of aging itself may be assured to vitamin E.

In 1972, vitamin E sales rose so rapidly as to rival those of the Pauling-popularized vitamin C.[176m] As the "latest nutrition fad,"[176n] priced between $5.00 and $7.00 per 100 capsules, vitamin E is being promoted by food faddists as a means of slowing down "the ravages of aging."[176o] In spite of these developments, evidence is not available that the American diet is sufficiently lacking in vitamin E to warrant intakes up to 30 times the Food and Nutrition Board's *Recommended Dietary Allowance*. Certainly, much more work will be required to support a role for vitamin E in pharmacologic doses in the prevention of the deleterious effects of aging among humans eating a conventional diet. Recent British studies[176p] point out the need for more accurate data on the vitamin E content of commonly eaten foods and also suggest that the vitamin E content of the same food may vary substantially from sample to sample. In general the British workers found, using laboratory analyses of diets to supply data, that the vitamin E content of the self-selected diets was less than recommended by British health authorities.[176q]

Water. Although potable water is available in most parts of the United States, it is an inexpensive nutrient which the aged, through custom or distaste, consume in less than optimum quantities. Water can be a useful aid in washing down partially masticated food which might otherwise prove too difficult to eat. When consumed in copious amounts, it reduces the osmotic work of the kidney. In patients subject to renal and vesical lithiasis, such as those confined to bed or paralyzed by accident or disease, water intakes as high as 4 liters daily are needed to prevent stone formation. Water has been suggested as a means of improving elimination.[177]

Water need not be taken in pure form. The aged often find it more acceptable in soups, juices, milk products, soft drinks, alcoholic beverages, tea and coffee. In prescribing such easily ingested and pleasant liquids, care must be taken to avoid overconsumption of pure appetite-satisfying calories and the consequent exclusion of protective foods from the diet.

The dangers of hypernatremia during tube feeding of obtunded and comatose patients with formulas prepared with insufficient water have already been mentioned (*v.s.*). Hyponatremia associated with apparent overhydration not infrequently complicates the courses of many chronic illnesses. While water restriction alone may be attempted in such cases, administration of a hypertonic solution of sodium chloride with dosage calculated on the basis of total body water is a more direct method of returning the deranged electrolyte pattern toward normal. Even so, water still must be restricted at the price of extreme thirst if the maneuver is to have a lasting effect. In chronic illnesses, in contrast to more acute situations, hypotonicity of body fluids have grave prognostic implications.

The water content of diets has received increasing attention with respect to its effect on the utilization of other nutrients by and on the body composition of growing animals.[178,179] Such effects have not been investigated in controlled studies in older animals or in aged man. Most research protocols have permitted *ad libitum* water intakes, thereby precluding any preliminary evaluation from work already completed. In view of the great variance associated with most parameters by which nutritional status is assessed in the aged, control of the water intake variable is recommended in future studies.

Calories. Calories have already received attention either in general discussion of nutrition and aging or under the respective headings of their components, protein, fat and carbohydrate. Mention has been made of the influence of under- or intermittent feeding on the aging of collagen. Note has been taken of the differences observed in many parameters when isocaloric diets are fed as three meals or taken as numerous small feedings throughout the day. Mention must be made also of the impressive role of caloric restriction in the prevention of chronic illness, well documented in man by the morbidity and mortality statistics among the over-weight.[180] In animals, calorie restriction has long been associated with greater longevity than has *ad libitum* feeding.[181,182a,b,c] Ross[182c] has recently demonstrated that the age of the rat at which dietary restriction begins is an important determinant of longevity. Restricting food intake from 21 to 70 days only, even though *ad libitum* feeding ensued throughout life, increased life duration. The adverse effects of *ad libitum* feeding early in life were partially overcome by restriction imposed at 70 days of age. Ross found the level of restriction most favorable for longevity to change with age. Rats severely restricted from age 21 days until death lived longest. When the same severe restriction was imposed later in life (300 days), life expectancy decreased; in somewhat older rats (365 days), life duration was drastically shortened. However, in these same older rats, the length of life could be extended when less severe degrees of restriction were imposed. Although not altering the morbidity from radiculoneuritis,[183] calorie restriction has afforded protection against almost every disease afflicting the rat.[184]

The control of overt obesity and its consequences is not the only reason for advocating calorie restriction throughout adult life. It may be advocated also for the millions not overtly obese who consume daily well into middle age calories in excess of those required for energy balance. They may show slow gains in weight and/or shifts in body composition. Premature changes in the islets of Langerhans, accumulation of lipids in arterial walls, increased load on the heart and the incompletely known effects of subjecting certain enzyme systems to excessive metabolic loads

increase the potential hazard of disease for all over-eaters. Volunteers on low-calorie diets have demonstrated greater mechanical efficiencies than similarly trained subjects on high-calorie regimens.[186]

Since calorie balance is dependent on thermodynamic equilibrium between food intake and energy expenditure, it is obvious that there should be a progressive decline in calorie ingestion to correspond with the progressive decline in physical activity beginning in the third decade and continuing throughout life if weight gain or, more important, an increase in the ratio of fat/nonfat tissue in the body is to be avoided. Not uncommonly, calorie intake in excess of calorie expenditure continues into middle age until death or some medical catastrophe intervenes. This situation strongly suggests the need of a carefully planned, intelligently presented, scientifically sound campaign conducted via all communication media to encourage regulation of calorie intake by all adults. A program of physical activity designed to meet individual requirements should be encouraged to take full advantage of the anabolic properties of exercise[124] and its ability to clear lipids from the blood.[185] In other words, even though restriction of calorie intake seems under average circumstances to be the most effective way to avoid calorie accretion, equilibrium still is the resultant of balanced forces, indicating that reasonable activity can be used effectively in achieving optimum calorie nutrition in the aging and even the aged.

CONCLUDING COMMENTS

This chapter has been designed to acquaint its readers with various aspects of gerontology that involve considerations of nutrition. Gerontology, the study of aging, is quite distinct from geriatrics, the treatment of disease in the aged. As long as knowledge of aging as a process is limited as it still is today, few clues exist as to methods of altering the process by nutritional means.[187] Most existing evidence reviewed here points to intrauterine and postnatal periods of life as those during which nutrition has most impact on aging as a biological process. For the moment, prevention of chronic illness by nutritional planning from youth through late maturity promises the greatest rewards in terms of a healthy, active old age. For the aged, recent moves by government and private sector agencies promise to relieve the burdens of hunger and poverty, leaving the elderly and their champions more opportunity to lend their support to the funding of investigation benefiting future aged but obviously not those who are old today. Hence, it may be safely concluded that for man the aging process cannot be substantially affected by nutritional measures. For the moment, prevention of chronic illness by nutritional planning in youth and late maturity promises the greatest rewards in terms of a healthy, active old age. Among the aged themselves, the large interindividual variation resulting from the lack of similarity among individuals in the temporal manifestation of aging patterns of the genome and the infinite variety of physical and emotional insults during long lives makes general recommendations for the aged as a class meaningless and mere grist for the mills of food faddists. Physicians informed in the role of nutrition in the management of health and disease who can offer the aged individualized medical care and a sympathetic understanding of the biologic and socioeconomic aspects of being old have no replacements. In a few years, as research in molecular biology unlocks the secret of aging, some more definitive role for nutrition in retarding the process *per se* may emerge. Those whose foresight has enabled them to be alive and well when that day arrives may be able to enjoy whatever benefits that role may then bestow.

BIBLIOGRAPHY

1. McWhirter and McWhirter: *The Guinness Book of World Records*, 13th Ed., London, Guinness Superlatives, Ltd., 1966.
1a.Watkin: Am. J. Pub. Health, *55*, 548, 1965.
1b.Schettlein—Gsell: Europa Medica, *1*, 177, 1964.
1c.Watkin: In *Proceedings of the Joint Meeting of the U.S. Veterans Administration Spinal Cord Injury Centers and the International Medical Society of Paraplegia*, Boston, October, 1971, (Talbot, H. S., Ed.) Washington, U.S. Veterans Administration, 1972.

1d.Watkin, D. M.: In *Proceedings of the Symposium on Changing Food Patterns*, Las Vegas, November, 1971, (Fine, P. Ed.). Chicago. American Medical Association. 1972.
1e.Vega and Robles: Salud Públ. Mex., *4*, 385, 1962.
1f.Cravioto: Am. J. Public Health, *53*, 1803, 1963.
1g.Ramos-Galván, Vega, and Cravioto: Bol. Med. Hosp. Infant. Mex., *21*, 157, 1964.
1h.Cravioto and Robles: Am. J. Orthopsychiat., *35*, 449, 1965.
1i.Cravioto, Delicardio and Birch: Pediatrics, *38*, 319, 1966.
1j.The Nutrition Foundation. *Proceedings of an International Conference on Malnutrition, Learning and Behavior*, Cambridge, Mass., Mar. 1–3, 1967.
1k.Barnes, Cunnold, Zimmerman, Simmons, MacLeod, and Krook: J. Nutrition, *89*, 399, 1966.
1l.Winick and Noble: J. Nutrition, *91*, 179, 1967.
1m.Hseuh, Augustin, and Chow: J. Nutrition, *91*, 195, 1967.
1n.Guthrie and Brown: J. Nutrition, *94*, 419, 1968.
1o.Howard and Granoff: J. Nutrition, *95*, 111, 1968.
1p.Knittle: J. Nutrition, *102*, 427, 1972.
1q.Roeder and Chow: In *Symposium on Nutrition and Aging*. Am. J. Clin. Nutr. *25*, 812, 1972.
1r.Kahn: In *Symposium on Nutrition and Aging*. Am. J. Clin. Nutr., *25*, 822, 1972.
1s.Barrows: In *Symposium on Nutrition and Aging*, Am. J. Clin. Nutr., *25*, 829, 1972.
1t.Watkin, Ferencz, Reh, Weswig, Pearson, Chichester, Kocher, Sheehy, *et al.*: Encuesta de Nutrición, República del Paraguay, Mayo-Agosto de 1965. Programa de Nutrición, Centro Nacional para el Control de Enfermedades Crónicas, Servicio de Salud Pública, Departamento de Salud, Educación y Bienestar de las EE. UU., Bethesda, Maryland, 1967, pp. 1–482.
1u.Chow, Blackwell, Blackwell, Hou, Anilane and Sherwin: Amer. J. Pub. Health., *58*, 668, 1968.
2. Mayer: Medical News, *1*, 11, May 22, 1966.
2a.White House Conference on Food, Nutrition and Health. Final Report and Addendum. Washington, D.C., Superintendent of Documents, U.S. Government Printing Office, 1969.
2b.————: pp. 62–64 plus Addendum pp. 1–5.
2c.Nutrition Subcommittee of the Domestic Council. White House Conference on Food, Nutrition and Health. Summary Report. Washington, D.C., Superintendent of Documents, U.S. Government Printing Office, December, 1970.
2d.Nutrition Subcommittee of the Domestic Council. White House Conference on Food, Nutrition and Health. Comprehensive Report. Washington, D.C., Dec., 1970.
2e.Watkin, D. M., Chairman. First Workshop to Recommend Steps to Implement Recommendations of the Panel on Aging of the White House Conference on Food, Nutrition and Health. Washington, D.C., August, 1970. Department of Health, Education and Welfare.

2f.Watkin, D. M.: Med. Clin North America, 54, 1589, 1970.

2g.White House Conference on Food, Nutrition and Health. Report of the Follow-Up Conference, Williamsburg, Va., February, 1971.

2h.Technical Committee on Nutrition, Watkin, D. M. Chairman. Issues. Chap V. Background and Issues: Nutrition. The White House Conference on Aging. March, 1971.

2i.Delegate Work Book. The White House Conference on Aging. Washington, D.C. November, 1971.

2j.Nixon, R. M.: Aging. Nos. 207–208, January-February, 1972. p. 3.

2k.Kennedy, E. M.: Aging. Nos. 207–208, January-February, 1972. p. 12.

2l.Committee on Labor and Public Welfare, U.S. Senate, 92nd Congress, 1st Session, Report No. 92–515, November 29, 1971.

2m.Committee of the Whole House on the State of the Union, U.S. House of Representatives, 92nd Congress, 1st Session, Report No. 92–726, December 9, 1971.

2n.Section on Nutrition. A Report to the Delegates from the Conference Sections and Special Concerns Sessions. 1971 White House Conference on Aging. Washington, D.C. December, 1971. pp. 23–26.

2o.Benet: New York Times Magazine, December 26, 1971, p. 3

2p.Division of Community Health Services, U.S. Public Health Service, in cooperation with Medical Care Section, American Public Health Association. Medical Care in Transition 1949–1962. Washington, D.C. Superintendent of Documents, U.S. Government Printing Office, 1964.

2q.Watkin, D. M.: Nutrition and aging in technically underdeveloped societies. In World Review of Nutrition and Dietetics (Rechcigl, M., Jr., Ed.), New York, S. Karger (in press).

2r.Watkin, D. M.: Nutritional problems today in the elderly in the United States. In Exton-Smith, A. N., and Scott, D. L., Eds. Vitamins for the Elderly: Report of the Proceedings of a Symposium held at the Royal College of Physicians, London, on 2nd May, 1968. Bristol: John Wright & Sons; Baltimore, Williams and Wilkins, 1968.

2s.Shock: In Age with a Future, p. 13, Copenhagen, Munskgaard, 1964.

2t.Oliver: In Geriatric Medicine, 2nd Ed. (E. J. Stieglitz, Ed.) Philadelphia, W. B. Saunders Co., 1949.

3. Yiengst, Barrows, Jr. and Shock: J. Gerontol., 14, 400, 1959.

3a.Brody: In Proceedings of the 7th International Congress of Gerontology, Vol. 8, Wien, Med. Akad. Wien, 1966.

3b.———: Proc. 9th International Congress of Gerontology Vol. 1 Kiev, p. 228, 1972.

4. Davies and Shock: J. Clin. Invest., 29, 496, 1950.

5. Watkin and Shock: (Abstract.) J. Clin. Invest., 34, 969, 1955.

6. Andrew, Shock, Barrows, Jr., and Yiengst: J. Gerontol., 14, 405, 1959.

7. Shock, Watkin, Yiengst, Norris, Gaffney, Gregerman, and Falzone, Jr.: J. Gerontol., 18, 1, 1963.

8. Pett and Ogilvie: Human Biol., 28, 177, 1956.

9. Norris, Shock, and Landowne: J. Gerontol., 13, 437, 1958.

10. Alvarez: Geriatrics, 15, 671, 1960.

11. Norris, Lundy, and Shock: Ann. N. Y. Acad. Sci., 110, 623, 1963.

12. Sagild: Scand. J. Clin. & Lab. Invest., 8, 44, 1956.

13. Allen, Anderson, and Langham: J. Gerontol., 15, 348, 1960.

13a.Shock: In Aging of the Lung (Cander and Moyer, Eds.), p. 1, New York, Grune and Stratton, 1964.

13b.Stone and Norris: J. Geront., 21 575, 1966.

13c.Rose: Hum. Develop., 8, 158, 1965.

14. Barrows, Jr.: Federation Proc., 15, 954, 1956.

15. Barrows, Jr., Yiengst, and Shock: J. Gerontol., 13, 351, 1958.

16. Falzone, Jr., Barrows, Jr., and Shock: J. Gerontol., 14, 2, 1959.

17. Barrows, Jr.: In The Biology of Aging (Strehler, B. L., Ed.), Symposium No. 6, p. 116, Washington, D.C., Am. Inst. Biol. Sci., 1960.

18. Barrows, Jr., Roeder, and Falzone, Jr.: J. Gerontol., 17, 144, 1962.

19. Barrows, Jr. and Roeder: J. Gerontol., 16, 321, 1961.

20. Rivlin and Knox: Am. J. Physiol., 197, 65, 1959.

21. Wulff, Quastler, and Sherman: Proc. Natl. Acad. Sci. U.S., 48, 1373, 1962.

21a.———: J. Gerontol., 19, 294, 1964.

21b.Wulff, Samis and Falzone: Adv. Gerontol. Res., 2, 37, 1967.

22. Fletcher and Sandai: J. Gerontol., 16, 255, 1961.

23. Shock: In Aging . . . Some Social and Biological Aspects (Shock, N. W., Ed.) Publ. No. viii, p. 241, Washington, D.C., Am. Assoc. Advance. Sci., 1960.

24. Medvedev: Usp. Sorrem. Biol., 51, 299, 1961.

24a.———: In Biological Aspects of Aging, (Shock, N. W., Ed.), p. 255, New York, Columbia University Press, 1962.

24b.———: In Biosynthesis of Proteins and Problems of Ontogenesis, p. 377, Moscow Gosudarstvennoe Izdatelstvo Meditsinskoy Literaturi, 1963.

24c.Ram: J. Gerontol., 22, 92, 1967.

24d.Cameron: Am. J. Psychiatry, 114, 943, 1958.

24e.Cameron, Salyom, Sved, and Wainrib: Recent Advances in Biological Psychiatry, Vol. 5, New York, Plenum Press, 1963.

24f.Cameron: Brit. J. Psychiatry, 109, 325, 1963.

24g.Cameron, Kral, Salyom, Sved, Wainrib, Beaulieu, and Enesco: In Macromolecules and Behavior, (Gaito, J., Ed.), New York, Appleton-Century-Crofts, 1966.

24h.Cameron: J.A.M.A. Medical News, 196, 29, 1966.

24*i*.Cameron and Brand: *Proceedings of the 4th World Congress of Psychiatry*, Sept. 1966, Madrid. Amsterdam, Excerpta Medica Foundation, 1967.

24*j*.Edelson: World Journal Tribune, Section 3, New York, April 9, 1967.

24*k*.Medvedev: Zhurnal Vsesouznogo Himicheskogo Obshchestva imeni D. I. Mendeleeva 8, 384, 1963.

24*l*.Medvedev: In *Advances in Gerontological Research* Vol. *1*, (Strehler, B. L., Ed.), p. 181. New York, The Academic Press, Inc., 1964.

24*m*.Medvedev: Ninth Ciba Foundation Lecture on Research on Aging. In *Aspects of the Biology of Ageing* (Woolhouse, H. W., Ed.), 21st Symp. Soc. Exp. Biol., *21*, 1, 1967, New York, Academic Press, 1967.

24*n*.von Hahn: J. Gerontol., *21*, 291, 1966.

24*o*.von Hahn: *Proceedings of the 7th International Congress of Gerontology, Vol. 8*, p. 243, Wien, Med. Akad. Wien., 1966.

25. Neuberger, Perrone, and Slack: Biochem J., *49*, 199, 1951.

26. Slack: Nature, *174*, 512, 1954.

27. Thompson and Ballou: J. Biol. Chem., *223*, 795, 1956.

28. Verzár: Sci. American, *208*, 104, 1963.

28*a*.Verzár: Exp. Gerontol., *3*, 69, 1968.

29. Chvapil, quoted by Verzár: Sci. American, *208*, 104, 1963.

30. McKay: In *Cowdry's Problems of Aging* (Lansing, A. I., Ed.), p. 139, Baltimore, Williams and Wilkins, 1952.

31. Holeckova, Chytil and Chvapil: Cas Lék ces., *100*, 612, 1961.

32. Chvapil and Holeckova: Physiol. Bohemoslov., *11*, 505, 1962.

33. Bjorksten, quoted by Verzár: Sci. American, *208*, 104, 1963.

33*a*.Piez: Ann. Rev. Biochem., *37*, 547, 1968.

34. Meyer and Verzár: Gerontologia, *3*, 184, 1959.

35. Gallop, Seifter, and Meilman: Nature, *183*, 1659, 1959.

36. Milch: Gerontologia (Basel), 7, 129, 1963.

36*a*.Milch and Murray: Proc. Soc. Exp. Biol. Med., *111*, 551, 1962.

36*b*.Milch, Murray, and Kenmore: Proc. Soc. Exp. Biol. Med., *111*, 554, 1962.

37. Dougherty: Federation Proc., *20*, Supp. *8*, 3, 1961.

38. Baily: Abstracts of Papers Presented at the International Collagen Symposium, The Hague (Scheveningen), The Netherlands, August 23–25, 1963.

39. Braams: Abstracts of Papers Presented at the International Collagen Symposium, The Hague (Scheveningen), The Netherlands, August 23–25, 1963.

40. Kountz, Hofstatter, and Ackermann: Geriatrics, *2*, 173, 1947.

41. ———: Geriatrics, *3*, 171, 1948.

42. ———: J. Gerontol., *6*, 20, 1951.

43. Kountz, Ackermann, Kheim, and Toro: Geriatrics, *8*, 63, 1953.

44. Schulze: Altersforsch, *8*, 64, 1954.

45. Schulze: In *Old Age in the Modern World*, 3rd Congr. Internat. Assoc. Gerontol, 1954., p. 127, London, E. and S. Livingstone, Ltd., 1955.

46. Watkin, Froeb, Hatch, and Gutman: Am. J. Med., *9*, 441, 1950.

47. Bogdonoff, Shock, and Nichols: J. Gerontol., *8*, 272, 1953.

48. Horwitt: J. Am. Dietet. Assoc., *29*, 443, 1953.

49. Food and Nutrition Board, National Research Council. *Recommended Dietary Allowances*, 7th Revised Ed., 1968, Publication No. 1694. Washington, D.C., Natl. Acad. Sci., 1968.

50. Morgan, Murai, and Gillum: J. Nutrition, *55*, 671, 1955.

51. Herbeuval, Cuny, Manciaux, and Hansen: In *Old Age in the Modern World*, 3rd Congr. Internat. Assoc. Gerontol., 1954, p. 574, Edinburgh, E. & S. Livingstone, Ltd., 1955.

52. Karel, Wilder, and Beber: Am. Geriat. Soc., *4*, 667, 1956.

53. Eastman: Am. Geriat. Soc., *10*, 633, 638, 1962.

54. Acheson and Jessop: Gerontologia, *6*, 193, 1962.

55. Reifenstein, Jr. and Albright: Clin. Invest., *26*, 24, 1947.

56. Kountz: Ann. Int. Med., *35*, 1055, 1951.

57. Ackermann, Toro, Kountz, and Kheim: J. Gerontol., *9*, 450, 1954.

58. Bogdonoff, Shock, and Parsons: J. Gerontol., *9*, 262, 1954.

59. Kountz, Kheim, Toro, Ackermann, and Toro: J. Am. Geriat. Soc., *7*, 757, 1959.

60. Watkin, Parsons, Yiengst, and Shock: J. Gerontol., *10*, 268, 1955.

61. Watkin: Ann. N.Y. Acad. Sci., *69*, 902, 1958.

62. Watkin: In *The Physician and the Total Care of the Cancer Patient*, p. 135, New York, Amer. Cancer Soc., 1962.

63. Watkin, Silverstone, and Shock: (Abstract) Federation Proc., *24*, 629, 1965.

64. Couch, Watkin, Rosenberg, Smith, Winitz, Otey, Birnbaum, and Greenstein: (Abstract) Federation Proc., *19*, 13, 1960.

65. Young, Scrimshaw, and Das.: (Abstract) Federation Proc., *26*, 629, 1967.

66. Mertz, Baxter, Jackson, Roderick, and Weis: J. Nutrition, *46*, 313, 1952.

67. Albanese, Higgons, Orto, and Zavattaro: Geriatrics, *12*, 465, 1957.

68. Tuttle, Swendseid, Mulcare, Griffith, and Bassett: Metabolism, *6*, 564, 1957.

69. Watts, Mann, Bradley, and Thompson: J. Gerontol., *19*, 370, 1964.

70. Watts, Tolbert, and Ruff: Canad. J. Biochem., *42*, 1437, 1964.

71. Rose: Federation Proc., *8*, 546, 1949.

72. Tuttle, Swendseid, and Bassett, (Abstract): Federation Proc., *19*, 11, 1960.

73. Tuttle, Swendseid, Mulcare, Griffith, and Bassett: Metabolism, *8*, 61, 1959.

74. Swendseid: In *Symposium on Protein Nutrition and Metabolism* (Kastelic, J., Draper, H. H., and Broquist, H. P. Eds.). p. 37, Spec. Publ. No. 4, Urbana, Illinois, Univ. of Illinois College of Agriculture, Agricultural Experiment Station, 1963.

75. Swendseid, Feelery, Harris, and Tuttle: J. Nutrition, *68*, 203, 1959.
76. Swendseid, Harris, and Tuttle: J. Nutrition, *71*, 105, 1960.
77. Clark, Yess, Vermillion, Goodwin, and Mertz: J. Nutrition, *79*, 131, 1963.
78. Tuttle, Bassett, Griffith, Mulcare, and Swendseid: Am. J. Clin. Nutr., *16*, 225, 1965.
79. Swendseid, Watts, Harris, and Tuttle: J. Nutrition, *75*, 295, 1961.
80. Swendseid and Tuttle: In *Progress in Meeting Protein Needs of Infants and Preschool Children*, Publ. No. 843, p. 323, Washington, D.C., Natl. Acad. Sci.-Natl. Res. Council, 1961.
81. Tuttle, Bassett, Griffith, Mulcare, and Swendseid: Am. J. Clin. Nutr., *16*, 229, 1965.
82. Rose: Nutr. Abstr. Rev., *27*, 631, 1957.
83. Reynolds, Steel, Jones, and Baumann: J. Nutrition, *64*, 99, 1958.
84. Swendseid, Griffith, and Tuttle: Metabolism, *12*, 96, 1963.
84a. Swendseid, Tuttle, Figueroa, Mulcare, Clark, and Massey: J. Nutr., *88*, 239, 1966.
85. Karlson: *Introduction to Modern Biochemistry*, p. 153, New York, Academic Press, 1963.
86. Swendseid, Villalobos, and Drenick, (Abstract): Federation Proc., *23*, 448, 1964.
87. Swendseid, Friedrich, and Tuttle, (Abstract): Federation Proc., *20*, 8, 1961.
88. Tuttle, Swendseid, Friedrich, and Griffith, (Abstract): Federation Proc., *21*, 395, 1962.
89. Drenick, Swendseid, Blahd, and Tuttle: J. Am. Med. Assn., *187*, 100, 1964.
89a. Swendseid, Yamada, Vinyard, Figueroa, and Drenick: Am. J. Clin. Nutr., *20*, 52, 1967.
89b. Miller: In *Amino Acid Pools* (Holden, J. T., Ed.), p. 708, New York, Elsevier, 1962.
89c. McMenamy, Shoemaker, Richmond, and Elwyn: Am. J. Physiol., *202*, 407, 1962.
89d. Swendseid, Tuttle, Drenick, Joven and Massey: Am. J. Clin. Nutr., *20*, 243, 1967.
89e. Munro: Scot Med. J., *1*, 285, 1956.
89f. Harris and Harris: Proc. Soc. Expt. Biol. Med., *64*, 471, 1947.
89g. Yearick and Nadeau: Am. J. Clin. Nutr., *20*, 338, 1967.
89h. Swendseid, Villalobos, Figueroa, and Drenick: Am. J. Clin. Nutr., *17*, 317, 1965.
90. Sharp, Lassen, Shankman, Hazlet, and Lendis: J. Nutrition, *63*, 155, 1957.
91. Tschudy, Bacchus, Weissman, Watkin, Eubanks, and White: J. Clin. Invest., *38*, 892, 1959.
92. Watkin: Am. J. Clin. Nutr., *9*, 446, 1961.
93. Bronte-Stewart, Keys, and Brock: Lancet, *2*, 1103, 1955.
94. Keys: Am. Med. Assn., *164*, 1912, 1957.
95. Ahrens, Jr., Tsaltas, Hirsch, and Insull, Jr.: J. Clin. Invest., *34*, 918, 1955.
96. Ahrens, Jr., Insull, Jr., Blomstrand, Hirsch, Tsaltas, and Peterson: Lancet, *1*, 943, 1957.
97. Jolliffe and Rinzler: Postgrad. Med., *29*, 569, 1961.
98. Jolliffe, Maslansky, Rudensey, Simon, and Faulkner: Circulation, *24*, 1415, 1961.
99. Brown and Page: J. Am. Med. Assn., *168*, 1989, 1958.
100. Keys, Anderson, and Grande: Lancet, *1*, 66, 1957.
101. Groen: Medicine, *38*, 1, 1959.
102. Albrink: Am. J. Med., *31*, 4, 1961.
103. Council on Foods and Nutrition, American Medical Association, Committee on Dietary Fat Levels (Hand, D. B., Chairman) J. Am. Med. Assn., *181*, 411, 1962.
103a. National Diet-Heart Study Research Group with the Approval of the Executive Committee on Diet and Heart Disease: The National Diet and Heart Study Final Report. American Heart Association Monograph Number Eighteen. Circulation, 37, No. 3, Supplement No. I, pp. I-1 through I-428, 1968.
103b. Page and Brown: Circulation, *37*, 313, 1968.
103c. Mellinkoff, Frankland, Schwabe, Kellner, Greipel, and McNall: Am. J. Clin. Nutr., *16*, 232, 1956.
104. Szilard: Proc. Nat. Acad. Sci. (U.S.A.), *45*, 30, 1959.
104a. Fredrickson and Lees: *The Metabolic Basis of Inherited Disease* (Stanbury, J. B., Wyngaarden, J. B., and Fredrickson, D. S., Eds.), 2nd Ed. p. 429–485, New York, The Blakiston Division-McGraw-Hill Book Company, 1966.
105. Passmore: In *Diet and Bodily Constitution*, (Wolstenholme, G. E. W., and O'Connor, M., Eds.), p. 59, London, J. and A. Churchill Ltd., 1964.
106. Smith and Shock: J. Gerontol., *4*, 27, 1949.
107. Silverstone, Brandfonbrener, Shock, and Yiengst: J. Clin. Invest., *36*, 504, 1957.
107a. Andres and Tobin: Proc. 9th International Congress of Gerontology Vol. 1. pp. 276–280, Kiev, 1972.
108. Pyke and Harrison: Lancet, *2*, 461, 1947.
109. Ohlson, Jackson, Bock, Cederquist, Brewer, Brown, Traver, Lott, Mayhew, Dunsing, and Tobey: Am. J. Public Health, *40*, 1101, 1950.
110. Vinther-Paulsen: J. Gerontol., *5*, 331, 1950.
111. Gustafsson, Quensel, Lanke, Lundquist, Grahenen, Bonow, and Krasse: Acta Odont. Scand., *11*, 232, 1954.
112. Ahrens, Jr., Hirsch, Oette, Farquhar, and Stein: Trans. Assoc. Am. Physicians, *74*, 134, 1961.
113. Himsworth: Lancet, *2*, 171, 1939.
114. Ellis: Quart. J. Med., *3*, 137, 1934.
115. Cohn, Joseph, and Allweiss: Am. J. Clin. Nutr., *11*, 356, 1962.
115a. Portman, Lawry, and Bruno: Proc. Soc. Exper. Biol. & Med., *91*, 321, 1956.
115b. Yudkin: Lancet, *2*, 155, 1957.
115c. Yudkin: Lancet, *1*, 1335, 1963.
115d. Yudkin and Roddy: Lancet, *2*, 6, 1964.
115e. Keys, Anderson, and Grande: J. Nutr., *70*, 257, 1960.
115f. Grande, Anderson, and Keyes: J. Nutr., *86*, 313, 1965.
115g. Cohen: Am. Heart J., *65*, 291, 1963.
115h. Antar, Ohlson, and Hodges: Am. J. Clin. Nutr., *14*, 169, 1964.

115*i*.Hodges and Krehl: Am. J. Clin. Nutr., *17*, 334, 1965.

115*j*.MacDonald and Braithwaite: Clin. Sci., *27*, 23, 1964.

115*k*.Kuo and Bassett: Ann. Int. Med., *62*, 1199, 1965.

115*l*.Yudkin: Am. J. Clin. Nutr., *20*, 108, 1967.

115*m*.Yudkin and Morland: Am. J. Clin. Nutr., *20*, 503,1967.

115*n*.Kaufman, Poznanski, Blondheim, and Stein: Am. J. Clin. Nutr., *18*, 261, 1966.

115*o*.Lopez, Hodges, and Krehl: Am. J. Clin. Nutr., *18*, 149, 1966.

116. Dallas and Nordin: Am. J. Clin. Nutr., *11*, 263, 1962.

116*a*.Smith and Frame: New England J. Med., *273*, 73, 1965.

116*b*.Saville and Whyte: Clin. Orthop., *65*, 81, 1969.

117. Nordin: Lancet, *1*, 1011, 1961.

118. Nordin: Am. J. Clin. Nutr., *10*, 384, 1962.

119. Whedon: Federation Proc., *18*, 1112, 1959.

120. Lutwak and Whedon: Borden's Rev. Nutr. Res., *23*, 45, 1962.

120*a*.Lutwak and Whedon: DM (Disease-a-Month), p. 1, April, 1963.

120*b*.Shorr and Carter: Bull. Hosp. Joint Dis., *13*, 59, 1952.

120*c*.Rich and Ensinck: Nature (London), *191*, 184, 1961.

120*d*.Rich, Ensinck, and Ivanovich: J. Clin. Invest., *43*, 545, 1964.

120*e*.Rich and Ivanovich: Ann. Int. Med., *63*, 1068, 1965.

120*f*.Cohen and Gardner: New England J. Med., *271*, 1129, 1964.

120*g*.Cohen and Gardner: J. Am. Med. Assn., *195*, 962, 1966.

120*h*.Bernstein, Sadowsky, Hegsted, Guri, and Stare: J. Am. Med. Assn., *198*, 85, 1966.

120*i*.Smith, Rizek and Frame: Amer. J. Clin. Nutr., *14*, 98, 1964.

120*j*.Rose: Proc. Roy. Soc. Med., *58*, 436, 1965.

120*k*.Exton-Smith: In *Symposium on Nutrition and Aging*, Am. J. Clin. Nutr. *25*, 853, 1972.

120*l*.Garn, Rohmann, and Wagner: Federation Proc., *26*, 1729, 1967.

120*m*.Garn, Rohmann, and Nolan: In *Relation of Development and Aging*, (Birren, J. E., Ed.), Springfield, Charles C Thomas, 1964.

121. Hegsted, Moscosco, and Collazos: J. Nutrition, *46*, 181, 1952.

122. Walker: Metabolism, *3*, 114, 1955.

123. Malm: *Calcium Requirement and Adaptation in Adult Men*, Oslo, Oslo University Press, 1958.

124. Calkins: Personal communication.

125. Ohlson, Roberts, Joseph, and Nelson: J. Am. Dietet. Assoc., *24*, 286, 1948.

126. Roberts, Kerr, and Ohlson: J. Am. Dietet. Assoc., *24*, 292, 1948.

127. Ackermann and Toro: J. Gerontol, *8*, 289, 1953.

128. Harrison: Federation Proc., *18*, 1085, 1959.

128*a*.Lutwak: J. Amer. Geriatrics Soc., *17*, 115, 1969.

128*b*.Henrikson, Krook, Bergman, *et al.*: Svensk. Tandlak. T., *63*, 323, 1969.

128*c*.Krook, Lutwak, Henrikson, *et al.*: J. Nutrition, *101*, 233, 1971.

128*d*.Lutwak, Krook, Henrikson, *et al.*: Isr. J. Med. Sci., 7, 504, 1971.

129. Weidmann: Biochem. J., *69*, 338, 1958.

130. Gitlin, Kamholtz, and Levine: J. Gerontology, *13*, 43, 1958.

131. Vose, Stover, and Mock: J. Gerontol., *16*, 120, 1961.

132. Harris: Federation Proc., *18*, 1100, 1959.

133. Watkin and Steinfeld: J. Natl. Cancer Inst., *33*, 169, 1964.

133*a*.Fletcher, Jones, and Morgan: Quart. J. Med., *32*, 321, 1963.

133*b*.Lutwak: Annual Lecture, New England Dairy and Food Council, Seekonk, Mass., November 16, 1971.

134. Arnold, Jr., Dean, Jay, and Knutson: Public Health Repts., *77*, 652, 1956.

135. U.S. Public Health Service, Public Health Repts., *71*, 963, 1956.

135*a*.Rich: J. Amer. Med. Assn. (Questions & Answers), *196*, 1165, 1966.

135*b*.Higgins, Nassim, Alexander, and Hilb: Brit. Med. J., *1*, 1159, 1965.

136. Fielding: Brit. Med. J., *5295*, 1800, 1962.

137. Leaf: New Engl. J. Med., *267*, 24, 1962.

138. Bondy: Year Book of Medicine, 1963–1964 Series, Chicago, Year Book Medical Publishers, 1963, p. 680.

139. Schneckloth, Dustan, and Corcoran: Metabolism, *6*, 723, 1957.

139*a*.Das: Ph.D. Thesis, MIT, Cambridge, Mass., 1967.

140. Stephenson, Penton, and Korenchevsky: Brit. Med. J., *2*, 839, 1941.

141. Wexberg: Am. J. Psychiat., *97*, 1406, 1941.

142. Jolliffe: J. Amer. Med. Assn., *117*, 1496, 1941.

143. Overholser: In *Geriatric Medicine*, 2nd Ed., (Stieglitz, E. J. Ed.). Philadelphia, W. B. Saunders Co., 1949.

144. Rafsky and Newman: Am. J. Med. Sci., *201*, 749, 1941.

145. ———: Gastroenterology, *1*, 737, 1943.

146. ———: Geriatrics, *2*, 101, 1947.

147. Horwitt, Liebert, Kreisler, and Wittman: Bull. Nat. Research Council (U.S.), *116*, 1948.

148. Lossy, Goldsmith, and Sarett: J. Nutrition, *45*, 213, 1951.

149. Schmidt: J. Gerontol., *6*, 132, 1951.

150. Schmidt: J. Gerontol, *6*, 369, 1951.

151. Watkin, Lang, Chow, and Shock: J. Nutrition, *50*, 341, 1953.

152. Chow, Lang, Davis, Conley, and Ellicott: Bull. Johns Hopkins Hosp., *87*, 156, 1950.

153. Watkin, Barrows, Chow, and Shock: Proc. Soc. Exp. Biol. Med., *107*, 219, 1961.

154. Beard, Pitney, and Sonneman: Blood, *9*, 789, 1954.

155. Mendelsohn and Watkin: J. Lab. Clin. Med., *51*, 860, 1958.

156. Mendelsohn, Watkin, Horbett, and Fahey: Blood, *13*, 740, 1958.
157. Weinstein, Weissman, and Watkin: J. Clin. Invest., *38*, 1904, 1959.
158. Weinstein and Watkin, (Abstract): Clinical Research, *8*, 219, 1960.
159. Boger, Wright, Strickland, Gylfe, and Ciminera: Proc. Soc. Exp. Biol. Med., *89*, 375, 1955.
160. Chow, Wood, Horonick, and Okuda: J. Gerontol., *11*, 142, 1956.
161. Gaffney, Horonick, Okuda, Meier, Chow, and Shock: J. Gerontol., *12*, 32, 1957.
161*a*.Hall and Finkler: J. Lab. & Clin. Med., *65*, 459, 1965.
161*b*.————: Blood, *27*, 611, 1966.
161*c*.————: Blood, *27*, 618, 1966.
162. Weinstein and Watkin: J. Clin. Invest., *39*, 1667, 1960.
163. Watkin and Weinstein, (Abstract): Federation Proc., *21*, 469, 1962.
164. Alexander, Lorenzen, Hoffman, and Garfinkel: Proc. Soc. Exp. Biol. Med., *65*, 275, 1947.
165. Sleisenger: New Engl. J. Med., *265*, 49, 1961.
166. Di Sant' Agnese and Jones: J. Amer. Med. Assn., *180*, 122, 1962.
167. Kirk and Chieffi: J. Nutrition, *36*, 315, 1948.
168. Yiengst and Shock: J. Gerontol., *4*, 205, 1949.
169. Birren, Bick, and Fox: J. Gerontol., *3*, 267, 1948.
170. Birren, Bick, and Yiengst: J. Exp. Psychol., *40*, 260, 1950.
171. Freeman, Rhoads, and Yeager: J. Lab. and Clin. Med., *31*, 480, 1946.
172. Bauer and Freyberg: J. Amer. Med. Assn., *130*, 1208, 1946.
173. Donegan, Messer, and Orgain: Ann. Int. Med., *30*, 429, 1949.
174. McCollum and McCallum: In *Food: The Yearbook of Agriculture, 1959.* (Stefferud, A., Ed.), p. 138, Washington, U.S. Government Printing Office, 1959.
175. Watkin, Van Itallie, Logan, Geyer, Davidson, and Stare: J. Lab. and Clin. Med., *37*, 269, 1951.
176. Mason: *The Vitamins, vol. 3*, (Sebrell, W. H., Jr. and Harris, R. S., Eds.) p. 514, New York, The Academic Press, 1954.
176*a*.Dam: Pharmacol. Rev., *9*, 1, 1957.
176*b*.Horwitt: Borden's Rev. Nutrition Res., *22*, 1, 1961.
176*c*.Herting: Am. J. Clin. Nutr., *19*, 210, 1967.

176*d*.Gordon and de Metry: Proc. Soc. Exper. Biol. & Med., *79*, 446, 1952.
176*e*.Gyorgy, Cogan, and Rose: Proc. Soc. Exper. Biol. & Med., *81*, 536, 1962.
176*f*.Horwitt, Harvey, Duncan, and Wilson: Am. J. Clin. Nutr., *4*, 408, 1956.
176*g*.Majaj, Dinning, Ozzam, and Darby: Am. J. Clin. Nutr., *12*, 374, 1963.
176*h*.Bunnell, Keating, Quaresimo, and Parman: Am. J. Clin. Nutr., *17*, 1, 1965.
176*i*.Horwitt: Vitamins & Hormones, *20*, 541, 1962.
176*j*.Dayton, Hashimoto, Rosenblum, and Pearce: J. Lab. & Clin. Med., *65*, 739, 1965.
176*k*.Harris and Embree: Am. J. Clin. Nutr., *13*, 385, 1963.
176*l*.Olson: Canad. J. Biochem., *43*, 1565, 1965.
176*m*.Cray: New York Times, February 13, 1972. p. F4.
176*n*.Rensberger: New York Times, March 13, 1972. p. 17.
176*o*.Newsweek, March 27, 1972, p. 63.
176*p*.Smith, Kelleher, Losowsky and Morrish: Brit. J. Nutrition., *26*, 89, 1971.
176*q*.*Recommended Intakes of Nutrients for the United Kingdom*, Department of Health and Social Security, Her Majesty's Stationery Office, London, 1969.
177. White: Geriatrics, *13*, 819, 1958.
178. Cizek: Am. J. Physiol., *197*, 342, 1959.
179. Keane, Smutko, Krieger, and Denton: J. Nutrition, *77*, 18, 1962.
180. Dublin and Marks: Human Biol., *2*, 159, 1930.
181. McKay: Am. J. Public Health, *37*, 521, 1947.
182. Ross: Federation Proc., *18*, 1190, 1959.
182*a*.Ross: J. Nutrition, *25*, 197, 1961.
182*b*.————: In *Diet and Bodily Constitution* (Wolstenholme, G. E. W., and O'Connor, M., Eds.), London, J. and A Churchill, Ltd., 1964, p. 90.
182*c*.Ross: In *Symposium on Nutrition and Aging*, Am. J. Clin. Nutr., *25*, 834, 1972.
183. Berg, Wolf, and Simms: J. Nutrition, *77*, 439, 1962.
184. Berg and Simms: J. Nutrition, *71*, 255, 1960.
185. Nikkilä and Konttinen: Lancet, *1*, 1151, 1962.
186. Watkin, Das, and McCarthy: *Abstracts of Papers Presented at the 23rd International Congress of Physiological Sciences*, Tokyo, September, 1965, p. 314.
187. Watkin: Eighth Ciba Foundation Lecture on Research on Aging. In *World Review of Nutrition and Dietetics* (Bourne, G. H., Ed.), *6*, 124, 1966, New York, S. Karger, 1966.

Chapter

26

Food and Nutrition Relating to Work and Environmental Stress

MAURICE E. SHILS

NUTRITIONAL REQUIREMENTS FOR WORK

It may be stated at the outset that the overwhelming majority of workers have nutritional requirements of the same order as those for individuals of the same sex and age in the general population. However, there is need for examination of the possible influences on nutritional requirements of activities and stresses imposed in various occupations, in order to know whether any changes occur that demand alterations in dietary practices. A corollary question concerns the effect of variations in dietary composition on work performance.

Calories. Assessment of energy expenditure at a given task may be measured most reliably by indirect calorimetry during performance of the task. If this technique is applied to each activity of daily living and the time spent on each activity is known, then the total caloric cost of the day can be estimated. Earlier workers, such as Voit, Atwater and others after them, estimated energy expenditure by analyzing diet records—a procedure open to a number of errors, including errors in the measurement of consumption, variations from the tables of food composition, variations in efficiency of food utilization and individual weight changes on given diets. The use of data obtained from indirect calorimetry for generalization also involves the problem of transferring data from a small group to a large population or to an untested individual; however, the error should be

smaller by far than that in the dietary method. Using tables based on calorimetric estimates, Passmore and Durnin[1] consider the more recent estimates of individual daily energy expenditure to be accurate within 10 per cent.

The Douglas bag has been used extensively for many years for collecting expired air but suffers from being bulky and unwieldy in confined spaces. The development of a light weight (8 lb) portable respirometer,[2,3] designated the Max Planck Institute respirometer or the Kofranyi-Michaelis respirometer, has facilitated the obtaining of data on energy expenditure by workers. This unit measures the volume of expired air directly and simultaneously diverts a small fraction into a rubber bladder for subsequent analysis. However, it has a limited sample storage capacity and offers considerable respiratory resistance at ventilation rates much above 25 to 30 liters/minute;[4] others consider it useful with ventilations up to 60 to 80 liters/minute.[5] A number of studies of various activities of industrial workers has been carried out using these techniqnes.[2,3,6–10] Wolff[11] has designed an instrument (the Integrating Motor Pneumotachograph) which measures instantaneous flow (rather than direct volume) which is integrated with respect to time; sampling is achieved by diverting a small fraction of air passing through the flowmeter and storing it for subsequent analysis. Its usefulness in physiologic studies in polar expeditions has been described.[12]

In addition to obtaining caloric expenditures for specific tasks, it is important to determine total daily energy expenditures of various individuals living under fairly unrestricted conditions. A limited amount of information has been obtained by a combination of respirometer measurements with time-motion studies,[13] diary technique[7,13] or by measurement of heart-rate, using small electrodes and telemetry.[14]

An excellent summary of various studies has been presented by Durnin and Passmore.[13] They have collected data from the literature and their own investigations on energy expenditures in sleep, personal care, walking, climbing, running, recreational activities, domestic and office work and a large variety of laboring activities, ranging from light to heavy and including agriculture, lumbering and fishing as well as industrial work. The reader is referred to published tables for data on energy expenditure in specific activities.[13,15]

Numerous efforts have been made to grade physical effort as a basis for estimating caloric needs. Burnet and Aykroyd,[16a] reporting for the Technical Commission of the Health Organization of the League of Nations in 1935, suggested an allowance of 2400 kilocalories (kcal) per day as adequate to meet the requirements of an adult male or female living an ordinary everyday life in a temperate climate and not engaged in manual work, with the following supplements for muscular activity: light work, up to 50 kcal per hour of work; moderate work, from 50 to 100 kcal per hour of work; hard work, from 100 to 200 kcal per hour of work; and very hard work 200 kcal and over per hour of work. Dill[16b] expressed levels of work in terms of the ratio of work metabolism to basal metabolism and defined moderate work as that in the range where the work metabolism is 1 to 3 times basal metabolism, and hard work as that in the range of 3 to 8 times. In the latter area lie most of the manual jobs in heavy industries, building trades, mining, and agriculture.

The Committee on Calorie Requirements of the Food and Agriculture Organization of the United Nations[17a,17b] developed formulas for calculating the caloric requirements of populations and population groups by estab-

lishing "reference standards" for men and women and adjusting the requirements of individuals differing from the reference in age, body size, environmental temperature and activity. The mean caloric requirements of the reference men and women involved in a degree of activity corresponding to an occupation in light industry are 3200 and 2300 per day, respectively. The Food and Nutrition Board of the National Research Council, beginning with its 1953 revision of the Recommended Dietary Allowances, adopted these references as a basis for caloric requirements. In successive revisions it has progressively changed the caloric requirements for the standard man and woman downward, so that they stand presently at 2800 and 2000 kcal, respectively.[17c] Having knowledge of the characteristics of a population group with respect to distribution as to age, body size, climate and activity, estimates of the caloric needs of that population can be reached.

Lehmann, Müller and Spitzer[6] classified hundreds of occupations into 10 groups of caloric requirements, ranging from 8/6 of basal metabolic rate (less than 2550 kcal) up to 17/6 and higher (greater than 5000 kcal). Christensen[18] suggested the following definitions of different grades of work:

Unduly heavy—
    energy expenditure over 12.5 kcal/min
Very heavy—
    energy expenditure over 10.0 kcal/min
Heavy—
    energy expenditure over 7.5 kcal/min
Moderate—
    energy expenditure over 5.0 kcal/min
Light—
    energy expenditure over 2.5 kcal/min

Passmore and Durnin[1] are in agreement with Christensen's definitions on the basis of their own work and urge their introduction into general use.

The energy expenditures of most of Christensen's grades apply only to rates of work which are carried on continuously for periods of a few minutes and must be interspersed with rest pauses. Hence, these definitions need to be considered in relation to work capacity in order to give information on average daily rates of work. Lehmann[8] and Müller[9] have considered this problem in the light of their studies on German workers. They set a figure of 4 kcal/min net or 5 kcal/min gross (*i.e.* including energy of basal metabolism) as the upper limit of energy available from foodstuff oxidation and they term this value the Endurance Limit. If more energy is needed anaerobic metabolism, with accumulation of lactic acid, results.

Work at 5 kcal/min gross for an 8-hour shift equals 2400 kcal and probably represents the upper rate of daily energy expenditure that can be maintained at a steady rate in heavy industry. Müller[9] estimated that only about 4 per cent of the 25 million workers in West Germany work to this degree and Passmore and Durnin[1] state that it is slightly higher than the rates recorded for British coal miners. At this rate of 5 kcal/min for 8 hours, if 500 kcal are allowed for 8 hours in bed and 1400 kcal for the additional 8 hours off work, the total 24-hour energy expenditure is 4300 kcal.

For work requiring expenditure above the endurance limit, increased rest pauses or increased absence from work occur. For such work Müller[9] makes the point that many small rest pauses relieve fatigue much more than a few long pauses.

Data are accumulating for those interested in regulating physical stress in chronic cardiac and pulmonary disease and in convalescence, and in correlating residual capacity with various demands of daily living in the orthopedically disabled. The energy costs of activities of the orthopedically disabled are high.[19a−c] For example, the requirements for ambulation by certain paraplegics for a period of only four minutes were comparable to those of a normal individual engaged in a 400-yard dash; unilateral above-knee amputees walking on level ground with a monaxial knee joint required 25 per cent more energy expenditure than normal subjects at the same speed.[19a]

Figures given in various tables of requirements, standards, or allowances are merely approximations of value as guides in estimating needs of groups. The requirements of the individual worker may vary greatly from the average for his occupation. This is exemplified in a study of coal miners where the average caloric expenditure for an eight-hour shift was 2002 kcal but the range was from 1587 to 2394.[10] To the factors of size, age, sex, and environment are added the variations in specific job situations and differences in activities among individuals on and off the job—all of which greatly influence the over-all calorie requirements.[13,19d]

Caloric deficiency resulting from inadequate food supply is one problem that the employed American has never had to face even in time of war. The so-called "food shortages" which have developed from time to time and which caused some difficulties in certain industries in World War II did not involve calorie insufficiency, but rather an inability on the part of workers to get certain types of foods to which they felt they were entitled or which they believed they needed. For the majority of workers shortages of *calories* in the form of the more expensive animal products such as meat, milk, and eggs could be met easily by increasing consumption of cereals and other plant materials. Such a shift in dietary pattern, particularly if it were a pronounced one, would raise the problems of insuring an adequate intake of other nutrients and, equally important, that of maintaining morale. Even mild, involuntary changes in the food pattern in this country are not taken lightly.

The effects of true deficiency in man have been studied under conditions of actual food shortages and in experimental situations, and a large literature exists.[20] In both acute starvation and semistarvation of some duration, physiologic, psychologic and some psychomotor changes sooner or later become marked while tests of intellective function show much less deterioration.[21−24] The degree of change in the various functions depends upon the severity of the calorie deficit, its duration, and the individual concerned. Young men performing hard work while deprived of food but receiving adequate water develop, within 24 hours, dehydration, hypoglycemia, and ketosis; these changes are accompanied by nausea, fatigue, poor work tolerance and impairment of speed and coordination.[20−23] Five hundred and eighty kcal/day as carbohydrate (with a supplement of 4.5 gm NaCl) prevented ketosis and liver damage, but failed to maintain adequate blood sugar values over a 12-day period. With 1010 kcal/day for 24 days satisfactory blood sugar levels were maintained.[23] It would appear that, when sufficient calories, NaCl, vitamins and water are provided to prevent ketosis, dehydration and hypoglycemia under conditions of moderate energy output and good motivation, performance capacity is well maintained up to a weight loss of 10 per cent of the original body weight. At some point between 10 and 16 per cent weight loss, rapid deterioration of maximum effort sets in.[23] Cardiovascular insufficiency, anemia and decreased strength and speed of muscular action in chronic semistarvation are additional limiting factors.[20]

With restriction of calorie intake in industrial situations, work output is curtailed accordingly. A demand for heavy work output during a period of serious calorie deficiency would not be tolerated by workers for more than a few days and then only under emergency conditions. An interesting example of the relation of productivity to food consumption was noted among German miners during World War II.[25] Young "cutters" in the coal mines had a daily output of 7.0 tons of coal per man on a total daily intake of 2800 kcal, about 1200 kcal above the estimated basal metabolic rate, or about 170 kcal per ton of coal mined. When 400 additional kcal were allowed, output increased to 9.6 tons per man or 155 work kcal per ton. At this rate the men lost, on the average, 1.2 kg of body weight in 6 weeks. The extra kcal were raised to 800, whereupon the output increased to 10 tons per man and the body weight slowly returned to normal. Additional data on caloric intake and productivity during the war and in postwar Germany tend to confirm a close relationship when food is limited.[25a]

The body adapts to certain degrees of chronic calorie restriction. In addition to a restriction of voluntary activity, there is decreased energy expenditure resulting from decreased basal metabolism and a decrease in the energy required to perform work. The reduction of basal metabolism is attributed to two factors, namely shrinkage of the metabolizing body mass and decrease of the cellular metabolic rate.[20,26,27] There is evidence that, in subacute caloric deficiency (approximately three weeks' duration), the decrease in basal metabolism results, for the most part, from the operation of the second factor,[27] whereas in chronic semistarvation the first factor is predominant.[20,26] The ability to preferentially metabolize body fat, to spare certain tissues and to decrease the work of the heart further aids in withstanding lack of calories. The calorie equivalent of weight change with calorie deficit is considered in Chapter 1.

The corollary question arises as to whether the composition of the low-calorie diet has any influence on the organism's resistance to the deficit. Only a few experiments concerning this question have been performed with laboratory animals and still fewer with man; definitive answers are still lacking, particularly for long-term situations. It has been demonstrated in short-term studies with rats[28] and dogs[29] that, when the caloric intake falls below 50 per cent of normal, dietary protein is used for energy purposes; in rats subsisting on low-calorie diets a moderately high-fat content (15 per cent) spares dietary protein to a much greater degree than low-fat diets.[28] With respect to healthy, active men, it would appear that, when the daily caloric intake is somewhat below 900 kcal, dietary protein is utilized as an energy source, producing a concomitant rise in urinary nitrogen.[30] At approximately 900 kcal, small amounts of dietary nitrogen (3 gm) partially decrease the negative balance; increasing the nitrogen does not improve the situation. Further increases in caloric intake result in improved nitrogen retention.

Water. Water exerts important effects in permitting maximal activity and the maintenance of body composition. It has been observed[31] that there is an increase in nitrogen excretion during dehydration. Active young men on a caloric-deficient–protein-free diet had marked increases in urinary nitrogen on 900 ml of water daily; even on 1800 ml the losses were greater than those on ad lib water intake. The increased urinary nitrogen, in turn, increased obligatory urine losses, accentuating the dehydration. The metabolic response was considered to be secondary to the stress of dehydration partly related to increased adrenal cortex activity. The importance of adequate water intake in improving performance in exhausting physical work has been shown with dogs.[32] Hilary has attributed the success of his Everest expedition to emphasis on maintenance of normal hydration during the last few days of the ascent.[33]

THE EFFECTS OF THE FREQUENCY AND COMPOSITION OF MEALS IN INDUSTRIAL WORKERS

Our custom of eating three meals a day probably is based more upon considerations of convenience than upon those of physiologic need. Experience in industry has shown the value to worker productivity of additional rest periods, particularly when associated with between-meal feedings. The view is widely held that between-meal snacks in themselves increase work performance and lessen fatigue. This may be true, but there is no proof that frequent feedings increase physiologic capacity to perform work. Undoubtedly, psychologic factors are important and account for some, if not all, of the beneficial results observed.

Haggard and Greenberg[34] found that high-carbohydrate intake increased muscular efficiency in laboratory exercises on the bicycle ergometer and that variations in efficiency were correlated with the length of time between meals. They then carried on experiments with employees in a shoe factory, in which productivity was measured during periods when 3 or 5 meals per day were eaten, and concluded that 5 meals a day resulted in superior work performance (about 40 per cent increase in productivity). Unfortunately, the laboratory findings of these investigators do not agree with data obtained by other workers and the reported changes in muscular efficiency have not been confirmed.[35–37] The study with shoe operators was not sufficiently well controlled to entirely rule out psychologic effects, as Ivy[38] has pointed out. These criticisms, of course, do not dispose of the finding that there was increased production with an increase in the number of meals. There have been similar

reports[39–41] of improved efficiency or well-being with increased meals but the "morale" factors have never been ruled out.

Haldi and Wynn[42] studied the productivity of seamstresses as influenced by different amounts and kinds of food consumed during the mid-morning and mid-afternoon rest periods. No differences were noted in work output when the caloric intake was varied from 80 to 650 kcal and the type of food from a soft drink to a small meal. Less definite evidence indicated that omitting all food during the rest period did not decrease production; this particular aspect of the problem could not be thoroughly assessed because the women objected to being denied the opportunity to partake of food during the rest period. In the Hawthorn experiment,[43] when women engaged in assembling telephones were given extra snacks their output increased; however, when they were given a rest period without food, their output also increased. Many other changes in working conditions increased output and it became apparent that a very important general factor influencing productivity was the knowledge on the part of the worker that management was concerned about her welfare and views. In a recent review Hutchinson[44] discusses the problem of meal habits and the frequency of meals and advocates a regimen of 6 meals daily. However, no convincing nutritional or physiologic evidence is given to support this proposal for the usual industrial situation.

Since an appreciable number of workers are believed to report for work without having eaten any breakfast or only a cup of coffee and toast or sweet bun, it is of some interest to note reports on attempts to assess the results of different types of breakfast and of no breakfast on test subjects. Tuttle and co-workers[45–47] found that maximum work output attainable on the bicycle ergometer within one minute or less was adversely affected on omission of breakfast or by the consumption of only black unsweetened coffee, as compared with performance with adequate breakfasts. The addition of mid-morning food intake when an adequate breakfast was eaten resulted in no advantage, but the mid-morning intake improved performance in one-half of the patients who omitted breakfasts.[48] Whatever the nature of the physiologic and/or psychologic basis of the results, the results would appear to warrant consideration of the practical applications.

A study of the short-term (2-day) effect of a "breakfast" consisting only of unsweetened black coffee showed the expected absence of a rise in blood sugar above the fasting level and a slight decline throughout the subsequent three-hour period.[48] Unfavorable subjective symptoms were often reported in the morning, including hunger, weakness, headache, and lassitude. When this type of breakfast was followed by a lunch consisting of a low-protein, low-calorie sandwich and coffee, a transitory high blood sugar developed which dropped by the third hour to levels below those found during fasting. This fall in blood sugar was accompanied by subjective symptoms of hypoglycemia. An intake of 360 kcal at breakfast decreased the blood sugar drop after the low-protein luncheon, and increasing amounts of protein and fat were associated with improved sense of well-being and flatter blood sugar curves. A similar type of experiment conducted over a period of weeks or months would be worthwhile in order to learn whether adaptation to omission of breakfast occurs. A study of the effect of omission of lunch and of three types of lunch (standard, high-fat and high-carbohydrate) on the ability of men to perform strenuous work revealed that the intake of meals affects performance and fatigue of visual functions.[49] No single type of meal (including no food at all) was superior or inferior for all of the functions measured in the fairly large battery of tests applied. However, it was concluded that, in general, the standard meal (carbohydrate 50 per cent, protein 12 per cent, and fat 38 per cent of the 1300 kcal) and the high-fat meal (fat supplying 83 per cent of the 1400 kcal) was preferable for this type of work.

Pyke, who has had considerable experience with industrial feeding in Great Britain, has summarized his experience and views on the subject of feeding individuals doing moderate work by concluding:[50]

"(a) Provided the daily diet supplies the full needs for nutrients, the number of meals into which it is divided does not appear to be crucial.

"(b) The nutritionist must always remember that industrial efficiency is influenced by very many factors other than diet."

Until more definitive experimental work demonstrates the contrary, we concur with this view.

EFFECTS OF SPECIFIC NUTRIENTS ON WORK PERFORMANCE

Proteins. Liebig's theory that protein was the fuel of muscular work was disproved in 1866; nevertheless the suggestion is still occasionally made that persons engaged in hard work require increased protein. As noted above, dietary protein is utilized efficiently for protein synthesis only when caloric intake is adequate. Chittenden, in 1904, noted that men receiving adequate calories performed hard work in good health on a daily protein intake of only 50 to 60 gm.[51] In 1926 and 1927 it was again demonstrated that, in hard work, there is only a small increase in nitrogen excretion, indicating little change in protein catabolism,[52,53] and even that change may have been an indirect one.[53] More recently, it has been shown that young men doing hard manual work over a period of two months accomplished as much and remained in as good physical condition with approximately 50 gm of protein daily as with approximately 160 gm.[54] Similarly, increasing the protein intake 50 per cent above the basic intake of 50 gm of protein per day during rehabilitation of semi-starved men did not improve work performance above that on the basic intake.[7]

Carbohydrate and Fat. While glucose has received wide publicity as the "quick-energy" sugar, the fact is that, normally, hydrolysis of disaccharides, such as sucrose, and also the more complex carbohydrates takes place so rapidly in the digestive tract that differences between the rates of absorption and utilization of different sugars and starches are of no practical importance to the healthy individual. On the other hand, the view is held[55] that a high-carbohydrate–low-protein meal is conducive to the development, within a short time, of hypoglycemia with its attendant symptoms of hunger, weakness, and fatigue and that high-protein meals maintain blood sugar level and a feeling of well-being. More recent studies have supported the view that the calorie intake and ratio of carbohydrate to protein in the breakfast meal influence the postprandial blood glucose curve, with the higher protein intakes being associated with lower peaks and slower return to fasting levels.[45-48,56] It is to be noted, however, that true hypoglycemic reactions were not observed. Haldi and his co-workers,[37,57] Lundbaeck[58] and others have challenged the acceptance of the idea of a hypoglycemic reaction as a normal response, since no hypoglycemic responses were observed in a large number of healthy individuals following high-carbohydrate meals. It may well be, however, that in a situation where an established eating pattern with 3 substantial meals per day is suddenly replaced by omission of breakfast and a low-calorie–low-protein lunch, then, for a while at least, a rapid fall in blood sugar may occur and symptoms of hypoglycemia result.[48]

The subject of the metabolism of sugar and fat in muscular work has likewise received much experimental attention.[29,35,59] When maximal work is being performed, a high-carbohydrate intake allows the work to be carried on for a longer period than does a high-fat diet.[60,61] However, this observation applies to continuous exhausting work of a type rarely met with in industry or everyday life. Although it has been found that carbohydrate is about 10 per cent more effective than fat as a fuel when the production of maximal work of some hours' duration is the criterion,[60,62] in maximal work lasting only a few minutes or in light or moderate work prolonged for a matter of hours there is apparently little difference in the efficiency of diets of varying fat or carbohydrate content. In short-term maximal work, such as short-distance speed swimming, Haldi and Wynn found no beneficial effect of high-carbohydrate diets nor did they find that a high-carbohydrate breakfast before exercise caused a hypoglycemic reaction.[36,37,57]

Since the recognition of the importance of plasma free fatty acids in the metabolism of lipids, various studies have suggested that they are a major substrate for the energy metabolism of tissues.[63,64] The energy derived from free fatty acids during exercise is about 50 per cent during light to moderate exercise: when the work load is increased, this percentage decreases.[65a] Hultman and his associates have emphasized the importance of muscle glycogen in the performance of heavy muscular work and the role of diet in its repletion.[65a] When subjects continued exercise to complete muscular exhaustion on a bicycle ergometer, muscle glycogen decreased on an exponential curve so that a very low glycogen content was present toward the end of exercise; however, the work could be continued for some minutes longer when glycogen was practially zero, probably due to an increase in fat oxidation, an increased uptake of glucose and compensatory work by less depleted muscles. Glucose infusion with maintenance of blood sugar between 200 and 600 mg per cent during hard work did not alter the glycogen decrease. It is concluded that energy release from glycogen breakdown is indispensable for heavy work.[65a] The character of the diet influenced the rate and level of glycogen resynthesis in exercised muscle and the ability to continue the work. When a carbohydrate-rich diet was given, glycogen was reformed to values much greater than the normal range. Fasting, a protein and fat diet or a mixed diet produced very slow and incomplete restoration of glycogen content.[65a,65b] A close correlation was also noted between the muscle content of glycogen and the ability to continue to maintain the pace in long-distance running; a special regimen which included a high-carbohydrate intake was superior in these respects to the same regimen with usual mixed diets.[65c] Potassium-magnesium aspartate given prior to exhausting exercise prolonged mean work time significantly as compared to that with placebos: the mechanism is uncertain.[65d]

Vitamins. It must be borne in mind in considering the information given below that, although practically all experimental work on the relation of nutrition to fatigue employs physical stress to produce fatigue, most modern industrial work fails to tax the physical endurance of the average worker.

The type of fatigue of greatest importance to industry is that involving the central nervous system, a type that has been the subject of relatively little scientific study.

The evidence leaves little room for doubt that the earliest symptoms of human deficiencies of those water-soluble vitamins about which we know most are those of easy fatigability, anorexia, irritability, and apathy. The ability to perform work efficiently is impaired in frank deficiency states, and adequate therapy will restore work capacity toward normal levels, as will the adequate treatment of other types of illness where permanent incapacity is not involved.

Simonson and co-workers[66] found no effect on 5 different types of muscular work from the addition of large amounts of the vitamin B complex to the usual diet of 12 healthy subjects. There was no beneficial effect of supplementation with 5 B complex vitamins and ascorbic acid on muscular ability, resistance to fatigue, or recovery from exertion of healthy young men subsisting on diets considered to be adequate.[67] In experiments lasting ten to twelve weeks and utilizing normal young men, it was found that intakes of thiamin at 4 different levels (from 0.23 mg per 1000 kcal daily up to 0.63 mg per 1000 kcal) exerted no beneficial effect on diets otherwise considered adequate. Muscular, neuromuscular, cardiovascular, psychomotor, and metabolic functions tested "were in no way limited—(and) clinical signs, subjective sensations and state of mind, and behavior were likewise unaffected."[68] A level of 0.96 mg of thiamin per 1000 kcal was allowed to the control subjects in these experiments. Supplementation with B complex vitamins of a diet considered adequate did not increase the endurance of several subjects operating a bicycle ergometer.[69]

An experiment with 86 volunteer military personnel exposed to a cold environment revealed no significant difference in physical and psychological performance in a ten-week test between supplemented and unsupplemented groups.[70] The supplementation consisted of large amounts of 7 B complex vitamins and ascorbic acid. The basal diets were presumed to be adequate except for a 3-week period of moderate caloric deficit.

The addition of varying amounts of ascorbic acid to diets already adequately provided with this vitamin has been found to exert no detectable effects in terms of general well-being, physical vigor, and efficiency for hard work.[71,72,72a]

From 1941 to 1943 a combined study of dietary habits, clinical status, and the effect of nutrient supplementation was conducted by Borsook and his associates on large numbers of aircraft workers in Southern California.[73–77] No significant specific therapeutic effects of a multiple vitamin-mineral supplement (vitamins A, D, C, B_1, riboflavin, niacinamide, and calcium) were observed. However, the supplemented group was reported to show decreases in unauthorized absences and turnover rate as compared with the group receiving a placebo.

This evidence supports the general opinion that, once the vitamin requirements of the organism are met, there is no value in additional supply, i.e., "super-nutrition" does not exist.

Effects of Low Nutrient Intake on Efficiency. Consideration of this topic involves one in a highly complex subject characterized by conflicting evidence and opinion. Johnson et al.[78] found that young men subjected to hard daily physical work and subsisting on a diet deficient in members of the B complex, notably thiamin, exhibited symptoms of easy fatigability, apathy, muscle and joint pains, anorexia, and constipation and a marked deterioration in work performance within one week. Another group on the same diet supplemented with thiamin exhibited only a few mild subjective symptoms, but their performance during hard work also deteriorated. Administration of yeast restored both groups to normal within four days.

Foltz, Barborka, and Ivy[79] studied the work performance on the bicycle ergometer of four medical students. When the thiamin intake was reduced from 0.43 to 0.59 mg per 1000 kcal of food to 0.33 to 0.38 mg per 1000 kcal, a decrease in appetite was noted within three weeks. After 1 month at this reduced thiamin intake a further decrease in thiamin intake was effected (0.17 to 0.21 mg per 1000 kcal) but no additional changes were noted until 4 weeks later, at which time a decided decrease in appetite and work output occurred, together with increased fatigue and muscle tenderness and a deterioration in mental attitude. The objective and subjective symptoms disappeared promptly after the addition of a yeast concentrate. Archdeacon and Murlin[80] noted a decrease in muscular endurance on the bicycle ergometer in two subjects on a diet low in the B complex vitamins (the thiamin intake being 0.27 mg per day or 0.09 mg per 1000 kcal), the effect being observed within 10 to 14 days on the diet. Addition of the B complex in the form of whole wheat bread or thiamin in pure form resulted in a marked improvement in endurance. Pyridoxine added in one experiment had a similar effect but riboflavin had none.

These results are in marked contrast to those of Keys and co-workers. In one experiment[68] already mentioned, no decrease in work performance was noted on diets containing 0.23 mg thiamin per 1000 kcal. In a later paper[81] the Minnesota investigators published the results of a study in which eight young men were studied before, during, and after a 2-week period during which five were on a basal diet providing on the average 0.16 mg of thiamin, 0.15 mg of riboflavin, and 1.8 mg of niacin per 1000 kcal. These men also received placebos while three control subjects were given the same basal diet plus capsules containing a yeast concentrate and synthetic B vitamins. With an energy expenditure of 4800 kcal during the experimental period, no differences were noted in endurance and in a variety of clinical, psychologic, and biochemical tests. The length of time on a low B complex intake (0.185 mg thiamin, 0.287 mg riboflavin, and 3.71 mg niacin daily per 1000 kcal) was extended to 161 days and again no impairment of work performance was noted at a calorie intake and expenditure of 3300 kcal.[82] A small increase in blood pyruvate indicated a borderline thiamin deficiency. Immediately thereafter the intake of two of the subjects (known as the restricted-deficient group) was restricted more severely to 0.008 mg thiamin, 0.013 mg riboflavin, and 0.1 mg niacin daily per 1000 kcal with a daily energy intake and

expenditure of 4000 kcal. Anorexia developed after the first week and by the end of the third week the subjects exhibited almost complete inability to take any food. Supplementation was begun with thiamin alone on the 24th day. Two additional men who had been on an adequate diet prior to ingesting the very deficient diet (the control-deficient group) exhibited anorexia to a lesser extent. Despite marked changes in general behavior and obvious signs of subjective distress, there were no significant changes in simple strength as measured by grip and back lift. Psychomotor tests of speed and coordination showed slight to marked deterioration. The restricted-deficient subjects showed a rapid and progressive deterioration and incapacity to perform brief severe work. Nausea developed on extreme exertion. Similarly this group was often unable to complete the prescribed daily exercise of moderately hard work, while the control-deficient group was able to perform both types of work. The administration of thiamin alone reversed the deterioration.

It is worth noting at this point that even severe thiamin deficiency does not cause any significant diminution in ability to perform intellectual tasks, although marked deterioration takes place in certain psychomotor and personality tests and endurance.[24,83,84]

Another experiment[85] bearing on this problem involved the maintenance of seven young men for 35 weeks on a diet that was low in vitamin B complex at a caloric level of approximately 3000. After 5 weeks, two of the subjects received supplements and acted as controls. In the subsequent period the latter showed no decrease in work performance or physical or psychologic appraisal, while the five experimental subjects showed definite deterioration in work performance after 15 weeks on a daily intake of 0.50 mg thiamin, 0.30 mg riboflavin, 5.8 mg niacin, low levels of the other B vitamins, and 45 gm of protein (94 per cent from non-animal sources). When the diet was supplemented with crystalline vitamins, improvement in physical performance tests occurred gradually. No evidence was obtained pointing to an outstanding effect of any one nutrient and improvement was more rapid in subjects receiving the complete group supplementation than in those receiving step-wise additions of nutrients.

One can only conjecture about the reasons for the discrepancy in results obtained in different laboratories with intakes of thiamin in the same range. There were obvious differences in the subjects, diets, and experimental conditions. It cannot be overemphasized that, in the study of the effects of nutritional deficiencies upon functions of the human subject, careful consideration must be given to both psychologic and physiologic factors which may influence the results. Since subjective reactions and individual variability are serious complicating factors in such experiments, one must exert the greatest caution in accepting the conclusions of experiments not rigidly controlled.

In the only report published on the effects of uncomplicated low-riboflavin intake on muscular performance, the Minnesota group[86] found no deleterious effects in three men after 84 days and, on another three men, after 152 days on a diet containing 0.99 mg riboflavin per day. This level of riboflavin will not cause the development of obvious clinical signs even over a period of 2 years in less active individuals.[87]

In a study[88] of experimental human ascorbic acid deficiency induced by a diet low in the vitamin, the first symptom was fatigue which appeared after 2 months. An impaired capacity for walking and running progressed during the 6-month deficiency period. A similar effect of vitamin C deficiency was noted by Farmer[89] in experiments with a group of young men existing for several months on a diet low in vitamin C.

In view of the ability of the body to store sufficient vitamin A so that deficiency signs may not occur for a year or more on an A-vitamin deficient diet,[90] it is not surprising that no decrease in ability to perform hard muscular exercise was noted in men kept on diets low in vitamin A for about six months.[91]

Do vitamin requirements increase as energy expenditure rises? From indirect data on human dietaries associated with the presence or absence of beriberi, and on the basis of animal experiments where the amount of activity or the environmental temperature was varied, or where experimental hyperthyroidism was induced, it has been concluded generally that the requirement for certain B complex vitamins, particularly thiamin, is related to total metabolism.

Although work ability is markedly diminished in severe vitamin C-deficiency states,[88,89] it is doubtful that hard work brings on scurvy more rapidly. Experiments in which both sedentary and working men were kept on scorbutic diets for eight weeks failed to show any difference between the groups.[72]

NUTRITION AND ENVIRONMENTAL STRESS

Influence of Cold Environment on Nutrient Requirements. This subject requires consideration of a number of factors. Caloric requirements and the general health of the individual will vary greatly depending on the degree of preotction against cold. The efficiency of arctic protective clothing and the availability of heated base camps and mechanical transportation have done much to provide a much less stressful microclimate. Hence, the usual responses to cold (cutaneous vasoconstriction and metabolic responses including shivering and non-shivering thermogenesis) are greatly minimized but not entirely overcome since face and extremities are subjected to cooling. Where possible much of the time is spent in shelter and caloric requirements will depend on the nature of the outdoor work and of the terrain. The weight and "hobbling" effect of arctic clothing adds to caloric needs.

A review of energy intake and expenditure in various polar expeditions indicates an average daily expenditure during 8- to 10-hour sledging operations of 5000 to 6500 kcal for men of 70 to 80 kg—usually associated with mild weight loss whereas in base camp daily expenditure is usually 1500 kcal less.[92] In an analysis of voluntary caloric intake by soldiers stationed in various climates, an inverse linear function was noted between caloric intake and temperature.[93] Average daily intake varied from 4400 kcal per man in the cold to 3200 kcal in the tropics. The proximate composition of the diets consumed was much the same regardless of environment.[92,93]

Other data were obtained with military units in Alaska[94] and northern Canada[95] and in a comparative study of troops performing similar tasks in areas with mean temperatures of −22.5, −7.3, 72 and 90° F.[96] These reports agree that caloric consumption in cold and temperate climates was similar, especially when calculated on an equal weight basis. A similar conclusion is reached by Consolazio in a review of these and other studies.[97]

Under arctic and subarctic living conditions there is a tendency for the majority of men to gain weight;[92,95] isolation, boredom and other abnormal living conditions predispose to excessive food intake.[95]

Considerable attention has been directed to the question of whether diet composition affects the ability of the organism to withstand exposure to cold when environmental protection is inadequate and protective physiologic mechanisms become prominent. In human studies the cooling of the internal tissues of the body was found to be most rapid on a high-protein diet (41 per cent of calories as protein) and least on a high-fat diet (73 per cent of calories), with a high-carbohydrate diet (66 per cent of calories) not quite so effective as a high-fat diet.[98] The least favorable method of feeding tested was the high-protein diet with 1 meal (20 per cent of the day's calories) served during an eight-hour exposure, and the most favorable method was the high-fat diet with 3 meals (20 per cent) served during eight hours of exposure. By a change from the first to the second diet plan, the decrement in rectal temperature was reduced by two-thirds (1.63° to 0.57° C) and the decrement in general psychomotor functioning by one half.[98a]

In an acute experiment at 7.5° C, semi-nude subjects were given test meals of 214 kcal as glucose, steak or glycine and sucrose, in an effort to determine whether specific dynamic action affected tolerance to cold. It was concluded that this was not effective.[99] An interesting and unexplained observation was a reduction of shivering in those subjects ingesting the glycine-sucrose test meal prior to cold exposure.

The problems related to development of survival rations in various environmental situations have been discussed by Johnson[100a] who stresses the fact that ketosis secondary to inadequate calories or lack of carbohydrate is exacerbated with cold exposure, presumably as the result of increased caloric requirements. Factors affecting the severity of ketosis have been considered[100b] and reemphasized in recent arctic survival studies.[100c]

Exposure to cold increases thermogenesis in experimental animals, as in man, with consequent hyperphagia. Various diets have been tested in efforts to determine whether any offer special protection. Beneficial effects of increased fat have been affirmed[101a,101b] and denied[101c] in rat experiments. With diets having 10 per cent fat, a level of protein of 40 per cent was appreciably more protective than those of 20 or 5 per cent.[102a,102b] Under severe cold stress, a purified diet also fed to rats conferred greater protection than did a commercial chow diet.[103]

In relation to the caloric expenditure occurring in cold climates, it is probable that vitamin requirements are not markedly altered from those in temperate climates. Troops in an arctic environment subsisting on a diet meeting the Recommended Allowances of the National Research Council did not appear to be noticeably benefited by vitamin supplements.[104] A short-term (3 month) study of performance of young men under cold stress during "borderline" and high intakes of thiamin and ascorbic acid did not reveal any significant differences attributable to these vitamins.[105] In conformity with the animal experiments of Dugal et al.,[106] a decreased ascorbic acid excretion was noted in the urines of these men during cold stress. Dugal[107] demonstrated the increased needs for ascorbic acid in rats, guinea pigs and monkeys exposed to cold.

Similar studies on the nutritional requirements for resistance by the rat to cold stress have indicated that there is significant impairment in deficiencies of thiamin,[108] riboflavin,[109] pyridoxine,[110] vitamin A[111] and pantothenic acid.[112] A contributing, but not the sole, factor in the decreased survival to cold is the impaired caloric intake by the deficient rats.[112]

These and other problems of cold acclimation have been recently reviewed.[113–115]

Requirements in Hot Environments. The altered nutritional requirements during exposure to heat are quantitative rather than qualitative and involve mainly water and sodium chloride. As the environmental temperature rises in relation to the body temperature, the flow of heat from the body to the environment is impeded. In an attempt to maintain its usual temperature, the body secretes sweat, the evaporation of which removes heat.

The capabilities of the body for sweat loss are great; for example, in one experiment in which young men were subjected to severe stress of temperature and work,[116] the maximum sweating rate was 4.2 liters per hour and some men completed four hours of work while sweating at rates of 3 liters per hour, a total amount equal to approximately 4 times the blood water. While this high rate is not met in industry except in exceptional short-term situations, the loss of 1 liter of water per hour for an eight-hour day occurs at times in certain heavy industries and, with this volume of water, a total of perhaps 10 to 20 gm of salt.

A number of investigators have demonstrated that, in a matter of a few hours, the physical status and performance of subjects in a hot environment and doing hard work deteriorate (proceeding under severe conditions to actual collapse) when water is withheld.[116–122] Administration of water under these circumstances enables the body to maintain lower rectal and skin temperatures, more normal pulse rates, and mental efficiency. Symptoms of acute water lack during hard work in a hot environment appear to be the most rapidly induced of any deficiency syndrome. Recovery from the effects of dehydration following water ingestion is even more rapid.

Thirst is a reliable guide to water needs under most circumstances. However, men sweating even at moderate rates do not tend to drink water as fast as they evaporate it, although they usually make up the deficiency after the day's work.[123] When the heat load is high and continued, thirst may fail to insure an adequate intake.[122,124,125] It has been recommended[124,126] that men working in the heat replace the water lost in sweat by hour-to-hour ingestion of amounts more than sufficient to keep thirst quenched at all times. Water balance is affected by dietary factors other than water intake, since renal function operates within certain physiologic limitations. Thus, as indicated below, salt depletion leads to body water loss, despite a good fluid intake. At the other extreme, diets imposing a high osmotic load on the kidney will increase the obligatory water loss. Starvation with its attendant metabolic changes leads to increased urine volume.[127] In short, a number of nutritional and metabolic factors influence renal function and the ability to utilize water efficiently.

The effects of salt deficiency among industrial workers were first pointed out by Moss[128] in connection with "miners' cramps." Since then it has been noted in a variety of occupations among workers exposed to elevated temperatures. The basis of this deficiency is failure to replace adequately the sodium chloride lost in sweat, while the water loss is made good. Symptoms may include nausea, vomiting, vertigo, mental apathy, exhaustion, painful cramps, and circulatory failure. It is important to note that heat exhaustion due to salt deficiency is not always associated with heat cramps.[129,130] Workers in hot environments should have ready access to water (preferably cool but not cold) at all times and they should be instructed as to the importance of frequent water and adequate salt intake. Since the average American's daily diet contains 10 to 15 gm of salt and since salt lost in sweat need not be replaced hourly, the salt consumed at mealtimes is adequate for most needs. It is desirable, however, for workers consuming more than 4 quarts of water daily to supplement their dietary salt intake by 1 gm of salt for each additional quart of water consumed. This is most satisfactorily supplied in the drinking water in concentrations not higher than 0.2 per cent.[124,126] The use of salt tablets is less desirable since they frequently cause gastric distress, nausea, and vomiting in some individuals, especially during hard work and, more importantly, there is no assurance that those needing salt most will take the tablets.

Acclimatization to work in the heat is associated with a decrease in the sodium content of sweat. In order for this adaptive change to occur there must be a salt deficit with its attendant changes. It has been postulated that mineralo-corticoid production is involved in this response. Recent detailed balance and physiologic studies have confirmed this view.[131] During acclimatization of young men in the heat, while subsisting on a salt intake leading to deficits of 140 to 320 mEq, renal and sweat sodium outputs were greatly reduced, plasma sodium fell and urinary tetrahydroaldosterone increased 3- to 6-fold. With this salt depletion and attendant water deficit, the subjects had lower sweat rates and skin temperatures, higher rectal temperatures and less efficient tissue heat conductance than during acclimatization with replacement of salt and water. When salt and water were replaced under the same conditions of heat and exercise, sodium was retained and plasma volume was believed to increase. There was no increase in urinary tetrahydroaldosterone or sodium and three of the five subjects had no reduction in sweat sodium. Thus, while severe prolonged salt depletion, especially in the heat, is dangerous, some degree of salt depletion accelerates acclimatization.

It has been concluded[97] that there is a definite increase in energy requirement of men living and working in a hot desert climate as compared to those carrying out similar activities in a temperate climate The increase has been attributed to the increased heat load imposed on the body by solar radiation; the extreme heat leading to increased blood flow, increased sweat gland activity, increased caloric loss associated with sweat vaporization and an increase in metabolic rate due to elevation in body temperature.

Johnson and his co-workers[132] found that varying the daily protein intake in successive two-month periods from about 100 to 150 to 75 gm and back to 100 gm had no deleterious effect upon ability to march on a treadmill for relatively short periods in humid heat or to perform very hard work of short duration in a temperate environment. These workers challenge the recommendation of

Lusk[133] that a high-protein diet is contraindicated in hard work, especially in hot weather. Certainly, the fact is well established that acclimatized men in tropical areas who have access to meat eat it and often in large amounts without obvious untoward reactions.

It has been stated above that water and salt are the substances of main concern where sweating is profuse and prolonged. However, this is not to be construed as meaning that other nutrients may not be lost in significant quantities. Dermal losses have been reviewed by Mitchell and Edman,[134] and further quantitative data on the content of sweat have been published.[135–139] Considerable quantities of nitrogen are lost under conditions that produce profuse sweating, with values averaging 149, 189 and 241 mg/hour during exposures to environmental temperatures of 70, 85 and 100° F for men performing moderate daily physical activities.[137] With acclimation at 100° F, nitrogen excretion in sweat decreased from 300 to 200 mg/hour. These sweat losses were not compensated after acclimation by decreased nitrogen losses from the kidneys and alimentary tract. As a result, the protein requirements should be increased appropriately to compensate for nitrogen losses in sweat.

Free amino acids are lost in sweat. It has been estimated that, with a sweat volume of 3 liters per day, the loss of essential amino acids is not likely to exceed 1.5 gm.[140] The data of Consolazio et al.[135] support this figure and indicate that approximately one-third of the weight of amino acids lost is made up of essential amino acids. Acclimation decreases the losses of amino acids to a moderate degree but they still approximate 13 per cent of the total nitrogen lost in sweat.

During profuse sweating at 100° F calcium losses via this route averaged 234 mg/day with evidence of decrease with acclimation.[136] In 7.5 hours at 100° F, sweat excretions averaged 0.601 gm/hour for sodium, 0.125 gm/hour for potassium, 2.3 mg/hour for magnesium, 0.13 mg/hour for iron and 0.45 to 0.81 mg/hour for phosphorus.[137] Thus, calcium, potassium and iron losses may be significant and this route of excretion must be appreciated in mineral balance studies, especially where profuse sweating occurs. It should be noted that, in these studies,[134–137] the composition of arm sweat was taken as representative of whole body sweat.

Whole body sweat during 1 hour of profuse sweating at 40 to 45° C at high humidity at 1.29 L/hr was found to contain an average of 41.2 micrograms per 100 ml of iron of which 29.8 was in the cell-free fraction;[138] iron loss per hour was 0.53±0.45 mg, considerably higher than that noted above. Calcium and magnesium losses were 0.33 and 0.13 mEq/L respectively and 0.42 and 0.16 mEq per hour, respectively.[139]

Although there are no well-established figures for optimal intakes of fat or carbohydrates and one cannot speak of actual requirements for these nutrients, it appears that the usual pattern of dietary intake need not be altered in hot climates in order to perform work.

At least two possibilities exist for changes in vitamin requirements of men at elevated temperature: losses in sweat and altered metabolic requirements. Losses of vitamins in sweat were studied in a number of laboratories during World War II.[141] The evidence supports the conclusion that, in absolute amounts and in comparison with the urinary excretion of the water-soluble vitamins, losses in sweat are not a significant factor in depleting the body's stores. There is no evidence that metabolic requirements are increased. On the contrary, the observed increased urinary excretion of pantothenic acid and ascorbic acid may mean a lowered requirement at elevated temperatures. Some popularization of the belief that the need for ascorbic acid is increased has resulted from reports[142,143] of benefits from large amounts of vitamin C given to workers and from reports[144] that, in hyperpyrexia of infective or artificially induced origin, plasma ascorbic acid levels are reduced. However, Osborne and Farmer[145] were unable to find any reduction in plasma ascorbic acid in patients exposed to a temperature of 102° F in fever cabinets, and Abt and co-workers[146] concluded from studies on infectious diseases that hyperpyrexia alone did not affect the vitamin C reserves or utilization. No bene-

ficial effect of large amounts of vitamin C was noted on the ability of young men to work in hot environments for short periods (three hours to four days) nor were there any apparent effects on temperature, vasomotor stability, psychomotor, or strength responses, or on resistance to heat exhaustion.[147]

Mills and co-workers[148,149] claimed that in a hot (91° F) moist environment the requirements for growth of rats for certain vitamins, specifically thiamin and choline, were increased over those at 75° F, while the requirements for riboflavin and other vitamins were not affected. It should be noted that, in this work, the vitamins were incorporated in the diet so that their intake varied directly with the quantity of the diet ingested. When thiamin in different amounts was administered to rats separately from the ration, it was found that an increase in environmental temperature resulted in a *decreased* thiamin requirement.[150,151] These authors believe that this decrease approximates the decrease in caloric requirement at the elevated temperature.

Anoxia and Low Pressure. Acute and subacute exposure to high altitudes with resultant oxygen deprivation is associated with anorexia, dehydration and decreased work capacity.[152a–c] The suggestion made in 1908[153a] that a high-carbohydrate diet would prove beneficial in alleviating symptoms of oxygen lack has been confirmed in rats[153b] and man.[152a,153c–e]

Significant gains in altitude tolerance for periods up to six hours could be accomplished in human subjects maintained at the equivalent of 15,000 to 17,000 feet by the ingestion of preflight and inflight foods of high-carbohydrate content, in contrast with performance after the omission of a meal, after a single meal high in protein, or after large amounts of fat.[153b–e]

A comparative study was performed with young men exercising at sea level and after abrupt transfer to 14,000 feet while subsisting on one of two liquid diets of the same caloric value. Each diet had 12 per cent calories as protein but differed in carbohydrate and fat. On the higher carbohydrate-lower fat intake (68 and 20 per cent of calories, respectively), the men had considerably better performance in heaviest work and less clinical symptoms at altitude as compared to those on the diet with 48 per cent of calories from carbohydrate and 40 per cent from fat.[152a] Significant increases in oxygen consumption occurred at the above altitude as compared to sea level for similar work. These increases suggest an increased caloric requirement during acute high altitude exposure which may be due to the increased metabolic cost of cardiac and respiratory work and/or to decreased efficiency of work performance.[152d] Other investigators have not found increases in oxygen consumption during various work performances at altitudes below 10,500 feet.

With pressurized cabins in commercial and military planes, this aspect of diet would appear to have little practical significance. With population groups subsisting at high altitudes, benefit may be derived from high-carbohydrate intake. The importance of food at very high altitudes has been emphasized.[33,155]

Pressurized cabins have also reduced the earlier problems of abdominal pain occurring as the result of expansion of intestinal gases following rapid ascent at low pressures. To minimize this problem advice has been given to avoid carbonated beverages and melons,[156] fried meat, beans, cabbage, green leafy vegetables and raw fruit[157] in the hours just preceding ascent. The problem of intestinal gases has assumed new importance with the advent of prolonged flight in a closed system; this is considered in the next section.

There is no evidence that mild vitamin deficiency states have any effect on human altitude tolerance.[154]

Nutrition and Food in Space Travel. A host of problems in this area stems from limitations in storage of food and water, weightlessness, closed space, regeneration requirements and a variety of pressure and temperature changes. The major problems in meeting dietary specifications to date have been related to food technology and packaging. In the earliest manned American Mercury flights, tubed semisolid foods were utilized; these demonstrated that weightlessness posed no problems in terms of chewing, swallowing and digestion. The last Mercury flight utilized bite-size precooked dehydrated foods

which were rehydrated by saliva as chewed. To these were added compressed bite-size foods and more recently, in the Apollo flights, thermostabilized wet meat products. Criteria for space foods and their development and testing have been summarized.[158–160] Daily intakes by Gemini[163] and Apollo[160] astronauts ranged widely from day to day and mission to mission and were less than the 2500 kcal provided. Low residue foods which minimized intestinal gas formation were fed before and during flight.

An effort was made to perform nitrogen and mineral balance studies before, during and after the 14-day Gemini VII flight.[164] Decreased in-flight food intake and other problems adversely affected the accuracy of the results and considerable interindividual variability was observed in all experimental indices. Calcium balances tended to be less during flight but were of little significance. The losses noted in phosphate, potassium and nitrogen may have reflected loss of muscle mass.

Because of potential bone demineralization associated with weightlessness much attention is being given to this problem.[162,165] Neuman finds reassurance in the absence of clinical changes in astronauts that might be expected if massive mobilization of calcium had occurred; on the other hand, he notes a marked and unexplained discrepancy between bone densitometry results indicating significant demineralization without the expected hypercalciuria. A summary of clinical, physiologic and biochemical aspects of the Gemini flights is available.[163]

The forthcoming manned orbiting space stations will provide opportunity for longer-term nutritional, metabolic and acceptability studies. Presumably, expendable food supplies will be available by periodic resupply vehicles and more sophisticated systems of rations and preparation will be tested. The need for the most efficient planning of diets will become increasingly important with prolonged flights. For example, an overestimate of 300 kcal per man day will waste 71 pounds of oxygen per man year while underestimates may shorten flight time.[166]

Present diets are not dissimilar to the pattern of customary American diets in terms of proximate composition and standards for vitamins and minerals. However, as flights become protracted and activities become less sedentary, new problems in nutrition and physiology will require answers. If food is to be stored, there will be an advantage to high-fat diets. The acceptability of and tolerance and safety of various diets differing markedly in proximate composition is beginning to be studied in man.[161] Regenerative cycling systems in a sealed ecology will be necessary for flights lasting years. Physicochemical regeneration systems now being studied appear most suitable for the production of carbohydrates from carbon dioxide and waste materials.[160,161,167] Bioregenerative systems, utilizing algae, higher plants, bacteria, fungi and animals would obtain their nutrients from human excreta. Preliminary studies with a hydrogen-fixing bacteria, H. eutrophia indicate that treated cells are digestible and nutritious for rats[167,169] but poorly tolerated by man.[170]

The energy requirement for work in space, which at first glance might be expected to be decreased because of zero gravity, may be increased over that required for similar tasks with the same equipment at one G environment.[163,171] This is largely related to the absence of gravitationally imposed friction; increased energy is expended in attempting to maintain position to order to accomplish a given task. "Anchoring" and other devices will undoubtedly minimize this problem.

Intestinal bacteria form the inflammable gases, hydrogen and methane, as well as a number of malodorous and toxic compounds which cannot be allowed to accumulate in a closed space. The problem of their removal will increase as flights become longer and crews become more numerous. Intestinal gas formation is affected by the type and abundance of microflora, the substrates and psychic and somatic conditions affecting the gastrointestinal tracts. Studies of the volumes of hydrogen and methane passed rectally and by pulmonary ventilation indicate that there are very large differences among individuals on the same diet. There is much less production when a bland formula of purified nutrients is consumed as compared to a Gemini-type diet of dehydrated or compressed foods. Appre-

ciably larger volumes of these gases are exhaled through the breath than are passed in flatus.[168]

It is intriguing to speculate on what man's ingenuity will produce in meeting these nutritional and metabolic problems of life maintenance imposed by independent space travel.

BIBLIOGRAPHY

1. Passmore and Durnin: Physiol. Rev., 35, 801, 1955.
2. Kofranyi and Michaelis: Arbeitsphysiologie, 11, 148, 1940.
3. Müller and Franz: Arbeitsphysiologie, 14, 499, 1952.
4. Montoye, van Huss, Reineke, and Cockrell: Internat. Z. angew. Physiol. einschl. Arbeitsphysiol., 17, 28, 1958.
5. Consolazio and Johnson: Fed. Proc., 39, 1444, 1971.
6. Lehmann, Müller, and Spitzer: Arbeitsphysiologie, 14, 166, 1949–50.
7. Garry, Passmore, Warnock, and Durnin: Med. Res. Council, Spec. Rep. Ser. No. 289, H. M. Stat. Off. 1955.
8. Lehmann: Praktische Arbeitsphysiologie, Stuttgart, Thiene 1953.
9. Müller: Quart. J. Exp. Physiol., 38, 205, 1953.
10. Humphreys, Lind and Sweetland: Brit. J. Indust. Med., 19, 264, 1962.
11. Wolff: Quart. J. Exper. Physiol., 43, 270, 1958.
12. Lewis and Masterton: Lancet, 1, 1009, 1963.
13. Durnin and Passmore: Human Energy Expenditure, London, Heinemann, 1966.
14. Bradfield, Huntzicker, and Fruehan: Am. J. Clin. Nutrition, 22, 696, 1969.
15. Kottke: In Metabolism, Altman and Dittmer, eds., Fed. Am. Soc. Exp. Biol., Bethesda, Md., 1968, pp. 355–361.
16a. Burnet and Aykroyd: Quart. Bull. Health Organ, League of Nations, 4, 323, 1935.
16b. Dill: Physiol. Rev., 16, 263, 1936.
17a. Report on Committee on Calorie Requirements: Food and Agriculture Organization of the United Nations. FAO Nutritional Studies No. 5, Washington, D.C., 1950.
17b. ———: FAO Nutritional Studies No. 15, Rome, 1957.
17c. Nat. Res. Council, Food and Nutrition Bd.: Recommended Dietary Allowances, 7th ed., 1968, Publ. #1694, Nat. Acad. Sci., Wash. D.C., 1968, pp. 1–2.
18. Christensen, E. H.: in Ergonomics Soc., Symposium on Fatigue; Floyd & Welford, editors, London, Lewis, 1953 pp. 93–108.
19a. Gordon: A.M.A. Arch. Int. Med., 101, 702, 1958.
19b. Molbeck: In Physical Activity in Health and Disease, eds., Evang and Andersen, Baltimore, Williams & Wilkins Co., 1966, pp. 146–155.

19c. Burk, Bonjer and van der Sluys: Ibid. p. 207.
19d. Durnin: Proc. Nutrition Soc., 25, 107, 1966.
20. Keys, Brozek, Henschel, Mickelsen, Taylor and Simonson: *The Biology of Human Starvation*, Minneapolis, University of Minnesota Press, 1950.
21. Henschel, Taylor and Keys: J. Appl. Physiol., 6, 624, 1954.
22. Taylor, Henschel, Michelsen and Keys: J. Appl. Physiol., 6, 613, 1954.
23. Taylor, Buskirk, Brozek, Anderson and Grande: J. Appl. Physiol., 10, 421, 1957.
24. Brozek: Am. J. Clin. Nutrition, 5, 332, 1957.
25. Kraut and Müller: Science, 104, 495, 1946.
25a. Keller and Kraut: Work and Nutrition in *World Review Nutrition and Dietetics*, G. H. Bourne, Editor, Vol. 3, New York, Hafner, 1962, pp. 67–81.
26. Taylor and Keys: Science, 112, 215, 1950.
27. Grande, Anderson, and Keys: J. Appl. Physiol., 12, 230, 1958.
28. Swanson: Fed. Proc., 10, 660, 1951.
29. Rosenthal and Allison: J. Nutrition, 44, 423, 1951.
30. Calloway and Spector: Am. J. Clin. Nutrition, 2, 405, 1954.
31. Grande, Anderson and Taylor: J. Appl. Physiol., 10, 430, 1957.
32. Young, Schafer and Price: J. Appl. Physiol., 15, 1022, 1960.
33. Hunt, J.: *A Conquest of Everest*, New York, E. P. Dutton & Co., 1954.
34. Haggard and Greenberg: *Diet and Physical Efficiency*, New Haven, Yale University Press, 1935.
35. Gemmill: Physiol. Rev., 22, 32, 1942.
36. Haldi, Bachmann, Ensor, and Wynn: Am. J. Physiol., 121, 123, 1938.
37. Haldi and Wynn: J. Nutrition, 33, 287, 1947.
38. Ivy: J.A.M.A., 118, 569, 1942.
39. Clarke, DeJongh, and Jokl: Manpower, 1, 30, 1943.
40. Haggard and Greenberg: J. Am. Dietet. Assoc., 15, 435, 1939.
41. Holmes, Pigot, Sawyer, and Comstock: J. Indust. Hyg. & Toxicol., 14, 207, 1932.
42. Haldi and Wynn: J. Appl. Physiol., 2, 269, 1949.
43. Roethlisberger and Dickson: *Management and the Worker*, Cambridge, Harvard University Press, 1946.
44. Hutchinson: Nutr. Abstr. Rev., 22, 283, 1952.
45. Tuttle, Wilson and Daum: J. Appl. Physiol., 1, 545, 1949.
46. Tuttle, Daum, Meyers, and Martin: J. Am. Dietetic Assoc., 26, 332, 1950.
47. Tuttle and Herbert: J. Am. Dietetic Assoc., 37, 137, 1960.
48. Orent-Keiles, and Hallman: Circ. No. 827, 1949, U.S. Dept. Agric., Washington, D.C.
49. Simonson, Brozek, and Keys: J. Appl. Physiol., 1, 270, 1948.
50. Pyke: *Industrial Nutrition*, London, Macdonald & Evans, 1950.

51. Chittenden: Physiological Economy in Nutrition, New York, Stokes, 1904.
52. Cathcart and Burnett: Proc. Roy. Soc., London, B 99, 405, 1926.
53. Garry: J. Physiol., 62, 364, 1927.
54. Darling, Johnson, Pitts, Consolazio, and Robinson: J. Nutrition, 28, 273, 1944.
55. Thorn, Quinby, and Clinton: Ann. Int. Med., 18, 913, 1943.
56. Coleman, Tuttle, and Daum: J. Am. Dietetic Assoc., 29, 239, 1953.
57. Haldi and Wynn: Am. J. Physiol., 145, 402, 1945–46.
58. Lundbaeck: Acta Physiol. Scand., 7, 29, 1944.
59. Keys: Fed. Proc., 2, 163, 1943.
60. Christensen, Krogh, and Linhard: Quart. Bull. Health Organ, League of Nations, 3, 388, 1934.
61. Christensen and Hansen: Skand. Arch. f. Physiol., 81, 160, 1939.
62. Krogh and Linhard: Biochem. J., 14, 290, 1920.
63. Andres, Cader and Zierler: J. Clin. Invest., 35, 671, 1956.
64. Friedberg and Estes: J. Clin. Invest., 41, 677, 1962.
65a. Hultman: Suppl. 1, Circ. Res., 20 and 21, 1–99, 1967.
65b. Bergström, Hermansen, Hultman and Saltin: Acta Physiol. Scand., 71, 140, 1967.
65c. Karlsson and Saltin: J. Appl. Physiol., 31, 203, 1971.
65d. Ahlborg, Ekelund and Nilsson: Acta Physiol. Scand., 74, 238, 1968.
66. Simonson, Enzer, Baer, and Brown: J. Indust. Hyg. & Toxicol., 24, 83, 1942.
67. Keys and Henschel: J. Nutrition, 23, 259, 1942.
68. Keys, Henschel, Mickelsen, and Brozek: J. Nutrition, 26, 399, 1943.
69. Foltz, Ivy, and Barborka: J. Lab. & Clin. Med., 27, 1396, 1942.
70. Ryer: J. Clin. Nutrition, 2, 97 and 179, 1954.
71. Johnson, Darling, Sargent, and Robinson: J. Nutrition, 29, 155, 1945.
72. Jokl, and Suzmann: Proc. Transvaal Mine Medical Off. Assoc., 19, 19, 1939.
72a. Gey, Cooper and Bottenberg: J.A.M.A., 211, 105, 1970.
73. Wiehl: Milbank Mem. Fund Quart., 20, 329, 1942.
74. Borsook, Alpert, and Keighley: Milbank Mem. Fund Quart., 21, 115, 1943.
75. Borsook: Milbank Mem. Fund Quart., 23, 113, 1954.
76. Borsook, Dubnoff, Keighley, and Wiehl: Milbank Mem. Fund Quart., 24, 99, 1946.
77. Borsook and Wiehl: Milbank Mem. Fund Quart., 24, 251, 1946.
78. Johnson, Darling, Forbes, Brouha, Egana, and Graybiel: J. Nutrition, 24, 585, 1942.
79. Foltz, Barborka, and Ivy: Gastroenterology, 2, 323, 1944.
80. Archdeacon and Murlin: J. Nutrition, 28, 241, 1944.

81. Keys, Henschel, Taylor, Mickelsen, and Brozek: J. Nutrition, 27, 485, 1944.
82. ———: Am. J. Physiol., 144, 5, 1945.
83. Brozek, Guetzkow, Mickelsen, and Keys: J. Appl. Psychol., 30, 359, 1946.
84. Brozek, J.: in Symposium on Nutrition and Behavior, Am. J. Clin. Nutrition, 5, 109, 1957.
85. Berryman, Henderson, Wheeler et al.: Am. J. Physiol., 148, 165, 1944.
86. Keys, Henschel, Mickelsen, et al.: J. Nutrition, 27, 165, 1944.
87. Horwitt, Hills, Harvey et al.: J. Nutrition, 39, 357, 1949.
88. Crandon, Lund, and Dill: New England J. Med., 223, 353, 1940.
89. Farmer: Federation Proc., 3, 179, 1945.
90. Vitamin A Subcommittee, British Accessory Food Factors Comm., Nature, 156, 11, 1945.
91. Wald, Brouha, and Johnson: Am. J. Physiol., 137, 551, 1942.
92. Edholm and Goldsmith: Proc. Nutrition Soc., 25, 113, 1966.
93. Johnson and Kark: Science, 106, 378, 1947.
94. Rodahl: J. Nutrition, 53, 575, 1954.
95. Le Blanc: J. App.. Physiol., 10, 281, 1957.
96. Welch, Buskirk, and Iampietro: Metabolism, 7, 141, 1958.
97. Consolazio: In World Review of Nutrition and Dietetics, G. H. Bourne, ed., New York, Hafner, Vol. 4, 1963, pp. 55–77.
98. Keeton, Lambert, Glickman et al.: Am. J. Physiol., 146, 66, 1946.
98a. Mitchell, Glickman, Lambert et al.: Am. J. Physiol., 146, 84, 1946.
99. Rochelle and Horvath: J. Appl. Physiol., 27, 710, 1969.
100a. Johnson: Fed. Proc., 22, 1439, 1963.
100b. Johnson, Passmore and Sargent: Arch. Intern. Med., 107, 43, 1961.
100c. Rogers, Setliffe and Buck: Aerosp. Med., 39, 585, 1968.
101a. Dugal, Leblond, and Therien: Canad. J. Research, 23, 244, 1945.
101b. LeBlanc: Canad. J. Biochem. and Physiol., 35, 25, 1957.
101c. Seller, You, and Moffat: Am. J. Physiol., 177, 367, 1954.
102a. Beaton, J. R.: Canad. J. Biochem. & Physiol., 41, 139, 1963.
102b. Beaton, Feleki and Stevenson: Canad. J. Physiol. and Pharmacol., 42, 533, 1964.
103. Heroux: Fed. Proc., 28, 955, 1969.
104. Blair, Urbush, and Reed: Quoted by Mitchell, and Edman, Reference 141.
105. Glickman, Keeton, Mitchell, and Fahnestock: Am. J. Physiol., 146, 538, 1946.
106. Dugal, and Therien: Canad. J. Research, 25, 111, 1947.
107. Dugal, L. P.: In Cold Injury, 2nd Conference, Macy, New York, 1952, p. 85.
108. Ershoff: Arch. Biochem., 28, 299, 1950.
109. ———: Proc. Soc. Exp. Biol. & Med., 79, 559, 1952.
110. ———: Proc. Soc. Exp. Biol. & Med., 78, 385, 1951.
111. ———: Proc. Soc. Exp. Biol. & Med., 79, 580, 1952.
112. ———: J. Nutrition, 49, 373, 1953.
113. Internat. Symp. Cold Acclimation: Fed. Proc. Suppl. 5, Dec., 1960.
114. Mosoro: Physiol. Rev., 46, 67, 1966.
115. Internat. Symp. Altitude and Cold: Fed. Proc., Suppl. 28, May-June, 1969.
116. Eichna, Ashe, Bean, and Shelley: J. Indust. Hyg. & Toxicol., 27, 59, 1945.
117. Gregory and Lee: J. Physiol., 86, 204, 1936.
118. Bean and Eichna: Federation Proc., 2, 144, 1943.
119. Brown: Chapter 13 in Adolph et al., Physiology of Man in the Desert, New York, Interscience Press, 1947.
120. Dill: Life, Heat and Altitude, Cambridge, Harvard University Press, 1939.
121. Lee and Boissard: Med. J. Australia, 2, 664, 1940.
122. Pitts, Johnson, and Consolazio: Am. J. Physiol., 142, 253, 1944.
123. Adolph and Dill: Am. J. Physiol., 123, 369, 1938.
124. Johnson: Gastroenterology, 1, 832, 1943.
125. Rothstein, Adolph, and Wills: Chapter 16 in Adolph, et al., Physiology of Man in the Desert, New York, Interscience Press, 1947.
126. Hastings and Guest: Bull. Food & Nutrition Board, National Research Council, 4, 167, 1944.
127. Gamble: Harvey Lectures, 42, 247, 1946–47.
128. Moss: Proc. Roy. Soc. London, B. 95, 181, 1923–24.
129. Ladell, Waterlow, and Hudson: Lancet, 2, 491, 1944.
130. Taylor, Henschel, Mickelsen, and Keys: Am. J. Physiol., 140, 439, 1943.
131. Smiles and Robinson: Am. J. Physiol., 31, 63, 1971.
132. Pitts, Consolazio, and Johnson: J. Nutrition, 27, 497, 1944.
133. Lusk: The Science of Nutrition, Ed. 4, Philadelphia, W. B. Saunders Co., 1931.
134. Mitchell and Edman: Am. J. Clin. Nutrition, 10, 163, 1962.
135. Consolazio, Nelson, Matoush, Harding, and Canham: J. Nutrition, 79, 399, 1963.
136. Consolazio, Matoush, Nelson, Hackler, and Preston: J. Nutrition, 78, 78, 1962.
137. Consolazio, Matoush, Nelson, Harding, and Canham: J. Nutrition, 79, 407, 1963.
138. Vellar: Scand. J. Clin. Lab. Invest., 21, 157, 1968.
139. Vellar and Askevold: Scand. J. Clin. Lab. Invest., 22, 65, 1968.
140. Hier, Cornbleet, and Bergeim: J. Biol. Chem., 166, 327, 1946.
141. Mitchell and Edman: Nutrition and Climatic Stress, Springfield, Charles C Thomas, 1951.
142. Anonymous: Science (Suppl.), 95, 12, 1942.
143. Holmes: Science, 96, 384, 1942.
144. Ershoff: Physiol. Rev., 28, 107, 1948.

145. Osborne and Farmer: Proc. Soc. Exper. Biol. & Med., *49*, 575, 1942.

146. Abt, Hardy, Farmer, and Maaske: Am. J. Dis. Child., *64*, 426, 1942.

147. Henschel, Taylor, Brozek *et al.*: Am. J. Trop. Med., *24*, 259, 1944.

148. Mills: Am. J. Physiol., *133*, 525, 1941.

149. ———: Arch. Biochem., *1*, 73, 1942.

150. Kline, Friedman, and Nelson: J. Nutrition, *21*, 35, 1945.

151. Edison, Silber, and Tennent: Am. J. Physiol., *144*, 643, 1945.

152a. Consolazio, Matoush, Johnson *et al.*: Fed. Proc., *28*, 937, 1969.

152b. Krzywicki, Consolazio, Matoush *et al.*: Fed. Proc. *28*, 1190, 1969.

152c. Chinn and Hannon: Fed. Proc., *28*, 944, 1969.

152d. Johnson, Consolazio, Daws, and Krzywicki: Nutrition Repts. Internat., *4*, 77, 1971.

153a. Boycott and Haldane: Am. J. Physiol., *37*, 355, 1908.

153b. Campbell: Quart. J. Exp. Physiol., *29*, 259, 1939.

153c. King, Bouvet, Crook *et al.*: Science, *102*, 36, 1945.

153d. Eckman, Barach, Fox *et al*: J. Aviat. Med., *16*, 328, 1945.

153e. Green, Butts and Mulholland: J. Aviat. Med., *16*, 311, 1945.

154. Friedemann and Ivy: Quart. Bull. Northwestern Univ. Med. School, *21*, 31, 1947. Harris, Ivy, and Friedemann: Ibid., *21*, 135, 1947.

155. Pugh and Ward: Lancet, *2*, 1115, 1956.

156. Blair, Dern, and Smith: J. Aviat. Med., *18*, 352, 1947.

157. Tillisch: Quoted by McFarland, *Human Factors in Air Transportation*, New York, McGraw-Hill Book Co., Inc., 1953.

158. Hollender, Klicka, and Smith: *In Symp. Nutrition of Man in Space*. Comm. Space Res. Life Sci. and Space Res. VIII, eds. Vishniac and Favorite, London, North-Holland Publ. Co., 1970, pp. 265–279.

159. Vanderveen: Ibid., pp. 280–285.

160. Fox: Ibid., pp. 287–294.

161. Calloway: Ibid., pp. 295–301.

162. Neuman: Ibid., pp. 309–315.

163. Berry and Curtis: *In Progress in Atomic Medicine*, Vol. 2, ed., Lawrence; New York, Grune & Stratton, 1968, pp. 217–264.

164. Lutwak, Whedon, LaChance *et al.*: J. Clin. Endocr. Metab., *29*, 1140, 1969.

165. Birge and Whedon: *In Hypodynamics and Hypogravics*, ed. McCally; New York, Academic Press, 1968, pp. 213–235.

166. Calloway: J. Am. Dietet. Assoc., *44*, 347, 1964.

167. Shapira, Mandel, Quattrone and Bell: *In* Comm. Space Res. Life Sci. Space Res. VII, eds. Vishniac and Favorite, Amsterdam-London, North-Holland Publ. Co., 1969, pp. 123–129.

168. Calloway and Murphy: Ibid., pp. 102–109.

169. Mandel and Shapira: Cited by Fox, ref. 160.

170. Waslien, Calloway and Margen: Nature, *221*, 84, 168.

171. Wunder: Life Into Space, Philadelphia, F. A. Davis Co., 1966, Chap. 10.

PART VI

Nutrition in the Prevention and Treatment of Disease

Chapter

27

Nutrition in Relation to Dental Medicine

James H. Shaw

AND

Edward A. Sweeney

Dental medicine is the specialty of medicine that is concerned with the welfare of the teeth and the soft tissues of the oral cavity and with the diagnosis of systemic diseases that have oral manifestations. During the past three or four decades, it has become increasingly evident that nutrition plays just as important a role in the development and maintenance of the oral tissues as in the development and maintenance of tissues elsewhere in the body. Indeed the tissue components of the mouth are little different from comparable tissues elsewhere in the body as far as their metabolic processes during development, growth and maintenance are concerned.

By reason of the specific location and function of the oral cavity, its tissues are subjected to a wider variety and probably a more stringent series of stresses than are tissues in other moist internal cavities of the body. Consider for example: the wide variety in physical texture of the food that has to be chewed into a form suitable for swallowing; the wide range of temperatures of common food components as ingested; the wide variety of chemical stimuli to which the tissues of the oral cavity are exposed periodically; and the ideal circumstances for the growth and multiplication of the wide spectrum of microorganisms that reside therein. The subdivision of food by the teeth and the buffering and diluting capacity of the saliva greatly reduce the intensity of some of these stresses before the food materials are passed

on to the lower areas of the gastrointestinal tract. The soft tissues are unusually susceptible to current metabolic abnormalities of nutritional origin. During the early years in which characteristic signs of individual nutrient deficiencies were recognized, the soft tissues of the oral cavity were particularly valuable by reason of their susceptibility to these nutritional disturbances and by reason of their ready accessibility for examination. The classical signs of nutritional deficiencies in oral tissues will not be discussed in this chapter since they are represented in detail in the chapters of this book that are concerned with the B complex deficiencies and with scurvy.

In contrast, the hard tissues of the oral cavity, the enamel, dentin and cementum, are much less influenced by post-developmental systemic disorders than by the systemic disorders which operate during the developmental period. To a certain degree, the dental hard structures are kymographs in which are recorded both physical and chemical evidence of the metabolic circumstances which were prevalent at the time the specific areas of these structures were elaborated and calcified. However, in addition the integrity of the teeth is influenced to a large extent by the oral environment which surrounds their external surfaces on a current basis. In any discussion of the relationship of a specific diet to the integrity of the hard structures, both the dietary influences upon oral environment and upon the nutritional status as mediated through one or more systemic pathways must be considered and integrated.

Over the past three or four decades, an appreciable change has occurred in the type of nutritional manifestation observed by clinicians. At the beginning of this period frank nutritional deficiencies, pellagra, beri-beri, and rickets, were commonly seen in dental practices in large urban areas and in rural communities alike. During this period, due to the widespread increase in the attention focused on nutritional problems, particularly in the oral cavity, a striking decrease in oral manifestations of nutritional deficiency diseases has been observed in the average practice. Hence our attention is being directed in an increasing degree to those nutritional abnormalities which occur during development or over prolonged periods of adult life, but which are not detected until long after the actual conditions of nutrient imbalance may have begun. Such studies need to be made in a variety of the chronic diseases that plague the human race.

The diseases of the oral cavity are particularly good examples of diseases which have delayed components. The incidence of tooth decay, in particular, has been shown to be related to specific nutritional abnormalities that occur during tooth development. The diseases of the periodontal tissues may likewise have nutritional components which are presently unknown or ill-defined, but the prevalence of these diseases should spur investigators to pursue more diligently the possible ways in which these influences are mediated.

Before a discussion of the oral diseases that result from nutritional abnormalities, let us consider some of the present knowledge about the structure of the teeth and surrounding tissues, the uniqueness of these calcified tissues, and some of the established facts concerned with the etiology of oral disease.

THE STRUCTURE OF TEETH

The teeth are composed of three highly calcified tissues: enamel, dentin and cementum (Fig. 27–1). Enclosed within these calcified tissues is a highly vascular connective tissue, the dental pulp, which is frequently called the "nerve" of the tooth because of its great sensitiveness to heat, cold and other stimuli. Around the periphery of the pulp, in contact with the inner surface of the dentin, is a layer of cells, the odontoblasts. These cells are responsible for the formation of the dentin and continue to lay down secondary dentin at a relatively slow rate throughout the life of the tooth. When these cells are stimulated by the proximity of a carious lesion, secondary dentin is formed more rapidly as a barrier between the lesion and the pulp. The odontoblasts are mesodermal in origin as are the cementoblasts which are responsible for the deposition of cementum around the outer surfaces of the roots of the tooth. In contrast, the enamel is of ectodermal origin, being formed by ameloblasts that persist as a portion of the enamel organ until the time the teeth begin to erupt into the oral cavity.

The teeth are retained in their bony sockets or alveolae by means of the highly fibrous tissue structure termed the periodontal membrane. The diseases which affect the integrity of this structure or the integrity of the bone surrounding the socket result in one or another phase of periodontal disease and may progress sufficiently to cause loosening and loss of the teeth.

Early anatomic studies of the enamel with the light microscope led investigators to postulate that the smallest structural units of enamel were inorganic prisms surrounded and cemented together by a sheath of interprismatic cementing substance. Only 2 or 3 per cent of organic matter is contained in the enamel. Almost the entire composition of the rest is inorganic substances. The tiny amount of organic matter present was originally believed to be contained in these interprismatic sheaths. However, recent observations made possible by the higher resolving power of the electron microscope indicated that this concept was unduly restricted. Instead, minute fibrils of organic matter have been observed to permeate each of the enamel prisms in extremely delicate and intimate fashion.[1] In addition, the interprismatic substance has been shown to have deposited

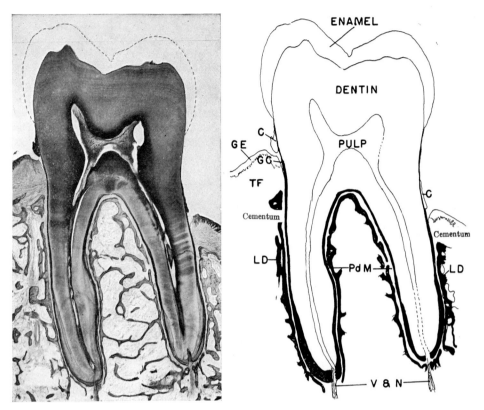

Fig. 27-1. Mesiodistal section of a lower molar tooth. (The enamel is disrupted by the evolution of gas bubbles during decalcification of the specimen.) Normally the gingival epithelium (*GE*) is in close apposition to the cervix of the tooth and acts as a barrier to decrease bacterial invasion of the underlying dermis. Transverse fibers (*TF*) form another barrier against bacterial penetration. In this case, a small amount of salivary calculus (*C*) was deposited and caused the formation of an abnormally deep gingival crevice (*GC*). This is the beginning of periodontoclasia which, at a later stage, causes destruction of the lamina dura (*LD*), a compact bony plate lining the alveolus as well as the periodontal membrane (*Pd M*) which attaches the entire tooth root to the surrounding bone. *V & N*, vessels and nerves supplying the dental pulp.

within it an appreciable number of inorganic crystals.

The dentin is traversed by tubules which radiate from the pulp to the dento-enamel junction. Organic processes from the odontoblasts actually penetrate the entire width of the dentin. It has been postulated that extracellular fluid may be transported from the pulp across the dentin by reason of these processes. The exact status of this hypothesis is indefinite at the present time. The organic content of dentin is much higher than for enamel and approximates the concentration of the long bones.

The time intervals involved in the development of teeth are important considerations in any discussion of the relationship of nutrition to tooth development and to the later caries susceptibility of the teeth. The life history of a tooth may be divided into three main eras: the period during which the crown of the tooth is forming and calcifying in the jaw; the period of maturation when the tooth is erupting into the oral cavity and its root or roots are forming; and the maintenance period while it is in full function in the oral cavity. The length of time during which a human tooth is developing and maturing prior to its functional responsibilities is often forgotten. As an example of the time interval involved let us consider the first secondary molar, the six-year molar, which is one of our more

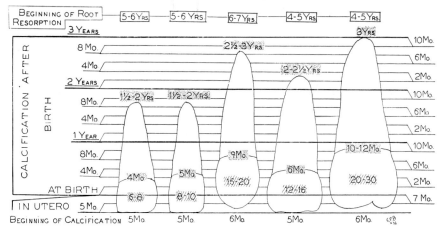

Fig. 27-2. Periods of calcification and eruption of the primary teeth. The portions of the teeth that are formed completely are seen below the lines. Figures in dotted areas, the time of completion of the crowns and roots, shaded figures, the time (in months) that the tooth appears normally in the mouth. Chart of the left upper jaw; this information applies approximately to the other teeth, with slight variations. (Adapted from Logan and Kronfeld.)

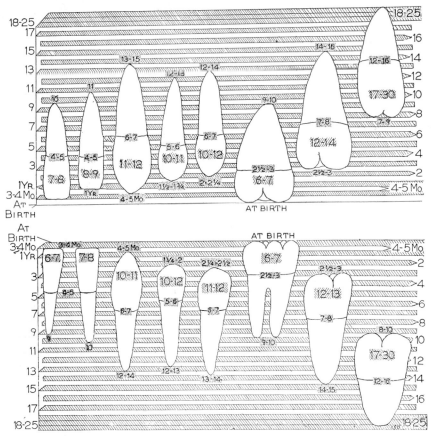

Fig. 27-3. Periods of calcification and eruption of the secondary teeth. The upper and lower first molars (sixth from the left) calcify at or soon after birth. The beginning of calcification of the other teeth and the average time of completion of their crowns and roots are indicated by figures in dotted areas. Shaded figures indicate when the crown appears normally in the mouth. This type of graph precludes drawing the teeth in correct anatomic form. (Adapted from Logan and Kronfeld.)

736

important teeth by reason of its large masticating surface. Its histologic primordia are elaborated about the time the infant is born. From then until $2\frac{1}{2}$ to 3 years of age, the organic frameworks of the enamel and dentin in the crown are being deposited and calcified. By the end of the third year, the crown has attained its adult size but is not yet fully calcified. Eruption into the oral cavity begins between 6 and 7 years of age and its roots are completed around 9 to 10 years of age. Thus almost 10 years elapse between the initiation of this tooth and the attainment of its final form. Comparable data for the primary teeth and the secondary teeth are presented in Figures 27–2 and 3.

THE UNIQUENESS OF THE DENTAL CALCIFIED STRUCTURES

In a discussion of nutritional influences upon teeth, we must recognize that at least three striking differences exist between the calcified tissues of the teeth and other tissues of the body. First, enamel contains no microscopically detectable capillary or lymphatic vessels to act as transport systems for nutrients. However, the intimate relationships between the organic and the inorganic components of enamel suggest that pathways for diffusion from saliva, and possibly blood, to the enamel and the rest of the body may readily exist, even though there is no evidence of any vascular or neural elements within enamel. The dentin likewise contains no formed vascular elements. However, its structure is such that it may lend itself more readily to a passage of extracellular fluids from the blood, by reason of dentinal tubules that traverse the dentin from the odontoblastic layer of the pulp to the dento-enamel junction.

Second, calcified dental tissues do not have a microscopically or chemically detectable ability to repair areas which are formed improperly or calcified inadequately during development, nor does the tooth have an ability to repair itself after a portion has been destroyed by tooth decay or by a mechanical injury. An exception to the latter statement may be the remineralization of those slightly decalcified superficial areas of the enamel where the organic matrix is intact, commonly referred to as "white spots." Lack of ability to repair dental tissues is in direct contrast to the long bones where the Haversian systems are continually being remodeled and replaced and where diseased or fractured areas heal. Yet, despite the above contrast, studies with radiotracer materials indicate that enamel and dentin are permeable to various inorganic ions. The inorganic elements of each area of mature teeth are capable of participating in an exchange process with comparable elements carried to the area by body fluids.[2] The observation in mature teeth that the interchange between normal and radioisotopic elements in the enamel took place by reason of the contact of enamel with saliva is particularly interesting and thought provoking. In contrast, the interchange in the dentin occurred by reason of the ions brought to the dentin by the blood supply in the pulp or the periodontal membrane. Thus, saliva acts as the pathway by which systemic nutritional influences are communicated to the enamel.

Third, unlike other tissues, the calcified tissues of teeth have a partial change of environment midway in their life history. During the developmental period, while the tooth is growing and calcifying, it has complete systemic contact through normal vascular and neural pathways. When the tooth begins to emerge into the oral cavity, the blood vascular supply to the enamel organ is severed, and the enamel surface comes in contact with that complex mixture of saliva, microorganisms, food debris, epithelial remnants, etc., which is typical of the oral cavity. Thus, instead of a systemic environment only, the tooth has, in addition, an oral or external environment. The effects of this environment have to be studied and evaluated whenever a change in incidence of tooth decay results from a postdevelopmental dietary manipulation.

MODERN CONCEPTS OF DENTAL CARIES

During recent years a number of facts have been clearly established about the etiology of dental caries. Some of these pertain to concepts which have been postulated for generations from human studies but which have been demonstrated now beyond reasonable doubt by definitive experimental trials with laboratory animals.

There can no longer be any question that microorganisms are required to cause the destruction of tooth substance in the characteristic fashion termed "tooth decay." This point was established in studies with caries-susceptible rats that were maintained throughout life under germ-free circumstances.[3] In this experimental environment, these animals did not develop tooth decay when fed a caries-producing ration. The germ-free technique provides the opportunity to evaluate which microorganisms or groups of microorganisms are responsible for the destruction of enamel and dentin in the characteristic manner defined as dental caries. In one study Orland and co-workers[4] inoculated germ-free caries-susceptible rats with a mixed culture of enterococci and found that characteristic carious lesions developed in the sulci of the molars. Mono inoculation by several different microorganisms caused carious lesions in more recent studies. Keyes[5] has demonstrated that under certain experimental conditions dental caries in rats and hamsters can be considered to be an infectious and transmissible disease. Fitzgerald and Keyes[6] have induced experimental dental caries in a strain of caries-inactive hamsters maintained under conventional caging conditions by oral inoculation of single or pooled cultures of streptococci that had been isolated from hamster carious lesions. Carious lesions have also been produced in rats that were maintained under germ-free conditions except for inoculation with a single strain of an oral streptococcus isolated from a rat[7] or with each of two strains of streptococci isolated from human carious lesions.[8] These cariogenic microorganisms stored intracellular iodophilic polysaccharide[9] and produced large quantities of extracellular non-dialyzable capsules that may be important in enabling the microorganisms to adhere to tooth surfaces.[8] Some strains isolated from human carious lesions were immunologically similar to strains isolated from oral cavities of rats and hamsters and were capable of causing carious lesions in rats and hamsters.[10]

Clinical observations have indicated that the salivary glands are of considerable importance in the maintenance of teeth. Where salivary glands are congenitally missing or are destroyed by radiation of the head and neck region, there is invariably an increased susceptibility to dental caries. Similarly, in experimental animals, the surgical removal of the major salivary glands results in spectacular increases in tooth decay.[11] Of the several salivary glands, the parotid and submaxillary glands have been shown to be most important in the rat, with the sublingual gland contributing relatively little to the maintenance of the teeth.[12] In human studies the quantity or consistency of the saliva has not yet been shown conclusively to have a definite relation to caries incidence except where xerostomia has been induced by surgical or radiological desalivation. The total amounts of certain salivary constituents secreted may be more important than the total volume in which they are secreted.[13]

The correctness of the old saying, "A clean tooth never decays," and the difficulty to obtain such a condition have been demonstrated by experiments in a series of rats where their diet was introduced directly into the stomach by a tube-feeding procedure.[14] The normal microbial oral flora were observed in those animals but no carious lesions developed. When the same caries-producing diet was eaten in the usual fashion by littermates, a high incidence of tooth decay was observed. Even when the supreme penalty of sialoadenectomy was imposed upon the tube-fed animals, no carious lesions developed. Of all the components of the diet, carbohydrate is essential in the oral cavity for the production of tooth decay. When a carbohydrate-free diet is fed for prolonged periods either to intact rats or to ones from which the principal salivary glands have been removed, no carious lesions develop.[15] If all the diet except the carbohydrate is introduced into the stomach by tube and only the carbohydrate ingested orally, carious lesions developed at approximately the expected rate for rats that consume the entire diet by the normal route.[16] Likewise, when caries-susceptible rats consume a liquid diet, they have appreciably less tooth decay than when their littermate control rats consume the same ration in solid form.[17]

Extensive studies have been conducted in human populations in a mental institution in Sweden, where sucrose was fed in several forms at high levels to inmates for relatively prolonged periods of time.[18] When high amounts of sucrose were fed in solution, the increase in dental caries incidence was barely perceptible. However, when sucrose was fed in the form of sticky candy such as caramels or toffees, there were tremendous increases in the incidence of tooth decay. Comparable amounts of sugar in chocolates or in bread caused intermediate increases in dental caries incidence. Provision of these sources of fermentable carbohydrate with the meals caused a lesser influence upon the dental caries incidence than the same supplements between meals. As soon as the supplements were stopped, the frequency of appearance of new carious lesions decreased to the pre-experimental level. These studies uniformly point toward the rate of oral clearance of carbohydrates and the frequency of their consumption as strong determining factors on the extent of tooth decay.

Mono- and disaccharides as the sole sources of carbohydrate in simple forms of purified diets usually cause a higher rate of dental caries incidence in experimental animals than the same quantities of starches or dextrins.[19] However, where natural diets are used, other carbohydrates have been shown to be equally or more cariogenic than sucrose. In some of the experiments by Hunt's group at Michigan State, finely ground rice has been shown to be more cariogenic than sucrose[20] and in other studies various forms of cooked cereals have been shown to be more cariogenic than sucrose.[21] Under some experimental conditions dietary sucrose permitted a more rapid progression of carious lesions than glucose and greater recoveries of cariogenic streptococci.[22] The latter microbiota produced large quantities of insoluble dextrans exclusively from sucrose which enabled the microorganisms to adhere to and metabolize on tooth surfaces.[23,24] Under some conditions, the inclusion of a dextranase preparation in the drinking water and diet of hamsters caused a major reduction in plaque

formation and caries activity.[25] These studies led to the hypothesis that sucrose was uniquely cariogenic and that its replacement by other disaccharides or by monosaccharides in the human diet would be beneficial. Unfortunately some laboratory data do not support that position. For example, in the rat, other carbohydrates such as glucose and maltose were as cariogenic as sucrose and the mixed flora in these rats was able to form insoluble dextrans from glucose and maltose.[26] In addition, dextranase was not effective in white rats.[27] Whether sucrose in man is uniquely cariogenic in any sense other than sucrose is the predominant simple sugar in human diets remains to be evaluated in clinical trials. Various antibiotic materials such as penicillin, tetracyclines, dibasic ammonium compounds and urea have been shown to cause a reduced incidence in tooth decay among experimental animals and in some cases also in human subjects.[28–30]

Strong genetic traits toward caries resistance or toward caries susceptibility have been reported in animal strains in laboratories.[31,32] The mechanism by which these hereditary tendencies are mediated is unknown. However, it is important to notice that both oral environmental and nutritional variations may modify the degree of manifestation of the genetic tendency. For example, if a strain of rats is highly susceptible to tooth decay, the incidence of dental caries may be greatly reduced by any one of a number of the above variations induced in the oral environment. In addition, various nutritional influences imposed during tooth development may reduce the incidence of tooth decay below that which would be expected in this caries-susceptible strain if these nutritional influences had not been brought to bear during tooth development. Likewise a caries-resistant strain of rats will have an increased incidence of tooth decay if the salivary glands are removed or if a particularly cariogenic ration is fed. An excellent description of the relationship between the genetic and environmental factors in experimental dental caries has been given by Larson.[33] The genetic determinism of the level of caries susceptibility in inbred strains of rats appeared to be very strong.[34] Offspring of caries-susceptible parents were able to establish a caries-producing microflora with ease after various attempts to prevent the parents from passing on their flora to the next generation. Likewise, massive oral inoculations of flora from caries-active rats into offspring of caries-resistant parents had little influence on their rate of caries activity. Probably the most striking evidence of a genetic factor was provided by a doublemating of female rats from a white caries-susceptible strain with males of the same strain and males of a black, less caries-susceptible strain.[35] Despite the identical environmental conditions, the heterozygotic offspring had a lesser dental caries incidence than the homozygotic littermates.

NUTRITIONAL INFLUENCES DURING TOOTH DEVELOPMENT

With this related background of information about the structure of teeth, the development of teeth, and the etiology of dental caries, let us examine some of the specific known relationships between nutrition and dental caries as they are encountered in the three eras in the life history of an individual tooth. Unquestionably the most striking of these influences occur by reason of imposition of nutritional deficiencies during tooth development. Three classic examples exist in which specific nutritional deficiencies adversely influence the development of various areas of the teeth in ways that are histologically discernible: avitaminosis-A, scurvy, and rickets attributable to deficiencies of vitamin D, calcium or phosphorus, or to a gross imbalance of the calcium-phosphorus ratio. In addition, inadequate levels of fluoride and disturbed calcium-phosphorus ratios during tooth development result in abnormalities of the chemical composition, at a submicroscopic level, which are related to caries susceptibility.

Vitamin A. Just as vitamin A deficiency influences the integrity of epithelial tissues throughout the entire body, this deficiency also influences the ameloblasts which are of epithelial origin. Early studies by Wolbach and Howe demonstrated that the deficiency of vitamin A in rodents resulted in degeneration and atrophy of the ameloblasts.[36,37] In the vitamin A-deficient animals, the first

histologically visible change in the teeth was observed in the odontoblasts. Since the ameloblasts are responsible for the organization of the odontogenic epithelium, it is believed that the first evidence of abnormality in the ameloblasts during the early stages of the development of vitamin A deficiency is the loss of the physiologic ability to stimulate the development and arrangement of the odontoblasts from the connective tissue in the vicinity. Thus, the odontoblasts are not stimulated to differentiate and do not arrange themselves in normal fashion. Later, profound anatomic changes in the ameloblasts are observed. In late stages of this deficiency, the cells exhibit such a degree of squamous metaplasia that virtually no recognizable ameloblasts can be found. Consequently a great reduction occurs in the rate at which the organic matrix of enamel is formed. Various degrees of abnormality occur in the formation of the matrix. Enamel hypoplasia is a prominent manifestation of severe and prolonged vitamin A deficiency in experimental animals. Since the proliferative activity of the odontogenic epithelium does not cease in vitamin A deficiency, chords of these undifferentiated epithelial cells invade the pulpal tissue where they form isolated cell masses. Some of these cells retain the ability to stimulate the neighboring mesenchyma to abortive attempts at dentin formation; in this fashion numerous calcified concretions occur in the pulp of the teeth.

Repair patterns in the teeth of rodents recovering from vitamin A deficiency are both straightforward and rapid. The odontogenic epithelium regains its function and morphologic appearance; this is followed by the formation of normal odontoblasts and the deposition and calcification of normal dentin. Where there has been an infolding of the odontogenic epithelium, recovery often results in tooth duplications and tumor-like formations.

Boyle has reported that similar changes occur in the developing dental tissues of a prematurely born vitamin A-deficient infant.[38] In additional cases of vitamin A deficiency in infants, Dinnerman has reported consistent abnormalities of structure and appearance in the enamel and the enamel-forming organs to those lesions observed in experimental animals.[39] In addition, the dentin was poorly calcified and contained scattered globules of unusual size; the predentin was extraordinarily wide. The other changes observed were entirely consistent with the descriptions in the literature for experimental animals.

No conclusive body of information indicates that enamel hypoplasia in human beings is directly attributable to vitamin A deficiency during tooth development. However, a linear enamel hypoplasia of deciduous incisor teeth has been reported as being present in as many as 50 per cent of children from some developing countries which commonly have endemic vitamin A and protein-calorie deficiencies.[40,41] The etiology of this perinatally timed enamel hypoplasia may have its basis in the malnutrition-infection interrelationships. With a cariogenic diet these affected teeth demonstrate a high susceptibility to a type of decay which has been called odontoclasia.

Repeated demonstrations have been made of influences of vitamin A deficiency on epiphyseal bone formation. These changes were primary results of the general deficiency syndrome, since they occurred sufficiently early in the deficiency to precede the cessation of over-all growth. The studies of Wolbach and Bessey have demonstrated that these are specific effects of vitamin A deficiency and that the nerve damage in these deficiency states is secondary to and caused by the bone changes.[42] Vitamin A is essential for the activity of the epiphyseal cartilage cells without which they are incapable of undergoing the normal sequence of growth, maturation and degeneration which is essential in the mechanism of endochondral or replacement bone growth. Since vitamin A deficiency suppresses the cartilage cell sequences, endochondral bone growth is retarded and finally ceases entirely in long-continued vitamin A deficiency. Remodeling sequences, involving concurrent resorption of bone with bone deposition and replacement of cancellous bone by compact bone, cease to operate. There is a greatly reduced rate of resorption of trabecular bone with retardation and failure of Haversian system forma-

tion which results in an arrestment of compact bone formation. Eventually all skeletal growth dependent upon replacement of endochondral bone formation ceases. Appositional growth of bone of periosteal origin continues until inanition intervenes at a rate in conformity to the normal growth pattern at each particular site. Presumably the fact that growth of bone of periosteal origin continues is evidence that there is no fundamental error of calcification in the vitamin A-deficient rodent.

These effects upon bone growth in vitamin A deficiency are of potential interest in the field of children's dentistry and orthodontics. There has never been any thorough investigation to determine whether orthodontic problems may be related to nutritional deficiencies during development. Since vitamin A deficiency causes such a profound influence on bone development, some of the inadequate growth patterns which result in orthodontic problems may have had their origin in prolonged periods of subclinical vitamin A deficiency during the developmental period of the child.

Vitamin C. Scurvy, the clinical entity which is attributable to vitamin C deficiency, has been described in detail in the chapter

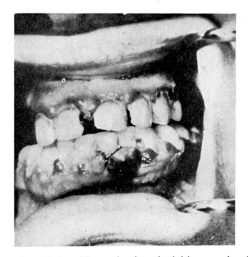

Fig. 27-4. Hemorrhagic gingivitis associated with avitaminosis C (scurvy). Note the swelling of the interdental papillae and the large hematoma between the lower left central and lateral incisors. (Cahn, L. R.: *Pathology of the Oral Cavity*, Baltimore, The Williams & Wilkins Co.)

concerned with ascorbic acid. In frank vitamin C deficiency, the lesions of the gingiva are particularly striking[43] (Fig. 27–4).

It is noteworthy that these occur only when teeth are present and that the condition is remarkably consistent. The gingival lesions begin on the interdental papilla, first as hyperemia with dilated thin-walled vessels which have a tendency to hemorrhage. Disintegration of the epithelium follows, and infection with ulceration, granulations and gangrene may result. The gums become inflamed and spongy and bleed easily. In cases of severe deficiency, these lesions become sufficiently extensive to obstruct mastication and are frequently accompanied by loosening of the teeth and tooth loss.

The deficiency of vitamin C primarily affects the ability of cells of connective tissue origin to elaborate their typical collagenous intercellular substances. The odontoblasts which form the dentin in developing teeth are of mesodermal origin and are readily affected by the deficiency of vitamin C. Wolbach and Howe have studied the pathogenesis of these changes extensively.[44] When guinea pigs are placed on a scorbutic diet, alterations soon appear in the odontoblasts which become atrophic and resemble the nearby pulp cells. There is a decrease in their orderly polar arrangement, a decrease in height, and eventually a complete disorganization. The decreased height of the odontoblasts in moderate deficiencies is believed to be sufficiently closely related to the vitamin C intake to permit this measurement to be used as a bioassay criterion.[45] At the same time, the rate of dentin formation is sufficiently closely related to the amount of vitamin C consumed that it also can be used as a criterion for the bioassay of the vitamin C content of the diet.[46] The dentin which is formed is laid down irregularly with the dentinal tubules lacking their normal parallel arrangement. In severe deficiencies, dentin deposition stops entirely and the predentin becomes hypercalcified. At late stages in the deficiency the ameloblasts atrophy and hemorrhages occur. These changes have been interpreted to be due to traumatic injury of the enamel organ as the result of inadequate support of the underlying dentin. Though these changes

occur readily in the developing teeth of experimental animals, evidence has not been presented yet to indicate a similar occurrence in human teeth as a result of scurvy during tooth development.

As would be expected there is a rarefaction of the alveolar bone comparable to what is seen in the ribs and bones of experimental animals and humans. The pathologic sequence in the destruction of the alveolar bone has been reported to closely resemble the changes observed in diffuse alveolar atrophy.[47] Weakness of the supporting bones, as well as the weakness of the collagen fibers in the supporting structures, allows for a greater mobility of the teeth and a decreased ability to withstand the mechanical stresses encountered in chewing.

The pathologic condition in the pulp and in the odontoblastic layer in human beings is nearly identical with the pathologic changes in the scorbutic guinea pig, according to Westin.[48] In the teeth of scorbutic adults the dentin is resorbed and porotic. The small amount of replacement dentin formed is of the osteodentin type. The pulp is atrophic and hyperemic. Degeneration of the odontoblasts, the formation of cysts, and foci of diverticuli-like regions of calcification were described.

Although the relationship of vitamin C deficiency to gingival changes and to bone pathology has been repeatedly demonstrated, there has never been a clear-cut demonstration of a relationship between scurvy and dental caries. A large experiment was conducted at an orphanage by Hanke where the usual orphanage diet was daily supplemented with a pint of orange juice and the juice of 1 lemon over a period of one year.[49] The experimental group of children evidently had a reduced incidence of new carious lesions in contrast to the control group of children which had had no citrus fruit supplementation. However, surveys by Westin,[50] Hess and Abramson,[51] and experiments by McBeath[52] and Grandison, Stott and Cruickshank[53] failed to demonstrate any difference in dental caries incidence between groups which received normal diets and those supplemented with considerable amounts of vitamin C.

Vitamin D, Calcium and Phosphorus.
The first experimental production of rickets to demonstrate an influence upon tooth development was reported by Lady May Mellanby in 1918.[54] She observed that a deficiency of a fat-soluble vitamin, later designated as vitamin D, in young puppies had a profound effect on the developing enamel and dentin of the secondary teeth, on the rate of eruption, and also on the position of the teeth in the jaw. When vitamin D deficiency was imposed upon a female dog during pregnancy, the primary teeth of the puppies had defects in structure and their eruption was delayed.[55] However, the puppies from comparable dogs supplemented with adequate amounts of the fat-soluble vitamin had normal deciduous teeth.

The changes that occur in teeth during the rachitic process are appreciably less complex than those in bones. The first and most prominent change observed in rickets in rats is a calciotraumatic line, a line of disturbed calcification in the dentin.[56] This is accompanied by retardation in the formation of predentin and a pronounced disturbance in the calcification of the dentin. The latter is no longer homogeneously basophilic but is stippled by an irregular deposition of inorganic salts. Calcification of the cementum is likewise retarded.

Enamel hypoplasia does not occur except in the more severe cases of rickets in the dog, whereas inadequate calcification of both the enamel and dentin can be demonstrated at relatively mild levels of the rachitic process. Enamel hypoplasia has not been described in the rat as a result of rickets, but it is likely that a sufficiently severe deficiency over a prolonged period would cause this abnormality even in this species. In human beings, there is likely to be more than one cause of

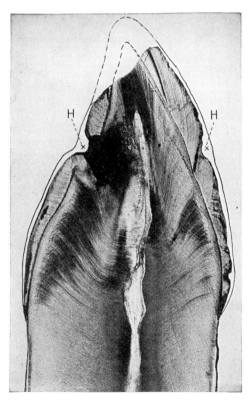

Fig. 27-5. Section of an upper canine tooth. A severe systemic disturbance, which occurred when the patient was about 3 years old, caused the hypoplasia of the enamel (*H*). As shown by poor calcification and rills in the subsequently formed enamel (near the cervix of the tooth), the condition improved but did not become normal. The solid line, extent of normal enamel; dotted lines, loss of tooth structure due to attrition.

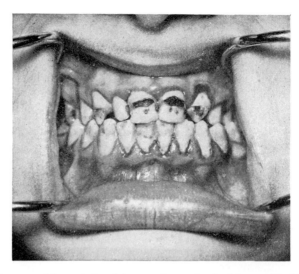

Fig. 27-6. Excessive enamel hypoplasia of the anterior teeth of a 16-year-old girl which may have been due to severe malnutrition in early childhood. The marked gingivitis on lower anterior gingiva cleared up quickly as a result of vitamin C therapy. (Cahn, L. R.: *Pathology of the Oral Cavity*, Baltimore, The Williams & Wilkins Co.)

enamel hypoplasia (Figs. 27–5 and 6). In a thorough survey of the case histories of individuals with enamel hypoplasia, Sarnat and Schour reported that only a small number of the cases had any evidence of a rachitic process during tooth development.[57]

The bony structures supporting the teeth develop changes that are characteristic of those in bone elsewhere in the body. Wide osteoid borders are found on the trabeculae of the alveolar bone, and the number and size of the trabeculae are greatly decreased.

Mellanby has conducted a wide variety of studies to determine to what extent there may be a correlation between the structure of human teeth as studied microscopically and the susceptibility to tooth decay.[58] In order to set up standards whereby such a comparison could be made, various stages of increasing severity of microscopic defects were described and correlated with the degrees of caries incidence in the same teeth. It should be clearly pointed out that the defects which Mellanby described and which have come to be referred to as Mellanby hypoplasia are only visible at a microscopic level and can only be clinically discerned by a careful exploration of the tooth surfaces with a sharp explorer. Thus this class of defects can be

readily differentiated from those major areas of hypoplasia which are grossly visible upon clinical examination. Mellanby reported that 78 per cent of deciduous teeth with well-calcified enamel and dentin were free from caries, while only 6 per cent of the teeth with appreciable degrees of microscopic abnormalities were free of tooth decay. Although these data have inherent assumptions, the over-all trend of the material suggests that there is a significant correlation between the structure of teeth as detected microscopically and the susceptibility to decay. However, this should not be interpreted to mean that grossly hypoplastic teeth will decay for that reason nor is the corollary true that teeth that appear to be microscopically perfectly calcified will never decay. It is noteworthy to recall from histologic studies that perfectly formed teeth are found very rarely in modern civilized populations. In contrast, the teeth of experimental animals rarely have developmental abnormalities unless a specific systemic disorder has been imposed during tooth development to alter the formation of organic matrix or the ability of the organic matrix to calcify properly. The rhesus monkey is a particularly good example of this for its teeth uniformly have a high degree of perfection in their formation that is seldom equaled and never excelled in human teeth. The studies on the correlation between Mellanby hypoplasia and caries incidence have been extended to clinical surveys in the schools of London, England where oral examinations were made in 1929, 1943, 1945, 1947, 1949, 1951 and 1955.[59] A consistently high correlation between good tooth structure and freedom from caries was observed.

The effect of vitamin D supplementation upon the initiation and progress of carious lesions has been studied a great deal more intensively than the effect of any other essential nutrient. Studies were conducted by Mellanby and co-workers in England in a series of experiments which lasted from 1923 through 1936. The most extensive of these experiments was conducted in three Birmingham children's institutions where the effect of supplements of cod liver oil and of irradiated ergosterol on dental caries incidence was evaluated.[60] The data obtained definitely pointed toward a lower incidence of new carious lesions and a lower rate of progress of existing lesions among the children in the group which received irradiated ergosterol and those in the group which received the cod liver oil supplement, than in the children who received no vitamin D supplement. The reduction in dental caries incidence among the fully erupted teeth in the vitamin D-supplemented groups was statistically significant.

This experiment was not conducted for sufficiently long to give definitive results about the effect of the vitamin D supplements on the caries susceptibility of the developing teeth. In the small group of teeth that partially developed during the experiment, there was a trend toward a lower caries experience for the groups of children given the vitamin D supplements. Data collected in clinical surveys have added supporting evidence that inadequate vitamin D during tooth development results in a higher caries incidence.

For a variety of reasons these studies have been criticized. If they stood as the only evidence that an adequate amount of vitamin D during childhood was beneficial with respect to caries incidence, or if these investigators had claimed that vitamin D was the only nutrient involved, there would be reason to question the validity of the conclusions. However, a variety of studies has been conducted in the United States and Canada which corroborate the original observations made by Mellanby and co-workers.[61-63] In only a few experiments where the effect of vitamin D supplementation was studied were negative results found. It is interesting to note that some of these negative studies were conducted in older groups of children than the remainder of the studies,[64] and that another one was conducted at such a high level of vitamin D supplementation as to raise a question as to whether the amount ingested was in the physiologic range of normalcy.[65] It is also noteworthy that none of the investigators who believed that vitamin D supplementation helped to reduce caries susceptibility claimed that this was the only reason for altered dental caries incidence, but rather that it was a partial means to cope with the problem.

Evidence from other types of studies also suggests that vitamin D is important for the maintenance of normal teeth in the child population. In a number of surveys efforts have been made to determine if there is any correlation between the dental caries incidence, the number of hours of sunshine in a given community, the latitude of the locality, and its winter temperature. For example, in a statistical evaluation by Mills, which was based on a large compilation of dental caries data collected by the United States Public Health Service, he reported that there was a definite increase of dental caries among 12- to 14-year-old boys as the latitude increased.[66] This increase amounted to approximately 15 carious lesions per 100 children for each degree of latitude. Increases were reported from 289 decayed, missing or filled (DMF) teeth per 100 children in the cities between 25° and 36° latitude in the southern states to approximately 491 DMF teeth per 100 children in the cities between 43° and 46° latitude just south of the Canadian border.

On the basis of the same dental caries data, East has shown that there is a definite correlation between the mean annual hours of sunshine and the average incidence of tooth decay.[67] He observed the following relationship: the average number of cavities per 100 boys was 290 in areas with 3000 and more hours of sunshine per year, and increased to a total of 486 in areas with less than 2,200 hours of sunshine annually. Other studies suggest that there is a correlation between the dental caries incidence and the mean winter temperature, with a greater incidence of tooth decay when the winter temperature is lower. The most likely explanation of these effects would be an increased exposure of the children to sunlight, with a greater amount of vitamin D being made available by reason of this exposure. Other more subtle factors than the simple irradiation of the skin may contribute to this end result. Although ethnic origin has been considered to some extent in these surveys, possible variations that might influence caries susceptibility on a regional basis have not been ruled out completely. In addition, variations in food patterns may influence the outcome and interpretation of the results. For example, throughout the southeastern states, where the caries incidence is generally lower than in the north, large amounts of a self-rising flour that contains appreciable supplements of inorganic phosphates are used. In the light of recent studies in experimental dental caries where the incidence of carious lesions was significantly reduced as a result of supplementation of the cariogenic diet with inorganic phosphates, the increased phosphate consumption through the use of self-rising flour may affect caries incidence materially.[68,69]

Studies in rodents have shown that the calcium-phosphorus ratio of the diet during tooth development is an important factor in determining the composition of the inorganic fraction of the enamel and dentin. Sobel observed that a diet with a high calcium-phosphorus ratio resulted in the formation of teeth in the white rat and the cotton rat whose inorganic components had a higher carbonate-phosphate ratio.[70,71] In contrast, the inorganic portion of the teeth of the animals which were fed a diet with a low calcium-phosphorus ratio during tooth development contained a much lower carbonate-phosphate ratio. In an experiment of this type conducted with cotton rats weaned at an early age, Sobel and co-workers reported

that the animals whose teeth had the high carbonate-phosphate ratio were more susceptible to tooth decay than the teeth of the animals with the lower carbonate-phosphate ratio.[72] It is unknown what relation these studies may have to human beings. The calcium-phosphorus ratios of the diets used by Sobel were appreciably more drastic than would ordinarily be encountered in human dietaries. The important contribution of these studies is the observation that the composition of the inorganic components of enamel and dentin varies depending upon the blood levels of the required elements which in turn are dependent upon the amounts supplied by the diet. It may well be that human teeth are more sensitive during development and calcification to abnormalities in the calcium-phosphorus ratio of the diet than the rat, or it may be that other circumstances in the developing, calcifying tooth determine the extent to which calcium and phosphorus variations in the blood stream are reflected in an alteration in the composition of the inorganic components of the enamel and dentin.

Fluorides. A further influence during the development of teeth upon which a great deal of emphasis is being placed currently is mediated through the ingestion of fluorides. No current chapter on the relation of nutrition to oral health would be complete without a discussion of the role of the fluorides in the etiology of dental caries. The fluorides are ubiquitous materials which occur in minute amounts in all foodstuffs and water supplies. Extensive surveys of the fluoride content of more than 130 foods are available. The majority of foods such as vegetables, meats, cereals and fruits contain between 0.2 and 1.5 ppm of fluorides. Outstanding exceptions to this lower range are the seafoods, the edible portions of which contain 5 to 15 ppm of fluoride, and tea leaves which contain 75 to 100 ppm of fluoride. A cup of tea will supply approximately 0.1 mg of fluoride. Reliable analyses of the fluoride contribution by foods in common human dietaries from areas as distant as Toronto, Minneapolis and Washington, D.C., indicate that an average diet supplies between 0.2 and 0.6 mg of fluoride daily, without the use of unusual amounts of either seafoods or tea.[73–75] Because of the widespread distribution of fluorides, it has not yet been possible to produce a diet that is completely deficient in this element. At the lowest levels of dietary fluoride yet available, no pathologic consequences, other than a high susceptibility to the development of carious lesions, have been noted in rats.[76]

In the data obtained from epidemiologic surveys in human populations and from rodent studies, there is a close correlation between the amount of fluoride ingested during tooth development and the amount of tooth decay that occurs in the teeth after development is completed. The first convincing evidence of such a relationship was provided by Bunting and co-workers in 1929, who reported the results of a survey in Minonk, Illinois.[77] The amount of tooth decay among the children born and raised in this community was a great deal less than in children who moved into Minonk after tooth development was complete. At the time of the survey, the investigators recognized that this striking difference must be related to the water supply, but the active agent was undefined. Later it was found that the drinking water contained 2.5 ppm of fluorides.

In 1939, more extensive information was provided by Dean and his collaborators as the result of a survey of 1,581 children in 4 communities in the Illinois area where the water contained varying amounts of fluorides.[78] Later a more comprehensive survey was reported for 4,425 children from 13 cities and 4 states by the same group of investigators.[79] The data from the latter study are presented in Table 27–1 in terms of the number of DMF permanent teeth observed in the 12- to 14-year-old children of these communities. Where the water contained 1 ppm of fluorides or more during tooth development, the children had a lower incidence of tooth decay than children in nearby communities where the water contained appreciably less than 1 ppm of fluoride. These findings have been corroborated by investigators in numerous areas of the United States, as well as in Canada, England, South Africa, Italy, Greece and Hungary. Although these studies were concerned with the secondary teeth of the children, the primary teeth, likewise, have been shown to benefit from the ingestion of fluoride-bearing waters during tooth development.[80] In addition, it has been shown that the beneficial effect from the consumption of fluoride-bearing waters during tooth development remains into adult life.[81] Surveys in the United States, Argentina, England and

Table 27-1. A Comparison of the Fluoride Content of the Drinking Water and the Amount of Tooth Decay among 4,425 Children, Twelve to Fourteen Years of Age in 13 Cities from 4 States. (Based on Reference 79)

	Fluoride Content (ppm)	Number of Children Examined	Children With No Tooth Decay (per cent)	Average Number of Diseased Teeth per Child
Colorado Springs, Colo.	2.6	404	28.5	2.5
Galesburg, Ill.	1.9	273	27.8	2.4
East Moline, Ill.	1.2	152	20.4	3.0
Kewanee, Ill.	0.9	123	17.9	3.4
Pueblo, Colo.	0.6	614	10.6	4.1
Marion, Ohio	0.4	263	5.7	5.6
Lima, Ohio	0.3	454	2.2	6.5
Middletown, Ohio	0.2	370	1.9	7.0
Zanesville, Ohio	0.2	459	2.6	7.3
Quincy, Ill.	0.1	330	2.4	7.1
Portsmouth, Ohio	0.1	469	1.3	7.7
Elkhart, Ind.	0.1	278	1.4	8.2
Michigan City, Ind.	0.1	236	0.0	10.4

Hungary have demonstrated that exposure to naturally borne fluorides during tooth development continues to manifest itself by a low incidence of tooth decay in adult life. Oh the basis of these and a great many other studies, there is no longer any doubt that water containing 1 ppm or more of fluorides has a definitely beneficial effect, when consumed during tooth development, upon the later caries susceptibility of the teeth. The ingestion of an optimal fluoride level during tooth development appears to be as effective in an area of relatively low caries incidence such as Hungary as in areas of high caries incidence such as England and the United States.

The fluoride content of the teeth developed in areas where different amounts of fluorides were present in the water supply closely parallels the amount of fluorides in the water.[82] Where drinking water contained zero to 0.3 ppm of fluoride, as in Washington, D.C., the teeth of the native continuous residents had approximately 0.010 per cent of fluorides in the enamel and 0.024 per cent in the dentin. Where the water supply contained 1.0 to 1.2 ppm of naturally occurring fluorides, as in Aurora, Illinois, the teeth of comparable residents contained 0.014 per cent fluorides in the enamel and 0.036 per cent in the dentin. Comparable increases in bone fluoride occurred as the fluoride content of the water supply increased.

Presumably the caries resistance of the teeth is somehow related to their fluoride content. The exact nature of this relationship is not known. In an x-ray diffraction study of bone samples with various levels of fluoride, Zipkin, Posner and Eanes[83] observed that increasing fluoride concentrations were associated with increased "crystallinity" of the hydroxyapatite as evidenced by larger crystal size and more nearly perfect crystals. These changes in "crystallinity" would reduce the effective surface area of the crystals in a given weight of bone, reduce the reactivity of the crystals and provide less area for deposition and surface orientation of carbon dioxide and citrate, in particular. The inverse relationship between fluoride concentration and the carbonate and citrate concentrations in bone has been demon-

strated.[84] Zipkin and Posner[85] postulated that, if this inverse relationship existed in enamel as well as in bone, a new concept could be introduced to explain the relationship between fluoride concentration in enamel and susceptibility to dental caries.

Further light is thrown upon this subject in studies by Jenkins and Speirs, who determined the level of fluoride content in various levels of the enamel.[86] They noted that the outer surface uniformly had a much higher fluoride level than the deeper layer. In addition, they observed that this difference in distribution was detectable in unerupted teeth as well as in erupted teeth. The latter observation indicates that this was a developmental arrangement of the concentration of fluoride, and not a distribution that took place after the teeth had erupted into the oral cavity by reason of contact with saliva. These observations have been corroborated by Brudevold and co-workers.[87,88] who also demonstrated a post-eruptive acquisition of fluoride by the surface layers of enamel, which increased in proportion to the amount of fluoride in the drinking water.

In view of the beneficial influence of inorganic fluorides as introduced into water supplies by nature, the next step was to determine whether the introduction of comparable inorganic fluorides into low-fluoride waters would be equally efficacious. The first survey was begun at Grand Rapids, Michigan, in January, 1945, where the fluoride content of the water supply was increased to 1.2 ppm under the joint sponsorship of the United States Public Health Service, the University of Michigan and the Michigan State Department of Health. Muskegon, Michigan, served as the control low-fluoride city. Soon after this, surveys were begun in a number of other cities. Some of the impressive data which are now available from the older surveys are presented in Table 27–2.[89] The over-all analysis of the data from these surveys indicates that the dental caries incidence in teeth formed during the survey period was on the average about 60 per cent lower than the caries incidence in otherwise comparable teeth formed prior to the increase in fluoride content of the water supply, or in those teeth

Table 27-2. Reduction in Tooth Decay Observed in Various Fluoridation Study Projects. (Based on Reference 89)

Community	Fluoridation		Age Group (year)	Reduction in Decay* (per cent)
	Date Started	Report Period (yr.)		
Grand Rapids, Mich.	Jan. 1945	8	6	70.8
			7	52.5
			8	49.2
			9	48.1
			13	39.7
Brantford, Ont.	June 1945	7	6	59.4
			7	69.5
			8	51.5
			9	46.2
			13	32.9
Newburgh, N. Y.	May 1945	7	6	69.4
			7	67.8
			8	40.4
			9	51.4
Evanston, Ill.	Feb. 1947	4	6	73.6
			7	56.4
			8	35.4
Sheboygan, Wis.	Feb. 1946	6	9–10 (4th grade)	35.3
			12–14 (8th grade)	29.7

* Decayed, missing and filled teeth.

formed in children in neighboring cities where the water supply did not have its fluoride content adjusted. As would be expected, the greatest benefits were in the youngest age groups and in the teeth of older children that were formed after fluoride adjustment occurred in the communal water supply. These facts are clearly shown in Figure 27–7 for the children of Newburgh and Kingston 10 years after fluoridation began in Newburgh.[90] The high similarity of the data to those in communities where the fluoride is naturally borne is most striking. It is also noteworthy that no comparable decreases in dental caries incidence were noted in the children of nearby communities where the fluoride content of the communal waters had not been increased. The latter was true despite the use even on a limited scale of various tooth pastes and other prophylactic measures which have been widely suggested as being highly beneficial for the reduction of dental caries incidence.

On the basis of present knowledge, it appears that the most sensitive tissue in the body to excessive ingestion of fluorides is the ameloblastic layer which forms the organic framework of the enamel. When the drinking water of a community contains 2.5 ppm or more of fluorides, a manifestation known as mottled enamel results.[91] This only occurs when the high fluoride ingestion is during the developmental period of the teeth and cannot occur after tooth development has been completed. The degree of mottled enamel may vary from slight nonaesthetically significant amounts to an extensive chalkiness of the surface with large opaque areas which may erode away rapidly and which in severe cases become heavily stained. As the fluoride content of the water increases, the severity and the extent of mottled enamel increase until at levels of 8 or 10 ppm in the communal water supply almost all of the individuals who grow up in the area have mottled enamel of such severity that it is aesthetically

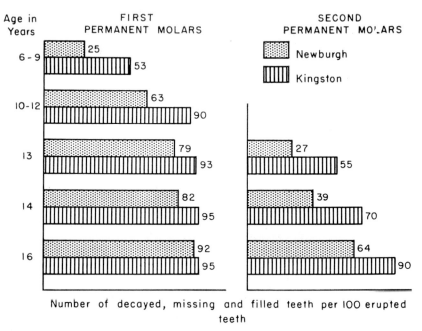

Fig. 27-7. The relation of added fluoride in the water supply for 10 years to the incidence of dental caries in first and second permanent molar teeth of children from 6 to 16 years of age. (Ast, Smith, Wachs and Cantwell,[90] courtesy of J. Am. Dent. Assoc.)

disfiguring. At fluoride levels from 2.5 ppm or more, the water supply is in need of treatment, either by the development of a new source, by adequate dilution with low-fluoride waters or by removal of the fluorides from the drinking water. However, on the basis of these epidemiologic surveys, fluorides contributing in the neighborhood of 1.2 ppm of fluoride to a water supply have definitely been shown to be of no detrimental public health significance with respect to the causation of mottled enamel in northern regions. In hotter climates where the water consumption is appreciably higher, the optimal level of fluoride ingestion is in the neighborhood of 0.6 to 0.7 ppm.[92] Controlled fluoridation at the recommended levels has not resulted in any aesthetically disfiguring mottling among the children of any community.

Abnormalities other than those caused in the developing teeth by excessively high fluoride ingestion have been sought in various surveys in the United States and elsewhere throughout the world. Probably the most important and extensive surveys in which general systemic influence of fluoride inges-

tion was sought were made in 1943 and 1953 in Bartlett and Cameron, Texas.[93] The former community had a water supply that contained approximately 8 ppm of fluoride, whereas the latter community, situated some 30 miles distant, had a water supply with about 0.4 ppm fluoride. In 1943 a series of inhabitants who had resided at least fifteen years in each community was selected at random and carefully examined by skilled physicians. A total of 116 was examined in Bartlett and 121 in Cameron. These individuals ranged from 15 to 68 years of age in 1943: 57.8 per cent of the Bartlett participants and 47.2 per cent of those from Cameron were over 55 years of age. X-ray films of various portions of the skeletal system and full case histories were taken. The data in these surveys indicated that there was no significant difference in any phase of health between individuals of one community and the other, with two exceptions. Many of the individuals who had resided in Bartlett during childhood had severely mottled teeth. In addition, a slightly higher incidence of cardiovascular disease was observed in Cameron. In all other regards, there were no detectable abnormalities that could be attributed to the different fluoride content of these two water supplies. Though this survey is undoubtedly the most intensive of all that have been conducted, many other surveys on different phases of the fluoride problem as related to systemic disease have been conducted. In all cases, levels of 1.0 ppm or more, up to as high as 8.0 ppm, in the United States have been shown to be negative with respect to any correlation of a systemic abnormality to the fluoride content of the water.

The case for both the dental benefits and the systemic safety of controlled fluoridation of public water supplies at recommended levels has been unequivocally established. Now new evidence is beginning to suggest that the ingestion of inadequate levels of fluoride over prolonged periods may be as disadvantageous for bone as inadequate levels of fluoride are for the development of caries-resistant teeth. Leone[94] reported the recognition of 279 cases of osteoporosis among 546 persons in a radiographic study in Framingham, Mass., where the water supply contains 0.1 ppm fluoride. In addition, a higher frequency of other bone abnormalities was noted than had been observed in either Bartlett or Cameron, Texas. He concluded that the data support "the hypothesis that disadvantageous effects on the bone structure of the adult population may be associated with the prolonged use of drinking water that contains an insufficient concentration of fluoride." Bernstein et al.[95] conducted a survey in two towns in North Dakota where the water supplies contained 4.0 to 5.8 ppm fluoride and in three towns where the water supplies contained 0.15 to 0.30 ppm fluoride. The prevalence of reduced bone density was much higher in the low-fluoride towns than in the high-fluoride communities. In addition, the males in the low-fluoride towns had a much higher frequency of calcification of the abdominal aorta. In addition, Rich and Ensinck[96,97] have reported improvements in calcium balance in 6 patients with osteoporosis and one with Paget's disease when small amounts of fluoride were given orally in several divided doses daily. The average improvement in calcium balance was 802 mg per week for these patients during the 10th to 14th weeks of therapy. Much more study needs to be given to this area of fluoride metabolism but these preliminary findings may indicate the existence of more widespread benefits of fluoride ingestion than had been previously expected.

It is noteworthy that over 3 million individuals in the United States have consumed natural fluoride-bearing waters in excess of 1.0 ppm for decades, and an additional 5 million individuals have consumed amounts between 0.5 and 1.0 ppm.[98] Already the fluoridation of community water supplies has been widely instituted throughout the United States and elsewhere in the world. As of December 31, 1970, fluorides were being added to the water supplies in cities and towns in the United States with a total population of 83,725,771.[99] Many other communities are in some phase of equipment purchase and installation. The water supplies in Chicago, the second largest city in the United States, have been fluoridated since August 1, 1956,[100] and New York City, the largest water installation in the United States, began fluoridation on September 30, 1965.[101] There has yet to be any evidence presented to indicate that any individual in any age group has been harmed by ingestion of these water supplies.

Uncharacterized Relations. Another example of a developmental influence upon the teeth may be obtained from the extensive dental caries statistics that were collected on the children of European countries during World Wars I and II. Studies representing a total of about 750,000 children from eleven countries have been summarized and evaluated in detail by Sognnaes.[102] It is noteworthy that the reduction in dental caries experience in all these studies did not occur concurrently with the reduction in refined foods and sugar. Possibly the most detailed data are available from the children in Norway where almost the complete reduction in carbohydrate intake from sugar and highly refined flours occurred in 1939. Yet the greatest increase in caries-free permanent teeth among 7-year-old children did not occur until 1945. Indeed, the reductions in 1940, 1941 and 1942 were relatively small. The attention of the reader should be drawn to the fact that all the teeth in this particular tabulation had been in the oral cavity for only 1 or 1½ years. Thus, there was a comparable length of exposure of the teeth in each particular group represented in the comparison. The teeth that erupted 6 to 8 years after hostilities enforced drastic changes in food habits were much more resistant to dental caries than the teeth that erupted during pre-war years and in the earlier war years.

In World War I the maximum reduction in caries incidence was not observed until 1922 and 1923; that is, after the cessation of hostilities and the partial return of fine foods and sugar to the European dietary. In the World War II period, the highest reduction in dental caries incidence was not reported until 1945. Thus, in both periods there was a 6- to 8-year lag in the attainment of the maximum caries resistance. In other words, the teeth that were benefited most were those that were just beginning to form when the war-time dietary change was imposed. This time lag obviously cannot be explained purely on the basis of alterations in the oral environment of teeth that have been in the oral cavity for short periods of time. Instead, these data point to strong effects of the diet during the war years on the development of teeth that are much more caries resistant than those teeth developed by children con-

suming the typical pre-war dietary foods. The fact that these reductions in dental caries incidence were so comparable for the two wars and in the several countries from which data are available suggests that the data have a very high degree of validity. The active factor or factors in this effect on dental caries incidence are unknown. Along with the greatly reduced incidence of dental caries, Toverud[103] has reported that the permanent teeth erupted much later and that the deciduous teeth were retained in the mouth longer during the war years than in the pre-war period.

Suggestions from other clinical surveys lend support to such developmental influences. In a survey conducted by Cohen[104] on a group of pre-school children in New England where the proneness to develop carious lesions is very high, it was noted that the 4- and 5-year-old children from families in the high socioeconomic group had a significantly lower incidence of dental caries than the children from the less favored groups (Table 27-3). This difference between groups reflects good prenatal and pediatric care, including diet counselling for the more favored groups. It is noteworthy that the dental caries experience among the pre-school children in the high socioeconomic group compared favorably with the caries index in children of the same

Table 27-3. Average Number of Decayed, Extracted and Filled Teeth in Pre-School Children of Different Socioeconomic Groups[104]

Socioeconomic Level	Age	Number of Children	Per Cent With One or More Defective Teeth	Average Number of Defective Teeth per Child
Low	4	135	84	3.90
	5	36	89	5.44
Medium	4	135	61	2.39
	5	36	69	3.06
High	4	77	53	2.03
	5	16	75	3.19
Total	4	347	68	2.89
	5	88	78	4.06

age in endemic fluoride areas and in areas where the communal water supplies have been fluoridated.

Similar results were observed in a clinic designed to give early pediatric care to children in two Norwegian communities. Toverud[105] reported that those children who received good care in the early years of their life had a significantly lower incidence of tooth decay than similar children in the community who did not receive the services of this clinic or who did not seek help until later in their development.

This type of clinical information has been greatly strengthened by investigations with rodents and monkeys.[106,107] The ingestion of diets composed of natural foodstuffs during tooth development resulted in teeth that were much more resistant than the teeth of comparable experimental animals that developed during maintenance of diets composed of highly purified ingredients. Although the natural diet contained significantly more fluorides than the purified diet, other studies with rats have indicated that the difference in fluoride content of the two diets was insufficient to cause the different incidence of tooth decay.[108] Further experiments to determine the active agent in this study have shown that the influence is a result of the different mineral components of the two diets. When the mineral components of the natural diet were fed as the sole source of minerals in the purified diet, an appreciably lower incidence of tooth decay resulted.[109]

NUTRITIONAL INFLUENCES DURING TOOTH MATURATION AND MAINTENANCE

The maturation period of a tooth is the era about which we know the least. There are several demonstrations in the literature that the caries susceptibility of the molar teeth of rodents decreases as the tooth age increases.[110–112] There are also clinical suggestions that, if a tooth is protected from decay during its early months in the oral cavity, it attains a greater degree of caries resistance and is less liable to be attacked by the carious process at later stages. These findings suggest a change in tooth structure

or in permeability of the tooth after emergence into the oral cavity.

Studies with radioisotopes show that the recently erupted tooth has a high ability to incorporate inorganic ions into its structure. The rate at which this occurs is between 10 to 20 times faster than the rate of exchange in teeth that have been in the oral cavity for appreciably longer periods of time.[113] In addition, the rate of exchange in recently erupted teeth is only about one-half the rate in developing crowns of teeth within the jaw. This small difference between unerupted and recently erupted teeth is in striking contrast to the concept that the enamel of erupted teeth is an inert region. Further radioisotope studies have shown that the inorganic components incorporated during maturation and during the maintenance period have their origin in the salivary secretions.

Another influence upon the maturation of teeth has been demonstrated in histologic studies. The teeth of rats that were exposed to a cariogenic diet during the early post-eruptive period had enamel that was much more permeable to histologic stains than comparable teeth in animals which were fed their entire ration by stomach tube.[14] These changes that take place during tooth maturation are influenced by the salivary secretions. In an experiment to study this relationship, rats were desalivated at various intervals after weaning.[114] The subjects in the several groups were maintained on a non-cariogenic diet until the rats in the last group were desalivated. Then all subjects were transferred on the same day to a cariogenic diet on which they were maintained for the same length of time. Under these circumstances, the rats which were sialoadenectomized at weaning had the highest incidence of carious lesions; their littermates which were sialoadenectomized after tooth maturation was complete had significantly less tooth decay. The mechanism by which this influence takes place is not known. Briner et al.[115] made an interesting observation concerning the presence of hypomineralized (and presumably developmentally immature) areas of the enamel in rat molars at the time of eruption. When a nutritionally adequate non-cariogenic diet was fed, these hypomineralized areas slowly mineralized to sound enamel. However, where a soft, cariogenic diet was fed, these hypomineralized areas increased dramatically and in time progressed to form gross carious lesions. Furthermore, we do not know whether variations in the composition of the saliva, or in the quantity of the saliva, may alter the rate or extent of maturation. This relationship between saliva, maturation of teeth and their caries susceptibility indicates a type of metabolic situation that could be altered by an adverse nutritional influence on the quantity or the quality of the saliva.

One of the most interesting areas for exploration in the dental caries field is the relation of systemic nutritional influences upon the teeth after their development and maturation are complete. Of this aspect, we know very little, and yet there are some recent experiments that suggest the definite importance of nutrition during the maintenance period. In post-developmental studies reported by Haldi and co-workers, two diets that were similar in their carbohydrate, protein and fat composition caused considerably different caries rates in the same strain of animals.[116] Uniformly, rats fed one of these purified diets had a much greater caries incidence than littermate rats fed the other purified diet. This post-developmental influence can be explained only on the basis of the operation of some systemic mechanism that is presently not understood. Since the composition and concentration of the three major components of the two diets were similar, this systemic influence must have been mediated by one or more of the several minor differences in the concentration of the minerals and the vitamins in the two diets. This influence may not have operated primarily through the teeth themselves, but possibly through the saliva or some other unrecognized pathway. In the latest study in this series, the investigators have reported that the salt mixture used in the less cariogenic of the two diets was capable of reducing the cariogenicity of the other diet when used in place of the other salt mixture.[117]

Another investigation conducted during the post-developmental period was described by Nizel and Harris in hamsters.[118] Subjects fed a diet composed of corn, grown in New England, and whole milk powder, prepared from milk produced in New England, had a high dental caries incidence. Comparable hamsters fed a diet composed of corn and whole milk powder produced in Texas had a significantly lower dental caries incidence. On the basis of chemical analyses, the New England and Texas diets had comparable carbohydrate, fat and protein contents; yet on this post-developmental basis, strikingly different caries experiences were produced by the two diets.

A third experiment of this general nature with equally striking results has been published by McClure and Folk.[119] When skim milk powders were heated mildly, appreciable increases in their caries-producing properties for rats were observed. Again, the carbohydrate, fat and protein percentages were identical before and after the heating process for each skim milk powder tested. Further studies have shown that these diets did not contain adequate amounts of lysine. When these diets and various heated cereal diets which were also inadequate in lysine were supplemented with lysine, sharp reductions in dental caries on the smooth surfaces were noted.[69,120] Supplementation of the diet with lysine was more effective than intubation.[120]

A fourth series of experiments has been reported by Constant et al.[112,121] in which the influence of various mineral supplements to low-mineral, highly cariogenic natural diets fed post-developmentally was appraised in cotton rats. Supplements of citrate, lactate or acetate salts did not alter the incidence of tooth decay. Supplements of calcium carbonate, disodium phosphate and various salt mixtures, with or without calcium, retarded the rate of development of caries in the erupted teeth. These investigators also noted that mature animals were quite resistant to tooth decay when fed the same low-mineral diet that caused extensive tooth decay in weanlings. Strälfors[68] has noted that the supplementation of cariogenic diets with phosphates caused major reductions in caries in the hamster. In addition, McClure[69] has demonstrated that supplementation of diets that cause smooth surface lesions with 1.6 per cent of dibasic sodium phosphate caused striking reductions in dental caries. Many additional studies on dietary phosphates and experimental dental caries have been conducted and are reviewed by Nizel and Harris.[122] While the influence of phosphates in reducing dental caries in laboratory animals has been consistent, human trials have been inconsistent; one indicated a good reduction[123] while two had negative results.[124,125] A recent study of a population normally consuming tortillas made from lime-soaked corn which contained large amounts of calcium and phosphate has shown a reduction in carious lesions in areas of the mouth which are not self-cleansing and where the susceptible enamel pits become plugged with calcified material.[126] A similar population primarily consuming bread served as a control group.

At present, there is no satisfactory explanation for the influences observed in these four types of experimental studies. However, somewhere in them valuable clues are contained which are needed to explain how and why such post-developmental differences influence the initiation and progression of carious lesions. Possibly this information may elucidate some of the seeming paradoxes seen in human populations.

In clinical investigations it is important, as well as difficult, during maturation and maintenance periods to attempt to evaluate the influence of a diet upon the dental caries incidence in terms of its two potential components: the oral environment and the systemic interrelationships. This evaluation is especially difficult in experiments or surveys with human subjects. A great variety of surveys has been conducted to determine the incidence of dental caries among primitive populations and to determine to what extent their dental caries experience has been modified as they came in contact with civilization. Among the most definitive of these surveys were the ones in which the incidence of tooth decay in about 3000 primitive and civilized groups of Eskimos in Greenland were studied.[127,128] The percentage of Eskimos with tooth decay in East Greenland varied from 4.3 for the males and 4.6 for the females at the isolated native settlements, up to 43.2 and 51.5, respectively, for the Eskimos residing in the neighborhood of trading stations. On the west side of Greenland, the

incidence was much higher and varied from 31.8 per cent for the males and 44.4 per cent for the females in native settlements up to 83.3 and 90.5 per cent, respectively, for those Eskimos who reside in the immediate neighborhood of the trading posts. It has been estimated than an average of 63 per cent of the total dietary intake of the western Greenlanders in 1930 was made up of imported foods, especially sugar and cereals, instead of the 17 per cent in 1901. In East Greenland, the natives in isolated settlements received relatively no imported food, and those at the trading stations, a great deal less than their contemporaries on the western side of the island. The data from this survey and numerous others point to the fact that the increasing use of foods associated with civilization has resulted in increased dental caries incidences among the populations using these diets. This increase has been widely interpreted to be mediated through changes in the oral environment. This may be true in the case of those who have adopted civilized foods after tooth development is complete. However, in the children of these areas, the consumption of the more refined foods during periods of tooth development probably has resulted in the formation of teeth that have a much higher caries susceptibility than the teeth of their ancestors. In addition, the teeth of the youngsters erupt into oral environments that are more cariogenic because of the greater availability of readily fermentable, adherent carbohydrates.

Numerous experiments have been conducted on the effect of the type and composition of the diet for children on their dental caries experience, in attempts to explore in specific terms why such remarkably large differences occur between the caries index of different population groups as described in the Greenland survey above. One of the longest series of studies was that conducted by Boyd and co-workers at the State University of Iowa, who became interested in this problem in the course of their studies on the dietary control of diabetic children.[129,130] These workers reported that where careful dietary control was maintained by the use of diets which were high in fat and protein, and low in carbohydrates, with ample supplies of all basic nutrients, there was much less tooth decay than in children of the same area who were not under such dietary regimentation. Many of their cases were studied for prolonged periods of time. These workers noted that non-adherence to the dietary recommendations resulted within a few months in an increased incidence of tooth decay. They believed that the low incidence of tooth decay which they observed in their diabetic children under dietary supervision was due to the general nutritional adequacy of the diet and not to the control of the diabetic process itself.

Similar studies were conducted by Drain and Boyd[131] and by McBeath[132,133] in children in other institutions for normal youngsters. When the customary diets were supplemented with milk, butter and eggs in the first case, and milk, eggs, wheat, meat, vegetables, oranges, butter and cod liver oil in the second case, they observed substantial reductions in the incidence of new cavities. In studies with outpatients, Howe and co-workers[134,135] and Livermore[136] reported a lower number of new carious lesions in the patients who were cooperative in accepting and following the recommendations made to them, but observed no reductions in uncooperative patients.

The general conclusions of these investigators implicated the nutritional improvement of the diets as the important factor in the causation of the reduced dental caries increments. They believed that the change in the oral environment occasioned by the relatively low carbohydrate content of their diets was less important than the improvement in their nutritional adequacy.

Other workers approached this subject from a different point of attack by the addition of various amounts of carbohydrate to the diets of institutionalized children without any attempt to maintain diets of comparable nutritional acceptance.[137,138] In one survey conducted in an orphanage, the incidence of tooth decay at the beginning of the experiment was very low, even though the amount of several nutrients in the diet was far below levels considered to be adequate. In the case of 51 orphanage children who received approximately 3 pounds of candy per week, definitely increased annual increments of tooth decay were observed during this period of high-carbohydrate ingestion. Unquestionably, the nutritional adequacy of the diet decreased by reason of the very large amount of candy provided for each child. At the same time, the oral environment must have contained a higher amount of readily fermentable carbohydrates during the period of carbohydrate administration than was the case prior to the experiment.

In experiments of either of the above two types, there is no practical way in which the degree of influence of the oral and systemic factors can be eliminated, one from another, on the basis of the most detailed published data. This is largely true because strict precautions were not taken to hold constant other factors than those under investigation. This comment obviously does not question the reliability of the results nor the efficacy of the procedures described for the control of dental caries. The probable conclusion that should be drawn from the two series of experiments is that both systemic conditions and the oral environment were influenced by the dietary changes. Hence, the altered initiation and development of carious lesions were the end product of changes in the two interrelated facets of the problem. However, from the results of the animal studies reviewed above, as well as from controlled clinical studies such as those at Vipeholm, Sweden,[18] there can be no question but that the excessive consumption of carbohydrate-containing foods, especially those that are retained on the tooth surfaces, is responsible to a large degree for a high dental caries incidence in caries-susceptible populations. It appears to be axiomatic now that carious lesions cannot occur without fermentable carbohydrates and the appropriate microbial flora. As the availability and frequency of carbohydrate consumption increase, the potentiality for the development and progression of caries increases.

LESIONS OF THE ORAL MUCOUS MEMBRANES AND OF THE SUPPORTING STRUCTURES OF THE TEETH

In the diagnosis and treatment of the various diseases of the oral mucous membranes, and of the supporting tissues of the teeth, it is desirable for the examiner to thoroughly evaluate all local oral conditions which might subject the oral tissues to excessive physical or chemical trauma, and to ascertain the presence of any systemic abnormality, whether nutritional, infectious, endocrine, constitutional or psychological which might alter the resistance of the oral tissues. Certainly a thorough visual examination of the oral tissues, as well as the eyes, hair, and skin, should be made to ascertain if any classical signs of nutritional deficiency are present. The various criteria of these deficiencies have been described in detail in the particular chapters of this book pertaining to the specific deficiencies. When none of these signs is found to exist as indications of frank deficiencies, evidence of subclinical dietary deficiency should be sought through discussions with the patient about his diet and also by laboratory tests and whatever clinical methods of evaluation are applicable in each individual case. Frequently such subclinical deficiencies may predispose

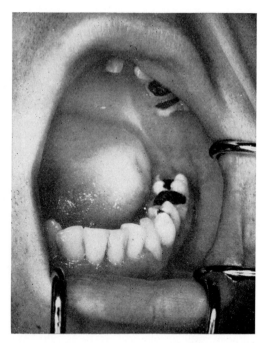

Fig. 27-9. Same patient as in Figure 27-8, 96 hours after oral administration of niacin at rate of 100 mg per day. No oral treatment was undertaken during this period. Note that the traumatic influences of badly broken-down molars in the upper and lower quadrants adjacent to previous site of lesion have not been altered. (Courtesy of Dr. David Weisberger.)

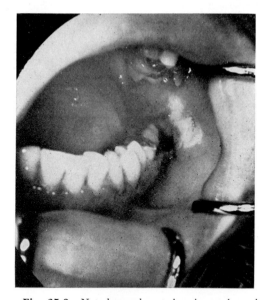

Fig. 27-8. Note large ulcerated region on buccal mucosa opposite the left first and second molars at the occlusal level. Smears of this area showed heavy concentrations of microorganisms of the fusospirochetal group. Extensive local treatment of the lesion had been ineffective. A dietary evaluation suggested a subclinical niacin deficiency. (Courtesy of Dr. David Weisberger.)

to a sufficiently low tissue tone, and resistance to traumatic or infectious processes that ordinarily tolerable oral conditions become overwhelming in their impact.

An example of the result of such a subclinical deficiency is shown in Figure 27–8, where a large ulcerated region is seen to exist on the buccal mucosa adjacent to the left molar teeth. Smears from this area were heavily laden with microorganisms of the fusospirochetal group. This patient was treated by a variety of local procedures for an appreciable length of time without any noticeable regression in the ulcerated area. Then a thorough evaluation of his dietary background suggested that he was likely to be in a state of subclinical deficiency in niacin, but there was no evidence of any of the classic signs of niacin deficiency. Hence niacin therapy was begun at a level of 100 mg per day with a quick resolution of the lesion being observed. Ninety-six hours after the beginning of this therapy, the lesion was completely resolved (Fig. 27–9). It will also be noted from this figure that the broken molars that were traumatizing the mucosa in that region had not been repaired. The trauma imposed by the broken-down molars may have precipitated the oral manifestation earlier than would otherwise have been the case.

There is an increasing concern among oral clinicians that many low-grade abnormalities of the oral tissues, such as mild gingivitis, are being dismissed as "normal" because of the frequency of their occurrence. The optimal goals to strive for are tissues that are healthy rather than any less satisfactory condition even though the latter is much more commonly observed in the population seen by an oral clinician.

An ideal example of healthy, adult oral tissue is shown in Figure 27–10. Based on clinical and histological features, the oral mucosa consists of the following 3 zones:

(a) the gingiva and the covering of the hard palate, the masticatory mucosa;

(b) specialized mucosa located on the dorsum of the tongue;

(c) the remaining oral mucous membranes.

The gingiva is divided into the following parts, as demonstrated in Figure 27–10:

(a) the marginal or free gingiva which surrounds the teeth in a collar-like fashion. A shallow depression separates this tissue from (b);

(b) the attached gingiva which is tightly connected to the underlying alveolar bone;

(c) the interdental papilla which extends interproximally and usually consists of both marginal and attached gingiva. The gingiva is demarcated from the alveolar mucosa by a clearly defined line, the mucogingival junction. The alveolar mucosa then blends imperceptibly with the buccal mucosa.

The maintenance of the integrity, physiology, and anatomy of the oral tissues is a goal that is too rarely seen or achieved by treatment in clinical practice.

Gingivitis. Gingivitis is an inflammation of the gingivae, including the interdental papillae. There are three main types of gingivitis: (1) hemorrhagic gingivitis, (2) ulcerative gingivitis, and (3) hypertrophic gingivitis.

Hemorrhagic Gingivitis. Hemorrhagic gingivitis which can be local or general is characterized by free bleeding, red gingiva and edematous interdental papillae. The epithelial lining of the gingival trough is thin and edematous and is usually infiltrated with polymorphonuclear leukocytes. Bordering the "rough" epithelium, numerous bacteria and fungi are found. The direct cause of hemorrhagic gingivitis is basically poor oral

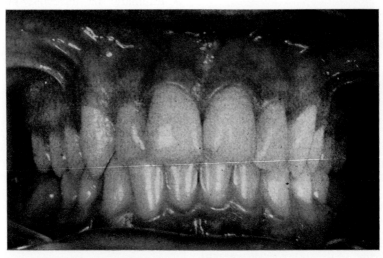

Fig. 27-10. An ideal example of healthy gingiva. Note the sharply pointed interdental papillae and the general appearance, arrangement and contours of the gingiva. (Courtesy of Dr. Paul Goldhaber.)

hygiene, but indirectly is dietary since the retention of food in the crevicular and interstitial areas favors an accumulation of those products of bacterial fermentation which can act as an irritant on the underlying tissues to produce typical inflammation and edema. Infrequent or poor dental care can contribute to the inflammatory process by failure to remove mineralized deposits which form from salivary calcium and phosphate on the teeth in the gingival area, and which serve as additional irritants for the initiation or progression of the gingivitis. Broken-down teeth, malformed and malplaced teeth, and traumatic occlusion act as physically debilitating circumstances or as food traps. Finally, iatrogenic factors must be included in this partial list of causes of gingivitis. Among these are improperly placed fillings, overhanging fillings, ill-fitting dentures and poorly constructed crowns and bridges. A predisposing systemic cause of hemorrhagic gingivitis occasionally appears to be avitaminosis C, although there unquestionably must be additional factors that are not presently recognized.

Acute Necrotizing Ulcerative Gingivitis (Trench Mouth, Vincent's Gingivitis). This is an acute and painful condition that is characterized by the loss of the interdental papillae (Figs. 27–11 and 12), pseudomembrane formation, bad breath, regional lymph node involvement, mild lymphocytosis (although not always), sometimes a rise in temperature, and anorexia. It is particularly characteristic that the first site of attack is the interdental papillae and that all are not attacked simultaneously. Instead, a variety of stages is noted with some papillae being very slightly involved and others, often close at hand, being completely destroyed (Fig. 27–12). When the process is allowed to go on without interruption, extensive loss of the interdental papillae is noted, with the formation of cup-like ulcers between the teeth. The lesion is characteristically sensitive to any pressure or instrumentation. Usually the rest of the gingiva is uniformly inflamed, and appears clinically as a reddened zone rather sharply demarcated from the subjacent alveolar mucosa. However, Vincent's disease is occasionally localized to a specific area or tooth with no involvement of the remaining oral tissues. While the direct cause of acute necrotizing ulcerative gingivitis is believed to be the fusospirochetal group of microorganisms, a variety of postulates has been made about underlying causes that predispose toward this rapidly fulminating disease entity. No underlying causes have been characterized in sufficient detail to justify a sound working hypothesis, but an association ap-

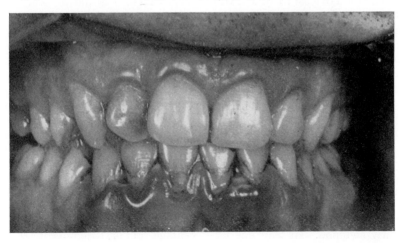

Fig. 27-11. Acute necrotizing ulcerative gingivitis. Note the varying degrees of destruction of the interdental papillae from a slight rolling of the margins and a blunting of the tip of the papilla between the lower central incisors, slight necrosis on the papilla between the right central and lateral incisors, and gross ulceration of the papillae between the right lateral incisor and canine and between the left central and lateral incisors. (Courtesy of Dr. Paul Goldhaber.)

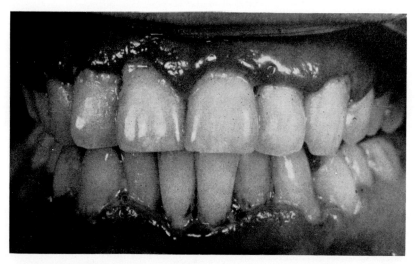

Fig. 27-12. Acute necrotizing ulcerative gingivitis. A more advanced case with extensive necrosis and ulceration of the gingiva throughout the anterior mandibular region and with a lesser amount of involvement but still relatively advanced effects on the maxillary gingiva. (Courtesy of Dr. Paul Goldhaber.)

pears to exist with psychological and emotional stresses such as those experienced by college students at examination times and during courtship difficulties. A complicating factor during such periods is the frequency of grossly abnormal dietary habits. In addition, abnormalities in the endocrine status during intensive stress are commonly involved. The most satisfactory treatment appears to be a thorough combination of local treatment with adequate diet and the alleviation of any psychologic stress or constitutional disorder that may be superimposed upon the condition.

Hypertrophic Gingivitis. This condition may exist either in the acute or in the chronic form. Acute hypertrophy of the gingiva is caused by a rapid influx into the gingiva of inflammatory cells, hemorrhage, or abnormal white blood cells. When confronted with the acute form of the disease, there is a necessity to think of, and to rule out wherever possible, an acute inflammation, such as periodontal abscess, scurvy, purpura, or leukemia. It is noteworthy that acute hypertrophic gingivitis is relatively rare. Chronic hypertrophy of the gingiva is fairly common. At least one factor that is involved in the causation of hypertrophic gingivitis is the lack of masticatory function. In Figures 27–13 and 14 is demonstrated a case of this syndrome before

and after treatment. At the first examination of the patient, a toothache in a lower left molar was recorded, and for the previous 10 months the patient had been chewing only on the right side. Examination revealed that the diffuse hypertrophic gingivitis was localized entirely on the left side of the mouth and that there was a deep carious lesion in the lower left first molar. Treatment consisted of providing a dental restoration of the first molar and active stimulation of the gingiva by having the patient chew wax 3 times a day. In Figure 27–14 the rapid return of the gingiva to normal size is recorded.

Conditioned gingival enlargement occurs when the systemic state of the individual is such to exaggerate the usual response to local irritation. Such a response is seen in patients experiencing hormonal change as for example in pregnancy and in both sexes at puberty. Exaggerated responses to local factors are also described in leukemia and vitamin C-deficiency states.

Neoplastic gingival enlargements, although accounting for a comparatively small percentage of oral tumors[139] (8 per cent), nonetheless comprise a rather sizable proportion of growths of the gingiva[140] (57 per cent). The remaining 43 per cent were shown to be inflammatory in nature. Early detection

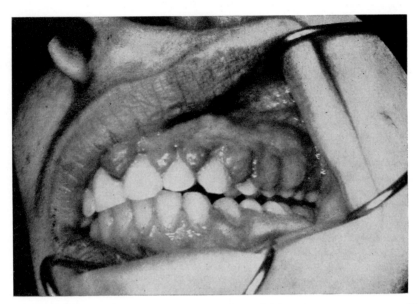

Fig. 27-13. Hypertrophic gingivitis. The chief complaint of this patient was sore gums. There was a prolonged history of toothache of a lower left molar necessitating chewing only on the right side. Examination revealed diffuse hypertrophic gingivitis localized on the left side of the mouth. (Courtesy of Dr. David Weisberger.)

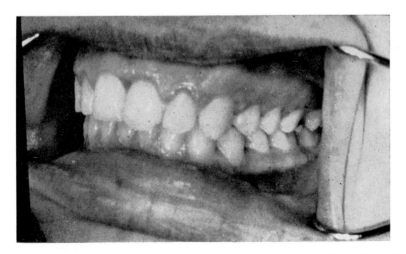

Fig. 27-14. Same patient as in Figure 27–13, after treatment that consisted of providing a dental restoration in the molar and active stimulation of the gingiva by chewing wax 3 times daily. (Courtesy of Dr. David Weisberger.)

and proper disposition in this field of oral diagnosis may indeed be life-saving.

Periodontitis. The commonest type of periodontitis is that familiarly known as pyorrhea alveolaris. This is in reality a rarefying osteitis of the supporting bone of the teeth and is accompanied by pocket formations that sometimes become infected with the evolution of a considerable amount of pus. This disease is usually a consequence of the failure to eliminate the gingivitis described in the preceding section. Local infection commonly plays an important role in the clinical course of the disease. There are two postulates as to how infection occurs. According to one school of thought, in order for there to be an infection in these areas, bacteria may have to pass two barriers of defense in order to form pockets in the al-

veolar bone (Fig. 27–15): first, the normal epithelial lining (Ep) of the gingival crevice; second, the strong transverse fibers (TF) over the crest of the alveolus. The latter appear to resist invasion, even after the gingivae have been destroyed. Figure 27–16 shows a case of periodontitis in which the epithelial papilla (Ep') had degenerated. The stroma (S) is inflamed and complete destruction of the transverse fibers has been achieved.

A more prevalent view today is the one supported by the findings of Weinmann,[141] which indicate that chronic infection of the gingiva progresses, following the course of the blood vessels, into the bone marrow spaces and on the periosteal side of the alveolar bone. According to this view the infection penetrates directly into the periodontal membrane only

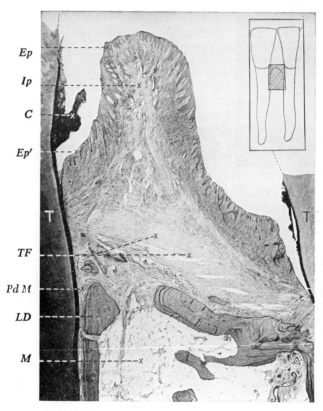

Fig. 27-15 Normal tissues between two teeth taken from area shown in insert. *Ep*, epithelium of the interdental papilla (*Ip*), and *Ep'*, epithelium in gingival crevice; *TF*, transseptal fibers which join the teeth together (*T-T*); *LD*, lamina dura and crest of alveolar bone; *M*, marrow; *Pd M*, periodontal membrane. Even though salivary calculus (*C*) is present, it has caused no inflammation.

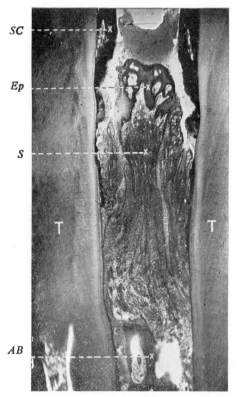

SC

Ep

S

T   T

AB

Fig. 27-16. Pathologic tissue taken from an area similar to that in Figure 27–15. Periodontoclasia resulting in destruction of the epithelium (*Ep*), severe inflammation of the stroma (*S*) and resorption of alveolar bone (*AB*). *SC*, salivary calculus; *T-T*, two adjoining teeth.

in exceptional cases. Resorption of the alveolar crest from the gingival side leads to destruction, first, of the supporting alveolar bone, and then of the lamina dura with its insertions of the periodontal membrane.

Although relatively little is known about the nature of systemic predisposing factors, it is likely that one or more systemic factors of nutritional and constitutional nature predispose toward the destruction of the tissues in this area. The main reason for believing in systemic influence of a presently unidentifiable nature is the observation that even after local conditions have been cleared up, periodontitis may continue to progress or may not regress. Various postulates concerning low-calcium intake, poor calcium utilization, avitaminoses C and D, deficiencies of the B complex and endocrine malfunction have been made. However, there is little evidence to support any of these hypotheses.

In experimental animals the only deficiency disease which has been reported to be comparable to periodontitis is scurvy in the guinea pig, in which Boyle and co-workers reported that prolonged vitamin C deficiency resulted in an absorption of the alveolar bone in a way that was characteristic of periodontitis in man.[47] However, clinical trials with human patients who had various degrees of periodontitis have not uniformly responded to vitamin C therapy, even though the tissues were saturated with vitamin C by administering doses of from 200 to 500 mg of ascorbic acid daily.

The only studies concerning vitamin D deficiency in relation to osteomalacia and to periodontitis have been ones reported from Indian surveys by Taylor and Day.[142] They examined 22 Indian women who were suffering from clinical osteomalacia by reason of diets deficient in calcium and in vitamin D, and found that 11 of them had severe cases of periodontitis. In view of the high incidence of periodontal diseases of all types in India, it is questionable whether the high incidence of periodontitis among these women with osteomalacia was attributable to the osteomalacia or was simply a manifestation that would have been expected in any group of Indian women of comparable age. However, more thorough clinical studies in this area are badly needed to provide definite information.

In the dog and in the monkey, various experiments in which B complex deficiencies were produced with resultant effects upon gingival inflammation and infection have been reported. Becks and Morgan described deficiencies in the filtrate fraction of the vitamin B complex, most likely pantothenic acid deficiency, and niacin deficiency in which severe abnormalities were reported in the supporting structures of the teeth of dogs.[143] Likewise, in monkeys fed diets deficient in the B complex, Chapman and Harris have produced severe gangrenous lesions of the gingival tissue and osteitis of the alveolar bone with exfoliation of the teeth.[144] These observations suggest that there are predisposing nutritional factors, when the deficiencies are particularly severe, to produce clinical entities comparable in some degrees to periodontal destruction. However, comparable observations are not available in human surveys.

For the best treatment of periodontitis, local irritating factors must be removed by proper procedures; an attempt must be made to restore the gingiva to normal physiologic form and function, and a program of home care to maintain the results of treatment must be conscientiously applied. For, without proper oral hygiene, all other measures are futile. The most satisfactory benefit from local treatment will be achieved when there is an accompanying improvement in systemic conditions. Though there are no specific dietary entities which have been clearly shown to be related to clinical periodontitis, improvement of the diet in all regards is strongly indicated. The best dietary prescription which can be given in these cases is the adherence to a fully adequate diet. Where there is reason to believe that one or more specific deficiencies exist in the patient, suitable therapeutic preparations should be given. Where there is no indication of specific deficiencies, general improvement of the diet will be found adequate, without supplementation by proprietary materials.

Noma (cancrum oris). This particularly catastrophic gangrenous lesion has its initial origin in the gingival area of the oral cavity even though it may ultimately involve the mucosa, cheeks, muscles and bone. Although the lesion is now rarely seen in Europe and North America, it is still prevalent in underdeveloped areas of the world where malnutrition and infection are major problems. Indeed, Tempest recently described over 250 cases that he has personally seen during only $3\frac{1}{2}$ years in Nigeria.[145]

The etiology of the lesion is somewhat obscure but usually involves a chronically malnourished child from 2 to 5 years of age who contracts an acute infection, often exanthematous such as measles or smallpox, which debilitates him further. Some days or a week after the precipitating systemic infection a gingival ulceration appears in the vicinity of the premolar-molar areas which within a few days spreads, becomes gangrenous, and can eventually slough leaving large defects in the cheeks, lips, and nose, often with large bony sequestra. Almost certainly the lesion is an extreme expression of Vincent's disease since the same fusospirochetal organisms are found in the tissues from the noma lesion. This is further borne out by the finding of the same organisms in extraoral lesions which also occasionally occur. It seems that an acute fusospirochetal infection of the oral cavity which ordinarily is kept within bounds by the host's natural defense may assume a rampant, explosive character in the malnourished debilitated child. Noma formerly had a mortality of 70 to 90 per cent, but with antibiotic therapy this has been reduced to under 15 per cent. However, the severe disfiguring sequelae present formidable surgical and psychosocial problems (Figure 27–17).

Relationships of Chewing Ability and Nutriture. Examples of an interrelationship between proper dentures and malnutrition have been reported. Mann and co-workers made a clinical study of 160 edentulous

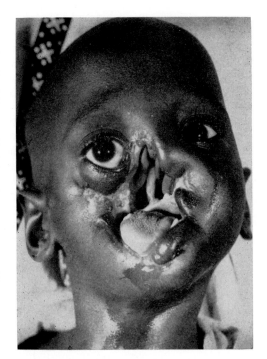

Fig. 27-17.   Disfigurement in a case of noma.

patients with a long-standing clinical record of multiple deficiency disease who had been under their observation for at least 3 years.[146] All had previous histories or present evidence of chronic pellagra, beriberi, scurvy, or riboflavin deficiency. The identity of these deficiencies was established by the presence of characteristic mucosal membrane lesions of pellagra, of the nutritional peripheral neuritis of beriberi, of the gingival lesions of scurvy, and of angular cheilosis and the ocular lesions of riboflavin deficiency.

The vertical dimension of the face had decreased in 140 out of the 160 cases. Fifty-seven of the 74 patients who had only 1 denture, or none, had perlèche. Fifty-two of the 66 patients who were wearing dentures with decreased vertical dimension gave evidence of perlèche. In contrast, only 7 of the 20 cases with a normal vertical dimension showed any evidence of angular cheilosis. Ninety-eight of the patients with a reduced vertical dimension complained of symptoms arising from the alimentary tract, "burning of the mouth and tongue, epigastric burning and pain, nausea and vomiting, intermittent

diarrhea, cramping and anorexia." Only 8 of the 20 patients with a normal vertical dimension mentioned these subjective symptoms. In the majority of these patients, artificial dentures had been constructed poorly or of inferior materials. This resulted in much irritation that was ultimately augmented by the unsanitary condition of these appliances. Under these circumstances in many of these patients, the consumption of adequate amounts of an adequate variety of foodstuffs was either difficult or impossible. When patients with a reduced vertical dimension were given riboflavin, there was a reduction in the cheilotic lesions, but at no time did these lesions disappear if a reduced vertical dimension was still present. Niacin and pyridoxine did not have any effect on angular cheilosis, although they aided in the reduction of other symptoms characteristic of these particular deficiencies.

These data indicate the necessity to restore adequate dental function by well-fitted dentures that restore the normal vertical dimension. Even dentures that are perfect when originally fitted must be examined periodically to determine whether or not the alveolar ridges have been resorbed sufficiently to alter the original normal relationships. If such a reduction in dental function is allowed to persist, perlèche may result from the decreased vertical dimension of the face and a complex nutritional deficiency disease may arise from the inability to masticate an adequate amount of food or an adequate variety of food.

In a continuation of these studies, Greene and co-workers made a survey of the incidence of impaired mastication ability in 446 consecutive patients at the Nutrition Clinic of the Hillman Hospital in Birmingham, Alabama.[147] Masticatory insufficiency was the term that was used to describe a variable clinical condition that resulted from one reason or another in the inadequate ability to chew food. A patient was considered to be in the state of masticatory insufficiency if any one of the following conditions prevailed: (1) no natural teeth and artificial dentures that were inadequate or painfully fitting; (2) no natural teeth and no artificial dentures or only one denture; or (3) less than 3 opposing serviceable natural masticating teeth and

3 opposing serviceable natural anterior teeth and no functional replacements in the form of dentures or bridges. Two hundred and sixty-eight of these patients had no natural teeth. Only 49 of these edentulous individuals had well-balanced functional artificial dentures. Of the 178 individuals who still had some natural teeth, only 96 had well-balanced dentitions. Thus, 301 of the 446 patients had various degrees of masticatory insufficiency, and only 145 had natural or artificial well-functioning dentitions according to the definitions laid down by the investigators. The incidence of masticatory insufficiency was observed to increase appreciably with age.

A further problem with patients who have been edentulous for prolonged periods is the difficulty in designing and making dentures that are comfortable and masticatorily efficient. After prolonged periods of edentulousness, the mucous membranes of the mouth and lips are sufficiently atrophied and altered that the wearing of plates is very difficult. In these cases in particular, there is a special necessity to correct the underlying nutritional disorders that have arisen over the edentulous period. Otherwise successful construction and fitting of the dentures in tissues with reduced viability and altered structure will increase the likelihood of unsatisfactory results.

Xerostomia (*Dry Mouth*). This is a rare condition, one form of which is believed to be induced by a prolonged avitaminosis A in a comparable fashion to that in which xerophthalmia is induced. In animals, besides atrophy of the lacrimal glands, occlusion of the main ducts of the salivary glands by desquamated epithelium has been observed. In human cases with completely dry cornea, there has been reported a lack of salivary secretion, and thickened, whitish mucous membranes of the mouth. These symptoms all disappear after administration of large doses of vitamin A. Xerostomia has also been reported to occur in the following conditions: aplasia of one or more of the salivary glands; systemic diseases with an accompanying high fever or inducing a state of dehydration; menopause; old age; psychic stimulation (fear, anxiety); certain drugs (atropine, anti-

histamines, rauwolfia alkaloids, sympathomimetic drugs); and post-radiation fibrosis of salivary glands.

Pain. Oral pain may vary from the annoyance of a "burning" sensation in the tongue to the excruciating manifestations of "tic douloureux." The "burning" tongue is one of the most difficult problems with which the dentist and physician must cope. Each case is a diagnostic problem in itself. The condition is usually localized in the lateral margins and the tip of the tongue and is described as a peppery feeling or a burning sensation. This is commonly an early sign of pernicious anemia, and also occurs early in pellagra, sometimes in diabetes, early pregnancy, and alcoholism. In all these situations a deficiency of one or more members of the vitamin B complex may be involved. If the diagnosis of the underlying factor can be made, the "burning tongue" is easily corrected. If there is suspicion of faulty absorption of nutrients, the parenteral route is advisable. In all cases, treatment is likely to be prolonged. Various claims have been made for specific effects of thiamin chloride and of pyridoxine hydrochloride. However, there are no data to corroborate these statements with any degree of accuracy, although isolated cases may have responded to therapy in this line. From available data, it cannot be deduced that these are specific for the treatment of such sensations as are described under the terms, "burning tongue" or "tic douloureux." In these conditions, it is important to remember to treat local conditions that may contribute to the breakdown of the adjacent tissues, but in addition, systemic conditions of a rather general nature must be considered and evaluated. It is relatively rare that individual nutrients will be found to be responsible for any of these manifestations.

By far, the better means of treating dietary abnormalities that may accompany or predispose toward these local lesions of the oral mucous membranes or of the supporting structures of the teeth is the prescription of a well-balanced diet composed of the four basic food groups with a general distribution of the foods generously among the several groups. In cases where there is clear-cut evidence of prolonged deficiency of one or more nutrients, there is obviously justification that these should be supplied in purified form in high enough amounts to replete the body supplies. However, by and large, this is neither necessary nor desirable. In addition, where there are cases of faulty absorption or excessive requirements by reason of peculiar constitutional circumstances or accompanying disease requirements, then supplementation also is in order. It is noteworthy too, in connection with postoperative healing, especially when there are extensive needs in the oral cavity, that a diet of generously adequate nature with respect to all the nutrients should be prescribed.

SUMMARY

Our knowledge about the relationships of nutrition to the diseases of the oral cavity has been rapidly expanding during the past decade. This is best exemplified by the increased factual information about the relationship of nutrition to the development, the maturation and the maintenance of the teeth and to the caries susceptibility of the teeth. Insofar as the influence of nutrition upon the lesions of the oral mucous membranes and of the supporting structures of the teeth is concerned, we still have a much smaller collection of established facts than is needed. It is not unreasonable to assume by reason of the rapidly expanding horizons in nutritional research that the next decade or two may well provide as many substantial answers to the latter category of oral problems as has been added to our pool of knowledge about tooth decay in the past decade or two. It is noteworthy, although not surprising in view of the chronic nature of most oral problems, that many of the nutritional problems of the mouth involve metabolic abnormalities which create predispositions to disease entities to be manifest years or decades later.

The best advice for any age group about the dietary regimen that will provide the best opportunity for normal oral tissues is simple and straightforward. Each of the basic four food groups should be represented liberally in each day's diet, and as many as possible in each of the day's three meals. The best selection of foods for dental health is one where as many of the foods as possible are purchased in their natural state without excessive refining and where the cooking procedures are such as to conserve the maximum of the original nutritive value. Attention should also be paid to the inclusion in the diet of a frequent and varied series of foods that require vigorous mastication as a means to stimulate and exercise the various tissues and organs involved in the comminution of food. In addition a liberal source of vitamin D should be provided daily throughout the entire period of an individual's growth and development. A minimum of sticky, adherent, high-carbohydrate foods with a low rate of clearance from the oral cavity should be consumed. After eating foods with a slow oral clearance, the teeth should be cleaned thoroughly by the procedure of choice to be recommended by the dentist. As in-between meal snacks, in place of sticky high-carbohydrate foods, fresh fruits, vegetables, fruit juices, milk and other dairy products are much to be preferred from a dental health standpoint. In the over-all nutritional planning for improved dental health, one of the most important facets to be considered is the fluoridation of public water supplies.

BIBLIOGRAPHY

1. Scott, Ussing, Sognnaes and Wyckoff: J. Dent. Res., *31*, 74, 1952.
2. Sognnaes and Shaw: J. Am. Dent. Assoc., *44*, 489, 1952.
3. Orland, Blayney, Harrison, Reyniers, Trexler, Wagner, Gordon and Luckey: J. Dent. Res., *33*, 147, 1954.
4. Orland, Blayney, Harrison, Reyniers, Trexler, Ervin, Gordon and Wagner: J. Am. Dent. Assoc., *50*, 259, 1955.
5. Keyes: Arch. Oral Biol., *1*, 304, 1960.
6. Fitzgerald and Keyes: J. Am. Dent. Assoc., *61*, 9, 1960.
7. Fitzgerald, Jordan and Stanley: J. Dent. Res., *39*, 923, 1960.
8. Gibbons, Berman, Knoettner and Kapsimalis: Arch. Oral Biol., *11*, 549, 1966.
9. Berman and Gibbons: Arch. Oral Biol., *11*, 533, 1966.
10. Zinner, Jablon, Aran and Saslow: Proc. Soc. Exp. Biol. & Med., *118*, 766, 1965.
11. Weisberger, Nelson and Boyle: Am. J. Orthodont. & Oral Surg., *26*, 88, 1940.

12. Schwartz and Shaw: J. Dent. Res., *34*, 239, 1955.
13. Afonsky: *Saliva and its Relation to Oral Health.* Birmingham, Univ. of Alabama Press, pp. 21–30, 1961.
14. Kite, Shaw and Sognnaes: J. Nutrition, *42*, 89, 1950.
15. Shaw: J. Nutrition, *53*, 151, 1954.
16. Haldi, Wynn, Shaw and Sognnaes: J. Nutrition, *49*, 295, 1953.
17. Anderson, Smith, Elvehjem and Phillips: J. Nutrition, *35*, 371, 1948.
18. Gustafsson, Quensel, Lanke, Lundqvist, Grahnen, Bonow and Krasse: Acta Odont. Scand., *11*, 232, 1954.
19. Schweigert, Shaw, Phillips and Elvehjem: J. Nutrition, *29*, 405, 1945.
20. Stewart, Hoppert and Hunt: J. Dent. Res., *32*, 210, 1953.
21. Constant, Phillips and Elvehjem: J. Nutrition, *46*, 271, 1952.
22. Krasse: Arch. Oral Biol., *10*, 215, 223, 1965.
23. Wood and Critchley: Arch. Oral Biol., *11*, 1039, 1966.
24. Gibbons and Banghart: Arch. Oral Biol., *12*, 11, 1967.
25. Fitzgerald, Keyes, Stoudt and Spinell: J. Am. Dent. Assoc., *76*, 301, 1968.
26. Shaw, Krumins and Gibbons: Arch. Oral Biol., *12*, 755, 1967.
27. Guggenheim, König, Mühlemann and Regolati: Arch. Oral Biol., *14*, 555, 1969.
28. Stephan, Fitzgerald, McClure, Harris and Jordan: J. Dent. Res., *31*, 421, 1952.
29. Phillips: J. Am. Diet. Assoc., *26*, 85, 1950.
30. Stephan and Miller: Proc. Soc. Exp. Biol. Med., *55*, 101, 1944.
31. Hunt, Hoppert and Erwin: J. Dent. Res., *23*, 205, 1944.
32. Hodge, Johansen, Hein and Maynard: J. Dent. Res., *32*, 654, 1953.
33. Larson: Chapter in *Environmental Variables in Oral Disease*, AAAS Pub. No. 181, Washington, D.C., 1966.
34. Shaw, Griffiths and Terborgh: Arch. Oral Biol., *7*, 693, 1962.
35. Larson and Simms: Science, *149*, 982, 1965.
36. Wolbach and Howe: J. Exptl. Med., *42*, 753, 1925.
37. ———: Am. J. Path., *9*, 275, 1933.
38. Boyle: J. Dent. Res., *13*, 39, 1933.
39. Dinnerman: Oral Med., Oral Surg., Oral Path., *4*, 1024, 1951.
40. Sweeney, Cabrerra, Urrutia and Mata: J. Dent. Res., *48*, 1275, 1969.
41. Sweeney, Saffir and deLeon: Am. J. Clin. Nutr., *24*, 29, 1971.
42. Wolbach and Bessey: Arch. Path., *32*, 689, 1941.
43. Dalldorf: In *The Vitamins*, Chicago, American Medical Association, Chap. XIX, p. 339, 1939.
44. Wolbach and Howe: Proc. Soc. Exp. Biol. Med., *22*, 400, 1925.
45. Crampton: J. Nutrition, *33*, 491, 1947.
46. Boyle, Bessey and Howe: Arch. Path., *30*, 90, 1940.
47. Boyle, Bessey and Wolbach: J. Am. Dent. Assoc., *24*, 1768, 1937.
48. Westin: Dent. Cosmos, *67*, 868, 1925.
49. Hanke: *Diet and Dental Health*, Chicago, University of Chicago Press, 235 pp., 1933.
50. Westin: *Uber Zahnveränderungen in Fällen von Skorbut bei Homo.*, Vol. 2, Stockholm, A. B. Fahlcrantz, 483 pp., 1931.
51. Hess and Abramson: Dent. Cosmos, *73*, 849, 1931.
52. McBeath: J. Dent. Res., *12*, 723, 1932.
53. Grandison, Stott and Cruickshank: Brit. Dent. J., *72*, 237, 1942.
54. Mellanby: Lancet, *2*, 767, 1918.
55. ———: Brit. Dent. J., *44*, 1031, 1923.
56. Weinman and Schour: Am. J. Path., *21*, 821, 1945.
57. Sarnat and Schour: J. Am. Dent. Assoc., *28*, 1989, 1941; *29*, 67, 1942.
58. Mellanby: Sp. Rep. Ser., Med. Res. Coun. No. 191, London, His Majesty's Stationery Office, 1934.
59. Mellanby, Coumoulos, Kelley and Neal: Brit. Med. J., *2*, 318, 1957.
60. Committee for the Investigation of Dental Disease: Sp. Rep. Ser., Med. Res. Coun., No. 211, London, His Majesty's Stationery Office, 1936.
61. Agnew, Agnew and Tisdall: J. Am. Dent. Assoc., *20*, 193, 1933; J. Pediat., *2*, 190, 1933.
62. McBeath: Am. J. Publ. Health, *24*, 1028, 1933.
63. McBeath and Verlin: J. Am. Dent. Assoc., *29*, 1393, 1942.
64. Anderson, Williams, Halderson, Summerfeldt and Agnew: J. Am. Dent. Assoc., *21*, 1349, 1934.
65. Day and Sedwick: J. Dent. Res., *14*, 213, 1934; J. Nutrition, *8*, 309, 1934.
66. Mills: J. Dent. Res., *16*, 417, 1937.
67. East: Am. J. Pub. Health, *29*, 777, 1939.
68. Strälfors: Svensk Tandläkare-Tidskrift, *49*, 108, 1956.
69. McClure: J. Nutrition, *65*, 619, 1958.
70. Sobel and Hanok: J. Biol. Chem., *176*, 1103, 1948.
71. ———: J. Dent. Res., *37*, 631, 1958.
72. Sobel, Hanok and Shaw: Abstracts, 124th Meeting American Chemical Society, Abst. No. 173, p. 72, 1953.
73. Armstrong and Knowlton: J. Dent. Res., *21*, 316, 1942.
74. Ham and Smith: Can. J. Res., *28*, 227, 1950.
75. McClure: Pub. Health Rept., *64*, 1061, 1949.
76. Maurer and Day: J. Nutrition, *62*, 561, 1957.
77. Bunting, Crowley, Hard and Keller: Dent. Cosmos, *70*, 1002, 1928.
78. Dean, Jay, Arnold, McClure and Elvove: Pub. Health Rept., *54*, 862, 1939.
79. Dean, Arnold and Elvove: Pub. Health Rept., *57*, 1155, 1942.
80. Dean: Pub. Health Rept., *53*, 1443, 1938.

81. Russell and Elvove: Pub. Health Rept., *66*, 1389, 1951.
82. McClure and Likins: J. Dent. Res., *30*, 172, 1951.
83. Zipkin, Posner and Eanes: Biochim. Biophys. Acta, *59*, 255, 1962.
84. Zipkin, McClure and Lee: Arch. Oral Biol., *2*, 190, 1960.
85. Zipkin and Posner: Int. Assoc. for Dent. Res. Preprinted Abstracts, 40th General Meeting, *28*, 103, 1962.
86. Jenkins and Speirs: J. Physiol. (Proc.), *121*, 21, 1953.
87. Brudevold, Gardner and Smith: J. Dent. Res., *35*, 420, 1956.
88. Isaac, Brudevold, Smith and Gardner: J. Dent. Res., *37*, 318, 1958.
89. Sognnaes, Arnold, Hodge and Kline: Washington, National Research Council, Publ. No. 294, 15 pp., 1953.
90. Ast, Smith, Wachs and Cantwell: J. Am. Dent. Assoc., *52*, 314, 1956.
91. Moulton, Ed.: *Fluorine and Dental Health*, Washington, American Association for the Advancement of Science, 101 pp., 1942.
92. Galagan and Vermillion: Pub. Health Rept., *72*, 491, 1957.
93. Shaw, Ed.: *Fluoridation as a Public Health Measure*, Washington, American Association for the Advancement of Science, 232 pp., 1954.
94. Leone: Arch. Indust. Health, *21*, 324 and 326, 1960.
95. Bernstein, Sadowsky, Hegsted, Guri and Stare: J.A.M.A., *198*, 499, 1966.
96. Rich and Ensinck: Nature, *191*, 184, 1961.
97. ———: Clin. Res., *10*, 118, 1962.
98. Hill, Jelinek and Blayney: J. Dent. Res., *28*, 398, 1949.
99. Fluoridation census, 1970 annual edition, Division of Dental Health, Preventive Practices Branch, Public Health Service, U.S. Department of Health, Education and Welfare, Bethesda, Md. Pub. PPB-25, May, 1971.
100. Editorial: News of Dentistry, J. Am. Dent. Assoc., *53*, 492, 1956.
101. Cover description, J. Am. Dent. Assoc., *71*, 1094, 1965.
102. Sognnaes: Am. J. Dis. Child., *75*, 792, 1948.
103. Toverud: The Millbank Memorial Fund Quarterly, *34*, 354, 1956; *35*, 127 and 373, 1957.
104. Cohen: Personal communication, 1954.
105. Toverud: Brit. Dent. J., *86*, 191, 1949.
106. Sognnaes: J. Am. Dent. Assoc., *37*, 676, 1948.
107. Shaw and Sognnaes: Unpublished data.
108. ———: J. Nutrition, *53*, 207, 1954.
109. Sognnaes and Shaw: J. Nutrition, *53*, 193, 1954.
110. Hodge: J. Dent. Res., *22*, 275, 1943.
111. Braunschneider, Hunt and Hoppert: J. Dent. Res., *27*, 154, 1948.
112. Constant, Sievert, Phillips and Elvehjem: J. Nutrition, *53*, 29, 1954.
113. Sognnaes, Shaw and Bogoroch: Am. J. Physiol., *180*, 408, 1955.
114. Fanning, Shaw and Sognnaes: J. Am. Dent. Assoc., *49*, 668, 1954.
115. Briner, Francis and Rosen: International Association for Dental Research Abstracts, 43rd General Meeting, Abstract 210, 1965.
116. Wynn, Haldi, Shaw and Sognnaes: J. Nutrition, *50*, 267, 1953.
117. Haldi, Wynn, Shaw and Sognnaes: J. Nutrition, *66*, 333, 1958.
118. Nizel and Harris: New England J. Med., *244*, 361, 1951.
119. McClure and Folk: Proc. Soc. Exp. Biol. Med., *83*, 21, 1953.
120. McClure: Proc. Soc. Exp. Biol., *96*, 631, 1957.
121. Constant, Sievert, Phillips and Elvehjem: J. Nutrition, *53*, 17, 1954.
122. Nizel and Harris: J. Dent. Res., *43*, 1123, 1964.
123. Strälfors: J. Dent. Res., *43*, 1137, 1964.
124. Ship and Mickelsen: J. Dent. Res., *43*, 1144, 1964.
125. Averill and Bibby: J. Dent. Res., *43*, 1150, 1964.
126. Sutfin, Sweeney, and Ascoli: J. Dent. Res., *49*, 772, 1970.
127. Pederson: Dent. Rec., *58*, 191, 1938.
128. ———: Deut. Zahn-., Mundt-., u. Kieferheilk, *6*, 728, 1939.
129. Boyd, Drain and Nelson: Am. J. Dis. Child., *38*, 721, 1929.
130. Boyd: Am. J. Dis. Child., *66*, 349, 1943.
131. Drain and Boyd: J. Am. Dent. Assoc., *22*, 155, 1935.
132. McBeath: J. Dent. Res., *12*, 723, 1932.
133. ———: J. Dent. Res., *13*, 243, 1933.
134. Howe, White and Rabine: Am. J. Dis. Child., *46*, 1045, 1933.
135. Howe, White and Elliott: J. Am. Dent. Assoc., *29*, 38, 1942.
136. Livermore: Dent. Surg., *18*, 1169, 1942.
137. Koehne and Bunting: J. Nutrition, 7, 657, 1934.
138. Koehne, Bunting and Morrell: Am. J. Dis. Child., *48*, 6, 1934.
139. McCarthy: J. Am. Dent. Assoc., *116*, 16, 1941.
140. Bernick: Oral Surg., Oral Path., Oral Med., *1*, 1098, 1948.
141. Weinmann: J. Periodont., *12*, 71, 1941.
142. Taylor and Day: Brit. Med. J., *2*, 221, 1940.
143. Becks and Morgan: J. Periodont., *13*, 18, 1942.
144. Chapman and Harris: J. Infect. Dis., *69*, 7, 1941.
145. Tempest: Brit. J. Surg., *53*, 949, 1966.
146. Mann, Mann and Spies: J. Am. Dent. Assoc., *32*, 1357, 1945.
147. Greene, Dreizen and Spies: J. Am. Dent. Assoc., *39*, 561, 1949.

Chapter

28

Nutrition in Diseases of the Gastrointestinal Tract

Section A   Nutrition in Diseases of the Stomach
Including Related Areas in the Esophagus and Duodenum

HARRY D. FEIN

The primary concern of the clinician is the appraisal and analysis of the complaints of his patient. This requires the fundamental knowledge on the part of the physician of the mechanisms operative in the production of the symptoms related to the various organ systems. First, there must be the appraisal of the site of the stimulus responsible for the symptom and the pathway of impulses to the area of manifestation, second, an appreciation and understanding of the pain threshold of the patient, and third, his reaction to the registered impulses both emotional and physiologic. This will help to determine functional and/or structural changes and choice of appropriate treatment of the patient. One recognizes the frequent association of functional disorders and symptoms related thereto with structural disease. The mechanism of the physiologic derangement may be purely local, secondary to the disease *per se*, but more often it is mediated through autonomic-hypothalamic-cerebral pathways as a result of the emotional trauma incidental to the presence of organic disease of a more or less serious nature. The stomach is the seat of dyspepsia, the symptom complex of disordered motility and the common denominator of most upper abdominal complaints. It may not be the lesion itself which produces the symptoms, but the gastric or gastrointestinal neuromuscular dysfunction which the lesion initiates. Distant diseases can pro-

duce the same disturbances of the stomach's neuromuscular activity and therefore the same symptoms. The trigger mechanism may lie elsewhere in the abdomen, in the emotions, or may be generalized throughout the body. Thus the patient with gastric cancer or pancreatic or biliary tract disease may have the same type of abnormal stomach sensations as the patient with peptic ulcer, nervousness, or some generalized systemic infection or disease. As far as stomach complaints are concerned, one hears from the patient as much about the way his stomach is reacting to the disturbing disease as about the disease itself. Various affections of the stomach may cause anorexia and consequent nutritional impairment due to restricted food intake. The stomach, in relation to its configuration and motility, is so complex that the proper interpretation as the result of its study is often difficult. This difficulty is reflected in the observation that opinion regarding diagnosis and treatment of stomach disease may vary from locality to locality and from gastroenterologist to gastroenterologist.

THE ROLE OF THE STOMACH IN NUTRITION

Cannon[1] has noted that Galen stated that the main functions of the stomach were to receive and retain the food during the processes of chemical digestion and then to pass the changed material onward. Beaumont's experiments in 1825 made it clear that this was indeed the case.[2] The stomach receives all types of food acting as the great reservoir in the first or salivary stage of digestion. It maintains the second or gastric stage where the ingested material is altered in such a way that the resultant chyme is discharged slowly and intermittently into the duodenum and small intestine without irritating those structures. This is accomplished by two types of motor activity, namely tonus and peristalsis. The mechanism that regulates gastric emptying and determines the rate at which food leaves the stomach is complex, subject to many influences, and as yet not fully understood.

The gastric juice represents a mixture of gastric secretion, saliva, and intestinal contents refluxed from the duodenum. Clinically, the gastric secretion is a complex and variable mixture of water, inorganic ions, including hydrogen ion, bicarbonate ion (when acid is absent) and a number of organic constituents. Among the latter are several active enzymes and their precursors, three or more different mucins and their degradation products, the intrinsic factor of Castle, and a variety of other substances derived in minute amounts from interstitial fluid and cellular degradation.[3] Recently immunoelectrophoretic studies seem to have confirmed the existence of four pepsinogens and four human pepsins.[4] The relative proportions of these may vary from person to person. In patients with normal gastric mucosa, the pepsin activity in gastric juice usually parallels the HCl output per unit of time. The function of pepsin in the stomach is to hydrolyze proteins to proteoses and peptones in preparation for further and more complete degradation in the intestine. Mucous products are produced by various cells in the stomach. These are mucoproteins composed of mucopolysaccharide and protein moieties. They exist in visible and dissolved forms. The visible mucus covers the entire lining of the mucosa and forms the first line of defense for the gastric mucosa against mechanical, thermal and chemical trauma.

Of special interest to the clinician are the hormones and drugs which exert a stimulating or inhibitory action on gastric secretion. The hormone gastrin (peptides I and II) produced by the antrum of the stomach in response to vagal stimulation, distention by food, and probably by exposure of the mucosa to the products of protein digestion, is the most potent stimulus to gastric secretion known. Histamine and its analogue, Histalog, are the best known available chemical stimulants of gastric secretion. The stomach, which receives most prescribed medications, is subject to erosion, ulceration, hypersecretion and intolerance to drugs. The anti-inflammatory agents such as the salicylates,[5] phenylbutazone, indomethacin, glucocorticoids and ACTH[6,7] may be particularly injurious. Colchicine, para-aminosalicylic acids, tolbutamide and caffeine seem to facilitate ulcer formation by reducing mucosal resistance. Caffeine may also increase acid-peptic secretion as do alcohol, aminophyllin, isonicotinic acid hydrazide, and reserpine. Caffeine sustains and potentiates other stimuli of hydrochloric acid secretion and reduces mucosal regeneration.

Different foods may influence gastric secretion as well as their pleasurable or indifferent anticipation Fatty foodstuffs exert an inhibitory effect on secretion by way of the gastrone mechanism. Carbohydrates, in the average diet, as a rule neither stimulate nor inhibit gastric secretion. Protein foods, such as meat, fish, chicken, cheese and milk are stimulants of gastric acidity. The protein renders the gastric contents neutral or nearly so and thus antral hormone is liberated.

The motor functions of the stomach are among the most important in the alimentary tract, they are complex and not fully understood. The tonic and peristaltic activity of the empty stomach stops abruptly during the ingestion of food thus permitting an increase in the intragastric volume under a relatively constant intragastric pressure (3 to 6 cm H_2O). Peristaltic activity resumes shortly thereafter with contractions limited to the pyloric region, followed in 5 to 10 minutes by waves originating higher in the fundus of the stomach. The mechanism that regulates gastric emptying and determines the rate at which food leaves the stomach is subject to many influences. There is a definite pattern of gastric emptying and under physiologic circumstances any variation in the rate of emptying results primarily from changes in stroke volume. At first the volume of the gastric meal decreases rapidly, and then with time more slowly with the result that a comparatively constant percentage of the remaining meal is evacuated per minute. Thus in the normal stomach several factors are known to influence gastric emptying. The hypertonic stomach tends to be hypermotile and to empty more rapidly than the hypotonic one. Liquids leave the stomach more rapidly than do semi-solids or solids whether ingested separately or not, and the rate of emptying is much greater with large-sized meals. This is all relevant to the occurrence of a dumping-like syndrome even in certain normals after large meals, and the beneficial effect of small meals in some and on the number of stools in patients with diarrhea. Carbohydrates leave the stomach sooner than proteins, and proteins leave more quickly than fats. Fats and fatty acids entering the intestine release enterogastrone which acts to delay the evacuation of the stomach and to suppress its secretion. Hypertonic and hypotonic solutions probably remain in the stomach longer than isotonic solutions to facilitate osmotic adjustment in the duodenum. A meal eaten at the time of marked hunger is generally evacuated more rapidly, probably because of increased tonus. Severe or protracted pain, especially of visceral origin, tends to decrease motor activity and evacuation. The emotional state may also markedly influence stomach activity. Generally, aggressive experiences are associated with increased motor activity, while depressive states result in decreased contractions and delayed evacuation of the stomach.

Disturbances of the vital functions of the stomach by disease, by partial or even total removal of the stomach invariably result in local or generalized symptoms of varying degree. Stomach emptying and function may thus be altered by a variety of physiologic states as mentioned above. In addition systemic disorders such as hypokalemia, diabetic acidosis and neuropathy, and uremia, as well as gastric ulcer itself may result in gastric retention and decreased gastric secretion. Obstruction in the region of the pylorus from whatever cause partially or completely impairs gastric emptying.

NUTRITION AND DIETARY TREATMENT IN SPECIFIC DISEASES OF THE STOMACH

The relation between nutrition and diseases of the stomach is a complex one. Diseases of the upper gastrointestinal tract may interfere with the actual intake of food by disturbing the appetite, inducing nausea and vomiting, evoking pain or producing mechanical obstruction. Traditionally, the medical therapy of disorders of the upper gastrointestinal tract has been in a large measure dietetic, though now there is some question as to the importance of rigid prolonged dietary restriction in diseases like peptic ulcer. Surgical therapy of the stomach may of itself lead to malfunction and nutritional disturbances requiring correction.

Dyspepsia. Dyspepsia may be defined as difficult or deranged digestion, a disordered state of the stomach in which its functions are disturbed. Ordinarily there is no awareness of digestive activity except a sense of satisfaction. In the dyspeptic from whatever cause, a characteristic variety of complaints referable to the upper gastrointestinal tract are present: aerophagy, bitter taste, bad breath, anorexia, nausea, heartburn, acrid or fetid eructions, a sense of fullness or bloating especially after meals, epigastric distress or pain, substernal discomfort or pain, regurgitation and vomiting, rumination, so-called cardiospasm and dysphagia. One should think then of dyspepsia under two main headings, (1) *Organic dyspepsia*, which arises directly from organic disease of the upper gastrointestinal tract, reflexly from other parts of the intestinal tract or from organic disease elsewhere in the body, and (2) *Functional dyspepsia*, which constitutes the majority of patients seen by the gastroenterologist, comprises well over 50 per cent of any group.

Dyspepsia of reflex origin is quite frequent. Disease of the biliary tract, liver disease, diseases of the pancreas, and enterocolonic disease for example, may all reflexly affect gastric function and digestion, thus giving rise to any or many of the symptoms previously mentioned. A careful search must be made for disease or dysfunction in organs or organ systems other than the stomach. Dyspepsia may be secondary to one of many systemic diseases other than that found primarily in the gastrointestinal tract; for example, atherosclerosis (generalized, coronary, or cerebral); hypertensive vascular disease; chronic renal disease, diabetes and other metabolic or endocrine disturbances; blood dyscrasias; collagen diseases; lymphomas; and other malignant diseases.

Most primary functional derangements of the gastrointestinal tract can be attributed to emotional tension. Visceral responses to emotional trauma have been observed in a variety of subjects by endoscopic examinations, balloon techniques and radiologic study. Disturbances of motility, tonus, secretion and vascularity have been noted. Personality patterns and their expressions are determined by experiences in early life, so that emotional behavior occurring in association with disease of physiologic derangement is the result of a complex series of interactions. Many conditioning factors will modify the character of the complaint. The disorders encountered as the result of emotional change may be classified into those due to, (1) hyperfunction, (2) hypofunction, and (3) mixed types. As the result of one or a combination of these physiologic disorders, one may find the patient complaining of a variety of symptoms, such as pain, pyrosis, dysphagia, abdominal fullness, anorexia, nausea, vomiting, and the other symptoms previously listed under dyspepsia. In this group there will be a variety of diagnostic types: the psychoneurotic, the infantile, the dependent, the aggressive and the frustrated. The treatment of this functional group of dyspeptics requires great skill on the part of the physician. He must be versed in the functional physiologic disorders so that he is able to dissect out and recognize the nature of the problem, and recognize the presence of emotional aberrations and physiologic effects. Treatment must be directed to the patient as a whole, with warm sympathetic understanding. One cannot treat such a patient simply by handing him a diet on a printed sheet or prescribing one or another type of medication. Treatment directed toward the involved organ *per se* is only palliative. A careful explanation of the mechanism for the production of the symptoms is of utmost importance. If no amelioration of emotional stress is achieved by specific therapy, or refractoriness is noted, psychiatric help should be sought.

TREATMENT OF THE PATIENT WITH DYSPEPSIA OF NERVOUS ORIGIN

Prudent Bland Diet. (cf Appendix, Table A-17). Such a diet covers the average nutritional needs; it avoids excessive amounts of saturated fats so characteristic of the average American diet; it avoids the highly spiced and seasoned foods and condiments; it provides for regularity of eating patterns. A general suggestion is the avoidance of stress at meals, haste in eating and bolting of food.

Tobacco, particularly cigarettes, is to be prohibited in such patients. It often causes pseudo-ulcer syndromes as well as interfering with appetite and normal digestion. Alcohol, as a general rule, is forbidden dyspeptic patients. There are some who can tolerate an occasional well-diluted alcoholic beverage and benefit from its relaxant effect. This may be permitted provided it is taken with food. The excessive use of coffee is likewise forbidden.

The management of the dyspeptic patient presents many problems and the approach is not primarily a dietary one. If organic disease is present, resulting in reflex dyspepsia, treatment for the underlying condition is of paramount importance. The patient with functional dyspepsia requires special and individual attention.

Hiatal Hernia. Herniation of part of the stomach through a diaphragmatic hiatus, the commonest of the diaphragmatic hernias, is one of the most important of the mechanical gastrointestinal diseases. It is probably the commonest pathologic condition affecting the upper gastrointestinal tract. It must be understood that hiatal hernia, like so many other mechanical defects of the gastrointestinal tract, causes illness in only a small proportion of the people it affects. The diagnosis of this condition is not synonymous with disease.

Heartburn or pyrosis is the most common complaint offered by these patients. Other manifestations in the order of decreasing incidence are regurgitation, which often accompanies pyrosis, substernal or xiphoid pain, which seems to be deep-seated, dysphagia, especially if the hernia is complicated by esophagitis with or without stricture, and bleeding with or without manifest anemia. Insufficiency of the gastroesophageal closing mechanism, regurgitation of gastric contents and motor dysfunction of the esophagus are the main pathophysiologic alterations that underlie the production of symptoms.

The treatment of hiatal hernias is a subject of controversy, usually depending on whether it is the medical or surgical point of view. Many internists are reluctant to urge early surgical repair, in the belief that most patients can be handled satisfactorily by medical means. The regimen to be suggested will depend upon the character of the hernia, the severity of symptoms and the presence or absence of associated diseases and complications. Any condition responsible for recurrent vomiting or episodes giving rise to sudden increases in intra-abdominal pressure may worsen the condition and bring about a complication. Chronic cough should be vigorously treated. Tight constricting abdominal supports or belts may be deleterious. Measures for the control of constipation are required to avoid straining at stool. Weight reduction is essential for the obese patient. The head of the bed should be elevated so that the patient sleeps in a semi-recumbent position. The usual recommendations are for a diet that is relatively bland, small frequent feedings, and a light evening meal to avoid distention particularly before retiring. Reclining after meals or physical effort after meals should be avoided. Alkalies and sedatives may be used as indicated.

In selected instances of painful attacks associated with spasm, one of the antispasmodic drugs may be used, as well as anticholinergic drugs when depression of vagal activity is desired provided that no gastric stasis results. If the attacks of pain are frequent or the hernia is complicated by esophagitis or peptic ulcer, the diet should be of the ulcer type and the patient treated as one does a peptic ulcer. The indications for operation may be present in many instances, yet surgery is often not advised initially. The risk of operation in many of the elderly patients is great, so that palliative treatment may be continued. Stricture when present has in many instances been successfully treated with bougie dilatation without resorting to surgery and should be tried. One may recommend a semi-solid balanced bland diet for the patient who has some degree of stricture and cannot tolerate solid foods. If the stricture is severe and even semi-solid foods cannot be taken, a balanced liquid formula or blenderized foods may be taken while treatment such as dilatation is employed or the patient is being prepared for surgical intervention.

Gastritis. This may be defined as an inflammation of the gastric wall, especially of the gastric mucosa. It is an anatomic designation of complex anatomic changes, usually called inflammatory, within the gastric wall. Gastritis is at least as common as gastric and duodenal ulcer combined. The thinking regarding diffuse gastric mucosal disease has in the past been confused, but is much less so now because of direct observation made feasible by the advances in gastroscopy, gastric photography, and gastric biopsy. There is little dispute about the aspects of acute gastritis. The concept of the more clinically important chronic gastritis, however, has been more actively studied and debated.

Acute gastritis may be divided into four types: (1) simple exogenous, (2) corrosive, (3) infectious (hematogenous), and (4) phlegmonous. The acute simple variety is frequent at any age and is characterized by malaise, anorexia, nausea and vomiting. It may be due to an infection with a specific microorganism or a virus. The disease may last from one to several days, and if food cannot be taken orally, the patient may be sustained by intravenous fluids. The immediate therapy of acute corrosive gastritis must combat collapse and consists of intravenous feedings until oral intake becomes feasible.

Acute infectious or hematogenous gastritis is a form of acute gastritis arising from toxins or bacteria entering the stomach from the blood stream. Avoidance of food may be helpful to the patient, but starvation must not be allowed. If oral intake can be instituted a bland diet should be given, otherwise intravenous feedings should be used. Acute phlegmonous gastritis is a rather rare purulent diffuse or localized inflammation of the gastric wall. General supportive measures and specific therapy for the underlying disease are indicated. At times surgery may be necessary.

Chronic nonspecific gastritis is clinically more important than the acute variety. Based on gastroscopic observations it may be divided into three types. (1) Superficial gastritis is a form in which the mucosa is reddened, edematous, and covered with adherent mucus; mucosal hemorrhages and small erosions are frequent. (2) Atrophic gastritis is characterized by a thinned, gray or greenish-gray hemorrhagic mucosa; the atrophy usually is distributed irregularly, but the entire stomach may be affected. (3) Hypertrophic gastritis presents a dull spongy or nodular appearing mucosa; the rugae are irregular, thickened, or nodular; hemorrhages and superficial erosions are frequent. Gastritis occurring after gastroenterostomy or partial gastric resection combines the manifestations of all three types. Menetrier's disease or giant gastric rugae are noted most commonly in the mid portion of the stomach along the greater curvature, although there may be diffuse involvement of the stomach.

The etiology and pathogenesis of chronic gastritis are not known. Dietary indiscretions, alcohol, tobacco, coffee, infections, and nutritional deficiencies have been implicated, but the evidence is inconclusive. All types of chronic gastritis are observed in association with peptic ulcer, but atrophy is more frequent in gastric than duodenal ulcer, whereas hyperplastic mucosa is more common in duodenal ulcer than in gastric ulcer. Atrophy of the gastric mucosa is invariably present with pernicious anemia and gastric polyposis, and not infrequently in patients with sprue, pellagra, and iron deficiency anemia. A possible immune mechanism in the development of gastric atrophy has been suggested.[8]

The consequences of chronic nonspecific gastritis are not known. The course seems to be persistent or recurrent with unpredictable variations in type, severity, and distribution in the same person. Minor surface alterations, such as erosions, hemorrhages, and hyperemia, usually heal completely. Severe and complete atrophy of the stomach generally tends to continue unchanged. In elderly patients, especially among women, deficiency of vitamin B_{12} may develop, but it does not progress to pernicious anemia. The associated clinical manifestations include weakness, loss of memory, mental depression, paresthesias, and abdominal discomfort with flatulence. These symptoms frequently respond to treatment with vitamin B_{12}. Deficiencies of iron and other vitamins also may be associated with atrophy of the gastric mucosa. The most frequent complaints are loss of appetite, fullness, belching, vague epigastric pain, nausea, and vomiting. These are also the symptoms of functional distress; they may be relieved by the use of a bland diet and antispasmodic drugs.

PEPTIC ULCER DISEASE

The general incidence of peptic ulcer approximates 15 per cent. It is more common in patients with rheumatoid arthritis, obstructive bronchopulmonary disease and possibly in patients with cirrhosis of the liver treated by portacaval shunt. The mechanisms involved are not known entirely. Duodenal ulcer appears to be more frequent in individuals with blood group O, especially those not secreting A, B, and H blood group factors in saliva and gastric juice. The significance of this relationship is not apparent, but suggests perhaps that duodenal ulcer represents the outcome of an interplay between environmental and hereditary factors. Constitutional factors are suggested by the occurrence of ulcers occasionally in families and in twins living separately.

Gastric ulcer resembles duodenal ulcer in its chronicity, recurrences, complications, and in its tendency to heal, especially when the acid content is neutralized or abolished.

Gastric ulcer differs from duodenal ulcer in its lower output of hydrochloric acid and the intermittency of the secretion, in its increased frequency in women, older age groups, and among the poorly nourished and impoverished social classes.

Peptic ulcer may be broadly described as the product of a pathologic physiology in which the mucosa fails to withstand the destructive action of the acid pepsin gastric juice. The local factors responsible probably include a diminution of cellular resistance, possibly a loss of protective intracellular substances, decreased cellular protection from an insufficient secretion of mucus, excessive secretion of hydrochloric acid, or a combination of these. The central nervous system probably plays a significant role, perhaps by producing hyperemia of the stomach and duodenum, possibly localized areas of ischemia, hypermotility, and hypersecretion, thereby increasing the vulnerability of the gastric mucosa to injury.

The controversy regarding physiologic gastric rest by dietary control in ulcer patients started during the nineteenth century. Some advocated an empty stomach, whereas others advocated hourly feedings of milk or milk combinations in an attempt to achieve neutralization of the free hydrochloric acid. The Sippy regimen of hourly milk combinations was interspersed with antacid powders.[9] The value of strict dietary control in the management of peptic ulcer is still highly controversial. Many dietary concepts have been examined, some endorsed and some condemned on the basis of individual experiences, controlled studies or statistical analysis. There has not evolved a basic dietary formulation acceptable to all physicians and to all patients, and applicable to all phases of ulcer disease.[10–12]

Most physicians agree that a dietary regimen of the Sippy type is unnecessary except in the acute phase of the active ulcer. There is some justification for the traditional dietary modifications recommended during the acute symptomatic period of the disease.

The overall aim of dietary control is to provide "physiologic rest" for the stomach, reduce mechanical trauma, minimize the effects of the ingesta on the chemical phase of gastric secretion and, more importantly, provide nutriment with maximum neutralizing capacity. Known stimulants of gastric secretion, such as alcohol and caffeine-containing beverages, should be avoided. Direct mucosal irritants, such as black pepper, chili, vinegar, mustard, pickles and irritating spices, should be eliminated entirely.

Small frequent feedings provide the most consistent buffering effects. In addition, total bulk is adjusted so as to avoid the distention stimulus to the antral gastric mechanism. Studies by Code et al. leave little doubt that all foods stimulate the production of gastric juice.[13] The secretory pattern for each food is rather characteristic, similar patterns being obtained with the bread and cereal group, fruit and vegetables, milk and dairy products and the meat, fish and egg group. Protein proved to be the most important acid-stimulating factor in the foods tested. The highest acid secretory equivalent values are found in the categories of meat, fish, and dairy products. The least stimulating foods, the carbohydrates and fats, are also the least neutralizing. The more effective neutralizers, amphoteric proteins, are the strongest secretogogues.

The following dietary principles should be acceptable in all instances relating to ulcers. The diet should be adequate to meet in full the nutritional needs of the patient with a margin of safety to compensate for various stresses, undernutrition, growth, development and normal physical activity. Caloric inadequacy for periods of 7 to 10 days during the management of the acute phase of ulcer disease presents no real nutritional deficiency or dietary problem. Obesity should be corrected because of its well-known harmful physical effects. Psychological factors should be recognized. The creation of the proper atmosphere at mealtimes certainly has favorable motor and secretory influences. Any concomitant diseases requiring dietary regulation, such as protein restriction in liver and renal disease, limitation of sodium, dietary control in diabetes, restriction of gluten in patients with gluten enteropathy, must obviously be taken into consideration.

The recent literature has emphasized the hazards of diets high in saturated fats and cholesterol in the high risk coronary-ulcer group. Excessive cholesterol and triglycerides in the blood may predispose to atherosclerosis and, therefore, increase the incidence of coronary artery disease and possibly cerebrovascular episodes. In studies of patients and of postmortem data, the incidence of myocardial infarction was found to be twice as high in patients with peptic ulcer who had been treated with a Sippy diet or milk products as it was in those who did not follow such a diet, or in control subjects without ulcer. The incidence of myocardial infarcts, in general, is higher in patients with chronic peptic ulcer disease than in subjects without ulcer. Studies have shown that diets in which 40 per cent of the calories are derived from fat, mainly saturated, produce high levels of serum cholesterol, whereas equicaloric polyunsaturated vegetable oil reduces serum cholesterol. The desirability of restricting saturated fat in the ulcer program is obvious.[14-20] Where it appears desirable to modify serum triglycerides and cholesterol, reference is made to Chapter 31 for diagnostic procedures, clarification of hyperlipidemias and their treatment.

The following dietary regimens are suggested, depending upon the phase of the ulcer disease.

Diet in Clinically Active Uncomplicated Ulcer. During the first 2 or 3 days the diet should be extremely bland, consisting of frequent feedings (hourly or two hourly) of milk interspersed with a nonabsorbable antacid preparation. (Diet I—see Appendix Table A-15.)

The patient may take additional feedings and antacids during the night, if awakened and exhibiting distress. If it is desirable to increase the fat content of such a dietary program without increasing the saturated fat, then add one of the polyunsaturated oils to the milk (1 ounce to a quart—flavor with decaffeinated coffee, syrup, or vanilla, if desired; sugar may be added to taste) and homogenize in a blender. Skim milk should be used when fat restriction and/or caloric restriction is desired. To relieve the monotony of plain milk, one may make up a mixture of milk with one of the many flavored prepared dried protein powders or use one

of the prepared liquid nutritional supplements. This will increase the nutritional and caloric value of the drink. Supplemental vitamins should be given at this time, if not included in adequate amounts in the commercial formula.

The average uncomplicated ulcer patient will be quickly relieved of his pain in a matter of a few days. Particularly if nocturnal pain has disappeared, the diet may be advanced to include cereal, toast, soft-boiled eggs, creamed soups, cottage cheese, pureed or well cooked vegetables, cooked or stewed fruits, jello, custard, plain puddings or plain crackers and cookies as tolerated (Diet II, see Appendix, Table A-16). If the patient remains symptom-free, he is advanced to a full bland or convalescent ulcer diet (see Appendix, Table A-17 for bland diet with between-meal feedings).

It is of the utmost importance that the ulcer patient does not allow long periods to elapse without having something to eat or drink. He must learn to take something between meals, the type of nourishment and amount can be regulated so as to gain weight if indicated, maintain his weight, or even lose weight if necessary.

Any strict diet for long periods of time may deprive the patient of nutrients, and many ulcer diets eliminating fresh vegetables, juices and fruits have induced borderline ascorbic acid deficiencies. This is less evident now with the administration of supplemental vitamins. Strict diets are self-defeating in many patients. When we prescribe a regimen, we want the patient to follow it, have the ulcer heal as thoroughly as possible, and not recur. In terms of these objectives, what are the effects of eliminating most tasty foods and insisting on minced and pureed foods? A few patients with the appropriate mental makeup may enjoy rigorous self-denial, but in most people one of two things happens; either they cheat on their diet and probably neglect to follow other restrictions, or they eat their food with a peculiar determination not conducive to the mental relaxation the ulcer patient needs. Most ulcer regimens are full of regulations; it is difficult for the patient to observe them for more than a few weeks or months. It is probably unsound, as well as unrealistic, to add to his difficulties by requiring observance of rigid dietary rules which have not been shown to be supported by sound rationale. Following a rigid dietary requirement for all time certainly has not been shown to prevent recurrences of the ulcer disease.

In the case of the acutely symptomatic active peptic ulcer a planned regimen may be desirable. It results in rapid improvement in over 80 per cent of the patients in a short time. Many ulcer patients improve within 24 to 48 hours with a change in environment. Regular administration of antacids, anticholinergics before meals, the longer-acting preparations at bedtime and the discrete use of sedatives should supplement the dietary regimen.

The Management of the Obese Patient with Ulcer Disease. The ulcer patient who is obese is subject to the same complications of degenerative disease that pertain to other overweight patients. In addition, he represents an additional serious risk if surgical intervention is contemplated for his ulcer or its complications. If one attempts too rapid a weight reduction by very sharp caloric restriction, there may be an exacerbation or recurrence of ulcer symptoms. During the course of weight reduction adjunctive measures such as the conventional antacid therapy (nonabsorbable alkalies) and the anticholinergic drugs should be employed, even though the ulcer may not be active or symptomatic. The use of frequent feedings high in protein, such as meat, gelatin, fish, pot or cottage cheese, will serve to control gastric acidity, ulcer pain, and limit the caloric intake. Modify a bland diet (Appendix, Table A-17) according to caloric needs.

Dietary Management of Upper Gastrointestinal Hemorrhage. Whatever may be the source of bleeding, the patient should be started on a diet close to normal as soon as nausea and hematemesis have stopped. Experience from many quarters has shown that bleeding patients progress more satisfactorily when fed than when starved. There is nothing to suggest that hunger contractions or the dyskinesias produced by blood in the stomach are any more beneficial to a bleeding patient than physiologic peristalsis. One should not forget that the empty stomach is far from a resting stomach. Early feeding should start with milk, custards, jello, and other bland foods as tolerated. This should be progressed rapidly to a full bland diet as soon as possible. The initial recommendations of early feeding in cases of hemorrhage were made by Lenhartz in 1904. He recommended the use of small hourly feedings during the first day, in an effort to neutralize the acid and facilitate healing of the ulcer. Meulengracht perpetuated and reinforced this regimen and, in 1934, he recommended the use of more sizable meals composed of high calorie pureed foods with between-meal feedings of milk.[21] He presented good evidence that hemorrhage may be controlled while feeding a patient an abundant diet. Thus, nutrition is maintained, loss of weight is prevented, convalescence is shortened and blood regeneration is favored. The patient does not complain of constant hunger, is more satisfied, and, above all, the mortality rate is lower than under the older starvation method.

If the bleeding has been more severe and patient tolerance is diminished, it may be desirable to limit the feedings during hemorrhage. A diet such as suggested for active peptic ulcer disease may be employed and rapidly progressed as tolerated. Pain is not a feature in hemorrhage, in fact pain, if it had been present, usually disappears or markedly diminishes with the onset of bleeding.

There is some question about the use of nonabsorbable antacids in the face of hemorrhage. Many clinicians use them as long as there is no nausea or vomiting. Others hesitate because of the danger of fecal impactions. These physicians feel that the hourly feedings act as adequate buffers. Anticholinergics do not appear to have any important place in the bleeding patient. Since they increase the heart rate, their use may make the evaluation of the patient more difficult especially in the event of possible surgery. In all likelihood the combined use of anticholinergics and nonabsorbable antacids increases the chances of fecal impaction and such a combination is best avoided.

Obstruction at the Pylorus and the Duodenal Bulb. This type of obstruction is both a medical and surgical problem. The cause may not be evident or certain initially and every effort must be made to relieve the obstruction, if possible, in order to make a positive diagnosis. Peptic ulcer disease is the commonest cause of pyloric obstruction and resulting gastric stasis, and accounts for approximately 80 per cent of the cases. The obstructing lesion is most often in the duodenum, but it may be in the pyloric channel or in the prepyloric antrum of the stomach. Next in order of frequency is gastric cancer, rarely pyloric muscle hypertrophy in the adult and on occasion prolapse of a gastric polyp into the duodenal bulb and malignant or inflammatory diseases of contiguous structures such as the biliary tract and pancreas.

The chief hazard for the patient with pyloric obstruction and consequent vomiting is the loss of fluid and electrolytes in the gastric secretions and the accompanying systemic imbalance. Advanced pyloric obstruction exhibits the classic findings of hypochloremic-hypokalemic alkalosis with hyperazotemia. The management of pyloric obstruction due to peptic ulcer disease must be undertaken in the following manner: (1) the restoration of fluid and electrolyte balance, (2) decompression of the dilated atonic stomach, and (3) the amelioration of the active ulcer disease. Since the secretions lost in pyloric obstruction result in essentially an isotonic contraction of body fluids, the administration of hypotonic solutions is dangerous and results in water intoxication. The need is for parenteral solutions of approximately isotonic concentration. The chief depletion is in Cl^- and K^+ but the latter should be given with caution and only after one is sure that satisfactory urinary output is present. It is best not to be too vigorous in attempts to restore fluid and acid-base balance and not to follow too rigid a schedule for correcting the calculated theoretical deficits.

The pyloric obstruction can be treated by intubation and constant suction. This should be maintained for no longer than 24 to 48 hours since prolonged gastric suction further depletes a patient who is already in electrolyte imbalance, has lost weight and requires nourishment. Wilkinson advocated alternate nasogastric feedings and drainage.[22] Brown also uses alternate feeding and drainage except that he suggests longer periods of feeding during the day and drainage during the night.[23] If the degree of obstruction is not too severe the stomach may be aspirated night and morning, i.e. before bedtime and on arising, and the amount of aspirate measured and recorded. This is preferable to intermittent or constant suction. The serial aspirations serve a twofold purpose, therapeutic and diagnostic. When the amount of accumulated fluid during the day is 250 ml or less, the night aspiration can be discontinued. Oral feedings can be started, with 30 to 60 ml of clear liquids given at hourly intervals. If this is well tolerated, the amounts can then be increased by small increments to 150 ml in each feeding.

As soon as feasible, frequently within 48 hours, the next step in the program is started, namely the treatment of the active peptic ulcer. The feedings are then changed to skim milk and, if tolerated, progressed to whole milk, alternating with nonabsorbable antacids given at hourly intervals as outlined under treatment for any case of active ulcer. Anticholinergic and antispasmodic drugs have no place in the face of obstruction and should not be employed. If the patient continues to improve on this prescribed regimen, the diet can be progressed to one that is bland and high in proteins and carbohydrates. Fats should be avoided since they are poorly tolerated in the face of obstruction. After 7 to 10 days of such treatment a repeat radiographic study should be made. If the obstructing lesion was due mainly to acute inflammation, spasm, and edema, there will be considerable radiographic improvement, indeed all signs of obstruction may be gone. However, if the obstruction was produced largely by thick cicatricial tissue the persistent distortion will remain. Throughout this period, correction of electrolyte imbalance, anemia if present, and maintenance of fluid intake must be accomplished by intravenous feedings. If the patient is badly nourished, has lost much weight, and would represent an especially poor surgical risk, jejunostomy feedings or parenteral nutrition (hyperalimentation) may be employed. The technique for the latter is covered in Chapter 36.

The patient who does not respond to a medical regimen will require surgery. Rarely is pyloric stenosis an emergency. Correction of fluid and electrolyte imbalance, improvement in the patient's nutritional state plus decompression of the dilated stomach must always precede surgical intervention. Most surgeons are now performing antrectomy with vagotomy. There may be hesitancy on the part of some to add the vagotomy considering the obstruction, but the latter is present because of the underlying ulcer disease and this is corrected at operation. The vagotomy is an especially important consideration when the acid output values are high. Less frequently is subtotal gastrectomy with or without vagotomy performed. In poor risk patients with long-standing peptic ulcer disease, in the older age group or those with concomitant diseases, gastroenterostomy may be performed with the added procedure of vagotomy, if feasible. In these cases it is desirable to do the simplest surgical procedure for relief of the patient's condition, fully aware that the gastroenterostomy stoma is left unprotected from the development of ulceration, if vagotomy is not performed. Pyloroplasty and vagotomy may have little place in pyloric obstruction for the thickened cicatrized tissue does not usually lend itself to a satisfactory pyloroplasty.

The peptic ulcer patient is not often presented for surgical intervention at the late date when he is so malnourished and in such a poor metabolic state that he must first be fed via a jejunostomy tube. Jejunostomy tube feedings if poorly formulated and given too rapidly may be ill tolerated and accompanied by diarrhea, distention and symptoms not unlike those found in the "dumping syndrome." In present practice jejunostomy feedings are resorted to only after some serious complication following abdominal surgery where the patient becomes a serious problem in maintaining nutrition. Fluid and electrolyte balance are maintained by the intravenous route until sufficient nutriment is tolerated via the jejunostomy. The patient is first tested with saline via jejunostomy tube and if tolerated, a diluted je-

junostomy formula is started by slow drip which then progresses to the full formula at a rate adjusted to prevent dumping symptoms (see Appendix, Table A-28). Jejunostomy feedings are preferable to total parenteral nutrition with its attendant dangers of catheter infection and septicemia.[24,25]

The principal effect of pyloric obstruction upon the prognosis at the present time is only the mortality that one might expect from an elective procedure, if the patient is in good surgical hands; that is, if the patient is properly prepared preoperatively by the correction of malnutrition, anemia, hyperazotemia, alkalosis and hypochloremia.

Management of the Patient Who Has Had Surgery for Peptic Ulcer Disease. Evaluation of the various surgical procedures for peptic ulcer disease is an ongoing study. Limited gastric resection of 40 to 50 per cent wtih removal of the antrum, combined with vagotomy, or pyloroplasty with vagotomy, are presently the procedures of choice in the treatment of duodenal ulcer. The unpleasant side effects and complications are minimal. Perhaps, in gastric ulcer, where surgery is indicated, subtotal resection is the operation of choice. By most criteria, 75 per cent subtotal gastrectomy is inferior to other procedures as an elective operation for duodenal ulcer. Vagotomy and pyloroplasty in the treatment of duodenal ulcer appear to be indicated as an emergency procedure in the poor risk patient, in underweight individuals, in young patients presenting for surgical management with complications of ulcer disease and in patients who have anatomic pathologic condition which makes resective surgery too hazardous.

Following surgery, how long should the patient remain on a restricted diet? There is no rationale for an indefinite period of rigid dietary restriction. A relatively bland diet is followed for several weeks postoperatively and then new foods are added as tolerated until a full regular diet is taken. Each patient must be individualized.

Diet in the Complications of Surgical Treatment. *The Dumping Syndrome.* It is generally recognized that the dumping or post-gastrectomy syndrome is the outstanding complication associated with substantial, partial or total surgical removal of the stomach, and occasionally after drainage operations. Clinically, the syndrome has its onset 10 to 15 minutes after the ingestion of a meal and is characterized by abdominal fullness and distention, followed by tachycardia, pallor, tachypnea, weakness, sweating and, in some instances, syncope. The intact stomach normally empties small quantities of food into the jejunum, permitting digestion of only small aliquots of food, and guards against a massive and acute change in osmotic load. Following gastric resection, the capacity of the stomach as a reservoir has been reduced and ingested material enters the intestine in larger quantities and more rapidly. There is evidence that the dumping syndrome is associated with a shift of plasma water to the intestinal lumen to equalize increased intraluminal osmotic pressure. This results in a marked and precipitous drop in plasma volume. The acute increase in osmotic pressure in the intestinal lumen results from the rapid entrance of small molecular components from the stomach.[26,27] It has also been postulated that dumping is the result of intestinal distention and increased intraluminal pressure. This has not been confirmed by balloon studies. The blood sugar has also been implicated in dumping; it may rapidly develop a rise to hyperglycemic levels then abruptly fall to hypoglycemic levels but these changes do not appear to coincide with the clinical symptoms of dumping. Occasionally a patient may have symptoms of hypoglycemia a few hours after a meal; symptoms referable to this should not be confused with the dumping syndrome. The fall in potassium and the sometimes-seen nonspecific electrocardiographic changes are not fully clarified, since they are not necessarily temporally related to the dumping syndrome. Some believe that the symptoms are brought on by excessive serotonin output.

Management of the Dumping Syndrome. Since most dumping symptoms are more easily produced by carbohydrates than by protein or fat and are related to the quantity of food ingested, dietary management is of great importance in treating the postgastrectomy syndrome. Carbohydrates are more rapidly hydrolyzed into smaller molecular

particles than either proteins or fat; thus the basis for the concept that carbohydrates are the least desirable food for the patient with the dumping syndrome.

The dietary regimen recommended is designed to consider the following: (1) type of food ingested, (2) total quantity of food taken at any one time, (3) daily caloric requirement, and (4) the physical form of the food ingested. Carbohydrate food should be limited. The diet should be high in proteins and fats with a caloric intake of 2000 to 3500 kcal per day. Feedings are recommended at frequent intervals, e.g. every 2 to 3 hours to avoid overloading the stomach. The diet should be a relatively dry one with restricted fluids at meals. Fluids may be taken more freely between meals. Sugar, sweets, candy, syrups and chocolate should be avoided. The patient with late postprandial dumping, in whom hypoglycemia is found, must shorten the intervals between meals, and increase the protein and fat content. The ingestion of a readily assimilable source of sugar at such time may be helpful. There are some patients who cannot achieve correction of their dumping syndrome by dietary means alone. If the symptoms are severe further surgical correction may be necessary.

Complications of Surgery. *Nutritional Impairment Following Gastric Surgery.* A nutritional defect following gastrectomy is the commonest undesirable sequela; the more extensive the gastric resection the greater the nutritional problem. This is generally seen as a failure to maintain or regain normal body weight or, more specifically, in a lack of one or more essential nutritional factors. These problems are now encountered in a relatively small group of patients and rarely in the partial-gastrectomized patient who enjoys a healthy appetite, appears to have almost normal gastric capacities, consumes an essentially unrestricted diet and has normal bowel function.

The causes of deficient nutrition will vary from patient to patient. The chief cause is simple reduction in caloric intake, because of either early satiety, reflecting a diminished gastric reservoir, or actual fear of eating because of the distressing postprandial symptoms. Others, as Goldstein,[28] implicate steatorrhea as a cause of weight loss, diarrhea, and malnutrition in a far higher percentage of patients than is generally recognized. These observers do not negate the importance of decreased caloric intake as a factor in postgastrectomy malnutrition, but emphasize the added detrimental effects of malabsorption. Decreased pancreatic secretion as a cause of malabsorption has been suggested, but this has not been shown to be a significant factor, neither has rapid intestinal transit. There is some evidence to suggest that faulty mixing of food with pancreatic juice and bile may be a factor in postgastrectomy steatorrhea. This, too, has not been proven. In some cases afferent loop stasis and bacterial overgrowth have been implicated as a cause of steatorrhea. This condition, if present, would apply in only a very small minority.

Anemia has been recognized as a complication of partial gastrectomy for many years with numerous reports concerning its frequency, course and possible etiology. Some months or even years after such surgery a varying percentage of individuals, up to 57 per cent, develops a mild iron deficiency anemia which usually responds to oral iron therapy. Women in their reproductive years develop this anemia oftener and sooner than postmenopausal women or men of comparable age. Some patients may develop a progressive fall in serum vitamin B_{12} levels as a result of impaired B_{12} absorption, but only a small number develop megaloblastic anemia. Occasionally megaloblastic anemia occurs as a result of folic acid deficiency. The incidence of postgastrectomy anemia due to both iron and vitamin deficiency seems to increase in the first postoperative decade. Inadequate food intake, chronic intermittent blood loss from the associated gastritis or gastrojejunitis and malabsorption of iron have each been blamed for the development of iron deficiency, while atrophy of the gastric mucosa is currently considered responsible for the development of most cases of vitamin B_{12} deficiency. Chronic malabsorption of calcium may lead to bone demineralization.

The management of the poorly nourished postgastrectomy patient is implied in the previous discussion. It is the designing of an acceptable, nutritious diet, along with a great deal of sympathetic understanding and encouragement, that is essential (though many patients improve spontaneously with time). If a problem such as dumping exists, every effort should be made to ameliorate this condition. If steatorrhea, other than the very mildest form, is present, it should be treated. Symptomatic measures, including anticholinergics, psychotropic drugs, dietary manipulation and pancreatic enzyme administration, should be tried. In those cases where there appears to be a true intolerance for fat, a mixture of medium-chain triglycerides may be used. The patient should be assured adequate calcium and vitamin D intake. In those cases with obvious deficiency of iron, B_{12} or folic acid, these substances should be administered. Anabolic agents and supplemental vitamins should also be considered. In the suspected afferent loop stasis with bacterial overgrowth, antibiotics should be given either in prolonged administration at reduced dosage or in repeated short courses. At best these cases are difficult to treat and every available means of nutritional and psychological support should be tried.

MISCELLANEOUS DISEASES OF THE STOMACH AND DUODENUM

Crohn's Disease. *Nonspecific Granulomatous Inflammation.* In 1950, Comfort *et al.*, in a report of 5 cases, established that nonspecific granulomatous inflammation of the stomach and the duodenum was the same condition as regional enteritis affecting other parts of the small intestine.[29] By 1967 approximately 62 cases had been recorded. Fielding *et al.* studied 12 patients with gastroduodenal involvement followed between the years 1944 and 1969.[30] In Comfort's original paper, patients with this condition exhibited the following symptoms: continuous or intermittent upper abdominal pain, made worse by food, systemic upset with fever, loss of weight, diarrhea, and finally a progressive stenosing lesion in the duodenum. Fielding and others found patients in whom the symptoms were relatively mild and when related to food were relieved by antacid therapy. Obstructive symptoms at some time during the course of the disorder were common and present in two thirds of the patients followed. There is no special dietary regimen other than the one used for the basic disease; i.e. a diet which is nutritionally balanced and easily tolerated without producing further gastrointestinal irritation and pain. Some patients with this disease do well on a regular selected diet, whereas others must follow a bland low residue diet.

Menetrier's Disease. *Menetrier's disease* or giant rugal hypertrophy is characterized by large, prominent gastric folds found diffusely throughout the stomach or localized to the body or antrum. Inflammation need not be present so that the term giant hypertrophic gastritis is a misnomer. The markedly elongated gastric glands secrete a thick viscous mucus. This secretion is high in albumin content and may lead to hypoalbuminemia, peripheral edema, and occasionally ascites. Menetrier's disease may be considered a protein losing gastropathy. There may be other symptoms such as vague dyspepsia, postprandial epigastric pain which may or may not be relieved by food and antacids. In some instances food may actually aggravate the pain. Anorexia, nausea, and sometimes vomiting may be present with marked weight loss as a prominent feature. The diagnosis is made by a combination of radiography, gastroscopy, peroral biopsy of the stomach, and cytology studies. Treatment is symptomatic with the administration of antacids and a high protein diet especially when hypoalbuminemia is present. Surgery may be necessary when intractable symptoms are present or if uncontrollable bleeding occurs.

Isolated Granulomatous Gastritis. An entity separate and distinct from Crohn's disease and sarcoidosis presents clinically as pyloric obstruction with radiologic features of antral narrowing simulating neoplasm. The treatment in these cases is that for pyloric obstruction or surgical intervention to establish a definite diagnosis if this is impossible with the other diagnostic means available.

Eosinophilic Gastritis. This is a rare disorder usually a part of a more diffuse process characterized by diffuse or circumscribed eosinophilic infiltration of the gastrointestinal tract. In both forms the stomach is the organ most commonly involved. In the diffuse form, symptoms are predominantly those of long-standing partial and intermittent pyloric obstruction. The circumscribed form presents as an eosinophilic granuloma anywhere in the gastrointestinal tract. When it is present in the stomach the symptoms are not as marked or as acute as in the diffuse variety. Biopsy is necessary for diagnosis and surgical resection of the isolated granuloma is curative. Steroids have been used with beneficial effect in the diffuse variety. No special dietary regimen is recommended other than avoiding foods to which the patient may be allergic. A selected balanced diet which the patient can tolerate without further gastrointestinal irritation is recommended. If dietary restrictions must be imposed, then supplemental vitamins are recommended.

BIBLIOGRAPHY

1. Cannon: Amer. J. Physiol., 1, 359, 1898.
2. Beaumont: Experiments and Observations on the Gastric Juice and the Physiology of Digestion. Plattsburg, F. P. Allen, 1833.
3. Hollander: What is meant by gastric mucus? Proc. World Congress of Gastroenterology, Washington, D.C., 1958.
4. Rapp, Aronson, Burton, and Grabar: J. Immunol., 92, 579, 1964.
5. Benson: Am. J. Dig. Dis., 16, No. 4, 357–362, 1971.
6. Kirsner: Acid-peptic disease. In *Textbook of Medicine*. Beeson and McDermott, Philadelphia, W. B. Saunders Co., 1967.
7. Wirts: Gastritis. In *The Stomach*. New York, Grune & Stratton, 1967.
8. Doniach, and Roitt: Seminars Hematology, 1, 313, 1964.
9. Sippy: in Musser and Kelly: *A Handbook of Practical Treatment*, Philadelphia, W. B. Saunders Co., 1912, Vol. 3.
10. Ingelfinger: Let the ulcer patient enjoy his food. In *Controversy in Internal Medicine*. Philadelphia, W. B. Saunders Co., 1966.
11. Roth: The ulcer patient should watch his diet. In *Controversy in Internal Medicine*, Philadelphia, W. B. Saunders Co., 1966.
12. Dietary Misconceptions: Nutrition Reviews, 26, 1, 1968.
13. Code et al.: Gastroenterology, 39, 1, 1960.
14. Sandweiss, et al.: Harper Hospital Bulletin 17, 2, 1959.
15. Briggs, et al.: Circulation, 21, 538, 1960.
16. Sterner, et al.: J.A.M.A., 181, 186, 1962.

17. Katz, *et al.*: *Nutrition and Atherosclerosis*, Philadelphia, Lea & Febiger, 1958.
18. Jolliffe: Circulation, *20*, 109, 1959.
19. Jolliffe, Rinzler, and Archer: Am. J. Clin. Nutrition, *7*, 451, 1959.
20. Christakis *et al.*: J.A.M.A., *198*, 597–604, 1966.
21. Meulengracht: Acta Med. Scandinav. (Suppl.), *59*, 375, 1934.
22. Wilkinson: Amer. J. Dig. Dis., *9*, 321, 1942.
23. Brown: Amer. J. Dig. Dis., *4*, 940, 1959.
24. Dudrick *et al.*: Med. Clin. N. Amer., *154*, 577, 1970.
25. Shils: J.A.M.A., *220*, 1721, 1972.
26. Roberts, *et al.*: Ann. Surg., *140*, 631, 1954.
27. Clarke, and Wimmer: Gastroenterology, *40*, 803, 1961.
28. Goldstein: Malabsorption following gastrectomy. In *The Stomach*, New York, Grune & Stratton, 1967.
29. Comfort, Weber, Baggenstoss, and Kiely: Amer. J. Med. Sci., *220*, 616–632, 1950.
30. Fielding, Toye, and Cooke: Gut, *11*, 1001–1006, 1970.

Chapter

28

Section B Nutrition in Diseases of the Intestines

Norman Zamcheck

AND

Selwyn A. Broitman

Because the intestinal tract, and, in particular, the small intestine, is the site of digestion and absorption of nutrients, diseases of the intestinal tract are promptly accompanied by alterations in host general nutrition. The dynamic interrelationship existing between the gut mucosal pathobiology and host nutrition has been elucidated largely in animals.[1]* In recent years, Dubos,[2] Donaldson,[3] Sprinz,[4] and others have emphasized the participation of the nutrition and metabolism of the gut flora in this complex dynamic interaction. Full understanding, therefore, of nutritional alterations in disease of the intestinal tract requires broad understanding of the biology of the gut itself, the nature of the previous diet of the patient, the gut flora, as well as knowledge of the normal and pathologic anatomy of the small intestine.

The influence of previous dietary experience on the enzyme activity, *i.e.* enzyme adaptation, has been widely appreciated by chemists,[5] and has recently been studied in the gut. Deren and associates[6] showed that feeding carbohydrate influenced the disaccharidase activity of the small bowel in rats. The significance of this aspect of "diet" with respect to clinical disaccharide disorders including malabsorption is only beginning to be appreciated (see below).

The most frequent clinical manifestations of disease of the intestine are diarrhea, steatorrhea and the consequent weight loss and

* Bibliographic numbers and references are grouped under the headings of specific subsections at the end of the chapter.

nutritional deficiencies. Some patients with steatorrhea, however, may have little diarrhea. The clinical evidence may be manifest elsewhere, *e.g.*, dermatitis and dementia (niacin deficiency); cheilosis and glossitis (riboflavin deficiency); bone marrow, *e.g.*, macrocytic anemia (folic acid and vitamin B_{12} deficiency), and tetany (calcium and/or magnesium deficiencies), to mention only a few.

A few disorders have been characterized in part biochemically. The elucidation of vitamin B_{12} malabsorption in pernicious anemia is described elsewhere. Gluten sensitivity, disaccharidase deficiencies, defect in tryptophan metabolism in Hartnup disease, agammaglobulinemic states, abetalipoproteinemia are examples. However interesting, this group provides a relatively small proportion of the patients seen clinically.

Most clinical disorders have in common an impairment in gut absorption apparatus. From the point of view of the nutritional consequences and nutrient needs, the specific pathologic process responsible for the impairment is less relevant. Thus we have the opportunity to make some limited generalizations. For successful treatment of the patient, however, nutritional management must be combined with a clear understanding of the site, etiology and extent of the gut disorder. Thus bacterial diarrhea requires appropriate antibiotic therapy; gut enzymatic deficiencies require the elimination of the non-utilizable substrate; regional enteritis and ulcerative colitis often respond to corticosteroid therapy; parasites may be eliminated by specific drugs.

The attempt is made in this chapter to allude only to those aspects of clinical nutrition which seem most pertinent to the disorders discussed. Limitations of space permit only a survey of the subject.

Diarrhea—General. The management of fulminant loss of the intestinal content presents one of the most challenging therapeutic problems in medicine. This is seen in cholera and other acute bacterial diarrheas, and in massive intestinal resection. The general principles of management, *i.e.*, fluid, nutrition, electrolyte, mineral, and vitamin replacement, apply similarly in all of these disorders. The more acute the diarrhea, the greater is the loss of water and electrolytes such as sodium, potassium, chloride, and bicarbonate. The fluid loss in acute inflammatory states tends to resemble plasma and accordingly the losses of protein as well as electrolytes become prominent. Quantitative aspects of replacement vary depending upon the severity, the location of the lesion, and the reduction of or interference with the absorbing apparatus. In the more chronic states, as in gluten enteropathy, steatorrhea tends to predominate because intestinal transit time is sufficiently slow to permit absorption of most of the other nutrients. Fat being the least easily absorbed, fat malabsorption and its consequences may be seen in those conditions in which malabsorption is least severe. In each section below specific deficits and their replacement will be discussed individually.

MASSIVE RESECTION OF THE SMALL BOWEL

The clinical state, par excellence, which represents a severe quantitative reduction in the absorptive apparatus is *massive resection of the small intestine*. Many of the nutritional and physiologic disturbances encountered in this condition also occur in many other malabsorptive disorders of the small intestine. For this reason a large proportion of this section is devoted to it.

Within the past 10 years the nutritional needs of these patients have been elucidated. In several painstaking metabolic studies[1-3] resection of 50 per cent of the small bowel or

less usually posed minimal difficulties. There are reports of patients surviving for long periods of time with as little as 8 to 18 inches of bowel remaining,[2,4] and Kinney *et al.* reported survival in one patient with only the duodenum and half the colon remaining.[2] The most common conditions requiring resection are mesenteric vascular occlusion, strangulated hernia or acute volvulus.

Absorptive Defects. The resultant absorptive defects depend upon the degree of resection, the area resected, the presence or absence of the ileocecal valve, and the state of the remaining bowel. Gastric hypersecretion, diminished bile salt reabsorption and pancreatic insufficiency contribute to the malabsorption.

Proximal Resections. Resection of up to 8 feet of proximal jejunum may result in minimal malabsorption of fat or protein since these can be handled by the large reserve capacity of the distal gut.[1] If the duodenum remains intact there is no defect in absorption of folic acid,[5] glucose,[6] calcium[7,8] and probably no defect in absorption of the fat-soluble vitamins.[1] The ileum can assume some of the functions of the upper small bowel. However, when proximal resections exceed 8 feet, fat and protein absorption are impaired and impaired absorption of calcium, magnesium and fat-soluble vitamins (A, D, and K) is encountered.

Distal Resections. A patient with a resected ileum who has an intact jejunum may require no specific diet therapy other than parenteral replacement of vitamin B_{12} and restriction of fat intake to 30 to 50 gm daily.[9] In the absence of the ileum, Booth[1] and Scheiner[9] have demonstrated the critical minimal amount of jejunum necessary for satisfactory absorption of water-soluble nutrients to be 1 to 4 feet. Since the ileum is the site of reabsorption of bile salts, its absence will cause fat malabsorption.[10,11] Rapid transit through the remaining jejunum contributes to losses of all nutrients, but particularly to losses of lipids. The longer the ileum remaining, the less rapid the transit. The presence of the ileocecal valve is of utmost importance in slowing the transfer of materials from the small to the large bowel. In the absence of the ileocecal valve, segments of small bowel have been reversed and interposed between the distal small bowel and the cecum.[12] The size of this antiperistaltic segment seems to be of prime import, although the findings to date have not shown this to be a complete substitute for an ileocecal valve.

Carbohydrate. Digestion of carbohydrate is simpler than that of fat and protein and, hence, it is absorbed best in these patients. The simple sugars are easily absorbed throughout the small bowel and are carried away by the portal circulation. Carbohydrate absorption may not be accurately reflected by the oral glucose tolerance test or by absence of sugars in the stool since gut bacteria and yeast metabolize them. The 3-0-methyl glucose absorption test has been of value in assessing the absorptive capacities of the small bowel following resection.[3] This methylated sugar is absorbed in the same manner as glucose; it is not metabolized and consequently all that is absorbed appears in the urine within 24 to 48 hours. It was previously shown to have little value as a diagnostic test of carbohydrate malabsorption[13] since it is virtually completely absorbed by even the diseased small bowel. In patients with resection the percentage excreted yields an approximate index of that amount of bowel remaining with carbohydrate absorptive capacity.

The question of compensatory increase in carbohydrate absorption by the remaining small bowel has been raised repeatedly but few quantitative data are available. Recently Dowling and Booth[14] have shown an actual increase in the absorptive capacity of the jejunum for glucose after distal resections.

Disaccharidase activity is present throughout the entire small bowel mucosa[15]; therefore, the disaccharides can be hydrolyzed into simple sugars for subsequent absorption at any level.

Impaired absorption of glucose, folic acid,[16] and xylose[4] has been reported in patients with only 20 cm of jejunum remaining.

Fat and Nitrogen. Fat and protein are mixed with pancreatic and biliary secretions and are emulsified before they are absorbed. Lipids are absorbed in the proximal small intestine under normal physiologic circumstances.[17,18] When the lipid load is increased,

the remaining lipid is absorbed by the ileum. Shortened exposure of lipid to a limited small bowel surface area, as in intestinal hurry, may contribute to steatorrhea, particularly in distal small bowel resections.

Studies in animals and in man identify the distal small bowel as the major site of bile salt absorption. The ileum has been shown to be the only intestinal site of active transport of both conjugated and unconjugated bile salts.[10]

Malabsorption of amino acids, accompanied by large losses of nitrogen in the feces, may occur in massive intestinal resection.[3] However, positive nitrogen balance can be maintained by a high protein intake if some part of the jejunum is present. This may be due in part to the reduction in urinary nitrogen, an attempt by the body to conserve tissue nitrogen.

Calcium and Magnesium. Calcium may be lost in large quantities initially following resection, but tetany is an infrequent and usually a late complication. Serum and urine calcium levels may remain normal for long periods. Magnesium losses parallel calcium losses since they share a similar transport system.[19] The effect of deficiency of this ion is discussed in Chapter 6, Section B.

Vitamins. Booth has shown that vitamin B_{12} is absorbed in the terminal ileum;[20] resection of that portion of the bowel will result in vitamin B_{12} malabsorption. Fat-soluble vitamins A, D and K are lost in large amounts in steatorrhea. The loss of vitamin D contributes to large calcium losses. Vitamin K losses may be reflected by a prolonged prothrombin time. Absorption of folic acid and other water-soluble vitamins is usually normal, providing 4 feet of proximal small bowel remains;[1] however, increased body needs may require supplements.

Electrolytes and Water. Excessive diarrhea leads to severe body potassium losses and to a lesser extent sodium, although serum values may be deceptively normal. Starvation leads to acidosis, and extensive water losses result in dehydration. These patients may show a delayed water absorption with nocturnal diuresis which is related to protein depletion.[21]

Plasma Protein. The small intestine is a

site of catabolism of albumin.[22] It has been postulated that the albumin half-life should be prolonged in cases of massive bowel resection, and, indeed, studies in our laboratory showed a prolonged albumin survival in two patients with massive bowel resection.[23] The gut also plays an important role in the metabolism of immunoglobulins, both in their synthesis and degradation.[24] If the gastrointestinal tract were the sole site of immunoglobulin synthesis, then reduction in bowel size by resection would tend to reduce the total body pool of these proteins. However, in 4 patients studied in this laboratory, Jabbari[25] found that IgG and IgA were high normal to elevated and IgM was normal. The half-life of IgG was normal in the three subjects tested. These observations suggested increased production rather than decreased catabolism. Accordingly, other important sites of production probably existed in these patients.

Gastric Secretion. Gastric hypersecretion has been observed in patients following extensive[3,26,27] bowel resection. Hypersecretion may worsen the patient's nutritional state by increasing the diarrhea and thereby interfere with absorption. The absorptive disturbance may be due in part to hypermotility and to alteration of gut intraluminal pH from that essential for optimal absorption. Vagotomy and pyloroplasty appear to improve the patient's clinical course following extensive intestinal resection.[26]

Clinical Course and Management. The clinical course of patients following massive resection may be divided into three phases: Phase 1 is the immediate postoperative period during which fluid electrolyte losses, diarrhea and infection may overwhelm the patient. During phase 2 fluid and electrolyte problems decrease, diarrhea starts to diminish, wounds heal and the patient becomes more active and desires food. It is during this phase that the absorptive defects become apparent. The degree of malabsorption and general and specific nutrient deficiencies which depend on the amount and area of bowel resected may now be assessed. Phase 3 is the period during which the patient attains a balance with his disability, and his weight stabilizes at a level

determined by the amount of nutrient absorbed by his remaining gut.

Metabolic balance studies indicate the loss of body nutrients. In general, the diet should contain 3500 to 4000 calories per day provided largely by carbohydrate, since it is most easily absorbed, and by protein. Metabolic needs consume at least 50 gm/day of protein. If only 50 per cent of protein intake is absorbed, then at least 100 gm must be ingested. Provided caloric intake is adequate, this level of protein is consistent with positive nitrogen balance while performing active work for prolonged periods without development of protein deficiency.

Since long-chain fatty acids are poorly absorbed, usual dietary fat is of limited usefulness in supplying absorbable calories. Fat intake should, therefore, be kept to the minimum needed to make the diet palatable. Medium-chain triglycerides (MCT) may be substituted for part of the dietary fat. Such supplements contribute to caloric intake and together with adequate carbohydrate intake, prevent further depletion of protein reserves.

For ordinary activity, 21 calories/lb of ideal body weight are necessary in order to maintain body weight. If the percentages of carbohydrate, protein and fat absorbed are known, then the caloric intake necessary to supply these requirements may be estimated. Initially, a deficit of 2000 to 3000 calories and later of 3500 or more will cause 1 kg weight loss. Vitamin and mineral requirements can be estimated from tables in the Appendix and the chapters on individual nutrients.

Phase 1. During this postoperative period replacement of large volumes of fluids, salts, potassium, calcium, magnesium and amino acids or plasma protein will be required. Adequate caloric replacement can be provided intravenously (see Chapter 36). Oral or tube feeding should be initiated as soon as possible. Tube formulas may be necessary for variable periods. Generally, these feedings are composed of amino acid hydrolysates, simple sugars, electrolytes, calcium, magnesium, and medium-chain triglycerides. Tube feeding can be given in a slow continuous 24-hour drip which allows for more complete absorption and diminishes the diarrhea produced by ingestion of large amounts of formula at one time. During this time, if low gastric pH and large volumes suggest gastric hypersecretion, and if diarrhea is excessive, and wound healing delayed, then vagotomy and pyloroplasty should be considered. If there is no evidence of gastric hypersecretion but diarrhea is uncontrollable by usual measures, then insertion of an antiperistaltic bowel segment may become necessary. The segment is most helpful in patients in whom the ileocecal valve has been resected.[12]

Phase 2. Generally the patients prefer ordinary foods rather than prepared formulas and, if allowed "guided" selection, they will consume more calories. At first the feedings should be small and frequent, every 2 hours, during the course of the day. Later, as the patient improves, the amount may be increased and the interval between feedings lengthened. Caloric intake should be as high as the patient will accept and consists largely of carbohydrate. Simple sugars should be used. Particular attention should be given to the patient's tolerance for milk. Extensive resection of the bowel results in a reduction of lactase activity whereupon ingestion of excessive lactose-containing foods may induce diarrhea. Decreased fluid intake will frequently decrease the volume of stool.

Restriction of fat intake to a minimum reduces steatorrhea and diminishes losses of fat-soluble vitamins, calcium and magnesium. It is difficult to maintain such restriction for long periods. Furthermore, the high caloric value of fat is desirable when it can be absorbed. Winawer *et al.*[3] reported a patient with massive intestinal resection who showed decreased steatorrhea, weight gain and improved calcium balance concomitant with MCT feeding.

Nitrogen balance improves during this phase. Calcium, magnesium and vitamin D losses parallel the degree of steatorrhea. Up to 3 gm of calcium per day may be required to maintain a positive calcium balance. Magnesium should be supplemented also either in small oral doses or by parenteral routes. Since they are absorbed similarly, administration of calcium or magnesium alone may enhance the loss of the other. A "cocktail" of the following may be given twice daily: 1 gm calcium, 20 mEq magnesium, 5000 U vitamin A and 500 U vitamin D and 30 mg of vitamin E. If the prothrombin time is prolonged, 10 to 20 mg vitamin K should be given by either the oral or the parenteral route, daily or as needed, to assure adequate blood coagulation. If malabsorption of vitamin B_{12} has been shown by the Schilling test, vitamin B_{12} (200 μgm) may be given parenterally every month to prevent combined system disease and anemia. Replacement of other water-soluble vitamins, folic acid, and iron is necessary only in extensive proximal resections. Use of pancreatic enzymes and bile salts should be avoided as they are of little benefit; in fact, they may be harmful. Complications in gastrointestinal function in undernourished patients may require total or supplementary parenteral feeding. This is discussed in Chapter 36.

Phase 3. Most patients succumb during the second phase. Those few who reach this stage usually have less extensive resections. They can be sustained more easily by the program worked out in the previous stage and require less management.

Complications and Prognosis. Postoperative wound infections, breakdown of anastomoses, gastric hypersecretion, fluid and electrolyte losses have been discussed. Calcium and magnesium imbalance may lead to tetany. Deficiencies of folic acid, iron or vitamin B_{12}, if not replaced, will lead to anemia. Recurrent abdominal distention and occasional renal stone formation occur. Food rejection and emotional problems are common. Tuberculosis is common.

MALABSORPTIVE SYNDROMES

The *diffuse disorders* of the small intestinal mucosa such as are seen in the flat bowel mucosa syndromes (Tables 28B–1 and 2) are variously termed primary or idiopathic steatorrhea, non-tropical sprue, adult celiac disease, celiac sprue and childhood celiac disease. The less severe disorders thereof are termed subacute atrophy. Creamer[1] concluded that the flat jejunal biopsy was not specific for adult celiac disease since this may be seen in a variety of other diseases (Table 28B–1). Others have ascribed some degree

Table 28B-1. Diseases Associated with Flat Jejunal Mucosa (Primary and Secondary Celiac Syndromes)*

A. Primary celiac syndrome
  (1) Gluten sensitive enteropathy (Celiac disease of children, adult celiac disease, idiopathic steatorrhea).

B. Secondary celiac syndrome
  (May or may not respond to gluten free diet.)
  (1) Carcinoma and lymphoma within and without the gut
  (2) Lactose toxicity in infants
  (3) Diabetes mellitus
  (4) Sarcoidosis
  (5) Sjögren's syndrome
  (6) Infectious hepatitis
  (7) Ulcerative colitis
  (8) Regional enteritis
  (9) Postgastrectomy states
  (10) Pancreatic disease
  (11) Giardia lamblia
  (12) Ankylostoma duodenale
  (13) Strongyloidiasis
  (14) Coccidiosis
  (15) Widespread dermatitis
  (16) Acne rosacea
  (17) Kwashiorkor
  (18) Rigid dieting in obesity
  (19) Experimental malnutrition in animals
  (20) Excessive ingestion of cathartics
  (21) Accompanying oral contraceptive agents
  (22) Tropical sprue
  (23) Hypo- and agammaglobulinemias
  (24) IgA deficiency

---

* From Creamer: Gut, 7,569, 1966.

of specificity to this group of disorders (Table 28B-2).

Determination of the extent, severity, and type of nutritional deficiency seen in any and all of these disorders requires investigation by a wide variety of absorption tests and tests for specific nutrients, as described elsewhere in this text.

Diagnosis dependent upon roentgenogram is often non-specific. The introduction of the peroral biopsy techniques[2] made possible the prompt pathologic diagnosis of small bowel disease, and provided a morphologic basis for evaluation of therapy.[3-5]

Gluten-Sensitive Enteropathy. Gluten-sensitive enteropathy is also called primary

idiopathic steatorrhea, non-tropical sprue, and adult celiac disease.

Although the cause of celiac disease is unknown, dietary elimination of wheat, oats, barley and rye has been used with dramatic relief since Dicke[1] first reported the relationship of wheat products to celiac disease. Subsequently, it was shown that the offending agent in wheat is confined to the protein moiety, gluten.[2] Precipitation of gluten with

Table 28B-2. Diagnostic Usefulness of Peroral Biopsy of the Small Intestine*

Diagnosable Lesions
  Celiac sprue
  Acanthocytosis (A-beta-lipoproteinemia)
  Whipple's disease
  Lymphangiectasia

Controversial Areas
  Amyloidosis
  Carcinoma (small bowel)
  Cholera
  Cirrhosis
  Cystic fibrosis
  Diabetes mellitus
  Disaccharidase deficiency
  Diverticulosis
  Hepatitis and other viral illnesses
  Hypogammaglobulinemia
  Iron deficiency anemia
  Lymphoma
  Parasitic diseases
  Peptic ulcer
  Scleroderma
  Tropical sprue

Alleged Abnormalities
  Neomycin malabsorption
  Gastrectomy
  Regional enteritis
  Ulcerative colitis

Miscellaneous—no significant mucosal pathology within proximal jejunum
  Pancreatic insufficiency
  Pernicious anemia
  Chronic gastritis
  Chronic idiopathic diarrhea
  Severe malnutrition
  Folate deficiency
  Systemic mast cell disease

---

* From Rubin and Dobbins: Gastroenterology, 49, 676, 1965.

70 per cent alcohol yields an alcohol insoluble portion—glutenin which is nontoxic, and an alcohol soluble fraction—gliaden which is toxic to the sensitive individual. As little as 3 gm per day of this latter fraction, fed to celiac patients in remission, produces diarrhea and steatorrhea. Reported attempts to further fractionate this portion enzymatically, and to purify the toxic component chemically are still the subject of considerable debate. Kowlessar, Warren and Bronstein[3] recently summarized these reports as well as studies concerned with mucosal cell enzymic defect, histochemical findings and immunologic phenomena in celiac disease. They offered the following hypothesis: the enzymic defect in celiac patients is one in which N-pyrrolidone peptides derived from intraluminal digestion of wheat protein enter the mucosal epithelial cell but cannot be further degraded. Increased intracellular levels of N-pyrrolidone peptides interfere with metabolism in such a way as to transform normal columnar to stratified squamous cells. The damaged mucosal epithelium is rendered permeable to wheat glycopeptides and other soluble wheat and milk proteins, which may be antigenic. Participation of these proteins in antigen-antibody reactions might thus account for high antibody titers to food proteins in the sera of celiac patients.[4] Transmucosal passage of food antigens across a damaged small bowel mucosa has also been suggested[5] to account for high titers of antibodies to milk proteins and gluten fractions in the serum found in a patient with systemic mast cell disease studied in this laboratory.

In adult celiac disease there may be diffuse involvement of the entire intestinal mucosa with more severe involvement of the upper small bowel than of the more distal small bowel.[6,7] The diminution of absorptive area may result in impaired absorption of all nutrients, principally fat, although sugar, protein, vitamin and mineral malabsorption may be present in varying degrees.[8]

The average age of onset is 35 to 40 years.[9–13] Sometimes the history of diarrhea may date to childhood but frequently will not. The disease is characterized by exacerbations and remissions. Pregnancy, infection and other stresses may precede the onset of symp-toms initially or precipitate exacerbations.[8,9] The presenting symptoms in over 75 per cent of the cases are weight loss, malaise and weakness and diarrhea.[10–12,14,15] Stools characteristically are bulky, light in color and foul smelling. Occasionally, however, a patient will complain of constipation. Physical examination reveals evidence of weight loss and malnutrition. Some patients may exhibit pallor, peripheral edema, hyperpigmentation, bleeding tendencies, clubbing and hypotension.[16] It is not uncommon to find evidence of hypofunction of all the endocrine glands.

Roentgenograms of the small bowel show hypomotility, dilatation, coarsening of the mucosal folds, puddling, segmentation, and flocculation of the barium.[14,17–19] This non-specific pattern seen in malabsorption is due to a variety of causes and is described more fully in Chapter 18.

Peroral biopsy of the small intestinal mucosa has confirmed the early observations of Sakula and Shiner[20] and Rubin and co-workers.[21] They reported varying degrees of villus change, abnormalities of the epithelial cells and inflammatory infiltration of the lamina propria. These changes, no longer considered specific for celiac disease, have been seen in many disease states (Table 28B-1).[22]

Marked histologic improvement of mucosal specimens usually occurs within the first few weeks of therapy, but months to years may be needed for return to normal state. Improvement in clinical parameters of absorption precedes the histologic improvement.[2,6,23–26]

Fecal fat and xylose tests, almost always abnormal in the untreated patient, are helpful in assessing the improvement in bowel function. In general, improvement parallels strictness of adherence to the gluten-free diet.[27,28] Disaccharide intolerance, particularly lactose, is common in this disease and milk ingestion may contribute to diarrhea. Oral tolerance tests of lactose, sucrose and starch may be normal or they may give a flat blood sugar response. Disaccharidase levels in the small intestinal mucosa are usually low. Disaccharide hydrolysis and subsequent monosaccharide absorption are usually diminished.[29–33]

Fat malabsorption is often accompanied by

deficiency of fat-soluble vitamins. Fatty acids released by bacterial action can contribute to influx of fluid into the gut lumen. Pancreatic and biliary secretions may be normal in celiac disease, and thus lipolysis of dietary fat to triglycerides and free fatty acids may be normal.[8] Subsequent micelle formation takes place but these lipids and bile salts are lost in the stool.

Hypocalcemia and hypomagnesemia lead to tetany, paresthesias and bone fractures.[34-36] Serum alkaline phosphatase[37] may be elevated. Electrolyte deficiencies due to excessive loss of potassium and sodium into the stool may occur in severe diarrhea.

Since the greatest morphologic and absorptive defects occur in the proximal intestine, folate deficiency may occur.[40] Depending upon the degree of injury to the terminal ileum, vitamin B_{12} absorption may or may not be adequate. Macrocytic red blood cells, hypersegmented polymorphonuclear leukocytes and a megaloblastic bone marrow may result from deficiency of folic acid alone or from a combination of both deficiencies. In cases of severe disease it may be reasonably assumed that the water-soluble vitamins are inadequately absorbed.

When the diagnosis is made, gluten is withdrawn from the diet. The successful treatment of this disease depends heavily on the dietician's ability to teach the patient how to select foods free of gluten-containing products and the patient's willingness to abide by this diet (see Appendix, Table A-18). The diet should contain as many calories as the patient can tolerate. A 3000 to 3500 calorie diet is recommended, high in carbohydrate and protein if the patient is underweight. Initially, fat intake should be restricted to approximately 40 to 60 gm/day. Fat intake can be increased as bowel function improves. Milk and products containing lactose should be limited initially if lactose intolerance is suspected.

Potassium supplements may be given in oral liquid form and continued as long as necessary if potassium depletion exists.

Initially, folic acid or folinic acid, 5 mg/day, may be given parenterally. Oral folic acid (15 mg/day) will suffice in many instances. The distal bowel is less severely affected in this disease than the proximal. Since the distal bowel heals first, vitamin B_{12} deficiency may not be a continuing problem. If the Schilling test demonstrates deficient absorption, vitamin B_{12}, 100 μg per month, should be given parenterally. Folic acid should not be given without vitamin B_{12} unless one is certain of adequate vitamin B_{12} absorption for fear of inducing acute combined system disease. Some degree of iron deficiency usually exists.[8] Parenteral preparations may be given when oral preparations are not tolerated. Iron is absorbed primarily in the duodenum[38,39] where the low pH of gastric acid converts ferrous iron to the ferric state. The addition of ascorbic acid either in the form of food, e.g., orange juice, or in tablet form at the time of iron ingestion facilitates its absorption.

Water-soluble vitamins, ascorbic acid, 100 mg/day, and B complex, may be given freely. If the patient is unable to eat, initial intravenous fluid therapy should contain vitamin supplements. As the condition improves these vitamins can be given by the oral route, preferably in liquid form. Many multivitamin preparations contain added minerals also. The quantity present, however, is not sufficient for adequate mineral replacement in the celiac patient. Calcium, 8 to 12 gm per day orally, is often required, given in 3 to 4 divided daily doses. When there is evidence of bone fracture or bone pain, the dose may be increased to 20 gm/day. One gram, given as a solution of calcium gluconate, may be administered slowly intravenously when tetany supervenes. As noted in Chapter 6 Section B, magnesium depletion should be suspected when serum calcium is depressed in a malabsorptive state. This should be checked and the deficiency treated if present with intravenous or intramuscular magnesium sulfate (2 to 4 gm daily) until normal serum levels are achieved and maintained on a normal diet. Vitamin D, 50,000 i.u. per day orally, is usually adequate where there is evidence of a pathologic bone condition.[41] When continued vitamin D therapy is required, or larger dosages are deemed necessary, careful monitoring of serum calcium levels is essential.

The principal therapeutic goal is the establishment of an effective gluten-free diet. Nutritional management usually becomes less demanding once the gluten-free diet is achieved. Although a gluten-free diet is usually effective in children, 15 to 25 per cent of adults will not respond satisfactorily. When further evaluation fails to reveal other causes for the disorder, corticosteroid therapy may be used.[42-44] The usual dosage is 40 to 60 mg of prednisolone per day in divided oral doses.[45] Parenteral preparations may also be used. Less is known about the effectiveness of ACTH in this disease. Within the first week of therapy the patient should show increased appetite, decreased diarrhea, and improved sense of well-being. The usual risks of corticosteroid therapy obtain; adequate potassium, magnesium, calcium and vitamin D should be provided. Osteoporosis and osteomalacia already present may be enhanced. Infection, handled poorly by the deficient patient, may be masked by this therapy.

Diuretics should be used cautiously, if at all, for the hypoproteinemic edema. The edema is usually not severe and responds to diet as the body protein stores are replenished. Diuretics tend to augment the potassium deficit already present and can precipitate hypokalemia and its consequences.

Testosterone or estrogen therapy may be useful in some children whose growth is retarded. Anabolic steroids may lend temporary support to some patients.

Patients should be observed closely for infections or bone fractures and treated promptly. Specific treatment for the decreased function of the pituitary, adrenal and thyroid glands is usually not necessary as these functions improve as metabolic deficits are replenished.

Tropical Sprue. Tropical sprue is a chronic recurrent afebrile disease of uncertain cause(s), occurring most commonly in the tropical and subtropical area such as Puerto Rico, Cuba, Hong Kong and India.[1] It is manifested clinically by diarrhea, steatorrhea, malnutrition, and usually macrocytic anemia resulting from the malabsorption of folic acid and/or vitamin B_{12}. Bacteria, viruses,[4] and parasites[5] have been implicated, but to date isolation and identification of a single causative agent have not been successful. Findings that well-nourished individuals arriving in the tropics from a temperate climate may acquire the disease within days or weeks of arrival,[6,7] the occurrence of epidemics in India and Burma[8-10] and the response to broad-spectrum antibiotics provide circumstantial evidence of an infectious component in the etiology.

Dammin[11] and Bayless and associates[12] studied the viral and bacteriologic flora in patients with tropical sprue, but these were inconclusive. Nadel and Gardner[13] tended to rule out bacterial involvement since over half of the patients studied had sterile intestinal fluid. However, the sampling techniques used at that time may have been inadequate.

Protein deficiency is chronic in the tropics and parasitic infestations of the intestinal tract are common; both conditions may be associated with altered gut morphology.[14] It is apparent that the small bowel reflects the numerous factors acting on it, *i.e.*, nutritional deficiencies, parasites, bacteria, viruses, etc., which alter gut morphology and further influence the absorption of available nutrients. This leads to an interacting cycle which is variously manifested clinically. Klipstein and Baker[15] editorialized that the syndrome of non-tropical sprue primarily involved impaired absorptive function of the gastrointestinal tract. Vitamin and mineral deficiencies and megaloblastic anemia were considered secondary to the malabsorptive state. Ghitis and co-workers[16] suggested that protein-calorie malnutrition may lead also to malabsorption but these individuals can be differentiated from non-tropical sprue patients by relatively normal values of serum folate and vitamin B_{12}. This distinction is not clear-cut since other workers[17] noted considerable overlap between the two groups. Gorbach and associates,[17] in studies of the small bowel microflora, observed that bacterial overgrowth was a frequent finding in non-tropical sprue and far less frequent in protein-calorie malnutrition. They documented bacterial interference with absorption in 80 per cent of the sprue cases but not in malnourished individuals. An additional point of differentiation was offered by Banwell *et al.*[18] who demonstrated that fluid secretion from the small intestinal mucosa was the usual event in non-tropical sprue but rarely occurred in protein-calorie malnutrition. In this regard the small bowel in tropical sprue patients has secretory characteristics similar to those observed in other chronic diarrheal diseases such as non tropical sprue,[19] scleroderma[20] and in the acute infectious diarrhea associated with *Vibrio cholera*[21] and *E. coli.*[22]

Physical examination reveals varying degrees of malnutrition: pallor, weight loss, submucosal and subepidermal hemorrhages, cheilosis, glossitis, hyperpigmentation of pressure points, generalized loss of muscle tone, and occasionally signs of posterolateral column involvement of the nervous system.

Intestinal structure may be normal or show flattening of the villi, increase in the crypt:villus ratio, and varying degrees of inflammatory reaction within the lamina propria.[2,3] The small bowel mucosa may differ histologically from that of celiac disease primarily in severity of lesion and in location. In tropical sprue the lesion is usually milder, but the mucosa is more uniformly involved than that of celiac disease in which the proximal bowel is more severely damaged and frequently markedly atrophic.

In tropical sprue the villi are frequently "leaf" shaped. Some villi which appear normal under the dissecting microscope may be found under light microscopy to contain a dense inflammatory infiltrate in the lamina propria, and the epithelial cells may be abnormal. Klipstein *et al.* attempted to distinguish tropical sprue from celiac disease on the basis of the location and distribution of lipid droplets in basement membrane and lacteals.[23] Swanson *et al.*[24] showed that with folate and with vitamin B_{12} repletion the villus structure improved.

Laboratory studies may reveal a macrocytic anemia and megaloblastic bone marrow, reduction in serum proteins, calcium, magnesium, phosphorus and potassium.[25] Quantitative stool fat analysis frequently demonstrates steatorrhea of a mild degree. Xylose absorption is impaired.[23] Hypoacidity or anacidity following gastric analysis has been demonstrated in 50 per cent of the cases.[26] The absorption of vitamin B_{12} with intrinsic

factor is usually impaired.[27] Absorption of folic acid and tissue stores[27] are decreased.[28] Smears of buccal and gastric epithelial cells reveal changes similar to those seen in untreated pernicious anemia.[29]

Jeejeebhoy found lowered serum vitamin B_{12} levels in 30 per cent of sprue patients studied, lowered folate levels in 70 per cent, and combined vitamin B_{12} and folate deficiency in 20 per cent. These deficiencies may occur in the presence or absence of steatorrhea. In the majority of persons with tropical sprue B_{12} malabsorption results from ileal malabsorption.[30] However Herbert and associates[31] demonstrated a lack of receptors for intrinsic factor B_{12} complex in morphologically normal ileal tissue obtained from several Puerto Rican expatriates in New York City. In others, reduced secretion of intrinsic factor has also been implicated in the vitamin B_{12} deficiency seen in these patients.[32] Development of folate deficiency in persons with tropical sprue may be related to two separate physiologic abnormalities of folate absorption: malabsorption of folate monoglutamate which appears to be related to the severity of the mucosal abnormality[33–35] and malabsorption of folate polyglutamate which may occur in patients with normal absorption of folic acid.[35]

Hypoalbuminemia and edema occur in approximately 25 per cent of patients with tropical sprue[36,37] resulting from an inadequate dietary intake, impaired albumin synthesis in the liver[39] and excessive protein leakage into the gastrointestinal tract.[40]

Hypocalcemia, a frequent finding in tropical sprue, has been considered a consequence of malabsorption and deficiency of vitamin D.[41] More likely, hypocalcemia may be induced by magnesium depletion rather than being secondary to vitamin D deficiency.[42] The presence of steatorrhea depends primarily upon the severity of the mucosal lesion.[43] Disaccharidase activity may be diminished in proportion to the severity of the gut mucosal lesion.[44,45] Oral absorption tests of disaccharides, especially lactose, give flat responses. Sucrosuria has been reported as a persistent finding. Steatorrhea is present more often in patients with severe malabsorption of vitamin B_{12}, suggesting involvement of distal bowel or a more diffuse lesion than that seen in patients with malabsorption of folic acid and d-xylose alone.

Treatment. A nutritious diet consisting of 2400 to 3000 calories, 100 to 150 gm of protein and an adequate dietary supply of folate is the primary requisite. If steatorrhea is a problem then the amount of fat may be reduced to 50 to 60 gm/day initially. Ingestion of lactose-containing foods in the presence of a relative lactase deficiency may augment diarrhea. Such substances should be deleted from the diet until improvement has occurred following therapy.

Intravenous electrolyte and fluid replacement is necessary in extremely ill patients; however, oral supplements of potassium, calcium, and vitamin D usually suffice. Occasionally, there will be an indication for parenteral magnesium. Multivitamin supplements may be given.

Clinical remission has been reported when the tropical sprue patient is treated with oral sulfonamides or broad-spectrum antibiotics.[23,41,46-48] Tetracycline and oxytetracycline (1 gm per day) in divided doses are commonly prescribed. Hematologic remission and symptomatic improvement have occurred with folic acid and/or vitamin B_{12} alone, although Sheehy reported that vague gastrointestinal symptoms and steatorrhea persisted in 60 per cent of patients treated with vitamins alone.[49] Klipstein[23] reported folate repletion occurring in some patients treated with tetracycline alone, and noted further clinical and histologic improvement with the addition of folic acid. At the present time, many prefer to treat with all three.

Crystalline folic acid, 15 mg per day orally, and 100 mcg, I.M., of vitamin B_{12} at monthly intervals are the usual doses. These may be continued until the respective serum levels and all absorption parameters return to normal. Guerra *et al.*[46] advocate continuing therapy until patients are at least morphologically stabilized. They also reported effective long-term results following treatment with 300 to 500 mg of oxytetracycline for 6 months.

Whipple's Disease (Intestinal Lipodystrophy). This previously fatal, chronic disorder is characterized by episodic fever,

arthritis and polyserositis, diarrhea progressing to steatorrhea, marked weight loss, anemia, hyperpigmentation, lymphadenopathy and, occasionally, splenomegaly.

The usual laboratory tests give evidence of malabsorption of fat, xylose, and vitamin B_{12}.[1] Loss of fat-soluble vitamins and hypocalcemia, hypomagnesemia and hypokalemia may result from excessive steatorrhea and diarrhea. Serum proteins, particularly albumin[2] and hemoglobulin, may be diminished. Radiologic changes in the small bowel are compatible with a malabsorption pattern. Stools are intermittently positive for blood, the actual mechanism for which has not been elucidated. The diagnosis of Whipple's disease is made histologically by peroral biopsy of the intestinal mucosa.[3] Macrophages of the lamina propria of the small intestinal mucosa contain PAS-positive staining material. Light and electron microscopy has shown this material to consist of bacilli.[3-5] Other tissues, especially lymph nodes, may also be involved. Following treatment with antibiotics or steroids the bacilli disappear from the lamina propria and to a large extent from the macrophages, only to reappear with clinical relapses. The lacteals may be distended with fat globules which are present in the lamina propria also. This derangement returns towards normal following therapy.[3,4] Vitale *et al.*[6] produced gastrointestinal lesions in primates similar to those observed in humans with Whipple's disease.

Numerous attempts have been made to culture the rod-like organisms present in the lamina propria of the bowel and in the lymph nodes. In one study[7] more than 30 identifiable strains were obtained from 8 biopsies in the same patient. The interpretation of this and other studies is rendered difficult because of the problems of gut luminal contamination. Charache[8] circumvented the problem by studying blood and lymph nodes obtained aseptically. Initial isolation revealed atypical bacterial forms—pleomorphic and rod-like gram-negative organisms—that reverted to β hemolytic, Lancefield Group D enterococcus on repeated subcultures. High serum antibody titer against this organism, 1:128, but a low titer against a variety of other organisms, was noted. Drug sensitivity correlated with the clinical response to therapy. The relationship of this or other organisms isolated from the blood to the pathogenesis of Whipple's Disease is still to be ascertained. A 30 per cent incidence of endocarditis in these patients at autopsy complicates the interpretation of blood cultures since these may represent an extension of the primary offender or represent secondary bacterial invasion. It is not known if patients with Whipple's disease have impaired bacterial resistance or if only one or more than one organism produces the clinical syndrome.[9]

Diet and replacement therapy are the same as those employed for other malabsorptive states and are based upon nutritional deficits, on-going needs and the specific absorptive defects.

Antibiotic therapy may bring about dramatic improvement.[1,3-5,10,11] Ruffin et al.[10] used procaine penicillin and streptomycin for a 10- to 14-day period followed by long-term (10 to 12 months) broad-spectrum antibiotics, such as tetracycline, or oxytetracycline alone, with success. Serial peroral intestinal mucosal biopsies have shown the gradual disappearance of the PAS-positive staining material.[1,3-5,10,11] Therapy should be continued as long as this material is detectable. Clinical recovery may antedate the histologic reversion to normal by months to years. Relapse does occur and responds to the reintroduction of antibiotic therapy.[4]

Adrenocorticotrophin and adrenocorticosteroid therapy are also reported to reverse the course of the disease in some patients.[12] Reasons for this effect are obscure and Pirola et al.[13] suggested that the use of corticosteroids be restricted to the critically ill patient, unresponsive to antibiotics.

Malabsorption Due to Bacterial Contamination of the Gut (Including Small Intestinal Diverticulosis, Blind Loop Syndrome and Scleroderma). Anatomical derangements of the small bowel resulting in stasis or inadequate propulsion of the bolus with subsequent bacterial proliferation may lead to a malabsorption of fat and vitamin B_{12} deficiency. Among these conditions are the long afferent loop of duodenum following gastric surgery (blind loop), strictures or fistulization of the bowel and small bowel diverticulosis. Small duodenal diverticula commonly seen on roentgen examination have not been shown to cause significant disease. Occasionally, a single very large diverticulum may result in malabsorptive problems. Since bacterial overgrowth is common to these conditions, they will be considered together.

Symptoms associated with a blind loop syndrome or with small bowel diverticulosis vary from vague abdominal pains, particularly after meals, flatulence, colicky pain postprandially, weight loss, diarrhea, constipation, nausea and vomiting. Physical examination may be normal or show varying degrees of malnutrition and evidence of vitamin B_{12} deficiency.

Clinical studies by Doig and Girdwood[1] and experimental studies by Donaldson[2-4] show that the intraluminal bacteria compete with the host for vitamin B_{12}. A wide variety of enteric microorganisms, both gram-positive and gram-negative, aerobic and anaerobic which may or may not require exogenous vitamin B_{12} for growth can bind vitamin B_{12}.[5] Competitive binding and/or utilization by the bacterial flora explains the vitamin B_{12} deficit leading to the macrocytic anemia. Antibiotic therapy interrupts this process: the exact mechanism, be it suppression or alteration of the flora or alteration of the host defense, is not yet clear.[6]

While competitive uptake by the luminal flora may deprive the host of vitamin B_{12}, a less direct mechanism appears to be involved in steatorrhea associated with conditions of stasis. Dawson and Isselbacher[7] first suggested that bacterial hydrolysis of conjugated bile salts may play a role in the pathogenesis of steatorrhea in the blind loop syndrome.

Conjugated bile salts promote fat absorption by aiding the emulsion of the fat in the intestine, by activating pancreatic lipase, by incorporating the products of lipolysis into micelles,[8] and by stimulating re-esterification within the epithelial cells. Free or unconjugated bile salts are either inactive or inhibitory to these processes under in vitro conditions simulating those in the intestine. Although current evidence points to a deficiency of conjugated bile salts as the explanation for steatorrhea in the blind loop syndrome, the toxic or inhibitory effects of unconjugated bile salts may be contributory. Free bile salts resulting from bacterial hydrolysis do not participate in micelle formation, perhaps because the lowered pH of the bacterially contaminated lumen may render the bile salts relatively insoluble.[6] Furthermore, free bile acids, particularly deoxycholic acid, inhibit the intestinal esterification of fatty acids during absorption. Portman showed that the intestinal flora is able to hydrolyze conjugated bile salts and to convert cholic to deoxycholic acid.[9] Donaldson noted unconjugated dehydroxy bile acids in a patient with a blind loop and in experimental animals[10] as did Kim and associates.[11] Rosenberg et al. demonstrated in 2 patients with blind loop syndrome that the total concentration of bile salts was normal.[12] They concluded that bacterial degradation of conjugated bile salts resulted in a concentration of unconjugated bile salts which inhibited a variety of in vitro transport systems.

Dietary treatment consists of abundant calories (2500 to 3500) high in protein, reduced fat, and bulk, i.e., a bland diet. Frequent small feedings are recommended. If lactose intolerance is noted, milk products should be excluded. Medical treatment is adequate in many patients. Surgical removal may be accomplished when the diverticula are confined to a short segment of gut or when they are large and empty slowly radiographically or when perforation, ulceration or hemorrhage occurs.

Iron supplements may be necessary if the duodenum is involved. Parenteral replacement, 200 μg of vitamin B_{12}, should be given each month. Therapy with a broad-spectrum antibiotic such as tetracycline or chlortetracycline in divided doses has been used successfully.[13] Intermittent therapy is desirable to minimize development of resistant organisms or overgrowth by yeasts. It is not known whether folic acid therapy is necessary or whether it is synthesized in adequate amounts by the gut flora.[14,15] Serum determinations should be performed when deficiency is suspected.

Scleroderma may involve the entire gastrointestinal tract. Histologically, atrophy and fragmentation of the muscular coat of the gastrointestinal tract with increased deposition of collagen and a largely intact mucosa are characteristic of this lesion.[16,17] Marked impairment of motility and development of dilated, static segments further contribute to bowel malfunction. The chief absorptive defect appears to be that of fat; vitamin B_{12} and xylose absorption are not consistently impaired.[17,18]

Impaired motility and stagnation within the small bowel favor abundant bacterial growth in the proximal small intestine. Salen et al.[19] suggested that the malabsorption pattern resulting from this bacterial overgrowth is similar to that seen in blind loop or intestinal diverticula.

Oral treatment with broad-spectrum antibiotics has been effective clinically. Maintenance of nutrition is hampered by the relentless course of this disease. However, reduction of fat in the diet will reduce the amount of diarrhea when steatorrhea is a problem. The patient should receive parenteral vitamin B_{12} therapy, 100 μg/month, oral supplements of water-soluble vitamins and minerals. Corticosteroid therapy or vitamins alone have been ineffective. When an isolated segment of the bowel is involved, surgical resection of that portion of the gut may lead to prolonged improvement.[18]

Mastocytosis. The skin lesions of systemic mastocytosis appear initially, but the disease may ultimately progress to involve many other organs including the intestine. Bank and Marks[1] reported one patient with systemic mastocytosis and malabsorption of carbohydrates, fat and vitamin B_{12}. Partial villous atrophy, with a prominent eosinophilic infiltrate of the lamina propria, was noted on surgical small bowel biopsy. They called attention to the lack of mast cells. Rubin and Dobbins reported similar findings.[2] Malabsorptive defects in association with systemic mastocytosis were studied by Broitman and associates[3] in a 61-year-old woman. Malabsorption of carbohydrates, fat and vitamin B_{12} indicated involvement of the entire small bowel. Surgical small bowel biopsy disclosed abnormal numbers of mast cells beneath the muscularis; a rectal biopsy disclosed abnormal numbers of mast cells in the lamina propria and submucosa. Peroral small bowel biopsy showed intense mucosal and submucosal round cell infiltrates containing large numbers of eosinophils. High titers of antibodies to gluten (fraction III), alpha lactalbumin and beta lactoglobulin indicated transmucosal passage of incompletely degraded food antigens. Sensitivity to gluten was demonstrated by a favorable response to a gluten-free diet, and prompt exacerbation of steatorrhea and diarrhea following gluten challenge. This was considered to be secondary to mast cell invasion of the gastrointestinal tract rather than to primary adult celiac disease unmasked by systemic mastocytosis. On a daily fat intake of 100 gm incorporated into a gluten-containing diet, the attacks of facial flushing, abdominal pain, tachycardia and explosive diarrhea ceased. This occurred coincident with a decrease in serum magnesium; restoration of magnesium levels to normal was followed by a recurrence of attacks. It was speculated that hypomagnesemia may promote degranulation and/or prevent regranulation of mast cells in man.

Although the symptoms were similar to those observed in other patients with mastocytosis, urinary histamine levels were normal. Histidine loading did not enhance symptoms or increase histaminuria above that of control subjects.

PROTEIN-LOSING ENTEROPATHIES

The gastrointestinal tract plays a prominent role in the metabolism and homeostasis of plasma proteins in normal and in pathologic states. Intact gamma globulin is absorbed in newborn animals; the gut synthesizes serum proteins, including immunoglobulins and lipoproteins, and degrades the plasma proteins. Serum proteins are normally lost into the gastrointestinal tract where they are degraded rapidly into their constituent amino acids for reabsorption and resynthesis of protein. Hypoproteinemia, therefore, develops when the rate of loss by excretion and catabolism exceeds the rate of nitrogen reabsorption and serum protein resynthesis.

Thus, diseases manifesting protein-losing enteropathy have no single common etiology and pathogenesis. Regardless of cause, patients exhibit reduced circulating and total body pool of albumin, a normal or slightly increased rate of albumin synthesis and a markedly shortened albumin survival determined by testing with radioactive labeled substances.[1]

Excessive protein loss into the bowel may result from numerous causes: (1) obstructed outflow of the gastrointestinal lymphatics with consequent loss of lymph and protein into the gut lumen (lymphangiectasia, intestinal lipodystrophy, lymphoma, carcinoma, constrictive pericarditis); (2) exudation through an inflamed or ulcerated mucosa (regional enteritis, ulcerative colitis, celiac sprue); (3) excessive secretion of mucus (atrophic gastritis, Menetrier's disease—hypertrophic gastritis and gastrointestinal cancer), or (4) excessive loss in other disorders (nephrosis, defective gamma globulin synthesis and some of the amino acidurias).

Mineral losses, as iron,[2] copper,[3] calcium,[4] and lipid loss[5] may accompany gastrointestinal protein loss. The constant finding of lymphocytopenia in patients with lymphatic channel abnormalities is suggestive of the loss of lymphocytes via the gastrointestinal tract.[1]

Clinically, the patient with protein-losing enteropathy may present with only edema and hypoproteinemia. In some, gastrointestinal complaints or symptoms of hypocalcemic tetany may prevail. Others may exhibit growth retardation. Occasionally, iron deficiency anemia, lymphocytopenia, eosinophilia or amino acidurias may be noted as well. A recent comprehensive review of this subject is provided by Waldmann.[1]

"Allergic Gastroenteropathy." Six infants were described by Waldmann[6] and Bookstein[7] with rhinitis asthma, eczema, growth retardation, periorbital edema, anemia, hypoalbuminemia, hypogammaglobulinemia and eosinophilia. The patients had precipitating antibodies to milk and Charcot-Leyden crystals in their stools. They exhibited a normal to increased rate of albumin synthesis, but a shortened albumin survival and increased fecal excretion of protein. Absorption tests showed no steatorrhea and minimal xylose malabsorption. Roentgenograms showed mucosal evidence of edema in

5 of the 6 patients, only one of whom showed segmentation and puddling of barium.

Biopsies performed on 5 patients revealed increased infiltration of the lamina propria with some eosinophilia. Two were normal. Serum levels of albumin and IgA and IgG were reduced. Elimination of milk from the diet of 3 patients ameliorated their symptoms and the disordered protein metabolism. Reintroduction of milk caused recurrence of symptoms and increased the protein losses. Corticosteroid therapy in 3 other patients reversed the protein loss. Eosinophilia and response to steroids support the suggestion of an allergic or hyperimmune state.[8]

Hypogammaglobulinemia, with multiple granulomatous ulcers in the terminal ileum and cecum associated with an increased gastrointestinal protein loss, was described by Holman[9] in a patient with repeated infections. Intestinal resection ameliorated the intestinal protein loss, but gamma globulin concentration continued to decrease. Another report[10] indicates that in some patients IgA and IgM may be decreased more than IgG. Biopsies of the jejunal mucosa have shown considerable variability, ranging from normal,[11,12] nodular lymphoid hyperplasia with a normal intervening mucosa and villus architecture[10,11,13] to partial or total villus atrophy.[11,14] The malabsorptive defect in these patients does not appear to be due to a single cause. In some patients giardial infestation in association with hypogammaglobulinemia was observed.[10,15] Elimination of the parasite was accompanied by cessation of diarrhea and steatorrhea in some.[10,11] In the absence of detectable pathogens in the stool, antibiotic therapy has been unsuccessful in alleviating steatorrhea.[14] Patients with total atrophy of the jejunal mucosa have been treated with a gluten-free diet with variable results.[11,14] Corticosteroids may be of some benefit in the management of patients with localized granulomatous disease.[11] While the enteric loss of protein may be ameliorated, and albuminemia may be corrected with the various therapeutic regimens listed above, gamma globulin synthesis remains unaffected. Waldmann[1] states that the primary disorder in these patients is defective gamma globulin synthesis, leading secondarily to gastrointestinal tract lesions and consequent loss of serum proteins via the gastrointestinal tract.

Cardiomyopathies. Excessive enteric protein loss occurs in congestive heart failure, especially in constrictive pericarditis,[16,17] in familial cardiomyopathies and in association with valvular and septal defects. Hypoproteinemia and edema are the chief presenting findings. Diarrhea and steatorrhea occur occasionally. In addition to the serum albumin decrease, the gamma globulins are also lowered. The total body protein pool is reduced, albumin survival time markedly shortened, and fecal protein losses excessive. Xylose tolerance tests have been reported to be normal.[18] Microscopically, dilatation of the submucosal lacteals and lymphatics in the small bowel have been described in two cases.[18,19]

A functional disorder of the intestine secondary to an increase in the central venous pressure has been suggested as the mechanism of protein losses into the gut associated with congestive heart failure.[20] Increased thoracic duct pressure and flow rate have been demonstrated in patients with constrictive pericarditis.[18,21]

Treatment is aimed at the cause. In congestive heart failure the usual measures are employed: digitalis, diuretics and low salt diet. Recovery from hypoproteinemia with disappearance of lymphatic dilatation has been reported following pericardectomy.[18,20,22–24]

Intestinal Lymphangiectasia. This syndrome in children or young adults is characterized by generally mild gastrointestinal symptoms, but occasionally by severe diarrhea and steatorrhea, nausea, vomiting, and abdominal pain, asymmetric edema, chylous effusions, hypoalbuminemia, hypogammaglobulinemia and lymphocytopenia.[1,9,25–28] Waldmann showed a decreased serum half-life of albumin and stated that this was the result of gastrointestinal protein loss. Subsequent studies by Herskovic et al. showed that trapping of ^{131}I labeled albumin in the edematous extremities contributes to the reduced circulating albumin.[29] Malabsorption of nutrients other than fat is uncommon.[25] The diagnosis is made by the demonstration of increased albumin loss and by the morphologic changes observed in small bowel biopsy, consisting of markedly dilated and telangiec-tatic lacteals and lymphatics in the lamina propria of the mucosa, submucosa, or serosa.[25]

Treatment of this disease has been unsatis-factory. Steroids and antibiotics have been unsuccessful.[30] Satisfactory resection of a lesion confined to a short segment of bowel has been reported in two studies[1,26] but poor results in another.[1] Dietary fat restriction decreases the "load" on the lacteals and reduces intestinal lymph flow and pressure, thereby diminishing retrograde enteric "leak-age." This effect is further enhanced by substituting medium-chain triglycerides for part of the dietary fat.[30–32]

CARBOHYDRATE INTOLERANCE

Carbohydrate "intolerance" or "dyspep-sia" has been recognized for a number of years. Bloating, abdominal discomfort, nau-sea, vomiting and explosive acidic diarrhea occur following ingestion of the offending sugar.[1]

At least 50 per cent of man's daily caloric in-take is provided by carbohydrate. Dietary starch and glycogen are hydrolyzed by alpha-amylase in the intestinal lumen to maltose (glucose-galactose) and isomaltose (glucose-glucose). Sucrose (glucose-fructose) from cane or beet sugar and lactose (galactose-glucose), milk sugar, are the major free dietary disac-charides. Further hydrolysis of disaccharide to monosaccharides is mediated by enzymes located in the brush border membrane of the intestinal villus.[2] Human jejunal mucosa contains up to five maltases, one or two sucrases and an alpha-dextrinase (an iso-maltase). Of the two lactases described only one has the properties of a digestive enzyme. It is specific for lactose, has a pH of 6.0 optima and is missing in patients unable to tolerate lactose. The second β-galactosidase can utilize substrates in addition to lactose, persists at normal levels in lactose-intolerant individuals and may not play a significant role in lactose digestion.[3]

Intolerance may occur to disaccharide or monosaccharides. Monosaccharide intoler-ance, a rare condition, is manifested at birth and requires prompt diagnosis for infant survival.[4] It appears to result from an altera-tion of the transport mechanism for glucose and galactose. Treatment consists of elimina-tion of glucose and galactose and replace-ment with fructose and addition of amino acid hydrolysates for caloric value.[5–7]

More commonly, intolerance may occur to any of the four disaccharides, lactose, sucrose, maltose or isomaltose, either singly or in combination.[7] Disaccharide intolerance oc-curs in infants and adults as a primary, in-herited enzyme defect,[8–10] or as an acquired defect secondary to other diseases of the small intestine (see Table 28B-3). Com-bined disaccharidase deficiencies may occur in any disorder of the small bowel epithelium such as celiac-sprue,[11–13] giardiasis,[1] acute enteric infections,[14] cystic fibrosis[15] and kwashiorkor.[16,17]

Lactose ingestion most frequently causes clinical symptoms. According to Haemmerli and associates[11] this may be due to the lesser amount of lactase activity normally found per gram of mucosal tissue compared to other disaccharidases. Deficiency of lactase is the most frequently reported isolated enzyme deficiency.[18] Isolated sucrose and combined sucrose-isomaltose intolerances have been re-ported in infants and children.[19,20] Appar-ently these intolerances are lost with age since only an occasional case has been re-ported in adults.[10] We have found no re-ports of isolated maltase deficiency. Among the congenital forms of disaccharide intoler-ance in infants, however, lactose intolerance seems to be the most common. Clinically symptomatic intolerance to lactose is seen even more frequently in the adult. There-fore, it must be either an inherited enzyme deficiency with delayed manifestation or an acquired deficiency. Cuatrecasas et al.[21] sug-gested that prolonged abstinence from milk and milk products results in lowered en-zymatic activity. However, there is no evi-dence to date that such a deficiency, clinically symptomatic, can be induced in man. Star-vation causes an equal lowering of activity of all the disaccharidases and all are raised equally by refeeding glucose alone. Knudsen suggests that this response is due to the caloric effect.[22]

Adaptive changes in rat gut mucosal disaccharidase activity in response to disaccharide feeding have been studied by Deren and associates.[23,24] Despite increases in lactase activity on lactose feeding, absorption was unchanged.[23] Diminished activity of this enzyme following weaning occurs commonly in many animals[25] except man. Sunshine and Kretchmer[26] have demonstrated complete absence of this enzyme in the sea lion pup, which from birth requires no milk.

Lactase deficiency in the North American adult population is reported to vary from 16 to 55 per cent, with the higher incidence in Blacks.[27,28] The incidence in children between the ages of 11 months to 11 years with similar eating habits and socioeconomic status varies from 10 per cent in Caucasians to 35 per cent in Blacks.[29] The increasing frequency of lactose-induced symptoms in Black children with advancing age suggests a gradual decline in enzymatic activity. Cook and Kajubi[30] reported significant variances in the tribal incidences of lactase deficiency in Uganda despite apparently similar diets.

Frequently, gut lactase activity may be the only abnormally low disaccharidase in an otherwise normal adult. While Scandinavians and West Europeans show the lowest incidence (2 to 8 per cent are lactose intolerant), Greek Cypriots, Arabs, and Ashkenazic Jews have an incidence of lactose intolerance of 60 to 80 per cent. Approximately 70 per cent of American Negroes and greater than 90 per cent of African Bantus, Japanese, Thais, Formosans and Filipinos are intolerant to lactose.[31,32] In general, the majority of adults the world over exhibit low gut lactase activity implying that low gut lactase may indeed be the "normal" situation. Recently, the variations in gut lactase activity in different populations has been the subject of anthropological studies.[33] The question posed by these findings is whether the inherited tendency of low gut lactase activity is the result of inadequate consumption of milk over many generations or whether inadequate consumption of milk was *due* to low gut lactase in these populations.

Lactose intolerance following gastric operaiton for peptic ulcer disease[11,34] has been attributed to pre-existing lowered lactase activity made symptomatic by the altered in-testinal anatomy and physiology.[10] Milk allergy, rapid delivery of a hyperosmotic load to the upper small bowel and inadequate lactose hydrolysis[35] may be contributing factors.

Intolerance to lactose and hypolactasia have also been reported in "irritable bowel syndrome,"[36] dermatitides,[37] ulcerative colitis,[38] and regional ileitis.[39]

When disaccharides are not hydrolyzed and absorbed, they remain within the gut lumen where they exert a hyperosmolar effect. As large volumes of water are drawn into the gut lumen distension and discomfort develop. The flora of the lower small bowel and colon metabolizes the sugar, forming lactic, butyric, and other irritant volatile acids causing cramps and diarrhea.[1]

Following ingestion of 100 gm of lactose, the normal individual shows a rise of at least 20 mg per cent glucose in serum.[40] In the presence of lactase deficiency, however, the blood glucose curve is "flat" and the patient develops clinical symptoms. If the patient is given equimolar amounts of glucose and galactose, however, the expected rise of at least 20 mg occurs. The stool of the lactase-deficient patient contains large amounts of lactic acid. The pH of the stool may not fall below 6 in the adult, but in children it may go as low as 4.5 in a matter of 1 to 2 hours. Peroral biopsy of the small intestine is usually normal; however, a flat mucosa on biopsy has been reported by Burke et al. in intolerant infants fed lactose[41] which reverted to normal on withdrawal of the sugar. In this instance lactose appeared to be toxic to the mucosa in a manner similar to gluten in celiac disease. Kern and associates reported steatorrhea in association with lactose intolerance in a woman.[42] A similar finding was noted by Welch in a small percentage of 100 patients with isolated lactase deficiency.[43] Assay of the small bowel mucosa for enzymatic activity by the method of Dahlqvist[44] in intolerant individuals revealed low or absent values for lactase and normal activity for the other disaccharidases. Welch suggested that the best single method of defining this group was on the basis of an increase in the sucrase: lactose ratio.[43]

Treatment in the infant is simple once the

Table 28B-3.   Classification of Disaccharide Intolerance.*

1. Lactose Intolerance
   a. Congenital physiological lactase deficiency in premature infants
   b. Congential lactase deficiency, presumably genetically determined (1) Some cases associated with lactosuria (? related to 1.-d-[2])
   c. Acquired lactase deficiency in children and adults, probably genetically determined
   d. Acquired: part of generalized disaccharidase deficiency and secondary to diffuse mucosal damage resulting from:
      (1) Celiac disease, tropical sprue, Whipple's disease, intestinal lymphangiectasia, etc.
      (2) Acute gastroenteritis (especially in infants)
      (3) Kwashiorkor
      (4) Administration of neomycin or PAS
      (5) Giardia lamblia infestation (presumed mucosal damage)
      (6) Post-bowel surgery in infants (presumed mucosal damage)
   e. Acquired: secondary to alteration in intestinal transit resulting from:
      (1) Small bowel resection (may decrease lactase level also)
      (2) Postgastrectomy or pyloroplasty (may unmask a pre-existing deficiency)
      (3) Lactose intolerance without lactase deficiency
   f. Suggested disease associations
      (1) Cystic fibrosis
      (2) Osteoporosis

2. Sucrose Intolerance.
   a. Congenital sucrase-isomaltase deficiencies: rare, genetically determined (63 cases as of 1965)
   b. Seemingly acquired sucrose intolerance, sucrase-isomaltase deficiency in adults, presumably also genetically determined and similar to the congenital deficiencies
   c. Acquired: secondary to diffuse mucosal damage

3. Glucose-Galactose Malabsorption
   a. Congenital, inherited inability to absorb these monosaccharides
   b. Acquired: secondary to diffuse mucosal damage in infants

* From Bayless and Christopher: Amer. J. Clin. Nutr. 22, 181, 1969.

offending sugar is identified. Numerous formula preparations contain sucrose and dextrins which can easily be substituted for lactose-containing preparations without losing calories. In sucrose-isomaltose malabsorption lactose is substituted. The older child or adult with sucrose-isomaltose intolerance requires thorough dietary education and diligent management. In the lactose-intolerant adult, elimination of lactose-containing foods results in prompt relief; for those who have had symptoms for many years without correct diagnosis this relief may be gratifying indeed.

METABOLIC DISORDERS

Diabetes. "Diabetic diarrhea" in some patients is associated with peripheral or autonomic neuropathy.[1,2] Steatorrhea, when present, is variable.

Abetalipoproteinemia (Acanthocytosis). A syndrome of severe hypolipidemia, progressive neuromuscular ataxia, atypical retinitis pigmentosa, and acanthocytosis in which there is a hereditary absence or deficiency of β-lipoprotein was described.[1-3] Steatorrhea was usually present and serum cholesterol, carotene and vitamin A were markedly reduced. Monosaccharide absorption was normal; however, lactose absorption and lactase activity within the intestinal mucosa were decreased as reported by Isselbacher. Peroral biopsy of the jejunal mucosa revealed large amounts of intraepithelial fat globules.[2]

During the process of fat absorption reesterification of triglycerides occurs within the mucosal epithelium (see Chapter 4). Triglycerides are then incorporated along with β-lipoprotein into the chylomicron. Isselbacher[4] suggested that this latter step may limit the rate of lipid movement across the mucosa into the lymphatic system. The impairment of protein synthesis by agents such as puromycin, acetoxycycloheximide, or ethionine reduced the absorption of long-chain fatty acids.[5,6] Consequently, in experimental animals so treated and given an oral load of fat, plasma triglycerides did not reach a normal elevation. Further, plasma β-lipoproteins decreased while α-lipoproteins were unaffected. Morphologically, the intestinal mucosal epithelium was engorged with triglyceride droplets.[5] The close parallel between these findings and those in congenital β-lipoprotein deficiency implicates defective β-lipoprotein synthesis in chylomicron formation.[2,7] Normally about 75 per cent of the total circulating lipid consists of β-lipoprotein.[8] Van Buchem and associates[9] suggested that in abetalipoproteinemia steatorrhea developed when the accumulation of intracellular fat reached a threshold value.

A convenient screening test for this disease, based upon autohemolysis of acanthocytic red blood cells, appears to be useful in assessing therapy.[10,11]

Isselbacher and associates[2] demonstrated weight gain and reduction in steatorrhea in patients following replacement of dietary fat with 30 to 45 gm of medium-chain triglycerides.

Amino Acid Anomalies. Steatorrhea is sometimes associated with congenital abnormalities of active transport of amino acids, initially described in the renal tubule and subsequently shown in the small bowel.[1]

PARASITIC INFESTATION

Diarrhea is a frequent symptom of parasitic infestation of the intestine. Absorptive defects for one or more nutrients may accompany excessive fluid and electrolyte loss. Knowledge of the life cycle of the parasite in the human host is a prerequisite for understanding the several mechanisms of malabsorption: (1) *competition with the host* for a particular nutrient, *e.g. Diphyllobothrium latum*,[1] the fish tapeworm, which consumes vitamin B_{12} within the gut lumen and deprives the host of this vitamin. (2) *Invasion of the gut mucosa, e.g. Strongyloides stercoralis*[2-4] attaches to the mucosa of the duodenum and

upper jejunum where it reduplicates. Mucosal disruption and inflammation may prevent optimal absorption.[2,5] In hookworm infestation the worm *Necator americanus* attaches to the tips of the intestinal villi, deriving nutrients from the host.[2] The resultant bleeding causes microcytic, hypochromic anemia which responds promptly to iron.[6] (3) *Interference with absorption* can be caused by large numbers of organisms such as *Giardia lamblia*.[7,8] Although there is some controversy as to the invasiveness of *Giardia*, mechanical interference with absorption by enormous numbers of parasites appears to be a factor. The parasite may also competitively deprive the host of nutrients and provoke inflammatory reaction in some individuals which accentuates absorptive defects.[7] Symptomatic infestation occurs most frequently in undernourished individuals and in those with impaired immune mechanisms. Some patients with symptomatic giardiasis have reduced immunoglobulin levels.[7,9]

Treatment of parasitic infections has been reviewed by Marsden, *et al*.[10,11] Diets high in calories, carbohydrates and protein and low in fats are used in patients with steatorrhea. Specific or multiple vitamin supplements are given as indicated. Iron preparations are given for iron deficiency anemia. During acute diarrhea, oral feedings may be withheld completely or clear liquids may be given.

ACUTE INFECTIOUS DIARRHEAS

An adequate discussion of this problem within the limited confines of this chapter is not possible. The reader is referred to extensive treatises on this subject, both general and specific.[1-3] Nutritional status influences susceptibility to, and the consequences of, bacterial infections.

Acute infectious diarrheas include, among others, salmonellosis, shigellosis, typhoid and paratyphoid fever, cholera, infantile diarrhea, *E. coli* diarrhea in adults, viral gastroenteritis, staphylococcal "food poisoning," and "traveler's diarrhea." In their more fulminant form these conditions are characterized by explosive diarrhea with immediate loss of fluid and electrolytes. Usually, however, they are self-limiting.

In general, therapy of infectious diarrheas is aimed at maintaining nutritional, fluid, and electrolyte balance while eliminating the causative microorganism. Eisenberg, Palazzola and Flippin[4] reported that as many as 74 per cent of adults with salmonellosis or shigellosis are afflicted with another or "primary" illness. Therapy, then, must be directed toward the primary illness as well as to the bacterial infection. Lindenbaum et al. showed evidence of malabsorption during and after recovery from acute intestinal infection in patients with acute enteritis, including cholera.[5,6] In infants with infectious enteritis Torres-Pinedo and associates[7] indicated that the volume and composition of diarrheal stools were partially determined by defective intestinal absorption of sugars. Following oral administration of glucose, fructose, lactose or sucrose, stool acidity markedly increased owing to an increase in organic acids. Presumably the latter was the result of bacterial fermentation. Additionally the accumulation of organic ions in the colon resulted in a cation-entrapment effect leading to increased losses of cations in the diarrheic stool.

Salmonellosis and Shigellosis. Salmonellosis, a major public health problem, is probably the most common cause of infectious gastroenteritis in the United States. During 1964, over 21,000 laboratory-confirmed human infections were reported.[1] Undoubtedly this represents but a small percentage of the total number of cases. In spite of its usual benign course in most adults, there may be serious manifestations such as peritonitis, endocarditis, pneumonia, osteomyelitis, urinary tract infection and meningitis.[2-4] The incidence of infection and the fatality rate with food salmonellae are highest in infancy and decline with age.[5] The prime vehicle of Salmonella transmission is food prepared from infected animals or contaminated during preparation. Virtually all types of food may comprise sources, especially those lightly cooked and subject to repeated handling.[6]

The acute gastroenteritis of salmonellosis may vary in severity from a mild infection to a serious systemic illness. Duration and severity of the diarrhea appear in some cases to be related to the acid secretory status of the host. Patients with salmonellosis and impaired gastric acid secretion exhibited a "cholera-like" diarrhea as compared to patients with normal gastric acid secretion who had mild diarrhea.[7,8] Salmonellae invade the small bowel mucosa, gain access to the general circulation via the small intestinal lymphatics and may ultimately favor sites such as joint spaces, kidney, and bone marrow. Small bowel mucosal changes may vary from minimal inflammation, and petechial hemorrhage, to frank ulceration and necrosis. These changes generally are most pronounced in the terminal ileum. Shigellosis is localized to the gut, occasionally involving the terminal ileum but mainly affecting the colon, with lesions ranging from congestion and erythema to extravasation of blood and pus, and occasionally ulceration and perforation. Chronic ulcerative colitis was considered to be a consequence of unusually severe shigellosis in approximately 15 per cent of cases by Felsen,[9] although the data were not conclusive.

Cholera. Cholera, caused by the *Vibrio cholerae*, exemplifies a fulminant form of infectious diarrhea prevalent in malnourished populations. The major symptom is profuse watery "rice water" diarrhea—isotonic with plasma. In the untreated case, vomiting and skeletal muscle cramping are early manifestations probably secondary to marked electrolyte imbalance. The patient is afebrile and the disease has an average duration of 4.2 days.[1] The mortality rate is as high as 60 to 80 per cent[1,2] in untreated cases. Adequate treatment reduces the mortality rate to essentially zero.[1]

The relationship of malnutrition to cholera is not clear. Unquestionably the highest incidence is found among the poor living under primitive conditions. There appears to be a selective affinity for individual members in a family,[3] more frequently the young. Cruickshank has suggested that malnutrition may similarly affect the course of cholera.[3] Rosenberg, however, found no evidence of specific vitamin deficiencies.[4]

Fluid loss during the 3 to 6 day illness may exceed 30 liters. The average electrolyte composition of the stool in severe adult cholera is as follows in mEq/L: Na^+ 140; K^+ 10; Cl^- 110; and HCO_3^- 40. Severe dehydration is evidenced by plasma protein concentrations as high as 14 gm/100 ml. Diarrhea appears to be related to the production of an enterotoxin by *V. cholerae* which increases small bowel intracellular cyclic AMP—stimulated directly by enterotoxin or via adenyl cyclase.[5-7] Associated with increased cyclic AMP is a reversal of chloride transport resulting in the net secretion of chloride. Sodium flux is also reduced to zero but the net absorptive flux of sodium can be increased again by the addition of an actively transported sugar or amino acid. Realization of these phenomena have provided a major adjunct to the therapy of acute cholera.[7] Glucose (56 mM) along with bicarbonate, potassium, sodium and chloride (in concentrations equal to those found in the stool), administered orally, stimulates absorption of intestinal fluid and results in a prompt decrease in the volume of stools.

In severe cases, however, vomiting and other symptoms resembling the "dumping syndrome" occur when fluids are given orally. In such cases, fluid replacement must be administered intravenously.

Phillips' method of treating cholera is well suited for use in epidemics and may be applied by unskilled technicians in uncomplicated cases.[9] It relies on measurement of plasma specific gravity by copper sulfate method.[10] Four ml of fluid replacement per kg body weight are given for each increase of 0.001 plasma specific gravity above normal (1.025). Children and infants require relatively more fluid replacement.

The standard intravenous fluid regimen consists of two parts isotonic saline to 1 part isotonic sodium lactate or bicarbonate.[8] After determining the state of hydration by determination of plasma specific gravity, rapid rehydration is accomplished by administering 100 ml/minute and infusions are continued thereafter at a rate equal to the measured gastrointestinal fluid losses.

Tetracycline, 1 gm/day in divided doses, halves the duration of the disease and decreases the fluid requirements.[1]

Traveler's diarrhea is usually far less severe than the acute bacterial diarrheas. Despite numerous studies to date, no satisfactory explanation has occurred for the transient diarrhea associated with movement about the surface of the earth. That it exists cannot be doubted; fortunately it is usually self-limiting and responds to simple preventive or therapeutic aids.

CHRONIC INFLAMMATORY BOWEL DISEASE

Granulomatous Inflammatory Diseases—Regional Enteritis, Granulomatous Ileocolitis, and Granulomatous Colitis. Regional enteritis is an inflammatory disease of unknown etiology usually affecting the terminal ileum, but occasionally extending throughout the small intestine.[1] Acute and/or chronic inflammation of the lamina propria with granuloma formation accompanies obstruction of the lymphatics. Regional enteritis occurs less frequently than ulcerative colitis, but the two diseases have certain similarities.[2,3] Like ulcerative colitis, it occurs most frequently in young adults, usually presenting between ages 16 and 30. It appears to be more common in patients of Jewish origin and it is relatively uncommon among Negroes.[4]

Regional enteritis is characterized by bouts of abdominal pain, fever and diarrhea. Weight loss, anorexia, anemia and steatorrhea may be present in the chronic state. Rectal bleeding is usually less prominent than in ulcerative colitis. Physical examination frequently reveals wasting and a right lower quadrant tender mass.

Complications may consist of internal and external fistulization, scarring with obstruction, perforation with abscess formation and hemorrhage. Abscesses, uveitis, iritis, arthritis, selective or diffuse malabsorption, osteoporosis and liver disease may accompany regional enteritis as well as ulcerative colitis.[5] Systemic amyloidosis is a rare complication[6] and development of carcinoma at the site of involvement has been reported in only a few instances.[7-10]

The nutritional deficit depends upon the extent, severity, and location of the diseased bowel. Because of the frequency of involvement of the terminal ileum, vitamin B_{12} uptake and bile salt reabsorption may be impaired and steatorrhea and macrocytic anemia may occur. Fistulization may take place with formation of a "blind loop" in which excessive bacterial proliferation occurs. Anemia may be enhanced by decreased iron intake, malabsorption of iron and chronic blood loss into the gut. Hypoproteinemia and edema result from inadequate dietary intake of protein, increased tissue catabolism, increased enteric protein loss, and malabsorption of amino acids. The net absorption of water and sodium may be diminished in the affected bowel.[11] Electrolyte losses, dehydration, folic acid deficiency, and mineral and fat-soluble vitamin losses parallel the severity of steatorrhea.

Maintenance of nutrition, allaying diarrhea, restoration of blood and fluid loss and control of infection are the aims of therapy.[12] Zetzel[3] recommended a high-calorie, high-protein, low-residue, low-fat, non-irritating diet with elimination of milk and milk products particularly if there is any suggestion of milk intolerance. High residue foods can cause obstruction in a narrowed ileum and must be avoided; one of Brown's patients had four episodes of obstruction, all precipitated by corn and all relieved by medical treatment.[13] In the case of bacterial overgrowth from fistulization and stasis in patients unable to undergo further surgery, *treatment* is similar to that outlined for blind loop syndrome and includes intermittent antibiotic therapy, parenteral replacement of vitamin B_{12}, supplemental vitamin and mineral therapy, and reduction of dietary fat.

Medications include replenishment of vitamins, especially the vitamin B group, vitamin K, and folic acid, and calcium, magnesium, iron and potassium. Sedatives, tranquilizers, antispasmodic-anticholinergic drugs, salicylazosulfapyridine (Azulfidine), and, when needed, broad-spectrum antibiotics. Adrenocorticotropic hormone and adrenocorticosteroids have been used in acute as well as long-term management with some success. Sparberg and Kirsner reported apparent beneficial suppression of symptoms in 217 cases treated on a long-term basis with 30 mg or more daily of prednisone or pred-

nisolone.[14] Perforation, abscess and sepsis, however, may be sequelae to such therapy and may further complicate management.

Patients with granulomatous disease may require surgical resection for palliation and control of obstruction, perforation and fistulization, and, rarely, cancer.

Granulomatous Colitis. In recent years, largely due to the combined efforts of English and American workers, granulomatous colitis has been recognized as a separate entity, clinically and pathologically, from non-specific ulcerative colitis.[15–21] With regional ileitis, it shares a tendency to form palpable masses, fistulae and strictures and obstructions. It less commonly involves the rectum, differing thereby from non-specific ulcerative colitis. In contrast to non-specific ulcerative colitis, malignancy is rare, toxic megacolon has not been reported and bleeding and chronic anemia are less frequent. The clinical course, not surprisingly, resembles that of severe regional ileitis. Two types of clinical course have been recognized. In one, the disease is low-grade and indolent and obstructive symptoms are often the indication for surgery and patients generally do well after operation. In another form, the clinical course is more severe, resembling severe regional ileitis and sharing its complications and surgical consequences.

The nutritional manifestations and treatment are similar to those described above.

With regard to the use of sulfonamides and corticosteroids Zetzel[22] commented that although these are less effective in patients with granulomatous disease of the bowel than in those with ulcerative colitis, they afford sufficient benefit during the initial medical treatment to warrant their usage—unless of course, their use is contraindicated by complications.

Ulcerative Colitis. Non-specific idiopathic ulcerative colitis is an acute and chronic febrile inflammatory and ulcerative disease of the colon and rectum[1] of unknown etiology. It is characterized by exacerbations and remissions and occasionally spontaneous recovery. Symptoms consist of abdominal pain, diarrhea, rectal bleeding, weight loss, and debilitation. There is an increased incidence of allergic manifestations, *e.g.*, asthma, hay fever and drug sensitivity. An allergic basis for the disease is further suggested by relief of symptoms after the elimination of certain foods, such as milk, wheat, eggs and tomatoes in some patients and exacerbations during the "pollen season" in others.

The concurrence of ulcerative colitis with (1) conditions associated with hypersensitivity states such as purpura, erythema nodosum, uveitis and arthritis, (2) the frequency of drug reactions, (3) the occasional elevation of serum alpha and gamma globulin, and (4) the favorable response to corticotropin and corticosteroid therapy lends support to the hypothesis that ulcerative colitis has as an immunologic basis the so-called delayed allergy or tuberculin type of hypersensitivity. It is associated with a number of other diseases including pyoderma gangrenosa, cirrhosis, nephrolithiasis, infections, osteoporosis and colonic carcinoma.[1-5]

Malnutrition is common because of increased tissue catabolism, decreased food intake, and excessive losses of nutrients, fluid and electrolytes. During exacerbations, loss of blood and plasma proteins occurs. Severe diarrhea leads to varying degrees of dehydration and losses of sodium, potassium and chloride. Steatorrhea and its sequelae (see above) may occur when the terminal ileum is involved. Anemia due to iron deficiency is frequent.

Non-specific jejunitis and jejunal villous atrophy have been reported by Salem and Truelove.[6] Flat curves following oral lactose tolerance tests and reduction in small bowel mucosal disaccharidase activity have been reported. After carbohydrate feeding, increased lactic acid and fatty acids occur in the stool.[7] (See Carbohydrate Intolerance.)

Nutritional management of ulcerative colitis is primarily supportive, symptomatic and non-specific. Elimination diets are employed widely, but despite occasional dramatic responses there is no controlled evidence that they are actually beneficial. The frequent failure of a specific food allergy regimen is attributed by some to structural bowel changes complicated by secondary infection. The "low residue" or "bland" diet is universally prescribed, but Kramer has pointed out the wide variation in these regimens.[8]

Kirsner[9] and Zetzel[10,11] have advocated the use of a diet devoid of the physical and chemical irritants contained in fruits, vegetables, fruit juices, condiments, alcoholic beverages, and excessively hot or cold foods. In the acutely ill patient Kirsner has recommended a limited diet consisting of toast, butter, soft boiled eggs, clear broth, tea, rice, jello, cream of wheat and custards. A diet containing meat and potatoes but without fruits and vegetables is used initially. Cooked vegetables and canned fruits may then be added when stools are consistently formed and free of blood.[9] Diet may be further liberalized as the patient improves.

Milk "allergy" has long been considered a factor in ulcerative colitis.[12,13] Hemagglutinins to the constituent milk proteins (lactalbumen) have been found in the serum of patients with ulcerative colitis by Taylor and Truelove,[14] but their origin and significance have not been satisfactorily explained. These same authors have observed that both the relapse rate and appearance of serial rectal biopsies were better while patients were on milk-free diet than when they were fed gluten-free and milk-free, or normal control diets. The histologic findings closely paralleled the clinical states. After maintenance on a milk-free diet many patients found that diarrhea ceased and that fruits and vegetables, which had previously been avoided, could again be eaten without symptoms. This response was noted particularly with the first attack of ulcerative colitis. Lactose has been suggested as the substance harmful in milk.[7] Lactase deficiency occurs more frequently in patients with ulcerative colitis than in the general population.[15]

Unreasonable restriction of diets can impose needless psychologic burdens on the patient. Success in overcoming the patient's disinterest in food requires patience on the part of the dietitian and of the physician to select attractive nutritious meals. Frequent small feedings are generally better tolerated than three regular ones. Not only is the patient less likely to consume as many calories when fed less frequently, but ingestion of larger volumes may stimulate bowel evacuation.

An intake of at least 2400 to 3600 calories

containing at least 125 to 150 mg of protein may be needed to restore positive nitrogen balance. Protein supplements in the form of prepared formulas may be added to the diet; however, good quality foods are preferred.

In patients with steatorrhea, restriction of dietary fat may be necessary to prevent further loss of nutrients and minerals. Reduction in the total pool of circulating bile salts may be one factor contributing to the steatorrhea. Substitution of a portion of the dietary fat with medium-chain triglycerides may be useful in the absence of adequate bile salts.[16] Kirsner[9] has emphasized that complete nutritional restoration may require at least 3 months or longer in the patient who has been acutely ill for a period of time.

Oral replacement of iron may cause gastrointestinal disturbances even when taken with meals and in such instances iron may be given by the parenteral route. If there is evidence of vitamin B_{12} malabsorption, then parenteral replacement in the amount of 100 to 200 μg per month should be given.

Potassium supplements are required only in exacerbations when excessive loss occurs. Anabolic steroid agents such as testosterone propionate have been prescribed to increase retention of nitrogen in tissue.

The goal is control rather than cure. Bed rest, sedation, tranquilizers, anticholinergics, anti-diarrheal agents and occasionally short term narcotics are used for control of symptoms.[9,10,17] Hospitalization frequently is necessary during acute exacerbations in order to remove the patient from stress in his environment, either known or unrecognized. As in any chronic disease state, tranquilizing drugs and particularly anti-depressive preparations may be effective in alleviating depression and anxiety. Antispasmodic and anticholinergic medications such as tincture of belladonna help suppress the gastrocolic reflex and sphincter spasm. Anti-diarrheal agents, e.g., Lomotil and paregoric, are useful in reducing bowel activity. Abdominal pain and tenesmus occasionally necessitate opiates but these should be avoided except for short-term usage since they may mask perforations and lead to addiction.

Antibiotic agents should be used in presence of fever, evidence of sepsis, etc. Long-term

therapy with sulfonamide preparations has been found to be particularly beneficial. The most commonly used preparation in the United States is salicylazosulfapyridine (Azulfidine).

While not curative, ACTH and corticosteroid therapy have decreased morbidity and mortality.[18] The efficacy of short-term treatment with corticosteroid therapy as opposed to long-term therapy has been amply borne out by Truelove and Witts.[19] In a well-controlled "double-blind" study, cortisone (25 mg BID) did not decrease the relapse rate. During the initial acute attack the results of treatment with cortisone, 50 mg QID P.O., or ACTH, 80 U/day IM, were essentially the same. In subsequent acute exacerbations, however, ACTH was superior to cortisone in bringing about complete clinical remission in the course of 6 weeks' treatment. The chance of subsequent relapse was greater following ACTH therapy, as was the risk of complications, thereby somewhat offsetting the beneficial results. It would seem that ACTH should be held in reserve. An occasional patient will necessitate long-term therapy. Prednisone, 10 to 15 mg/P.O., is most frequently used. Hydrocortisone enemas have been employed with success not only during an acute episode, but also on a long-term basis. Corticosteroid therapy is not without risk. When used for prolonged periods, calcium depletion with osteoporosis and ready fractures must be watched for. Perforations of diseased bowel may be masked.

In acute fulminant ulcerative colitis general supportive measures may prove inadequate and operation is required in order to control hemorrhage. Excessive fecal water potassium and sodium losses lead to hypotension, prostration, renal impairment and oliguria, muscle flaccidity and cardiac arrhythmias.

"Toxic dilatation" of the colon is a state of rapid deterioration manifested by high fever, anorexia, nausea, vomiting, and increasing prostration accompanied by colonic distention and tenderness. The diarrhea may decrease and bowel sounds cease. The transverse colon radiographically shows progressive distention. Perforation and sepsis may supervene. The exact mechanism is not known. The *treatment* recommended is cessation of all oral feeding, continuous gastric aspiration, restoration of blood, plasma, fluids and electrolytes, and parenteral antibiotics. A continuous intravenous drip of ACTH is recommended. If the patient does not show prompt response, surgery may be warranted.

The incidence of colonic carcinoma has been reported to be increased up to 20 times in ulcerative colitis. The appearance of cancer parallels the duration of the disease rather than its severity.[5]

Based on the hypothesis that ulcerative colitis is an "autoimmune" disease, a few preliminary reports suggested that the use of immunosuppressants such as azathioprine may be beneficial.[20] The efficacy of this therapy awaits further investigation. In the interim, Kraft and Kirsner[21] cautioned on the indiscriminate use of immunosuppressive treatment in inflammatory bowel disease. They emphasized the hazards of suppressing host defenses in patients who are vulnerable to many local and systemic risks including infection and the possibility of development of primary neoplasms as lymphoma and reticulum cell sarcoma as noted in a small number of individuals given azathioprine therapy along with renal transplants. Additionally immunosuppressive drugs may enhance oncogenic viruses, alter host immunological homeostasis, repressing immunological mechanisms for the normal surveillance and rejection of malignant cells.[22]

OTHER COLONIC DISEASES

Colonic Diverticulum. A new concept has emerged in the treatment of diverticular disease of the colon based on a better understanding of the pathophysiology.[1] Development of pulsion diverticula has been attributed to increased intraluminal pressure. The hypertrophied musculature of the sigmoid bowel wall exhibited motor activity to various stimuli in excess of that seen in normal controls.[2-4] With simultaneous intraluminal pressure recordings and cineradiography, Painter and Truelove[2] demonstrated that contraction of the thickened sigmoid muscle led to narrowing and "blocking" of very short segments of the colon which caused high intracolonic pressures. These high pressures contributed to the formation of diverticula. Almy[1] suggested that a larger fecal mass in the sigmoid would prevent the close approximation of the colonic walls, hence, he recommended that the traditional low residue diet be supplanted by one with large amounts of bulk, and be supplemented with hydrophilic colloids. Since morphine sulfate increased intraluminal pressures whereas Meperidine did not, the latter drug is recommended for relief of pain in episodes of exacerbation of diverticular disease. Antibiotics are used when there is evidence of systemic infection manifested by fever and elevation of the white blood count.

Diverticulosis of the large bowel does not usually present nutritional complications until it is complicated by inflammation, formation of abscesses or fistulae, perforation, or obstruction.

Villous Adenoma. Garis in 1941 reported a case of prerenal azotemia due to fluid and electrolyte loss[1] accompanying a villous adenoma, but the relationship was not fully recognized until 1954 when McKittrick and Wheelock described the electrolyte depletion, dehydration, hypotension and azotemia.[2] Additional reports have appeared subsequently.[3,4]

In the normal colon there is a continuous exchange of water and electrolytes across the mucosa, the result being the efflux of water, sodium and chloride from the lumen and a net transfer of potassium and bicarbonate into the lumen to maintain isotonicity.[5] The normal fecal sodium output approximates 3.1 mEq/24 hours and the potassium 9.0 mEq/24 hours.[6] In patients with villous tumors large volumes of protein-rich mucosal fluid (3 to 4 L/24 hour) may be passed containing up to 160 mEq sodium and up to 70 mEq potassium per 24 hours. Such losses lead to lowered serum electrolyte concentrations.[7] Salem suggested that the sodium losses in this condition are quantitatively greater than potassium losses, but because potassium balance is more precarious than sodium balance, the symptoms of hypokalemia are encountered more frequently than those of hyponatremia. The fecal potassium losses are due to the increase in stool volume rather than an increased fecal potassium concentration. Therapy consists of colloid, fluid and electrolyte replacement. Sufficient bleeding may occur to warrant transfusion and protein losses may result in the lowering of serum protein values.[8]

This uncommon lesion, usually found in the rectum of older patients, may occur anywhere in the colon. Malignant change occurs in 30 to 74 per cent of the cases.[9,10] Surgical extirpation is the only definite therapy, but villous adenomas tend to recur.

USE OF MEDIUM-CHAIN TRIGLYCERIDES IN MALABSORPTION

Fat digestion and absorption entail (1) hydrolysis by pancreatic lipase catalyzed by bile salts; (2) micelle formation of the fatty acids and monoglycerides and bile salts; (3) passage into the epithelial cell by an as yet undefined mechanism; (4) re-esterification of fatty acids of ten or more carbon atoms to triglycerides within the intestinal mucosa; with shorter chain fatty acids, esterification is not obligatory; (5) the re-esterified triglycerides are subsequently incorporated with phospholipids, cholesterol and protein into a beta-lipoprotein moiety, the chylomicron, and (6) the lipid so packaged continues its movement across the mucosa into the lymphatic system.[1]

In contrast, medium-chain triglycerides (MCT) and short-chain fatty acids appear to be absorbed about four times as efficiently as long-chain triglycerides (LCT) in experimental animals.[2] Although the rate of intraluminal lipolysis of MCT occurs faster than that of LCT,[3] a portion of the MCT enters the mucosal cell intact and undergoes intracellular hydrolysis.[4] Medium-chain fatty acids derived in this manner as well as medium-chain fatty acids liberated within the intestinal lumen and absorbed are transported without esterification to the liver via the portal vein.[1] Thus diversion of pancreatic enzymes does not prevent hydrolysis of MCT[5] since extensive mucosal hydrolysis occurs. In conditions in which there are diminished concentrations of bile salts, less impairment of absorption of MCT occurs than of absorption of long-chain triglyceride

since bile salts are not required for dispersion of MCT in water. Clinically, in patients with pancreatic disease and biliary atresia MCT is absorbed[6] more efficiently than LCT. Additional evidence that MCT are relatively well absorbed despite low bile salt concentrations was provided in normal individuals with cholestyramine-induced steatorrhea. Substitution of MCT for LCT abolished steatorrhea and no interference with cholestyramine sequestration of bile salts by MCT could be demonstrated.[7]

Both short-chain[8] and medium-chain triglycerides may be absorbed in part from the colon.[9] In the dog colon, Pihl, Glotzer and Patterson[10] demonstrated the absorption of 6-, 8- and 10-carbon fatty acids.

The differences between LCT (in which form most dietary fat occurs) and MCT (fractionated from coconut oil) make the latter useful in disorders of fat absorption. Commercial MCT is a bland oil composed primarily of the triglycerides of C_8 and C_{10} fatty acids (Appendix, Table A-6).

Recent clinical observations have indicated that MCT are useful in treating patients with cystic fibrosis of the pancreas,[11,12] pancreatic insufficiency,[13-15] carcinoma of the pancreas,[12] extra hepatic biliary tract obstruction,[14] biliary atresia, bile fistula,[6] gastrectomy steatorrhea,[12,15-17] massive small bowel resection,[18,19] regional enteritis,[16] intestinal lymphangiectasia,[20,21] abeta-lipoproteinemia,[15,22] cholestyramine-induced steatorrhea,[23] and cirrhosis.[16,24]

Senior[6] pointed out that MCT may play an important supplementary role in accelerating recovery from malabsorption treated by other therapies, including (1) gluten-free diets in celiac disease, (2) antibiotics in bacterial overgrowth of proximal gastrointestinal tract and (3) with Whipple's disease on long-term antibiotic therapy, (4) with pancreatic insufficiency responding partially to enzyme and bicarbonate replacement, but still fat intolerant, (5) with tropical sprue during treatment with folic acid and antibiotics, (6) with intestinal parasitism under specific therapy (7) with "bile salt diarrhea" with cholestyramine-produced steatorrhea.

In most cases diarrhea and steatorrhea decreased in patients responsive to MCT. To date, weight gain in patients given MCT supplements has been variable.[18] In this regard, it is interesting that the early clinical use of MCT was in the control of obesity.[26]

Saunders[27] called attention to the fact that the widely used van de Kamer[28] assay method did not completely extract MCT from stools. And indeed, the initial disillusionment during the clinical studies could be traced to the use of inappropriate methodology for quantitating the degree of steatorrhea following MCT-containing diets.[6] Less than 60 per cent of fatty acids such as octanoic can be recovered using the van de Kamer method. Braddock et al.[29] modified this by altering the ratio of ether and ethanol used in saponification and extraction of MCT and observed reliable results. Senior,[30] however, pointed out that the conventional van de Kamer method may give a reasonable estimation of fecal fat in patients given MCT since the error of underestimation (owing to incomplete extraction of octanoic acid) is compensated for by an error of overestimation when the fatty acid equivalent of 284 is used instead of 144 in the van de Kamer formula. The latter would be appropriate for MCT fatty acids as octanoic. To circumvent these difficulties, Broitman et al. in this laboratory[31] urged the use of a fecal fat assay based on the principle of electrical capacitance.[32]

Despite evidence of clinical improvement in patients, long-term MCT feeding has not been entirely successful. Crampy abdominal pain and increased diarrhea have been reported with its use.[16] Increased steatorrhea has also been observed following the use of the oil preparation of MCT in one patient with short bowel syndrome.[16]

MCT is available as the purified oil or as the major fat constituent in the commercially available powdered diet, Portagen (Appendix, Table A-23). Recipes are available for its use in cooking.[30] It may be substituted for long-chain fats in oral or tube formulas fed to patients with serious fat malabsorption.

It has been suggested[16] that MCT should not be used in patients with decompensated cirrhosis because short-chain fatty acids inhibit oxidative phosphorylation[33] and may exert a narcotic effect on the central nervous system.[34] In cirrhotics, particularly those with hepatic encephalopathy, blood levels of short- and medium-chain fatty acids are increased.[35,36] MCT feeding may accentuate these effects. MCT are indicated in patients exhibiting continual nutritional caloric deterioration where all therapy has been unsuccessful in reversing the course of the malabsorptive disease, particularly in those instances where increased time for recovery and gain in body weight may result in spontaneous or therapeutic reversal of the initial problem. This is particularly relevant in infants in whom nutritional considerations are critical.[6]

For additional information concerning biochemical and physiologic consideration and the clinical application of MCT the interested reader is referred to several excellent reviews.[25,30,37,38]

DIET AND THE CLINICIAN

The "diet" recommended by a physician is usually influenced by personal prejudice, mores, and local dietary habits, many of which are carried over from times when little was known about the causes of gastrointestinal disorders and even less about specific medical therapy.

Weinstein et al.[1] and Donaldson[2] noted the need for more scientific information on the effect of diet in gastrointestinal diseases. The importance of using diets of proven usefulness is stressed. These include: (1) avoidance of gluten in gluten-sensitive enteropathy;[3] (2) omission of disaccharides, e.g., lactose, in lactase-deficient patients;[4] (3) substitution of fructose in infants unable to actively transport glucose and galactose;[5] (4) substitution of artificially prepared medium-chain triglycerides for long-chain dietary lipids in patients with diminution or absence of pancreatic enzymes or bile salts,[6] and with other malabsorptive disorders, and (5) restriction of dietary fat in patients with steatorrhea in order to prevent further aggravation of steatorrhea with consequent loss of nutrients and minerals.

Dietotherapy otherwise should be concerned with maintenance of nutrition or replacement of patient's losses. This is not an easy task and involves patience, imagination, time and much manipulation of foods. Perusal of diet manuals reveals great preoccupation with and wide variation in foods constituting so-called "bland," "high," and "low residue" diets. Kramer[7] has pointed out the disparities in descriptions of "high and low residue" diets which allegedly alter the intestinal contents or excreta. He advocates eliminating the word "residue," preferring "roughage" or "bulk" when referring to foods containing material resistant to chemical digestion. Cereals such as bran, vegetables, fruits, and nuts contain the largest amount of "roughage." Foods which increase the moisture content of excreta should be referred to as "laxative" food or "juices," such as prune juice. Foods containing significant proportions of hemicellulose and/or cellulose, e.g. in fruits and vegetables, would, therefore, be included in both categories.

The presence of large amounts of undigestible material or "bulk" within the intestinal lumen presumably acts as a mechanical stimulant in aiding evacuation. Bacterial action forming volatile acids within the colon also results in a laxative effect.[8]

Kramer studied the effect of foods commonly incriminated as causing alteration of bowel habits in otherwise healthy patients with ileostomies.[9] Excreta were checked for water content, wet and dry weights and electrolyte concentration following diets containing baked beans, cabbage, corn, prune juice, orange juice, pepper, milk and fried foods in amounts normally ingested. Cabbage increased the volume and weight in two thirds of cases and baked beans increased dry weight only. The only substance he found consistently to increase stool weight and water content was prune juice, which contains diphenylisatin, a chemical laxative.[10] Water loading in this same group of patients by 6 to 8 glasses of water per day above the control intake did not appreciably alter the volume of ileal excreta, which remained at about 500 ml per day.[9] This apparently contradicts the common practice of prescribing increased water ingestion for the treatment of constipation. Whether his data are equally valid for the patient with a diseased colon or ileum remains to be studied.

BIBLIOGRAPHY

Nutrition and Disease of the Intestinal Tract

1. Zamcheck: Fed. Proc., *19*, 855, 1960.
2. Dubos, Shaedler, Costello, and Stevens: Fed. Proc., *22*, 1322, 1963.
3. Donaldson: New Eng. J. Med., *270*, 938, 1964.
4. Sprinz: Fed. Proc., *21*, 57, 1962.
5. Spencer, and Knox: Fed. Proc., *19*, 886, 1960.
6. Deren, Broitman, and Zamcheck: J. Clin. Invest., *46*, 186, 1967.

Massive Resection of the Small Bowel

1. Booth: Postgrad Med. J., *37*, 725, 1961.
2. Kinney, Goldwyn, Barr, and Moore: J.A.M.A., *179*, 153, 1962.
3. Winawer, Broitman, Wolochow, *et al.*: New Eng. J. Med., *274*, 72, 1966.
4. Jarnum, Schwartz, Thing, and Thorsoe: Acta Chir. Scand., *122*, 428, 1961.
5. Cox, Meynell, Cooke, and Gaddie: Gastroenterology, *35*, 390, 1958.
6. Shay, Gershon-Cohen, and Fels: Amer. J. Dig. Dis., *6*, 335, 1939.
7. Harrison, and Harrison: J. Biol. Chem., *188*, 83, 1951.
8. Nicolaysen: Acta Physiol. Scand., *22*, 260, 1951.
9. Scheiner, Shils, and Vanamee: Amer. J. Clin. Nutr., *17*, 64, 1965.
10. Lack, and Weiner: Amer. J. Physiol., *200*, 313, 1961.
11. Hardison, and Rosenberg: New Eng. J. Med., *277*, 337, 1967.
12. Gazet, and Kopp: Surgery, *56*, 565, 1964.
13. Fordtran, Clodi, Soergel, and Ingelfinger: Ann. Int. Med., *57*, 883, 1962.
14. Dowling, and Booth: Lancet, *2*, 146, 1966.
15. Dahlqvist, and Borgstrom: Biochem. J., *81*, 411, 1961.
16. Harrison and Booth: Gut, *1*, 237, 1960.
17. Booth, and Jones: Gut, *2*, 23, 1961.
18. Borgstrom, Dahlqvist, Lundh, and Sjovall: J. Clin. Invest., *37*, 1521, 1957.
19. Alcock, and MacIntyre: Biochem. J., *76*, 19P, 1960.
20. Booth, and Mollin: Lancet *1*, 18, 1959.
21. Klahr, Tripathy, Garcia, *et al.*: Amer. J. Med., *43*, 84, 1967.
22. Waldmann: Gastroenterology, *50*, 422, 1966.
23. Winawer, Herskovic, Goldsmith, *et al.*: Amer. J. Dig. Dis., *12*, 753, 1967.
24. Taylor: Gastroenterology, *51*, 1058, 1966.
25. Jabbari, Winawer, and Zamcheck: Unpublished observations.
26. Frederick, Sizer, and Osborne: New Eng. J. Med., *272*, 509, 1965.
27. Osborne, Sizer, Frederick, and Zamcheck: Amer. J. Surg., *114*, 393, 1967.

Malabsorptive Syndromes

1. Creamer: Gut, 7, 569, 1966.
2. Sakula, and Shiner: Lancet, *2*, 876, 1957.

3. Yardley, Bayless, Norton, and Hendrix: New Eng. J. Med., 267, 1173, 1962.
4. Rubin, Brandborg, Flick, et al.: Gastroenterology, 43, 621, 1962.
5. Bayless, Yardley, and Hendrix: Arch. Int. Med., 111, 83, 1963.

Gluten-Sensitive Enteropathy

1. Dicke: *Investigation of the harmful effects of certain types of cereal on patients with celiac disease.* Thesis, Utrecht, 1950.
2. Dicke, Weijers, and van de Kamer: Acta Paediat., 42, 34, 1953.
3. Kowlessar, Warren, and Bronstein: In *Progress in Gastroenterology*, Vol. II, Ed. Glass, New York, Grune & Stratton, Inc. 1970.
4. Kivel, Kearns, and Liebowitz: New Eng. J. Med., 271, 769, 1964.
5. Broitman, McCray, May, et al.: Amer. J. Med., 48, 382, 1970.
6. Rubin, Brandborg, Flick, et al.: *Intestinal Biopsy.* pp. 67–83, Eds. Wolstenholme and Cameron, Boston, Little, Brown & Co., 1962.
7. MacDonald, Brandborg, Flick, et al.: Gastroenterology, 47, 573, 1964.
8. Adlersberg: *The Malabsorption Syndrome.* New York, Grune & Stratton, 1957.
9. Green and Wollaeger: Gastroenterology, 38, 399, 1960.
10. Cooke, Feeney, and Hawkins: Quart. J. Med., 22, 59, 1953.
11. Snell: Ann. Intern. Med., 12, 1632, 1939.
12. Adlersberg and Schein: J.A.M.A., 134, 1459, 1947.
13. Suarez: Ann. Intern. Med., 12, 529, 1938.
14. Thaysen: *Non-tropical Sprue. A Study in Idiopathic Steatorrhea.* London, Humphrey Milford, 1932.
15. Manson-Bahr: *The Dysenteric Disorders.* 2nd Ed., Baltimore, The Williams & Wilkins Co., 1943.
16. Bossaak, Wong, and Adlersberg: In *The Malabsorption Syndrome*, Ed. Adlersberg, New York, Grune & Stratton, 1957.
17. Adlersberg, Marshak, Colcher, et al.: Gastroenterology, 26, 548, 1954.
18. Laws, Booth, Showdon, and Stewart: Brit. Med. J., 1, 1313, 1963.
19. Marshak, Wolfe, and Eliasoph: In *The Malabsorption Syndrome*, Ed. Adlersberg, New York, Grune & Stratton, 1957.
20. Sakula, and Shiner: Lancet, 2, 876, 1957.
21. Rubin, Brandborg, Phelps, and Taylor: Gastroenterology, 38, 28, 1960.
22. Creamer: Gut, 7, 569, 1966.
23. Rubin, Brandborg, Flick, et al.: Gastroenterology, 43, 621, 1962.
24. McCarthy, Borland, Kurtz, and Ruffin: Amer. J. Path., 44, 585, 1964.
25. McDonald, Brandborg, Flick, et al.: Gastroenterology, 74, 573, 1964.
26. Yardley, Bayless, Norton, and Hendrix: New Eng. J. Med., 267, 1173, 1962.
27. Benson, Kowlessar, and Sleisenger: Medicine, 43, 1, 1964.

28. Sleisenger: New Eng. J. Med., 265, 49, 1961.
29. Plotkin, and Isselbacher: New Eng. J. Med., 271, 1033, 1964.
30. Shmerling, Auricchio, Rubino, et al.: Helv. Paediat. Acta, 19, 507, 1964.
31. Nordio, Lamedica, Vignok, and Berio: Ann. Paediat. (Basel), 204, 3, 1965.
32. Lifshitz, Klatz, and Holman: Amer. J. Dig. Dis., 10, 47, 1965.
33. Arthur: Arch. Dis. Child., 41, 519, 1966.
34. Ashley, and French: Brit. J. Radiol., 24, 321, 1951.
35. Anderson, Ashley, French, and Gerrard: Brit. J. Radiol., 25, 298, 1952.
36. Balint, and Hirschowitz: New Eng. J. Med., 265, 631, 1961.
37. Cooke, Fore, Cox, et al.: Gut, 4, 279, 1963.
38. Granick: J. Biol. Chem., 164, 737, 1946.
39. Stewart, Yuile, Claiborne, et al.: J. Exp. Med., 92, 375, 1950.
40. Cox, Meyrell, Cooke, and Gaddie: Gastroenterology, 35, 390, 1958.
41. Hartley: In *The Malabsorption Syndrome*, Ed. Adlersberg. New York, Grune & Stratton, 1957, p. 172.
42. Badenoch, and Callender: Lancet, 1, 192, 1960.
43. Kelley, Logan, and Christ: New Eng. J. Med., 252, 658, 1955.
44. Taylor, Wollaeger, Comfort, and Power: Gastroenterology, 20, 203, 1952.
45. Colcher and Adlersberg: In *The Malabsorption Syndrome*. Ed. Adlersberg. New York, Grune & Stratton, 1957.

Tropical Sprue

1. Frazer: *In* Proc. World Cong. Gastroenterology, Baltimore, The Williams & Wilkins Co., Vol. 1, p. 619, 1959.
2. Swanson, and Thomassen: Amer. J. Path., 46, 511, 1965.
3. Butterworth, and Perez-Santiago: Ann. Intern. Med., 48, 8, 1958.
4. Bayless, Guardiola-Rotger, and Wheby: Gastroenterology, 51, 32, 1966.
5. Milanes, Curbelo, Rodrigues et al.: Gastroenterology, 7, 306, 1946.
6. Bayless, Wheby, and Swanson: Amer. J. Clin. Nutr., 21, 1030, 1968.
7. O'Brien, and England: Brit. Med. J., 2, 1157, 1966.
8. Avery: Trans. Roy. Soc. Trop. Med. Hyg., 41, 377, 1948.
9. Keele, and Bound: Brit. Med. J., 1, 77, 1946.
10. Mathan, and Baker: Amer. J. Clin. Nutr., 21, 1077, 1968.
11. Dammin: Fed. Proc., 24, 35, 1965.
12. Bayless, Guardiola-Rotger, and Wheby: Gastroenterology, 51, 32, 1966.
13. Nadel, and Gardner: Amer. J. Trop. Med., 5, 686, 1956.
14. Creamer: Gut, 7, 569, 1966.
15. Klipstein, and Baker: Gastroenterology, 58, 717, 1970.

16. Ghitis, Tripathy, and Mayoral: Amer. J. Clin. Nutr., *20*, 1206, 1967.
17. Gorbach, Banwell, Jacobs, *et al.*: Amer. J. Clin. Nutr., *23*, 1545, 1970.
18. Banwell, Gorbach, Mitra, *et al.*: Amer. J. Clin. Nutr., *23*, 1559, 1970.
19. Fordtran, Rector, Locklear, and Ewton: J. Clin. Invest., *46*, 287, 1967.
20. Phillips, and Schmid: Gut, *10*, 440, 1969.
21. Banwell, Pierce, Mitra, *et al.*: J. Clin. Invest., *49*, 183, 1969.
22. Banwell, Gorbach, Mitra, and Pierce: Gastroenterology, *58*, 925, 1970.
23. Klipstein, Schenk, and Samloff: Gastroenterology, *51*, 317, 1966.
24. Swanson, Wheby, and Bayless: Morphologic effects of folate on the jejunal lesion of tropical sprue. (Proc. 63rd Ann. Meeting Amer. Assoc. Pathol. and Bacteriol., Cleveland, Ohio), 1966.
25. Haddock, Vega de Rodriquez, Flock, and Cintron-Rivera: Amer. J. Dig. Dis., *7*, 967, 1962.
26. Rodriquez-Olleros, and Hernandez-Morales: Puerto Rico J. Pub. Health & Trop. Med., *15*, 274, 1940.
27. Meyer, Suarez, Buso, *et al.*: Proc. Soc. Exp. Biol. Med., *83*, 681, 1953.
28. Girdwood: Lancet, *2*, 53, 1953.
29. Graham, and Rheault: J. Lab. Clin. Med., *43*, 235, 1954.
30. Klipstein: Scand. J. Gastroent. (Suppl), *6*, 93, 1970.
31. Herbert: Amer. J. Clin. Nutr., *21*, 1115, 1968.
32. Wheby, and Bayless: Blood, *31*, 817, 1968.
33. Anderson, Belcher, Chanarin, and Mellin: Brit. J. Haemat., *6*, 439, 1960.
34. Klipstein: Blood, *21*, 626, 1963.
35. Hoffbrand, Necheles, Maldonado, Horta, and Santini: Brit. Med. J., *2*, 543, 1969.
36. Baker, and Mathan: Tropical Sprue in Southern India. In *Tropical Sprue*. The Wellcome Trust. London, Churchill and Sons, 1970.
37. Jeejeebhoy, Desai, Borkar, Deshpande, and Pathare: Amer. J. Clin. Nutr., *21*, 994, 1968.
38. Tandon, Iyenger, Deo, and Saraya: J. Assoc. Physicians India, *14*, 197, 1966.
39. Jeejeebhoy, Samuel, Singh *et al.*: Gastroenterology, *56*, 252, 1969.
40. Rubini, Sheehy, Meroney, and Louro: J. Lab. Clin. Med., *58*, 902, 1961.
41. Haddock, Del, and Vasquez: J. Clin. Endocrin., *26*, 859, 1966.
42. Shils, M. E.: (Personal communication) 1972.
43. Jeejeebhoy, Desai, Marokha, *et al:* Gastroenterology, *51*, 333, 1966.
44. Bayless, Walter, and Barker: (Abstr.) Clin. Res., *12*, 445, 1964.
45. Desai, and Jeejeebhoy: Indian J. Path. Bact., *10*, 107, 1967.
46. Guerra, Wheby, and Bayless: Ann. Intern. Med., *63*, 619, 1965.
47. Klipstein: Ann. Intern. Med., *61*, 721, 1964.
48. French, Gaddie, and Smith: Quart. J. Med., *25*, 333, 1956.
49. Sheehy, Baggs, Perez-Santiago, and Flock: Ann. Intern. Med., *57*, 892, 1962.

Whipple's Disease

1. Bobruff, DiBianco, Loebel, and Groisser: Gastroenterology, *45*, 108, 1963.
2. Laster, Waldmann, Fester: Whipple's disease, Proc. Amer. Gastroenterological Assoc., New York, April 27, 1962.
3. Sugarman, Bigman, and Jarkowski: J.A.M.A., *174*, 2192, 1960.
4. Trier, Phelps, Eidelman, and Rubin: Gastroenterology, *48*, 684, 1965.
5. Yardley, and Hendrix: Bull. Johns Hopkins Hosp., *109*, 80, 1961.
6. Vitale, *et al.*: Personal communication.
7. Kok, Dybkaer, and Rostgaard: Acta Path. et Microbiol. Scandinav., *60*, 431, 1964.
8. Charache, Bayless, Shelley, and Hendrix: Trans. Assoc. Amer. Physicians, *79*, 399, 1966.
9. Bayless: Adv. Int. Med., *16*, 171, 1970.
10. Ruffin, Kurtz, and Roufail: J.A.M.A., *195*, 476, 1966.
11. England, French, and Rawson: Gastroenterology, *39*, 219, 1960.
12. Holt, Isselbacher, and Jones: New Eng. J. Med., *264*, 1335, 1961.
13. Pirola, Miskel, and MacDonald: Med. J. Australia, *2*, 985, 1967.

Malabsorption Due to Bacterial Contamination of the Gut

1. Doig, and Girdwood: Quart. J. Med., *29*, 333, 1960.
2. Donaldson, Carrigan, and Matsios: Gastroenterology, *43*, 282, 1962.
3. Strauss, Donaldson, and Gardner: Lancet, *2*, 736, 1961.
4. Donaldson: Gastroenterology, *43*, 271, 1962.
5. Giannella, Broitman, and Zamcheck: J. Clin. Invest., *50*, 1100, 1971.
6. Donaldson: Ann. Intern. Med., *64*, 1948, 1966.
7. Dawson, and Isselbacher: J. Clin. Invest., *39*, 730, 1960.
8. Hofmann and Borgström: J. Clin. Invest., *43*, 247, 1964.
9. Portman: Fed. Proc., *21*, 896, 1962.
10. Donaldson: J. Clin. Invest., *44*, 1815, 1965.
11. Kim, Spritz, Blum, *et al.*: Clin. Res., *13*, 255, 1965 (Abstr.).
12. Rosenberg, Hardison, and Bull: New Eng. J. Med., *276*, 1391, 1967.
13. Tabaqchali, and Booth: Lancet, *2*, 12, 1966.
14. Klipstein, and Samloff: Amer. J. Clin. Nutr., *19*, 237, 1966.
15. Hoffbrand, Tabaqchali, and Mollin: Lancet, *2*, 1339, 1966.
16. Heins, Steinberg, and Sackner: Ann. Intern. Med., *59*, 822, 1963.
17. Hoskins, Norris, Gottlieb, and Zamcheck: Amer. J. Med., *33*, 459, 1962.

18. McBrien, and Lockhart-Mummery: Brit. Med. J., 2, 1653, 1962.
19. Salen, Goldstein, and Wirts: Ann. Intern. Med., 64, 835, 1966.

Mastocytosis

1. Bank and Marks: Gastroenterology, 45, 535, 1963.
2. Rubin and Dobbins: Gastroenterology, 49, 676, 1965.
3. Broitman, McCray, May, et al.: Amer. J. Med., 48, 382, 1970.
4. Jarnum and Zacharie: Gut, 8, 64, 1967.

Protein Losing Enteropathies

1. Waldmann: Gastroenterology, 50, 422, 1967.
2. Ulstrom and Krivit: Amer. J. Dis. Child., 100, 509, 1960.
3. Waldmann, Morell, Wochner, and Sternlieb: J. Clin. Invest., 44, 1107, 1965.
4. Milhaud and Vesin: Nature, 191, 872, 1961.
5. Mistilis, Skyring, and Stephen: Lancet, 1, 77, 1965.
6. Waldmann, Gordon, Dutcher, and Wertlake: In *Plasma Proteins and Gastrointestinal Tract in Health and Disease.* Copenhagen, Ejnar Munksgaards Forlag, 1962.
7. Bookstein, French, and Pollard: Amer. J. Dig. Dis., 10, 573, 1965.
8. Waldmann, Wochner, Laster, and Gordon: New Eng. J. Med., 276, 761, 1967.
9. Holman, Nickel, and Sleisenger: Amer. J. Med., 27, 963, 1959.
10. Hermans, Huizenga, Hoffman, et al.: Amer. J. Med., 39, 476, 1966.
11. Waldmann and Laster: J. Clin. Invest., 43, 1025, 1964.
12. McCarthy, Austad, and Read: Amer. J. Dig. Dis., 10, 945, 1965.
13. Allen and Hadden: Brit. Med. J., 2, 486, 1964.
14. Collins and Ellis: Amer. J. Med., 39, 476, 1965.
15. Hoskins, Winawer, Broitman, et al.: Gastroenterology, 53, 265, 1967.
16. Paul, Castleman, and White: Amer. J. Med. Sci., 216, 361, 1948.
17. Gimlette: Brit. Heart J., 21, 9, 1959.
18. Petersen and Hastrup: Acta Med. Scand., 173, 401, 1963.
19. Kaihara, Nishimura, Aoyagi, et al.: Jap. Heart J., 4, 386, 1963.
20. Davidson, Waldmann, Goodman, and Gordon: Lancet, 1, 899, 1961.
21. Petersen and Ottosen: Acta Med. Scand., 176, 335, 1964.
22. Díaz, Linazasoro, López-Garcia, and Guedes: Rev. Clin. Esp., 77, 252, 1960.
23. Oeff and Lerche: Klin. Wschr., 39, 100, 1961.
24. Plauth, Waldmann, Wochner, and Braunwald: Pediatrics, 34, 636, 1964.

Intestinal Lymphangiectasia

25. Waldmann, Steinfeld, Dutcher, et al.: Gastroenterology, 41, 197, 1961.

26. Jeejeebhoy: Lancet, 1, 343, 1962.
27. Marshak, Wolf, Cohen, and Janowitz: Radiology, 77, 893, 1961.
28. Schwartz and Jarnum: Lancet, 1, 327, 1959.
29. Herskovic, Winawer, Goldsmith, et al.: Pediatrics, 40, 345, 1967.
30. Steinfeld, Davidson, and Gordon: Amer. J. Med., 29, 405, 1960.
31. Jeffries, Chapman, and Sleisenger: New Eng. J. Med., 270, 761, 1964.
32. Holt: Pediatrics, 34, 629, 1964.

Carbohydrate Intolerance

1. Durand: In Durand (Ed.), *Disorders Due to Intestinal Defective Carbohydrate Digestion and Absorption.* Rome, Il Pensiero Scientifico, 1964.
2. Miller and Crane: Biochim. Biopsys. Acta, 52, 293, 1961.
3. Gray: Gastroenterology, 58, 96, 1970.
4. Laplane, Polonovski, Etienne, et al.: Arch. franc. Pediat., 19, 895, 1962.
5. Schneider, Kinter, and Stirling: New Eng. J. Med., 274, 305, 1966.
6. Lindquist and Meluwisse: Acta Paediat., 51, 674, 1962.
7. Abraham, Levin, Oberholzer, and Russell: Arch. Dis. Child., 42, 592, 1967.
8. Littman and Hammond: Gastroenterology, 48, 237, 1965.
9. Ferguson and Maxwell: Lancet, 2, 188, 1967.
10. Sonntag, Brill, Troyer, et al.: Gastroenterology, 47, 18, 1964.
11. Haemmerli, Kistler, Ammann, et al.: Amer. J. Med., 38, 7, 1965.
12. Welsh, Rohrer, Drewry, et al.: Arch. Int. Med., 117, 495, 1966.
13. Weser and Sleisenger: Gastroenterology, 48, 571, 1965.
14. Welsh, May, Drury, and Walker: (Abstr.) Clin. Res., 13, 32, 1965.
15. Sunshine and Kretchmer: Pediatrics, 34, 38, 1964.
16. Cozzetto: Pediatrics, 32, 228, 1963.
17. Bowie, Brinkman, and Hansen: Lancet, 2, 550, 1963.
18. Dahlqvist: J. Clin. Invest., 41, 463, 1962.
19. Weijers and van de Kamer: Acta Paediat., 51, 371, 1962.
20. Auricchio, Dahlqvist, Murset, and Parker: J. Pediat., 62, 165, 1963.
21. Cuatrecasas, Lockwood, and Caldwell: Lancet, 1, 14, 1965.
22. Knudsen, Bellamy, Lecocq, et al.: (Abstr.) Clin. Res., 14, 300, 1966.
23. Broitman, Thalenfeld, and Zamcheck: (Abstr.) Clin. Res., 15, 229, 1967.
24. Deren, Broitman, and Zamcheck: J. Clin. Invest., 46, 186, 1967.
25. Heilskov: Acta Physiol. Scand., 24, 84, 1951.
26. Sunshine and Kretchmer: Science, 144, 850, 1964.
27. Bayless and Rosensweig: J.A.M.A., 197, 968, 1966.

27

28. Littman and Hammond: Gastroenterology, *48*, 237, 1965.
29. Huang and Bayless: New Eng. J. Med., *276*, 1283, 1967.
30. Cook and Kajubi: Lancet, *1*, 725, 1966.
31. Bayless and Christopher: Amer. J. Clin. Nutr., *22*, 181, 1969.
32. Gilat, Kuhn, Gelman and Mizrahy: Amer. J. Dig. Dis., *15*, 895, 1970.
33. Simoons: Amer. J. Dig. Dis., *15*, 695, 1970.
34. Welsh, Shaw, and Walker: Ann. Intern. Med., *64*, 1252, 1966.
35. Hellemans: Acta Med. Scand., *148*, 367, 1954.
36. Weser, Rubin, Ross, and Sleisenger: New Eng. J. Med., *273*, 1070, 1965.
37. Paton, Murray, and Watson: Brit. Med. J., *1*, 459, 1966.
38. Schneider, Carter, and Goodhart: Lancet, *1*, 503, 1966.
39. Struthers, Singleton, and Kern: Ann. Intern. Med., *63*, 221, 1965.
40. Dunphy, Littman, Hammond, *et al.*: Gastroenterology, *45*, 477, 1963.
41. Burke *et al.*: Paediat. J., *1*, 147, 1965.
42. Kern, Struthers, and Attwood: Gastroenterology, *45*, 477, 1963.
43. Welsh: Medicine, *49*, 257, 1970.
44. Dahlqvist: Anal. Biochem., *7*, 8, 1964.

Metabolic Disorders—Diabetes

1. Rundles: Medicine, *24*, 111, 1945.
2. Wruble and Kalser: Am. J. Med., *37*, 118, 1964.

Abetalipoproteinemia

1. Salt, Wolff, Lloyd, *et al.*: Lancet, *2*, 325, 1960.
2. Isselbacher, Scheig, Plotkin, and Caulfield: Medicine, *43*, 347, 1964.
3. Sobrevilla, Goodman, and Kane: Amer. J. Med., *37*, 821, 1964.
4. Isselbacher: Gastroenterology, *50*, 78, 1966.
5. Sabesin and Isselbacher: Science, *147*, 1149, 1965.
6. Hyams, Sabesin, and Isselbacher: Fed. Proc., *24*, 671, 1965.
7. Gotto, Levy, John, and Fredrickson: New Eng. J. Med., *284*, 813, 1971.
8. Eder: Amer. J. Med., *23*, 269, 1957.
9. van Buchem, Pal, de Gier, *et al.*: Amer. J. Med., *40*, 794, 1966.
10. Simon and Ways: J. Clin. Invest., *43*, 1311, 1964.
11. Ways and Simon: J. Clin. Invest., *43*, 1322, 1964.

Amino Acid Anomalies

1. Milne: Lancet, *1*, 327, 1964.

Parasitic Infestation

1. Von Bornsdarff: Parasitological Reviews, *5*, 207, 1956.

2. Faust, Russell, and Jung (Eds.): *Craig and Faust's Clinical Parasitology*, 8th Ed., Philadelphia, Lea & Febiger, 1970.
3. Amir-Ahmadi, Braun, Neva, *et al.*: Amer. J. Dig. Dis., *13*, 959, 1968.
4. Milner, Irvine, Barton, *et al.*: Gut, *6*, 574, 1965.
5. Stemmermann: Gastroenterology, *53*, 59, 1967.
6. Sheehy, Meroney, Cox, and Saler: Gastroenterology, *42*, 148, 1962.
7. Hoskins, Winawer, Broitman, *et al.*: Gastroenterology, *53*, 265, 1967.
8. Yardley, Takano, and Hendrix: Bull. Johns Hopkins Hosp., *115*, 389, 1964.
9. Hermans, Huizenga, Hoffman, *et al.*: Amer. J. Med., *40*, 78–89, 1966.
10. Marsden and Hoskins: Gastroenterology, *51*, 701, 1966.
11. Marsden and Schultz: Gastroenterology, *57*, 724, 1969.

Acute Infectious Diarrheas

1. Morgan: In Dubos and Hirsch, *Bacterial and Mycotic Infections in Man*, Philadelphia, J. B. Lippincott Co., 1965, p. 610.
2. Watt: Shigellosis: In Sartwell, *Preventive Medicine and Public Health*, 9th Ed., New York, Appleton-Century-Crofts, 1965.
3. Raffensperger: Intestinal Infections, In Bockus, *Gastroenterology* 2, 787; Philadelphia, W. B. Saunders Co., 1964.
4. Eisenberg, Palazzola, and Flippin: New Eng. J. Med., *253*, 90, 1955.
5. Lindenbaum, Alam, and Kent: Brit. Med. J., *2*, 162, 1966.
6. Lindenbaum: Brit. Med. J., *2*, 326, 1965.
7. Torres-Pinedo, Rivera, and Rodriguez: Ann. N.Y. Acad. Sci., *176*, 284, 1971.

Salmonellosis and Shigellosis

1. Communicable Disease Center: Morbidity and Mortality weekly rep., *14*, 393, 1965.
2. Saphra and Winter: New Eng. J. Med., *256*, 1128, 1967.
3. Isenberg: Amer. J. Med. Sci., *229*, 497, 1958.
4. Black, Kunz, and Swartz: New Eng. J. Med., *262*, 811, 1960.
5. Cruickshank: Med. Clin. N. Amer., *51*, 643, 1967.
6. Bowmer: Jour. Milk and Food Tech., *28*, 74, 1965.
7. Giannella, Broitman, and Zamcheck: Amer. J. Dig. Dis., *16*, 1001, 1971.
8. Ibid: Amer. J. Dig. Dis., *16*, 1007, 1971.
9. Felsen: In Conn, *Current Therapy*, Philadelphia, W. B. Saunders Co., 1945.

Cholera

1. Phillips: Ann. Intern. Med., *65*, 922, 1966.
2. Gordon, Feeley, Greenough, *et al.*: Ann. Intern. Med., *64*, 1328, 1966.
3. Cruickshank: Med. Clin. N. Amer., *51*, 643, 1967.

4. Rosenberg, Greenough, Lindenbaum, and Gordon: Amer. J. Clin. Nutr., *19*, 384, 1966.
5. Carpenter: Amer. J. Med., *50*, 1, 1971.
6. Field: New Eng. J. Med., *284*, 1137, 1971.
7. Greenough, Carpenter, Bayless, *et al.*: In Glass: *Progress in Gastroenterology II*, New York, Grune & Stratton, 1970.
8. Taylor, Hirschhorn, and Phillips: (Abstr.) Fed. Proc., *26*, 384, 1967.
9. Phillips: In Conn: *Current Therapy*, Philadelphia, W. B. Saunder Co., 1964.
10. Phillips, Van Slyke, Hamilton *et al.*: J. Biol. Chem., *183*, 305, 1950.

Chronic Inflammatory Bowel Disease

1. Crohn, Ginzburg, and Oppenheimer: J.A.M.A., *99*, 1323, 1932.
2. Zetzel: New Eng. J. Med., *254*, 990, 1956.
3. Zetzel: In *Cecil-Loeb Textbook of Medicine*, 11th Ed., Philadelphia, W. B. Saunders Co., 1963.
4. Mendeloff, Monk, Siegel, and Lilienfeld: Gastroenterology, *51*, 748, 1966.
5. Soren: Arch. Int. Med., *117*, 78, 1966.
6. Werthen, Schapira, Rubinstein, and Janowitz: Amer. J. Med., *29*, 416, 1960.
7. Weingarten, Parker, Chazen, and Jacobson: Arch. Surg., *78*, 483, 1959.
8. Ginzburg, Schneider, Dreizen, and Levinson: Surgery, *39*, 347, 1956.
9. Atwell, Duthie, and Goligher: Brit. J. Surg., *52*, 966, 1965.
10. Berman and Prior: J. Mt. Sinai Hosp., *31*, 30, 1964.
11. Atwell and Duthie: Gastroenterology, *46*, 16, 1964.
12. Kirsner: J.A.M.A., *169*, 433, 1959.
13. Brown and Daffner: Ann. Int. Med., *49*, 595, 1958.
14. Sparberg and Kirsner: Amer. J. Dig. Dis., *11*, 865, 1966.
15. Lockhart-Mummery and Morson: Gut, *1*, 87, 1950.
16. Lindner, Marshak, Wolf, and Janowitz: New Eng. J. Med., *269*, 379, 1963.
17. Crohn and Yarnis: J. Mount Sinai Hosp., *33*, 503, 1966.
18. Marshak, Lindner, and Janowitz: Gut, 7, 258, 1966.
19. Lockhart-Mummery and Morson: Gut, *5*, 439, 1965.
20. Jones, Lennard-Jones, and Lockhart-Mummery: Gut, 7, 448, 1966.
21. Morson: Proc. Roy. Soc. Med., *61*, 79, 1968.
22. Zetzel: New Eng. J. Med., *282*, 600, 1970.

Ulcerative Colitis

1. Truelove: Postgrad. Med., *22*, 132, 1957.
2. Korelitz and Coles: Gastroenterology, *52*, 78, 1967.
3. Wright, Lunsden, Luntz, *et al.*: Quart. J. Med., *34*, 229, 1965.

4. Deren, Parush, Levitt, and Khilnani: Ann. Int. Med., *56*, 843, 1962.
5. Goldgraber and Kirsner: Cancer, *17*, 657, 1964.
6. Salem and Truelove: Brit. Med. J., *1*, 827, 1965.
7. Frazer, Hood, Montgomery, *et al.*: Lancet, *1*, 503, 1966.
8. Kramer: Gastroenterology, *47*, 649, 1964.
9. Kirsner: J.A.M.A., *169*, 433, 1959.
10. Zetzel: New Eng. J. Med., *271*, 891, 1964.
11. Zetzel: In *Cecil-Loeb Textbook of Medicine*, 11th Ed., Philadelphia, W. B. Saunders Co., 1963.
12. Wright and Truelove: Brit. Med. J., 2, 142, 1965.
13. Dudek, Spiro, and Thayer: Gastroenterology, *49*, 544, 1965.
14. Taylor and Truelove: Brit. Med. J., 2, 926, 1961.
15. Struthers, Singleton, and Kern: Ann. Intern. Med., *63*, 221, 1965.
16. Iber, Hardoon and Sangree: (Abstr.) Clin. Res., *11*, 185, 1963.
17. Wright and Truelove: Brit. Med. J., 2, 138, 1965.
18. Korelitz and Lindner: Gastroenterology, *46*, 671, 1964.
19. Truelove and Witts: Brit. Med. J., 2, 1041, 1955.
20. Wright: Gastroenterology, *58*, 875, 1970.
21. Kraft and Kirsner: Gastroenterology, *60*, 922, 1971.
22. Kirsner: Scand. J. Gastroenterology 6, (Suppl.), *63*, 1970.

Other Colonic Diseases—

Colonic Diverticulum

1. Almy: Gastroenterology, *49*, 109, 1965.
2. Painter, Truelove, Ardran, and Tuckey: Gastroenterology, *49*, 169, 1965.
3. Painter and Truelove: Gut, *5*, 201, 1964.
4. Arfwidsson: Acta Chir. Scand. (Suppl.) 342, 1964.

Villous Adenoma

1. Garis: Ann. Intern. Med., *15*, 916, 1941.
2. McKittrick and Wheelock: *Carcinoma of Colon*, Springfield, Charles C Thomas, 1954.
3. Goldgraber and Kirsner: Gastroenterology, *35*, 36, 1958.
4. Davis, Seavey, and Sessions: Ann. Surg., *155*, 806, 1962.
5. Levitan, Fordtran, Burrows, and Ingelfinger: Clin. Invest., *41*, 1754, 1962.
6. Dempsey, Caroll, Albright, and Henneman: Metabolism, 7, 108, 1958.
7. Salem, Prokipchuk, and Hendrix: Bull. Johns Hopkins Hosp., *117*, 69, 1965.
8. Masson, Heremons, and Dive: Gastroenterologia, *105*, 270, 1966.
9. Scarborough and Klein: Amer. J. Surg., *76*, 723, 1948.
10. Wheat and Ackerman: Ann. Surg., *147*, 476, 1958.

Medium-Chain Triglycerides in Malabsorption

1. Isselbacher: Gastroenterology, *50*, 78, 1966.
2. Bennett: Quart. J. Exp. Physiol., *49*, 210, 1964.
3. Greenberger, Rodgers, and Isselbacher: J. Clin. Invest., *45*, 217, 1966.
4. Playoust and Isselbacher: J. Clin. Invest., *43*, 878, 1964.
5. Bennett and Holt: Clin. Res., *13*, 535, 1965.
6. Senior: Amer. J. Med. Sci., *257*, 75, 1969.
7. Zurier, Hashim, and Van Itallie: In *Recent Advances in Gastroenterology*. Tokyo, Third World Congr. Gastroenterology, 1967, Vol. 2, 281, 1967.
8. Dawson, Holdsworth, and Webb: Proc. Soc. Exp. Biol. Med., *117*, 97, 1964.
9. Linscheer, Castelli, Moore, *et al.*: (Abstr.) J. Clin. Invest., *43*, 1280, 1964.
10. Pihl, Glotzer, and Patterson: J. Appl. Physiol., *21*, 1059, 1966.
11. Kuo and Huang: J. Clin. Invest., *44*, 1924, 1965.
12. Holt, Hashim, and Van Itallie: Amer. J. Gastroenterology, *43*, 549, 1965.
13. Hashim, Roholt, and Van Itallie: (Abstr.) Clin. Res., *10*, 394, 1962.
14. Iber, Hardoon, and Sprague: (Abstr.) Clin. Res., *11*, 185, 1963.
15. Law: (Abstr.) Clin. Res., *14*, 48, 1966.
16. Greenberger, Ruppert, and Tzagournis: Ann. Intern. Med., *66*, 727, 1967.
17. Pinter, McCracken, Lamar, and Goldsmith: Am. J. Clin. Nutr., *15*, 293, 1964.
18. Winawer, Broitman, Wolochow, *et al.*: New Eng. J. Med., *274*, 72, 1966.
19. Zurier, Cambell, Hashim, and Van Itallie: New Eng. J. Med., *274*, 490, 1966.
20. Holt: Pediatrics, *34*, 629, 1964.
21. Herskovic, Winawer, Goldsmith, *et al.*: Pediatrics, *40*, 345, 1967.
22. Isselbacher, Scheig, Plotkin, and Caulfield: Medicine (Balt), *43*, 347, 1964.
23. Zurier, Hashim, and Van Itallie: Gastroenterology, *49*, 490, 1965.
24. Linscheer, Patterson, Moore, *et al.*: J. Clin. Invest., *45*, 1317, 1966.
25. Tantibhedyangkul and Hashim: Bull. N.Y. Acad. Med., *47*, 17, 1971.
26. Kaunitz, Slanetz, Johnson, *et al.*: J. Nutr., *64*, 513, 1958.
27. Saunders: Gastroenterology, *52*, 135, 1967.
28. van de Kamer, ten Bokken Huinink, and Weyers: J. Biol. Chem., *177*, 347, 1949.
29. Braddock, Fleisher, and Barbero: Gastroenterology, *55*, 165, 1968.
30. *Medium Chain Triglycerides*, Eds. Senior, Van Itallie and Greenberger, Philadelphia, Univ. of Pennsylvania Press, 1968.
31. Broitman, Pizzolante, and Zamcheck: Unpublished observations.
32. Wolochow, Broitman, Williams, and Zamcheck: J. Lab. Clin. Med., *65*, 334, 1965.
33. Samson and Dahl: J. Clin. Invest., *35*, 1291, 1956.
34. Hird and Weidemann: Biochem. J., *98*, 378, 1966.
35. Muto and Takahaski: Postgrad. Med., *37*, A158, 1965.
36. Zieve: Arch. Int. Med., *118*, 211, 1966.
37. Holt: In *Progress in Gastroenterology*, Ed. Glass. New York, Grune & Stratton, 1968, pp. 277–298.
38. Greenberger and Skillman: New Eng. J. Med., *280*, 1045, 1969.

Diet and the Clinician

1. Weinstein, Alson, Van Itallie, *et al.*: J.A.M.A., *176*, 935, 1961.
2. Donaldson: Gastroenterology, *52*, 897, 1967.
3. Dicke, Weijers, and van de Kamer: Acta Paediat., *42*, 34, 1953.
4. Littman and Hammond: Gastroenterology, *48*, 237, 1965.
5. Lindquist and Meenwisse: Acta Paediat., *51*, 674, 1962.
6. Iber, Hardoon and Sprague: Clin. Res., *11*, 185, 1963.
7. Kramer: Gastroenterology, *47*, 649, 1964.
8. Williams and Olmsted: Ann. Intern. Med., *10*, 717, 1936.
9. Kramer, Kearney, and Ingelfinger: Gastroenterology, *42*, 535, 1962.
10. Baum, Sanders, and Straub: J. Am. Pharm. Assn., *40*, 348, 1951.

Chapter

28

Section C Nutrition in Diseases of the Pancreas

Phani Dhar, Norman Zamcheck,

AND

Selwyn A. Broitman

THE SYNDROME OF PANCREATIC INSUFFICIENCY

Advanced chronic pancreatitis or, less commonly, neoplastic obstruction of the pancreatic duct may result in a syndrome characterized by steatorrhea and weight loss with or without diabetes mellitus and/or pancreatic calcification.[1-5] When chronic inflammation is the underlying cause, the pancreatic parenchyma shows atrophy and fibrous replacement, the ducts show areas of dilatation and obstruction ("chain of lakes" appearance) and deposits of calcium may be found both in the parenchyma and within the ductal system. Malabsorption results from impaired secretion of pancreatic juice. When the underlying disease is a tumor, malabsorption results largely from obstruction to the out-flow of pancreatic juice even though the acini are intact. Digestion is impaired to the extent to which availability of pancreatic juice is compromised. The spectrum of insufficiency ranges from subclinical abnormalities detectable only by secretory tests to overt steatorrhea characterized by pale bulky, malodorous stools and marked wasting and emaciation. Diabetes mellitus accompanies the above syndrome when the islands of Langerhans are destroyed and is one of the common clinical manifestations of pancreatic insufficiency.[2,4,6-8]

Inadequate digestion may be accompanied by malabsorption of the lipid-soluble vitamins A, D, E, and K. Steatorrhea may thus be complicated by manifestations of hypovitaminosis. Functional integrity of the pancreas is also necessary for the absorption of vitamin B_{12}.[9-11] Toskes *et al.* have reported that deficiency of this vitamin is reversible on pancreatic substitution therapy, both in pancreatectomized rats and in patients with exocrine pancreatic insufficiency.[12,13] Low duodenal pH in the absence of pancreatic bicarbonate may encourage excessive iron absorption and lead to hemosiderosis.[14-16] A clinically significant defect in iron metabolism however does not occur frequently in patients with pancreatic insufficiency.[17]

Other, less frequent causes of pancreatic insufficiency are surgical resection of the pancreas, gastrectomy, cystic fibrosis, protein-calorie malnutrition and Zollinger-Ellison syndrome.[18-20]

ROLE OF PANCREAS IN NORMAL NUTRITION

The human pancreas secretes 1500 to 4000 ml of juice per day of a pH between 7.5 and 8.5, containing 6 to 12 gm of enzymes necessary for the digestion of protein, fat and carbohydrate. Secretion of this juice is initiated by vagal stimulus and subsequently maintained by the hormones, secretin and pancreozymin. Secretin is released from the duodenal mucosa following contact with the acid contents of the stomach; it stimulates the secretion of water and electrolytes, mainly bicarbonate.

Pancreozymin, released from the small bowel mucosa in response to contact with peptones and other products of gastric digestion, stimulates the secretion of enzymes. Secretion of both the aqueous and the enzymatic components of the pancreatic juice is stimulated by gastrin, released from the antrum in response to distension. Of the dietary stimuli for pancreatic secretion, protein and fat are most potent.

There are 3 main classes of pancreatic enzymes:

(1) The proteolytic enzymes consist of trypsinogen, chymotrypsin, procarboxypeptidases A and B and proelastase. In addition, there are two nucleolytic enzymes, ribonuclease and deoxyribonuclease. Produced in the ribosomes of the acinar cells, the proteases are encased in lipid membranes by the golgi apparatus and secreted into the pancreatic ductules as inactive precursors. In the duodenum trypsinogen is activated to trypsin by enterokinase in the presence of calcium. Trypsin, in turn, initiates the hydrolysis of ingested proteins, activates other proteolytic enzymes, and autocatalyzes the conversion of inactive trypsinogen into trypsin. The proteases, thus released, hydrolyze the ingested proteins to dipeptides and amino acids. Hydrolysis of dipeptides to amino acids is completed by dipeptidases of the intestinal mucosal cells. Approximately 70 to 80 per cent of dietary proteins are digested and absorbed by the time they reach the ileum.

(2) The pancreatic lipolytic enzymes consist of lipase, phospholipases A and B and cholesterol esterase. Emulsification of dietary fat, ingested mainly as water-insoluble triglycerides, is achieved by bile salts aided by lysolecithin; the latter is derived from the action of pancreatic lecithinase-A on the dietary and biliary lecithins. Pancreatic lipase, working at the water-lipid interfaces, hydrolyzes triglycerides to diglycerides and fatty acids. with liberation of glycerol. Monoglycerides, which constitute 70 to 75 per cent of the hydrolyzed fat, are then incorporated into the bile salt micelles and transported across the mucosa by mechanisms incompletely understood. Chey et al. suggest that in addition to causing lipolysis, pancreatic secretions may also assist in the absorption of fatty acids.[21] Digestion and absorption of specific dietary lipids are discussed in Chapter 4.

(3) The amylolytic component of pancreatic juice, alpha amylase, hydrolyzes starch to oligosaccharides, disaccharides and small amounts of monosaccharides. Further hydrolysis of disaccharides is accomplished by the disaccharidases of the intestinal mucosal cells.

COMPENSATORY DIGESTIVE MECHANISMS IN PANCREATIC INSUFFICIENCY

The reserve potential of the digestive system is well appreciated. Davenport has made the point that fat malabsorption is clinically recognized in only 15 per cent of subjects with impaired pancreatic secretions and that pancreatic trypsin may be reduced by 90 per cent or more before malabsorption becomes apparent.[18] Kalser et al. found completely normal fat assimilation in a patient with 75 per cent pancreatectomy.[22] Several other workers have observed that frank steatorrhea occurs only occasionally even in patients with long-standing pancreatic disease.[2,4,23] In the absence of pancreatic enzymes, a number of alternative digestive mechanisms may contribute to normal digestion. Digestion of dietary starch may be carried out by the salivary and the intestinal mucosal amylases. Limited lipolysis may be accomplished by the human gastric juice independent of the influence of acid or regurgitated duodenal contents.[24] Lipase is also present in desquamated mucosal cells but its physiologic role is not understood. One class of dietary fats, the medium-chain triglycerides (MCT), can be absorbed without prior lipolysis.[25]

Of the dietary proteins, 10 to 15 per cent may be hydrolyzed to amino acids in the stomach. In dogs 22 to 85 per cent of the ingested proteins can be absorbed in the total absence of pancreatic secretions. Following total pancreatectomy, 46 and 62 per cent of 75 gm of proteins fed daily were absorbed by a patient described by Davenport.[18] Thus overt malabsorption in patients with chronic pancreatic disease is relatively infrequent because of an impressive reserve capacity of the pancreas and the presence of a number of compensatory digestive mechanisms.

DIAGNOSIS OF PANCREATIC INSUFFICIENCY

Patients with pancreatic insufficiency may present themselves with either the symptoms of pancreatic inflammation or those of the consequent digestive disturbances. Symptoms suggestive of both may coexist, but it is uncommon for pain, steatorrhea, diabetes and pancreatic calcification to be present all in the same patient.[2] One thus has to demonstrate maldigestion in patients with obvious pancreatic disease (characteristic pain and hyperamylasemia with the background of alcoholism, biliary calculi or other predisposing causes) or, conversely, to establish the presence of pancreatic disease in patients with obvious malabsorption (weight loss, diarrhea, steatorrhea, etc.). Steatorrhea, however, may not be obvious even when pancreatic lipolysis is impaired;[26] it is completely obscured in patients who avoid dietary fat for relief from diarrhea and flatulence. Nutritional deficiency in such patients may be attributed erroneously to alcoholism, undernutrition, occult neoplasm or to other un-

related causes. Error can also be made in assuming that malabsorption in patients with pancreatic disease is always exclusively the consequence of pancreatic dysfunction. Indeed in the alcoholic patient defect in absorption may frequently result from subclinical protein malnutrition[27,28] or from bile salt abnormalities,[29-31] or from other digestive disturbances that often accompany alcoholism.[32,33] Consideration must also be given to other diagnostic possibilities, such as defects of the small bowel, metabolic and endocrine disorders and postoperative states, all of which can impair absorption with or without pancreatic disease.[20,26,34] Thus, lactase deficiency may complicate pancreatic dysfunction in cystic fibrosis[35] and render patients refractory to usual therapy. Steatorrhea in diabetics may suggest pancreatic insufficiency in patients who, in fact, have celiac disease or bacterial overgrowth due to reduced intestinal motility.[34] Special laboratory tests are invaluable in defining the pathophysiology and for objective assessment of therapy.

The tests listed in Table 28C-1 are available at most hospitals and are well standardized and therefore readily interpretable. They do not measure the secretory capacity of the pancreas; instead they help to demon-

Table 28C-1. Tests Commonly Used for Differential Diagnosis of Malabsorption

Test	Findings in Pancreatic Insufficiency
(1) Stool Examination:[36]	Gross: pale bulky, loose and greasy. Microscopic: >10 meat fibers per coverslip. >6 fat globules per low power field (>8 globules after acid and heating).
Chemical analysis[37-39]	>2.5 gm Nitrogen per day. >5-7 gm Fat per day.
(2) Serum Carotene	<50 μg/100 ml (<20 μg/100 ml usually in small bowel malabsorption)[40]
(3) Fasting blood sugar and glucose tolerance test	Diabetic curve in about 66% of patients.[41]
(4) D-xylose test (with 25 gm oral D-xylose)	>4.5 gm excretion of D-xylose in 5-hour urine collection (decreased in small bowel diseases and bacterial overgrowth syndromes).
(5) Upper gastrointestinal roentgen examination with small bowel follow-through	Normal small bowel pattern. (Pancreatic calcification and extrinsic duodenal abnormalities in relation to the head of the pancreas may sometimes be present)

strate pancreatic pathologic condition indirectly by characterizing the digestive disturbance. In pancreatic disease, both fat and nitrogen contents of stool increase since isolated enzyme deficiency is rare. This finding serves to distinguish pancreatic disease from bile salt abnormalities in which only fat is malabsorbed.[20] Fecal fat determination quantitates the degree of fat malabsorption, while the D-xylose test and upper gastrointestinal radiography with or without small bowel biopsy help to exclude lesions of the small bowel. Serum carotene measurement is a relatively insensitive test but continues to be used primarily because of the ease with which it can be performed. Simple microscopic examination of the stool with the patient on a diet containing 75 to 100 gm of fat per day is still useful in screening for steator-

rhea. Drummey *et al.* found definite microscopic evidence of increased fecal fat in 75 per cent of patients with 6 to 10 per cent and in 94 per cent of patients with 11 to 15 per cent fecal excretion of the dietary fat.[42] Moore *et al.* using slightly different technique found a lower percentage of positive results, but concluded that this method compared favorably with other screening techniques.[36]

In addition to the above techniques a number of others are sometimes employed for evaluating pancreatic function (Table 28C-2). Their routine use is limited at present.[43,44]

Other tests which do not measure digestive disturbance but help indirectly by establishing or excluding the presence of pancreatic disease include measurement of sweat electrolytes (increased in cystic fibrosis), operative or duodenoscopic pancreatography, selective ar-

Table 28C-2. Other Tests for Malabsorption and Pancreatic Dysfunction

Test	Findings in Pancreatic Insufficiency
(1) Stool Enzymes	—Trypsin: <20 μg/gm of stool[45] —Chymotrypsin: <74 μg/gm of stool[45] or <165 units/kg body weight/24 hrs.[46] *Note:* Positive results more frequent in cystic fibrosis.[43] Enzymes get partially bound to insoluble debris in ileum.[47]
(2) Serum Enzymes[23] (Evocative test)	—Peak serum amylase value of >159 units or a rise in serum amylase by >72 units following secretin/pancreozymin stimulation. *Note:* Positivity reflects ductal obstruction. Percent positivity varies widely from series to series.[48]
(3) Analysis of Duodenal Contents following Secretin (1 unit/kg body weight, I.V.) stimulations.[49]	—Total volume: <2 ml/kg body weight —Bicarbonate concentration: <90 mEq/liter —Total amylase: <6 units/kg body weight. *Note:* The only test directly measuring pancreatic exocrine function. —Reagents vary in potency requiring extensive standardization possible only at specialized laboratories.[43] —Various modifications include "augmented secretin test,"[50,51] use of Pancreozymin[52] with determination of total protein output,[44,53] use of test meal instead of hormones,[54,55] use of inert markers to assess accuracy of collection[51] and cytologic studies on the apirate.
(4) Tests using labeled fats (administered orally) [131]I Triolein and ^{131}I oleic acid	—Normal serum radioactivity with oleic acid but low with Triolein —High stool radioactivity after Triolein. (5–5.6% of ingested dose).[36,56] *Note:* Measurement of fecal radioactivity is considered better than that of blood. However, studies comparing this method with the chemical fat determination show widely variable correlations.[36,57,58]

teriography, scintiscanning and serum carcinoembryonic antigen determination (positive results are found in 85 per cent of patients with pancreatic cancer).[59,60]

TREATMENT OF PANCREATIC INSUFFICIENCY

Nutrition in Acute Pancreatitis. Proper alimentation of patients with acute pancreatitis is essential and often difficult. This is specially so when the inflammation is prolonged or is complicated by pseudocyst or abscess formation. Pre-existing nutritional deficiencies, attendant nausea and vomiting and massive loss of fluid, electrolytes and albumin in the inflammatory exudate constitute a heavy metabolic load. Nasogastric suction further compounds the nutritional problem. Attempts to meet this metabolic demand must be made through the parenteral route and replacements made in proportion to the losses incurred.[61,62] Rehydration is monitored by skin turgor, moistness of tongue, urine output, hematocrit and occasionally by central venous pressures. Sodium and potassium lost in vomiting and calcium lost by precipitation as soaps of fatty acids and by other mechanisms[62,63] have to be replaced according to the clinical and electrocardiographic signs and the serum levels. Initial hematocrit is usually high due to hemoconcentration. If on rehydration it falls to anemic levels as in acute hemorrhagic pancreatitis or in pancreatitis complicated by gastrointestinal hemorrhage whole blood should be transfused.[64] Infusion of colloids, *e.g.* albumin or plasma, may be indicated if the hematocrit is adequate, but the attack is severe, prolonged or complicated by exudative ascites or drop in the level of serum albumin. Elliott *et al.* have shown that prompt and adequate replacement of colloid losses may be life-saving during a fulminant attack of pancreatitis.[65] The use of systemic protease inhibitors, *e.g.* Trasylol, however, continues to be disputed.[66,67] It has not been shown to change the course of disease once the necroinflammatory activity is established. Rosenberg *et al.* suggest that Trasylol in the dosage of 150,000 to 320,000 units per day,

given by the intravenous route early in the course of disease, may be useful.[68]

Impairment of carbohydrate metabolism is encountered in almost all patients with acute pancreatitis but it is transient and only rarely requires treatment with insulin.[69]

Nutrition in the Phase of Recovery. The average patient with uncomplicated pancreatitis is free from pain, nausea and vomiting usually within 2 to 3 days on a regimen consisting of intravenous alimentation and nasogastric suction with or without anticholinergics and/or antibiotics.[1] By this time normal bowel sounds return and serum amylase too declines to normal range. The nasogastric tube is clamped now for about 12 hours and gastric acids are neutralized by hourly administration of an antacid. If the patient continues to be asymptomatic the tube may be removed and an "ulcer-type" diet started. Diets rich in protein and fat which stimulate pancreatic secretion should be avoided in preference to carbohydrates.[70] By the end of the first week most patients are able to tolerate a 6 meal bland diet.

Nutrition in Patients with Acute Complications. When acute illness persists longer than a few days with persistent or recurrent elevation in serum amylase, continued abdominal pain and ileus or when cessation of nasogastric suction is followed by return of symptoms, the presence of a complication such as pancreatic abscess, pseudocyst or obstruction to main pancreatic ducts is suspected. Oral feeding has then to be curtailed for longer periods of time and nutrition has to be maintained by the intravenous route; total parenteral nutrition may be necessary (Chapter 36).

Treatment of Chronic Pancreatic Insufficiency. The object of therapy in such patients is to prevent further damage to the pancreas, forestall further attacks of acute inflammation, alleviate pain, treat steatorrhea and correct malnutrition. Large meals must be avoided; the frequency of attacks may be reduced by substituting for these frequent small feedings of a low-fat diet. All gastric stimulants such as coffee, tea, spices and condiments should be avoided. Specific treatment of pancreatic maldigestion consists of manipulation of the diet and enzyme replacement therapy. A number of complete and supplementary synthetic diets and formulas are available (see Appendix, Tables A-23, A-26). They may substitute for regular diet in the subacute phase of the disease or supplement the restricted diet recommended for patients with chronic pancreatitis. MCT-containing diets (*e.g.* Portagen) low in lactose may be particularly useful in patients with cystic fibrosis complicated by lactase deficiency.

Protein absorption can be readily increased by increasing protein intake. The same, however, is not true for dietary fat which, when undigested, causes flatulence and diarrhea. Fat intake must be restricted to 50 to 70 gm a day or less and protein and carbohydrate correspondingly increased to as much as 120 and 450 gm respectively.[5] Appropriate dietary patterns are given in the Appendix, Table A-19.

To improve fat absorption, two approaches may be used:

Enzyme Replacement Therapy. Desiccated extracts of porcine and bovine pancreas (pancreatin, pancrelipase) are commercially available as tablets, powder or capsules.[71] The active ingredients are contained either in the core of enteric coated tablets or in the form of acid-resistant granules. Giulian *et al.* tested the in vitro lipolytic activity of 15 commercial preparations, and found greatest activity in Cotazym (Organon), Lipan (Spirt & Co.), Panteric granules (Parke, Davis and Co.) and Viokase (Vio Bin Corp.).[72] The usual daily dose of 10 to 20 gm may be given in 3 divided doses with or immediately after meals.[73] Jordan and Grossman found better therapeutic results by administering 0.66 gm of Viokase every hour for 12 hours every day.[74] Kalser *et al.*, however, did not find any advantage of hourly doses over conventional thrice-daily doses.[22] Schneider *et al.* recommended that the powder be sprinkled directly on the food immediately before eating.[75] Therapeutic results can sometimes be improved by the addition of antacids, *e.g.* bicarbonate or aluminum hydroxide gel, to the regimen. The antacids prevent gastric inactivation of pancreatic supplements[76] and, in the absence of pancreatic bicarbonate, restore optimum *p*H in the duodenum for the action of pancreatic enzymes. Knill-

Jones *et al.* found that fat absorption could be significantly improved by the addition of proteolytic enzymes from pineapple stem (bromelains) to the pancreatic extract (Nutrizym, Merck).[77] However, bromelains given alone did not improve fat absorption in patients with pancreatic insufficiency. Varying opinions regarding the ideal enzyme preparation, dose requirements and administration schedule presumably arise from both differences in methods of assessment and variability among the patients. The studies of Kalser and Warren and their colleagues[22,73] provide ample justification for initiating therapy in all patients with 1 to 2 gm of pancreatic extract (*e.g.* Viokase) administered thrice daily with meals. The regimen may then be modified according to individual patient's response.

Use of Medium-Chain Triglycerides. Medium-chain triglycerides (MCT) are neutral lipids which contain fatty acid molecules with chain lengths varying from 6 to 12 carbon atoms. Substantial quantities of such lipids may be hydrolyzed in the stomach and the intestine in the absence of pancreatic lipase. Small quantities of MCT enter the mucosal cells without prior hydrolysis.[25] Substitution of dietary fat by MCT in patients with pancreatic insufficiency may relieve steatorrhea and lead to gain in weight.[25,78] References regarding preparations and administration of MCT can be found in Chapter 28, Section B on diseases of the intestines. To avoid monotony fish, chicken and lean meat may be included in the menu several times a week within the limits of toleration for long-chain triglycerides. Inclusion of other low-fat foods, such as apples, bananas, lettuce, celery and rice, may further improve the palatability of the diet.[79] The usual side effects of MCT, namely nausea, vomiting, abdominal distention, cramps and diarrhea, seen in about 10 per cent of the patients, can be avoided by initiating therapy with small supplements of a palatable preparation. Use of MCT is contraindicated in patients with cirrhosis of the liver, especially when complicated by encephalopathy.[25,79]

Diabetes Mellitus in Association with Pancreatic Disease.[69] Almost all patients with acute pancreatitis have impaired glucose tolerance with glycosuria in about 11 per cent. This abnormality is transient and may represent the combined effect of several factors including (a) increased glycogenolysis resulting from increased serum amylase activity, (b) increased insulin degradation and (c) general reaction of the body to stress. Specific treatment in the acute phase is seldom necessary. In patients with chronic pancreatitis the incidence of diabetes mellitus varies from 13 per cent in those without calcification to 45 per cent in those with. It is usually mild and labile and is only rarely complicated by retinopathy or glomerulosclerosis.

Mild carbohydrate intolerance may be controlled by low-carbohydrate diet with or without oral antidiabetic drugs. If the above fails, therapy with insulin is indicated. Strict precautions against insulin overdose are necessary, especially in the alcoholic patient, for death from irreversible hypoglycemia is well documented in such individuals.[41]

MANAGEMENT OF SPECIFIC CONDITIONS

Alcohol-Induced Pancreatitis. Chronic pancreatitis is usually associated with excessive consumption of alcohol.[1,3-5,80,81] A number of pathogenetic mechanisms have been postulated including (a) stimulation of pancreatic secretion with obstruction to the outflow,[82,83] (b) direct toxicity of ethanol to pancreatic parenchyma,[84-86] (c) regurgitation of infected duodenal contents[87] and (d) malnutrition.[23,27] Strict avoidance of alcohol is recommended since this alone may reduce the frequency of painful attacks in such patients. However, the damage caused by alcoholic pancreatitis is irreversible and "no degree of repentance" can "resolve the original sin" (Spiro).[81] Diet and enzyme therapy for chronic pancreatic insufficiency have been described above. In addition, supplements of folic acid and thiamin which are poorly absorbed in alcoholic patients[88,89] and of other B vitamins and ascorbic acid which may be deficient on account of reduced dietary intake should be prescribed. Other alcohol-related problems[32,33] that may contribute to nutritional depletion should be simultaneously diagnosed and treated.

Protein-Calorie Malnutrition. There is convincing evidence in the literature that both exocrine and endocrine pancreatic insufficiency may occur in association with protein-calorie malnutrition (Chapter 21). Pancreas of rats fed ethionine (thus functionally methionine deficient) develop marked acinar atrophy and fibrosis, and secrete diminished amounts of trypsin, chymotrypsin and lipase.[90] Tandon et al. have reported reversible impairment of pancreatic exocrine functions in patients taking protein-deficient diets.[91] Clinical examples of "trophopathic pancreopathy"[92] are also seen in children with kwashiorkor[93] and in adults with alcoholism.[27] Shaper has suggested that if malnutrition is prolonged the reversible functional changes may be followed by extensive fibrosis and calcification within the pancreas.[7] Pancreatic calcification has indeed been reported in 6 to 13.3 per cent of young diabetic patients from areas of the world where chronic protein-calorie malnutrition is common.[94]

Therapy is directed to correction of nutritional deficiencies. Complete clinical recovery may be achieved in a period of 12 to 14 weeks by feeding patient a diet providing 50 calories per kg body weight, containing 1.5 gm per kg of protein, 80 gm of fat and the remainder of carbohydrates.[91] Supplements of iron and vitamins may be given as needed. Specific therapy with enzymes and/or insulin is indicated only in patients with irreversible pancreatic damage. Infections, especially tuberculosis and malaria, parasitic infestations and cirrhosis, when present, must also be treated.

Pancreatitis with Biliary Calculi. The dramatic onset of pancreatitis due to biliary calculi leads to its prompt diagnosis and management; this probably accounts for the low incidence of associated chronic pancreatic insufficiency.[81,95] Careful exclusion of biliary tract disease is mandatory in all patients with acute pancreatitis. Contrast studies should best be done 4 to 6 weeks after the acute attack after pancreatic edema and transient liver function abnormalities have subsided.

SURGICAL CONDITIONS

Postgastrectomy Patients (Chapter 28A). Surgery of the upper gastrointestinal tract occasionally results in uncovering of latent defects in absorption or in the de novo appearance of malabsorption.[20,34] This may be a consequence either of inadequate mixing of chyme with the enzymes or of diminished secretion of the enzymes due to interruption of normal physiologic stimuli, *e.g.* low acid, resected antrum, bypass of duodenum, etc.[96] Diagnostic possibilities are multiple and in addition to pancreatic insufficiency include undernutrition due to small stomach, dumping syndrome, afferent loop dysfunction,[97] inadvertent gastroileostomy and unmasked gluten enteropathy. Pancreatic dysfunction, when suspected, must be confirmed by laboratory tests. Conservative therapy for pancreatic insufficiency often fails,[98] necessitating surgical procedures to restore normal digestive anatomy and physiology.

Patients with Pancreatic Resection. Patients with massive pancreatic resection frequently develop both exocrine and endocrine insufficiencies and thus require treatment for maldigestion, as well as diabetes mellitus.[22,73] Requirements of patients vary according to the proportion of pancreas resected, the state of the remaining pancreas and associated conditions. Therapy should thus be individualized using glucose tolerance and fat absorption as guidelines.

Cystic Fibrosis. Pancreatic insufficiency is a common consequence of cystic fibrosis, seen mostly in children and sometimes in young adults. There is widespread involvement of the exocrine glands but the principal manifestations occur in the respiratory and the digestive systems.[35] Diagnosis is established by demonstration of increased chloride in sweat. Meticulous therapy for bronchiolar abnormalities with aerosols, mucolytic agents and antibiotics is essential to prevent morbidity and mortality from recurrent infections.[99] The nutritional abnormalities are mainly secondary to pancreatic insufficiency but may sometimes be complicated by small bowel malabsorption and hepatic abnormalities. Treatment with high-protein, low-fat diet with adequate supplements of fat-soluble vitamins and enzyme preparations often helps. The dose requirement of pancreatic enzymes is relatively high in the range of 0.1 to 0.3 gm pancreatin/kg body weight per day.[71] Disaccharidase (mainly lactase) deficiency may coexist requiring elimination of milk products from the diet.[35] Good results have been reported with the use of MCT preparations. Portagen which, in addition to having MCT, has a low-lactase content, may be of special value in selected patients.

Zollinger-Ellison Syndrome. Malabsorption in Z-E syndrome probably results from a number of factors:[20,100] (1) The increased acidity may cause an irreversible denaturation of the pancreatic enzymes in the proximal small bowel, (2) low duodenal pH may deconjugate the bile acids and thus impair micellar solubilization of fat, and (3) structural and functional changes of the intestinal mucosa itself may depress absorption. Daily fecal excretion of fat averages 26 ± 3.6 per cent of the dietary intake. Xylose absorption is only slightly depressed and vitamin B_{12} absorption is usually normal. In addition to maldigestion and malabsorption, diarrhea and hypokalemia may result from hypermotility secondary to increased intestinal fluid volumes and increased vagal activity.[34] Alkalinization of duodenal contents may prevent inactivation of pancreatic enzymes[101] but uncontrolled gastrin release by the tumor defeats this effort. Continuous nasogastric suction along with vigorous intravenous alimentation and replacement of fluid and electrocyte losses are necessary to maintain life in the seriously ill patient. Definitive therapy consists of total gastrectomy, or rarely, resection of an isolated pancreatic adenoma.

Pancreatic Cancer. Maldigestion in patients with cancer of the pancreas, specially of the head, generally results from interruption of the flow of pancreatic juice to the duodenum. Steatorrhea seldom occurs presumably because of reduced food intake. Therapy with sufficient dosage of pancreatic enzymes may improve digestion in the pre- and postoperative patient.

BIBLIOGRAPHY

1. Comfort, Gambill, and Baggenstoss: Gastroenterology, 6, 239, 376, 1946.

2. Gambill, Baggenstoss, and Priestley: Gastroenterology, *39*, 404, 1960.
3. Dreiling, Janowitz, and Perrier: *Pancreatic Inflammatory Disease. A Physiologic Approach.* New York, Harper & Row, 1964.
4. Marks, Bank, and Louw: In *Progress in Gastroenterology*, Glass (Ed.). New York, Grune & Stratton, 1968, p. 412.
5. Berk and Guth: Med. Clin. N. Amer., *54*, 479, 1970.
6. Zuidema: Trop. Geogr. Med., *11*, 70, 1959.
7. Shaper: Lancet, *1*, 1223, 1960.
8. Gee Verghese, Pillai, Joseph, and Pitchumoni: J. Ass. Physns., India, *10*, 173, 1962.
9. Veeger, Abels, Hellmans and Niewig: New Engl. J. Med., *267*, 1341, 1962.
10. Editorial: "Releasing Factor" and Vitamin B$_{12}$ Absorption. New Engl. J. Med., *268*, 955, 1963.
11. Jeffries: New Engl. J. Med., *284*, 666, 1971.
12. Toskes, Hansell, Cerda and Deren: New Engl. J. Med., *284*, 627, 1971.
13. Toskes and Deren: J. Clin. Invest., *51*, 216, 1972.
14. Davis: Lancet, *2*, 749, 1961.
15. Biggs and Davis: Lancet, *2*, 814, 1963.
16. Benjamin, Cortell and Conrad: Gastroenterology, *53*, 389, 1967.
17. Balcerzak, Peternel, and Heinle: Gastroenterology, *53*, 257, 1967.
18. Davenport: *Physiology of the Digestive Tract. An Introductory Text.* 2nd ed. Chicago, Year Book Medical Publishers Incorporated, 1966.
19. Isselbacher and Senior: Gastroenterology, *46*, 287, 1964.
20. Wilson and Dietschy: Gastroenterology, *61*, 911, 1971.
21. Chey, Shay, and O'Leary: Gastroenterology, *45*, 196, 1963.
22. Kalser, Leite, and Warren: New Engl. J. Med., *279*, 570, 1968.
23. Fitzgerald, Fitzgerald, Fennelly, McMullin, and Boland: Gut, *4*, 193, 1963.
24. Cohen, Morgan, and Hofman: Gastroenterology, *60*, 1, 1971.
25. Greenberger and Skillman: New Engl. J. Med., *280*, 1045, 1969.
26. Kirsner: Med. Clin. N. Amer., *53*, 1169, 1969.
27. Mezey, Jow, Slavin, and Tobon: Gastroenterology, *59*, 657, 1970.
28. Adibi and Allen: Gastroenterology, *59*, 404, 1970.
29. Kalant: Gastroenterology, *56*, 380, 1969.
30. Rosenberg, Hardison, and Bull: New Engl. J. Med., *276*, 1391, 1967.
31. Gracey, Burke, Oshin, Barker, and Glasgow: Gut, *12*, 683, 1971.
32. Small, Longarini, and Zamcheck: Amer. J. Med., *27*, 575, 1959.
33. Dinoso, Chey, Padow, Rosen, Ottenberg, and Lorber: Amer. J. Gastroent., *56*, 209, 1971.
34. Jeffries, Weser, and Sleisenger: Gastroenterology, *46*, 434, 1964.
35. Di Sant' Agnese: Cystic Fibrosis and Other Genetic Pancreatic Diseases in Childhood. In *The Exocrine Pancreas.* p. 227, Editors, Beck and Sinclair. London, J. & A. Churchill, 1971.
36. Moore, Englert, Bigler, and Clark: Amer. J. Dig. Dis., *16*, 97, 1971.
37. Wallaeger, Comfort, and Osterberg: Gastroenterology, *9*, 272, 1947.
38. Van De Kamer, Huinink, Ten, and Weyers: J. Biol. Chem., *177*, 347, 1949.
39. Wolochow, Broitman, Williams, and Zamcheck: J. Lab. Clin. Med., *65*, 334, 1965.
40. Ingelfinger: In *Year Book of Medicine*, 1967–1968 series, p. 466, Chicago, Year Book Medical Publishers. 1967.
41. Marks and Bank: S. Afr. Med. J., *37*, 1039, 1963.
42. Drummey, Benson, and Jones: New Engl. J. Med., *264*, 85, 1961.
43. Brooks: New Engl. J. Med., *286*, 300, 1972.
44. Hanscom: Med. Clin. N. Amer., *52*, 1483, 1968.
45. Haverback, Dyce, Gutentag, and Montgomery: Gastroenterology, *44*, 588, 1963.
46. Muller, Wisniewski, and Hansky: Aust. Ann. Med., *1*, 47, 1970.
47. Roy, Campbell, and Goldberg: Gastroenterology, *53*, 584, 1967.
48. Shay, Sun, Chey, and O'Leary: Amer. J. Digest. Dis., *6*, 142, 1961.
49. Dreiling: Investigation of Pancreatic Function, In *The Exocrine Pancreas.* p. 154, Eds., Beck and Sinclair. London, J. & A. Curchill, 1971.
50. Hartley, Gambill, and Summerskill: Gastroenterology, *48*, 312, 1965.
51. Lagerlof, Schutz, and Holmer: Gastroenterology, *52*, 67, 1967.
52. Sun: Gastroenterology, *45*, 203, 1963.
53. Hanscom and Littman: Gastroenterology, *45*, 209, 1963.
54. Lundh: Gastroenterology, *42*, 275, 1962.
55. Thaysen, Mullertz, Worning, and Bang: Gastroenterology, *46*, 23, 1964.
56. Wormsley: Gut, *4*, 261, 1963.
57. Cox: Gastroenterology, *44*, 275, 1963.
58. Rufin, Blahd, Nordyke, and Grossman: Gastroenterology, *41*, 220, 1961.
59. Ona, Dhar, Moore, Kupchik, and Zamcheck, Clin. Res. (Abstract), *20*, 463, 1972.
60. Moore, Kupchik, Marcon, and Zamcheck: Amer. J. Digest. Dis., *16*, 1, 1971.
61. Nugent: Med. Clin. N. Amer., *53*, 431, 1969.
62. Banks: Gastroenterology, *61*, 382, 1971.
63. Turner-Warwick: Lancet, *2*, 546, 1956.
64. Elliott: Arch. Surg. (Chicago), *75*, 573, 1957.
65. Elliott, Zollinger, Moore, and Ellison: Gastroenterology, *28*, 563, 1955.
66. Beck, Mekenna, Zylberszac, Solymar, and Eisenstein: Gastroenterology, *48*, 478, 1965.
67. Grozinger, Hollis, and Artz: J.A.M.A., *178*, 652, 1964.
68. Rosenberg and Janowitz: Gastroenterology, *48*, 350, 1965.

69. Williams: *Textbook of Endocrinology*, 4th Ed. Philadelphia, W. B. Saunders Co., 1968.

70. Snodgrass: Diseases of Pancreas, Ch. 334, In *Harrison's Principles of Internal Medicine.* New York, McGraw-Hill Book Co., 1970.

71. Editorial. Today's Drugs: Pancreatic Extracts. Brit. Med. J., 2, 161, 1970.

72. Giulian, Singh, Mansfield, Pairent, and Howard: Ann. Surg., 165, 564, 1967.

73. Warren, Poulantzas, and Kune: Ann. Surg., 164, 830, 1966.

74. Jordan, and Grossman: Gastroenterology, 36, 447, 1959.

75. Schneider, Sammons, and Beale: Brit. Med. J., 2, 735, 1970.

76. Heizer, Cleveland, and Iber: Bull. Hopkins Hosp., 116, 261, 1965.

77. Knill-Jones, Pearce, Batten, and Williams: Brit. Med. J., 4, 21, 1970.

78. Iber, Hardoon, and Sangree: Clin. Res. (Abstract), 11, 185, 1963.

79. Holt: Gastroenterology, 53, 961, 1967.

80. Mayday and Pheils: Med. J. Australia, 1, 1142, 1970.

81. Spiro: In *The Exocrine Pancreas*, p. 212, Eds., Beck and Sinclair. London. J. & A. Churchill, 1971.

82. Gross and Hallenbeck: Gastroenterology, 38, 919, 1960.

83. Pirola and Davis: Aust. Ann. Med., 1, 24, 1970.

84. Janowitz and Bayer: Ann. Int. Med., 74, 444, 1971.

85. Darle, Ekholm and Edlund: Gastroenterology, 58, 62, 1970.

86. Sarles, Lebreuil, Tasso, Figarella, Clemente, Devaux, Fagonde, and Payan: Gut, 12, 377, 1971.

87. McCutcheon: Gut, 9, 296, 1968.

88. Halsted, Griggs, and Harris: J. Lab. Clin. Med., 69, 116, 1967.

89. Tomasulo, Kater, and Iber: Amer. J. Clin. Nutr., 21, 1341, 1968.

90. Libre and McFarland: Proc. Soc. Exp. Biol. Med., 8, 452, 1964.

91. Tandon, Banks, George, Sama, Ramachandran, and Gandhi: Gastroenterology, 58, 358, 1970.

92. Coppo and Cavazzuti: Gastroenterology, 99, 145, 1963.

93. Davies: Lancet, 1, 317, 1948.

94. Ramalingaswami: Lancet, 2, 733, 1969.

95. Sarles, Sarles, Camatte, Muratore, Gaini, Guien, Pastor, and LeRoy: Gut, 6, 545, 1965.

96. Lundh: Gastroenterology, 42, 637, 1962.

97. Wirts and Goldstein: Ann. Intern. Med., 58, 25, 1963.

98. Marks, Bank, and Airth: Gut, 4, 217, 1963.

99. Lobeck: In *The Metabolic Basis of Inherited Disease*, 3rd ed., p. 1605, Eds., Stanbury, Wyngaarden and Fredrickson. New York, McGraw-Hill Book Co., 1972.

100. Moshal, Broitman, and Zamcheck: Am. J. Clin. Nutr., 23, 336, 1970.

101. Vogel, Weinstein, Herskovic, and Spiro: Ann. Intern. Med., 67, 816, 1967.

Chapter

28

Section D Diseases of the Liver

CHARLES S. DAVIDSON

Diet therapy is generally accepted as an important, if not the most important, factor in the management of patients ill with diseases of the liver.[1,2] When one inspects the scientific evidence for this conclusion many data are still wanting, but, until proven otherwise, this form of therapy is advised, as it has stood the test of time and may, in fact, turn out to be as important as it seems. In certain specific instances, alterations of the diet have a proved relationship to some of the complications of liver disease, specifically, to ascites formation and hepatic coma.

The part played by ill-balanced diets and secondary nutritional disorders in the pathogenesis of hepatic diseases in man is presently the center of controversy and experiment.

Everyone seems to agree that malnutrition can and does produce functional, structural and clinical alterations of the liver in kwashiorkor and other types of "fatty" liver. But, many deny that nutritional hepatic injury alone causes cirrhosis in man.

NUTRITIONAL FACTORS IN EXPERIMENTAL LIVER DISEASE IN ANIMALS

The two important liver lesions produced in the experimental animal by feeding an abnormal diet are fatty change and massive necrosis. Both may lead to scarring, usually a typical cirrhosis from fatty liver and so-called postnecrotic scarring from massive hepatic necrosis.[3,4]

Best and his colleagues, in their classic experiments, found that fatty livers developed in pancreatectomized dogs maintained on insulin.[5] It was later shown that this effect was largely, if not entirely, due to a deficiency of the external secretion of the pancreas which failed to promote the proper digestion and absorption of protein and thus of the essential amino acid, methionine. Choline was likewise found to prevent and cure this fatty liver. Methionine was shown to act as a methyl donor, allowing the synthesis of the essential nutrient choline from ethanolamine. A protein-deficient diet or, more particularly, one deficient in methionine and choline will regularly produce fatty liver in experimental animals (chiefly rats) and, if continued long enough, will lead to cirrhosis in most animals. Deficiency of other amino acids and, in some studies, of other substances will also lead to fatty liver, but the most severe fatty liver, and the one most likely leading to cirrhosis, results from protein-choline-methionine deficiency. The place of vitamin B_{12} in fatty liver production is under investigation.

The massive necrosis observed in rats is produced by an entirely different dietary means. The diets usually have been high in protein mostly furnished by torula yeast and have been deficient in sulfur-containing amino acids and vitamin E. In addition, a third factor is necessary to produce this lesion, trace quantities of organic selenium, an element which, in somewhat larger amounts in the diet, will *induce* liver disease.

These lesions have been considered the prototypes of hepatic disease in man, the former resembling the cirrhosis in alcoholics. The massive hepatic necrosis and postnecrotic scarring resemble somewhat, although distantly, the massive hepatic necrosis and so-called postnecrotic cirrhosis or postnecrotic scarring of man.

A note of caution is proper at this time to those eager to transfer concepts based on dietary hepatic disease in rats to the interpretation of hepatic disease in man. Elias has shown that the microscopic structure of the liver of the rat is different from that of man. Moreover, fatty liver in the rat has been produced in many circumstances apparently unrelated to nutritional disturbances. For example, fatty liver has been produced by alcohol ingestion in spite of an adequate diet.

NUTRITIONAL ASPECTS OF LIVER DISEASE IN MAN

Introduction. In man, the following nutritional factors and possibly many others must be considered in the etiology of liver disease: a low-protein diet, which is otherwise adequate in calories (kwashiorkor)[6]; increased iron intake, probably associated with a low-protein diet, seems clearly of primary importance in hemochromatosis and hemosiderosis; toxic substances may produce additional damage if diet is poor (carbon tetrachloride), and some toxic substances in the diet, either resulting from the ingestion of hepatotoxic plants or hepatotoxic fungi, may contribute to the etiology of liver disease.[7] Alcohol can by no means be excluded.[8]

Once the liver is severely damaged, there is no doubt that the general nutritional welfare of the body suffers and the majority of patients with chronic liver disease come to the physician nutritionally bankrupt. Their nutritional disturbances may be multiple, in some cases due to deficient intake from anorexia or caused by altered or impaired digestion and absorption of nutrients or, finally, produced by abnormalities of intermediary metabolism which may occur in established liver disease.

NUTRITIONAL ASPECTS OF VIRAL HEPATITIS

Infectious hepatitis usually refers to a specific disease, transmitted presumably by the fecal-oral route and leading to what is almost always a self-limited disease. Serum hepatitis, although often less severe in onset, seems less often self-limited, but sometimes appears to progress to chronic hepatitis. Together these are called viral hepatitis. It is well to remember that other viruses (*e.g.*, yellow fever), bacteria (*e.g.*, brucellosis), spirochetes (*e.g.*, syphilis), fungi (*e.g.*, histoplasmosis), protozoa (*e.g.*, amebiasis), and helminths (*e.g.*, schistosomiasis) may also cause liver disease. In Western civilizations infectious hepatitis is the most common hepatic disease seen in clinical practice. It affects the young, the healthy and the well-nourished.

Unfortunately, the nutritional aspects of most infectious diseases involving the liver have not been studied, except for infectious and serum hepatitis. These have been studied thoroughly because of their high incidence in military populations. Two broad questions need consideration with regard to these two kinds of hepatitis:

1. Are malnourished, non-immune individuals more liable to infection with these viruses than well-nourished individuals?

2. Does diet therapy affect the course of these diseases?

Few critical studies have been done on rates of infection in malnourishd populations infected with hepatitis. After World War II there were no reports of overwhelming epidemics in prisoner-of-war camps. During the war, the attack rate of infectious hepatitis in well-nourished, meat-eating Indian soldiers was no different from that observed in ill-nourished, vegetarian, Indian soldiers who eschewed meat on religious grounds.

Capps[9] was the first to suggest that convalescence might be prolonged in soldiers with viral hepatitis if food intake was inadequate. The study was a particularly difficult one because wartime conditions made strict control impossible. A later study in which better control was possible indicated that optimal dietary intakes did shorten convalescence, but the effect was not a large one.[10] The food consumed daily by these soldiers provided approximately 40 calories per kg body weight. Protein was about 13 per cent of the calories and fat 30 to 35 per cent. This partition of nutrients is similar to that in the food consumed each day by healthy active soldiers studied by Johnson and Kark.[11]

Dietary Management of Uncomplicated Infectious Hepatitis. The Army experience indicates that the best results are obtained when the full dietary regimen is instituted as soon as possible. Anorexia is a cardinal symptom of infectious hepatitis, particularly in the early stages. During this time, occasionally it may be necessary to feed patients with glucose intravenously pending return of appetite. As soon as appetite has begun to return, simple foods may be eaten as desired, with emphasis on a well-balanced normal diet.

Usually frequent small feedings of attractive meals at regular intervals are best tolerated. Three large meals a day may only serve to make the patient nauseated. Many patients say that during this stage they are hungry, but as soon as they have eaten a little, anorexia and even severe nausea may occur. For these patients, a tasty liquid formula in small quantities at frequent intervals is sometimes well tolerated.

During convalescence from acute hepatitis, a well-balanced, nutritious, mixed diet contains all the essential nutrients needed. This may be provided by attractive meals served at regular intervals, when the patient is most likely to be hungry, and by interval feedings of milk shakes or eggnogs.

If the above measures do not insure an adequate intake of food, then food may be given by tube feedings (Appendix, Tables A-23, A-27, A-28). Intravenous feedings of glucose will rarely be needed if the patient is urged to eat.

An adequate protein intake of 1 gm/kg body weight or above is usually easily obtained from a well-planned, mixed diet. The protein should come from both animal and vegetable sources. Adequate supplies of protein, choline, inositol, methionine, and other amino acids and vitamins are provided in mixed protein-containing foods, such as meats, fish, eggs, dairy products, and cereals. Amino acid supplements are unnecessary, as digestion and absorption of protein seem satisfactory in this disease. Moreover, supplements of vitamins, choline, inositol, methionine, etc., are also unnecessary unless food intake is drastically altered from normal, as adequate quantities are in a good mixed diet.

In a few susceptible individuals with severe hepatitis, usually those with massive necrosis, high or even normal protein intake may induce the syndrome of hepatic precoma or coma (see below). When protein in normal amounts is poorly tolerated and leads to this syndrome, it is an extremely poor prognostic sign. It is probable that the protein ingested has not further damaged the liver, but only that, because of the severity of the liver disease, it is poorly tolerated by critically ill patients. In this circumstance, the regimen for hepatic coma given below should be carefully followed.

There is no need to restrict fat intake in patients ill with infectious hepatitis, unless it leads to disturbances of digestion. Some patients will have steatorrhea from high-fat diets and even anorexia and nausea may sometimes be produced. High-fat diets are not necessary, but 30 to 40 per cent of the calories per day from fat certainly adds palatability to the diet, carries fat-soluble vitamins, and is generally well tolerated, certainly during convalescence. In general, it is wiser to provide fat through dairy products and egg rather than fried foods and, particularly, fatty meats.

An adequate carbohydrate intake is readily obtained, provided that a well-balanced diet is consumed in accordance with the principles noted above. It has been the custom of many physicians to provide hard candy *ad libitum* to patients ill with infectious hepatitis. This should usually not be done, as sweets, particularly between meals, disturb the appetite and provide an unbalanced source of calories.

In infectious hepatitis the plasma prothrombin level is often reduced. This is usually the result of disturbed liver function. The damaged liver is unable to synthesize prothrombin, and it is therefore unable to use vitamin K. However, intrahepatic biliary obstruction does occur in infective hepatitis, and occasionally the exclusion of bile from the gut will interfere with absorption of vitamin K. Under these conditions, parenteral vitamin K, or oral, water-soluble vitamin K will effectively raise prothrombin levels. In 1940, Kark and Souter showed that the degree of response of prothrombin levels to vitamin K therapy was a good index of hepatic function. This has been accepted as an excellent test of liver functional impairment.

Usually, gross sodium and water retention does not complicate infectious hepatitis. Although it is true that recovery from infectious hepatitis is often ushered in with a diuresis, it is only in the severely ill patient that sodium retention needs to be treated through strict dietary regulation of salt and sodium-containing foods. When this is necessary, the low-salt regimen, prescribed for the treatment of cirrhosis, should be followed.

Liquid Preparations for Complete or Between-Meal Feedings. For supplementary or for complete feeding, palatable liquid formulas may be useful (Appendix, Tables A-23, A-24, A-26).

It should be remembered that formulas high in milk products may be poorly tolerated by some patients. This would be especially true if intestinal lactase deficiency is present. When poorly tolerated the quantity given may be reduced, the mixture somewhat diluted until the patient is able to take the full mixture or low-milk formulas used.

A number of powdered supplementary foods (easily reconstituted by adding water or milk) are marketed. Sustagen or better various "instant breakfasts" are excellent in many respects. They are bland, "balanced" foods fortified with vitamins at a therapeutic level, and cost per gram of protein is not excessive.

The palatability of all these drinks depends to a great extent on the thoroughness of mixing of the preparation. Electric milk-shake mixers are ideal, but hand beaters are satisfactory if used with care and thoroughness. The milk shakes should be made up fresh each day and kept refrigerated from preparation until service.

When low-sodium supplementary or in-between-meal feedings are necessary, a low-sodium drink is suggested (Appendix, Tables A-24, A-27).

When the patient with infectious hepatitis comes under medical care, much of the damage within the liver is done, and diet therapy serves to allow or hopefully to hasten healing and regeneration of the hepatic cells.

There are grave doubts that optimal diet therapy prevents the relentless march to cirrhosis which develops in occasional patients with hepatitis (less than 1 per cent); nor does it seem able to prevent laboratory and clinical relapses. In infancy and childhood, fortunately, infectious hepatitis nearly always runs a benign course.

When infectious hepatitis or serum hepatitis develops in the third trimester of pregnancy, the prognosis for mother and child is less benign, while in the first trimester no ill effects usually ensue provided that treatment is vigorous. Hepatitis which appears during the second trimester of pregnancy is a more serious complication than hepatitis which develops earlier. It is not known whether endocrinologic, metabolic, or nutritional factors are responsible for the malignant nature of hepatitis which occasionally occurs in the terminal stages of pregnancy.

The complications of infectious hepatitis require modifications of dietary management. The most common complications are nausea and vomiting, which may have to be managed with tube feedings or intravenous feedings. The other complication is progression toward severe hepatic insufficiency which requires separate consideration, as indicated under the section Hepatic Coma Syndrome. The dietary management of chronic hepatitis is no different from that of cirrhosis and is discussed below under this heading.

Tube or Gavage Feeding. When anorexia, nausea or vomiting is severe enough to limit caloric intake, tube feeding should be instituted without delay. One of the most significant advances in therapeutics in the past years has been the recognition that thin polyethylene or nylon tubing can be used for gavage feeding of individual patients for weeks at a time, without causing distress to the patient and without damage to the mucous membranes of the upper respiratory or gastrointestinal tract. When once passed, it can usually be left in place. The patient can eat his usual meals without discomfort during the day with the tube in position, and during the night, while he sleeps, a tube feeding can be run into his stomach or duodenum. In pre-coma or in comatose patients, the danger of aspiration pneumonia as a result of regurgitation of stomach contents must be kept in mind.

Intravenous Feeding. The indication for intravenous feeding is vomiting. Intravenous feeding may also be used as a supplement to oral or gavage feeding, especially to supply low-sodium amino acid supplements to low-protein diets. Techniques and formulas for intravenous feeding are given in Chapter 36.

THE HEPATIC COMA SYNDROME

Physicians from Galen's age to ours have recognized a connection between hepatic dysfunction and cerebral function. Kinnear Wilson was the first to describe pathologic lesions of the brain in patients ill with cirrhosis, and histologic abnormalities have been observed in the brains of patients who have died from hepatic coma, which can be stated to be the cause of the neurologic and psychic manifestations of liver disease.

The manifestations of pre-coma and coma have been clarified by various clinical observations.[12–21] Walshe describes as part of the clinical picture of coma: confusion, apathy, personality changes, spasticity, muscle spasms, choreiform movements, athetoid postures, lead pipe and cogwheel rigidity of the arms, flexion withdrawal of the legs, and cholemic crying. Ankle clonus with plantar flexor Babinski responses was rather characteristic.[13]

The neurologic findings are not uncommonly complicated in the alcoholic by delirium tremens; by hemorrhage into the brain as a result of prothrombin or fibrinogen deficiency; by other types of hemorrhagic disturbances, such as scurvy; and by Wernicke's encephalopathy, the result of thiamin deficiency.

The neurologic signs and symptoms of hepatic coma and pre-coma have been observed in Eck-fistula dogs given meat, in patients with portacaval or portarenal shunts, in patients with portal vein occlusion, and in patients with a wide variety of hepatic disorders ranging from Chiari's syndrome to acute hepatitis. In many of these persons, attacks have been precipitated by oral feedings of meat, high-protein diets, casein

hydrolysates, amino acid mixtures, amino acids, ammonium chloride, ammonium citrate, urea, cation exchange resins containing ammonium and particularly after gastrointestinal bleeding.

It also appears that methionine or amino acid mixtures given by mouth will regularly precipitate neurologic signs in some patients ill with liver disease. It has been shown that the administration of oral, broad-spectrum antibiotics will inhibit the neurologic ill effects of protein feeding in patients who are in a state of impending coma. The observations and data on hand suggest that nitrogenous substances from the bowel—presumably the result of bacterial action on protein foods or nitrogenous chemicals—produce the neurologic and mental changes described above. This can occur when blood is shunted directly from the portal system into the systemic system, even in the presence of normal hepatic function—the toxic substance being carried directly from the bowel to the brain (portal-systemic encephalopathy of Sherlock). The hepatic coma syndrome is more commonly seen when the liver is damaged. Presumably the healthy liver detoxifies or utilizes the toxic nitrogenous material as it passes up the portal vein. When the hepatic cells are damaged (anoxia, fatty infiltration, infection, etc.) or when vascular shunts develop within the liver, the toxic nitrogenous materials also pass into the systemic blood stream.

TREATMENT OF HEPATIC COMA AND PRE-COMA

Consumption of an adequate diet with at least normal protein content is recognized as an essential part of the therapy of many forms of liver disease, but may precipitate hepatic pre-coma or coma. In the nutritional therapy of patients with liver disease, the physician and the patient must walk a tightrope. Too much protein may induce hepatic coma, too little protein may even prolong a patient's illness. A proper balance can usually be achieved by careful observation of the patient for the signs of impending coma. Treatment with broad-spectrum antibiotics, such as neomycin, should be instituted when the

syndrome appears. If the syndrome progresses or the patient is first seen when in
coma, protein administration should be
omitted altogether.

At each visit to the sickroom the patient
must be asked to cock up his hands; if the
"flapping tremor" is noted or mental confusion is found, antibiotics should immediately be prescribed. At this stage it is usually
not necessary to reduce the protein content
of the diet; at least not below the Recommended Dietary Allowance of approximately
1 gm per kg of body weight per day.

If the patient cannot eat, nutrition may be
maintained as described above utilizing less
protein.

THE FATTY LIVER

The association of fatty liver with pellagra,
with starvation, with diseases of inanition—
such as ulcerative colitis and tuberculosis—
and with alcoholism is well known. Many
believe that fatty liver is the forerunner of
some forms of dietary cirrhosis, of tropical
cirrhosis, and of alcoholic Laennec's cirrhosis.
The exact progression to cirrhosis from the
fatty liver is still cloaked in mystery. Recent
studies in Africa and elsewhere would seem
to indicate that in man cirrhosis may not
develop as a result of nutritional deficiency
alone (see kwashiorkor below). Should this
be correct, it would seem that cirrhosis
associated with alcoholism and other nutritional disturbances, such as ulcerative colitis,
may not be the result simply of nutritional
deficiency, but could be due to toxic factors
which cause hepatic cellular necrosis, or,
possibly, autoimmune responses which produce further damage.

Workers in several laboratories have recently explored the causes of the alcoholic
fatty liver.[22,23,24] It has been assumed that
the accumulation of fat was on the basis of the
nutritional deficiency so common among
alcoholics. Probably deficiency of nutrients
(protein, choline, methionine) contributes,
perhaps it is most important. The metabolic
effects of alcohol must, however, be considered. Large amounts, acutely given, appear to mobilize fat from adipose tissue to the
liver as do some other stressful situations,
operating through the pituitary and the
adrenals. Lesser amounts, more in keeping
with the usual alcoholic's drinking habits, exert an important effect upon the liver itself,
increasing the synthesis of fat in this organ.
It has been possible, in experimental animals
and in man, to induce fatty change in the
liver when alcohol is substituted for sucrose
in an otherwise adequate diet.[23]

KWASHIORKOR

Until recently, Western physicians did not
recognize that primary malnutrition—due to
an unbalanced diet—produced fatty liver
disease in man as it does in the laboratory
animal. As a result of clinical studies in the
past three decades, it has become clear that
primary, nutritional, fatty liver disease is
widespread in the tropics and is perhaps, after
caloric deficiency, the most common nutritional disease of man.

Kwashiorkor is a disease of widespread
tropical geographic distribution.[6] Patients
with the disease have been found in Central
and South America, Africa, India and South-
east Asia. Occasional instances have been
reported from Europe during famines (Mehlnährschaden). It is rare in the United States.
Kark[25] reported a case in a 10-month-old
Negro child in Chicago in 1950; and Davies,[26]
who examined the collected pathologic material at Duke University in North Carolina
in 1949, found only 1 case among the children
who had been autopsied at Duke University
in the past 20 years. This syndrome is discussed more fully in Chapter 21.

TOXIC HEPATITIS AND CIRRHOSIS

Opie and others have clearly indicated
that the resistance to and repair of hepatic
damage by toxic agents, such as carbon tetrachloride, is enhanced by diet therapy.
Iatrogenic jaundice may be the result of
endocrine therapy (methyl testosterone jaundice), some oral contraceptives, psychochemo-
therapy (chlorpromazine and iproniazid jaundice), and other drugs. Acute toxic hepatitis
should be managed on regimens suitable for
patients with infectious hepatitis, and those

ill with chronic toxic hepatitis or cirrhosis should be treated as are patients with Laennec's cirrhosis.

The development of toxic liver diseases other than those described above has also been related to nutritional factors. Senecio cirrhosis is seen in South Africa. It is the result of eating bread and other foods made from flour contaminated with the crushed seeds of species of *Senecio*, a plant which grows in the wheat fields of the Cape Province. In North America, Senecio poisoning is one cause of cirrhosis in cattle. Selzer[27] and her colleagues have shown that Senecio cirrhosis develops in rats only when the weed is added to an experimental diet poor in protein. An adequate protein intake protects the animals. These experiments may bear on the problem of infantile hepatic necrosis in Indians, and on Jamaican infantile veno-occlusive hepatitis which resembles Senecio cirrhosis and which occurs in weanlings living on low-protein diets and fed decoctions of local plants.

CIRRHOSIS AND FIBROSIS OF THE LIVER[27]

Cirrhosis is a common disease in the tropics, in those who are alcoholics, and occurs occasionally in individuals who have had attacks of hepatitis. It also is part of the pathologic changes in patients suffering from other disorders, such as hemochromatosis, biliary cirrhosis, cholangiolitic jaundice, and hepatolenticular degeneration. It may appear after infection with brucella abortus, spirochetes, and amoebae; after infestation with schistosomes; or as a result of metabolic or cardiac diseases. While diet therapy is used to treat the cirrhosis which develops in all these conditions, outstanding success is not attained in all instances. It is true that many alcoholics with Laennec's cirrhosis can be restored to and kept in good health by diet therapy, provided that they do not drink. Among the remainder, far too many patients with cirrhosis progress slowly or rapidly towards death in hepatic failure, or as a result of rupture of esophageal varices, for us to be too sanguine about the long-term results of present-day diet therapy. Nevertheless, manipulations of diet have constituted a major advance in our attack on the problem. Diet therapy is only one part of the therapeutic regimens found to be of benefit for patients ill with cirrhosis. In essence, the regimen consists of bed rest during acute phases, absolute prohibition of all forms of alcohol, protection of the patient from hepatotoxic drugs and chemicals, and provision of a diet rich in protein, calories, and other nutrients. Salt or sodium restriction is used when necessary. Supplementations to the diet of salt substitutes and intravenous and water-soluble vitamins are made as indicated. Particular attention is paid to actual daily dietary intake, to simple supportive psychotherapy, and to the daily weight of the patient. When specific deficiencies coexist with cirrhosis, the patients should be treated immediately with a good diet and parenteral water-soluble vitamins. After the lesions have gone away, extra vitamins are not necessary to treat the cirrhosis, if a well-balanced diet is consumed each day.

Klatskin and Gabuzda have shown that marked improvement occurs in alcoholic cirrhotic patients even when they are given a minimal dietary regimen, provided alcohol intake is stopped.

Intravenous albumin, methionine, choline, the B complex vitamins, and liver extract do not seem to confer any special benefits.

With regard to the treatment of cirrhosis in alcoholics, preventive teetotalism must be the goal.

Dietary Treatment of Edema and Ascites in Cirrhosis. Hidden water retention, frank edema, and ascites are common complications of cirrhosis.[28] They are usually associated with nutritional, endocrinologic, and secondary metabolic disorders. The signs of malnutrition commonly seen are loss of flesh and a raw, beefy tongue—both due to protein wastage—scurvy, pellagra, cheilosis, and other signs of B complex deficiency. Endocrinologic changes consist in the main of spider nevi, liver palms, loss of libido, testicular and prostatic atrophy, loss of hair on the chest, gynecomastia, and amenorrhea or menorrhagia. These latter findings are related to the lack of production of hormones due to malnutrition and also to the inability of the damaged liver to conjugate and deactivate normally circulating hormones. Metabolic defects are hypoalbuminemia, depressed levels of prothrombin and cholinesterase in the serum, and electrolyte imbalance. The retention of water has been related to raised portal pressure, increased antidiuretic hormone, secondary aldosteronism, hypoalbuminemia, and tissue permeability defects, among others. Restriction of dietary sodium to levels about equal to that lost by the body from the skin, stool, and urine (200 mg per day) prevents further ascites accumulation. Repair of tissue mass is also associated with a slow, steady loss of excess water as the restoration of protein nutrition moves the patient's tissue from depletion towards the normal state. With tissue repair, a long-term, slow, steady diuresis occurs, and eventually the kidney is once again able to handle the sodium load of a normal salt-containing diet.[29,30,31]

Restriction of Sodium. Restriction of sodium has been a most useful procedure in the delivery of ascitic and edema fluid, in preventing the re-accumulation of ascites following paracentesis, and in restoration of tissue in malnourished cirrhotics. The difficulties encountered in therapy are mainly economic, for repair of tissue wasting and restoration of hepatic integrity may take many months. In addition, the diet is made up of expensive protein foods, some of which have to be processed commercially to remove sodium.

With the use of modern diuretics, particularly chlorothiazide and spironolactone, severe restriction may not be necessary at all times, and may in some instances, particularly when a good proportion of the ascites has gone, be harmful. Once the ascites and edema have gone, or are minimal, cautious removal of diuretics can be tried. If this is tolerated without gain in ascites (best measured by gain in weight) sodium can cautiously be added to the diet.

Hidden sources of sodium in intravenously administered plasma and whole blood (sodium citrate) transfusions, in the diet—such as is contained in bread or drinking water which has been artificially softened, or in some oral and parenteral drugs may cause an unexpected re-accumulation of fluid in patients who are "dry."

An instance of the effects of adding sodium to the diet is shown in an experiment on the cirrhosis patient J. D. (Fig. 28D–1) in which 10 gm of salt (170 mEq of sodium) were added each day for three days to his low sodium diet at a time when he was "dry" and when his weight was steady. As a result of this, he gained 5 pounds of weight in four days, and it took a week for him to lose this extra water bound in his body by the excess sodium. The rapid weight gain induced by deliberate salting during therapy with low sodium diets and the length of time required to restore equilibrium are exceedingly useful methods for demonstrating to the individual patient the good effects of a low sodium regimen and the ill effects of straying from the regimen. It may sometimes be wise for the physician to demonstrate to the patient and his family the value of sodium restriction by deliberate salting of diets for short periods of time.

To control the level of sodium intake in the diet, it is necessary to weigh the patient *each day* or to have him weigh himself, preferably the first thing in the morning. These weights should be charted. Rapid gain in body weight means that water is accumulating because of sodium retention and too much sodium in the diet. On the other hand, a slow, steady gain of weight which is associated with clinical improvement is usually due to restoration of tissue mass. Rarely, rapid gain in body water and body weight are the result of "low salt syndrome."

When patients have been on the low-sodium diet for some months and when clinical improvement is obvious, the daily output of sodium in their urine begins to increase and eventually they can return to a diet containing moderate or normal quantities of salt. The decision to increase the amount of sodium in the diet should be implemented by a trial of salt feeding. This must be controlled by daily weighing. If, for example, 5 gm of salt are added each day to the diet and if the weight increases each day at a rapid rate, then the patient has not recovered his ability to excrete sodium and to handle the excess salt. Obviously, he must remain on his low-sodium diet for a further period of therapy until it is considered wise to attempt a second trial of salt feeding. Measurement of 24-hour urinary sodium excretion is worthwhile at this time.

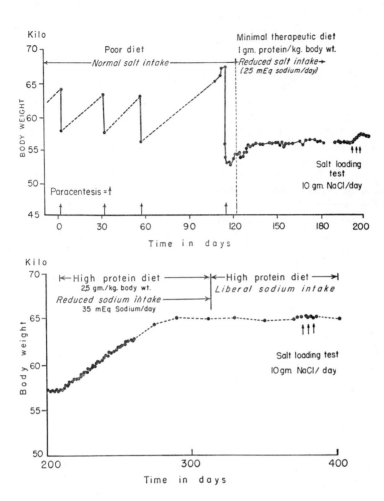

Fig. 28D-1. The effect of various diets on body weight and ascitic fluid accumulation in patient J. D., ill with alcoholism, cirrhosis, and ascites.

1. From day 0 to 110 patient was treated at home by repeated paracenteses. At this time his diet was poor; he had a normal salt intake, and he re-accumulated fluid rapidly.

2. On day 111, a paracentesis was done, and he began to re-accumulate water. He was placed on a minimal therapeutic diet (1 gm of protein per kilogram body weight, and basal plus 150 per cent calories). Sodium was reduced to 25 mEq per day. On this regimen he stopped collecting fluid, but did not gain weight. On day 190 a salt-loading test was started. He was unable to handle sodium, and re-accumulated water.

3. On day 200, the diet was changed by increasing the protein to 2.5 gm per kg body weight per day. This addition of protein raised the sodium intake to 35 mEq per day. On this regimen there was a rapid restoration of body tissue, with reduction in liver size. Spider nevi disappeared. The steady gain in tissue was associated with a concomitant loss of water.

4. On day 310, his regimen was changed to a diet containing liberal amounts of salt. He did not gain water, and on day 376 when a salt-loading test was administered, there was no re-accumulation of water. Restoration of tissue mass and regeneration of liver tissue allowed the kidney to handle sodium normally.

Hazards of Sodium Restriction. Sodium restriction is not without hazard. In those patients in whom chronic renal disease coexists with cirrhosis, the untoward manifestations of severe sodium depletion are the result of high urinary output and failure of the kidneys to reabsorb sodium. In such patients, sodium is removed from the body at a relatively faster rate than water. The blood plasma and extracellular fluid become hypotonic; presumably, the tissues lose potassium; the individual cells are damaged; sodium enters the cell from the extracellular space, and an acute cellular hydration develops. The patient subjected to continued loss of electrolytes becomes weak and lethargic. If the electrolyte loss is not corrected, he becomes confused and may have convulsions. Muscular cramps and pain—especially abdominal pain or cramps—often occur early during the development of the "low salt syndrome." In these patients serum sodium is usually low (below 120 mEq sodium per liter of serum), the blood urea rises and the carbon dioxide-combining power of the plasma drops. The patient eventually dies in uremia, if not treated with hypertonic saline infusions. The exact relation of potassium deficiency to this syndrome has not been clarified.

A similar syndrome has been reported in cirrhotic patients who, while living on a low-salt diet, are treated with diuretics or repeated paracenteses. These patients do not suffer from chronic renal disease. In them repeated diuresis and paracentesis deplete the body stores. Patients undergoing frequent paracentesis repeatedly "bleed" electrolytes and water (an ultrafiltrate of plasma) into the peritoneal cavity. If water is replaced without sodium, cellular overhydration with generalized hypotonicity of body fluids develops and a "low salt syndrome" appears.

Restoration of the salt balance of cirrhotic patients rarely needs to be vigorous. Moderate hyponatremia is frequent and, although not ideal, is not accompanied by dire effects. When sodium depletion or overhydration has been rapid in onset, related to renal disease, over-vigorous diuresis or paracentesis, therapy is sometimes necessary, particularly if symptoms related to this state appear.

Restriction of water intake to 1 to 1.5 liters per day frequently will suffice. In critical situations parenteral infusion of hypertonic saline is necessary. Fluid intake must be restricted when hypertonic saline solution is given.

In view of the dangers of salt depletion, it is most important to test renal function before initiating low-sodium diet therapy in cirrhosis. When the dietary regimen is started, measurements of nonprotein nitrogen—and, when possible, plasma carbon dioxide-combining power and serum sodium and potassium—should be made at least once a week for the first few weeks after treatment has been instituted. The physician should watch for the development of cramps, abdominal pain, or unusual drowsiness.

If renal function is moderately disturbed, salt restriction may be instituted, but starting rather cautiously and allowing an initial intake of between 50 and 60 mEq of sodium per day, thereafter increasing or decreasing the sodium intake as indicated by changes in body weight, urine output, the clinical conditions of the patients, and biochemical data.

Nutrient Intake With Low-Sodium Diet.[32] Most patients ill with cirrhosis, and especially those who have ascites, show the ill effects of long-continued protein and caloric starvation. In them, part of the cellular protein has been replaced by water and possibly by electrolytes. This chronic cellular waterlogging may be clinically occult, but contributes to edema and ascites when they develop. With low-sodium and high-protein intakes even non-edematous patients deliver water and salt and lay down tissue protein. Moreover, patients ill with cirrhosis and ascites frequently improve on a diet which is "well balanced" by present concepts, and provides 1 gm of protein per kg of body weight. Sample low sodium diets are given in the Appendix (Table A-10).

When a nutritionally well-balanced, low-sodium, adequate protein diet is offered and consumed day after day by the cirrhotic patient, supplementation of the diet with choline, methionine, and vitamins is not necessary. In our hands, intravenous injection of liver extracts has not been of value in the management of cirrhotic patients. Its exact usefulness awaits further evaluation. When patients with cirrhosis present themselves initially for examination, they are often ill with vitamin deficiency syndromes, but these are not as commonly seen now as in the prewar years. When deficiency states are noted, treatment with water-soluble vitamins should be vigorous. It is our custom, when we diagnose vitamin deficiencies in our cirrhotic patients, to give a B complex vitamin mixture, or an intramuscular injection of a water-soluble B complex mixture, once a day for several days or until the patient is eating well.

Many alcoholics, especially those with liver disease, are deficient in folic acid, judging from the megaloblastic anemia which responds to folic acid[33] and the low blood levels of this vitamin which have been found.[34] Thus, folic acid should be given not only when it is proven to be deficient, but always should be included in the vitamin B complex mixture used. It is important to note that many manufactured vitamin B complex mixtures do not contain folic acid because of its masking effect in pernicious anemia. Folic acid must then be given separately.

To replace the taste of salt which is missing in the diet, patients may use a salt substitute. This may be sprinkled *ad libitum* over the food, as it contains no sodium. Recently, we have used two sodium-free glutamic acid flavoring agents, ammonium glutamate and calcium glutamate. These condiments certainly add zest to low-sodium diets. A few drops of lemon squeezed on meat add much to the flavor.

NUTRITIONAL ASPECTS OF BILIARY TRACT DISEASE

Onions and French fried potatoes, and other cooked fatty foods, are anathema to most patients who are dyspeptic and who also suffer from chronic cholecystitis, biliary stones, or other disease involving the biliary tract. This is not surprising, since a number of nutrients affect the quality and quantity of bile, the motility of the gallbladder, and the tone of the sphincter of Oddi. Moreover, the bile is essential for proper absorption of fats, fat-soluble vitamins, and a number of hormones and metabolic substances which cycle

through the enterohepatic circulation during consumption and digestion of food.[31,38] However, it is surprising to find that only 5 to 10 per cent of patients with gallstones are dyspeptic.

Effects of Diet on the Biliary Tract and Bile. High-protein diets and, to a lesser extent, high-fat diets increase bile production. Dehydration and high-carbohydrate diets decrease bile formation. Fatty food cholagogues—such as cream, egg yolk, and olive oil—cause the sphincter of Oddi to relax and initiate contraction of the gallbladder. This process is thought to be initiated by food through the hormone cholecystokinin, which is released from the upper intestinal wall into the blood stream and is carried to the gallbladder and sphincter of Oddi. Thus, at mealtimes a store of gallbladder bile is released into the duodenum when it is most needed to help in the digestion and absorption of fats.

Many clinicians suspect that aberrations of this mechanism are responsible for initiating biliary or pancreatic disorders. It has been postulated that, following large meals high in fat and protein, the gallbladder may contract against an unrelaxed sphincter of Oddi (achalasia of the sphincter of Oddi) or against a spastic sphincter of Oddi (biliary dyskinesia). This may result in acute or recurrent biliary colic, and obstructive jaundice may develop. If an anomalous pancreatic duct opens directly into the biliary duct, then, when the situation described above develops, bile may regurgitate into the pancreas, and acute or relapsing chronic pancreatitis may ensue.

Nutrition and the Development of Gallstones and Cholecystitis.[39,40,41] Recent studies have clearly demonstrated that neither bile nor gallstones nor gallbladder wall from patients with gallstones or cholecystitis is infected with organisms. This and other investigations strengthen the concept that cholecystitis is not an infectious disease, but is the result of a chemical inflammation of the wall of the gallbladder. Thus it seems that the genesis of cholecystitis and gallstones (except pigment stones resulting from hemolytic phenomena) must be sought in that rather vague but important field of medical endeavor which relates body build, race, and other genetic factors to environmental, endocrinologic, and nutritional abnormalities. Cholecystitis—and in particular, gallstones—varies in incidence from country to country; appears to be high in those who live on a high-calorie, high-fat diet; is rarely seen among the Japanese; is common in Jewish people; appears in families and in the obese and fair; becomes troublesome at the menopause; and occurs more commonly in females than in males. The development of cholecystitis and gallstones appears to be related to cardiovascular disease, to familial hypercholesterolemia, to pancreatic disease, and to diabetes.

While there is no proof at present that dietary habits are the prime cause of cholecystitis and gallstones, the data collected thus far are highly suggestive. What is needed are world-wide studies on the incidence of gallbladder diseases in populations consuming different diets—studies which would be similar to those made in different parts of the world which relate degenerative heart disease with high-fat diets and high blood cholesterol levels.

Dietary Management of Patients with Dyspepsia, Gallstones, and Cholecystitis.[42, 43] A cholesterol-free diet cannot be regarded as a means of preventing gallstones. On the other hand, prescription of a low fat-containing diet is a time honored dietary regimen for patients with chronic flatulent dyspepsia who have, in addition, physical signs or radiologic evidence of chronic cholecystitis or gallstones. Greasy or fried foods, eggs, mayonnaise, salad dressings, cheese and pork products, and high fat-containing pastries rich in cream or suet should be avoided. Many patients recognize that they cannot tolerate onions, sauerkraut, cabbage, radishes, turnips, cucumbers, and spicy foods such as chili con carne and curry. Vegetable fats, such as olive oil or corn oil which are rather unsaturated, seem to be beneficial when the gallbladder is functioning normally, as they stimulate bile flow. Their employment in the regimen must depend on the patient's ability to tolerate them.

When acute cholecystitis develops, no fried food should be given by mouth, and the patient may need to be fed parenterally. Immediately after an acute attack, the diet should be limited to small amounts of carbohydrate foodstuffs such as fruit juices, pureed potatoes, rice, and tapioca. Later, more solid cereals can be added, together with skim milk, broiled fish, and lean broiled meats. Non-fat white chicken or turkey meat may also be employed.

Chronic Obstructive Jaundice. Chronic obstructive jaundice is most commonly seen as a result of postoperative traumatic stricture of the bile ducts, congenital lesions of the bile ducts, undetected calculi, carcinoma of the pancreas or hepatic ducts, cysts in the head of the pancreas, biliary cirrhosis, and cholangiolitis.[45] In all these lesions, the nutrition and metabolism of the body are disturbed by acholia. In essence, the main pathophysiological disturbance is steatorrhea with resulting malnutrition due to loss of calories, fat-soluble vitamins, and minerals. Loss of dietary calories raises the demand for calories from protein sources, with resultant development of fatty liver and impaired production of plasma proteins. Medium-chain triglycerides permit better fat absorption and, hence, more calories. Failure to absorb vitamin K produces prothrombin deficiency, manifested by needle puncture hematomata, spontaneous bruising, and a hemorrhagic tendency. The loss of calcium and vitamin D produces osteomalacia, with demineralized bone, kyphosis, fractures, collapse of vertebrae, and herniation of the intervertebral disc into the vertebral bodies (Schmorl's nodes). In addition, osteoporosis may be present, perhaps due to protein deficiency and reduced steroid output as a result of malnutrition. Vitamin A deficiency produces night blindness and hyperkeratosis, while failure of absorption of unsaturated fatty acids may result in eczematous-like skin lesions. Vitamin E deficiency may produce muscle weakness.[46] Loss of potassium may cause potassium nephropathy, atony of the bowel, and typical muscle weakness.

Prevention of the ill effects of chronic obstructive jaundice consists of providing a regimen sufficient in calories and rich in protein. Fat is poorly tolerated and badly absorbed and should be limited to 40 grams daily.

The failure to absorb fat normally is due primarily to the lack of bile salts in the intestine. Bile salts are necessary for fat absorption, at least in part to form micelles with fat.

If prothrombin levels are low, vitamin K may have to be given by intramuscular injection each day until the deficiency is corrected. Bone lesions, if present, may have to be treated vigorously with vitamin D, 100,000 units a week. A maintenance dose of 6 gm of calcium gluconate per day should be taken in addition to skim milk, buttermilk, and other high calcium-containing foods. If there is severe osteomalacia, the calcium should be increased to 2 to 3 times the maintenance dose per day.

There is some evidence that the anemia of chronic obstructive jaundice is the result of iron deficiency, and, if there is no response to vitamin B complex medication, ferrous sulfate grains, $7\frac{1}{2}$ per day, may have to be continued indefinitely. Occasionally, intravenous iron therapy or transfusions may be necessary.

The development of cirrhosis in chronic obstructive jaundice needs special dietary attention as described above.

BIBLIOGRAPHY

1. Patek and Post: J. Clin. Invest., 20, 481, 1941.
2. Symposium on Liver Disease. Am. J. Clin. Nutr., 21, 1325, 1968.
3. Hartroft: In Diseases of the Liver, Philadelphia, J. B. Lippincott Co., 1963.
4. Himsworth: Liver and Its Diseases, Cambridge, Harvard University Press, 1950.
5. Best and Ridout: Ann. Rev. Biochem., 8, 349, 1939.
6. Brock and Autret: World Health Org. Monog. Ser. 8 and Bull., 5, 1, 1952.
7. Davidson: Ann. N.Y. Acad Sci., 104, 1026, 1963.
8. Rubin and Lieber: Ann. Intern. Med., 69, 1063–1067, 1968.
9. Capps and Barker: Ann. Intern. Med., 26, 405, 1947.
10. Chalmers: J. Clin. Invest., 34, 1163, 1965.
11. Johnson and Kark: Science, 105, 378, 1947.
12. Walshe: Lancet, 1, 1075, 1953.
13. Walshe: Quart. J. Med., 20, 421, 1951.
14. Adams and Foley: Tr. Am. Neurol. A., 74, 271, 1949.
15. McDermott and Adams: J. Clin. Invest., 32, 587, 1953.
16. Davidson and Gabuzda: New Engl. J. Med., 243, 779, 1950.
17. Phillips, Gabuzda and Davidson: J. Clin. Invest., 31, 351, 1952.
18. Sherlock, Summerskill, White and Phear: Lancet, 2, 453, 1954.
19. Murphy, Chalmers, Eckhardt and Davidson: New Engl. J. Med., 239, 605, 1948.
20. Gabuzda, Phillips and Davidson: New Engl. J. Med., 246, 124, 1952.
21. Phillips, Schwartz, Gabuzda and Davidson: New Engl. J. Med., 247, 239, 1952.
22. Lieber and Davidson: Amer. J. Med., 33, 319, 1962.
23. Lieber, Jones and DeCarli: J. Clin. Invest., 44, 1009, 1965.
24. Isselbacher: Psychosomatic Med., 28, 424, 1966.
25. Kark and Pirani: Illinois State Med. J., 98, 292, 1950.
26. Teowell, Davies and Dean: Brit. Med. J., 2, 796, 798, 1952.
27. Selzer, Parker, and Sapeicka: Brit. J. Exper. Path., 32, 14, 1951.
28. Eisenmenger, Ahrens, Blondheim and Kundel: J. Lab. & Clin. Med., 34, 1029, 1949.
29. Kark, Keeton, Calloway, et al.: Arch. Int. Med., 88, 61, 1951.
30. ———: J.A.M.A., 159, 1257, 1955.
31. Davidson: Liver Pathophysiology. Boston, Little, Brown & Co., 1970.
32. Davidson (Ed.) Nat. Ac. Sci.: Nat. Res. Council Pub. 325, 1954.
33. Jandl: J. Clin. Invest., 34, 390, 1955.
34. Herbert, Zalusky and Davidson: Ann. Intern. Med., 58, 977, 1963.
35. Friedman, Kannel, and Dawber: J. Chron. Dis., 19, 273–292, 1966.
36. Small and Rapo: New Engl. J. Med., 283, 53–57, 1970.
37. Boucher: Lancet, 1, 711–715, 1971.
38. Williams and Fish: In Diseases of the Liver, 3rd Ed., L. Schiff (Ed.), Philadelphia, J. B. Lippincott Co., 1969.
39. Small: New Engl. J. Med., 279, 588–593, 1968.
40. Comess et al.: New Engl. J. Med., 277, 894–898, 1967.
41. Sampliner et al.: New Engl. J. Med., 283, 1358–1364, 1970.
42. McDermott and Brown: In Nardi and Zuidema (Eds.) Surgery, 2nd Ed., Boston, Little, Brown & Co., 1965.
43. Taylor (Ed.): The Biliary System, Philadelphia, F. A. Davis Co., 1965.
44. Smith and Sherlock: Surgery of the Gall Bladder and Bile Ducts, London, Butterworths, 1964.
45. Ahrens, Payne, Kunkel, et al.: Medicine, 29, 299, 1950.
46. Klatskin and Krehl: J. Clin. Invest., 29, 1528, 1950.

Chapter

29

Diet in the Treatment of Diabetes Mellitus

GERALD J. FRIEDMAN

The scientific progress in the field of metabolism since the discovery of insulin has profoundly influenced the concepts of the etiology of diabetes mellitus, but the cause (or causes) of it remains a mystery.

DEFINITION OF DIABETES MELLITUS

The old concept of insulin deficiency as the basic mechanism in the development of diabetes in man has seen a revival during recent years.[1] However, there is still a wide diversity of opinion as to the definition of diabetes mellitus.[2-5] Root and Bailey considered the simplest definition to be: "diabetes is a disorder in blood sugar regulation."[4] Such a statement could imply the possible operation of all the many factors, genetic, endocrine, and others, known to influence the level of the blood sugar. The disturbance might therefore depend upon diet, primary or secondary failure of the beta cells of the islets of Langerhans due to one or more hereditary defects, or to any of the other factors that influence insulin synthesis, secretion, transport, and action in responsive tissues.[6] Regardless of the mechanisms involved, diabetics young or old with mild or severe disease suffer from a subnormal ability to retain glucose in their systems.[7] From the clinical point of view, idiopathic or primary diabetes mellitus may be defined as a hereditary disease of metabolism in which there is an inadequate supply of effective insulin, characterized by disturbances of carbohydrate, fat, and protein homeostasis and by macroangiopathic, microangiopathic and neuropathic changes.

In enlarging upon definitions of primary diabetes, two types are generally recognized:

1. *Growth-Onset* (Juvenile; Ketosis-Prone). Growth-onset diabetes is an unstable or labile type. Juvenile diabetics account for 5 per cent of the total diabetic population with an additional 5 per cent being brittle adult diabetics.

Growth-onset diabetes usually, but not always, arises during childhood or puberty; is abrupt in onset; is symptomatic; occurs usually in undernourished patients; has wide variations in blood sugar values in response to small changes in insulin dose, exercise, or infection; is difficult to control; and is frequently associated with ketosis. While insulin production may be normal at the onset of the disease it usually becomes nonexistent within a few years.[8] The essential abnormalities in juvenile diabetes are related to absolute insulin deficiency. Vascular complications and degenerative changes are infrequent until diabetes has been present for 5 years.

2. *Maturity-Onset* (Ketosis-Resistant). The obese maturity-onset-type patient accounts for 80 per cent of the diabetic population while the nonobese stable, adult type makes up 10 per cent of the diabetics.

The ketosis-resistant diabetic has a gradual onset of the disorder, usually after the age of 35 years; is usually overweight; may have minimal to no symptoms; may have narrow variations in blood sugar; may be relatively easy to control especially if the patient adheres to his diet; rarely develops ketosis except in the presence of unusual stress or severe infection; and has a plasma-insulin response that is adequate, although delayed or diminished, but not absent. Vascular complications and degenerative changes are common and frequent.

Diet is essential in the treatment of both the juvenile and maturity-onset types. Insulin is necessary for all of the juvenile type and for about 30 per cent of the maturity-onset type. Oral agents are not efficacious for the juvenile type.

NATURAL HISTORY OF DIABETES MELLITUS

Primary or genetic diabetes may be classified into four stages:

Prediabetes. The first stage is *prediabetes* or "diabetes pre-mellitus."[8] It exists prior to the onset of identifiable diabetes mellitus. It is that period of time from conception until the development of impaired glucose tolerance in an individual predisposed to diabetes on genetic grounds. It can be suspected in an identical twin of a diabetic; or in the offspring of two diabetic parents; in the presence of diabetes-like vascular lesions; and, in the woman with a history of large babies or frequent miscarriages.

The prediabetic state is characterized by normal glucose tolerance, but there is a delayed or decreased elevation in plasma insulin secretion following glucose or amino acid stimulation.[1,9,10] This also occurs in other nondiabetic relatives of diabetic patients,[11] and is similar to the defect present in clinical diabetes mellitus. The disappearance rate of intravenously administered glucose (k-value) is significantly lower than in the control group although still within the normal range. Cerasi and Luft[12] have postulated that a diminished insulin response to glucose is the basic pathogenic factor in the development of the different stages of the diabetic syndrome. The presence of low insulin response in healthy monozygotic twins of diabetic patients indicates that this insulin deficiency is inherited and antedates the appearance of decreased glucose tolerance.[13] The combination of normal glucose tolerance and decreased insulin response to glucose characterizes the so-called "prediabetic" state.[1] Thickening of the capillary

basement membrane of muscle has been found in a large percentage of patients with a genetic predisposition towards diabetes.[14]

Subclinical Diabetes. The second stage is *subclinical diabetes*.[15] The fasting blood sugar and glucose tolerance tests are normal, but islet cell decompensation can be demonstrated by an abnormal cortisone-glucose tolerance test. The glucose tolerance test may be abnormal during pregnancy ("gestational diabetes") or stress.

Latent Diabetes. The third stage is *latent (or chemical) diabetes*. In this group the diagnosis is made by the presence of an abnormal glucose tolerance test in the absence of symptoms of diabetes.

Overt Diabetes. The fourth, and most advanced, stage of diabetes is *overt (or clinical) diabetes*. The classical symptoms, as well as fasting hyperglycemia and glycosuria, are present.

In the natural history of diabetes, progression or regression from one stage to another may occur slowly over many years, may be rapid, or may never occur.[16] Fluctuations in carbohydrate metabolism are common. Reversion from abnormal to normal glucose tolerance with regression from the latent stage to the prediabetes stage and even from overt, ketotic diabetes to prediabetes has been reported.[17-19] On the other hand, Fajans and Conn[16] have reported rapid progression from prediabetes to overt diabetes without going through the latent stage.

The carbohydrate intolerance of maturity-onset diabetes may show no change in severity over the course of many years. Many have shown the nonprogressive course of carbohydrate intolerance of the maturity-onset type of diabetes, which may exist in asymptomatic states for years or decades, in those middle-aged individuals in whom the occurrence of occlusive vascular disease or neuropathy is the presenting complication of their maturity-onset type of diabetes mellitus. Growth-onset diabetes was thought to be characterized by a rapid deterioration of insulin reserves. However, in 1960 Fajans and Conn reported latent (asymptomatic) diabetes in children and adolescents manifested only by an abnormal glucose tolerance test.[20]

DIETARY MANAGEMENT OF DIABETES

The principal objective in the treatment of patients with diabetes mellitus is to permit the diabetic to lead a normal life in good health. The treatment program should be designed to correct defects in metabolism, preserve pancreatic functions, prevent chronic diabetic complications, and promote psychosocial adjustment.[21] Diet, hypoglycemic agents, and exercise are the major modalities in treatment. Proper dietary management still remains the most important factor in the practical treatment of diabetes mellitus.

The basic nutritional requirements for patients with diabetes mellitus are, in general, the same as those for all individuals and include adequate quality and quantity of all nutrients.[22] In addition, diabetic patients have special nutritional requirements that should be met by dietary prescription. Such a dietary program should be an integral component of broad, general health care for the diabetic that includes periodic medical examinations, regular exercise, avoidance of cigarette smoking, attendance to personal hygiene, and prevention of infection.

Total Calories

The single most important objective of dietary treatment of diabetic patients is control of total caloric intake to attain the ideal body weight, since most diabetics (80 per cent) are obese. The Food and Drug Administration (FDA) in its final labeling for the sulfonylurea drugs and for phenformin included a special warning that stated: "Diet and reduction of excess weight are the foundations of initial therapy of Diabetes Mellitus. When the disease is adequately controlled by these measures no hypoglycemic drug therapy is indicated." The "indications" section of the labeling approved recently by FDA for all oral hypoglycemic drugs says: "Oral hypoglycemic drugs are indicated in the treatment of adult onset, non-ketotic diabetes mellitus only when the condition can not be controlled adequately by diet and reduction of excess weight alone."

Thus in the obese patient the first aim of dietary therapy should be the provision of a diet that is restricted in calories and that is nutritionally adequate.[23] The caloric requirements of the diabetic will depend on his activity, age, sex, body weight, and the climate. Patients who are sedentary and overweight seldom need more than 20 kcal per kilogram of ideal body weight per day. If they are overweight and performing moderate activity they require 30 kcal per kilogram per day. Those who are overweight and perform strenuous activity require 35 kcal per kilogram per day. Those who are normal weight and doing sedentary work require 30 kcal per kilogram per day. For moderate activity 35 kcal per kilogram per day are required, and for marked activity 40 kcal per kilogram per day. Underweight diabetics require 35 kcal per kilogram per day for sedentary work, 40 kcal per kilogram per day for moderate activity, and 45 to 50 kcal per kilogram per day for strenuous activity. Active adolescent boys during their peak growth period need from 3100 to 3600 kcal per day, and adolescent girls from 2400 to 2700 kcal per day. In general, children require 1000 kcal per day plus an additional 100 kcal for every year of age.

"Achievement of this goal [of weight reduction] may be associated with the reduction or disappearance of the requirement for exogenous insulin, improvement or correction of fasting hyperglycemia and glucose intolerance, and reduction of known risk factors for atherosclerotic vascular disease such as obesity, hypertension, hyperlipidemia and hyperglycemia."[23] The finding of an abnormal glucose tolerance in the presence of an elevated plasma insulin level suggests that the patient is insensitive to his own insulin. This situation is commonly seen in the obese, adult-onset type of diabetic and is corrected by weight reduction which will enhance sensitivity to endogenous insulin and will tend to normalize the glucose tolerance. Even in nondiabetics, the obese have a greater output of insulin after a carbohydrate meal than do thin nondiabetics. The increased output of insulin has been explained, in part, by the insulin-resistant state of the tissues, particularly the adipose tissues of the obese individual.[24]

Obese individuals not only have hyperinsulinemia following a glucose load, but also have high basal levels of insulin. The combination of a high fasting insulin level and an exaggerated increase of insulin above baseline may result in a total insulin output that is markedly greater than for a slender person.[25] It has been postulated that the hyperinsulinemia is due to overstimulation of the pancreas and leads to insular exhaustion, thus accounting for the higher incidence of diabetes in the obese. The belief that the hyperinsulinemia of obesity is solely a secondary response to insulin antagonism has been questioned by Grey and Kipnis,[26] who suggest that the hyperinsulinemia of obesity is also a result of dietary factors rather than exclusively a secondary adaptation to insulin resistance. They postulate that the insulin antagonism that develops with obesity might actually represent an adaptive mechanism to protect the obese person from hypoglycemic episodes resulting from excessive intake of carbohydrates.

Populations characterized by obesity have a high incidence of abnormal glucose tolerance and clinical diabetes. Those characterized by slimness have a low incidence of diabetes. A worldwide diabetic survey demonstrated a decrease in glucose tolerance with increasing obesity, increasing sugar consumption, increasing dietary fat and protein, and increasing economic status.[27]

Carbohydrate Requirements

There has been, and continues to be, a great disagreement among workers in the field of diabetes as to the relative merits of a high-carbohydrate versus a low-carbohydrate diet in the treatment of diabetes.[28] Wood and Bierman have recently published an excellent review on the history of this subject.[29] The discovery of insulin in 1921 made it possible to liberalize the carbohydrate intake, and some investigators have given large amounts. In 1923 Geyelin of Columbia University began to prescribe high-carbohydrate diets to diabetic patients treated with insulin. In 1935 after reviewing 10 years of his experience with the high-carbohydrate, low-fat diet, he concluded that the increased effectiveness of insulin that consistently followed the institution of a high-carbohydrate diet was "chiefly dependent on the degree to which fat is curtailed." M. Rabinowitch of McGill University was another advocate of the high-carbohydrate, low-fat diet. His goal was to keep his patients five to ten pounds under their average body weight. He suggested even less fat be included in the diet than previous observers (i.e., less than 50 grams a day) and believed that the restriction of dietary fat would help lower the incidence of cardiovascular-renal disease. He also observed that "potential diabetes can be activated and mild diabetes can be made severe by too rigid restriction of carbohydrates."

Himsworth[30] demonstrated that diets high in carbohydrates improved glucose tolerance in normal persons. These observations of the effects of high-carbohydrate diet on oral glucose tolerance in normal subjects have recently been confirmed by others.[31-33]

A number of dietary surveys have been made in conjunction with studies of the prevalence of diabetes. The Zulus consume about 85 per cent of their calories as carbohydrates but they are thin and virtually free of diabetes. In the same area of the world, the Masai who live on meat, milk, and blood and eat only 20 per cent of their calories as carbohydrate also remain thin and are spared from diabetes.[34] Henry et al.[35] have shown that various American Indian tribes who have remained relatively homogeneous have a very high incidence of abnormal glucose tolerance and clinical diabetes. Like other low-income Americans their diets contain high-carbohydrate and fat contents with the result that over half the population exceeds 125 per cent of the optimal weight. The diabetes is maturity onset in nature and is associated with a high incidence of large-vessel disease. On the other hand, Mouratoff et al.[36] found two other groups, the Eskimos and the Athabaskan Indians in Alaska, who have been spared from diabetes and atherosclerosis on a high-fat, low-carbohydrate diet (less than 50 grams per day). Both of these groups have a low incidence of obesity. The Indians in India have a low incidence of diabetes on a high-carbohydrate, low-caloric diet. However, those who migrated to South

Africa have a high incidence of maturity-onset diabetes and vascular disease. The major change in the group that migrated to Africa was an increase in the caloric intake of the diet; the carbohydrate percentage remained high and there was an increase in obesity.[34] Other changes that have occurred with migration have been found in the Yemenite Jews who migrated to Israel and adopted the European diet high in calories and carbohydrates in place of their former diet, which was a high-fat, low-caloric diet; showed an increased incidence of diabetes and obesity has been observed.[34]

Albrink and Davidson feel that the most important fact that emerges from clinical and epidemiologic studies is the deleterious effect of obesity on diabetes.[22] They indicate that the fewest vascular complications are found when the habitual dietary intake results in leanness regardless of the proportion of carbohydrate or fat in the diet.

A difference of opinion exists as to the optimal proportion of carbohydrate and fat to be recommended to the diabetic who is of normal weight or underweight. There has been a gradual liberalization in the recommended carbohydrate intake since the discovery of insulin. At the present time most clinics allow 40 per cent of the total calories to be carbohydrate, close to the normal average of the United States population in whom 45 per cent of the calories ingested are in the form of carbohydrates. There are two schools of thought in regard to the proportion of carbohydrate and fat intake. One group feels that carbohydrate intake should not be liberalized in either the insulin-dependent or insulin-independent diabetic on the grounds that a high-carbohydrate intake will accentuate postprandial hyperglycemic peaks. Hyperglycemic peaks should be avoided in the diabetic, since Gabbay[37,38] has shown that with decreased insulin activity and hyperglycemia, glucose is converted via the insulin-independent polyol pathway to sorbitol and fructose which accumulate in nervous tissue in experimental diabetic neuropathy. In addition to osmotic swelling, a number of other concomitant functional changes have been described. In human and experimental diabetic neuropathy the earliest clinical ex-

pression of demyelinization is a decrease in nerve conduction velocity. Correction of hyperglycemia, by diet or hypoglycemic agents, in diabetic patients has resulted in improvement in the delayed nerve conduction velocity.[39] Clinical studies have shown a greater effect of ingested glucose than of its equivalent as starch upon the rise of circulating glucose and insulin.[40] Yudkin has suggested that a high intake of refined carbohydrate results in an increased incidence of atherosclerosis and diabetes,[41a] but this has been contradicted.[41b,41c]

Brunzell and his colleagues[42] reported an improved glucose tolerance with high-carbohydrate feedings in mild diabetes. Glucose and immunoreactive insulin levels were measured in normal persons and subjects with mild diabetes maintained on basal (45 per cent) carbohydrate and high (85 per cent) carbohydrate diets in order to evaluate the effect of increased dietary carbohydrate in diabetes mellitus. Fasting blood glucose levels fell in all subjects and oral glucose tolerance improved significantly after 10 days of high-carbohydrate feeding. Fasting insulin levels also were lower on the high-carbohydrate diet. However, insulin response to oral glucose did not change significantly. These data suggest that the high-carbohydrate diet increased the sensitivity of peripheral tissues to insulin. Preliminary data[43] suggest that patients with moderate and severe diabetes, following treatment with oral drugs or insulin, respond to the same carbohydrate diet in a manner similar to those with mild diabetes. Insulin, either endogenous or exogenous, must be available to obtain this effect. This short-term study is in agreement with the long-term effect of a high-carbohydrate diet noted by Stone and Connor.[44] These investigators are of the opinion that in mild diabetes, regardless of weight, a high-carbohydrate, low-fat diet improves glucose tolerance as well as decreasing cholesterol levels and therefore should be used for diabetic management.

The Committee on Food and Nutrition of the American Diabetes Association in their 1971 dietary recommendations[23] for patients with diabetes mellitus stated: "There no longer appears to be any need to restrict disproportionately the intake of carbohydrates in the diet of most diabetic patients. Increase of dietary carbohydrate, even to extremes, without increase of total calories, does not appear to increase insulin requirement in the insulin treated diabetic patient. In the less severe typically obese diabetic, substitution of carbohydrate for fat does not appear to elevate blood glucose or worsen glucose tolerance. . . . The average proportion of calories consumed of carbohydrate in the U.S. population as a whole approximates 45 per cent; this proportion or even higher appears to be acceptable for the usual diabetic patient as well."

Fat Requirements

The epidemiologic and experimental evidence relating circulating lipids to atherosclerotic cardiovascular disease also appears to apply to the diabetic patient.[45,46] Since persons with diabetes are particularly susceptible to atherosclerosis and its complications, it seems prudent, on the basis of current information, for such patients to consume a diet that will favor the lowest serum levels of cholesterol and triglycerides. Diabetic patients who already have hyperlipidemia are more prone to develop atherosclerosis and require particular attention to dietary management. Reduction of serum lipids can be accomplished in usual situations by limitation of the intake of calories, saturated fat, and cholesterol. Since most diabetics are obese, hypertriglyceridemia, when present, responds to caloric restriction as it does in nondiabetic patients. Diabetics appear to respond to reduction of saturated fat and cholesterol intake with a lowering of circulating cholesterol, as do nondiabetic persons.

Present views on the relation between hyperlipoproteinemias and atherosclerosis are given in Chapter 31 together with classification of phenotypes and recommendations for diet therapy. It is recommended that all diabetics have lipoprotein phenotyping.

The low-saturated-fat diet used in the dietary treatment of patients with Type II hyperlipoproteinemia (hypercholesterolemia) may be obtained in one of two ways. The

fat calories may be replaced by carbohydrate so the total fat intake is low and the calories are made up by a high-carbohydrate intake. Alternatively, the saturated fat calories may be replaced by polyunsaturated fats so the total fat approximates the national average of about 40 per cent of calories. Concern has been expressed for diabetics receiving the high-carbohydrate diet for fear that it will produce hypertriglyceridemia as in Type IV hyperlipidemia or will have a deleterious effect on the diabetes.[22] Stone and Connor,[44] however, found neither of these complications in nonobese, insulin-dependent diabetics on a low-fat (20 per cent), low-cholesterol (100 mg/day) diet at the end of 12 months. The use of a low-saturated-fat diet supplemented with large amounts of polyunsaturated fat resulted in an additional cholesterol-lowering effect. This supplementation made the diet easier to follow, permitted greater variety, and did not have the disadvantage of the possible triglyceride-raising effect of the high-carbohydrate diet. In two well-controlled studies on the effect of this diet in nondiabetics, the reduction of serum cholesterol was 8 to 10 per cent in persons who did not lose weight.[47,48]

Type IV hyperlipoproteinemia is a very common type and is often associated with abnormalities of glucose tolerance. The pattern and treatment have been reviewed in Chapter 31.

For diabetic patients with malabsorption, medium-chain triglycerides may be more efficiently absorbed than the naturally occurring long-chain fats.[49] However, the medium-chain triglycerides may induce clinically significant hyperketonemia in certain insulin-dependent diabetic patients.[50]

Protein Requirements

The requirements for protein at different ages have been considered in Chapter 2A and the recommended allowances are set forth in the Appendix, Table A-1. The diabetic patient is likely to require extra protein to offset losses from the excessive gluconeogenesis and ketogenesis that are associated with impaired glucose utilization. The presence of infection, pregnancy, and debilitating disease also requires additional protein. Patients with nephrosis or malabsorption may suffer appreciable losses of protein in the urine or feces and require replacement. Uremia and hepatic coma, on the other hand, usually dictate decreased amounts of protein. Thus, in diabetic patients whose hepatic and renal status permits, an additional allowance of protein ranging up to 0.5 grams per kilogram per day should be considered depending upon the metabolic condition of the individual concerned.

Vitamin and Mineral Requirements

Diets for diabetic patients under good control usually contain the adequate amounts of vitamins that are recommended by the Food and Nutrition Board (Appendix, Table A-1). However, in those with poorly controlled diabetes, infection, malabsorption, or other complications, vitamin supplementation may be necessary.

Diabetic patients with poorly controlled disease usually develop deficits of water, sodium, potassium, and chloride. This is especially true when diuresis or excessive sweating occurs. It is dramatically demonstrated in a patient in diabetic ketoacidosis. Deficiencies of certain electrolytes can also occur in prolonged diarrhea, renal disease with abnormalities of tubular absorption, as well as in diabetic ketoacidosis. Prolonged use of certain diuretics may produce electrolyte and acid-base disturbances. Large doses of insulin, which cause hypoglycemia, will lower blood potassium. At times the diabetic patient must restrict sodium and potassium because of associated renal, hepatic, or cardiovascular disease. During acute illnesses especially when anorexia, vomiting, or diarrhea occurs, the patient must be observed closely so that water and electrolyte balance may be maintained. Intravenous fluids may be necessary, but patients should be changed to more normal diets as soon as possible. The control of fluid and electrolyte balance has been considered in Chapter 7.

The maintenance of adequate amounts of calcium, phosphorus, iron, copper, iodine, manganese, cobalt, and zinc usually presents no problem to the well-controlled diabetic. There have been some reports of slow healing of diabetic ulcers thought to be due to a zinc deficiency, but this point requires further investigation. Trivalent chromium, a glucose-tolerance factor for rats, may also improve the glucose tolerance for a small number of people with diabetes mellitus. Glinsmann and Mertz studied the effect of supplementing a diet with 60 to 1000 mcg of chromium ion, administered orally three times a day with meals, for periods ranging from 15 to 133 days and found that there was an improvement in the glucose tolerance in 3 out of 6 patients studied.[51,52] The chromium ion supplementation had no effect on the glucose tolerance of normal individuals. After chromium administration was stopped, glucose tolerance of the responsive diabetic patients reverted to the prechromium state.

Alcohol

Alcohol in moderation may be added to the diabetic diet provided that the intake is small and the caloric values of alcoholic beverages are considered in the calculation of the diet (Appendix, Table A-4).

CALCULATION OF THE DIABETIC DIET

1. Estimate the ideal body weight in pounds by referring to a standard height/weight table (Appendix, Table A-3). A rough approximation may be made by allowing 105 lb for the first 5 feet of height and 5 lb for each additional inch over 5 feet; for medium and heavy frames add 5 to 10 lb. For example, a patient with a normal frame who is 5'6" tall will have an ideal body weight of 135 lb.

2. Convert the ideal body weight from pounds to kilograms by dividing the pounds by 2.2.

3. Calculate the *total amount of kcal* the patient needs per day for each kilogram of ideal body weight on the basis of body weight and activity as follows:

	Sedentary	Moderate	Marked Activity
Overweight:	20–25	30	35
Normal:	30	35	40
Underweight:	35	40	45–50

4. Composition: (A) *Protein:* Consider 1.5 grams per kilogram of ideal body weight as the protein requirement for the diabetic patient whose hepatic and renal status permits. (B) *Carbohydrate:* In the absence of carbohydrate-induced hypertriglyceridemia Type IV the carbohydrate allowance may be 40 to 50 per cent of the total calories. In the presence of this type of hypertriglyceridemia the carbohydrate allowance should be between 125 and 150 grams per day. (C) *Fat:* The remaining calories should be given in the form of fat. The saturated fat intake should be limited and polyunsaturated fats substituted for them. Most clinics recommend a limitation of total fat calories to 35 per cent or less of the total caloric intake, with a polyunsaturated-to-saturated fat ratio of 2.5.

5. Translate the calculated diet into food servings and distribute as desired among three meals plus extra feedings. Examples of such diets are given in the Appendix, Tables A-7 to A-9. All patients receiving insulin must have a bedtime feeding. Children should have midmorning and mid-afternoon feedings as well.

Individualization and Meal Spacing

The diabetic patient who requires insulin therapy must adjust not only his caloric intake but his eating habits as well. Food intake should be spaced in a fashion that takes into account administered insulin and physical activity in order to avoid intermittent hypoglycemia. Regularity of food intake and regularity of exercise are of paramount importance. Any dietary program, to be practical and effective, must be based on appropriate patient motivation coupled with diagnostic evaluation, dietary instruction, and follow-up by the physician and dietitian.

Diet therapy in the diabetic must be adapted to the specific needs of individual patients. Patients with hyperlipoproteinemia must be typed and treated depending on their type. It is essential that the diet for the diabetic patient take into account his individual food preferences, background, economic status, and the setting in which he eats his meals.[49] The rationale of the diet must be carefully explained to the patient in an effort to enlist his full cooperation.

That this is a complex situation is emphasized by the results of surveys. Tunbridge and Wetherill[53] repeated a study in 1968 similar to that done in 1948 to determine whether the patients were adhering to their prescribed diets. In both surveys less than one-third of the patients were keeping within 10 per cent of such diets. There was considerable fluctuation in intake from day to day with no particular pattern discernible during the week; variability was noted even in patients who were adhering closely to the prescribed diet. The extreme example of such variation was in a patient with caloric range from 1265 to 2850 kcal per day within a week. Based on single but searching interviews, Bloom found that 17 out of 111 insulin-dependent diabetics adhered strictly and regularly to their prescribed diets, 60 adhered in a "general" way, and the other 34 were unable to follow regular diets.[54] It was found that the average blood sugar levels observed in the diabetic clinic were unrelated to the standard of dietary adherence and were similar in all groups. He also reported a significant relationship between dietary control and the severity of hypoglycemic reactions and noted that patients who did not adhere to the diet were much less likely to have severe reactions. Tunbridge and Wetherill also were unable to find any obvious relation between dietary regulation and diabetic control.[53]

It must be noted that half the diabetics in the United States have incomes of $4,000 or less per year. It has been pointed out that the cost of the diabetic diet may be much greater than the cost of normal diets for certain groups and may play a role in the lack of dietary adherence.[52] The increased consumption of food as the symbol of success by persons who have recently escaped poverty also plays a factor in dietary adherence.

Between-meal snacks, including a small meal before bedtime, are often essential for the diabetic. It is particularly important to children, adolescents, and certain adult patients who have a high daily requirement for calories. Short-term clinical studies have shown improved glucose tolerance with a schedule of 10 feedings compared to 3 meals or a single isocaloric feeding.[55] In epidemiologic surveys, in which men were grouped according to habitual meal frequency, those who ate 3 meals or less per day showed significantly more obesity, higher serum cholesterol levels and diminished glucose tolerance. Multiple frequent feedings, avoiding large evening meals, are far less detrimental to the diabetic.

Insulin-dependent diabetics must eat multiple meals in order to avoid hypoglycemia. Their meals must be spaced according to the type of insulin they are taking and the period of peak action. The basic pattern of caloric intake must be individualized to promote maximum cooperation from the patient for day-to-day consistency. This consistency may result in a greater safety from hypoglycemia and the avoidance of hyperglycemia.

Diet instructions should be as simple as possible while the monotony of diet can be avoided by teaching the patient to use suitable food exchanges. The patient must be taught the foods he must limit and those he can consume in unlimited quantities.

The diet must be tailored to the patient. For example, if a patient becomes physically ill when forced to eat breakfast, the insulin injections must be readjusted, as well as midmorning snacks, without upsetting the patient or the overall adequacy of the diet. Since diabetes is frequently associated with other medical disorders which may require special dietary treatment or restrictions, the basic diet must be altered accordingly. Restriction of the intake of sodium may be necessary for those who have heart and kidney disease; the composition and consistency of the diet may be varied for patients with gastrointestinal disorders, e.g., peptic ulcer, gallbladder disease, or colitis; the fat content may have to be reduced for those with gallbladder disease and protein restriction may be necessary in those with either renal or advanced hepatic insufficiency.

SUMMARY OF GENERAL CONSIDERATIONS AND RECOMMENDATIONS

1. The patient must be made aware that, in many instances, adequate weight reduction will convert his abnormal glucose tolerance test to normal and make treatment with hypoglycemic agents unnecessary. It will also reduce his risk of developing certain serious complications of diabetes such as coronary heart disease.

2. The physician or nutritionist must be prepared to consult frequently with the patient and to make adjustments to fit the patient's needs and preferences. The planning of a diabetic diet for a child requires free communication with physician, dietitian, mother, and child. The diet must be interesting, palatable, and flexible.

3. It is not necessary to buy special foods. The diet should be selected from the same foods purchased for the rest of the family. The diet should conform with the eating habits of the patient's family and his own tastes. Simplicity of dietary prescriptions is desirable.

4. When a diabetic patient, especially an insulin-dependent one, is unable to take his usual feedings, the carbohydrate content of the diet must be replaced with a sweetened beverage, e.g., ginger ale or orange juice, or with parenteral glucose in order to prevent insulin reactions.

5. Caloric requirements depend upon age, weight, height, rate of growth, sex, exercise, and general condition of the patient.

6. The diet must frequently be adjusted to the insulin dose.

7. Controlling the diabetic's diet requires persistence and caring about the patient on the part of the physician.

BIBLIOGRAPHY

1. Cerasi and Luft: Diabetes, *21* (Suppl. 2), 685, 1972.
2. Fajans: Med. Clin. N. Amer., *55*, 793, 1971.
3. Waife (ed.): *Diabetes Mellitus* 7th Ed. Indianapolis, Lilly Research Laboratories, p. 1, 1969.
4. Root and Bailey: *In Modern Nutrition in Health and Disease.* Wohl and Goodhart (eds.) 4th Ed. Philadelphia, Lea & Febiger, p. 782, 1968.

5. Goldner: *In Diabetes Mellitus: Diagnosis and Treatment*. Vol. 2. New York, American Diabetes Association, p. 39, 1967.
6. Williams and Ensinck: Diabetes, *15*, 623, 1966.
7. Renold: *In Pathology of Diabetes*, Warren, LeCompte, and Legg (eds.). 4th Ed. Philadelphia, Lea & Febiger, p. 124, 1966.
8. Conn and Fajans: Amer. J. Med., *31*, 839, 1961.
9. Colwell and Lein: Diabetes *16*, 560, 1967.
10. Floyd, Fajans, Conn et al.: J. Clin. Endocr., *28*, 266, 1968.
11. Rull, Conn, Floyd and Fajans: Diabetes, *19*, 1, 1970.
12. Cerasi and Luft: Diabetes, *16*, 615, 1967.
13. Pyke, Cassar, Todd and Taylor: Brit. Med. J., *4*, 649, 1970.
14 Siperstein, Unger and Madison: J. Clin. Invest., *47*, 1973, 1968.
15 Conn and Fajans: Amer. J. Med., *31*, 839, 1961.
16. Fajans and Conn: *In On the Nature and Treatment of Diabetes*. Leibel and Wrenshall (eds.). New York, Excerpta Medica Foundation International Congress Series, 84, Chap. 46, pp. 641–656, 1965.
17. Kahn, Soeldner, Gleason, Rojas, Camerini-Davalos and Marble: New Eng. J. Med., *287*, 343, 1969.
18. O'Sullivan and Hurwitz: Arch. Intern. Med., *117*, 769, 1966.
19. Peck, Kirtley and Peck: Diabetes, *7*, 93, 1968.
20. Fajans and Conn: Diabetes, *9*, 83, 1960.
21. Knowles: *In Diabetes Mellitus: Diagnosis and Treatment*. Vol. II. New York City, American Diabetes Association, p. 79, 1967.
22. Albrink and Davidson: Med. Clin. N. Amer., *55*, 877, 1971.
23. Committee on Food and Nutrition, Amer. Diabetes Assoc.: Diabetes, *20*, 633, 1971.
24. Salans, Knittle and Hirsch: J. Clin. Invest., *47*, 153, 1968.
25. Bierman and Porte: Ann. Int. Med., *68*, 929, 1968.
26. Grey and Kipnis: New Eng. J. Med., *285*, 827, 1971
27. West and Kalbfeisch: Diabetes, *19*, 656, 1970.
28. Fajans: Diabetes, *21*, (Suppl. II), 678, 1972.
29. Wood and Bierman: New Concepts of Diabetic Dietetics. Nutrition Today, p. 4, May-June, 1972.
30. Himsworth: Brit. Med. J., *2*, 57, 1934.
31. Wales, Viktora and Wolff: Amer. Med. Sci., *254*, 499, 1967.
32. Ford, Bozian and Knowles: Amer. J. Clin. Nutr., *21*, 904, 1968.
33. Anderson, Herman and Zakin: Amer. J. Clin. Nutr., *21*, 529, 1968.
34. Cleave, Campbell and Painter: *Diabetes, Coronary Thrombosis and the Saccharine Disease*. 2nd ed. Bristol, John Wright and Sons, Ltd , 1969.
35. Henry, Burch, Bennett and Miller: Diabetes, *18*, 33, 1969.
36. Mouratoff, Carroll and Scott: Diabetes, *18*, 29, 1969.
37. Gabbay, Mierola and Field: Science, *151*, 209, 1966.
38. Gabbay: Diabetes, *18*, 336, 1969; *20*, 331, 1971.
39. Ward, Barnes, Fisher, Jessop and Baker: Lancet, *1*, 428, 1971.
40. Swan, Davidson and Albrink: Lancet, *1*, 60, 1966.
41a.Yudkin: Lancet, 2, 4, 1964.
41b.Burns-Cox, Doll and Ball: Brit. Heart J., *31*, 485, 1969.
41c.Howell and Wilson: Brit. Med. J., *31*, 485, 1969.
42. Brunzell, Lerner, Hazzard, Porte and Bierman: New Eng. J. Med., *284*, 521, 1971.
43. Brunzell, Lerner, Porte et al.: Diabetes, *19*, Suppl. 1, 379, 1970.
44. Stone and Connor: Diabetes, *12*, 127, 1963.
45. Cornfield and Mitchell: Arch. Environ. Health, *19*, 382, 1969.
46. Intersociety Commission for Heart Disease Resources: Primary Prevention of the Atherosclerotic Diseases. Circulation, *42*, A53, 1970.
47. Dayton, Pearce, Hashimoto, Dixon and Tomeyasu: *In Preventing Complications of Atherosclerosis*. Monograph 25. New York, American Heart Association, 1969.
48. The National Diet Heart Study Final Report. Monograph 18. New York, American Heart Association, 1968.
49. Van Itallie and Campbell: *In Diabetes Mellitus: Diagnosis and Treatment*. Vol II. New York, American Diabetes Association, p. 91, 1967.
50. Bergen, Hashim and Van Itallie: Diabetes, *15*, 723, 1966.
51. Glinsmann and Mertz: Metabolism, *15*, 510, 1966.
52. Anon.: Nutr. Rev., *25*, 49, 1967.
53. Tunbridge and Wetherill: Brit. Med. J., *2*, 78, 1970.
54. Bloom: Proc. Roy. Soc. Med., *60*, 149, 1967.
55. Fabry and Tepperman: Amer. J. Clin. Nutr., *23*, 1059, 1970.

Chapter

30

Nutrition and Cardiovascular-Renal Diseases

ROBERT M. KARK

AND

JOSEPH H. OYAMA

GENERAL CONSIDERATIONS

The kidneys, particularly the proximal convolutions of the nephrons, are the guardians of the nutritional wealth of the body. Each day, for example, nearly 2 kg of ascorbic acid are filtered through the walls of the glomerular tufts into the renal tubules and all but a few milligrams are returned to the blood stream. The excretion of ascorbic acid in the urine, like that of many other water-soluble nutrients, is said to be determined by its plasma level, the rate of glomerular filtration, and the maximum rate of its tubular reabsorption;[1] and of these functions, the latter is crucial in preventing urinary wastage of the vitamin.* The efficiency of the proximal convolutions in defending the body against loss of such water-soluble substances as ascorbic acid, glucose, amino acids and other nutrients is more than matched by the lower reaches of the nephron which act to conserve water and electrolytes. Even

* The extraordinary reabsorptive capacity of the proximal convolutions of the tubules in both health and disease is one reason why measurement of the urinary output of the water-soluble vitamins is of little value in the diagnosis of the classic deficiency diseases. Forty years ago we thought differently; 40 years ago the vitamins were just beginning to be synthesized and most clinicians interested in nutrition were seeking methods of diagnosing pellagra, beriberi, and scurvy in the laboratory. The so-called subclinical forms of these diseases were thought to be common and important, and we believed that a vitamin deficiency might be brought to light by measurement of its urinary excretion, particularly after injection of a test dose.

in chronic renal disease or in diabetes insipidus, when large amounts of dilute urine are passed each day, there is little or no excessive loss of ascorbic acid, and conditioned deficiencies of ascorbic acid, or of other water-soluble vitamins, must be extremely uncommon complications of chronic renal failure. Nevertheless, renal wastage of nutrients does occur. Excessive urinary loss of water, electrolytes, calcium and phosphorus, as well as protein and amino acids, is common.

Prevention and treatment of these nutritional deficiencies are one side of the coin the physician has to deal with; on the other side of the coin he finds renal retention of nutrients and their toxic metabolic products. Elimination and control of bodily excesses of water, of water and sodium (edema); of potassium, phosphorus, chloride and protons, and of the nitrogenous-and-sulfur-containing metabolites of protein are necessary and can often be achieved by diet. Frequently, powerful drugs and complicated dialyzing devices must be used and these, in turn, may also disturb the nutritional economy of the body.

THE CHEMICAL COMPOSITION OF THE KIDNEY[2]

The kidneys weigh about 300 gm in adults, being approximately 0.3 per cent of total body weight. Eighty per cent of the organ is water and 5 per cent is fat. Half of this fat consists of phosphatides, which is high when compared to other organs, save the brain. Protein, including mucoprotein, make up 13 per cent. There is little carbohydrate present, approximately 1 per cent being found. This includes small amounts of glycogen which may be increased in severe diabetes. Variable but considerable amounts of urea, uric acid, serum albumin and other organic substances, such as oxalates, may be present, depending on the state of health. Urea and other substances, together with electrolytes, are highly concentrated in the papilla and become less concentrated as one moves from the papillary tip through the medulla to the cortex. This layering relates to the counter-current multiplying system of Wirtz which finally forms the urine.

With regard to vitamins, ascorbic acid and the B complex vitamins, particularly niacin, riboflavin, and thiamin, are present in considerable amount compared to other organs. As far as electrolytes and trace elements are concerned, chloride is most abundant, being 200 mg/100 gm fat-free wet weight (F.F.W.W.) of tissue. Sodium and potassium are less abundant (each 175 mg/100 gm. F.F.W.W.) and are followed by magnesium, calcium and phosphorus (from 20 to 14 mg/100 gm F.F.W.W.).

The ranges of metal concentration of eighteen "essential" and "nonessential" elements have been studied by Perry and his colleagues[3] (Table 30-1). It is of interest that, of all the trace elements, cadmium is abundant in the kidney compared to its low level in other organs. Cadmium has generally been considered to serve no physio-

Table 30-1. Ranges of Metal Concentration in the Kidney and Liver of American Adults (frozen tissue)[*3]

| Metal | 10th and 90th Percentiles | |
	Liver	Kidney
Essential		
Mg	340–750	360–680
Ca	55–170	130–430
Mn	1.0–4.0	0.82–2.7
Fe	95–430	72–200
Cu	5.0–21	3.0–5.4
Zn	34–92	49–120
Mo	0.33–1.5	0.21–0.50
Nonessential		
Sr	0.008–0.040	0.033–0.14
Ba	<.001–0.015	<.001–0.029
Al	0.62–4.4	0.51–3.0
Ti	<.1–0.33†	<.1–0.12†
V		
Cr	<.002–0.071	<.002–0.087
Ni	.09–0.19†	<.09–0.19†
Ag	0.0091–0.030	<.0009–0.0093†
Cd	0.53–3.0	13–45
Sn	0.041–0.62	0.042–0.39
Pb	0.29–1.2	0.21–1.1

* Concentrations are expressed as micromoles of metal per gm of tissue ash. Values cited are tenth and ninetieth percentiles of the sample except where < occurs, in which case values cited are limit of detectability and ninetieth percentile. Therefore < indicates that less than 90 per cent of the values equaled or exceeded the minimum measurable concentration of a particular metal.
† Indicate that less than 50 per cent of the values, and blanks indicate that less than 10 per cent of the values, equaled or exceeded the minimum measurable concentrations.

logical function and its presence in tissues has been explained in the past by contamination.

Recently, Valee and his colleagues[4] have extracted a protein from the cortex of horse kidneys which they named "metallothianen." This protein is rich in cadmium, zinc and sulfur. Vander reported in 1962 that cadmium acts directly on the kidneys to enhance sodium and water reabsorption. At present, no other substance, save aldosterone, is known to enhance reabsorption of sodium. It is possible, therefore, to speculate that cadmium might play an important part in renal tubular transport of sodium and, thereby, play a role in the genesis of some forms of hypertension or edema.

Of interest is the occurrence of "ouch-ouch" disease commonly seen in Toyama City on Japan's Island Sea. This illness characterized by proximal tubular dysfunction of the Fanconi syndrome and hypercalciuria results in osteomalacia with extreme bone pain from which the disease derives its name. The etiology has been attributed to the high concentrations of cadmium found in the local rice and soybean which resulted from contamination of the soil by a nearby cadmium mining plant.[5] Cadmium nephropathy is also characterized by a specific type of proteinuria in which albumin molecules of small molecular weight (minialbumins) are excreted.[6]

Although conventional biochemical techniques provide data on the enzyme activity or content of the kidney as a whole, they do not usually yield information of specific physiologic importance because the individual functional units of the nephron cannot be studied by these techniques. Histochemical staining techniques are useful for orientation but are not quantitative. Detailed knowledge of the activities of specific enzymes in the individual anatomical and structural units of the nephron of man in health and disease is needed to provide exact data on the enzymatic and other cellular mechanisms active in the processes of tubular reabsorption and secretion. The enzyme topography of the nephron has been described for a number of enzymes not only for man but for monkeys, dogs, rats, rabbits, frogs, and toadfish.[7-9] The data thus far collected reveal wide differences in activi-

ties of enzymes between structures and between species, emphasizing again the hazards of applying directly to man facts collected on animals.

STRUCTURE, FUNCTION, AND METABOLIC ACTIVITIES OF THE KIDNEYS

The anatomy of the kidney is extraordinarily complex, particularly the intertwining of tubules and blood vessels. In 1843, Bowman clearly related filtration of plasma and secretion of urine to the intimate relationship of blood-filled glomeruli and the tubular capsule which envelops them. Since then it has become more and more apparent that structure subserves function.

Function. Broadly, the kidney has three functions.* These are (1) the urinary functions of the kidney; (2) their homeostatic and metabolic functions; and (3) their endocrine activity. The first is concerned with expulsion of excess water, solutes, waste products of metabolism (including protons), dead and dying renal cells, minute amounts of proteins—particularly renal mucoproteins—and ingested poisons. The second function is related to the first. It deals with the maintenance of normal nutrition and acid-base and electrolyte balance and the water economy of the body. The third deals with hormones secreted by the organ. Among these are *renin* (see below), and *erythropoietin*, which balances hemoglobin and red cell production. A third hormone (or group of hormones—the prostaglandins) is present in the kidney of dogs and may be secreted by the medulla in man. It may act to preserve normal blood pressure, and regulate sodium transport in man.

Metabolic and Synthetic Activities. The metabolic and synthetic activities of the

* No comprehensive account of renal function can be given here. For those who need to refresh their memories, we suggest they browse in the following: R. F. Pitts, *Physiology of the Kidney and Body Fluids; An Introductory Text*, 2nd edition, Chicago, Year Book Publishers, 1968; L. G. Welt, *Clinical Disorders of Hydration and Acid-Base Equilibrium*, 3rd edition, Boston, Little, Brown & Co., 1971; D. A. Black (Ed.), *Renal Disease*, 3rd edition, Philadelphia, Blackwell Davis Co., 1972.

kidney are second only to the liver. The formation of ammonia in the renal tubules from glutamine and other amino acids is a well-known and well-studied function, but the kidney is also an active site of glucose formation. In addition, it synthesizes protein, mucoproteins and fats, and uses energy to transport and secrete innumerable organic and inorganic substances. The kidney has the highest oxygen consumption of any organ save the minute carotid chemoreceptors. The oxygen consumption of the renal cortex is the highest of any tissue, while its respiratory quotient is one of the lowest. The studies of Lee et al.[10] indicate that the oxidation of fatty acids is the principal energy-yielding process in the cortex's highly aerobic metabolism, but the cortex is capable of utilizing a variety of substrates, including glucose, fructose, mannose, pyruvate, and acetate. The oxygen consumption of the renal medulla is about one-sixth that of the cortex, and it is primarily dependent on glucose to supply energy for its predominantly anaerobic glycolytic metabolism.

The older investigators believed that three-fourths of the theoretical work of the kidney was involved in excreting urea and advised restriction of dietary protein intake to "rest" the kidney injured by disease. It is true that dietary protein is restricted in the treatment of certain renal disorders but not, as we shall see, to "rest" the kidney. Although we do not know exactly what the kidney does with most of the energy released by its metabolism, we now know that little is expended on the medullary countercurrent mechanism which concentrates urine. Most of the energy released appears to be used in the active reabsorption of solutes and nutrients such as sodium[11] in the proximal and distal (cortical) convolutions of the tubule.

RENAL DISORDERS IN ANIMALS FOLLOWING CONSUMPTION OF INADEQUATE DIETS

Experimental. In animals, disturbances of renal function and structure have been produced with some difficulty by dietary manipulations. Nocturia, hematuria, renal calculi, and tubular abnormalities have de-veloped as a result of inadequate food intake. Thus far, deficiencies of ascorbic acid, vitamin K, vitamin A, alpha tocopherol, linoleic acid, choline, potassium, magnesium and chloride have been shown to affect the kidneys of animals—usually the tubules.[12] The pathologic changes have not always been clear-cut, and this is, perhaps, due to present-day difficulties in interpreting structural abnormalities in tubular cells by tinctorial techniques.

The older literature—what little there is of it—deals in the main with the effects of high- or low-protein diets on renal hypertrophy and repair after nephrectomy, or on short-term effects of different diets on renal function, and has been completely reviewed by Smith.[13]

It has been known for some time that an excessive intake of vitamin D can produce hypercalcemia, hypercalciuria and metastatic calcification in the kidney, which may lead to either fatal or reversible renal failure. Dietary imbalance, with a high-calcium, low-phosphorus diet, has been shown to promote renal lithiasis.[14] In recent years, it has been suspected that an excessive intake of common salt was a factor in the production of essential hypertension. The relationships between sodium intake and the kidney have been explored by Meneely and his colleagues[15] who produced renal lesions and hypertension in rats by diets containing large amounts of salt.

Best and Hartroft[16] have produced hypertension and renal disease in adult rats by an acute deprivation of choline during their infancy; the rats being fed at a luxus level during their life span. This observation, coupled with Hartroft's finding of glomerulo-sclerotic-like deposits in the kidneys of choline-deficient rats,[17] raises again the question of the intestinal origin of the vascular complications of the diabetes, long suspected of being dietary in origin. It is interesting to recall the investigations of Burr and his associates[18–20] on linoleic acid deficiency and renal lesion in rats and to speculate that imbalances of fat intake may be a factor in producing hardening of the arteries, in the kidney, not only in diabetic patients but in many others.

Naturally Occurring Disorders. Although renal calculi, some presumably of nutritional origin, have been reported in animals, there are no commonly known nutritional disorders which affect the kidney of domestic and wild animals. Renal diseases are quite common in beasts as in man, but are, in the main, infections. Pregnant sheep develop a disease which has been related to human eclampsia but, at present, this seems rather far-fetched to us.

RENAL FUNCTION, DIET AND EXPERIMENTAL NUTRITIONAL DYSFUNCTION IN MAN

Although the kidneys of man hardly ever suffer permanent damage as a result of dietary deficiency, function is affected by food and meals and, on occasion, manipulation of diet and water can produce functional disturbances which may be quite profound.

Maintenance of Normal Hydrogen Ion Concentration. In health, the renal tubules, together with the lungs, play a central role in maintaining the normal hydrogen ion concentration of plasma and extracellular fluids. Each day the nutritional and metabolic activity of the body produces an excess of acid metabolites. These consist mainly of 20 mol of carbonic acid which is volatile and eliminated by the lungs, and 50 to 100 mEq of hydrogen ion as fixed acid (phosphate, sulfate, etc.) which must be excreted by the kidney. In the urine, the excess hydrogen ions are excreted as titratable acids and as ammonium. Most of the titratable acidity is present as acid phosphate (NaH_2PO_4 and KH_2PO_4) together with small amounts of organic acids like citric acid. Normally, this accounts for 20 to 24 mEq of hydrogen daily, while ammonium, which represents the larger part of the metabolic fixed acid excreted, amounts to 30 to 50 mEq daily. Within the tubular cells, glutaminase and other amino-oxidases produce ammonia. The fat-soluble ammonia diffuses freely into the tubular lumen where it is ionized to the ammonium (NH_4^+) ion by combining with an H^+ ion from carbonic acid, thus releasing bicarbonate ions (HCO_3^-) which are reabsorbed into the blood to replenish the

"alkali reserve" while the ammonium is excreted in the urine.

The net effect of both phosphate and ammonium excretion is to replenish the plasma bicarbonate level while excreting hydrogen ions. It has been shown that there is a reciprocal relationship between urinary potassium and pH; this has been interpreted to indicate that hydrogen and potassium ions are exchanged during some of the above reactions, particularly phosphate excretion. It should be noted that hydrogen ion is also exchanged for sodium in many of these reactions. When acidosis occurs in individuals with healthy kidneys, acid phosphate excretion can increase relatively little, but ammonium output may rise tenfold. The potential ability of the kidney to synthesize ammonium to take care of excess protons produced by severe exercise or disease is considerable. When patients become acidotic, for example, during diabetic ketosis, the ammonium synthetic mechanism undergoes an adaptive hypertrophy and the tubular cells can produce and secrete 10 times the amount they normally present to the urine. This also occurs during consumption of the high-fat "ketogenic diet" and during consumption of culinary and other chemicals which produce acidosis (*e.g.*, methanol, ammonium chloride).

Renal tubular acidosis (RTA) is a condition in which there is a defect in renal excretion of hydrogen ion, or reabsorption of bicarbonate, or both, which occurs in the absence of, or out of proportion to, an impairment in the glomerular filtration rate. RTA can be divided into two forms: (*a*) proximal RTA, caused by a defect in proximal tubular reabsorption of bicarbonate; (*b*) distal RTA, resulting from an inability to establish adequate H^+ ion gradients between blood and distal tubular fluid.

Urinary pH. As with other renal functions, healthy kidneys can produce urine with a wide range of pH (between 4.5 and 8) but the pooled daily specimen is usually acid (pH 6). This has led to a misleading tendency among some writers to call urine pH from 6 to 7 "alkaline," which is manifestly inaccurate and misleading. Immediately following a meal, the urine becomes less acid (the "alkaline tide") and a few hours later it becomes acid again. During sleep, decreased pulmonary ventilation causes respiratory acidosis and the urine becomes highly acid. Because of these physiologic facts, the urinary pH varies widely in health.

Ingestion of different foods, various diets, and culinary chemicals (such as bicarbonate of soda) also affects the urinary pH. The usual diet of Western man, rich in animal protein, produces an acid urine. Predominantly vegetable diets, such as are commonly consumed in the East, in the tropics, and by economically depressed individuals, produce an alkaline urine.

Effect of Diet on Renal Function. Studies on renal function with low-protein and high-protein diets on healthy individuals have been made by a number of individuals using modern techniques, but no gross changes were observed.[21-23] Brod believes that, with a high-protein intake, there is a rise in filtration rate resulting from renal hyperemia and he stressed the importance of protein in the daily rhythm of glomerular filtration which parallels the rhythm of the metabolic processes of the body. The most exhaustive studies of the effects of diet on renal function of healthy young men have been made by Johnson and Sargent, and as yet have been only briefly presented in the literature.[24] They showed that many alterations can be provoked in renal function by nutritional imbalance, caloric deficit, dehydration, physical work and extremes of temperature.

In these investigations, the experiments involved all possible combination of water deprivation, salt deprivation and protein deprivation, thus producing the three commonly recognized varieties of hydropenia; i.e., pure water depletion hydropenia, pure salt depletion hydropenia and mixed salt and water hydropenia. In the chronically and severely dehydrated subject, an ingested water load was retained only when the osmolar excretion exceeded 700 milliosmols/day. Therefore, without knowledge of the rate of osmolar excretion, one cannot conclude that a subject is well hydrated merely because he excretes a copious volume of dilute urine after a water load.

They found that ketonuria was easily produced by nutritional imbalance and aggravated by exposure to cold or hard work. Transient albuminuria could be produced by an unbalanced diet or vigorous exercise, and exposure to cold accentuated this phenomenon. Microscopic hematuria and cylindruria could also be produced by starvation or unbalanced diets, especially pure carbohydrate. When a predisposition existed, moderate exercise could accentuate the microscopic hematuria and cylindruria.

They also found that a combination of chronic dehydration and a diet containing over 12 gm of nitrogen per day increased the concentrations of urea, creatinine and nonprotein nitrogen in the serum. Caloric deficiency decreased creatinine and urea clearances. Gross variations in diet could produce large alterations in the clearance values for sodium, chloride and total osmolar active substances.

Factors Influencing Urinary Findings. Johnson and Sargent reviewed their findings in healthy men as they relate to the sick. They stressed the need for the physician to recognize that abnormal urinalyses and tests of renal function in patients might not be the result only of parenchymal renal disease. They might well be the result of dietary imbalance (oral or parenteral); dehydration or over-hydration; fever or hypothermia; activity or rest, and these effects of illness or treatment must be taken into consideration when reviewing laboratory data on blood and urine. Teschan and his colleagues[25] recently described increased excretion of white cells and cylindruria with exercise in young recruits They also described decreased osmolalities and decreased free-water clearance with severe exercise. Johnson and Sargent, and Schedl and his colleagues,[26] have shown the need for close dietary control when measuring the urinary creatinine clearance and osmolar clearance. In the former test, the 24-hour excretion of endogenous creatinine is influenced adversely by a low-protein diet. The latter test is only of value when solutes are available to the kidney for clearance and erroneous results may be obtained when patients are tested while consuming a low-sodium diet or any other diet low in solutes.

THE COMMON NUTRIENTS
AND RENAL DISORDERS

Below we describe some of the more common nutritional disturbances seen in patients with renal and associated disorders. These will be categorized briefly in terms of the individual nutrients, and later, some are discussed in greater depth when one deals with the common clinical situations in which they occur.

Water. Excessive renal loss of water is seen: in the absence of antidiuretic hormone (diabetes insipidus); when the renal tubules are unable to react to diuretic hormone (nephrogenic diabetes insipidus); in many established cases of chronic renal failure and during the diuretic phase of recovery from acute renal failure. It may also be apparent when osmotic agents such as glucose (diabetes mellitus, intravenous infusion), mannitol or urea produce a diuresis and, also, when diuretic drugs are used. Excessive retention of water (without salt) is most often the result of injudicious infusion of glucose and water during and after operations, the surgeon at the same time withholding sodium. The syndrome of inappropriate ADH secretion with water retention has been associated with many conditions and been recently reviewed. This frequently produces water intoxication, a condition which may also be operative in preeclampsia of pregnancy.

Calories. Caloric deficiency is a major problem in uremia from any cause. In uremia, vomiting as well as loss of appetite interferes with food intake and diarrhea with absorption. Caloric deficiency is also a major problem in nephrotic patients and is aggravated by edema of the gastrointestinal tract and by ascites. Occasionally, polycystic kidneys can be so large as to press on the stomach and mechanically interfere with eating.

Caloric excess and obesity are difficult to deal with in patients with renal disease who are treated with steroids, particularly if they are adolescent girls. Obesity has been stated to be a cause of proteinuria but we have not been able to confirm this.

Protein and Amino Acids. Protein deficiency is universal in the nephrotic syndrome and manifests itself by tissue protein deple-

tion, hypoalbuminemia and fatty metamorphosis of the renal tubules and sometimes of the liver. Long-term treatment of renal disease with steroid hormones also results in tissue protein wastage. Proteinuria appears to condition malnutrition only if large amounts of albumin are lost each day with the urine and the nutritional economy does not appear to be seriously compromised when other plasma proteins are lost as, for example, when large quantities of myeloma protein are excreted. Amino acids are lost in the urine in renal tubular disorders and may precipitate as stones (cystinuria). When disease processes, such as acute hepatic necrosis, raise the blood levels of amino acids, these may exceed tubular reabsorptive capacity and overflow into the urine. Excessive urinary loss of amino acids may also account for hepatic disease and bone and tissue changes which are sometimes associated with renal tubular defects.

Genetic defects produce inborn errors of metabolism which result in excessive urinary loss of amino acids and other nitrogenous and non-nitrogenous substances in the urine. Among these are cystinuria, cystinosis, alkaptonuria, maple-syrup urine disease, citrullinuria, benign fructosuria and pentosuria. With the tremendous and explosive interest in human genetic disorders, no doubt many more inborn errors of metabolism will be uncovered which involve the kidney. Some, such as galactosuria, phenylketonuria and cystinuria, are being successfully treated by dietary manipulation (see Chapter 39).

At present, there is no evidence that an excessive or luxus protein intake *per se* harms the kidney. But the kidney has to deal with the catabolic products of protein metabolism. Intrinsic and extrinsic protein metabolic products include polypeptides, amino acids, amines, urea, uric acid, ammonium ions, protons, and a host of known and unknown organic and inorganic fragments. Some of these produce clearly delineated renal diseases. One such is gouty nephropathy, the result of deposition of uric acid in the renal medulla and papillae.

On the other hand, in uremic poisoning, which is the common manifestation of renal failure, it is still not clear which protein breakdown products are responsible for symptoms. Studies have implicated a wide variety of products to be responsible for some of the hematologic and neurologic disturbances associated with uremia.[27] Substances such as phenolic acids and guanidino-succinic acid are felt to be, in part, responsible for the bleeding abnormality of uremia.[28]

Carbohydrate. Excessive consumption of certain fruits, like plums, and vegetables, like Jerusalem artichokes, allows escape in the urine of the uncommon carbohydrates the plants contain but they produce no ill effects. Losses of carbohydrates also occur in genetic disorders, as we stated before. With renal tubular disorders, such as renal glycosuria of the Fanconi syndrome, sufficient glucose can be lost to produce symptoms of hypoglycemia. Glucose intolerance is a common feature of renal failure, even when those patients with diabetic nephropathy are excluded. Carbohydrate and insulin metabolism in renal failure has recently been reviewed.[29,30] There is a rough correlation of the intolerance with retention of nitrogen. Glucose intolerance appears to be associated with a dialyzable antagonist, not yet identified, to the peripheral metabolic action of insulin.[31] Improvement in intolerance occurs with repeated dialysis. Some other factors important in glucose intolerance frequently seen in renal failure may be inadequate calorie intake, potassium depletion and chronic acidemia. Glucose intolerance is clearly undesirable and measures to improve correctable factors should be taken where possible. Occasionally, the hyperglycemia may require exogenous insulin for control. Tolerance of fructose, galactose and sorbitol is apparently normal in renal failure.[32]

Lipids. No clear-cut data are available in man on the effects of fat consumption nor of disorders of lipids which bear on the nutrition of the kidney and its vessels. There is a rare familial disorder (first described by Fabry and named for him) involving the kidney in which the cells of the glomerular tuft are filled with lipid but this does not appear to have nutritional consequences. Recently, disorders of lipid metabolism have been described in patients with chronic renal failure, particularly patients on chronic hemodialysis.[33–35]

The observation of lactescent or milky blood flowing through dialysis tubing during hemodialysis suggested that abnormalities in triglyceride metabolism were present in chronic uremia. Most regularly dialyzed patients have elevated triglyceride levels. Many dialyzed, non-nephrotic uremic patients were also found to have abnormal triglyceride levels. Hypertriglyceridemia, therefore, appears to be a feature of chronic renal failure itself, which is more marked in dialyzed patients.

Since work of Ahrens[36] and Dole[37] it has become obvious that carbohydrate and lipid metabolism are very intimately related. As described above, uremic patients have glucose intolerance often associated with greater than normal basal insulin levels. Triglyceride and immunoreactive insulin levels have been found to be directly related suggesting that increased synthesis of triglyceride-rich lipoprotein contributes to the triglyceride elevation in uremia.[34]

Triglyceride removal is believed to be mediated by the lipoprotein lipase enzyme system. Impaired removal may result in accumulation of both dietary and endogenous triglyceride. Post-heparin lipolytic activity, an indirect measure of lipoprotein lipase activity, has been reported to be subnormal in both dialyzed and undialyzed uremic subjects.[35]

Lewis et al.[38] suggest that serum alpha lipoprotein levels may be regulated by renal tissue. They found alpha lipoproteins to be greatly decreased in anephric patients on dialysis. The beta lipoprotein levels were normal. After renal transplantation alpha lipoprotein levels became normal and remained normal as long as the kidney functioned well. If the kidney was rejected and removed, alpha lipoprotein levels again decreased to low levels.

Hypercholesterolemia is, of course, a hallmark of the nephrotic syndrome and is further discussed below. Berlyne[39] has recently shown that ischemic heart disease is a complication of nephrotic syndrome that occurs with a frequency about 85 times that of the general population of the same age group.

Every effort should be made to return plasma lipid values to normal in the nephrotic patient.

Sodium. Consumption of sodium in excess has been claimed to be related to the development of high blood pressure and is, perhaps, genetically mediated, as we shall see below. Retention of sodium with water as a result of functional or structural abnormalities of the kidney is common and is present in acute glomerulonephritis, in acute renal failure, as well as in the nephrotic syndrome. Renal loss of sodium may be the result of functional disturbances of the tubule— Addison's disease is one example—but sodium wasting is more common with tubular damage as in chronic renal failure and chronic pyelonephritis and in the diuretic phase of acute renal failure. Preeclampsia is commonly thought to be the result of excess consumption of sodium but there is evidence that too little salt early in pregnancy may precipitate the disorder. Diets low in salt, diuretics and repeated paracenteses may produce serious deficits of salt and consequent reduction of plasma volume and interfere with renal function. The blood urea nitrogen may be spectacularly increased when this happens.

Chloride. In general, nutritional lack or excess of chloride parallels the state of sodium nutriture. When mercurial diuretics are given, there may be excessive loss of chloride. Hypochloremia with alkalosis is seen during potassium deficiency and prolonged gastric suction. There is a urinary retention of chloride by the bowel relative to sodium in patients with ureterostomies, and hyperchloremia frequently develops. Hyperchloremic acidosis is a common biochemical manifestation of chronic uremia.

Potassium. Potassium retention is common in chronic and acute renal failure. Potassium deficiency is seen in functional or organic renal disorders such as renal tubular syndromes, chronic pyelonephritis or hyperaldosteronism. It develops commonly as a result of treatment with diuretic agents and steroid hormones and may follow self-induced diarrhea. Chronic deficiency results in kaliopenic nephropathy.

Calcium and Phosphorus. Small amounts of calcium are normally deposited in the kidney. Primary and secondary hyperparathyroidism, excess intake of vitamin D, neoplasms, immobilization, the milk-alkali syndrome, sarcoidosis and hyperthyroidism may all produce hypercalcemia, hypercalciuria, nephrocalcinosis, and sometimes renal calculi. A low serum calcium is common in chronic renal failure; osteomalacia and deformities of bones may result from calcium wastage in renal tubular disorders (Fanconi). In the nephrotic syndrome, hypocalcemia is often related to the low serum protein levels.

Phosphorus is retained in both acute and chronic renal disease and is rather toxic. With renal tubular disorders, hyperparathyroidism, and some other states of hypercalcemia, phosphaturia occurs and a low serum phosphorus is noted. Uremic bone disease and the effects of calcium, phosphate and vitamin D are discussed below.

Vitamin D. A great deal of recent research has uncovered much of the mechanism of vitamin D metabolism. It is now known that vitamin D is converted in the body to metabolically active forms; these forms have greater activity than the parent compound in initiating intestinal calcium transport and bone mineral mobilization.[40] One metabolite is 25-hydroxycholecalciferol (25-OHCC). The liver appears to be the organ responsible for this step in hydroxylation. Another metabolite, 1,25-diOHCC, appears to be the functionally active vitamin form, and this is thought to be generated exclusively in kidney tissue.[41] This observation explains much of the abnormality associated with decreased calcium absorption and vitamin D resistance in chronic renal failure. Moreover, Avioli[42] has shown that there are abnormalities in the metabolism and excretion of vitamin D_3 in chronic renal failure. Vitamin D is discussed in Chapter 5B.

Other Minerals. In Wilson's disease, in which there is a tubular defect and excess tissue copper, renal wasting of copper and other nutrients may occur. Treatment with a copper-free diet has been used. Magnesium deficiency has been observed in aldosterone-producing tumors and in alcoholism. It is not clear whether deficiency of magnesium affects the kidney. Some animal work suggests magnesium deficiency does affect renal function.[43] Injection of magnesium has been used to treat eclampsia and, also, the muscle-twitching of uremia. This is a pharmacologic not a nutritional use of the element.

Iron. Occasionally, with gross hematuria from the urinary tract, as in Bilharzia, acute glomerulonephritis, and tumors, iron-deficiency anemia may be seen. Anemia due to lack of erythropoietin is much more common in chronic renal failure than iron deficiency and does not respond to specific treatment with vitamins or iron; however, every now and then one sees patients with chronic renal failure, particularly female patients with iron-deficiency anemia, which responds to appropriate treatment.

Mixed Disturbance of Nutriture. In clinical situations, isolated deficiency or excess of any single one of the above nutrients is most uncommon for renal disorders, as with most clinical situations. Disturbances of nutriture in renal disease involve many rather than few nutrients.

DEFICIENCY DISEASES AND RENAL DISORDERS IN MAN

Until the description of kaliopenic nephropathy, there had been no real evidence on hand to indicate that deficiencies of major nutrients *seriously* affected renal structure and function in man. This is surprising, since the kidneys must pursue vigorously their synthetic activities and other biochemical functions which serve the body. Despite their need for protein and nutrients to carry on their varied metabolic activities, they appear to be relatively resistant to the effects of nutritional deprivation. Their immunity to nutritional disease is probably related to their unique position in the nutritional economy of the body. They are small organs, but in an active man, they receive over 1,700 liters of blood each day—one-fifth of the cardiac output and one-fifth of the circulating nutrients. Some of the alterations in renal function during nutritional deficiency are discussed below.

Protein-Calorie Malnutrition. In severe chronic caloric malnutrition, renal function is disturbed and reduced. The most commonly described features have been polyuria, nocturia, and hyposthenuria.[44] The pathophysiologic effects of starvation on the metabolic and excretory functions of the kidney recently have been greatly elucidated by several investigators.

Metabolic Alterations During Starvation. During prolonged starvation the body tends to protect its protein stores by decreasing protein catabolism and relies primarily upon utilization of fat stores for energy. Urea nitrogen, ordinarily the major nitrogenous end product, rapidly diminishes to low basal excretion levels and ammonium nitrogen represents a greater proportion of total urinary nitrogen excretion. The reduction of urea nitrogen reflects the decreased gluconeogenesis from protein sources.

Owen *et al.*[45,46] have shown that the kidneys are very active metabolically during prolonged starvation. Oxygen consumption increases and CO_2 production increases. Various substrates, *e.g.* lactate, pyruvate, β-hydroxybutyrate, amino nitrogen, glycerol and fatty acids, are extracted across the renal bed. There is increased renal production of glucose and acetoacetate. Of the total amount of glucose synthesized daily during starvation, the kidney contributes 45 per cent, the liver contributing the other 55 per cent. Analysis of individual amino acid concentration, in arterial and venous renal blood has shown there is net uptake of glycine, alanine and proline with net release of serine during starvation.

The altered metabolic activity of the kidney during starvation is reflected in the constituents of the urine. Ketone bodies, principally β-hydroxybutyrate, are greatly increased; urea is diminished and ammonium is increased. Of the amino acids present in urine glycine is excreted in greatest amounts. Ammonium production by the kidney has been shown to be closely tied to gluconeogenesis, and is promptly stimulated by conditions of acidosis.[47] During starvation the increased ammonium is needed to balance the increased excretion of β-hydroxybutyrate. During starvation the kidney thus reflects the change in metabolism of the body, *i.e.* the decrease in protein catabolism, the utilization of lipids for energy, and plays a major role in the daily production of glucose.

Dilution and Concentration Ability During Starvation. It has long been recognized that during starvation subjects excrete copious dilute urine. The structural and functional characteristics of the counter-current multiplier system of the kidney have been well described.[48] Essential to the elaboration of a concentrated urine is the maintenance of an osmotic gradient in the deep medullary portion of the kidney. It has long been recognized that high protein feedings increase the concentrative ability of the kidney. Studies by Klahr et al.[49] suggest that the mechanism of decreased concentrative ability in malnutrition is secondary to the failure to establish a hyperosmolar medullary gradient due to the diminished urea concentration in the medullary regions. The concentrative defect was restored in malnourished individuals by the intravenous administration of urea. Manitius et al.,[50] however, postulated that the enhanced concentrating ability on protein feeding was related to increased Na and K in the renal papilla.

Acid-Base Balance in Starvation. The kidneys play a primary role in the regulation of electrolyte and hydrogen ion homeostasis. Acid loads are poorly handled by malnourished patients. Klahr et al.[51] found that the inability to excrete hydrogen ion loads was due to a diminished titratable acid excretion. Ammonia production was elevated in starvation but titratable acid was diminished primarily due to the decreased urinary excretion of phosphate. When malnourished patients were provided with phosphate ions, by intravenous or oral supplementation, the ability to excrete acid loads and increase titratable acids in the urine was restored.

Sodium Homeostasis in Starvation. It has long been recognized that despite the virtual absence of sodium intake there is a continuing natriuresis associated with starvation.[52–54] This natriuresis can be abolished by feeding of small amounts of carbohydrates, whereas fats do not have this sodium-sparing effect. Epstein et al.[55] recently showed that protein or carbohydrate feedings but not fat would abolish the natriuresis of starvation. They postulate the loss of sodium to be the

consequence of continuing breakdown of protein tissue with release of electrolytes and that this breakdown is diminished with protein and/or carbohydrate feedings.

Urinary Excretion of Vitamins During Starvation. Consolazio et al.,[56] Keys et al.,[57] and others have studied urinary excretion of vitamins during prolonged starving. Vitamin excretion rapidly diminishes during caloric restriction, but did not reach zero level during a 10-day period in the studies by Consolazio. Keys et al. had reported increased excretion of riboflavin during starvation.

Structural Alteration During Starvation. When patients die of starvation, little is found in the kidney but atrophy. Gross structural changes are not often seen in kidney of malnourished infants and children coming to autopsy. Some histologic alterations have been reported.[58] These consist of intense fatty metamorphosis of the convoluted tubules. Perhaps more detailed studies such as electron microscopy and enzymatic analysis can shed further light.

Vitamin Deficient States. There are no characteristic renal structural or functional changes in pellagra and beriberi while scurvy and hemorrhagic hypoprothrombinemia are the only deficiency states known to produce hematuria. Eales[59] has described some changes in renal function in 14 patients with florid scurvy, but these changes may have been due to the associated anemia and slight protein depletion. Thiamin and pyridoxine deficiencies have been implicated in the experimental production of renal stones, but their significance with regard to man is not clear.[60,61]

Mineral Deficiency States. The effects of deficiencies of sodium and potassium on renal function have been recently reviewed[62] and will not be extensively described here. The well-known effects of sodium deficit are reduction of plasma volume with consequent reduction of renal blood flow and glomerular filtration rate. Sodium-preserving homeostatic mechanisms come into play with reduction of urinary excretion of sodium and increased tubular reabsorption. No permanent structural alterations related to chronic hyponatremia have been described.

Chronic hypokalemia can permanently alter the function and structure of the kidney[63] and is described in further detail below.

The effects of deficiencies of other minerals such as magnesium, calcium and phosphate on renal function have not as yet been clearly defined, but there is some experimental evidence in animals to suggest that magnesium deficiency may alter renal function.

CLASSIFICATION OF RENAL DISORDERS

There seems to be no end to the number of classifications of renal diseases one reads about. Even today, each person who deals with the problem comes to it with little knowledge of the exact etiology and less of the natural history of each renal disorder. Although the pathology of the kidney seen post mortem has been worked out, more or less to everybody's satisfaction, classification based on autopsy findings is not too accurate. When patients die of renal disorders, the prosector in the dead house sees, in the main, sclerotic "end-stage" kidneys. These, more often than not, are called by him "chronic glomerulonephritis," "chronic pyelonephritis" or "arteriolonephrosclerosis." He is frequently unable to find clues to lead him back to the original disease process, and it is even more difficult for him to determine how the disease process progressed during life to reach its final scarred state. Serial renal biopsies, during life, give a dynamic picture of renal pathology and allow us to make exact histologic diagnoses early in disease. This technique has been used only for a decade or so and, as yet, not enough evidence has been collected to allow one to make a firm histologic classification, let alone an etiologic one, which is, of course, most satisfactory.

Classification can be simple. For example, one can classify renal disorders into two classes: (1) intrinsic renal diseases, and (2) generalized disease processes involving the kidney. But classifications can be very complex. Usually, in any single classification, we find that the author has to mix his categories. In one instance, the nomenclature is histologic, *e.g.* glomerulonephritis; in another, it names a clinical entity, *e.g.* the nephrotic

syndrome; it may describe a metabolic disorder, "renal glycosuria," or a specific etiology—"leptospirosis of the kidney." To clarify the discussion of the nutritional aspects of renal disorders, a classification is given in Table 30–2. One hopes it might be useful to the reader, even if it is not academically satisfactory.

Nutrition and Hypertension. Hypertension by itself is not a disease. Rather, it is a sympton complex that may manifest itself in the course of many disorders and whose development may be based on one of several mechanisms. It may occur as a symptom in the course of such diseases as acute or chronic glomerulonephritis, pyelonephritis, lesions of the brain (notably tumors), renal arterial stenosis, polycystic renal disease, congenital anomalies of the kidneys, hyperthyroidism, coarctation of the aorta and tumors of the adrenal glands, such as pheochromocytoma and aldosteronoma. When hypertension occurs in the course of any of these conditions, management of the secondary hypertension is directed, for the most part, toward diagnosis and treatment of the primary condition unless the blood pressure elevation is extreme or accelerating as in the "malignant" phase.

In addition to patients who have these forms of hypertension, for which known causes exist, many patients suffer from well-recognized, persistent, chronic hypertensive disease. By far the most common form of this latter type of elevated blood pressure is primary hypertension, or diffuse arteriolar disease with hypertension, the cause of which is still unknown even though it was first described by Richard Bright in 1827.[64]

It has been known for many years that both genetic and environmental factors appear to play a role in hypertension, particularly in that form of hypertension formerly named "essential" and nowadays called "primary." In the following consideration of the nutritional aspects of hypertension, only primary hypertension and hypertension associated with renal disease (renal hypertension) will be discussed.

The present concepts of the pathogenesis are not agreed upon and the investigations into hypertension have emphasized different mechanisms. A recent conference on Hyper-

Table 30-2.   Classification of Some Renal Diseases and Disorders

Acute Glomerulitis . . . .: *e g.* Lupus Nephritis; Rheumatoid Arthritis.

* The Acute Glomerulonephritides . . . .: *e.g.* Post-Streptococcal; Henoch-Schönlein; Necrotizing.

* Persistent Asymptomatic Proteinuria.

* The Nephrotic Syndrome (see Table 30–5)

* The Chronic Glomerulonephritides . . . . .: *e.g.* Post-Streptococcal; Diabetic Nephropathy; Lupus Nephritis.

* Hypertension . . . .: *e.g.* Renovascular Hypertension; Pre-eclampsia; Primary or "Essential"; Endocrine.

Arteriolonephrosclerosis.

* Chronic Pyelonephritis.

* Interstitial Nephritis . . . .: *e.g.* Kaliopenic Nephropathy; Analgesic Abuse; Scarlet Fever.

* Acute Renal Failure . . . .: *e.g.* Transfusion Reaction; Crush Syndrome; Postoperative.

Infections of the Kidney . . . .: *e.g.* Acute Pyelonephritis; Tuberculosis.

* Renal Tubular Defects (see Table 30–8)

* Genetic Disorders . . . .: *e.g.* Polycystic Disease; Hereditary Nephritis; Primary Hyperoxaluria; Cystinosis.

* Endocrine Disorders . . . .: *e.g.* Juxtaglomerular Apparatus Hypertrophy; Diabetes Insipidus.

Obstructive Uropathy . . . .: *e.g.* Renal Calculi; Prostatic Hypertrophy; Retroperitoneal Fibrosis.

* Renal Calculi . . . .: *e.g.* Uric Acid; Cystine.

---

* Dietary treatment or nutritional abnormalities are or may be important.

tensive Mechanisms[65] brought together investigations with three main approaches—autonomic neurophysiologic control of blood pressure, renal-adrenal control of the circulation, and classicial circulatory physiology. Contributors discussed catecholamine turnover and excretion, ultrastructure of vasomotor nerves and role of the autonomic nervous system as well as many other facets of hypertension. The results of these papers do not indicate any specific etiology and it is not clear how many of the phenomena described are cause or effect.

Richard Bright long ago agreed the kidney was intimately involved with the production and maintenance of chronic hypertension. In the 1930's his observations were substantiated by investigations of Goldblatt *et al.* which placed on firm experimental basis evidence for renal pressor agents. The issue now is at an extremely interesting stage with informed opinion varying as to the view whether the renin-angiotensin system is significant in many types of hypertension. Moreover, antipressor substances have been isolated from renal tissue and their role is still speculative. Finally, the interrelationships between the autonomic system, renin-angio tensin system, and circulatory volume are only now beginning to become unraveled.

At the present writing the accumulated evidence appears to suggest the following chain of reactions: multiple factors → stimulation of receptors in the juxtaglomerular apparatus of the kidney → increased secretion and release of renin → increased circulatory angiotensin II →increased peripheral vascular resistance → hypertension. The multiple factors involved with initiation of this sequence may be neuro-mediated, humoral-mediated, pressure-mediated or volume-mediated. In addition, angiotensin II is known to stimulate the adrenal cortex to secrete aldosterone which promotes renal tubular reabsorption of sodium and thereby affects the electrolyte economy of the body, the plasma volume and presumably the blood pressure.[66]

Aldosterone, moreover, acts on cell membranes throughout the body to affect sodium transport. Tobian[67] and others[68] have shown that there is a much higher sodium content in the arteries of patients and animals with hypertension and that these levels return to normal when the hypertension is relieved. There is also some evidence that the sodium in the arteries, presumably bound to acid mucopolysaccharides in the wall, provides the setting for vascular response to vasoactive substances, presumably making the vessel more sensitive to hypertensive agents.

These complex interrelationships are all very well but they do not explain specific differences in response of blood pressure to high salt intake. Moreover, in man, while some hypertensive patients respond to treatment with low-sodium diet and natriuretic drugs, many do not. It is obvious then that intake of salt and genetic sensitivity can be logically worked into a pathogenetic mosaic.

For example, there is a low incidence of hypertension in several primitive ethnic groups living under different conditions— Greenland Eskimos, aboriginal tribes in mountains of China, Cuner Indians of Panama and aboriginal Australians. Dahl[69] suggests a common factor of these widely differing groups living under widely differing environmental conditions is a very low salt intake (1 to 2 gm/day) as opposed to the usual 10 to 15 gm/day in Western civilized populations. By contrast, the population in Northern Honshu in Japan has an extremely high salt intake in the diet (mean 26 gm/day). The incidence of hypertension and death from cerebral hemorrhage is probably the highest known, approximately 40 per cent of the population being hypertensive. Explanations other than salt intake have also been suggested.[70] Schroeder[71] has been collecting evidence which implies that trace minerals, perhaps cadmium derived from canned foods, as etiologically connected with human hypertension.

Furthermore, strong genetic factors are involved in view of the experimental evidence accumulated by Dahl which shows a direct quantitative unequivocal relationship between dietary salt and hypertension in the laboratory rat. By selective inbreeding, Dahl[72] has been able to produce two strains that breed true. One strain is extremely sensitive to salt and readily develops hypertension. The other strain is resistant and never develops hypertension no matter how much salt is consumed. Young animals are most susceptible and the longer salt is eaten the more severe the effect. Hypertension, once established, is usually self-sustained when salt is removed. In addition, the salt-resistant strain is also resistant to the well-known hypertensive effects of treatment with DOCA or clipping a renal artery. The sensitive animals respond exquisitely to these experimental procedures. Neither group develops hypertension on basal nonsalted ration.

This demonstration of genetic variability in susceptibility to salt hypertension is proposed as paralleling the variation in human familial predisposition to hypertension. One can speculate, therefore, that in man individuals who are sensitive to salt intake will readily develop hypertension when consuming large amounts of salt or when renal artery stenosis or other forms of renal damage release vasoactive substance. Those who are resistant will not develop hypertension despite consuming large amounts of salt or will not get hypertension with renal damage of the same order. In addition, patients with primary or renal hypertension may be divided into two groups—those who respond to salt withdrawal and those who do not.

Recently a debate has centered around the implications of the high salt intake of the very young because of addition of salt to baby foods by manufacturers.[73] Controversy surrounds the question whether high salt intake of infants disposes them to high salt appetites in later life with its possible role of maintaining hypertension.[74]

Types of Primary Hypertension. The scope of this presentation does not allow for detailed description of the classification and clinical characteristics of the types of essential hypertension. In general, essential hypertension is divided into four types (groups I, II, III and IV) on the basis of clinical and retinal findings: groups I and II represent respective degrees of severity of so-called benign hypertension; group III represents a transitional form, or "early malignant" hypertension; and group IV encompasses malignant hypertension. It should be emphasized that a significant proportion of patients in groups III and IV, and even some in group II, has recently been shown to have unilateral or bilateral renal arterial occlusive disease susceptible to surgical treatment with return of the elevated blood pressure to normal or nearly normal levels. Therefore, appropriate diagnostic procedures must be carried out before the severely hypertensive patient is classified as an advanced stage of "essential" hypertension indicating only medical management. Benign hypertension usually develops insidiously and gradually, runs a prolonged or chronic course and rarely produces symptoms until the condition has existed for some time when secondary changes may occur in the heart, kidneys, central nervous system and peripheral arterioles. Little change is seen in the ocular fundi of patients who have benign hypertension except for retinal arteriolar narrowing, focal constrictions and varying degrees of arteriolar sclerosis depending on the chronicity of the disease. Malignant hypertension, as a rule, develops more suddenly, although in many instances benign hypertension of long standing suddenly may develop the characteristics and severity of the malignant type. Malignant hypertension usually occurs in younger patients; the blood pressure reaches extreme heights and the clinical course is punctuated by rapidly progressing symptoms of cardiac failure, renal insufficiency or cerebral vascular changes. Examination of the ocular fundi reveals, in addition to advanced arteriolar changes, hemorrhages and cotton-wool exudates, and, in patients who have severe malignant hypertension (group IV), papilledema in varying degrees.

As indicated by the foregoing, the kidneys appear to play a central role in hypertension. It is not surprising, therefore, that renal disease is very often associated with hypertension. Hypertension and renal failure are found together in three conditions: acute renal failure, chronic renal failure, and malignant hypertension. It is difficult to estimate the prevalence of hypertension in chronic renal failure, but among patients selected for chronic hemodialysis programs hypertension is common.[75] The most frequent causes of renal failure in this group are chronic glomerulonephritis, chronic pyelonephritis, polycystic kidneys and malignant-phase hypertension without previous evidence of renal disease.

In the majority of patients with hypertension and chronic renal failure, the hypertension is controllable with dietary manipulations (principally of salt intake), antihypertensive agents and regular dialysis. A small number of patients, however, have uncontrollable hypertension which may even worsen with dietary restriction of salt or regular dialysis. Bilateral nephrectomy can reduce blood pressure in this group of patients.[76]

Patients with hypertension and chronic renal failure often walk a narrow line between excess salt and exacerbation of hypertension and salt deficiency with reduction of renal function. Nevertheless, with careful monitoring Hunt[77,78] has shown that appropriate salt restriction assists greatly in controlling blood pressure in renal disease with hypertension.

TREATMENT

Caloric Restriction. Obesity is common in patients who have essential hypertension although there is no direct relationship. For this reason, the total caloric intake should be restricted in such patients. Great fluctuations in blood pressure often occur after the ingestion of large meals because of decreased efficiency of vasomotor regulation in patients who have essential hypertension. Furthermore, it is known from experience with all types of myocardial insufficiency that filling of the stomach may result in embarrassment to the heart. The heart then labors under the double load of hypertension and obesity.

For information in regard to calorically restricted diets applicable to hypertensive patients who are obese, the reader is referred to the chapter on Obesity (Chapter 22) and to the Appendix (Tables A-7–A-9). As a general rule, a diet restricted to 1,000 to 1,200 calories daily will bring about desired results without harm to the patient. In most cases, reduction of excessive weight is not accompanied by more than a mild decrease in blood pressure, but in some cases the drop in blood pressure is notable or even striking. Even when blood pressure is not lowered, improvement in subjective symptoms, such as fatigue and dyspnea, may be noted in a degree concomitant with the loss in weight.

Although reduction of caloric intake and exercise in moderation are indicated in the treatment of obese patients who have uncomplicated hypertension, dietary restriction should not be too severe or be carried out over too prolonged a period. To impose unnecessary or too drastic restrictions on pations suffering from uncomplicated early hypertension is frequently productive of more harm than good.

Less frequently, hypertensive patients are greatly underweight and undernourished. No evidence exists to support the thesis that hypertension is benefited by undernutrition; hence, in these patients it is important to restore weight and nutrition to as nearly normal levels as possible. However, reduced intake of food with due consideration for a properly balanced diet may have a beneficial effect in the hypertensive patient entirely apart from blood pressure level, *e.g.* in the latent diabetic, in subjects with elevated blood lipid levels or hyperuricemia.

In summary, the best interest of either the overweight or underweight patient is served by the adjustment of caloric intake in such a manner as to bring the weight of the patient to a normal level.

Protein. For years, sharp restriction of protein was widely used in the treatment of essential hypertension among some members of the medical profession and laity alike. This belief was inculcated so firmly in the minds of the laity that many patients who had hypertension literally had a phobia concerning meat and its supposedly harmful effects.

In fact, some patients voluntarily, or by a physician's order, made such drastic restriction of protein in their diets that they experienced symptoms and signs of deprivation of protein, namely, weakness, wasting, hypoproteinemia with edema, and anemia. Up to the present time, evidence does not exist that ingestion of protein plays any role in the production or aggravation of hypertension. Therefore, adequate justification is not present for rigid restriction of protein in the diet of hypertensive patients as long as the ability of the kidneys to excrete nitrogen remains adequate. Protein restriction in chronic renal failure is discussed below. As is the case with all foods in the diet of hypertensive patients, moderation should be exercised in the amount of protein eaten, but there should be no objection to a reasonable amount of meat and the temperate use of other protein foods.

Intake of Fluid. In the absence of symptoms and signs of cardiac or renal insufficiency, the hypertensive patient should be allowed a normal intake of fluids of the usual variety. Some restriction is useful during dietary reduction of weight in the obese patient to prevent "plateauing" of the weight curve and discouragement of the subject.

No evidence exists that alcohol as such plays any part in the causation or aggravation of hypertension; consequently, the temperate use of alcoholic beverages by patients who have uncomplicated hypertension is not contraindicated. However, because of the other effects of alcohol, the use of these beverages in quantities other than strictly moderate should be discouraged. The use of coffee or tea in moderation is probably harmless to most patients who have essential hypertension. However, their use in patients who suffer from extreme nervousness, irritability or insomnia should be restricted.

Restriction of Salt. The belief that restriction of the intake of salt is beneficial to patients who have essential hypertension, as well as other forms of cardiovascular renal disease, is not new but appears to have arisen as the result of the work of Ambard and Beaujard[79] in the early part of the present century. These investigators were the first to record the observation that deprivation of salt may result in decrease in blood pressure in persons who have essential hypertension. In 1922, Allen and Sherrill[80] found that diets sharply restricted in salt were effective in lowering the blood pressure of some hypertensive patients. Like Ambard and Beaujard and others, Allen and Sherrill were of the opinion that restriction of chloride rather than of sodium was the effective feature of a low-salt regimen.

The introduction by Kempner,[81] in 1944, of the rice-fruit diet constituted one of the major and heroic attempts at control of essential hypertension by dietary means. This diet, made up solely of rice, fruit and fruit juice, gives approximately 20 gm of protein per day; it contains no protein of animal origin and gives approximately 0.2 gm of sodium per day. Kempner explained the beneficial results of such a program in the treatment of hypertension on the assumption that hypertension produces functional impairment of tubular epithelium in the kidneys because of a decreased supply of oxygen to these cells. In his early reports, Kempner[82] observed objective improvement in almost two-thirds of 500 patients; this improvement was evidenced by significant decrease in blood pressure, reduction in cardiac size, reversal of abnormal electrocardiographic patterns, return to normal or near normal values for urea and other retained metabolites in the blood, and regression of characteristic hypertensive changes in the ocular fundi. The diet caused loss of weight in most of his patients and in his hands did not induce negative nitrogen balance.[83] However, it has been shown since this early work of Kempner that strict adherence to a rice-fruit diet for some time will induce negative nitrogen balance in some patients;[84] this observation, plus the loss of weight, has led to the suggestion that the rice-fruit diet is, in reality, a semistarvation diet.[85] Most of Kempner's earlier claims have been questioned by other investigators in the field. Most workers doubt that the diet exerts a specific antipressor or depressor effect on the blood pressure of hypertensive patients; others consider that the frequent occurrence of the salt-depletion syndrome in some patients consuming the rice-fruit diet indicates a great need for discrimination in its use. Under rigid metabolic dietary control[86] it will result in a decrease of blood pressure in some hypertensive patients. However, it does not provide the clinician with a practical means of treating patients with essential hypertension. The advent of the "thiazides" and potent antihypertensive drugs has made the Kempner regimen obsolete.

While Kempner has ascribed the therapeutic effect of the rice-fruit diet to the nature and amount of protein allowed, it is probable that drastic restriction of salt is the responsible factor. The exact relationship between sodium chloride and the genesis of essential hypertension is, at the present time, unknown. It would appear to be extremely complex; any attempt to analyze it into component parts would necessitate specific knowledge regarding the relation of the kidneys to hypertension, the relation of the adrenal glands to salt balance and the relation of other unknown influences to the adrenal glands themselves.

Grollman and his associates[87] observed a striking decrease in the blood pressure of 6 patients who had essential hypertension and who were treated with a diet that was more liberal than the rice-fruit diet but that provided less than 0.5 gm of sodium (1.3 gm of sodium chloride) daily. They considered the basis for the success of this form of treatment to be the drastic restriction of sodium chloride in the diet and state that the employment of moderate rather than drastic restriction of sodium in the diet may account for many of the therapeutic failures reported. This point of view has been generally accepted and has led to avoidance of the severe protein restriction of the Kempner diet. The availability of virtually sodium-free milk has enhanced both the nutritional value and the palatability of the extremely low-sodium diet.

In general, neither the rice-fruit diet nor a weighed low-sodium (0.2 gm) diet has been strikingly effective in reducing blood pressure in the majority of patients who have severe essential hypertension; other observers have reported similar results.[88-90] For this reason, the extremely low-sodium type of diet, with or without reduction of protein, was reserved in the past for the group of patients suffering from severe advanced hypertensive disease who have not responded to various medical means of controlling blood pressure and who have been adjudged unsuitable candidates for surgical treatment. The fantastic development of potent antihypertensive drugs in the last two decades—the rauwolfia alkaloids, hydralazine, the ganglionic blocking agents and other adrenergic blockers or competitive inhibitors of catecholamine vasoconstrictors, the monoamine oxidase inhibitors, and the benzothiadiazines—has revolutionized the treatment of hypertension and relegated rigid dietary sodium restriction to a purely historical interest. It is essential to remember, nevertheless, that the effectiveness of these drugs is considerably enhanced by moderate restriction of sodium while the chronic depletion of potassium (which all the diuretic agents among them produce) is likely to be aggravated by a high-salt intake. Therefore, in most hypertensive patients and in the absence of heart failure, the amount of sodium permitted in the diet will range from 2.0 to 0.5 gm daily, depending on the individual response to the antihypertensive agents in regard to relief of symptoms and lowering of blood pressure (see Appendix Table A-10). The development of hypotensive reactions is an indication for reduction in the dosage of the one or more of the drugs rather than for an increase in the salt intake. Potassium supplements are often necessary as part of the regimen when the diuretic drugs are used continuously.

Appropriate sodium restriction assists greatly in control of blood pressure in renal disease and hypertension. However, when patients have renal failure, particular care must be taken to avoid sodium restriction so severe as to cause depletion of extracellular volume. It is critical that blood pressure not be decreased too severely because this can cause further reduction of glomerular filtration. Thiazide diuretics and antihypertensive medications must be monitored with exquisite care to prevent further renal insufficiency. In advanced renal failure control of blood pressure may need to be sacrificed for expansion of plasma volume to increase glomerular filtration and avoid damage to target organs. Such hypertension should be permitted only long enough to establish dialysis or transplantation if the patient is suitable for such a program. A number of patients with advanced renal disease and hypertension may require bilateral nephrectomy and maintenance on chronic dialysis for control of hypertension. In such nephrectomized patients significant correlation between total exchangeable body salt and blood pressure in the renoprival state has been reported.[91] In such patients salt intake is important in maintenance of acceptable blood pressures.[92]

In summary, no dietary treatment is known that has any specific favorable effect on the course of essential hypertension. The patient who has essential hypertension should eat as much as is necessary to maintain strength and nutrition but should avoid excesses. This restriction of the quantity and quality of the diet should be extended to total calories, total volume of fluids, protein and salt. Special modification of the diet for the patient with hypertensive vascular disease may be indicated because of coincidental or associated disturbances in lipid, carbohydrate or purine metabolism. *Moderation* as a watchword should apply to the diet as well as to all other aspects of treatment.

PREECLAMPSIA OF PREGNANCY

Hypertension, proteinuria and edema are the cardinal clinical features of preeclampsia of pregnancy in which the glomeruli are enlarged, swollen and ischemic. Edema of the cells of the glomerular tuft is the most prominent pathologic feature, and the glomerular change is widespread through the kidney, all glomeruli being equally affected. Clinically, the unusual spasm of the retinal arteries and the increase in the level of the serum uric acid are valuable criteria for distinguishing preeclampsia from hypertensive vascular disease in pregnancy.

The clinical pattern and the geographic distribution of preeclampsia remind one of primary nutritional disorders, particularly pellagra. Epidemic outbreaks occur in various parts of the world. The disease is endemic in some areas, and the sporadic cases which we see in large cities tend to appear in the poor and the ignorant and in those whose nutrition has been disturbed by food fads or for other reasons. Theobald[93] was among the first to draw attention to its peculiar geographic distribution and to relate its appearance to nutritional factors. He recalls that when he was in charge of the largest obstetric service in the city Bangkok, Siam, he saw only 8 cases of eclampsia from 1926 to 1929. When he moved to Ceylon, the situation was quite different. The incidence there was 28 per thousand live births and was probably the highest in the world. On returning to Great Britain, he found that the mortality rates were higher in Scotland than in Wales. He also noted that the incidence of eclampsia doubled in Hong Kong during 1941 when gross malnutrition was rife as a result of the war. On the other hand, preeclampsia increased in Belgium and Holland after their liberation from German occupation, at a time when food became more plentiful.

There is a marked variation in the incidence of preeclampsia in different areas of South Africa.[94] In Cape Town, where four groups of people live under distinct social and economic conditions, eclampsia is common in the Cape Malays and less common among Bantu, Cape colored and European population groups.[95] The Cape Malays are Moslems, artisans and fishermen. They are descendants of slaves brought to South Africa from Java and Malaya in the 18th century, and they have an unusual pattern of food intake,[96] as well as characteristic methods of preparing their diet.[97]

Wachstein and others have suggested that the metabolism of vitamin B_6 is altered in pregnancy,[98] but it does not appear that a simple deficiency of this vitamin is responsible for the specific lesion of the kidney in preeclampsia. It appears more likely that the lesion may be the result of a very complex metabolic disturbance involving abnormal hormone activity and an unbalanced dietary intake, particularly an abnormal intake of salt.

Although most investigators have felt that the disease is precipitated by excess salt consumption, this concept has not been documented. Recent reports cast grave doubt on this concept and there is a real question of efficacy, and safety, of strenuous salt restriction or diuretic therapy. Sarles[99] has found that after a control period of 10 to 12 days on a 120 mEq sodium diet, the excretion of a 25 gm sodium chloride load was identical in normal pregnant patients and preeclamptics. Schewitz[100] suggests that preeclamptics on low-salt diets are salt depleted and retain it avidly when given, accounting for the often reported decreased sodium excretion after an acute load of sodium. In normal pregnancy, renin levels are found to be very high as well as the aldosterone secretion rates, suggesting to some that there is a physiologic need for sodium retention in normal pregnancy.[101] A thorough dietary investigation of salt intake early in pregnancy by Robinson[102] demonstrated a high incidence of preeclampsia in women taking *small* amounts of salt compared to those taking large amounts of salt. A series of detailed studies on salt intake in pregnant rats by Pike and her colleagues[103] indicate that the physiologic disturbances in the animal on low-salt intake parallel those in pregnant women with preeclampsia. These studies strengthen the concept of chronic water intoxication as the pathophysiologic change in preeclampsia. All of these studies indicate that much work is still required to clarify the nutritional aspects of preeclampsia.

Where the disorder has appeared, the traditional therapy has been a low-salt diet, antihypertensive drugs and natriuretic agents. The evidence cited above calls into question this traditional approach. Schewitz[100] has recommended high-protein, high-vitamin and a high- or, at least, unrestricted salt intake. Thiazide diuretics are not recommended. Hypertension is treated if above 180/120 mm Hg. Sedation and bed rest are the most important measures.

Rigid salt restriction has been associated with vascular collapse during labor or immediately post-delivery. When thiazide diuretics are used, it is imperative to see that adequate amounts of potassium are given to prevent hypokalemia. It is, therefore, imperative to see that adequate amounts of potassium (3 gm of potassium chloride or its equivalent) are given when these diuretics are used. Of great interest is a recent paper by Perey and his colleagues[104] who have induced multiple cysts in the kidneys of fetal rabbits by producing potassium deficiency in the pregnant does. If this work is confirmed, it may well have fundamental bearing on the problem of congenital renal disease in man.

There is no deficiency of magnesium in preeclamptic women. Parenteral magnesium sulfate is commonly used by obstetricians to treat preeclampsia and eclampsia. This, as we have said, is a pharmacologic not a nutritional usage.

KALIOPENIC NEPHROPATHY[63,105,106]

Potassium depletion produces functional and structural derangements in the kidneys of man and animals. If the deficiency is severe in degree and prolonged in nature, the kidneys are liable to be permanently damaged. What is distressing, however, is the development of renal disease in a number of people depleted of potassium for a relatively short period of time. These individuals, like the large majority of patients we see with potassium deficiency and healthy kidneys, are, in the main, brought to this state by the injudicious use of powerful hormones or diuretic agents. These useful and life-saving drugs produce kaliopenia unless the physician employing them takes pains to see that the potassium lost in the urine is replaced each day by potassium-containing medicines. It is not enough to prescribe foods rich in potassium. Patients, unfortunately, are more impressed with drugs than diets.

Since the advent of steroid hormones, like prednisone and particularly the thiazide diuretics, kaliopenic nephropathy has become a common disorder. Previously, it was rarely seen. In fact, the relationship of renal disease to potassium depletion was not clearly recognized until 1950 when Perkins, Petersen and Riley[107] first described renal lesions in patients with potassium deficiency due to chronic diarrhea. We now recognize that potassium depletion may develop as a result of many disorders producing either a renal or a gastrointestinal loss of the element. Pure dietary deficiency in man has only been produced experimentally,[108] but loss of appetite

Table 30-3. Causes of Kaliopenia and Kaliopenic Nephropathy in Man

1. *Dietary Deficiency*
   (*a*) Experimental

2. *Gastrointestinal Loss*
   (*a*) *Diarrhea:* particularly ulcerative colitis; regional colitis and ileitis; dysentery; malabsorption syndrome; acute infectious diarrhea
   (*b*) *Purgatives:* usually self-induced
   (*c*) *Enemas or Colonic Lavage:* often self-induced
   (*d*) *Uterosigmoidostomy*
   (*e*) *Fistulas:* particularly small bowel drainage
   (*f*) *Vomiting*
   (*g*) *Combinations of above*

3. *Urinary Loss*
   (*a*) *Endocrine Disturbances:* aldosterone tumors; primary hyperaldosteronism; Cushing's syndrome; primary and secondary hypertrophy of the juxtaglomerular apparatus; diabetic coma
   (*b*) *Renal Diseases:* renal tubular dysfunction; chronic pyelonephritis; interstitial nephritis; chronic renal failure; diuretic phase of acute renal failure

4. *Iatrogenic*
   (*a*) Diuretic drugs
   (*b*) Steroid hormones

and other causes of inadequate intake of dietary potassium such as anorexia nervosa contribute to depletion in many instances. (See Table 30-3.) Of course, potassium loss is common in wasting disorders such as cirrhosis, but these losses occur *pari passu* with nitrogen wasting which has different effects from loss of potassium alone. The best-known effects of potassium depletion— aside from its potentiation of digitalis action and its effects on the electrocardiogram— are nocturia, muscle weakness or paralysis, vasopressin-resistant failure to concentrate the urine, and inability to acidify the urine. Table 30-4 outlines some of the effects of potassium depletion on the kidney. In most instances, these changes appear quite rapidly and are easily reversible with ingestion of adequate amounts of potassium by mouth (3 gm of potassium chloride or its equivalent per day). Infusion of potassium ions is necessary at times but may be fraught with

Table 30-4. Effects of Potassium Depletion on the Kidney

1. *Biochemical Changes in Renal Tubules*
   (a) Intracellular acidosis
   (b) Decreased capacity to accumulate para-aminohippurate
   (c) Increased glutaminase, D-amino oxidase and carbonic anhydrase activity
   (d) Increased lactic dehydrogenase activity in the collecting tubules
   (e) Decreased lactic dehydrogenase activity in the loop of Henle

2. *Functional Changes of Renal Tubules*
   (a) Vasopressin-resistant hyposthenuria or isos-thenuria
   (b) Impaired para-aminohippurate extraction and excretion
   (c) Inability to establish minimal urinary pH; relative increase in urinary ammonia
   (d) Decreased urinary citric acid and other organic acids
   (e) Impaired capacity to conserve sodium when consuming a low dietary sodium intake
   (f) Phosphaturia

3. *Structural Changes in Renal Tubules*
   (a) Vacuolar (hydropic) nephropathy of proximal tubules
   (b) Granular degeneration and atrophy of cells in distal and collecting tubules
   (c) Increased intercalated cells in the collecting tubules
   (d) Alterations in mitochondria of the collecting tubules

4. *Structural Changes in Interstitial Tissues*
   (a) Edema
   (b) Fibrosis

danger as levels in the blood can pile up rapidly and cause cardiac arrest.[109]

Histologic Changes. Striking vacuolization of the cells of the proximal and distal convolutions of the tubules with basal displacement of the nuclei is characteristic of potassium depletion in man. This histologic change is completely reversible with potassium repletion, but the development of interstitial fibrosis is a progressive lesion and is the forerunner of full-blown interstitial nephritis or chronic pyelonephritis.

Muehrcke and McMillan[110] have reviewed cases from our clinic and from the world literature. They point out that the patients with gastrointestinal loss of potassium usually seek medical advice because of diarrhea, dehydration or other symptoms. Their electrolyte disorders are diagnosed and effectively treated early in the course of their potassium depletion. Consequently, irreversible histologic changes are less frequent with gastrointestinal disorders than in patients with renal loss of potassium who may have had hypokalemia for many years without symptoms. Moreover, in these patients the renal tubular cells are the actual site of potassium loss and suffer greater functional and structural damage than when they are actively conserving potassium, which is what they do when the gastrointestinal tract is the site of potassium loss.

It is a curious fact that, once the irreversible destructive process of interstitial nephritis or pyelonephritis has developed in potassium-depleted patients, we have noted that their kidneys are peculiarly prone to continue to lose potassium, not withstanding the original site of loss.

These studies, like others, indicate that the renal tubular cell needs adequate supplies of potassium to preserve its integrity. The physician using agents such as steroids and diuretics which deplete the body of this electrolyte must be aware of the possibilities of damaging the kidney by his actions, and of involving the organ in a secondary permanently harmful renal infection.

Symptoms. Moreover, the physician must be on the lookout for clues to the diagnosis of potassium deficiency such as nocturnal frequency, fatigue, weakness of the limbs, and early changes in the electrocardiogram. Exact diagnosis comes with measurement of serum potassium but the degree of depletion is often difficult to assess and may require metabolism studies for exact knowledge.

For prevention and treatment, enteric-coated tablets of potassium chloride were commonly used. As patients may get abdominal cramps from the hypertonic solution formed during fragmentation of the tablet in the gut or, as sometimes happens, the tablets may cause dangerous bowel disease, including bowel perforation, we prefer a liquid formula, using a concentrated solution of potassium gluconate or potassium citrate, flavored with syrup of orange, and given in half a glass of water 3 times a day. If intravenous potassium is used, 20 mEq per liter of fluid, given slowly, are usually adequate.

ACUTE GLOMERULONEPHRITIS

Etiology. Many disorders produce the classic clinical picture of acute nephritis—hematuria, edema and hypertension—and the histologic picture of glomerulonephritis with involvement of glomeruli, tubules and interstitial tissue. Among these are Henoch-Schönlein purpura, lupus nephritis, necrotizing lesions such as seen in Goodpasture's syndrome, and even, on rare occasions, acute hemorrhagic pyelonephritis. But most of the cases and most studies have involved the rather common and usually benign disease of childhood, post-streptococcal nephritis. Of the children who are admitted to hospital, from 85 to 95 per cent make a complete recovery, but when adults are sick enough to be admitted, only 50 per cent get completely well. The complications which concern us from a nutritional point of view are edema, hypertension, massive persistent proteinuria with or without nephrotic edema, oliguria or anuria (acute renal failure) and chronic renal failure.

Protein Intake. This disorder is surrounded by controversies. The nutritional controversy concerns the use of a low-protein diet. Those who used to use boiled rice and fruit juice to treat children and adults with acute nephritis based their regimen of care on the erroneous concepts of Addis,[111] Newburgh[112] and Von Rohrer[113] who believed that most of the work of the kidney was applied to dealing with the waste products of protein breakdown. Thus, they sought to limit dietary protein to "rest" the organ and so speed repair. We now know that this is an incorrect concept. As we have seen above, the chemical energy supplied to the kidney is mainly used in active transport of electrolytes in the convoluted tubules, and not in discharging urea.

Modern clinical studies have indicated that protein restriction is without value. Illingsworth and his colleagues[114] treated 42 patients by allocating them at random to two dietary regimens—strict protein restriction and the ordinary diet of the children's ward. The children were observed for a year and strict criteria were used to assess cure. No advantage was found by restricting protein.

Mortensen[115] treated 44 patients with either low- or high-protein diets. Evaluation of health and renal status 2 years after discharge from hospital indicated that those on the high-protein diet did better than those on the low-protein diet.

There is, therefore, no rational reason or need to restrict protein in acute post-streptococcal nephritis unless oliguria or anuria develops. When this complication appears in children, it usually lasts from 36 to 72 hours and a conservative regimen for acute renal failure is called for (see below). In adults, and occasionally in children, severe and very prolonged anuria develops. This is usually fatal despite the use of all measures available at present.

With regard to salt, this is not restricted, unless hypertension, edema or oliguria are judged to be potential hazards. Thus, in most patients with acute post-streptococcal glomerulonephritis, dietary management is not crucial and bed rest and drugs are central to treatment.

THE NEPHROTIC SYNDROME

The metabolic, nutritional and clinical consequences of continued massive albuminuria constitute the nephrotic syndrome. Florid cases are readily recognized from infancy to extreme old age, and the diagnosis can be confirmed rapidly in the laboratory by urinalysis and simple biochemical studies of the blood.

Biochemical Changes. The well-known metabolic hallmarks of the nephrotic syndrome are proteinuria, hypoalbuminemia and hypercholesterolemia.[116] But the full-blown picture presents many more biochemical aberrations than this. Albumin is the major protein lost in the urine, accounting for approximately 70 per cent of the total. As can be seen from Table 30–5, other nutritionally important plasma proteins, such as ceruloplasmin, also run to waste in the urine.

Table 30-5. Some Biochemical Changes in the Urine of
Patients with the Nephrotic Syndrome

Increased	Decreased	Variable
Albumin	Sodium	Glucose
Alpha globulin	Chloride	Potassium
Beta globulin		Amino acids
Gamma globulin		Nitrogen
Protein-bound iodine		
Ceruloplasmin		
Siderophilin		
Antidiuretic substance		
Complement		
Prothrombin		
Antithrombin		
Proconvertin		

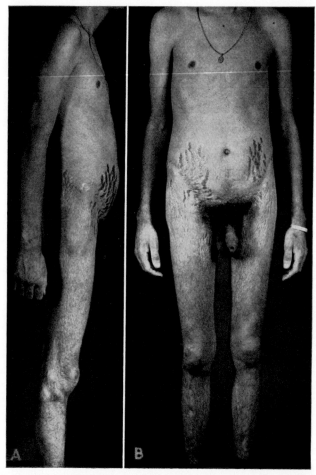

Fig. 30-1A and B. Patient R. H., aged 18 years. *Nephrotic Syndrome, Malnutrition,* and *"Lipoid Nephrosis."*
Photographs show severe tissue wasting and abdominal striae following diuresis and weight loss from 223 to
125 pounds in this 6-foot, previously husky youth who had ascites, severe pedal edema, and massive proteinuria.

The continued drain of nitrogen in the urine also compromises the tissue and cellular stores of protein, and the clinical consequences of this impoverishment are tissue wastage, malnutrition (see Figs. 30–1A and 1B), fatty metamorphosis of the liver, sodium retention, hydremia and edema.[117] Depletion of complement makes the nephrotic patient particularly susceptible to infection, and loss of specialized protein, such as those which bind thyroid hormone and iron, explains satisfactorily the apparent hypothyroidism and tendency to anemia. More difficult to explain is the marked increase in circulating serum lipids[118] and relatively large plasma proteins such as cholinesterase and fibrinogen (Table 30–6).

These changes may develop as a result of disturbance in the transport of fats, or they may be the result of some as yet unidentified mechanism. We have speculated elsewhere[119,120] that the metabolic changes seen in the nephrotic syndrome are the result of increased hepatic synthesis of protein and fats, called forth by depletion of hepatic albumin and made evident by the retention of large molecular protein molecules in the blood stream and the loss of the small ones in the urine. Be this as it may, studies on nephrotic rats and man have clearly demonstrated that infusion of large amounts of serum albumin can restore both the protein and the lipid abnormalities in the plasma to normal.

Massive loss of albumin in the urine is not invariably accompanied by all the clinical or biochemical stigmata of the nephrotic syndrome. The loss of protein may not be sufficient to overwhelm the body's homeostatic mechanisms, and clinical edema may never appear. These patients with subclinical forms feel well, and rarely appear in the clinic unless proteinuria is detected on routine examination. In other formes frustes the serum lipid levels are normal or decreased in amount. The reasons for this are not clear. In our experience, low or normal levels of serum cholestrol may accompany the nephrotic syndrome in generalized disease processes, *e.g.* systemic lupus erythematosus, and may well indicate a poor prognosis.

Treatment. Treatment in the nephrotic syndrome should be directed toward the patient's principal complaint of edema, to the malnutrition, to the underlying renal condition, and to the specific etiologic factors when these can be determined. At present, much of the treatment is necessarily of a nonspecific nature, although with increasing accuracy in diagnosis, this situation will change.

Salt Restriction. Salt restriction is one of the most important of the measures designed to prevent edema and to initiate diuresis, and while low-salt diets are widely prescribed, little attention is paid by many clinicians to ensuring that these are sufficiently low in sodium. An intake of less than 10 mEq/day (580 mg sodium chloride) almost always prevents the accumulation of edema and will often start a diuresis, even without

Table 30-6. Some Biochemical Changes in the Blood of
Patients with the Nephrotic Syndrome

Increased	Decreased	Variable
Total lipid	Albumin	Alpha globulin
Triglycerides	Protein-bound iodine	Gamma globulin
Phospholipids	Siderophilin	Alpha lipoprotein
Free cholesterol	Ceruloplasmin	Sodium
Cholesterol esters	Complement	Chloride
Beta lipoprotein	Osmotic Pressure	Calcium
Alpha globulin	Plasma volume	
Beta globulin		
Fibrinogen		
Cholinesterase		
Aldosterone		

other forms of therapy. Limitation of salt intake to this level is now relatively easy with low-sodium milk powders (Lonalac), or low-sodium fresh milk, as the diet can be given mainly in the form of drinks or, in severely edematous subjects with poor appetites, by intranasal drip feeding. Modern diuretic agents are most useful in producing natriuresis but, as discussed above, may produce potassium deficiency. See Appendix, Tables A–10, A–27 and A–28 for low-sodium diets and formulas.

The use of diuretics is based on symptomatic relief of edema and does not affect the underlying process per se. Since most nephrotics exhibit features of secondary hyperaldosteronism, spironolactone (an aldosterone-blocking agent) is frequently effective in initiating a diuresis.

Protein Intake. The level of protein intake required by these patients has been the cause of much argument. High-protein diets of 150 gm per day or more were originally advocated by Epstein and employed with considerable success. Later writers, however, observed a rise in the urinary protein loss on such diets and interpreted this as deterioration in the renal condition. On the basis of animal studies, it was also argued that high-protein diets were undesirable as the prognosis in nephrotoxic serum nephritis was worse when high-protein diets were given. Also the kidney was said to be required to do more "work" in excreting the additional urea load. Neither of these hypotheses is tenable, as it has been shown that increased proteinuria is to be expected with small rises of serum proteins and, as discussed previously, the work load caused by the excretion of urea is a very small fraction of that required by other tubular secretory processes in the kidney either normally or in the nephrotic syndrome. The demonstration on high-protein diets of prolonged positive nitrogen balances, at times amounting to 500 gm nitrogen in some patients with proteinuria of many months' duration, suggests the presence of a severe body deficit of protein of which the reduced serum proteins are only one manifestation. In adult patients, no maximal level of protein intake could be observed other than that set by the patient's appetite, and positive nitrogen balances were recorded with protein intakes ranging from 65 to 200 gm, higher intakes leading to higher positive balances. Since this body nitrogen deficit seems of fundamental importance in the patient with prolonged proteinuria, it would appear advisable to replace protein as rapidly as possible; in practice, it had been found that intakes of 120 gm per day for the average adult, with high-caloric intakes (50 to 60 cal/kg), have provided satisfactory repletion without unpalatable diets. Higher levels may be obtained on occasion with continuous tube feeding, and there seems to be no contraindication to their use. It is, of course, essential to ensure that patients actually take such diets; too often, high-protein, high-caloric diets are advised but not consumed. The poor appetite of the edematous patient requires constant supervision and coaxing to ensure that adequate intakes are obtained. Bananas supply a palatable, acceptable source of calories low in sodium.

Calcium and Potassium Deficiency. In some patients with severe and prolonged proteinuria deficiencies of both calcium and potassium may occur, with resulting bone rarefaction. Avioli[42] has recently shown the loss of active vitamin D metabolites in proteinuric states. What role this loss may play in calcium deficiency is not certain. Both these defects are corrected by high-protein, high-vitamin diets, with the use of low-sodium milk or milk powder described, although additional potassium may be required in the early stages of treatment.

Hyperlipidemia. The nephrotic syndrome is characterized by high serum cholesterol levels, as well as phospholipids and triglycerides. Berlyne[39] has recently shown that nephrotic patients have an increased incidence of coronary artery disease and death. He suggests that measures to decrease hyperlipemia (*e.g.* unsaturated fats in diet, use of hypocholesterolemic agents) be taken in chronic nephrotic patients.

Steroid Therapy. The precise value of steroid therapy in the nephrotic syndrome is still to be determined since the nephrotic syndrome has so many causes (Table 30–7); moreover, there has been considerable con-

Table 30-7. Causes of the Nephrotic Syndrome

(1) *Heredofamilial*
Microcystic disease

(2) *Infective*
Syphilis
Malaria
Subacute bacterial
endocarditis
Tuberculosis*
Diphtheria*

(3) *Toxins*
Organic mercurials*
Inorganic mercurials
(teething powder)
Tridione, Paradione*
Bismuth*
Gold*
Trichlorethylene*

(4) *Allergic*
Poison oak*
Bee sting
Pollens and dust
Serum sickness

(5) *Mechanical*
Renal vein thrombosis
Constrictive pericarditis
Congestive cardiac failure
Tricuspid valve disease
Thrombosis or obstruction of inferior
vena cava

(6) *Generalized Disease Processes*
Amyloidosis—primary
Amyloidosis—secondary
Myelomatosis
Systemic lupus erythematosus
Diabetic glomerulosclerosis
Schönlein-Henoch purpura
Arteriolar nephrosclerosis
Progressive systemic sclerosis
Sickle cell anemia*

(7) *Intrinsic Renal Disease*
Membranous glomerulonephritis
Proliferative glomerulonephritis
Mixed membranous and proliferative
glomerulonephritis
Tubular degeneration, no glomerular
lesions (lipoid nephrosis)
Tubular degeneration, minimal glomerular
lesions

* These causes have not been thoroughly validated.

fusion in the type of steroid used in different reports.

Unfortunately, there are still too few patients for whom specific treatment can be given for the nephrotic syndrome, but it is to be hoped that better methods of diagnosis will result in better treatment. Constrictive pericarditis, congestive cardiac failure and, possibly, lupus nephritis are among the conditions in which treatment may be directed toward a specific cause with satisfactory improvement in the nephrotic syndrome.

DIABETIC NEPHROPATHY[121,122]

In the United States, nodular glomerulosclerosis has been found in 17 to 36 per cent of diabetic patients dying in hospitals, and diffuse glomerulosclerosis and arteriolar hyalinization are even more common. Most of the pathologic lesions of diabetes, including the specific renal lesions, can be explained on the hypothesis of widespread deposition, particularly in and around the blood vessels, of protein carbohydrate complexes which are present in abnormal amounts in the blood of patients with the disease. The problem is to decide whether the lesions are complications of diabetes which might be avoided by diet or whether they are concomitant changes, the tendency towards which is inherited separately. Unfortunately, there is as yet no clear-cut answer. We know of no incontrovertible evidence that specific renal lesions of diabetes can be prevented by strict control of the disease. The rarity of glomerulosclerosis in "acquired diabetes" such as Cushing's syndrome, and the difficulty of producing it in experimental animals are points against it being a complication and in favor of its being a concomitant of "idiopathic" diabetes. Against this view and in favor of the complication theory are the apparent rarity of glomerulosclerosis before 1923, the year of the introduction of insulin, and the fact that our studies indicate that the incidence of renal involvement differs considerably in different parts of the world. For example, in a series of 200 diabetic patients attending a university teaching hospital in East Africa, no cases were found of established renal disease, and only one of gangrene. Of 145 diabetic patients attending the Tohoku University Hospital in Japan, 26.8 per cent had persistent proteinuria, and 8.6 per cent had the Kimmelstiel-Wilson syndrome. These latter figures are comparable to what might be found in the United States. The typical Japanese diet (low fat, high carbohydrate) is similar to that of East Africans and differs from that of Americans. The common feature distinguishing the Americans and Japanese from East Africans appears to be the availability of insulin, which raises the possibility that the lesions are caused by the kidney's reaction to injections of exogenous insulin. Insulin antibodies are frequently present in serum of patients taking exogenous insulin. Anti-insulin antibodies have in some cases been found in glomerular lesions and raises the question whether diabetic nodular glomerulosclerosis may be an antigen-antibody complex-initiated process. However, we have found nodules in sections of renal biopsies from patients who, we were quite sure, had never received insulin. There are also a number of reports in the literature of patients with typical nodular lesions in whom the diagnosis of diabetes was not made during life; presumably they, too, had never received insulin.

A frequent clinical finding has been that requirements for insulin often fall as renal failure worsens. The exact mechanisms remain to be determined, but the normal kidney plays an active role in insulin metabolism. With renal failure the urinary excretion of insulin diminishes and the half-life in serum is prolonged.[124] These as well as other factors may account for the clinical phenomenon.

The whole question of diet in relation to diabetic nephropathy must remain sub judice. Treatment of the nephropathy by diet is similar to dietary treatment of either the nephrotic syndrome or of chronic renal failure; with, of course, the added problem of use of insulin or oral antihyperglycemic drugs.

CHRONIC RENAL FAILURE

In patients with chronic renal failure, few functioning nephrons remain. These are usually hypertrophied and functioning at the upper limits of their activity. They have little reserve left to deal efficiently with new catabolic loads which may appear as a result of infection, trauma, and overenthusiastic treatment with diets and drugs. Moreover, during the slow development of chronic renal failure, the cells of the body are bathed in an abnormal fluid and, in many cases, appear to have come into a new homeostatic equilibrium with the altered humoral environment. It is important to recognize that changing personally established patterns of fluid intake and diet (which so often occur when these patients are admitted to hospital for any cause) may do more harm than good. Under these circumstances, establishing new dietary regimens—if this is what the physician wants to do—must be done cautiously and with circumspection.

Aims of Treatment. In chronic renal failure, the aims of treatment are to minimize protein catabolism; to avoid dehydration and overhydration; to control electrolyte and fluid loss from vomiting and diarrhea; to maintain electrolyte levels within normal limits as far as possible; to gently correct acidosis, and finally, to treat complications such as hypertension, bone pain, and central nervous system abnormalities. In these patients, nutritional status is nearly always below par and one must try to maintain it at a reasonable level.

Sodium. With regard to nutrition, at present the major error perpetrated by the practitioner in dietary care of the uremic patient is to prescribe a diet too low in sodium. Many patients with chronic renal failure do not retain sodium and, in fact, some waste salt excessively in their urine. This occurs particularly in cystic disease of the medulla and in chronic pyelonephritis, but is not uncommon in any form of chronic renal failure.

Therefore, a common dietary complication seen in hospital is a low-salt syndrome from diets, diuretics, diarrhea, vomiting and the misguided use of intravenous fluids which are low in sodium or, perhaps, contain no electrolyte. Most of these patients need 4 to 5 gm of salt each day, and some may require massive amounts of sodium. This requirement can be determined by measurement of 24-hour urinary electrolyte output.

Water. The patient with chronic uremia is also under continuous osmotic diuresis from the high level of urea in the glomerular filtrate. His obligatory water output is high and he can easily become dehydrated. Moreover, as he fails, fewer and fewer nephrons remain and, terminally, the urinary output may be very small. The patient may, therefore, be in danger of water intoxication on the one hand and dehydration on the other, and the physician must steer him between these extremes. Charting the daily weight and an accurate measurement of urinary output are excellent guides to care. Serum electrolyte levels should be drawn at least once or twice per week and, on occasion, more frequently.

Protein. If tissue protein catabolism could be controlled by drugs or other means, the problem of uremia could be solved. As far as diet is concerned, there are no accurate figures on optimum intake of protein or, for that matter, on caloric, fat or carbohydrate requirements in uremia. Burnett believes that, if patients are allowed to self-select their diets, they will eventually choose one suitable for their personal protein needs. Others believe in rigid protein restriction, ranging from 0 to 20 gm per day.

The minimum requirement for protein for healthy active males is about 0.5 gm per kg body weight, and therefore, many clinicians empirically prescribe such a diet for uremic or azotemic patients, making sure they eat mainly animal protein of high biologic value, with appropriate fat and carbohydrate intakes at a level of 3 to 4 gm of carbohydrate and 1 to 2 gm of fat per kg body weight per day.

As the disease progresses, many patients develop symptoms related to a high-phosphorus, high-potassium and low-calcium blood

level. On occasion, it is possible to alleviate symptoms and prolong their life with a low-phosphorus, low-protein diet. In the few patients who can tolerate such a diet, one sometimes can achieve a worthwhile delay of the inevitable.

Giordano[125] reported on the use of synthetic diets containing small quantities of amino-nitrogen (2 gm/day) in the form of the essential amino acids. He stated that this diet produced a positive nitrogen balance by utilizing ammonia from urea (formed from protein catabolism) for the synthesis of the nonessential amino acids. His work has been amply confirmed by Berlyne[126] and others[127-130] who have shown with isotopically labeled tracers the re-utilization of endogenous urea and incorporation into proteins and tissue. Richards et al.[131] have speculated on the non-protein diet for uremics, by providing the keto analogues of essential amino acids. American and English modifications of the Giordano-Giovannetti diet (see Appendix, Table A-12) have demonstrated that many patients with chronic renal failure may have improvement of general well-being, disappearance of many uremic symptoms, and perhaps, prolongation of life of improved quality. Hyperkalemia and metabolic acidosis are not always prevented by these diets and additional dietary modifications or medications may be necessary.

In many instances, however, the remaining renal function is so minimal (creatinine clearances less than 2 ml/min) that dialytic measures are necessary to maintain these patients. Dialysis, acute and chronic, introduces many factors that require dietary modification and are discussed further below.

BONE DISEASE IN CHRONIC RENAL FAILURE[132-134]

Bone disease is probably more common in patients with chronic renal failure than previously thought, but the symptoms are not specific. Severe and sometimes disabling bone pain exists for years before the diagnosis is made. Even though the underlying renal disease is usually incurable, the symptomatic relief which can often be afforded patients with this condition is so striking that all patients with chronic renal failure (blood urea greater than 70 mg per 100 ml) should be screened for it.

Although the exact pathogenesis of uremic osteodystrophy has yet to be determined, enough evidence has accumulated to propose a schema of events.[135] As nephron damage occurs, GFR falls. Phosphate is retained and there is a reciprocal fall in blood calcium. The fall in calcium is sensed by the parathyroid gland which is stimulated to secrete PTH. PTH affects renal tubular cells to promote phosphate excretion, and to normalize serum phosphate and calcium.

Phosphate concentrations and calcium concentrations are maintained near normal throughout much of the natural course of the disease. As the disease advances, however, a point is reached (generally when GFR falls to 30 per cent of normal) where maximal phosphaturia per nephron is not sufficient to permit maintenance of normophosphatemia; persistent hyperphosphatemia occurs and hypocalcemia becomes permanent. Thus the stimulus to PTH secretion becomes increased further. The maintenance of normocalcemia in the early stages of renal failure is effected by increased levels of PTH. Increased levels of PTH have been found in early renal insufficiency and extremely high levels found in end stage renal failure.[136]

Of course, at whatever stage in the disease, vitamin D resistance can occur and results in decreased intestinal absorption of calcium potentiating hypocalcemia. Calcium absorption from the intestine is apparently mediated by a specific calcium-binding protein. There is mounting evidence that vitamin D exerts its effect by mediating the synthesis of the specific calcium-binding protein.[139] Of considerable importance is the recent finding that the kidney may be responsible for the production of the specific metabolite of vitamin D that mediates intestinal absorption of calcium.[138] Vitamin D resistance may also be the result of abnormal metabolism of vitamin D in chronic renal failure, loss of active metabolites in the urine, or true resistance to the vitamin at receptor sites. Chronic metabolic acidosis has also

been postulated to be a factor in the pathogenesis of uremic bone disease.[137]

The sum total of these events are increased bone reabsorption and defective mineralization of bone which may present clinically as osteitis fibrosa or osteomalacia.

Treatment. Prevention and management of uremic bone disease can be successful only with full knowledge of the clinical condition, metabolic balance studies and bone pathology. Calcium, phosphorus, alkaline phosphatase and x-ray films of bones are followed as guides. The goal is to try to maintain as near normal levels of calcium and phosphate as possible, while maintaining acid-base balance and clinical well-being, thereby preserving the skeleton and preventing extraosseous calcification. Hyperphosphatemia can be prevented by reducing phosphate in diets or by reduction of absorption of phosphate with phosphate-binding antacids. Calcium intake should be generous (at least 500 mg per day) and since so many foods contain phosphate as well as calcium, calcium may be supplied as the carbonate, lactate or gluconate.

Vitamin D therapy should be restricted to patients with proven osteomalacic features. In such patients, the dosage required may vary widely. The initial dose may be 10,000 to 50,000 units daily and slowly increased if no response is apparent in a month; occasionally 10 to 50 times the usual doses are required. Careful monitoring of calcium, phosphate and alkaline phosphatase is required. It may take a year or more before healing occurs. The action of vitamin D is prolonged and to prevent vitamin D intoxication, reduction of dosage should be considered when improvement appears.

When osteitis fibrosa is present and the calcium phosphorus product above 75, vitamin D should not be used. Such patients may require subtotal parathyroidectomy for control of symptoms. The exact indications are yet unsettled, but with newer techniques of directly measuring PTH levels and the response to dietary and drug therapy, it may soon be possible to select patients on a rational basis. Moreover, specific vitamin D metabolites may become available for therapeutic usage.

RENAL TUBULAR DEFECTS

In 1956, Dent and his colleagues[140] described in the Hartnup family a hereditary pellagra-like skin rash with unusual aminoaciduria and bizarre biochemical features. They speculated that the findings might be the result of abnormal metabolism or requirements for niacin. In addition, a renal tubular defect was found, and this is of particular interest to us because tubular defects fail to conserve filtered nutrients and are a prime renal cause of deficiency diseases.

Fanconi first proposed the concept that a defect in the function of the tubular cells could account for the clinical syndrome which bears his name.[141] Children afflicted with this disease have a genetically inherited abnormality in which a histologic defect in the proximal tubule is associated with defective tubular reabsorption and wastage of glucose, amino acids and phosphates. The

Table 30-8. Proximal Tubular Syndromes*

A. *Tubular Syndromes due to Congenital Disorders*
  1. Inborn Errors of Metabolism with Secondary Tubular Involvement
    (1) Cystinosis
    (2) Wilson's disease
    (3) Galactosemia
    (4) Lowe syndrome
    (5) Hartnup syndrome
    (6) Glycogen storage disease
  2. Syndromes of Possibly Primary Tubular Origin
    (1) Idiopathic de Toni-Debre-Fanconi syndrome
    (2) Incomplete tubular syndromes
  3. Malformations of the Urinary Tract Associated with Tubular Dysfunctions

B. *Tubular Syndromes due to Acquired Disorders*
  1. Syndromes caused by poisons and toxins (accidental and experimental)
  2. Kidney diseases associated with tubular syndromes
  3. Idiopathic renal tubular acidosis
    (1) Infantile form (Lightwood)
    (2) Late form (Butler-Albright)

* After Bickel, H., p. 347 in Black, D. A. K.: *Renal Disease*, Oxford, Blackwell Scientific Publications, 1962.

latter disturbance leads to rickets or osteomalacia (Milkman's syndrome),[142,143] depending on the age of the patient. Fanconi's name has become generally used as an eponym to describe the various types of "tubular failure," such as "the adult Fanconi syndrome" and "the secondary Fanconi syndrome" which occur in patients ill with renal disorders such as pyelonephritis or multiple myeloma. A wide variety of clinical syndromes have been described as a result of failure of the tubules to reabsorb nutrients (see Table 30-8), and further additions to the list may be anticipated. It is possible that the whole spectrum of primary nutritional diseases could be mimicked by renal wastage of specific nutrients, and it is quite possible that, in some instances, the inherited genes may be lethal. Proximal renal tubular defects can be classified in many ways. Often they present multiple biochemical and structural defects, or a single substance (renal glycosuria; renal phosphaturia) or related substances (amino-aciduria) may be involved.

Treatment of these disorders is not satisfactory at this time and consists of attempts to restore blood levels of involved nutrients by diet or pills. For example, phosphate or potassium supplements are given if either of these nutrients is at a low level in the blood. Frequent carbohydrate feedings may be necessary in occasional patients with gross hypoglycemia and symptoms. Some patients, particularly those with phosphate diabetes, are thought to have vitamin D resistance and may respond to treatment with massive doses of the vitamin. No satisfactory dietary treatment exists for most of the genetic or hereditary forms of tubular disorders and, as yet, treatment of the secondary forms of tubular defect, such as Wilson's disease, is experimental and described elsewhere in this volume.

ACUTE RENAL FAILURE

The causes of oliguria or anuria are legion. Acute obstruction of the urinary tract, dehydration, and various types of water and electrolyte disturbance, such as prolonged and severe water intoxication, may disturb urine formation and urine flow. Insults to the body remote from the kidney, such as an acute myocardial infarct, may reduce glomerular filtration to such low levels that little or no urine is formed. And finally, nephrotoxins, parenchymatous renal disease, endotoxins, hemolytic crises, renal vascular damage and acute allergic or immunologic reactions may disturb the function of the kidney, damage its cells and produce acute renal failure.

Aims of Treatment. The aims of treatment of acute renal failure are: to discover the cause and deal with it and its consequences; to keep endogenous protein breakdown to a minimum; to maintain nutritional status; to meticulously control water and sodium balance; to treat symptoms of acidosis or alkalosis; to prevent or treat hyperkalemia, hypocalcemia and uremia as they arise; and last but not least, to protect the patient from infection, which is the main cause of death.

Course of Illness. The course of the illness may be short or long and can be divided into four phases: onset, oliguric or anuric phase, and early and late diuretic phase. The disorder may be mild or severe and, while the course can often be predicted initially from the type of disorder which has precipitated the failure, in at least 30 per cent of the cases no diagnosis is made. The slope of the daily rise in the blood urea nitrogen is a good index of tissue breakdown and is one measure of mildness or severity. Potassium intoxication and pulmonary edema from sodium and water overload are the chief dangers in the early part of failure and depletion of water, potassium and salt in the diuretic phase.

Treatment. Treatment may be conservative: mannitol and furosemide may be used to prevent and treat the internal hydronephrosis of transfusion reactions or, the physician may elect to use peritoneal or extracorporeal dialysis. The indications for one form or another of treatment will not be discussed here. It is important, however, to state that there is a trend to earlier and more frequent dialyses, while at the same time providing limited meals to maintain nutrition and morale at optimum levels.

Dietary Management. In conservative management when, for example, it is pre-dicted that the course is to be a short one, the aims of dietary treatment are to prevent accumulation of water and salt, to prevent and treat hyperkalemia and to limit the accumulation of nitrogenous end products to a minimum. This is done by measuring and charting each day the total fluid output from dejecta (urine, stool, vomit, sweat, gastric suction) and from body surfaces (burns, fistulas, wounds). The next day, the patient is given that amount of fluid, plus 300-ml water. This 300-ml water, plus the preformed water of metabolism, balance the insensible water loss. As a further control, the patient is weighed accurately each day and the weights are charted. He should lose steadily approximately 0.25 to 0.5 kg per day. Fluid and food by mouth are preferable to infusions by vein. If the serum sodium concentration falls below 130 mEq/liter, fluid intake is restricted. If the serum sodium goes above 140 mEq/liter, fluid may be increased somewhat. A weight loss of greater than 0.5 kg/day suggests the need for more fluid, while a stable or increasing weight indicates overhydration.

Potassium. Potassium intoxication results from release into the blood stream of potassium from pus, pockets of blood, hemolysis, dead and dying tissue and tissue protein catabolism. The effects of high levels of potassium on the myocardium are aggravated by other factors such as hyponatremia, hypocalcemia and acidosis. It is vital to recall that there is no correlation between the changes in the electrocardiogram and the level of serum potassium during intoxication. In caring for the patient, both electrocardiography and measurement of electrolytes should be used. The patient's intake of potassium should be reduced to a minimum and the ion should be removed from the gut by sodium-containing polystyrene sulfonate resins, taken by mouth (10 gm, 4 times a day) and, preferably, mixed with sorbitol. The latter acts as a mild purgative and facilitates passage of the resin through the gastrointestinal tract. In addition, sorbitol removes water by producing diarrhea. Forty gm of the resin, with sorbitol, should also be given by rectal tube once a day or twice a day. If electrocardiographic changes appear, 50 to 200 ml of an intravenous solution of hypertonic sodium bicarbonate are given over 15 minutes. Thereafter, 200 to 300 ml of 20 to 50 per cent glucose in water are given over 6 hours, and one unit of regular insulin per 5 gm of glucose is added to the solution. This drives potassium from the circulation into the cells. This may suffice, or dialysis may be needed.

Carbohydrate. It was popular to feed patients ill with acute renal failure with emulsion of peanut oil, glucose and vitamins, but these mixtures usually nauseate the patients and cause vomiting.[144] The central aim of previous and present dietary care is to try to prevent endogenous tissue protein breakdown and there are clear-cut data that intakes of at least 100 gm of carbohydrate each day must be consumed to achieve some protection by dietary means. Johnson and Sargent,[145] on the other hand, studying men in artificial survival situations, indicate that nitrogen wastage is slowed down by intakes of up to 3,000 calories per day from carbohydrate. Since body fat stores usually suffice to provide some calories for the relatively short time conservative management is used, the main problem is getting in the mandatory calories from carbohydrate by mouth and at the same time using a limited supply of fluid. Ginger ale and corn syrup, in equal parts, taken in small amounts throughout the day, may be tolerated and butterscotch candies are acceptable to some. But vomiting and nausea may force one to resort to parenteral feeding. Perhaps, under these circumstances, it may be better to switch to dialysis or to transfer the patient to a dialysis center, as peritoneal dialysis—simple as it seems—requires the employment of individuals skilled in its use and completely trained in the complexities of water and electrolyte disturbances.

Protein. Berlyne and his co-workers designed a low-protein diet on the principles developed by Giordano and Giovannetti. This low-protein diet contains about 2.6 gm of nitrogen which provide the minimal daily requirements of the essential amino acids. It also provides 2,000 calories, 9 mEq of sodium and 15 mEq of potassium a day. When compared with conventional carbohydrate diets used to treat acute renal failure, it was well accepted; patients vomited

less, and their general health and tissue nutriture were better maintained. However, with the diet it was not possible to decrease the frequency of dialysis when the daily rise in blood urea nitrogen was only 12 mg/100 ml/day as compared with 34 mg/100 ml/day when the patient consumed the conventional all-carbohydrate diet.[146]

Diuretic Phase. During the diuretic phase, rapidly rising rates of urinary flow may be associated with further increases in the serum urea nitrogen as well as electrolyte depletion. Careful attention to fluid balance and electrolyte output and serum levels is vital. If the uremia is mild and the patient can eat, one allows a "normal" diet and fluids. This is usually all that is needed. If the situation is not straightforward, the basic rules of treatment and control used during the management of oliguria continue to apply. Physicians must not use diuretics or otherwise attempt to speed convalescence by "forcing fluids" over and above that required to be replaced day by day.

Diet. If one elects to embark on early repeated dialysis, then, whenever possible, an attractively presented, appealing diet is prescribed and the patient is encouraged to eat. The sodium, protein and potassium content should be limited by omitting, for example, those fruits and fruit juices which are rich in potassium and by limiting protein to 0.5 gm to 0.75 gm per kg body weight. Salty foods and salt are not used in preparing meals. Multiple small feedings are required as the limitation of fluid intake is mandatory and presents difficulties to the dietitian and to the patient's deglutition. The patient should be encouraged to eat by all who come in contact with him—the physician in charge should consult frequently with the dietitian and she should prepare and chart each day a "caloric count" of both oral and intravenous intake for the physician.

Excessive amounts of vitamins do no good, but a daily supplement should be given either by mouth or parenterally. Certain drugs such as norethandrolone are supposed to reduce protein catabolism in patients and are of value, particularly in acute renal failure.

Parenteral Nutrition. When oral intake of essential nutrients is contraindicated or impossible because of nausea, vomiting, debilitation, coma, etc., then parenteral nutrition should be considered part of the overall metabolic management of such patients. The use of intravenous carbohydrates, amino acids, and fat emulsions as part of the therapeutic regimen in many surgical and medical problems is now well established.

Initially, it was felt that intravenous fluid volume restrictions would prevent the use of parenteral nutrition in acute renal failure. However, with the present application of dialytic methods, the problems of fluid balance are easily overcome. Moreover, it is now possible to make up mixtures of concentrated carbohydrates and amino acids in small volumes of fluid which can maintain patients in positive nutritional states without overhydration.

We have used, with success, a regimen of providing protein and calories intravenously concomitantly with frequent dialyses in acute renal failure. The mixture can be made with readily available protein hydrolysates or purified amino acids and hypertonic glucose and administered as a constant infusion through a central venous catheter, as described by Wilmore and Dudrick.[147] These workers have described[148,149] the use of essential amino acid mixtures and hypertonic glucose in small fluid volumes to treat acute renal failure. They have shown that such patients can be maintained in positive nitrogen balance while urea nitrogen remains stable or decreases. European workers[150,151] have shown that fat emulsions and amino acid solutions are effective in maintaining nutritional balance in patients with acute renal failure.

Too rapid administration of such hypertonic solution can result in hyperglycemia and occasionally hyperosmolar coma. This form of nutrition therapy, therefore, requires careful monitoring, but has proven itself invaluable and life-saving in many cases. Various aspects of parenteral nutrition are considered in Chapter 36.

NUTRITION AND DIALYSIS

Dialytic therapy, peritoneal or hemodialysis, acute or chronic, has now become commonplace in the treatment of renal failure. Many patients now undergo regular hemodialyses on a long-term basis. The intervention of such techniques have required modifications in the dietotherapy of such patients.

Peritoneal Dialysis. The technique, indications, and hazards of peritoneal dialysis are covered elsewhere[152] and will not be discussed here. Peritoneal dialysis is associated with significant loss of protein, chiefly as albumin, IgG and amino acids. The loss of protein may be as great as 20 to 60 gm depending on the duration of dialysis.[153] Berlyne[154] has reported losses of 5 to 10 gm of amino acids during peritoneal dialysis. In the undernourished uremic patients these losses of albumin and amino acids can result in persistent hypoproteinemia, wasting, and increased susceptibility to infections. Detailed studies of plasma amino acids in such patients indicate a pattern similar to that found in patients known to have chronic protein deficiency.[155] The losses of proteins and amino acids should be replaced with increased dietary proteins or by parenteral plasma or amino acid solutions. It has been shown that addition of amino acids to the dialysate can reduce the loss of amino acids.[156]

All the B vitamins are water-soluble and have molecular weights which render them dialyzable. Folic acid is also lost during peritoneal dialysis, but there is no significant loss of vitamin B_{12}, perhaps due to its tight protein binding.[157] Deficiency states attributable to loss of B complex vitamins and folic acid during peritoneal dialysis have been reported.[158] It is suggested that daily vitamin supplements and folic acid supplement be given patients who are regularly dialyzed.

Hemodialysis. The successful development of a hemodialysis machine has revolutionized the care of the terminal renal failure patient. Maintenance of life with chronic intermittent hemodialysis is now well established and new centers are continuously being developed. The dialyzer has its limitations, however, particularly when one considers the metabolic and reabsorptive capacity of a normal kidney.

Contrasted to peritoneal dialysis, very small amounts of protein are lost during hemodialysis. Proteins are large molecules and do not pass through the dialyzer membrane. However, smaller molecules, electrolytes, vitamins, folate and amino acids pass readily through the membrane. The loss varies with type of dialyzer and various flow characteristics and other factors, but losses of free amino acids of 1.1 gm/hr and total amino acids of 3 gm/hr of dialysis have been found by Giordano.[159] Comparable or greater losses have been reported by others.[160,161]

If patients are not given supplements of high quality protein, the nitrogen losses are not made up and patients can become progressively malnourished. Indeed, when plasma aminograms were studied in a group of chronically dialyzed, undernourished patients, a pattern very similar to that found in kwashiorkor has been found.[162] A number of studies have commented on the need for increased dietary nitrogen in chronically dialyzed patients. Approximately 0.75 gm/kg per day of high biological value protein is necessary to maintain nitrogen balance in anephric patients who undergo twice weekly dialyses.[161]

Megaloblastic anemia with low folate levels, presumably secondary to loss of folate in the dialysate, has been reported.[163] Low B vitamin levels and ascorbic acid depletion have also been reported in dialysis patients.[164]

The loss of electrolytes is prevented by dialysis against a bath with added electrolytes. Similarly the addition of amino acids to the bath fluid can reduce the loss of amino acids. This hardly seems practicable, however, when additional dietary protein will do just as well.

Impairment of fat metabolism has been found in dialysis patients. Hyperlipidemias, especially hypertriglyceridemia, perhaps due to impaired lipoprotein lipase activity, have been described. Chronic dialysis patients have been found to have higher basal insulin levels which correlate strongly with high triglyceride levels.

Bone disease is a frequent and often serious complication of chronic renal failure; it appears to be of even greater importance in patients undergoing long-term hemodialysis. Since essentially all patients receiving hemodialysis have progressed beyond the end-stage renal failure phase of their disease, the severity and duration of their uremia are, on the whole, much more severe and much longer than those with chronic renal failure who are manageable without dialysis.

The need for greater amounts of protein results in greater amounts of phosphate and serum phosphate levels can be extremely elevated in dialysis patients. The hyperphosphatemia may be resistant to dietary measures, dialysis and phosphate-binding gels. Secondary hyperparathyroidism and manifestations of bone disease may appear and seem to increase as duration of dialysis is extended. The treatment for bone disease in dialysis patients is similar to that outlined above for chronic renal failure.

Transplantation. The complete excretory, metabolic, synthetic activities of a kidney can only be recovered with an adequately functioning kidney. Successful transplantation can lead ultimately to restoration of a normal state of health if no permanent sequelae of renal failure have occurred in other organs.

With an adequately functioning transplanted kidney, diet and therapy will be governed by considerations other than nitrogen retention, e.g. obesity, underweight, etc. Many transplanted kidneys, however, will suffer episodes of rejection which may sufficiently compromise the function so that restrictions on protein, salt, etc. may again be necessary.

In some instances, hyperparathyroidism may persist after transplantation.[165] Hypercalcemia may result and damage the transplanted kidney. In such cases, evidence of hyperparathyroidism should be carefully sought in kidney-transplanted patients and adjustments of vitamin D, calcium and phosphate made as required. In some of these patients parathyroidectomy may be necessary.

NUTRITION AND RENAL CALCULI

Renal calculi are a common and serious malady. They were well known to Hippocrates and Galen and the ancient Arabic physicians described instruments for breaking up stones. Nutritional factors have long been suspected in their pathogenesis and throughout the centuries various strange and expensive diets have been advised. It has been, however, only since the latter half of the 19th century when the chemical composition of the stones became known that serious research and a rational approach to the nature and treatment of calculus disease have been undertaken.

Recent estimates show that one in every thousand persons in the U.S. requires hospitalization for kidney stones.[166] Autopsy studies have shown an incidence of stones in 1.12 per cent of cases, with 0.38 per cent of the deaths related to presence of calculi.[167] In the "stone belt" of the Middle East the disease can reach epidemic proportions. In those areas about 80 per cent of the stones are vesical and over 50 per cent are found in children.

Renal lithiasis is not a single entity. Stones are found under a variety of conditions with many factors contributing to their formation. An extensive review of renal stones has recently appeared in print.[168] Stone pathogenesis can be considered under two broad headings:

1. Local factors which promote stone formation, such as infection, obstruction and urinary tract abnormalities;
2. Metabolic processes which result in increased excretion of stone components, e.g., hyperoxaluria; cystinuria; hypercalciuria.

Chemical Composition. The chemical composition of stones is not constant and statistics vary, but in general the chief cation is calcium. In more than half the cases, stones are mixtures of calcium, ammonium, magnesium, phosphates and carbonates. Oxalate is also an important anion. Table 30-9[169] gives the chemical composition of some 10,000 urinary stones. Uric acid makes up

Table 30-9.[169]　Chemical Composition of Urinary Stones

	Number of Specimens	Per-centage	
Calcium oxalate monohydrate	3,136	31.69	Oxalates
Calcium oxalate dihydrate	4,094	41.37	73.06
Magnesium ammophosphate hexahydrate	912	9.22	
Carbonate apatite	444	4.49	
Hydroxyl apatite	228	2.31	
Calcium hydrogen phosphate dihydrate	131	1.34	Phosphates 17.51
Tricalcium phosphate	13	0.13	
Magnesium phosphate octahydrate	1	0.01	
Diammonium calcium phosphate	1	0.01	
Uric acid	740	7.48	
Sodium acid urate	4	0.04	Uric acid
Ammonium acid urate	8	0.08	and
Calcium acid urate	1	0.01	urates
Calcium magnesium urate	1	0.01	7.63
Dicalcium urate	1	0.01	
Hematin	26	0.26	
Fibrin	55	0.55	
Mucine	3	0.03	
Steatin	4	0.04	
Cystine	88	0.88	
Xanthine	1	0.01	
Indigo	1	0.01	
Sulfonamides	2	0.02	
Total	9,895	100	

about 5 to 10 per cent of stones and cystine stones represent less than 1 per cent of the total.

Calcium-containing Stones. Hypercalciuria is the most frequently found metabolic abnormality in nephrolithiases. The study of renal excretion of calcium is a complex problem and involves consideration of protein binding, inhibitors, chelations, hormonal influence, relationship to other electrolytes and as yet undefined conditions. Hypercalciuria is often related to hyperparathyroidism, bone disease, ingestion of milk and alkali, sarcoidosis and renal tubular acidosis. However, the most common abnormality is idiopathic hypercalciuria which was present in about 42 per cent of a recent series of stone-forming patients.[170]

The underlying pathogenesis of idiopathic hypercalciuria is not yet known but most investigators attribute the hypercalciuria to disordered renal tubular cell handling of calcium. Some alteration in handling of dietary calcium in these patients, however, has also been found. Normally, about one-third of dietary calcium is absorbed and subsequently excreted in the urine with two-thirds excreted in fecal material. These ratios are reversed in the idiopathic hypercalciuric patient; two-thirds of dietary calcium may be absorbed and subsequently excreted in urine.[171] Urinary calcium varies over a fairly wide range on normal diets with values of 250 mg daily for women and 300 mg daily for men considered upper normal values. Values in excess of 400 mg daily are often found in idiopathic hypercalciuria. This disorder is largely confined to males. There were only 24 females in a total of 186 patients with idiopathic hypercalciuria in a recent series.[170] The hypercalciuric female with kidney stones has an even chance of having primary hyperparathyroidism, whereas the hypercalciuric male with stones has somewhat less than 10 per cent chance of having parathyroid overactivity.

Oxalate-containing Stones. Oxalate is present in about two-thirds of renal stones. Primary hyperoxaluria is a rare hereditary disorder transmitted in an autosomal recessive pattern, which results in calcium oxalate deposition in many tissues frequently leading to progressive renal failure and death from nephrolithiasis and nephrocalcinosis. The disorder is characterized by increased urinary excretion of oxalic and glycolic acids, as a result of an impairment of metabolism of glyoxylic acid.

Several acquired disorders are known in which hyperoxaluria can occur. Certain foods are very rich in oxalates such as rhubarb, spinach, chocolate, dandelion greens, asparagus, cranberries, etc. Instances of oxalate poisoning secondary to rhubarb gluttony have been reported, but they are not well documented. Oxalate calculi have been produced in animals by the administration of large doses of soluble oxalate. Ethylene glycol is metabolized to oxalic acid and hyperoxaluria is a feature of ingestion of anti-freeze (of which ethylene glycol is the major constituent).

Hyperoxaluria occurs in experimental pyridoxine deficiency in animals and man and may occasionally play a role in nephrolithiases.[172] Thiamin deficiency in rats has been associated with accumulation of glycolate in blood and tissues. Magnesium deficiency, experimentally, has been associated with hyperoxaluria and stone formation.[172] The primary defect, however, is altered metabolism with increased endogenous production of oxalate.

Uric Acid Stones. Uric acid stones are fairly common and in many cases are secondary to increased cell turn over as in leukemia, and chemotherapy of cancer. There appears, however, to be a group of patients with a genetic predisposition to hyperuricemia. In general, these patients appear to have increased uric acid pools and increased rates of conversion of glycine to uric acid. In addition, these patients have undue persistent acidity of urine chiefly due to a defect in ammonium excretion, presumably from a disordered metabolism of glutamine by the renal tubules.

The main dietary source of uric acid is purine, chiefly in high-protein foods. Dietary restriction of high-protein foods is commonly prescribed in uric acid stone forms but probably plays a small role in prevention of recurrence.

Starvation is associated with high uric acid

levels in serum and urine as a consequence of mobilization of body protein stores and inhibition of uric acid excretion by lactic acid and other acidic products of starvation.

Cystine Stones. Cystine stones are rare. Cystinuria is a hereditary defect of transport of cystine, lysine, arginine and ornithine. There appears to be at least two forms; in one the pattern is recessive and the heterozygote shows no noteworthy excess of cystine in the urine. In the other, the inheritance is incompletely recessive and the heterozygote may have intermediate degrees of cystinuria and may rarely form stones. Cystine is very poorly soluble in acid solution and stone formation is generally associated with acid urine.

Treatment. Nephrolithiasis is a chronic condition and in most cases the patient may have recurrences throughout his life. Therapeutic measures and dietary therapy, where useful, are therefore part of a long-term program. Since most studies show that concentration of urine and saturation of urine with minerals favor stone formation, the simple expediency of drinking large quantities of fluid (3,000 to 4,000 cc daily) to dilute the urine is perhaps the most important prophylactic measure. Since deficiencies of magnesium, pyridoxine and thiamin have been associated with the development of stones, it is obvious that a nutritionally well-balanced diet is important.

Unfortunately, specific dietary measures aimed at restricting the calcium and oxalate intake in food are frequently ineffective in preventing recurrences of stones. However, although dietary calcium has little effect on urinary calcium, excretion of calcium may be reduced in patients with idiopathic hypercalciuria by varying the calcium intake. Low-oxalate diets have not proved to be particularly successful in preventing oxalate stones. However, since excretion of oxalate does increase after ingestion of high-oxalate foods, avoidance of these foods does have some rationale.

In recent years, the use of inorganic orthophosphate has been shown to be effective in preventing calcium oxalate stones. This requires the administration of sufficient amounts of sodium or potassium phosphate to supply 1 to 3 gm elemental phosphorus per day. Phosphate ingestion results in diminished urinary calcium excretion and increased urinary pyrophosphate excretion. The thiazide diuretics can cause a marked sustained reduction of urinary calcium and has been reported to be successful in preventing recurrences of calculi. Cellulose phosphate inhibits absorption of calcium and results in lowered urinary calcium.[123]

Prevention of uric acid stones is readily accomplished in most instances by high fluid intake and administration of alkali to keep urine pH above 6.5. Dietary restriction of foods high in purine (sweetbreads, brain, liver, anchovies) is advisable, but drastic reduction of protein has not been shown to be effective. The xanthine-oxidase inhibitor drug—allopurinol—which prevents the synthesis of uric acid has been highly successful in the treatment and prevention of uric acid stones.

The combined use of fluids and alkali is also quite effective in most cases of cystinuria. The urine pH should be maintained above 8.0. Low-protein diets have not been effective, but avoidance of foods high in methionine and cystine may be beneficial. The management of the difficult patients who do not respond to these measures has been facilitated by the demonstration that d-penicillamine can combine with cystine to form a soluble disulfide. Its use results in marked lowering of urinary cystine excretion. Unfortunately, d-penicillamine does have toxic effects and its use must be carefully supervised.

In summary, therapeutic diets are used less often now in treating renal calculi, but dietary modification continues to be a sound preventive measure against recurrence of stones, particularly in conjunction with a program of high-fluid intake and judicious use of specific drugs.

CONGESTIVE HEART FAILURE

The basic aims in the management of cardiac disease are (1) to reduce the exercise work load of the organ as much as possible, and (2) to diminish the work of the heart at rest. Ingestion of food increases cardiac work. Moreover, it is also probable that the heart functions at a disadvantage after a heavy meal because, with distention of the stomach, the diaphragm is elevated and the heart is displaced upward. *Obesity* constitutes a handicap to circulation and respiration that, in the presence of cardiac failure, may become a serious factor due to elevation of the diaphragm, decrease in volume of the lungs and change in position of the heart. Adiposity of the cardiac muscle may be another factor in the impairment of adequate myocardial function. Furthermore, it has been shown that obesity increases the work of the heart during exertion. Therefore, one of the foremost aims of a dietary program for cardiac disease, particularly if the patient is suffering from cardiac failure, is reduction in body weight if the patient is obese. It calls for a diet low in calories that will serve not only to eliminate excess weight but also to maintain cardiac work at as low a level as possible.

Since it is known that undernutrition decreases bodily consumption of oxygen with resultant decrease in cardiac work, one would expect a diet low in calories to be especially useful in the treatment of *acute* congestive cardiac failure, in line with the previously stated basic aims in the management of heart disease. Physicians were aware of the fact that calorically restricted diets were of value in the treatment of cardiac failure long before the theoretic basis for such diets was understood. Karell,[173] in 1866, introduced the diet that bears his name and that consists solely of 800 ml of milk daily. Such a program frequently has been found to result in great diuresis, remarkable improvement in myocardial efficiency and alleviation of symptoms. Some workers have advocated institution of the Karell diet for 3 to 7 days in the early stages of congestive cardiac failure, followed by a diet restricted to 800 to 1,200 calories per day; with its duration determined by the progress of the patient and the amount of weight to be lost.

Although no indication exists for drastic reduction of the intake of protein in the diet, the effect of the specific dynamic action of protein with the resultant extra demand for energy placed on the heart requires that the intake of protein for an adult patient of aver-

age size suffering from congestive cardiac failure should be moderate, 60 to 70 gm daily.

In congestive cardiac failure, the myocardium fails to perform adequately its function of propelling blood through the circulatory system. Consequently, a disproportionate amount of blood is usually present in that part of the vascular system concerned with the right side of the heart; venous return is retarded and stasis results. In turn, fluid is diffused from the blood stream through the walls of the blood vessels into tissue spaces of the lungs and liver and into the peripheral tissues—in fact, into all parts of the extracellular fluid compartment of the body. Impaired excretion of sodium by the kidneys results in retention of salt and water in these tissues.

Warren and Stead,[174] in well-controlled studies, were able to produce edema in patients who had recovered from previous episodes of congestive cardiac failure by adding an excessive amount of salt to their diets. Under these circumstances, typical symptoms and signs of congestive cardiac failure again developed. These investigators concluded that the edema is due to inadequate cardiac output. The kidneys are unable to excrete salt and water adequately (because of impaired renal hemodynamics and hormonal factors) and the excess of sodium and water is stored in tissue spaces as edema fluid. As a result of this series of events, the other symptoms and signs of cardiac decompensation develop. In essence, the renal dysfunction is at the beginning of the line of events stemming from "forward" cardiac failure. A great deal of human and animal research in the last 20 years has supported this concept; but the exact intermediate steps in the chain between the inefficient heart and renal hemodynamics, glomerular-tubular balance, renin and angiotensin induction, sodium reabsorption-regulating hormones (aldosterone and other adrenal steroids) and neurohormonal factors are still under intensive and productive study. The probable involvement, in heart failure, of some of the same mechanisms concerned with hypertension of renal vascular origin, is a striking example of Nature's economy.

Despite the fact that controversy continued for years regarding the pathogenesis of congestive cardiac failure, between proponents of the "forward" or the "backward" theory, the work of Warren and Stead served to focus attention on the importance of the sodium ion in the genesis of cardiac edema. For years, it has been known that patients suffering from cardiac disease have difficulty in excreting sodium in a normal manner, although the value for sodium in serum does not increase. However, renewed interest in the use of diets low in salt for patients suffering from congestive cardiac failure was brought about by the observations of Barker,[175] by the work of Warren and Stead, and by the studies of Schroeder,[176] Schemm,[177] Wheeler and associates[178] and others who have advocated an acid-ash diet sharply restricted in salt but with an abundant allowance of fluid. This form of treatment, in conjunction with the administration of digitalis in one of its various forms, the use of mercurial diuretics and, in recent years, the "thiazides," and the employment of other commonly accepted measures in the management of congestive cardiac failure, proved to be quite efficacious and gained widespread acceptance.

Further studies have indicated that restriction of ingested salt to 1.5 to 2.0 gm daily is the most important feature of the program (see Appendix, Table A-10). Clinical experience further has shown that diuresis may be enhanced by the free ingestion of fluid, depending on the desire of the patient, up to 2,500 to 3,000 ml daily. It has been our practice to employ such a diet in the majority of hospitalized cases, that is, to allow approximately 0.5 gm of sodium (1.3 gm of sodium chloride) daily with unrestricted fluid in the management of patients who have congestive cardiac failure with edema. Increasingly, patients with cardiac failure are encountered in whom edema, both pulmonary and peripheral, appears to be refractory to treatment. Usually such a situation is observed in patients who have far-advanced myocardial disease; many such patients have had repeated episodes of congestive cardiac failure. In these patients, it may be found that diuresis will not proceed satisfactorily or clinical improvement ensue until the amount of sodium in the diet is re-duced to 0.2 gm (0.5 gm of sodium chloride) daily. Fluid intake should be limited to prevent dilution hyponatremia. Contrariwise, ambulatory patients are encountered in whom cardiac failure is more than usually amenable to treatment; in such instances, diuresis may be accomplished and clinical improvement obtained with a more liberal dietary program containing 2.0 gm of sodium (5.0 gm of sodium chloride) daily. Sodium intake may be "titrated" to some extent against diuretic dosage or frequency of use.

The acid-ash diets advocated in the past by Barker, Schemm and others were helpful in enhancing mercurial diuresis, but their lack of palatability led to early replacement by the oral administration of acid-forming salts, such as ammonium chloride and calcium chloride; more recently, also, by lysine or arginine monohydrochloride, given orally as an adjuvant to mercurial diuresis in the more resistant cardiac edemas. The risk of serious metabolic acidosis in certain patients with renal or hepatic impairment must be guarded against. Potassium chloride, orally, is now frequently used where both hypochloremia and potassium deficiency require compensation, e.g. with the continued administration of thiazides over prolonged periods.

The development of newer potent diuretics, especially furosemide and ethacrynic acid, has greatly enhanced the treatment of refractory edema. These agents often work when renal function is depressed or when hyponatremia is present. They are, however, extremely potent and when used injudiciously may result in serious salt depletion, especially when salt intake is curtailed.

Dilution Hyponatremia. In advanced congestive heart failure, especially when the patient's general and cardiac condition has deteriorated due to acute infection, over- or underdigitalization, excessive use of potent diuretics or other stresses, unusual retention of water develops on a low-sodium diet and unrestricted fluid intake. This leads to dilutional lowering of extracellular sodium concentration, although the total body sodium content is usually excessive.[179] In this state, refractoriness to diuretics is common and the administration of salt is useless and often dangerous. Restriction of fluids is urgently indicated along with appropriate treatment for the underlying causes of the aggravated circulatory failure. Restoration of serum sodium concentration after spontaneous water diuresis may then occur, with improvement in the patient's general status.

Depletion of Salt. Any diet in which the amount of salt is drastically restricted is associated with the risk of harmful effects that may result from deficiency of sodium or chloride, especially if a defect is present in the resorptive function of the renal tubules, preventing adequate conservation of salt. This is particularly true in older patients with congestive cardiac failure on a hypertensive or arteriosclerotic basis, because of the loss of salt that accompanies therapeutic diuresis. The clinician who employs such a regimen must be constantly on the alert, especially in elderly patients with little gross edema, in evaluating complaints of weakness, lassitude, anorexia, nausea and vomiting, mental confusion, abdominal cramps and aching in skeletal muscles as possible indications of impending disaster in the form of depletion of salt. Patients consuming such diets must be kept under frequent and close observation, especially in warm weather, when excessive amounts of salt may be lost through perspiration, or during periods of gastrointestinal upsets. The blood urea nitrogen and serum electrolytes should be checked.

In *summary*, the diet in the treatment of congestive cardiac failure should be adjusted to maintain the dry body weight at normal or slightly below normal levels; it should be well balanced, light and nutritious, with adequate easily assimilated carbohydrates, a moderate amount of protein, sufficient fat to meet caloric needs, and an adequate content of vitamins and graded restriction of salt as indicated.[180] In the selection of food, consideration should be given to the patient's likes and dislikes. Fried and greasy foods should be avoided, as should excessive amounts of spices and condiments, and foods tending to produce flatulence. Meals should be eaten slowly and thoroughly masticated. In many cases, 5 or 6 small meals daily are to be preferred to 3 large ones. Constant vigilance should be maintained against symptoms of depletion of salt in all patients who are to be maintained for a prolonged period on a diet restricted in salt. Potassium depletion on the current diuretic agents is prevalent and must be constantly checked and treated.

ACUTE MYOCARDIAL INFARCTION

Early in the course of acute myocardial infarction, the type of diet indicated must be governed by the extent of myocardial damage and the condition of the patient. *Absolute rest in bed* is of prime importance; the patient's output of energy should not be taxed in any way during the early stages, and he should be maintained at conditions that are as near basal as possible. He should not be allowed to feed himself or to roll over in bed unassisted. The bowels should be kept as regular as possible by means of mild laxatives or enemas if necessary; straining at stool should be avoided. Whether a bedpan or a bedside commode occasions the lesser degree of exertion is a moot question, and its solution must be left to the judgment of the clinician.

In the first 2 or 3 days, the diet must be light. In most cases, a liquid diet with a volume of 1,000 to 1,500 ml per day is indicated, but in some patients, critically ill, no food should be given. Such a patient may wish only small amounts of fluid at a time— water, ginger ale, low-sodium milk or tea. Care should be taken to avoid abdominal distention in patients who do not tolerate milk well. When milk is tolerated, the Karell diet (200 ml of milk 4 times daily) may be employed for 2 or 3 days. Even in the absence of congestive cardiac failure, the intake of sodium should be restricted. In the event of persistent and distressing vomiting in the early days after acute myocardial infarction, small amounts (50 to 100 ml) of hypertonic solution of dextrose (10 to 20 per cent) may be given intravenously with caution at regular intervals during the day, or by very slow continuous drips, to provide adequate fluid and carbohydrate. Large intravenous infusions of any sort are contraindicated because of the extra load they impose on a damaged myocardium and the hazard of precipitating pulmonary edema.

BIBLIOGRAPHY

1. Selkurt: Am. J. Physiol., *142*, 182, 1944.
2. Long, (Ed.): *Biochemists' Handbook*, New York, Van Nostrand, 1961.
3. Perry, Tipton, Schroeder and Cook: J. Lab. & Clin. Med., *60*, 235, 1962.
4. Kagi and Vallee: J. Biol. Chem., *236*, 2435, 1961.
5. Emmerson: Ann. Int. Med., *73*, 854, 1970.
6. Leading article: Lancet, *1*, 133, 1968.
7. Bonting, Pollak, Muehrcke and Kark: Science, *127*, 1342, 1958.
8. ———: J. Clin. Invest., *39*, 1381, 1960.
9. Mattenheimer, Pollak and Muehrcke: Nephron, *7*, 144, 1970.
10. Lee, Vance and Cahill: Am. J. Physiol., *203*, 27, 1962.
11. Lassen, Mauck and Thaysen: Acta Physiol. Scand., *51*, 37, 1961.
12. Follis: *The Pathology of Nutritional Disease*, Springfield, Charles C Thomas, 1948.
13. Smith: *The Kidney: Structure and Function in Health and Disease*, New York, Oxford University Press, p. 472, 1951.
14. McCarrison: Brit. Med. J., *1*, 1009, 1931.
15. Meneely, Tucker, Darby and Auerbach: Ann. Intern. Med., *39*, 991, 1953.
16. Best and Hartroft: Fed. Proc., *8*, 610, 1949.
17. Hartroft: Am. J. Path., *31*, 381, 1955.
18. Burr and Burr: J. Biol. Chem., *82*, 345, 1929.
19. ———: J. Biol. Chem., *86*, 587, 1930.
20. Borland and Jackson: Arch. Path., *11*, 687, 1931.
21. Pullman, Alving, Devor and Landowne: J. Lab. & Clin. Med., *44*, 320, 1954.
22. Nielsen and Bang: Acta Med. Scand., *130*, 382, 1948.
23. ———: Scand. J. Clin. & Lab. Med., *1*, 295, 1949.
24. Sargent and Johnson: Am. J. Clin. Nutr., *4*, 466, 1956.
25. Schrier, Hano, Keller *et al.*: Ann. Int. Med., *73*, 213, 1970.
26. Bleiler and Schedl: J. Lab. & Clin. Med., *59*, 945, 1962.
27. Symposium on Uremic Toxins. Arch. Int. Med., 126, Nov. 1970.
28. Giovannetti, Cioni, Balestri, Biagini: Clin. Sci., *13*, 141, 1968.
29. Rubenstein and Spitz: Diabetes, *17*, 161, 1968.
30. Spitz, Rubenstein, Bersohn *et al.*: Quart. J. Med., *39*, 201, 1970.
31. Hampers, Soeldner, Doak and Merrill: J. Clin. Invest., *45*, 1719, 1966.
32. Luke, Briggs, McKiddie and Kennedy: *In: Nutrition in Renal Disease*, ed. Berlyne, Baltimore, Williams & Wilkins Co., 1968, p. 170.
33. Bagdade, Porte and Bierman: New Eng. J. Med., *279*, 181, 1968.
34. Bagdade: J. Clin. Nutr., *21*, 426, 1968.
35. Tsaltas and Friedman: Am. J. Clin. Nutr., *21*, 430, 1968.
36. Ahrens, Tsaltas, Hersch and Intull: J. Clin. Invest., *34*, 918, 1955.
37. Dole: J. Clin. Invest., *35*, 150, 1956.
38. Lewis, Zueheke, Nakamoto *et al.*: New Eng. J. Med., *275*, 1097, 1966.
39. Berlyne and Malliek: Lancet, *2*, 399, 1969.
40. DeLuca: Fed. Proc., *28*, 1678, 1969.
41. DeLuca: New Eng. J. Med., *284*, 554, 1971.
42. Avioli, Birge, Lee and Slatopolsky: J. Clin. Invest., *47*, 2239, 1968.
43. Anonymous: Nutrition Reviews, *28*, 72, 1970.
44. McCance: Med. Rs. Council Spec. Rep. Ser. No. 275, His Majesty's Stationery Office, London, 1951.
45. Owen, Felig, Morgan *et al.*: J. Clin. Invest., *48*, 574, 1969.
46. Felig, Owen, Wahren and Cahill: J. Clin. Invest., *48*, 584, 1969.
47. Alleyene: Rush-Pres. St. Luke Hosp. Bull., *9*, 84, 1970.
48. Berliner and Bennett: Am. J. Med., *42*, 777, 1967.
49. Klahr, Tripathy, Garcia *et al.*: Am. J. Med., *43*, 84, 1967.
50. Manitius, Pigeon and Epstein: Am. J. Physiol., *205*, 101, 1963.
51. Klahr, Tripathy, Lotero: Am. J. Med., *48*, 325, 1970.
52. Bloom: Arch. Int. Med., *106*, 321, 1960.
53. Gamble: Harvey Lectures Ser., *42*, 247, 1947.
54. Hervey and McCance: Proc. Roy. Soc., London, Ser. B, *139*, 527, 1952.
55. Katz, Holingsworth and Epstein: J. Lab. Clin. Med., *72*, 93, 1968.
56. Consolazio, Matoush, Johnson *et al:* Am. J. Clin. Nutr., *20*, 672, 1967.
57. Keys, Brozek, Henschel, *et al.*: *Human Starvation*, Minneapolis, Univ. of Minn. Press, 1951.
58. Davies: Am. J. Clin. Nutr., *4*, 539, 1956.
59. Eales: Am. J. Clin. Nutr., *4*, 529, 1956.
60. Gershoff, Faragalla, Nelson and Andrus: Am. J. Med., *27*, 72, 1959.
61. Liang: Biochem. J., *82*, 429, 1962.
62. Schwartz and Relman: New Eng. J. Med., *276*, 383, 452, 1967.
63. Conn and Johnson: Am. J. Clin. Nutr., *4*, 523, 1966.
64. Bright: Reports of Medical Cases, *Selected with a View of Illustrating the Symptoms and Cure of Diseases by a Reference to Morbid Anatomy*, vol. I, p. 14, London, Longman, Rees, Orme, Brown & Green, 1827.
65. Am. Heart Assoc. Monograph number 32, Am. Heart Assoc. New York, 1970.
66. Bull, Hillman, Cannon and Laragh: Circ. Res., *27*, 953, 1970.
67. Tobian and Binnion: J. Clin. Invest., *33*, 1407, 1954.
68. Headings, Rondell, and Bohr: Am. J. Physiol., *199*, 783, 1960.
69. Dahl: *In: Essential Hypertension*. ed. K. D. Bock and P. T. Cottier. Berne, Springer-Verlag, 1960, p. 530.

70. Schroeder: *In: Essential Hypertension*, ed. Bock and Cottier, Berne, Springer-Verlag 1960, p. 83.
71. Schroeder: J.A.M.A., *187*, 358, 1964.
72. Dahl, Heine and Tassinari: J. Exp. Med., *115*, 1173, 1962.
73. Dahl: Am. J. Clin. Nutr., *21*, 787, 1968.
74. Guthrie: Am. J. Clin. Nutr., *21*, 863, 1968.
75. Brown, Duesterdieck, Fraser *et al.*: Brit. Med. Bull., *27*, 128, 1971.
76. Kolff, Nakamoto, Poutasse *et al.*: Circ., *30*, Supp. no. II, p. 23, 1964.
77. Hunt, Strong, Harrison *et al.*: Am. J. Cardio., *26*, 280, 1970.
78. Hunt, Novak and Nelson: Rush-Pres. St. Luke Hosp. Bull., *9*, 96, 1970.
79. Ambard and Beaujard: Arch. gén. de méd., *1*, 520, 1904.
80. Allen and Sherrill: J. Metab. Res., *2*, 429, 1922.
81. Kempner: North Carolina Med. J., *5*, 125, 1944.
82. Kempner: North Carolina Med. J., *6*, 61 and 117, 1945.
83. Kempner: Am. J. Med., *4*, 545, 1948.
84. Schwartz: J. Clin. Invest., *27*, 406, 1948.
85. Chapman: Medicine, *29*, 29, 1950.
86. Watkin *et al.*: Am. J. Med., *9*, 428, 1950.
87. Grollman *et al.*: J.A.M.A., *129*, 533, 1945.
88. Ayman: J.A.M.A., *141*, 974, 1941.
89. Bryant: Proc. Soc. Exp. Biol. Med., *65*, 227, 1947.
90. Landowne *et al.*: J. Lab. and Clin. Med., *34*, 1380, 1949.
91. Carlberger and Collste: Scand. J. Urol. Nephrol., *2*, 151, 1968.
92. Wilkinson, Scott, Uldale *et al.*: Quart. J. Med., *39*, 377, 1970.
93. Theobald: The Toxemias of Pregnancy in Women. In Ciba Foundation Symposium, Philadelphia, The Blakiston Company, p. 23, 1950.
94. Chrichton: Toxemia in South Africa. Trans. Internat. Congress of Obstetricians and Gynaecologists, Dublin, 1947.
95. Brock: Personal communication, 1956.
96. duPlessis: *The Cape Malays*, Cape Town, Maskew Miller, 1944.
97. Gerber: *Traditional Cookery of the Cape Malays*, Cape Town, A.A. Balkema, 1957.
98. Wachstein and Gudaitis: Am. J. Clin. Path., *22*, 652, 1952.
99. Sarles, Hill, LeBlanc *et al.*: Am. J. Obstet. Gyn., *102*, 1, 1968.
100. Schewitz: Med. Clin. N. Amer., *55*, 47, 1971.
101. Brown, Davies, Doak *et al.*: Lancet, *2*, 900, 1963.
102. Robinson: Lancet, *1*, 78, 1958.
103. Kirksey and Pike: J. Nutr., *77*, 34 and 43, 1962; *78*, 325, 1962; and *80*, 421, 1963.
104. Perey, Herdman, Vernier and Good: J. Lab. Clin. Med., *70*, 881, 1967.
105. Schwartz: New Eng. J. Med., *253*, 601, 1955.
106. Milne, Muehrcke and Heard: Brit. Med. Bull., *13*, 15, 1957.
107. Perkins, Petersen and Riley: Am. J. Med., *8*, 115, 1950.
108. Black and Milne: Clin. Sci., *11*, 397, 1952.
109. Black: *Essentials of Fluid Balance*, Oxford, Blackwell Scientific Publications, 1960.
110. Muehrcke and McMillan: Ann. Int. Med., *59*, 427, 1963.
111. Addis: *Glomerular Nephritis: Diagnosis and Treatment*, New York, The Macmillan Co., 1948.
112. Camera, Reimer and Newburgh: Univ. Michigan Med. Bull., *18*, 285, 1952.
113. Von Rohrer: Arch. f. ges. Physiol., *109*, 375, 1905.
114. Illingsworth, Philpott and Rendle-Short: Arch. Dis. Child., *29*, 551, 1954.
115. Mortensen: Acta Med. Scand., *129*, 321, 1947.
116. Kark, Pirani, Pollak *et al.*: Ann. Int. Med., *49*, 751, 1958.
117. Squire: Am. J. Clin. Nutr., *4*, 509, 1956.
118. Baxter: Arch. Int. Med., *109*, 742, 1962.
119. Voorhaus and Kark: Am. J. Med., *14*, 707, 1953.
120. Soothill and Kark: Clin. Res. Proc., *4*, 140, 1956.
121. Kark and Gellman: *In: Diabetes*, Williams, ed., New York, Paul B. Hoeber, 1960. p. 563.
122. Gellman, Pirani, Soothill *et al.*: Medicine, *38*, 321, 1959.
123. Dent, Harper, and Parfitt: Clin. Sci., *27*, 417, 1964.
124. Rabkin, Simon, Steiner and Colwell: New Eng. J. Med., *282*, 182, 1970.
125. Giordano: J. Lab. Clin Med., *62*, 231, 1963.
126. Berlyne, Gaan, and Ginks: Am. J. Clin. Nutr., *21*, 547, 1968.
127. Giovannetti and Maggiore: Lancet, *1*, 1000, 1964.
128. Giordano, DePascale, Balestrieri *et al.*: Am. J. Clin. Nutr., *21*, 394, 1968.
129. Robson, Kerr, and Ashcroft: *In: Nutrition in Renal Disease*, ed. Berlyne, Baltimore, The Williams & Wilkins Co., 1968, p. 71.
130. Fürst, Josephson, Virnars: *In: Nutrition in Renal Disease*, ed. Berlyne, Baltimore, The Williams & Wilkins Co., 1968, p. 99.
131. Richards, Houghton, Metcalfe-Gibson *et al.*: *In: Nutrition in Renal Disease*, ed. Berlyne, Baltimore, The Williams & Wilkins Co., 1968, p. 93.
132. Pollak, Schneider, Freund and Kark: Arch. Int. Med., *103*, 200, 1959.
133. Stanbury: Medicine, *41*, 1, 1962.
134. Symposium-Divalent Ion Metabolism and Osteodystrophy in Chronic Renal Failure. Arch. Int. Med., *124*, nos. 3, 4, 5, 6, 1969.
135. Bricker, Ogden, Schreiner, Walser: Invited Discussion. Arch. Int. Med., *124*, 292, 1969.
136. Reiss, Canterbury, Kanter: Arch. Int. Med., *124*, 417, 1961.
137. Lennon: Arch. Int. Med., *124*, 557, 1969.
138. Fraser and Kodicek: Nature, (Lond.), *228*, 764, 1970.
139. Wasserman and Taylor: J. Bio. Chem., *243*, 3987, 1968.

140. Baron, Dent, Harris *et al.*: Lancet, *271*, 421, 1956.
141. Fanconi: Jahrb. Kinderh., *147*, 299, 1936.
142. Milkman: Am. J. Roentgen, *24*, 29, 1930.
143. Albright, Burnett, Parson *et al.*: Medicine, *28*, 399, 1946.
144. Lowe and Valtin: Am. J. Clin. Nutr., *4*, 486, 1956.
145. Sargent, Sargent, Johnson and Stolpe: WADC Technical Report 53–484, Part II. Vols. I and II. Wright Air Development Center, Dayton, Ohio, 1955.
146. Berlyne, Bazzard, Booth *et al.*: Quart. J. Med., *36*, 59–84, 1967.
147. Wilmore and Dudrick: Arch. Surg., *98*, 256, 1969.
148. Wilmore and Dudrick: Arch. Surg., *99*, 669, 1969.
149. Dudrick, Steger and Long: Surg., *68*, 180, 1970.
150. Wretlind: *In: Nutrition in Renal Disease*, ed. Berlyne, Baltimore, The Williams & Wilkins Co., 1968, p. 199.
151. Lee, Hill, Ginks and Pohl: *In: Nutrition in Renal Disease*, ed. Berlyne, Baltimore, The Williams & Wilkins Co., 1968, p. 216.
152. Dunea: Med. Clin. N. Amer., *55*, 155, 1971.
153. Berlyne, Jones, Hewitt, and Nitwarangkur: Lancet, *1*, 738, 1964.
154. Berlyne, Lee, Giordano *et al.*: Lancet, *1*, 1339, 1967.
155. Young and Parsons: Clin. Sci., *97*, 1, 1969.
156. Glessing: Lancet, *2*, 812, 1968.
157. Sevit and Hoffbrand: Brit. Med. J., *2*, 18, 1961.
158. Palmer, Newell, Gray, and Quinton: New Eng. J. Med., *274*, 248, 1966.
159. Giordano, DePascale, Cristofaro *et al.*: *In: Nutrition in Renal Disease*, ed. Berlyne, Baltimore, The Williams & Wilkins Co., 1968, p. 23.
160. Young and Parson: Clin. Sci., *31*, 299, 1969.
161. Ginn, Frost and Lacy: Am. J. Clin. Nutr., *21*, 385, 1968.
162. Gulassy, Peters, Lin and Ryan: Am. J. Clin. Nutr., *21*, 565, 1968.
163. Whitehead, Comty, Posen and Kaye: New Eng. J. Med., *279*, 970, 1968.
164. Sullivan and Eisenstein: Am. J. Clin. Nutr., *23*, 1339, 1970.
165. Hampers, Katz, Wilson and Merrill: Arch. Int. Med., *124*, 282, 1969.
166. Boyce, Garvey and Strawcutter: J.A.M.A., *161*, 1433, 1956.
167. Bell: *Renal Calculi in Renal Diseases*, 2nd ed. p. 414, Philadelphia, Lea & Febiger, 1950.
168. Smith: Amer. J. Med., *45*, 649, 1968.
169. Herring: J. Urol., *88*, 545, 1962.
170. Yendt: Canad. Med. Assoc. J., *102*, 479, 1970.
171. Henneman, Benedict, Forbes, and Dudley: New Eng. J. Med., *259*, 802, 1958.
172. Gershoff and Prien: Am. J. Clin. Nutr., *20*, 393, 1967.
173. Karell: Arch. gén. de méd., *2*, 513, 1866.
174. Warren and Stead: Arch. Int. Med., *73*, 138, 1944.
175. Barker: J.A.M.A., *98*, 2193, 1932.
176. Schroeder: Am. Heart J., *22*, 141, 1941.
177. Schemm: Ann. Int. Med., *17*, 952, 1942.
178. Wheeler, Bridges and White: J.A.M.A., *133*, 16, 1947.
179. Weston, Grossman, Borun and Hanenson: Am. J. Med., *25*, 558, 1958.
180. Leiter: Arch. Int. Med., *105*, 825, 1960.

Chapter

31

Diet, Hyperlipidemia and Atherosclerosis

ROBERT I. LEVY AND NANCY ERNST

Arteriosclerosis is a general term for the degeneration of the arteries, resulting in thickening and hardening of the arterial wall. Atherosclerosis, one type of arteriosclerosis, is characterized by accumulation of lipids (primarily cholesterol, but also phospholipid and triglycerides) in the walls of medium and large arteries. Atherosclerosis is a disorder that underlies most arteriosclerotic heart disease (coronary artery disease) and, in addition, plays a major role in cerebrovascular disease.[1,2]

It is hard to overemphasize the enormity of atherosclerosis as a disease. Cardiovascular disease accounts for more deaths each year than all other causes of death combined. In 1967 (the latest year for which complete figures are available) over 1 million Americans died of cardiovascular disease. Over 50 per cent of these deaths were due to atherosclerotic heart disease. While deaths from hypertensive and rheumatic heart disease have been decreasing over the past 20 years, those attributable to coronary heart disease have not. It has been suggested, in fact, that the mortality from coronary atherosclerosis has reached epidemic proportions.[3] In 1967 there were 573,000 deaths due to coronary heart disease, almost 160,000 of these deaths occurred in subjects under 65. It is estimated that over 4 million Americans have definite evidence of coronary artery disease, 2.1 million in the age group under 65. This *premature* heart disease in the otherwise well, potential wage earners creates a tremendous socioeconomic problem. The total economic impact of atherosclerotic cardiovascular disease, affecting those under 65

years of age, was estimated at a national cost of 17.8 billion dollars for the year 1967.[4]

It has become increasingly evident that further inroads against the excessive morbidity and mortality from coronary heart disease must come from advances made in defining susceptibles in the community, and not in improvements in hospital care.[5] Perhaps this point is best made by noting that over a 14-year period of observations in a sample of persons from Framingham, Massachusetts, 65 per cent of deaths from coronary heart disease before age 65 occurred *outside* the hospital.[6] In 51 per cent of these cases, death occurred suddenly within 1 hour of onset of the terminal event. Moreover, approximately one-third of these cases of sudden death in the community occurred in persons *without prior evidence* of coronary heart disease.

Attention has now focused on defining those habits or traits which are felt to convey an increased "risk" for premature coronary heart disease. The recent report of the Intersociety Commission for Heart Disease Resources has designated hypercholesterolemia, hypertension, and cigarette smoking as major risk factors.[3] Inherent to the risk factor approach is the concept of decreasing risk through appropriate medical intervention. Unfortunately, despite numerous studies it is not yet clear whether modifications of risk factors will substantially reduce coronary heart disease mortality. Intervention trials of better design, employing adequate numbers of patients are clearly needed. Presumptive evidence at this time would suggest, however, *the clinical modification, when possible, of all detected risk factors.*

895

RISK FACTORS

Numerous studies evaluating the prevalence or incidence of atherosclerosis in various populations have been conducted over the past 25 years. They have helped to define apparent biological, demographic and social differences between "normal" and coronary-prone subjects. From these studies have emerged several exogenous and endogenous variables, which may be correlated with an increased risk of developing premature coronary heart disease. Among those factors felt to convey increased risk are elevated blood lipids, cigarette smoking, hypertension, obesity, hyperglycemia (diabetes), sedentary living, psychosocial tensions, and a positive family history of premature atherosclerotic disease.

Environmental Factors

It is theorized that environmental factors are responsible for the findings that the cardiovascular death rate for migrants, particularly men, is, in most cases, closer to the cardiovascular mortality in the U.S. than that of the country of birth.[7]

Diet, cigarette smoking, stress and tension, and patterns of physical activity are influential environmental factors and often confuse the intrepretation of endogenous variables.

Diet. Over the past century, man has become more reluctant to accept deterioration of coronary arteries and subsequent development of atherosclerosis as a necessary accompaniment of the aging process or of his personal being or so-called constitution.

In a search for associated factors from his mode of life, diet became one of the focal points of inquiry. No one could challenge the observations that cholesterol-supplemented animals developed high serum cholesterols, that dietary constituents could and did influence serum lipids, and that these cholesterol elevations were associated with an increased rate of coronary heart disease.

Gradually, the question became not whether diet could be associated with coronary heart disease, but to what extent diet influences the development of coronary heart disease in man. Was diet a preventive measure? Could diet improve deteriorating coronary status? If intensive investigations proved diet change commendable—was it feasible to undertake dietary change in those individuals at predictable risk for coronary heart disease?

Review of the nutritional literature, unfortunately, does not provide answers to all these questions. It is possible to see that diet and atherosclerosis were, from early investigational days, marked by numerous conflicting observations and controversies.

In the early 1900's, investigators[8] demonstrated that by feeding large amounts of cholesterol to rabbits, it was possible to produce arterial lesions similar to those found in human atherosclerosis. These observations were significant at the time and instigated a closer look at the cholesterol picture. The role of diet—specifically the effect of cholesterol feeding on serum cholesterol—was demonstrated in other laboratory animals by several investigators. The accepted concept at that time was that plasma cholesterol was primarily controlled by the cholesterol in the diet.[9] However, the possibility of cholesterol synthesis by the animal body was soon considered. In 1925 evidence[10] was presented that cholesterol is synthesized in the animal organism. Supportive and clarifying data soon followed.[11,12]

Today, it is recognized that in most animals, except primates, the lipoprotein spectrum is different from that of man. Man has more low-density lipoprotein and less high-density lipoprotein (see later section) than laboratory animals such as rats, rabbits, sheep, and dogs, and there appear to be differences in lipid transport functions. Recently a well-controlled study of primates (Rhesus monkey) revealed that atherosclerotic lesions which developed after 17 months of high cholesterol feeding regressed after 40 months of cholesterol-free chow.[13]

Dietary Cholesterol. Dietary studies in man have flourished; unfortunately they have produced much conflicting and often confusing evidence. In the early 1950's, many investigators were contending that dietary cholesterol did not influence serum cholesterol levels. Keys,[14] one of the early opponents of cholesterol restriction, stated that the blood cholesterol was independent of the cholesterol intake over a wide range. Keys argued that the plasma cholesterol concentration will respond to a zero intake of cholesterol—such as the rice diet, but that administration of large doses of cholesterol produces only small and trivial changes in the plasma cholesterol of man. In 1956, Keys reported dietary experiments and population survey findings which he considered "definitive" that cholesterol in the natural diet had no effect, if the other elements in the diet are held constant.[15] At this time, Kinsell[16] and Ahrens[17] were in agreement with this theory.

Recent studies have contributed substantial data indicating that, contrary to previous thought, dietary cholesterol does affect serum cholesterol.[18–20] Connor[21] observed that the effect of a given intake of dietary cholesterol was independent of the fat composition of the diet. Keys et al.[22] repeated these findings. He further suggested that "other things being equal, the serum cholesterol appears to be a linear function of the square root of the cholesterol in the daily diet." It is probable that some of the earlier conflicting data regarding dietary cholesterol were in error, due to the fact that the cholesterol had not been fed in a form suitable for absorption. Cholesterol must be dissolved in or closely associated with other fats in order to be absorbed.[22]

Dietary cholesterol has thus been shown to have an undeniable hypercholesterolemic effect. Furthermore, although it was initially thought that man's maximum daily absorption of dietary cholesterol, despite greatly increased cholesterol loads, could not exceed 300 to 500 mg/day,[23,24] it is now clear that cholesterol absorption is proportional to cholesterol ingestion at all levels of cholesterol intake. Borgstrom[25] has found that absorption of dietary cholesterol is directly related to the dosage given. Quintao et al.[26,27] added supportive data demonstrating that absorption of dietary cholesterol increases with increased intake. Patients fed as much as 3 gm/day absorbed up to 1 gm of cholesterol.

Total Dietary Fat. By the mid-1950's some investigators were labeling the intake of dietary fat—and not cholesterol—as the dietary factor related to coronary heart diseases. Epidemiologic studies were reviewed[28] citing evidence that atherosclerosis varied in different populations and could in many instances be correlated to levels of fat intake. In populations where the fat intake was low there was a low incidence of coronary heart disease, whereas populations having a high-fat intake had a high incidence of coronary heart disease. Similarly, it was shown that diets low in fat led to a highly significant decrease in plasma cholesterol.[29–31] Several studies also reported that adding vegetable fat to the low-fat diets resulted in increases in plasma cholesterol to levels exhibited on a normal mixed diet.[14,29,32]

Polyunsaturated Fatty Acids. In 1952 Kinsell et al.[16] reported that formula diets containing large amounts of vegetable fat produced a major and sustained fall in serum cholesterol while, in contrast, a formula containing the same proportion of animal fat produced cholesterol levels comparable to a normal, mixed diet. This report was initially met with skepticism; however, further studies by Kinsell,[33] Ahrens[17,34] and Beveridge[35] added further collaborative and undeniable evidence, refuting earlier reports that a high-fat diet *per se* is always associated with an increase in serum cholesterol. These new studies showed that the polyunsaturated oils (safflower, corn, cottonseed, for example) produce decreases in serum cholesterol, while isocaloric amounts of the saturated fats (butter, coconut oil, and palm oil) increase levels of serum cholesterol. Keys[36] ultimately concluded that polyunsaturated fatty acids have half the effect per gram on decreasing serum cholesterol concentrations as do saturated fatty acids acting in the opposite direction. The principal polyunsaturates in the diet are linoleic (C_{18}:2) and linolenic (C_{18}:3) which are most abundant in oils of grains, seeds, and nuts. Longer chain, highly unsaturated acids are present in fish oils.

Saturated Fatty Acids. Saturated fat is present in the diet in animal products, such as meat, egg yolk, dairy products, and in certain vegetable products, such as coconut oil and hydrogenated shortenings and margarines. Saturated fatty acids vary in their degree of cholesterol influences. For example, stearic acid (C_{18}) has little or no effect on serum cholesterol,[37–40] while the saturated acids lauric (C_{14}), and palmitic (C_{16}) dramatically increase cholesterol concentrations.[37,38] Since palmitic is more abundant in food than lauric or myristic, it may be the primary fatty acid affecting cholesterol concentrations.[37] Saturated fatty acids containing 10 carbons or less (MCT) have not been shown to have any effect on cholesterol levels.[41,42]

Monounsaturated Fatty Acids. The most abundant monounsaturated fatty acid in the diet is oleic acid (C_{18}:1) which is found in all food fats and is especially high in olive oil. Dietary studies have shown that monounsaturated acids have no effect on serum cholesterol concentrations.[43–45]

Hydrogenated Oils. Hydrogenated oils have been reported to produce higher serum cholesterols than the corresponding unhydrogenated oils.[40,44,45] Oils are treated with hydrogen to increase their stability and to produce the degree of hardness required for shortenings and margarines.

Dietary Carbohydrate. The influence of dietary carbohydrate on the pathogenesis of coronary heart disease has received considerable attention in recent years. It has been shown that carbohydrate influences serum lipids, particularly triglycerides.[46,47] The normal response to a high-carbohydrate diet is an increase in triglycerides by approximately 50 to 100 per cent. In some lipidemic subjects, a high-carbohydrate intake produces more intense lipemia with triglyceride levels increasing by 1,000 mg per cent or more.[48]

The intake of sucrose has attracted particular interest. Yudkin[49] reported a significant positive correlation between the intake of refined sugars and the incidence of coronary heart disease among the populations of various countries. In support of the concept that the consumption of refined sugars is an important factor in coronary heart disease are the reports by Yudkin et al.[50,51] that patients with occlusive vascular disease consume more sugar than control subjects. These results have not been confirmed by other investigators.[52,53]

The possible relationship between the kind of dietary carbohydrate consumed and serum lipid levels has recently been reviewed by McGandy.[54] Several studies cite findings that substitution of the simple sugars for starch results in increased concentrations of serum triglycerides and often in serum cholesterol.[55–59] Others report that, at a level of carbohydrate intake comparable to many western diets, sucrose has only a slight if any effect on serum lipids.[60] McGandy[61] concluded that the effects of dietary carbohydrate on serum lipids are of much smaller magnitude than the effect of dietary fat.

It is clear that the significance of an increased intake of refined sugars on the development of coronary heart disease remains unsettled. The previously cited studies suggest that there is a very individualistic variability in lipid response to carbohydrate feeding. It appears that interchanging different sugars for starch will produce significant change in triglyceride and cholesterol concentrations only in certain individuals.

Diet Trials. Several studies have been conducted to determine whether changing the composition of the diet will affect the atherosclerotic process and the incidence and mortality from coronary heart disease.

In a study of survivors from myocardial infarction, Lyon et al.[62] compared 155 patients receiving a low-fat, low-cholesterol diet with 125 controls. They reported that after a 3- to 4-year period, there were fewer reinfarctions and resulting fatalities in the diet group. Nelson[63] reported a lower mortality in patients with coronary heart disease or cerebrovascular disease who adhered to a low-fat diet than in a comparative control group following no diet. Collecting data from an early diet trial begun in 1946, Morrison[64,65] reports that survivors of myocardial infarction following a low-fat, low-cholesterol diet and a control diet manifested lower serum cholesterol levels and less mortality from atherosclerosis than a control group. Bierenbaum et al.[66] compared male subjects with documented myocardial infarctions following a 30 per cent fat diet, moderately high in polyunsaturated fatty acids with a nondietary-treated coronary group. Results indicate a statistically lower incidence of reinfarction and mortality in the experimental diet group.

These findings have not always been confirmed by other studies. A low-fat diet trial involving 265 men under the age of 65 who had survived a first myocardial infarction was conducted in London from 1957 to 1963.[67] It concluded that a low-fat diet did not improve prognosis.

Rose et al.[68] reported that although serum cholesterol was lowered in patients receiving a low-saturated-fat diet supplemented with corn oil, the incidence of myocardial infarction was unchanged from the control group. Hood et al.,[69] reporting a Swedish trial with patients with essential hypercholesterolemia, found that a low-saturated-fat, low-cholesterol diet with added polyunsaturated oils did not change the total rate of myocardial infarctions between dieters and matched controls; however, mortality rates were 4 times higher in subjects who did not adhere to the diet when compared to those who did. Another study among a group of investigators in London[70] involved testing a diet high in unsaturated fat in male survivors of myocardial infarctions: Here the experimental diet induced some differences in relapse rate but not in mortality rate.

Additional dietary intervention studies dealing with prevention of coronary heart disease have been reported recently.[71-75] The diets in these studies were low in saturated fat and cholesterol with a moderately high intake of polyunsaturated fat. All of these studies have reported a decrease in the incidence of new coronary events in treated as compared with the respective comparison groups.

All of the dietary trials summarized above as well as the National Diet-Heart Feasibility Study 1960–1967[76] show that cholesterol concentrations can be effectively lowered by 8 to 18 per cent with diet. None of the studies has conclusively proven, however, that this cholesterol lowering will prevent or delay coronary heart disease or coronary mortality. Most of the dietary studies can be criticized in terms of study design, observer bias or improper and often "soft" end points.[77] The cost of carrying out an effective dietary trial in the United States today is enormous, requiring a large number of subjects (and paramedical personnel) and prolonged time intervals to gain statistically valid differences in coronary morbidity and mortality.[78] Without such studies, however, arguments for lowering cholesterol through diet in coronary-prone patients remain primarily circumstantial.

Cigarette Smoking. Cigarette smoking is one of the most important exogenous factors which tend to increase incidence of coronary heart disease. Indeed, it has been found that the incidence of myocardial infarction is 3 times greater and death from coronary heart disease 5 times greater in smokers than in nonsmokers.[79] There are those, however, who feel that cigarette smoking has no cumulative or permanent effect on the development of coronary heart disease.[79-82] Other data indicate that cigarette smoking has a cumulative effect and that the coronary disease risk for ex-smokers does not revert as quickly to nonsmoker levels as was once emphasized.[83] There is general agreement in these studies that risk is proportionate to the number of cigarettes smoked and that pipe and cigar smokers (qualified by Kahn[83] to 4/day) suffer no greater mortality than nonsmokers.

Psychological and Social Findings. A recent review[84] cited findings from over 160 papers, the majority of which report a relationship between coronary heart disease and such psychological or social variables as education, religion, income, occupation, social mobility, personality traits, and the like.

There seems to be a clinical impression that stress is associated with sudden death and probably development of coronary heart disease.[85] However, the Framingham study reported that some aspects of stressful living such as extremes of family size, marital stress, degree of affluence, and heavy consumption of coffee and tea (indirect measurement of stress) were not associated with increased risk of coronary heart disease.[82]

Physical activity is one of the variables which has been studied within occupational groups, thereby minimizing possible effects of socioeconomic variations. Data collected in these studies[86-88] support the hypothesis that men in the more sedentary occupations have more fatalities from coronary heart disease than men in occupations requiring at least moderate activity. The Framingham study revealed that the more sedentary individuals developed an excess of lethal attacks; however, not of angina pectoris (arm and chest pain produced by effort and secondary to insufficient coronary blood flow). Physical activity also was related to ability to survive an attack.[82] The thought has been expressed that activity improves collateral coronary circulation,[82] but it is also hypothesized that the sedentary individual may choose less exercise due to general poor health.[75] Epidemiologists have pointed out that methodological inadequacies of many psychosocial studies impair interpretation as to absolute correlation with coronary heart disease.[82]

Endogenous Factors

Endogenous factors, perhaps by being more readily stratified, have been extensively studied, and the presence of hypertension, hyperlipidemia, obesity, and diabetes is generally accepted as an index for increased susceptibility to coronary heart disease. Other determinants such as age, electrocardiographic abnormalities, increased uric acid levels and a positive family history also have associations of varying significance with increased atherogenesis.

Hypertension. Hypertension has been correlated with both an increased rate of new myocardial infarction and sudden death.[89] A positive correlation has been established between coronary heart disease and elevations in both systolic and diastolic blood pressures.[82,90]

The Framingham study reported a 2.6-fold increase in risk in hypertensive men, ages 40 to 59, and a 6-fold increase in hypertensive women of the same age.[91] Another study reported that hypertensives 60 to 70 years of age had an increased rate of angina pectoris.[92] Seasonal variations in blood pressure[90] have been documented and should be recognized in interpretation of long-term epidemiologic studies.

Diabetes Mellitus. The association of diabetes mellitus and increased incidence of coronary heart disease has long been recognized. The person with diabetes is reported to have a coronary heart disease occurrence rate 2 times that found in normals[89] and diabetics are noted to be more susceptible to a lethal outcome.[82] In a large industrial population[93] the risk of myocardial infarction in diabetic men, ages 25 to 64, was 2.55 times

higher than in nondiabetics. For the individual with diabetes who survives the initial myocardial infarction, long-term prognosis after myocardial infarction is poor. Statistics relate 5-year post-heart-attack survival rates for diabetics that are significantly below those of nondiabetics.[94]

An impaired glucose tolerance, even in the absence of overt diabetes, has been associated with coronary heart disease.[95] Epstein[96] reviews data suggesting that hyperglycemia, expressed not only as diabetes mellitus, but also in lesser degrees of glucose tolerance, should be recognized as a predictive indication of coronary heart disease. The Tecumseh study[97,98] found a greater prevalence of coronary heart disease when hyperglycemia was present than when glucose tolerance was normal; this finding was independent of blood pressure and blood cholesterol levels.

Obesity. Morbidity and mortality are significantly higher in the overweight when compared to those of normal weight, with the death rate from heart and circulatory disorders at least 1.5 times that of non-overweight subjects.[99] In the Framingham study,[82] obesity was associated with increased risk of angina pectoris and sudden death but not of myocardial infarction. Data from the Tecumseh population[97] support this evidence, concluding that relative weight has an effect on incidence of coronary heart disease that is independent of blood pressure and blood sugar levels.

Obesity is often associated with diabetes, hyperlipidemia, and hypertension. There is no doubt that obesity increases coronary heart disease risk in subjects with hypertension, diabetes, or hypercholesterolemia. Certain data[92,99,100] indicate that the relationship of coronary heart disease and obesity has no statistical significance, when the association with the previously mentioned risk factors are discounted.

Positive Family History. Serum lipid levels, blood pressure, and blood sugar levels are under both genetic control and environmental influences. Coronary heart disease apparently occurs in families. The question is whether this is because of the genetic variables mentioned above or due to other possible genetic mutations. Disagreement on interpretation of data arises when exogenous factors such as diet, smoking and other family habits are not satisfactorily excluded.[101]

Although there is no cogent proof that coronary heart disease is itself familial, there is evidence that coronary heart disease tends to aggregate among blood relatives.[102] Epstein[103] reviews data that the coronary heart disease pattern is family clustered, but reports this trend is largely confined to the younger age groups. Further evidence collected in the Tecumseh, Michigan study[104] revealed fatal coronary heart disease to be commonest in those individuals whose parents died of coronary heart disease before age 65 and fatal coronary heart disease to be rarer when parental death was due to other causes.

Electrocardiographic Abnormalities. Certain electrocardiographic abnormalities, in particular left ventricular hypertrophy (LVH) and intraventricular block (IVB), have an association with increased morbidity to coronary heart disease.[82] A definite ECG-LVH finding is correlated with a 3-fold increase of coronary heart disease after adjustment for the effect of coexisting hypertension.[105]

Other Factors, Multiplicity of Risk Factors and Age. Other factors associated with increased risk of coronary heart disease, but yet in need of supportive data, are hemoglobin levels exceeding 17 gm,[100] elevated uric acid levels, rapid pulse at rest, and low vital capacity.[82]

The effect of any given risk factor or combination of factors increases with age, signifying that *age* itself must be considered a factor of risk in the forecast of coronary heart disease. This trend is reflected in the study of eight periodic health examination programs[105] where the incidence rate per 1,000 man-years was 2.1 at age 30 to 39, increased to 8.1 at ages 40 to 41 and 17.4 at age 50 to 59. Furthermore, those individuals having multiple risk factors are especially prone to the development of coronary heart disease— *the risk being proportional to the number of factors found.* The *additive* effect of risk factors is evident in all the studies and aptly summarized in the Framingham report.[82] The individual who had any one of three risk factors (hypercholesterolemia, hypertension,

or cigarette smoking) had a risk 1.5 times that of a man having none of these factors. The presence of two factors increased the risk to approximately 3 times normal and the combination of three factors was associated with an 8 times greater risk than a man at the same age[30,59] having no risk factors.

HYPERLIPIDEMIA

Hypercholesterolemia, the most extensively measured lipid, is strongly associated with coronary heart disease. The degree of risk rises in proportion to the concentration of cholesterol,[82,92] the effect of cholesterol being greatest at younger ages,[100] and usually manifested by myocardial infarction rather than angina pectoris[92] with the risk gradient remaining even when adjustment is made for other factors related to coronary heart disease risk and to blood lipids.[106]

Hypertriglyceridemia has also been associated with increased prevalence of coronary heart disease.[107,108] The problems relating to accurate measurement of triglyceride levels and the frequent association of hypertriglyceridemia with hypercholesterolemia have presented difficulties in the clear identification of hypertriglyceridemia alone as an indication of susceptibility to premature coronary heart disease.

Neither cholesterol or triglyceride circulates in solution in free form. All of the blood lipids (cholesterol, phospholipid, triglyceride) circulate bound to specific proteins. These proteins (lipoproteins) serve to solubilize the otherwise insoluble lipid and transport them into and out of the plasma. Serum lipoprotein determinations were proposed as predictors of coronary heart disease in the early 1950's.[109,110] However, it was argued that a simple cholesterol determination was as useful as the more difficult lipoprotein measurements in determining those at risk.[111] In time we have learned that although cholesterol may provide an easily measured indication of those persons "at risk," *it fails to provide* the clinical insight needed for useful patient management. It is now clear that cholesterol or triglyceride measurements are non-specific, and that hypercholesterolemia is just a sign of a heterogenous group of dis-

orders differing in clinical signs, prognosis
and responsiveness to therapy. Some subjects with hypercholesterolemia, in fact, are
not at all at risk for coronary heart disease.[112]

Visualization of hyperlipidemia in terms
of the vehicles of lipid transport—the lipoproteins—allows one to apply more specificity
and definition to the study and understanding of lipid transport and its disorders.[113] Hypercholesterolemia or hypertriglyceridemia
must be translated into hyperlipoproteinemia

if specific risk of coronary heart disease is to
be defined. Only by separating the hyperlipidemias metabolically in terms of specific
lipoprotein aberrations can one offer a patient
effective diagnosis and treatment.[112]

Classification of Lipoproteins[113]

There are four major lipoprotein families
normally found in the plasma (Fig. 31-1).
The various techniques for separating and

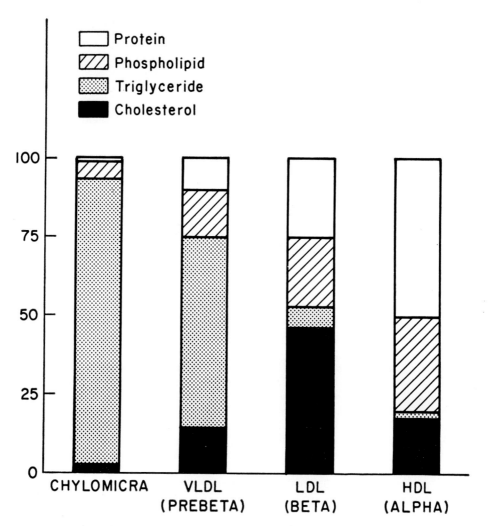

APPROXIMATE % COMPOSITION OF LIPOPROTEINS

Fig. 31-1. Schematic representation of the four lipoprotein families as defined by paper electrophoresis and
analytical ultracentrifugation. (Courtesy of J. Am. Dietet. Assoc., *58*, 406, 1971.)

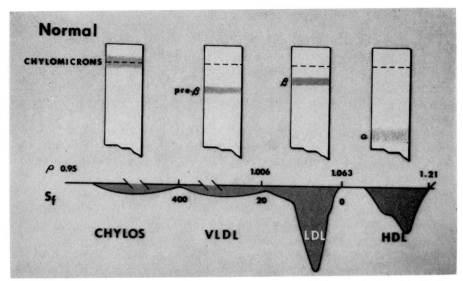

Fig. 31-2. Representation of approximate percentage of lipoproteins. (Courtesy of Progress in Cardiovascular Disease, *14*, 341, 1972.)

classifying them are based on either electrophoresis or ultracentrifugation. The lipid-containing proteins are lighter and less dense than other proteins; the ultracentrifuge may therefore be used to separate sequentially chylomicrons, very-low-density lipoproteins (VLDL), low-density lipoproteins (LDL), and high-density lipoproteins (HDL). A comparatively simple and inexpensive technique employing electrophoresis on paper or agarose gel allows separation of the lipoproteins, according to their charge. The classes thus defined are a nonmigrating, a beta-migrating, a prebeta-migrating, and an alpha-migrating lipoprotein.[114] These two systems of nomenclature are, fortunately, essentially exchangeable. The lipid-rich particles remaining at the electrophoretic origin correspond to the centrifugally defined chylomicrons, the beta-migrating lipoprotein fraction with LDL, prebeta with VLDL, and alpha with HDL (Fig. 31-2). Each of the lipoprotein families defined by these techniques contains—in varying proportions—cholesterol, phospholipid, triglyceride, and protein (Fig. 31-1).

Chylomicrons, the largest of the lipoproteins, consist chiefly of triglycerides (80 to 95 per cent), with lesser amounts of cholesterol (2 to 7 per cent), phospholipid (3 to 6 per cent), and protein (0.5 to 1 per cent).

They are synthesized in the intestine and serve to transport dietary glycerides from the intestinal mucosa via the thoracic duct into the plasma and ultimately to sites of utilization in the tissues. It is presumed that the majority of the glyceride is removed from chylomicrons by heparin-activated lipoprotein lipase, a collective group of enzymes located in the adipose tissue, heart, and skeletal muscle. Chylomicron remnants are then completely removed by the liver[115] (Fig. 31-3). Chylomicrons can be detected by their adherence to the electrophoretic origin on paper or agarose gel or perhaps most simply by the presence or absence of a "cream layer" over plasma stored at 4° C. Chylomicrons are cleared rapidly from the plasma (6 to 12 hours) after a fatty meal. Therefore, the presence of chylomicrons (observable as a cream layer) in fasting plasma 12 to 14 hours after a meal is abnormal and indicates defective handling of dietary fats.[116]

VLDL, the next smallest and lightest of the lipoproteins, are also composed predominately of triglyceride (60 to 80 percent). The remaining composition being cholesterol (5 to 13 per cent), phospholipid (5 to 18 per cent), and protein (5 to 15 per cent). In contrast to the chylomicrons, VLDL transports triglyceride primarily of hepatic origin;

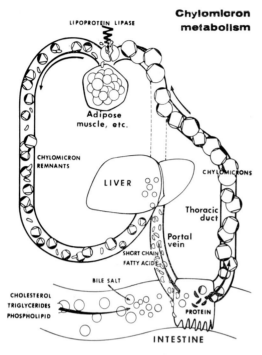

Chylomicron metabolism

Fig. 31-3. Schematic view of the metabolism and transport of chylomicrons (dietary fat). For explanation see text.

synthesized from various precursors such as fatty acid and carbohydrates. The clearance of VLDL involves removal of triglyceride and conversion into smaller, more soluble lipoproteins. Lipoprotein lipase appears to play a significant role in this metabolic sequence.[116]

A small amount of VLDL is normally present in fasting plasma. VLDL in increased concentrations may produce turbid plasma, but no cream layer. In the absence of chylomicrons, increased levels of VLDL correlate directly with increased plasma levels of triglyceride.

LDL by weight is approximately 25 per cent protein and 45 per cent cholesterol. It normally carries from one-half to two-thirds of the total plasma cholesterol. The high-cholesterol content and smaller size of LDL may account for its greater atherogenic potential as compared to VLDL and chylomicrons. LDL appears to be derived in part, if not completely, from the intravascular breakdown of VLDL.[117] At present, its

exact function is unknown. LDL does not produce turbidity, even when present in greatly increased concentrations.

HDL, the fourth and smallest of the lipoprotein species, contains 45 to 50 per cent protein, 30 per cent phospholipid, and 20 per cent cholesterol. Neither it nor LDL carries much glyceride. There is some evidence that HDL serves to stabilize VLDL and is involved in transporting cholesterol and other lipids from plasma back into the tissues.[118]

Physiology of Lipid Transport[113,116,118,119]

Present-day concepts consider the lipoprotein moiety (protein, cholesterol, and phospholipid) as the vehicle for the transport of glyceride, a neutral fat with a turnover rate of 100 to 150 gm per day. Kinetic studies demonstrate that the turnover of phospholipid and cholesterol is quite slow—both less than 1 to 2 gm a day. On a normal diet, from 70 to 150 gm of glyceride enter from the intestine each day and are cleared by the periphery; an additional 10 to 50 gm glyceride can enter each day from the liver. In any state in which too much triglyceride is mobilized from the liver or intestine or too little cleared, glyceride-rich lipoprotein accumulates in the plasma. Thus, a major determinant of plasma lipoprotein levels is the demand for glyceride transport.

Exogenous glyceride transport is relatively easy to visualize (Fig. 31–3). The fat ingested is broken down into smaller fragments by the bile acids, acting as detergents, and the enzymes, esterases and lipases, in the intestine and pancreatic juices. The absorbed fat is then esterified and joins with protein in the cells of the intestine to form chylomicrons which enter the blood stream via the lymphatics. A small amount of fatty acids of C_{10} length or less enters the circulation directly via the portal system.

Exogenous hypertriglyceridemia can occur because of an increased intake of glyceride or because of inadequate peripheral clearance. Exogenous hyperlipemia is a daily phenomenon. Associated with each meal we consume, there is a tide of exogenous glyceride or chylomicrons. Following a standard 100 gm fat meal in a normal person, chylomicrons will appear (triglycerides and cholesterol increase) and reach a peak after approximately 4 hours. In the normal subject, the chylomicrons will be cleared approximately 8 to 12 hours after the last meal. This exogenous triglyceride, then, is an important factor to be aware of in evaluating patients. In testing an individual for a lipid transport disorder, the blood sample should be taken approximately 12 to 16 hours after the last meal, when the normal chylomicron tide will have cleared.

Endogenous hyperglyceridemia is more difficult to visualize. The liver synthesizes glycerides *de novo* from carbohydrate entering from the intestine, from fatty acid mobilized from adipose tissue, and from a number of different two-carbon sources (Fig. 31–4). If the liver is synthesizing glyceride at too rapid a rate, or if it is not being cleared, endogenous glyceride (prebeta lipoprotein, VLDL) will accumulate in the plasma. Endogenous hyperglyceridemia is a common phenomenon. It can be produced in normals by a high-carbohydrate diet. Although carbohydrate ingestion is accompanied by an increase in triglycerides as a normal phe-

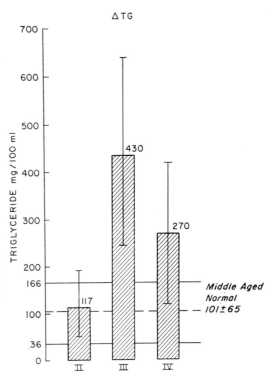

Fig. 31-5. Triglyceride response in different types of hyperlipoproteinemia to a diet high in carbohydrate (greater than 7 gm carbohydrate per kg per day). Values are expressed as increments in triglycerides above the baseline level (Δ triglycerides). (Courtesy of Diabetes, *18*, 739, 1960.)

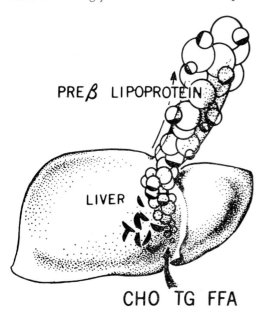

Fig. 31-4. Schematic view of endogenous glyceride production in the liver. (Courtesy of J. Am. Dietet. Assoc., *58*, 406, 1971.)

nomenon, some patients demonstrate increased sensitivity to carbohydrate, which may result in higher and persistently elevated triglyceride levels (Fig. 31–5).

Both exogenous and endogenous glycerides must be cleared from the plasma. This occurs predominantly in the liver, adipose tissue, and muscle where the glycerides are stored or metabolized. At these sites of glyceride clearance, lipoprotein lipase is probably active in the breakdown of the large glyceride-containing moieties into smaller, more soluble lipoproteins and fatty acids. The adipose cell, the storage vat for fat, does not have the capacity for synthesizing lipoprotein. Therefore, glyceride cannot be released into the plasma. Rather, the only lipid leaving the adipose cell is fatty acid, which produces glyceridemia only secondarily; the fatty acid returns to the liver and then stimulates endogenous glyceride release. Thus, hyperglyceridemia can occur because of too much glyceride entering from the intestine, too much glyceride production by the liver, or too little glyceride clearance by the periphery.

A much less dynamic but important factor in controlling the plasma levels of lipoprotein is the state of cholesterol balance. The average American eats too much cholesterol. There are two sources of plasma cholesterol—the exogenous cholesterol, *i.e.*, the cholesterol in the diet, and the cholesterol made *de novo* predominantly in the liver and intestine.[120] Cholesterol entering from the intestine seems to exert a negative feedback and inhibits the cholesterol production in the liver. If the exogenous load of cholesterol is decreased, the liver will synthesize more cholesterol. Fortunately, or unfortunately, for the average American, if less cholesterol is consumed (less than 300 mg/day), plasma cholesterol will fall considerably despite the increase in endogenous cholesterol synthesis. Bile acids are the major degradation products of cholesterol. Much of the bile acids is reabsorbed and constantly recycled in what is called the enterohepatic cycle (Fig. 31–6).

Other determinants, which are more difficult to measure but which play a significant role in controlling the concentration of lipoproteins in the plasma, include the availability of carbohydrates and proteins and the action of a number of hormones, including insulin, thyroxin, glucagon, epinephrine, and adrenal and pituitary factors. These hormones act primarily by increasing or decreasing lipogenesis and/or lipolysis in the liver and adipose tissue. Insulin tends to maintain glyceride in adipose tissue. A number of hormones, *e.g.* epinephrine, the catecholamines, and glucagon, influence the breakdown of glyceride in adipose tissue, resulting in their release as fatty acids into the plasma, thereby giving rise to a secondary form of endogenous hyperlipemia. Other factors even more difficult to measure are involved in controlling lipoprotein concentrations. Age is a factor not really understood; it is known that in Americans the levels of all the lipids and lipoproteins increase with age. What is considered abnormal for a 20-year-old does not necessarily hold for a 50-year-old person.

Emotion and stress can both affect plasma lipid concentrations, and this is important

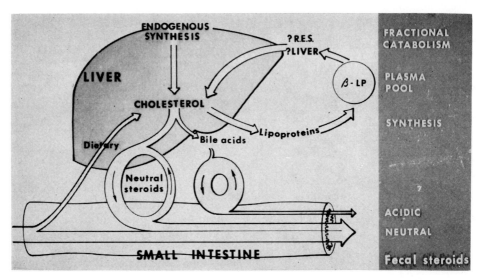

Fig. 31-6. Schematic view of the dynamics of hepatic cholesterol metabolism. Liver cholesterol comes from three sources: endogenous synthesis, lipoprotein catabolism and the diet. Hepatic cholesterol leaves the liver via the blood stream on lipoproteins and via the biliary tree as neutral and acidic sterols. As shown here the acidic and neutral sterols constantly recirculate between the liver and intestine in what is known as "the enterohepatic cycle."

to keep in mind when evaluating the efficacy of a drug or diet. The importance of sampling an individual in a steady state cannot be overemphasized. After a heart attack, for example, triglycerides usually increase and plasma cholesterol concentrations often decrease markedly. One must sample an individual either before or 4 or more weeks after a heart attack to know whether he has a lipid transport abnormality.[121]

Classification of Hyperlipoproteinemia[113,116]

Lipoprotein concentrations are controlled by many different metabolic and genetic factors. Thus, hypercholesterolemia may be due to many different abnormalities. At present, five lipoprotein patterns or types have been delineated in the hyperlipoproteinemias (Table 31–1). Each is classified in terms of the abnormal accumulation in plasma of one or more lipoprotein species. No lipoprotein pattern or type is unique. Each may result from a primary, inherited disorder or may be secondary to other pathologic states with a variety of different mechanisms responsible for the hyperlipoproteinemia.

Type I. This lipoprotein pattern is indicative of an inability to clear dietary fat (chylomicrons). It is nearly always familial, and in its severe form is a rare disorder. The patients are usually young and have creamy plasma, lipemia retinalis, hepatosplenomegaly, eruptive xanthomas, and bouts of abdominal pain associated with ingestion of dietary fats. After standing in the cold a discrete cream layer forms in the plasma of these patients. Plasma cholesterols may be normal or elevated; triglyceride concentrations are grossly elevated (often above 5,000 mg per cent). The familial disorder is recessively transmitted and is characterized by a deficiency in one or more of the enzymes involved in the clearance of fat from the circulation.

Type II (Hyperbetalipoproteinemia). This is a common pattern found at all ages. It is characterized by a marked increase in otherwise normal beta lipoproteins (LDL). Though the plasma is almost always clear, cholesterol levels are often in the 300 to 600 mg per cent range with normal or only modestly elevated

plasma triglycerides. Type II patients may have xanthelasma, arcus juvenilis, and tendon and tuberous xanthomas. Of note is the associated premature coronary artery disease and the often striking family history of early death. This makes it important for all physicians to recognize that the Type II abnormality is often familial and is transmitted as a dominant trait with essentially complete penetrance. Secondary causes of the Type II pattern such as excessive dietary cholesterol intake, myxedema, myeloma, liver disease or nephrosis can be quickly evaluated. When secondary causes have been ruled out, a Type II patient's family should be screened because the patient's mother or father and 50 per cent of the patient's siblings and children (diagnosable as early as age 1) will have hyperbetalipoproteinemia. Therapy for all of the secondary hyperlipoproteinemias should be directed at the acquired problem, i.e., thyroid replacement for myxedema. When this is not possible or when the disorder is primary, specific therapy should be directed at the hyperlipoproteinemia.

Type III. This is a relatively uncommon pattern associated with the presence in the plasma of abnormal betalipoprotein forms. Patients may have clear, cloudy, or milky plasma with elevations of both cholesterol and triglyceride concentrations into the 350 to 800 mg per cent range. These patients often present in the third or fourth decade of life with planar xanthomas (orange-yellow lipid deposits in the creases of the palms of the hands) as well as tuberoeruptive (elbow, knees, and buttocks) and tendon xanthomas. Commonly, both premature coronary and peripheral arterial disease occurs. This type is usually familial and is apparently transmitted as a recessive trait.

Type IV. This is a very common lipoprotein pattern, most frequently seen after the second decade of life and often associated with diabetes mellitus and premature atherosclerosis. It is characterized by an isolated increase in endogenous triglyceride (prebetalipoproteins or VLDL). The plasma may be clear, cloudy, or milky depending upon the triglyceride concentration. Cholesterol levels are frequently normal. The patients usually have no external stigmata.

The pattern sometimes reflects a familial disorder transmitted as a dominant trait with delayed expression. It may be that several different mutations are responsible. It is often, however, secondary to other metabolic disorders, stress, or alcohol, and whether primary or secondary is usually exacerbated by obesity.

Type V. This is frequently seen secondary to acute metabolic disorders like diabetic acidosis, pancreatitis, alcoholism, and nephrosis but may be familial. The patients usually become symptomatic after age 20 and may have all the features of Type I: creamy plasma, hepatosplenomegaly, and bouts of abdominal pain often with frank pancreatitis. They often have multiple abdominal scars after years of occult abdominal pain. They appear to be intolerant to both dietary and endogenous fat and have triglycerides in the 1,000 to 6,000 mg per cent range with mildly to markedly elevated plasma cholesterols on an unrestricted diet. Abnormal glucose tolerance and hyperuricemia are frequently associated.

Although hyperlipidemia is present in all five types of hyperlipoproteinemia, *only* three are associated with premature atherosclerotic heart disease. These are the types designated as Types II, III and IV.[122]

Screening for Hyperlipoproteinemia

Observations of the plasma may be used as a first step in screening for an abnormal lipoprotein pattern. A floating "cream" layer in a plasma sample which has been refrigerated overnight at 4° C identifies the presence of chylomicrons. This observation suggests either a non-fasting subject or an abnormality worthy of further investigation. A turbid infranate is caused by increased concentrations of VLDL. A clear infranate may contain elevated concentrations of LDL, since these molecules are small, completely soluble and do not refract light. Using these guidelines, a cream layer plus a clear infranate suggest a Type I pattern. Turbid plasma without evidence of chylomicrons indicates Types III and IV. In Type III one may often notice a scant cream layer of chylomicrons. In Type II, the plasma may be clear or slightly turbid if VLDL is elevated in addition to LDL.

The combination of cholesterol and triglyceride determination will detect hyperlipoproteinemia in most cases.[123] Increases in cholesterol concentrations generally reflect either increased LDL or VLDL or both. Increases in plasma glycerides indicate increased VLDL or chylomicrons (Fig. 31–2). These determinations coupled with the observation of the plasma standing overnight at 4° C should always be done in the laboratory approach to hyperlipoproteinemia and may obviate more expensive, time-consuming procedures.

Normal values of plasma lipid and lipoprotein concentrations are listed in Table 31–2. Normal values are at best arbitrary. Lower values may be more desirable—especially in considering cholesterol as a factor of heart disease risk where, in appropriate individuals, values above 220 mg per cent are associated with increasing risk.[124]

Diagnosis and Treatment of Hyperlipoproteinemia: *Types I and V* (Table 31–3). Types I and V are disorders characterized by a fat-induced hyperlipidemia due to the inability to dispose of triglyceride of exogenous origin. In Type I, this is due to the absence of lipoprotein lipase activity. The cause of the defect in Type V is still unclear. Both are associated with episodic abdominal pain, often secondary to pancreatitis and hepatosplenomegaly. A later age of onset, abnormal glucose tolerance, hyperuricemia, and an exaggerated response in VLDL to dietary carbohydrate clinically distinguish patients with Type V from those with Type I. Despite enormous elevations in plasma lipid levels, patients with Types I and V show no propensity for premature coronary heart disease.[116]

Type I. *Diet Therapy.*[125] This has the objective of reducing dietary fat to a level where the patient becomes asymptomatic and free of abdominal pain. The diet for Type I is extremely low in fat (25 to 35 gm) and is dry, unpalatable and lacks satiety value. All separable fats and oils are eliminated. The major source of dietary fat is lean trimmed meat. The meat is restricted to 5 ounces per day and contributes approximately 15 gm of fat. The fat in the basic diet (from skim milk,

Table 31-1. The Five Types of Primary Hyperlipoproteinemia

Features	Type I	Type II	Type III	Type IV	Type V
Incidence	Very rare	Common	Relatively uncommon	Common	Uncommon
Appearance of plasma	Cream layer over clear infranate on standing	Clear	Clear, cloudy or milky	Slightly turbid to cloudy, unchanged with standing	Cream layer over turbid infranate on standing
Cholesterol	Normal or elevated	Elevated	Elevated	Normal or elevated	Elevated or normal
Triglyceride	Markedly elevated	Normal or slightly elevated	Usually elevated	Elevated	Elevated to markedly elevated
Clinical presentation	Eruptive xanthomas, hepatosplenomegaly, abdominal pain, lipemia retinalis	Xanthelasma, tendon and tuberous xanthomas, juvenile corneal arcus, accelerated atherosclerosis	Xanthoma planum; tuberoeruptive and tendon xanthomas; accelerated atherosclerosis of coronary and peripheral vessels	Accelerated coronary vessel disease, abnormal glucose tolerance, hyperuricemia	Eruptive xanthomas, hepatosplenomegaly, abdominal pain, hyperglycemia, hyperuricemia, lipemia retinalis
Origin; possible mechanism	Genetic recessive; deficiency in lipoprotein lipase	When genetic, dominant, sporadic; decreased catabolism of betalipoprotein	Genetic mode of transmission unclear; sporadic	When genetic, dominant, sporadic; excessive endogenous glyceride synthesis or deficient glyceride clearance?	Probably genetic, dominant, sporadic
Age of detection	Early childhood	Early childhood (in severe cases)	Adulthood (over age 20)	Adulthood	Early adulthood
Conditions to be excluded	Dysgammaglobulinemia, insulinopenic diabetes	*Dietary* cholesterol *excess*, myxedema, myeloma, nephrosis, porphyria, obstructive liver disease	Myxedema, dysgammaglobulinemia	*Diabetes*, glycogen storage disease, nephrotic syndrome, pregnancy, Werner's syndrome	*Diabetic acidosis*, nephrosis, *alcoholism*, *pancreatitis*, myeloma, dysproteinemias

Table 31-2. Plasma Lipid and Lipoprotein Cholesterol Concentrations:
"Normal Limits" Based on Washington Area Population Sample.[116]

Age of Subjects	Plasma Cholesterol mg%	Very-Low-Density Lipoproteins mg%	Low-Density Lipoproteins mg%	High-Density Lipoproteins		Plasma Triglyceride mg%
				mg%	mg%	
Newborn				M	F	
"Cord Blood"	50–95	0–15	20–45	30–55	30–55	10–65
1–9 yrs.	120–230	5–25	50–170	30–65	30–65	10–140
10–19	120–230	5–25	50–170	30–65	30–70	10–140
20–29	120–240	5–25	60–170	35–70	35–75	10–140
30–39	140–270	5–35	70–190	30–65	35–80	10–150
40–49	150–310	5–35	80–190	30–65	40–85	10–160
50–59	160–330	10–40	80–210	30–65	35–85	10–190

"Normal limits," as defined here, are not necessarily "safe" or "acceptable" limits.

The "normal" ranges exhibited by this population sample do not necessarily hold for other countries or even for other regions of the United States.

bread, cereals, and so on) contributes an additional 10 to 20 gm. Individuals may have difficulty following this regimen and maintaining weight, particularly when energy requirements are high. It has been observed that dietary adherence is usually related to the severity of the bouts of abdominal pain which the patient experiences with ingestion of fat.

Informing the patient regarding cooking with herbs, wine, and other seasonings is helpful. The flavor of many meats and vegetables is enhanced by marinating with such items as bouillon, tomato juice, and vinegar. Wrapping meat with aluminum foil helps retain moisture during cooking. To make the diet more palatable, an oil-containing medium-chain triglyceride (MCT) may be prescribed. The use of MCT permits a fat intake without chylomicron formation, since the medium-chain fatty acids are transported directly via the portal system to the liver (Fig. 31–3). If MCT is prescribed, caloric requirements are more easily achieved, cooking methods and menu items are not as limited, and the patient's acceptance of the diet is better.

Diet in Children. Since this disorder may manifest itself in the first year of life, diet therapy for the infant and child is important. After the diagnosis has been established, a very-low-fat formula may be used as a maintenance diet for small infants.

The composition of the suggested maintenance formula is: fat 14 per cent of the calories, protein 16 per cent of the calories, and carbohydrate 70 per cent of the calories. Skim milk—2½ cups; whole milk—½ cup; corn syrup—5 tablespoons; vegetable oil—1 teaspoon; vitamin supplements (including A and E).

Add about 1 cup of water or bring up to a total volume of 1 quart. Beat the mixture with an egg beater or use a food blender. The oil may separate somewhat on standing. Shake the bottle to mix formula before feeding. This provides: kcal/quart–633; kcal/ounce = 20; composition/100 ml of formula: protein, 2.7 gm; fat, 1.0 gm; carbohydrate, 11.5 gm.

A low-fat powder mixture and a powdered formula with MCT are also available commercially.

As the infant's food consumption is increased with solid food, the fat in the formula should be lowered proportionally. The diet recommended for the child with Type I is restricted to 10 to 15 gm of fat per day. In practical terms this is proportionally the same restriction as recommended for adults. Obviously this diet varies from the diet of the average American child. Such foods as hot

Table 31-3. Therapy for Hyperlipoproteinemia

Factor	Type I	Type II	Type III	Type IV	Type V
Dietary prescription	low-fat, 25–35 gm.	low-cholesterol, polyunsaturated fat increased	low-cholesterol; approximately: 20% calories protein, 40% calories fat, 40% calories carbohydrate	controlled carbohydrate (approximately 40% calories); moderately restricted cholesterol	restricted-fat (30% calories); controlled carbohydrate (50% calories); moderately restricted cholesterol
Calories	not restricted	not restricted	achieve and maintain "ideal" weight, i.e., reducing diet if necessary	achieve and maintain "ideal" weight, i.e., reducing diet if necessary	achieve and maintain "ideal" weight, i.e., reducing diet if necessary
Protein	total protein intake not limited	total protein intake not limited	high protein	not limited other than control of patient's weight	high protein
Fat	restricted to 25–35 gm.; kind of fat not important	saturated fat intake limited; polyunsaturated intake increased	controlled to 40% calories (polyunsaturated fats recommended in preference to saturated fats)	not limited other than control of patient's weight (polyunsaturated fats recommended in preference to saturated fats)	restricted to 30% calories (polyunsaturated fats recommended in preference to saturated fats)
Cholesterol	not restricted	less than 300 mg, or as low as possible; only source of cholesterol is meat	less than 300 mg.; only source of cholesterol is meat	moderately restricted to 300–500 mg.	moderately restricted to 300–500 mg.
Carbohydrate	not restricted	not restricted	controlled; most concentrated sweets eliminated	controlled; most concentrated sweets eliminated	controlled; most concentrated sweets eliminated
Alcohol	not recommended	may be used with discretion	limited to 2 servings (substituted for carbohydrate)	limited to 2 servings (substituted for carbohydrate)	not recommended
Current drug therapy	none effective at present	1. cholestyramine 16–32 gm/day 2. D-Thyroxine 3–8 mg/day 3. Nicotinic acid	1. Clofibrate 2 gm/day 2. Nicotinic acid 3–6 gm/day 3. D-Thyroxine	1. Clofibrate 2 gm/day 2. Nicotinic acid 3–6 gm/day	1. Nicotinic acid 3–6 gm/day 2. Clofibrate

dogs, cheese, ice cream are excluded with lean meats and skim milk being substituted. This is a difficult diet to make palatable and satisfying. The use of MCT provides a means to more interesting food preparation.

Drug Therapy. None of the presently available hypolipidemic drugs has any sustained effect on this type of hyperlipoproteinemia.

Type V. *Diet Therapy.*[125] The first objective is achieving and maintaining ideal weight. The maintenance diet is planned to avoid excesses of fat or carbohydrate. The caloric distribution is 25 to 30 per cent modified fat (lower in saturates and higher in polyunsaturates), 50 per cent carbohydrate and 20 to 25 per cent protein. Most concentrated sweets are eliminated, and alcohol is not recommended. The dietary plan is rigid and is similar in form and food groups to the familiar diabetic diet plans.[126] Cholesterol intake is restricted to 300 to 500 mg.

Both fat and carbohydrate may contribute to increased triglycerides in the patient with Type V. It is impractical, however, to restrict both fat and carbohydrate in the diet. Since these patients have bouts of abdominal pain after consuming increased amounts of dietary fats, fat rather than carbohydrate is reduced. If pain persists or recurs, it may be necessary for the patient to temporarily follow the Type I very-low-fat diet.

Drug Therapy. Nicotinic acid (3 to 6 gm/day) is the most effective drug and may be added to the diet for maintenance therapy.[112]

Diagnosis and Treatment of Hyperlipoproteinemia: Types II, III and IV

These appear to be associated with an increased risk of coronary heart disease; although the degree of risk, modes of inheritance, age of detection, and responsiveness to therapy vary[116] (Tables 31–1 and 31–3).

Type II. Familial Type II hyperlipoproteinemia is inherited as a highly penetrant, autosomal dominant trait. Early expression of the genotype makes the diagnosis possible in childhood and even at birth on samples of umbilical cord blood. Incidence studies suggest that Type II may occur in 1 of every 150 to 200 live births.[127] Cholesterol concentrations above 230 mg per cent in any

patient below age 20 should make one suspect this disorder.[128] In patients under 20 with a family history of premature coronary heart disease, screening for hyperlipoproteinemia is mandatory. Heterozygotes for the disorder demonstrate (1) increased concentrations of LDL based on age-corrected norms, and (2) a first-degree relative with hyperlipoproteinemia, or (3) tendon xanthomas.

In the familial disorder, increased quantities of LDL accumulate in the blood probably due to its decreased catabolism.[129] Dietary cholesterol excess is probably the most common secondary cause of Type II. Analysis of an individual's lipid status is incomplete without knowledge of his dietary habits. Appropriate tests should also be done to rule out myxedema, obstructive liver disease, nephrosis, dysproteinemia and porphyria.

The physical examination is usually not revealing in the patient with Type II below age 20. Adults may manifest characteristic thickening of the Achilles tendon as well as extensor xanthomas of the hand. Tuberous xanthomas on the elbows, knees and tibia occur less frequently. Corneal arcus senilis may be significant before age 45. Unfortunately corneal arcus senilis and xanthelasma are visible markers that are rarely specific for familial Type II in the adult. Neither hyperuricemia nor diabetes occurs frequently in Type II.[130]

Type II and Vascular Disease. In the homozygous Type II patient, cholesterol concentrations will often be in the 600 to 900 mg per cent range and sudden cardiac death before age 20 is not unusual.[116] Postmortem examination reveals marked superficial xanthomatosis and severe atherosclerotic changes involving cardiac valves as well as coronary arteries.[131]

Incidence and prevalence studies of coronary heart disease in families with Type II emphasize the importance of early diagnosis. Harlan and co-workers, however, examining a large group of American kindred with hypercholesterolemia and xanthomatosis, reported no differences in mortality between affected and non-affected members.[132] This is in contrast with a 20-year follow-up of 12 Danish kindreds which documented an impressive incidence of early death from coronary heart disease in the relatives with high plasma cholesterol levels.[133] In addition, Slack's study[134] of first-degree relatives of patients with Type II disclosed that 20 out of 30 biochemically affected male relatives developed coronary heart disease at a mean age of 43.8 years. In the NIH Clinical Center experience, only 1/117 patients with familial Type II below age 20 had coronary heart disease; however, greater than 20 per cent of those between ages 20 to 29 had coronary heart disease, and by age 50 over 50 per cent of the diagnosed Type II males had sustained a coronary event.[116]

Diet Therapy. Effective diet therapy[125] should produce falls in plasma cholesterol levels of 15 to 25 per cent in Type II subjects. This dietary regimen is as low in cholesterol as is practical. It is also low in saturated fat with an increased proportion of dietary fat supplied as polyunsaturated fats and oils. Cholesterol content of foods are listed in Table A-5 in the Appendix. Data on the fatty acid composition of common fats and oils are given in Table A-6 in the Appendix. Restriction of carbohydrate is unnecessary. The composition of the diet will vary, depending on the low-cholesterol food preferences. The cholesterol intake can be expected to range from 100 to 250 mg/day. Meat is the primary source of cholesterol; other foods contribute insignificant amounts. The P/S ratio (gm of polyunsaturated to gm of saturated fatty acid) will vary from 1.8 to 2.8. The distribution of calories will vary: protein, 10 to 20 per cent; fat, 25 to 40 per cent; and carbohydrate, 40 to 65 per cent.[135] Serum cholesterol in Type II subjects usually does not respond to weight reduction (unless triglyceride is also elevated) and, therefore, total caloric level is not stressed for lipid lowering.

The diet is planned to restrict cooked lean meat to no more than 9 ounces/day with beef, lamb, ham and pork being limited to a 3-ounce portion 3 times a week. This restriction controls the level of saturated fat. Nine ounces of meat have not proven to be a restriction in quantity for most people. However, the limitation of beef, lamb, pork and ham is difficult and not popular.

An intake of at least 1 teaspoon of fat or oil high in polyunsaturates (linoleic acid) is recommended for every ounce of meat. This is a small amount of fat; because the amount is not limited, it is expected (and should be encouraged) that more will be consumed. If an individual only consumes 1 teaspoon per ounce, total fat intake would be expected to be low, approximately 20 to 25 per cent of calories.

The Type II diet presents change for the average person, but the restrictions have not been found to be too difficult for the individual who enjoys experimental or creative cooking. It is more difficult for the person who is not interested in cooking and wants to use convenient foods. Optimal dietary control is also difficult to achieve for the person who must or chooses to eat most of his meals in restaurants.

Diet in Children. Since Type II is dominantly inherited and is so readily diagnosed in the first or second year of life, it is likely that the diet will be instituted at a very early age. The diet for the child with Type II is the same diet as that recommended for adults. Dietary cholesterol is restricted to 100 to 150 mg/day, in practical terms this is the same restriction as recommended for adults. Early diet adaptations are advantageous because the child is establishing eating patterns which include lean meats, fish, poultry and skim milk while learning to avoid such foods as hot dogs, cheese, and egg yolk. Such principles are easier established in childhood than attempting to change an adult's typical American diet.

Drug Therapy. Most Type II patients will require additional therapy to normalize LDL levels. The current drug of choice in familial Type II is cholestyramine, an anion exchange resin which sequesters bile acids in the intestine and leads to their increased excretion.[112] Turnover studies suggest that LDL catabolism is increased by cholestyramine treatment.[129,136] The combination of a low-cholesterol, increased polyunsaturated fat diet and the drug, cholestyramine, will allow the normalization of lipids in the majority of Type II subjects. Ileal bypass,[137] a surgical procedure that short-circuits the bile acid-absorbing portion of the terminal ileum, has been recommended as an alternate to drug therapy. It is hard to recommend this procedure in patients who can tolerate drugs. Furthermore, this surgical procedure is ineffective in other types of hyperlipoproteinemias.

Type III. Type III is usually a familial disorder, although the exact mode of inheritance is unclear. This disorder is characterized by abnormal beta-VLDL lipoprotein forms which migrate on paper electrophoresis as a broader band than normal beta lipoprotein. An elevated cholesterol and triglyceride of approximately the same proportions should make one suspect this disorder. Diagnosis, however, may be confirmed only by demonstrating the abnormal beta-VLDL in the supernatant of a sample centrifuged at density 1.006 gm/ml in the preparative ultracentrifuge.

Physical examination may provide valuable diagnostic clues for Type III. Planar xanthomas found in the creases of the palmar surface of the hand are almost pathognomonic. Tuberoeruptive xanthomas with characteristic reddish, inflammatory appearance are also seen on the elbows, buttocks and knees. Metabolic abnormalities are frequently seen.[130] The Type III patient manifests sensitivity to dietary carbohydrate with an exaggerated rise in the plasma triglyceride level. Abnormal glucose tolerance is present in 40 per cent of those tested. Hyperuricemia is seen in about 20 per cent.

Type III and Vascular Disease. Type III is associated with an increased risk of peripheral vessel disease as well as coronary heart disease.[138] Males frequently present with intermittent claudication or angina pectoris between ages 25 to 35. In females, signs and symptoms of the disorder may not be expressed for 15 to 20 years later. One autopsy finding of a 57-year-old female with Type III revealed 70 to 100 per cent occlusions of major coronary vessels by collections of foam cells with deposits of fibrous tissue.[131]

Diet Therapy.[125] Endogenous hyperglyceridemia is *most effectively controlled by caloric restriction.* During periods of weight reduction, the glyceride and cholesterol concentrations in essentially all patients with Types III, IV and V hyperlipoproteinemia can be normalized. Therefore, the first step in the management of such patients is *weight reduction.* Any reducing plan based on good nutrition can be used; however, for convenience and simplicity, low calorie diets of the NIH Clinical Center are planned using unsaturated fat and limiting cholesterol. Many subjects with Types III, IV and V are overweight and caloric restrictions can be aimed at achieving "ideal" weight (Table 31–3).

The patient with Type III will respond well to specific therapy. The maintenance diet prescribed after the desired weight loss is composed of 20 per cent protein, 40 per cent carbohydrate, and 40 per cent fat with a cholesterol intake of less than 300 mg/day. Most concentrated sweets are restricted, and alcohol is limited. The dietary plan is rigid and similar in form to the Type V diet previously discussed. Since diet therapy alone will frequently normalize the blood lipids, patient motivation is often high.

Drug Therapy. Clofibrate in doses of 2 gm daily has an additive effect which allows the maintenance of low normal lipids. With this prescribed therapy, xanthomatosis regresses completely and peripheral blood flow improves both objectively and subjectively.[112,138]

Type IV. When familial, this type is transmitted as a mendelian dominant trait with delayed expression and penetrance. It is not clear whether the primary defect is one of overproduction[139] or diminished clearance.[140] Detection of this disorder is rarely made before age 25. The individual with an abnormal glucose tolerance and elevated uric acid level is suspect for the disorder; however, secondary causes such as stress, diabetes, obesity, alcoholism and birth control pills may explain the associated hyperprebetalipoproteinemia.

Type IV patients appear to be sensitive to carbohydrate, although the subsequent increase in triglyceride is actually less than that seen in Type III. Glucose tolerance is impaired in 70 per cent. Approximately one-third of Type IV patients tested have immunoreactive insulins that are high, one-third are normal and one-third are low.[130]

Type IV and Vascular Disease. Although few studies have dealt specifically with primary Type IV, several have noted the high preva-

lence of the Type IV pattern.[108,141] Studies
of populations with documented coronary
heart disease by coronary angiography report a sizable prevalence of Type IV pattern, similar to the prevalence of the Type II
pattern.[142-144] On the other hand, one study
of familial Type IV revealed a lack of coronary heart disease in members below age 70
which was attributed to the absence of obesity
and diabetes mellitus in the kindred.[145]
Interpretation of these studies is made difficult by the imprecise criteria often used in
defining the Type IV phenotype, as well as the
frequency with which secondary causes of
the pattern appear.

Diet Therapy.[125] For the patient with
Type IV the objective is *always* weight reduction until ideal weight is attained. This
alone will often result in complete normalization of blood lipids.[112] The maintenance
diet consists of a controlled carbohydrate
intake to approximately 40 per cent of
calories and limiting cholesterol intake to
300 to 500 mg/day. Most concentrated
sweets are restricted and alcohol is limited.
Protein and fat are not restricted, but saturated fat is restricted, as in the Type III
plan. The success of this diet may be measured by the blood lipids and the maintenance of ideal weight. If the patient needs a
stricter regimen or more explicit instructions
for weight control, the Type III diet may be
used (Table 31-3).

Drug Therapy. Neither cholestyramine,
which may cause triglyceride levels to increase, nor clofibrate appears to be clearly
efficacious in Type IV. Nicotinic acid may
be effective, though problems with glucose
intolerance and hyperuricemia make its use
with this type difficult.

THE CENTRAL ROLE
OF DIET THERAPY

Diet is the cornerstone of therapy for any
of the primary lipid transport disorders.
Diet therapy should always be tried before
any drug is used. Often dietary manipulations alone will allow normalization of plasma
lipid levels. If the addition of drugs proves
necessary, diet should be continued since
the effect of diet and drugs is additive and

more effective than either alone. Though the
evidence that dietary intervention in the
coronary-prone patient will actually decrease
coronary morbidity and mortality is still
primarily presumptive, logic demands an active and aggressive approach to the high risk
patient.

The success of dietary management depends on the rapport of the doctor, dietitian,
and patient. The physician should explain
the significance of the lipids to the patient.
The dietitian should understand the patient's
disease and dietary needs and counsel him on
its practical aspects. Frequent return visits,
teaching aids, and family dietary counseling
are all of benefit. The patient should be encouraged to call or write for additional information. The patient's motivation and
understanding of the diet are essential in
dietary management. Successful management of the high risk patient with hyperlipoproteinemia depends on a close and enthusiastic working relationship between the
physician, dietitian and patient.

BIBLIOGRAPHY

1. Getz, Vesselinovitch, and Wissler: Amer. J.
   Med., *46*, 657, 1969.
2. Fredrickson: "Atherosclerosis and other forms
   of arteriosclerosis." Chapter 267, in Wintrobe,
   Thorn, Adams, Bennett, Braunwald, Isselbacher, and Petersdorf (Eds.), *Harrison's Principles of Internal Medicine.* New York, McGraw-
   Hill Book Co., 1970, pp. 1239–1252.
3. Report of inter-society commission for heart
   disease resources. Primary prevention of the
   atherosclerotic diseases. Circulation, *42*, A-55,
   1970.
4. Data from heart disease and stroke control
   program and chronic respiratory disease control
   program, Division of Chronic Disease Programs,
   U.S. Public Health Service, 1967.
5. Lown and Ruberman: Mod. Conc. of Cardio-
   vas. Dis., *39*, 97, 1970.
6. Gordon and Kannel: J.A.M.A., *215*, 1617,
   1971.
7. Kreuger and Morijama: Amer. J. Public
   Health, *57*, 496, 1967.
8. Anitschkow: "A history of experimentation on
   arterial atherosclerosis in animals." Chapter 2,
   in *Cowdry's Atherosclerosis—A Survey of the Problem.*
   2nd Ed. Blumenthal (Ed.), Springfield, Charles
   C Thomas, 1967, pp. 21–44.
9. Ahrens: Amer. J. Med., *23*, 928, 1957.
10. Randles and Knudson: J. Biol. Chem., *66*,
    459, 1925.

11. Schoenheimer and Breusch: J. Biol. Chem:, *103*, 439, 1933.
12. Rittenberg, and Schoenheimer: J. Biol. Chem., *121*, 235, 1937.
13. Armstrong, Warner, and Connor: Circ. Res., *27*, 59, 1970.
14. Keys, Mickelsen, Miller, and Chapman: Science, *112*, 79, 1950.
15. Keys, Anderson, Mickelsen, Adelson, and Flaminio: J. Nutr., *59*, 39, 1956.
16. Kinsell, Partridge, Boling, Margen, and Michaels: J. Clin. Endocrin. Metab., *12*, 909, 1952.
17. Ahrens, Tsaltas, Hirsch, and Insull: J. Clin. Invest., *34*, 918, 1955.
18. Steiner, Howard, and Akgun: J.A.M.A., *181*, 186, 1962.
19. Erickson, Coots, Mattson, and Kligman: J. Clin. Invest., *43*, 2017, 1964
20. Connor, Hodges, and Bleiler: J. Clin. Invest., *40*, 894, 1961.
21. Connor, Stone, and Hodges: J. Clin. Invest., *43*, 1691, 1964.
22. Keys, Anderson, and Grande: Metabolism, *14*, 759, 1965.
23. Kaplan, Cox, and Taylor: Arch. Path., *76*, 359, 1963.
24. Wilson and Lindsey: J. Clin. Invest., *44*, 1805, 1965.
25. Borgstrom: J. Lip. Res., *10*, 331, 1969.
26. Quintao, Grundy, and Ahrens: J. Lip. Res., *12*, 221, 1971
27. Quintao, Grundy, and Ahrens: J. Lip. Res., *12*, 233, 1971.
28. Keys: J. Chron. Dis., *4*, 364, 1956.
29. Mayer, Connell, Dewolfe, and Beveridge: Amer. J. Clin. Nutr., *2*, 316, 1954.
30. Wilmot and Swank: Amer. J. Med. Sci., *223*, 25, 1952.
31. Starke: Amer. J. Med., *9*, 494, 1950.
32. Hildreth, Mellinkoff, Blair, and Hildreth: J. Clin. Invest., *30*, 649, 1951.
33. Kinsell, Michaels, Partridge, Boling, Balch, and Cochrane: J. Clin. Nutr., *1*, 224, 1953.
34. Ahrens, Blankenhorn, and Tsaltas: Proc. Soc. Exper. Biol. Med., *86*, 872, 1954.
35. Beveridge, Connell, Mayer, Firstbrook, and DeWolfe: Circulation, *10*, 593, 1954.
36. Keys, Anderson, and Grande: Lancet, *1*, 787, 776, 1957.
37. Keys, Anderson, and Grande: Metabolism, *14*, 1965.
38. Hegsted, McGandy, Myers, and Stare: Amer. J. Clin. Nutr., *17*, 281, 1965.
39. Horlick and Craig: Lancet, *2*, 566, 1957.
40. Ahrens, Insull, Bloomstrand, Hirsch, Tsaltas, and Peterson: Lancet, *1*, 943, 1957.
41. Grande, Anderson, and Keys: J. Nutr., *74*, 420, 1961.
42. Hashim, Arteaga, and Van Itallie: Lancet, *1*, 1105, 1960.
43. Keys, Anderson, and Grande: Proc. Soc. Exper. Biol. Med., *98*, 387, 1958.
44. Keys, Anderson, and Grande: Metabolism, *14*, 747, 1965.
45. Anderson, Grande, and Keys: J. Nutr., *75*, 388, 1961.
46. Antonis and Bersohn: Lancet, *1*, 3, 1961.
47. Antonis and Bersohn: Lancet, *1*, 998, 1962.
48. Anderson: Amer. J. Clin. Nutr., *20*, 168, 1967.
49. Yudkin: Lancet, *2*, 4, 1964.
50. Yudkin, and Roddy: Lancet, *2*, 6, 1964.
51. Yudkin and Morland: Amer. J. Clin. Nutr., *20*, 503, 1967.
52. Burns-Cox, Doll, and Ball: Brit. Heart J., *31*, 485, 1969.
53. Howell, and Wilson: Brit. Med. J., *3*, 145, 1969.
54. McGandy, Hegsted, and Stare: New Eng. J. Med., *277*, 186–192; 245–277, 1967.
55. MacDonald and Braithwaite: Clin. Sci., *27*, 23, 1964.
56. Groen, Balogh, Yaron, and Cohen: Amer. J. Clin. Nutr., *19*, 46, 1966.
57. Antar and Ohlson: J. Nutr., *85*, 329, 1965.
58. Kuo and Bassett: Ann. Intern. Med., *62*, 1199, 1965.
58a.Kuo, P. T.: *In* Cardiac and Vascular Diseases. Conn and and Horwitz (Eds.) Philadelphia, Lea & Febiger, 1971.
59. Kaufmann, Poznanski, Blondheim, and Stein: Amer. J. Clin, Nutr., *18*, 261, 1966.
60. Dunnigan, Fyfe, McKiddie, and Crosbie: Clin. Sci., *38*, 1, 1970.
61. McGandy, Hegsted, Myers, and Stare: Amer. J. Clin. Nutr., *18*, 237, 1966.
62. Lyon, Yankley, Gofman, and Strisower: Calif. Med., *84*, 325, 1956.
63. Nelson: North W. Med., *55*, 643, 1956.
64. Morrison: J.A.M.A., *159*, 1425, 1955.
65. ———: J.A.M.A., *173*, 884, 1960.
66. Bierenbaum, Green, Florin, Fleishman, and Caldwell: J.A.M.A., *202*, 1119, 1967.
67. London Hospital Research Committee: Low fat diet in myocardial infarction. Lancet, *2*, 501, 1965.
68. Rose, Thomson, and Williams: Brit. Med. J., *I*, 1531, 1965.
69. Hood, Sanne, Orndahl, Ahlstrom, and Welin: Acta Med. Scand., *178*, 161, 1965.
70. Controlled trial of soya-bean oil in myocardial infarction: Lancet, *2*, 693, 1968.
71. Leren: Acta Med. Scan., Suppl. 466, 1966.
72. ———: Circulation, *42*, 935, 1970.
73. Rinzler: Bull. N.Y. Acad. Med., *44*, 936, 1968.
74. Turpeinen, Miettinen, Karvonen, Roine, Pekkarinen, Lehtosuo, and Alivirta: Amer. J. Clin. Nutr., *21*, 255, 1968.
75. Dayton, Pearce, Hashimoto, Dixon, and Tomiyasu: Circulation, *39* and *40*, Suppl. 2, 1969.
76. The National Diet-Heart Study Final Report, Circulation, *37*, Suppl. 1, 1–428, 1968.
77. Cornfield and Mitchell: Arch. Environ. Health, *19*, 382, 1969.
78. Report of the National Heart and Lung Institute. Task Force on Arteriosclerosis. Vol. 1, June, 1971.

79. Doyle, Dawber, Kannel, Heslin, and Kahn: New Eng. J. Med., *266*, 796, 1962.
80. Doyle, Dawber, Kannel, Kinch, and Kahn: J.A.M.A., *190*, 886, 1964.
81. Shapiro, Weinblatt, Frank, and Sager: J. Chron. Dis., *18*, 527, 1965.
82. Kannel, Castelli, and McNamara: J. Occup. Med., *9*, 611, 1967.
83. Kahn: NCI Monograph, *19*, 1, 1966.
84. Jenkins: New Eng. J. Med., *284*, 244, 307, 1971.
85. Doyle: Mod. Conc. Cardiovasc. Dis., *35*, 81, 1966.
86. Breslow and Bull: J. Chron. Dis., *11*, 421, 1960.
87. Kahn: Amer. J. Public Health, *53*, 1058, 1963.
88. Taylor, Klepetor, Keys, Parlin, Blackburn, and Puchner: Amer. J. Public Health, *52*, 1697, 1962.
89. Stamler, Lindberg, Berkson, Shaffer, Miller, and Poindexter: J. Chron. Dis., *11*, 405, 1960.
90. Paul, Lepper, Phelan, Dupertuis, McMillan, McKean, and Park: Circulation, *28*, 20, 1963.
91. Kannel, Dawber, Kagan, Revotskie, and Stoke: Ann. Intern. Med., *55*, 33, 1961.
92. Chapman and Massey: J. Chron. Dis., *17*, 933, 1964.
93. Pell and D'Alonzo: J.A.M.A., *185*, 831, 1963.
94. Partamian and Bradley: New Eng. J. Med., *273*, 455, 1965.
95. Epstein, Francis, Hayner, Johnson, Kjelsberg, Napier, Ostrander, Payne, and Dodge: Amer. J. Epid., *81*, 307, 1965.
96. Epstein: Circulation, *36*, 609, 1967.
97. Epstein, Ostrander, Johnson, Payne, Hayner, Keller, and Francis: Ann. Intern. Med., *62*, 1170, 1965.
98. Ostrander, Francis, Hayner, Kjelsberg, and Epstein: Ann. Intern. Med., *62*, 1188, 1965.
99. Marks: Bull. N.Y. Acad. Med., *36*, 296, 1960.
100. Dunn, Ipsen, Elsom, and Ohtani: Amer. J. Med. Sci., *259*, 309, 1970.
101. Murphy: Canad. Med. Assoc. J., *97*, 1181, 1967.
102. Bloor: Circulation Suppl., IV to Vol. 39 and 40, IV-130, 1969.
103. Epstein: Israel J. Med. Sci., *3*, 594, 1967.
104. Deutscher, Ostrander, and Epstein: Amer. J. Epid., *91*, 233, 1970.
105. Kannel, Gordon, Castelli, and Margolis: Ann. Intern. Med., *72*, 813, 1970.
106. Kannel, Castelli, Gordon, and McNamara: Ann. Intern. Med., *74*, 1, 1971.
107. Albrink, Meigs, Wister, and Mann: Amer. J. Med., *31*, 4, 1961.
108. Brown, Kinch, and Doyle: New Eng. J. Med., *273*, 947, 1965.
109. Jones, Gofman, Lindgren, Lyon, Graham, Strisower, and Nichols: Amer. J. Med., *11*, 358, 1951.
110. Tamplin, Strisower, DeLalla, Gofman, and Glazier: J. Gerontol., *9*, 403, 1954.
111. Technical Group of Committee on Lipoproteins and Atherosclerosis and Committee on Lipoproteins and Atherosclerosis of National Advisory Heart Council. Circulation, *14*, 691, 1956.
112. Levy and Fredrickson: Postgrad. Med., *47*, 130, 1970.
113. Fredrickson, Levy, and Lees: New Eng. J. Med., *276*, 32, 94, 148, 215, 273, 1967.
114. Hatch and Lees: Adv. Lipid Res., *6*, 4, 1968.
115. Redgrave: J. Clin. Invest., *49*, 465, 1970.
116. Fredrickson and Levy: "Familial hyperlipoproteinemia," Chapter 28, in *The Metabolic Basis of Inherited Disease*, 3rd Ed., Stanbury, Wyngaarden, and Fredrickson (Eds.), New York, McGraw-Hill Book Co., 1972.
117. Levy, Bilheimer and Eisenberg: The structure and metabolism of chylomicrons and very low density lipoproteins (VLDL), in *Plasma Lipoproteins*. Biochem. Soc. Symp. No. 33, 1971. R. M. S. Smellie (Ed.). London and New York, Academic Press, 1971.
118. Fredrickson, Gotto, and Levy: "Familial hypolipoproteinemia," Chapter 26, in *The Metabolic Basis of Inherited Disease*, 3rd Ed., Stanbury, Wyngaarden, and Fredrickson (Eds.), New York, McGraw-Hill Book Co., 1972.
119. Nikkila: Adv. Lipid Res., 7, 63, 1969.
120. Dietschy and Wilson: New Eng. J. Med., *282*, 1128, 1179, 1241, 1970.
121. Fredrickson: Circulation, *39* and *40*, IV-99, 1969.
122. Stone and Levy: Progr. Cardiovasc. Dis., *14*, 341, 1972.
123. Fredrickson, Levy, Kwiterovich, and Jover: New York: Plenum Publish. Corp. from Drugs Affecting Lipid Metab. 307.
124. Page and Stamler: Mod. Conc. Cardiovasc. Dis., *37*, 119, 1968.
125. Fredrickson, Levy, Jones, Bonnell, and Ernst: *A Handbook for Physicians*, U.S. Dept. of Health, Education and Welfare, Pub. Health Ser., Washington, D.C., U.S. Govt. Printing Off., 1970, p. 83.
126. Meal Planning with Exchange Lists. Chicago: Amer. Dietet. Assn., 1950.
127. Glueck, Heckman, Schonfeld, Skiner, and Pierce: (Abstr.), Circulation, Suppl. III, *42*, 11, 1970.
128. Kwiterovich, Levy, and Fredrickson: (Abstr.), Circulation, *42*, III, 11, 1970.
129. Langer, Strober, and Levy: J. Clin. Invest., *48*, 49a, 1969.
130. Glueck, Levy, and Fredrickson: Diabetes, *18*, 739, 1969.
131. Roberts, Levy, and Fredrickson: Arch. Path., *90*, 46, 1970.
132. Harlan, Graham, and Estes: Medicine (Baltimore), *45*, 77, 1966.
133. Jensen, Blankenhorn, and Kornerup: Circulation, *36*, 77, 1967.
134. Slack: Lancet, *2*, 1380, 1969.
135. Levy, Bonnell, and Ernst: J. Amer. Dietet. Assoc., *58*, 406, 1971.
136. Levy and Langer: New York Acad. Sci., *179*, 475, 1971.
137. Gomes, Bernatz, Kotlke, Juergens, and Titus: Mayo Clinic, Proc., *45*, 229, 1970.

138. Zelis, Mason, Braunwald, and Levy: J. Clin.
     Invest., *49*, 1007, 1970.
139. Reaven, Lerner, Stein, and Farquhar: J. Clin.
     Invest., *46*, 1756, 1967.
140. Quarfordt, Frank, Shames, Berman, and Stein-
     berg: J. Clin. Invest., *49*, 2281, 1970.
141. Gibson: CVD Epidemiology Newsletter, No.
     10, Amer. Heart Assoc., New York, 1971, p. 7.
142. Heinle, Levy, Fredrickson, and Gorlin: Amer.
     J. Cardiol., *24*, 178, 1969.
143. Blankenhorn, Chin, and Lau: Ann. Intern.
     Med., *69*, 21, 1968.
144. Kuo: Ann. Intern. Med., *68*, 449, 1968.
145. Schriebman, Wilson, and Arky: New Eng. J.
     Med., *281*, 981, 1969.

Chapter

32

Nutrition in Diseases of the Bones and Joints

THEODORE B. BAYLES

INTRODUCTION

"Collagen diseases," "group diseases," and "connective tissue diseases" are synonyms used to describe several diseases of unknown etiology. They have certain similarities, similar sites of pathologic involvement, and, barely possible, a common pathogenesis. Clinically, the conditions involved are rheumatic fever, rheumatoid arthritis, periarteritis nodosa, lupus erythematosus disseminatus, scleroderma, dermatomyositis, and perhaps malignant nephrosclerosis. Rich[1] has suggested a common etiologic basis of tissue sensitization, but most observers agree that the similar pathologic findings may be explained by a similar response of connective tissue to a variety of insults. Connective tissue has a limited spectrum of response to injury.

In this poorly understood group of connective tissue diseases, nutrition has not been proved to be of *specific etiologic or therapeutic importance;* but debility, chronic disease state, muscle wasting, fever, gastrointestinal or kidney involvement (nephritis), poor appetite, etc., make the matter of proper, adequate, and full nutrition a problem of real moment to the patient and the clinician.

Rheumatic Fever. The evidence strongly suggests that the immunologic insult of hemolytic streptococcus (Group A) infections to the susceptible human acts as the trigger in the onset of rheumatic fever. The part played by dietary or metabolic factors in rendering the human susceptible has not been proved. Once the rheumatic process has been established in the patient, there is no evidence

that dietary factors can influence its course. On the other hand, common sense dictates attention to dietary intake. For children,[2] the following diet has been recommended— low in fat; high in protein and carbohydrate, including 1 quart of skim milk; unlimited water; 5000 units vitamin A; 400 units vitamin D; 100 mg vitamin C; double the standard allowance of vitamin B complex; and 15 mg of iron. When rheumatic carditis and/or congestive heart failure is present, sodium intake should be restricted to 1 to 2 gm daily.

There is no positive evidence that a vitamin deficiency is a direct or indirect eitologic agent in rheumatic fever.[3] A study of experimental scurvy[4] led to the conclusion that there was "only a superficial morphologic similarity between the articular lesions of scurvy and those of either rheumatoid arthritis or rheumatic fever." The importance of vitamin C in rheumatic fever has been lessened by the findings that ascorbic acid blood levels in rheumatic fever subjects and normals were the same on the same intakes.[5] The unexplained observation by Massell[6] that large doses of ascorbic acid (4 gm/day) apparently depressed rheumatic activity has not been confirmed or amplified.

A great deal of investigation has attempted to relate the rheumatic process to hypersensitivity initiated by hemolytic streptococcus (Group A) infections, but even so, Fischel[7] concluded "there is, as yet, no clinical test for the detection of an allergic reaction in rheumatic individuals that does not occur in patients recovering from a streptococcal infection or certain other diseases." Certainly the effect of nutrition on this type of biologic reaction is far from clear at the present time.

Studies on the social and hygienic factors in host susceptibility seem to incriminate crowding with consequent greater exposure to the hemolytic streptococci rather than the inadequate or substandard diets provided in substandard homes. Nevertheless, Massell[8] states that clinical practice at the House of Good Samaritan, Boston, dictates a high protein diet with fresh fruit daily.

Rheumatoid Arthritis. The patient's question, "What kind of diet do you recommend?" is too often incorrectly answered by the physician, either with a peremptory remark that it does not matter what the patient eats or, at the other extreme, by the imposition of a rigid program based on the physician's own dietary fetish. No dietary deficiency has been causally related to rheumatoid arthritis, but we are dealing with a chronic, progressive, inflammatory tissue disorder in which good nutrition of the individual is of fundamental importance. The victim of rheumatoid arthritis has a known negative nitrogen and calcium balance, muscle atrophy, decalcification of bone, and, in the active state of the disease, decreased carbohydrate tolerance.[9] We must point out that the active stage of the disease, with remissions and exacerbations, may go on for many years, and even a patient in apparent complete remission is subject to a relapse. It has been said, "Once an arthritic, always an arthritic." With this lugubrious yet correct viewpoint, to disregard nutrition in this chronic disease is bad medical practice. *The patient with rheumatoid arthritis has a systemic disease and is a sick individual.*

Attempts to relate this disorder to specific dietary factors have not been successful. Bayles, Richardson and Hall[10] found no evidence of significant dietary deficiency preceding onset of the disease. Bauer[11] reviewed and discarded the various diets suggested in the past as not specific and perhaps harmful. The decreased carbohydrate tolerance is probably related to the chronic inflammatory state rather than to a fundamental dyscrasia in sugar metabolism;[12]

therefore, carbohydrate intake need not be decreased except to enhance protein ingestion. The lowered serum albumin and elevated globulin may indicate hypersensitivity, chronic inflammation, or inanition.

The diet which we prescribe is a nutritious well-balanced diet with caloric content dependent on ideal weight and activity.

Vitamins, over and above those furnished by a good diet, have not been proved to alter the course of rheumatoid arthritis, despite some evidence that absorption and utilization may sometimes be below normal in this chronic disease. It has been established that vitamin A,[13] vitamin B complex (thiamin hydrochloride, niacin, riboflavin),[14] vitamin C,[15] E or K, when studied directly, did not alter the symptoms or course of the disease.

Administration of vitamin D in concentrated high dosage is potentially dangerous and of little or no value. The toxic effects have consisted of polydipsia, polyuria, muscle weakness, headache, drowsiness, nausea, vomiting, and diarrhea—in decreasing frequency. Hypercalcemia may cause metastatic calcification in soft tissues and, more seriously, in the kidney.[16]

The anemia of rheumatoid arthritis is partially hemolytic in character;[17] it is not primarily due to iron deficiency, nor to inhibition by a "toxin" from the disease of the normal hematopoietic process in the bone marrow. Hence, once any concomitant iron deficiency has been corrected by oral administration of iron, further oral iron will not improve the anemia. Sinclair and Duthie[18] obtained satisfactory rises in hemoglobin with intravenous iron in 38 of 51 cases, but 13 cases remained refractory. Supportive blood transfusions have only a transitory effect on the anemia of rheumatoid arthritis. Cobalt therapy, in our experience,[19] has not corrected the anemia.

In elderly patients with mild rheumatoid arthritis—and this disease may often start in the sixth or seventh decade—supplementing the diet with liver by mouth often has a salutary effect, but certainly this cannot be considered specific at the present time.

Degenerative Joint Disease (Osteoarthritis). Degenerative joint disease or hypertrophic arthritis is more amenable to a nutritional approach than is rheumatoid arthritis.[20] Degenerative joint changes in weight-bearing joints, specifically the hip and knee, are the most serious clinical and crippling problem in this disease. While the joint damage may be secondary to a slipped femoral epiphysis, poor posture, marked bowleg, or knock knee deformity, it is often aggravated by obesity. Obesity can be corrected by placing the patient on a subcaloric diet. Weight loss almost invariably alleviates the symptoms to a greater or lesser extent. However, there is nothing intrinsic in the diet that produces the favorable effect. Most patients with degenerative joint disease lose weight more happily on a moderately high protein and moderately low fat, and carbohydrate diet; the amount of fat and carbohydrate will vary, but I try to give 80 to 100 gm of protein, 50 to 60 gm of fat, and 100 to 150 gm of carbohydrate.

A typical diet for an obese patient with degenerative joint disease of the knees or hips will contain approximately 100 to 150 gm of carbohydrate, 80 to 100 gm of protein, 50 to 60 gm of fat and 1,200 to 1,500 calories. In my experience this dietary program has resulted in weight loss, relatively satisfactory satiety, general well-being, an improvement in both weight-bearing and non-weight-bearing joints. However, other factors, such as thyroid function, menopausal hormone imbalance, and the mechanical stresses and strains involved in degenerative joint disease, make the evaluation of the effect of diet very difficult.

Gout. Gout is a metabolic disease of unknown etiology manifested by (1) an increase in the serum uric acid concentration, (2) recurrent attacks of the characteristic type of acute arthritis, (3) deposits of sodium urate monohydrates which appear chiefly in and around the joints of the extremities and may lead to joint destruction and severe crippling, (4) renal disease involving glomerular, tubular, and interstitial tissues (sometimes including deposits of urate crystals) and blood vessels and in which hypertension and urolithiasis and kidney stones are common.[21] The normal serum uric acid varies from 2 to 6 mg per 100 ml of plasma or serum. Patients

with gout have levels of 6 to 10 and rarely up to 20 mg per 100 ml of serum or plasma.

As Hall et al.[22] have pointed out in a recent epidemiological study of gout and hyperuricemia, there is a direct correlation between the percentage of patients developing gouty arthritis and the serum uric acid level. The study shows that with a serum uric acid under 6.0 mg per cent only 1.1 per cent of men develop gouty arthritis. Between 6.0 and 6.9 mg per cent, 7.3 per cent of men develop gouty arthritis. Between 8.0 and 8.9 mg per cent uric acid in the blood, 18.7 per cent of men develop acute gouty arthritis and of those with a serum uric acid level greater than 9.0 mg per cent, 83 per cent develop acute gouty arthritis. This indicates the importance of proper control of the serum uric acid level in this metabolic disease, gout. Hyperuricemia is transmitted by a single dominant autosomal gene which is not sex-linked; only a portion of the heterozygotes for this factor develops gouty arthritis.[23] Stecher, Hersh and Solomon[24] estimated penetrance of 84 per cent in the heterozygous male and 12 per cent or less in the female relatives. Familial hyperuricemia is usually not present in males under the age of sixteen, or in women until after the menopause. The mechanism of hyperuricemia has been ascribed to (a) overproduction of uric acid in the body or (b) diminished destruction of uric acid in the body or (c) decreased renal excretion of uric acid. None of these theories has been conclusively proved. Recently a variety of isotopically labeled compounds have been administered to birds, rats, and man. When the isotope tracer is identified in various positions in excreted uric acid and in purines isolated from tissues, it becomes apparent that the metabolic precursors of uric acid may be relatively simple compounds readily available from the "metabolic pool."[25-27] It seems likely that glycine is the nucleus about which carbon and nitrogen atoms become associated in the biosynthesis of uric acid.[28]

This incontrovertible experimental evidence that simple available compounds in the body, such as carbon dioxide, glycine, and ammonia, may be synthesized into uric acid makes the dietary treatment of gout less vital than former authorities in this field thought.

Whether the above facts preclude the possibility of dietary factors altering human uric acid metabolism is not as yet decided.

A large fluid intake is helpful in eliminating uric acid, in preventing renal calculi, and in retarding progressive involvement of the kidney. Treatment of the azotemia associated with chronic gouty nephritis is similar to the treatment of azotemia due to other causes. A high carbohydrate diet has a tendency to increase uric acid secretion, whereas a high fat diet tends to retard it and may in some patients precipitate gouty attacks. Only those protein foods containing nucleoproteins whose end product in breakdown is uric acid need be considered. A diet restricted to 100 mg of purine a day permits a 3-oz serving of meat, fish, seafood, peas, beans, or lentils a day. Foods of high purine content may be excluded but with modern therapy diet plays no significant role. Of course, under no circumstance should the caloric intake of the diet be such as to increase the weight of a patient above his ideal. During the *acute* attack a soft diet high in carbohydrate and low in fat and protein is recommended.

During the period between attacks, the diet should be varied, well-balanced and adjusted to the desired weight of the patient and, as pointed out, should not allow overweight. It should include adequate skim milk and 2 quarts of water or sweet liquids. Alcohol should be eliminated or taken sparingly and diluted, *i.e.*, highballs.

The methylxanthines (caffeine, theophylline, and theobromine) of coffee, tea, and cocoa are metabolized to methyl-urates and are not deposited in the gouty tophus;[29] therefore, these common beverages need not be avoided.

In this chapter an evaluation of general medical treatment is not made, but it should be mentioned that Benemid (probenecid), a uricosuric agent, was, about 1950, perhaps the first significant advance in the treatment of gout since colchicine was introduced to clinical medicine 300 or more years ago. Benemid is a relatively non-toxic, continually active tubular reabsorption blocking agent which lowers, and keeps low, the large miscible pool and stored uric acid and urates in the body of gouty subjects. Recently allopurinol has been added to our resources in the treatment of gout. This is an analog of hypoxanthine and was first reported in 1957[30] to be a potent inhibitor of xanthine oxidase. This is the enzyme that catalyzes the oxidation of hypoxanthine to xanthine and xanthine to uric acid. The administration of this drug to man results in a striking reduction in plasma and urinary concentrations of uric acid, with a simultaneous increase in plasma and urinary concentrations of hypoxanthine and xanthine.[31,32] The administration of allopurinol results in the high rate of renal excretion of oxypurines, predominantly xanthine. Xanthine is a sparingly soluble compound and its concentration in urine reaches values which in subjects with a metabolic disease called xanthinuria have led to xanthine stone formation. This can be somewhat counteracted by an increased fluid intake. At the present time allopurinol has been used in large numbers of patients for the treatment of gout, particularly those who do not respond to Benemid and the more classic methods. There has been minimal toxicity.[33]

Miscellaneous. *Ochronotic arthritis* is a rare condition resulting from a hereditary disorder, alkaptonuria, which is characterized by the presence of homogentisic acid in the urine. This substance when oxidized gives a brownish-black color to the urine. When homogentisic acid is deposited in joint cartilage, it leads to rapid disintegration of the cartilage and subsequent joint disease. In 1958 LaDu and others[34] demonstrated the absence of the enzyme homogentisic acid oxidase in the liver of a patient with alkaptonuria and ochronotic arthritis. The absence of this enzyme prevents the normal breakdown or metabolism of homogentisic acid with the resultant piling up of this substance in the body. Presently it is not feasible to compensate for the enzyme deficiency, but recently Holdsworth[35] has shown that a diet low in phenylalanine-tyrosine will reduce the amount of homogentisic acid excreted in the urine and may produce clinical improvement.

Infectious arthritis, as classified by the American Rheumatism Association, refers to the specific infections of joints by known bacteria, spirochetes, viruses, filterable agents, and the like.

Postmenopausal senile osteoporosis of the spine may be confused with spondylitis or degenerative joint disease of the spine, but here radiographic study will soon reveal the true diagnosis. Senile osteoporosis requires a high protein diet, adequate calcium intake, and small amounts of vitamin D (2000 units daily) to increase calcium absorption. The administration of male hormone and estrogens leads to increased deposition of protein matrix, thus enhancing bone recalcification.

The term *rheumatism* indicates all the aches and pains of the musculoskeletal system which cannot be more accurately diagnosed as bursitis, rheumatoid arthritis, gout, etc. Many such syndromes are of psychogenic origin, while others are manifestations of an organic nature which we do not as yet understand. I do not believe that any specific diet is useful in these conditions.

Neuropathic Arthropathy — Charcot's Joints. Rapid degenerative changes in joints may be due to lack of trophic impulses, as Charcot postulated, or due to microtraumata resulting from the loss of the normal proprioceptive senses; the latter theory is more widely accepted. Clinical conditions which may produce this type of joint disease are tabes dorsalis, syringomyelia, trauma to spinal cord or posterior nerve roots, cord tumors, spinal caries from tuberculosis, malignant tumors, myelitis, poliomyelitis, leprosy, yaws, diabetic neuritis, toxic neuritis, and hemiplegic states.

Dietary regimens are not helpful in these conditions except to reduce body weight and improve nutrition of and to the peripheral nerves and joint structures.

Allergic arthritis as such does not exist, but joint inflammation and urticaria have been reproduced in certain patients by certain foods or other substances. The elimination of the allergens from the diet is obviously indicated in the treatment of such patients.

BIBLIOGRAPHY

1. Rich: Harvey Lectures, 42, 106, 1947.
2. Jackson: J.A.M.A., 141, 439, 1949.
3. Glover: Ann. Rheumatic Dis., 5, 126, 1946.
4. Pirant, Bly, and Sutherland: Arch. Path., 49, 710, 1950.
5. Wilson and Lubschez: J. Clin. Invest., 25, 428, 1946.
6. Massell, Warren, Patterson, and Lehmus: New Eng. J. Med., 242, 614, 1950.
7. Fischel: Am. J. Med., 7, 772, 1949.
8. Massell: Personal communication.
9. Webb and Bayles: Unpublished observations.
10. Bayles, Richardson, and Hall: New Eng. J. Med., 229, 319, 1943.
11. Bauer: J.A.M.A., 104, 1, 1935.
12. Holsti: Acta Med. Scand., Supp. III, 137, 1943.
13. Hall, Bayles, and Soutter: New Eng. J. Med., 223, 92, 1940.
14. Bayles, Palmer, Massod, and Judd: New Eng. J. Med., 242, 249, 1950.
15. Hall, Darling, and Taylor: Ann. Int. Med., 13, 415, 1939.
16. Paul: J. Iowa Med. Soc., 36, 141, 1946.
17. Freireich, Ross, and Bayles: J. Clin. Invest., 36, 1043, 1957.
18. Sinclair and Duthie: Lancet, 2, 646, 1949.
19. Bayles, Colpoys, and Gardner: Unpublished observations.
20. Bayles: Med. Clin. North America, 34, 1435, 1950.
21. Wyngaarden, J. B.: Etiology and Pathogenesis of Gout. In *Arthritis and Allied Conditions,* Hollander, J. L., Ed., 8th Ed., Philadelphia, Lea & Febiger, p. 1071, 1972.
22. Hall, A. P., Barry, P. E., Dawber, T. R. and McNamara, P. M.: Am. J. Med., 42, 27, 1967.
23. Smyth, Cotterman, and Freyberg: J. Clin. Invest., 27, 749, 1948.
24. Stecher, Hersh, and Solomon: Ann. Int. Med., 31, 595, 1949.
25. Heinrich and Wilson: J. Biol. Chem., 186, 447, 1950.
26. Karlson and Barker: J. Biol. Chem., 177, 597, 1949.
27. Barnes and Schoenheimer: J. Biol. Chem., 151, 123, 1943.
28. Shemin and Rittenberg: J. Biol. Chem., 167, 875, 1947.
29. Wolfson, Huddlestun, and Levine: J. Clin. Invest., 26, 995, 1947.
30. Feigelson, P., Davidson, J. D. and Robins, R. K.: J. Biol. Chem., 226, 993, 1957.
31. Wyngaarden, J. B., Rundles, R. W., Silberman, H. R. and Hunter, S.: Arth. and Rheum., 6, 306, 1963.
32. Rundles, R. W., Wyngaarden, J. B., Hitchings, G. H., Elion, G. B. and Silberman, H. R.: Trans. Assoc. Amer. Phys., 76, 126, 1963.
33. Wyngaarden, J. B., Rundles, R. W., and Metz, E.: Ann. Intern. Med., 62, 842, 1965.
34. LaDu, B. N., Zannoni, V. G., Laster, L., and Seegmiller, J. E.: J. Biol. Chem., 230, 251, 1958.
35. Holdsworth, D. E.: Personal communication.

Chapter

33

Allergy and Diet

VINCENT J. FONTANA

AND

M. B. STRAUSS

THE IMMUNOLOGY OF FOOD ALLERGY

Rosenau and Anderson[1] (1906) were probably the first to demonstrate that sensitization could be produced through the digestive tract, by passage of proteins through the gastrointestinal mucous membranes. Walzer's experiments[2,3] showed that in 90 per cent of normal human beings undigested protein could be absorbed through the mucous membrane of the intestine and be demonstrated in the blood.

In those cases in which allergic symptoms apparently occur on the first ingestion of a food, Zinsser[4] feels that active sensitization may have occurred *in utero* by passage of the exciting agent (antigen) from the mother through the placenta, and Ratner[5] suggests that pregnant and nursing mothers with allergic histories should refrain from using large quantities of foods with high sensitizing capacity, such as fish and eggs, and that milk should be thoroughly boiled. Infants are rarely born hypersensitive, for the skin-sensitizing antibodies are apparently unable to pass through the placenta and the fetus is never passively sensitized to an antigen.

The gamma E globulins exhibit all the properties of the reaginic antibody. They fix to human skin; they combine with allergens that can neutralize them; and they are heat labile. The association between reaginic antibody and a unique immunoglobulin class IgE or gamma E is now firmly estab-lished.[5a] There is available evidence that histamine release from leukocytes by white cell-bound gamma E globulin upon antigen contact may make the mucosa of the shock organs of the allergic individual more vulnerable to antigenic stimulation.[5b]

Skin sensitizing antibodies are found in the blood of a child of known allergic parentage before the child itself begins to exhibit allergic symptoms.[6] Thus, the clinical form of allergy would not seem to be determined by the mere presence in the blood of skin-sensitizing antibodies. There must exist, as a necessary attribute for clinical sensitization, some sensitized tissue area, or "shock organ."[7] There is conclusive evidence of the ability of normal persons to absorb proteins from the gastrointestinal tract apparently unaltered and in sufficient quantities to sensitize human beings.[8–12] The absorption of proteins through the intestinal wall occurs with greater regularity than is generally believed.[13] By feeding milk to normal guinea pigs one is able to demonstrate sensitization in these animals by intravenous injection of milk. Fink and Quinn[14] studied antibody production in inbred strains of mice and found that younger mice produced much less antibody than more mature animals. Cannon and Longmire[62] showed that 5 to 10 per cent of skin grafts exchanged between pairs of newly hatched chicks of different breeds are tolerated and survive into adult life but the percentage of successes falls rapidly as the age at which the chicks are operated upon increases. It reaches zero if the operation be delayed to the end of the second week.

Even more striking results were obtained when antibody response was studied in the prenatal period. A group of English workers led by Medawar[63] found that mice never develop, or develop only to a limited degree, the power to become sensitized to foreign homologous tissue cells to which they have been exposed sufficiently in fetal life. Burnet[64] discusses the possibility that during early, embryonic life, an animal may accept foreign cells and develop a lasting tolerance to them; its ability to recognize the difference between "self" and "not-self" does not come until later, some time before birth. This would make one wonder if it would not be advantageous, by means of a widely varied maternal diet, to expose the fetus at a very early age to as many foods as possible so that they be accepted as "self," no antibody formation being elicited upon later contact with them. This effect would depend, of course, upon the passage of sufficient food protein into the maternal circulation and through the placenta.

Glaser and Johnstone[15] suggested that a physiological immunologic immaturity exists in the early months of post-natal life and that the absorption of unaltered proteins from the intestinal tract produces sensitization and clinical symptoms in potentially allergic children. They fed soybean from birth to infants whose antecedents included one parent or sibling with allergic disease. Only 14 (15 per cent) of this group showed major allergic diseases, compared with 42 (64 per cent) of the sibling control group and 91 (52 per cent) of a non-related control group of comparable ages. Their experiments showed that 4 times as many infants in the control groups developed major allergic conditions as in the experimental group where the foreign food, cow's milk, was withheld from the infant diet, and a non-antigenic casein hydrolysate, soybean, substituted. Apparently, therefore, practically all individuals, non-allergic, allergic, and potentially allergic, are exposed to prolonged parenteral contact with undigested foreign protein. That all individuals are not clinically sensitive to foods indicates, as Cooke[16] has suggested,

that intimate exposure to the foreign protein is not, of itself, a sufficient cause. There must be some predisposing mechanism present, some capacity for sensitization mediated, at least in part, by a hereditary factor.[17,18] It would seem, therefore, prudent to expose the infant, especially if potentially allergic, to the least possible quantity of those food antigens notorious for their high sensitizing potential (such as milk, egg, fish, and nuts), whether ingested directly or transmitted in the breast milk[19,20] of a nursing mother eating these foods, perhaps excessively.

THE CLINICAL MANIFESTATIONS OF ALLERGY

Allergic reactions may occur in any area of the body, since antibody is distributed throughout the various cells and tissue fluids. There are sites, however, characteristic for each clinical allergic malady, in which the tissues are thought to have a greater concentration of antibody, and which therefore show greater allergic activity upon exposure to the invading specific antigen. These sites may be the portals of entry where the primary invasion of antigen occurs. Often, however, the sites of the greatest allergic activity are distant from the portals of entry, the antigen being transported to them by the blood and lymph. For instance, in the individual asthmatic to horse dander, the symptoms result from allergic activity in the respiratory tissues, which are also the site of invasion of the airborne antigen. In the individual asthmatic to a food such as egg, symptoms also result from allergic activity in the respiratory tissues, but here the antigen has been transported from its portal of entry, the intestinal membrane.

The various clinical forms of allergy may be classified according to the major systems of the body in which the sensitized tissue areas chiefly involved in the allergic response are found. These major systems are (a) respiratory, (b) alimentary, (c) cutaneous, (d) neural, (e) cardiovascular, (f) genitourinary, and (g) articular. Since tissue areas in several major systems may be sensitized to the same antigen, several manifestations of clinical allergy may result in an individual from a single type of invading antigen. In the individual sensitive to clams, for instance, the ingestion of his specific excitant may result simultaneously in coryza, bronchial asthma, pruritus, urticaria, tracheal edema, abdominal cramps and diarrhea, due to activity in various sensitized areas of the respiratory, cutaneous, and alimentary systems.

Cooke[21] pointed out that the allergic response may be either of an immediate reaction type, occurring within 4 hours after contact with the antigen, or a delayed type, requiring from 4 to 72 hours for the appearance of the symptoms. Both types may be present in a single patient, but to different excitants; a person may develop asthma immediately upon contact with horses, but urticaria only after a delay of 24 hours following the eating of egg. Furthermore, a food antigen may cause immediate symptoms in one patient, delayed in another. While the length of the reaction time may vary from person to person and from cause to cause, it is always a constant in any one individual to any given antigen. The immediate type is also termed the skin-sensitive, or wheal type, since the immediately positive skin test, with typical wheal formation, may be obtained in sensitive individuals on application of the extract of the specific excitant by intracutaneous or scarification procedures. The delayed reaction type is also designated as the skin-negative, non-wheal type, due to its behavior upon skin test. An attempt to classify the varieties of clinical allergy is shown in Table 33–1.

THE CLINICAL MANIFESTATIONS OF FOOD ALLERGY

Food allergy may produce any of the various manifestations of sensitivity previously enumerated, with the exception of

Table 33-1. The Clinical Forms of Allergy

1. Skin-sensitive—Wheal (Immediate Reaction Type)
    (a) Hereditary: Spontaneous
        Allergic coryza, seasonal (hay fever), nonseasonal; bronchial asthma
        Causes: Airborne; pollens, dusts, fungi; foods
        Urticaria; angioedema of skin or alimentary tract; allergic headache; allergic nerve disorder
        Causes: Foods
    (b) Nonhereditary: Induced, physiologic, anaphylactic, serum sickness, therapeutic accidents
        Causes: Heterologous serum, antibiotics, insulin, organ extracts, toxoids, virus vaccines (egg media), helminths, serum conjugates
    (c) Physical allergy: Asthma, urticaria, angioedema, purpura, headaches
        Causes: Heat, cold, sunlight

2. Skin-negative—No wheal (Delayed Reaction Type)
    (a) Noninfective:
        Hereditary: Allergic coryza, bronchial asthma, urticaria, angioedema, dermatitis, allergic headaches, allergic nerve disorders
        Causes: Foods, some drugs
        Nonhereditary: (1) Drug allergy; allergic coryza, bronchial asthma, urticaria, angioedema, dermatitis, vascular allergy
        Causes: Aspirin, quinine, sulfonamides, mercury, serum conjugates
        Nonhereditary: (2) Contact dermatitis
        Causes: Natural and synthetic oils, resins; chemicals; drugs; foods
    (b) Infective:
        Hereditary: Allergic corzya, bronchial asthma; urticaria; angioedema of skin or alimentary tract; dermatitis; sinusitis
        Causes: Bacterial and fungal products
        Nonhereditary: Tuberculin type sensitization; periarteritis; vascular allergy; rheumatoid arthritis
        Causes: Bacterial products

pollenosis, which is always due to plant pollens; bacterial allergy; and physical allergy. It may be the sole or a contributing cause, producing symptoms of the immediate or delayed type, acute or chronic, mild or severe. Sensitivity to foods may manifest itself in the respiratory system as coryza, conjunctivitis, bronchitis, bronchial asthma and sinusitis; in the alimentary system as manifestations of gastroenteritis, such as herpes, stomatitis, bad breath, "bilious" attacks, gingivitis, nausea, vomiting, flatus, abdominal distention and pain, colitis, diarrhea, constipation, pruritus ani; and in the cutaneous system as pruritus, dermatitis, urticaria, angioedema, purpura; in the neural system as headache, peripheral neuritis, optic neuritis, vertigo, allergic labyrinthitis; in the cardiovascular system as tachycardia; in the genitourinary system as hematuria, pruritus vulvae; in the articular system as arthralgia; in the ocular system as conjunctivitis, corneal ulcers. It must be emphasized that food sensitivity is only an occasional or rare cause of many of these manifestations. The symptoms of food allergy may mimic those of many other clinical conditions. It is often difficult, even impossible, to demonstrate its presence and to prove its etiologic significance. The classification of food allergy is shown in Table 33–2.

Psychosomatic factors may be important in activating and altering latent allergic symptoms. To the chore of collecting data on the incidence of food allergy by history or by trial-and-error methods may be added the difficulties of comparing the results of skin testing by different investigators, using food extracts of varying potencies, and employing varying skills and methods of testing. Even

Table 33-2.   Classification of Food Allergy

1. Skin-sensitive—Wheal (Immediate Reaction Type)
   Antibody: Skin-sensitizing
   A. Hereditary: Spontaneous, abrupt, obvious, often severe symptoms, involving all major systems of the body
      Portal of entry:
      (a) Alimentary mucosa
          Causes: Foods by ingestion
      (b) Respiratory mucosa
          Causes: Inhaled dusty airborne food dusts and volatile food odors by inhalation (rare)
      (c) Skin
          Causes: Foods by percutaneous absorption (rare)
      (d) By parenteral injection
          Causes: Therapeutic agents containing food excitants
   B. Nonhereditary: Induced, anaphylactic, often severe symptoms involving all major systems of the body
      Portal of entry:
      By parenteral injection
          Causes: Sensitizers such as organ extracts, viral vaccines (egg media)
2. Skin-negative—No wheal (Delayed Reaction Type)
   Antibody: Unknown
   A. Hereditary: Deliberate, obscure symptoms involving all major systems of the body
      Portal of entry:
      (a) Alimentary mucosa
          Causes: Foods by ingestion
   B. Nonhereditary: Induced (contact dermatitis), rare, involving respiratory and cutaneous systems
      Portal of entry:
      (a) Intact oral and buccal mucosa and skin
          Causes: Foods, essential oils of foods and spices

when standardized extracts and techniques of skin testing are a constant, as with a single investigator, the results may be unsatisfactory since approximately one-half of the authentic food allergic cases fail to give positive skin tests.

The majority of cases of food sensitiveness occur in early life. From a study of 200 cases of bronchial asthma,[23] it was found by intracutaneous and clinical testing that only individuals of 3 years or younger developed symptoms from foods alone. Inhalant substances, such as pollens, dusts, and animal danders, gradually replace the food allergies, so that by the age of 5 to 10 years the majority of patients were no longer clinically food-sensitive, although the skin test reaction often persisted. In only 5 per cent of adult asthmatic patients could a food allergy be demonstrated as the sole excitant.

It is generally agreed that the incidence of food allergy depends greatly on age. In the infant, sensitization to various foods is relatively high and ranks in importance with infection, while after the age of 5 years there is a tendency towards spontaneous disappearance of food allergy. Therefore, according to Chobot[23] the incidence of clinical food allergy is low, in relation to that caused by inhalant substances and infection. On the other hand, Rinkel[24] feels that there is a higher incidence of food allergy in adults than in children, although it is less readily demonstrable. The comparative simplicity of the diet in childhood makes the diagnosis of food sensitivity easier.

FOOD ALLERGY IN CHILDREN

It is not known why some infants develop a specific sensitization shortly after birth, although heredity may play a dominant role. Spain and Cooke[18] have shown that where both parents are allergic, as indicated by the occurrence of bronchial asthma and/or hay fever, approximately 70 per cent of the offspring will develop a clinical allergic condition by the age of ten years. Where there is an antecedent unilateral history of bronchial asthma and/or hay fever, 50 per cent of the offspring will develop clinical allergic symptoms by the age of 30 years. It would seem,

therefore, that both incidence and age of onset of clinical allergic conditions are influenced by the strength of the inherited trait. Infections, focal or constitutional, and changes in the general health of the patient may play an important part in predisposing to the development or precipitation of allergic manifestations.

It is significant that Rowe and Rowe[25] and Stoesser[26] found allergy to food most important in asthma of early childhood, while inhalants were more significant in the latter part of the preschool period. It is of interest that Ratner and Untracht[27] found that 5 per cent of 500 allergic children were sensitive, clinically and by skin test, to a single food— egg. In the child, as in the adult, the allergic process can affect any of the body systems.

Types of Sensitizing Foods. Milk and egg are usually the first foods to which the infant becomes sensitive, probably because they are among the initial foods comprising his diet. In Clein's series of 140 allergic infants,[28] 1 out of every 15 was sensitive to cow's milk. Among the conditions they developed were eczema, pylorospasm and colic, while some felt "unhappy all the time." Less common symptoms were cough, choking and gasping, nose colds, constipation, asthma, anorexia, attacks of sneezing.

Heiner has reported a syndrome found in infants that includes intestinal blood loss in a hypochromic microcytic anemia thought to be due to milk allergy.[28a] Iron therapy and blood transfusions correct the anemia but do not alleviate the fetal blood loss thought to be milk induced. Ingestion of cow's milk, therefore, must cause the occult loss of significant quantities of blood in the gastrointestinal tract of some children with hypochromic microcytic anemia. This syndrome should be considered in any infant or child with occult fecal blood losses, especially in the presence of a family history of allergy.

The symptoms produced by a food allergy may involve any tissue of the body. The possibility of a food allergy should be considered in a child with constitutional or generalized signs of easy fatigability, irritability, insomnia, poor work in school or intermittent headaches and stomach aches. These children oftentimes find it difficult to get along with their siblings or peers. If these children have a positive family or personal history of allergy and are experiencing the constitutional tension-fatigue symptoms described, a thorough investigation for a food allergy should be undertaken.

Direct skin testing by either the scratch or intradermal methods is rarely employed in such cases because of the threat of a possible violent reaction to the use of an excitant of high potency. The diagnosis is usually established by the history, the indirect skin test method, the food diary, and trial-and-error procedures.

Sensitization to milk presents a considerable though essential replacement problem. In the case of other foods, simple removal is sufficient, but where milk is to be avoided, some substitute that fulfills the nutritional and mineral requirements must be given to the infant and young child. Such proprietary products as Mullsoy, Soybean, Soyalac, or Isomil are often satisfactory milk substitutes, unless the infant is sensitive to soybean in which case Nutramigen or a meat base formula may be tried. In cases of disaccharide intolerance, a disease which may mimic milk allergy or soybean sensitivity, the use of a meat base formula or carbohydrate-free (Borden) formula will be helpful in making a diagnosis. After alleviation of the patient's symptoms, special formulas containing milk, soybean or disaccharide may be tried individually to elicit the true etiological cause of the patient's symptoms. Specifications for their use are supplied by the makers of all these substances. Goat's milk, fresh or canned, often offers a highly satisfactory replacement, although an allergenic factor common to both cow's and goat's milk may prevent its use.

The infant or child highly allergic to egg must avoid all traces of it. In those with a more moderate degree of sensitization, the white of egg may be the excitant, the yolk being readily tolerated as well as poultry. Fortunately, most infants and children do not demonstrate an exquisite degree of food intolerance, and can satisfactorily follow a diet which need not be too restricted, provided heat-treated or cooked items are used. Rat-

ner[30] has offered such a diet which has proven helpful.

Malnutrition and Allergic Conditions. Cannon[32] has emphasized the fact that intracellular globulin, including antibody globulin, acts as a protein reserve which can be called upon to replenish plasma proteins, and with which these tend to remain in equilibrium. Low protein diets, or any interference with the rebuilding of protein reserves, leads to hypoproteinemia and progressive exhaustion of antibody reserves. This is true in conditions with severe tissue protein depletion, such as starvation, sprue, intestinal tuberculosis, and ulcerative colitis. Such exhaustion of antibody reserves explains the increased susceptibility to infection.[32] Kolmer[33] suggests that the peculiar increased tendency to infection in some cases of diabetes mellitus may be due to deficiency in the synthesis of antibody-globulin by the cells of the reticuloendothelial system. The diabetic is less able to form antibody than the normal individual due to an increased neoglucogenesis and, as a consequence, a large protein deficit may occur.[34-36] Wohl et al. have shown that low antibody response to antigenic stimulation in diabetics appears to bear a relationship to blood protein levels rather than to fasting blood sugar levels; furthermore, oral supplementation with casein concentrate or lactalbumin hydrolysate enhanced antibody formation.[37]

While most of the studies on the effect of malnutrition on antibody formation have concerned immune types of antibody, this same mechanism would also be apt to influence the skin-sensitizing antibody of the allergic individual. The diminution or temporary disappearance of allergic symptoms such as urticaria, dermatitis, headache, and bronchial asthma, reported in individuals suffering from wartime malnutrition, might conceivably be explained on this basis. Not only is the degree of exposure to the specific protein probably decreased, but there may be a deficiency in the reserves of antibody globulin necessary for the reaction with antigen to produce allergic symptoms. The temporary lessening or loss of sensitization effects during acute illness, however, cannot be explained upon this basis. Relief from allergic symptoms, even those of intractable bronchial asthma[38] and allergic dermatitis,[39] occurs frequently during acute intercurrent infections, such as lobar pneumonia,[40] Kaposis' varicelliform eruption,[41] and measles.[38] Such remissions would seem to be due to the mobilization of endocrine defense mechanisms during fever,[42] an ACTH-like effect resulting from the release of steroid hormones.[43]

Severe allergic conditions may have an adverse effect upon nutrition. The individual with uncontrolled bronchial asthma is frequently undernourished, since he has come to realize that the lightest of meals may cause embarrassed digestion and abdominal distention, with a consequent heightening of the asthmatic distress. Anorexia, nausea, flatus, diarrhea, and constipation may result from apprehension concerning his health and from nervous tension caused by fear of precipitating an attack by the unwitting ingestion of some highly potent excitant, unidentifiable in some food preparation. Anemia, avitaminosis, underweight and, in the child, lack of proper growth, with a reduced vital capacity, are the evidences of impaired nutrition. The interruption of sleep, respiratory or intestinal symptoms, or irritability and tension due to antiasthmatic stimulating drugs, such as ephedrine, may intensify the problem. One of the first evidences of an improved allergic status and success in allergic management is a gain in weight.

In forms of severe food allergy, such as urticaria, dermatitis, gastroenteritis, colitis, and headaches, evidences of malnutrition often result from self-inflicted, but usually unjustified, curtailment of the diet. The whims, fads, and phobias regarding food allergy which plague many persons, both allergic and non-allergic, force upon the physician the added responsibility of attempting to re-educate the patient, to reassure him, and to encourage him to adopt an adequate diet.

Food Allergy. *History taking.* The presence of a food allergy is often simple to identify in the immediate type, but frequently difficult to locate in the delayed type. It may be established by (1) the history, (2) cutaneous tests, (3) food diary, and (4) clinical tests employing trial-and-error methods and restric-

tive diets. History taking is the most important of all diagnostic procedures, and should be completed first. It may provide information of great consequence, not only as to the specific food causes, but also as to the degree to which they affect the patient. With such knowledge, the investigator is forewarned, and may avert what might have been a hazardous exposure of the hypersensitive patient to the active food excitant by routine skin testing or clinical trial. In the immediate reaction type, where symptoms follow so swiftly upon exposure to the exciting food, the patient is usually fully aware of at least the more obvious and more potent food factors and the extent of disturbance they produce. The individual who describes the prompt development of edema of the lips and tongue upon accidental contact with traces of egg, nut, or fish, or who reports asthma from the inhalation of their odors, is not a candidate for further exposure to such foods by skin test or by ingestion experiments. Until the history and the degree of sensitivity can be verified, testing should be scrupulously avoided with those food excitants described as producing swift, severe symptoms; this is especially the case when the route of contact is by surface exposure of mucosa or skin, or by inhalation of food odors, such as those of fish, meat, celery, banana, or onion. Cases with a history of such a high degree of sensitivity should be investigated by the passive transfer method.

A comprehensive investigation of the occurrence of allergic conditions in the patient and his family should be obtained, since the presence of bronchial asthma, allergic coryza, or hay fever in the antecedent or collateral members of the family furnishes evidence of the inherited nature of sensitivity[17,18] and strongly suggests that cutaneous tests will be of value. An inherited capacity for vigorous allergic response is usually present in food-sensitive cases with an immediate reaction time. Sensitivity in any form may show itself in other members of the family, and at times the same specific food cause and the same pattern of symptoms may persist through many generations. In La Roche's case,[44] members in 4 generations of a family developed acute gastrointestinal symptoms from the ingestion of eggs, and Spain[65] had a case where gastrointestinal allergy to milk was present in 3 successive generations.

A point of diagnostic importance is the character of the symptoms. They may be acute, explosive in nature, and even hazardous to life in the immediate reaction type; insidious and obscure, although severe, in the delayed reaction type. A description should be obtained of the frequency, intensity, and duration of the symptoms, their paroxysmal or continuous character, their relation to meals, and to the daily, weekly, or monthly routine of the patient. Such correlations may usually be established through the maintenance of a food diary. Usually, the more acute the attack, the more brief the reaction time. The length of the symptom-free periods between attacks depends upon the frequency of exposure to the food excitant. The attacks may be of a cumulative nature, as when a food eaten regularly, usually daily, becomes irritating only when the limit of tolerance is reached.

A characteristic of food allergy of the immediate reaction type is the fact that symptoms of overwhelming intensity may result from exposure to minute amounts of the food factor; here the symptoms speedily reach a crucial stage, marked by almost instantaneous nausea, vomiting, diarrhea, and asthma, and by ominous attacks of urticaria and angioedema. Individuals subject to attacks of such great intensity live in a continual state of dread and apprehension, due to the threat of sudden diarrhea, or of edema which may swiftly involve an area of such vital importance as the tongue or larynx. Such persons are usually quite aware of the inciting food cause, such as egg, nut, or a seed, but may be unable to avoid it completely, due to its presence in sauces, salads, or in a multiplicity of commercially prepared food mixtures. An exquisite degree of sensitiveness to egg has forced one patient to avoid all food and drink outside the home, and to use china and silverware kept constantly segregated from that employed in the household, for fear of contamination with egg in washings and handling. Such patients, fortunately rare, may have multiple abdominal scars, the results of repeated emergency operations necessitated by acute intestinal episodes, usually due to edema of the gut. In their abruptness and severity, the symptoms successfully mimic those of the acute surgical abdomen resulting from such varied causes as volvulus, intussusception, mesenteric thrombosis, biliary colic, and acute appendicitis. The surgeon, even if he is aware that the symptoms may be due to a food allergy, may be forced to operate in order to resolve the dilemma of whether food allergy or a surgically correctable crisis is responsible.

Both severity and periodicity of symptoms of food allergy may be influenced by other associated and intimately linked allergic conditions. Attacks of hay fever or bronchial asthma, for instance, may intensify the attacks of a food allergy or activate a latent food allergy. It is a frequent observation that hay fever patients are able to ingest without allergic discomfort such foods as peaches, melon, sweet corn, chocolate, or seafood, except during the hay fever season when they are contending with intense and disturbing symptoms of pollenosis. At these times, such food excitants may causes dermatitis, urticaria, bronchial asthma, or increased coryza. The skin tests are often positive to the exciting foods not only during the pollen periods, but nonseasonally.

In food allergy, as in other types of sensitivity and, indeed, in many other entirely different maladies, the frequency and severity of symptoms may be influenced by worry, anxiety, and states of physical stress. In searching for a diagnosis, the physician must be fully aware of the complexities produced by such psychosomatic factors. These are obviously operative in many individuals and may well prove an obstacle to improvement even where the physical factor, the offending food, is known. A young housewife whose urticarial attacks were identified by positive skin test as due to celery was able to eat it without ill effect once the problems of her household budget were solved. Occasional attacks occurred when celery was eaten at the first of the month, when the question of payment of bills was acute. Considerable time, effort, and patience must be expended by both physician and patient in collecting data on the dietary habits and reactions to food of the patient being studied. No filling of blank history forms, no pattern of routine questioning is sufficient, since problems in food allergy differ so considerably among themselves. Questioning and cross-questioning is essential, especially in those cases with a delayed reaction time and negative skin test results.[22] Such inquiry may offer the only clue to possible food factors. Foods notorious for their outstanding antigenic activity and for their high incidence as excitants should be particularly suspected. These are, in most instances, ingested uncooked, hence with their characteristic proteins unaltered by heat. They are: milk; eggs; seafood; nuts; seeds, as mustard; chocolate; orange; tomato. However, not only these but the individual items in all food groups, such as meats, seafood, fruits, vegetables, cereals, beverages, and spices, must be considered separately and in detail.

FOODS EATEN TO EXCESS. Patients may eat immoderate amounts of a food because of food fads, efforts to gain or lose weight on unbalanced diets, or to economize. Milk, tomato juice, orange juice, and chocolate are common offenders. A candidate for the football squad may drink several quarts of milk daily to gain weight; a dowager may consume excessive quantities of orange or tomato juice to lose weight; a stenographer may eat many chocolate bars to save lunch money. Such extremes may lead to food intolerance, where a moderate and less monotonous intake of the same foods would cause no discomfort.

FOODS EATEN THOUGH DISLIKED. Dislike of a food may be only a whim or a fancy, but it should be regarded as significant until proven otherwise. Aversion to egg or milk in children may be the result of Nature's protective effort, often misinterpreted by parents.

FOODS EATEN THOUGH CAUSING RECOGNIZED MILDLY RELATED ALLERGIC SYMPTOMS. A patient may be fully aware that a food, such as chocolate, may cause stomatitis, without realizing that it also produces his allergic headaches. Any food described as causing mildly associated effects should be placed on the suspect list.

FOODS EATEN THOUGH KNOWN TO HAVE CAUSED EARLIER, NOW ABSENT, FORMS OF SENSITIVITY. A patient may remember that in childhood a severe chronic dermatitis disappeared when a food such as egg was eliminated from the diet although its return to the diet in recent years was not followed by a reappearance of the dermatitis. It is not realized that the present allergic manifestation, such as colitis, may be the result of a less obvious sensitization to the same food.

FOODS EATEN THOUGH KNOWN TO CAUSE ALLERGIC SYMPTOMS IN ANOTHER MEMBER OF THE FAMILY. A familial allergy to a food such as egg or milk, in an antecedent or collateral member of the family, directs suspicion against this food as a cause of the patient's symptoms.

Such prolonged investigative procedures, applied to all types of foods, may often prove pleasurable and exciting to the patient who delights in discussing his diet, but they may prove wearisome to the physician; they are certainly not adaptable to mass production methods. Each patient is a separate and different problem, upon whom adequate information cannot be obtained in a few minutes or at a single visit. Only after the expenditure of considerable time and effort can satisfactory data be obtained.

The Immediate Reaction Type of Food Allergy. In this type, due to the brief interval between ingestion of the disturbing food and the occurrence of symptoms, the patient is able to inform the investigator at least partially of the exciting causes and of the degree to which they affect him. He may, however, be unaware of the importance of related, but possibly less disturbing food substances, or that certain preparations may contain a food he knows to be an offender. Thus, an individual may be conscientiously avoiding egg as such, while continuing to eat food mixes containing egg.

Upon skin test, definitely positive results are usually obtained with the extracts of those foods known to the patient for their immediate effect. As previously stated, such tests may be hazardous and should usually be avoided. Skin tests should be completed, however, with the extracts of other foods which may cause a definite but less obvious allergic disturbance.

Cutaneous Testing Procedures. *The Direct Method.* Whether the scarification or the intradermal technique be employed, the diagnostic skin testing procedure should not be attempted until the history has been completed. A full discussion of the methods of cutaneous testing of foods is not pertinent to this chapter and may be readily found in many textbooks on allergy. It should be mentioned, however, that frequently foods suspected and subsequently proven by clinical test to be authentic causes of immediate symptoms cannot be identified by skin test. Such negative effects are due in many instances to the disparity between the food as eaten, often altered by cooking, and the extract of it which is prepared from unheated material. Then, too, it may well be that many food extracts are rendered ineffective by changes resulting from the chemical manipulations essential to their preparation, and by changes occurring during storage. Also frequent are false positive reactions, due to nonspecific irritation of the cells of the skin.

The Indirect Method. Direct testing of the skin may be contraindicated due to wishes of the parents; the presence of eczematous or lichenified skin; or the threat of an extreme degree of sensitization. The sera from allergic persons of the immediately reacting type usually contain skin-sensitizing antibodies responsible for the development of the wheal characteristic of the positive test.[45] Such antibodies may be shifted to the skin of a normal individual by intracutaneously injected deposits of the allergic serum, conferring temporary and local sensitization to the food excitants which are disturbing to the patient. This phenomenon can usually be shown by the positive results upon testing the serum sites with specifically offending antigens. This procedure has its limitations, but is usually safe, although systemic reactions (vertigo, faintness, diarrhea, and oppression of the chest) have been known to occur in normal recipients in whom sites, made with serum from an exquisitely sensitive patient, were tested with extracts or excessive high potency.

The Specifically Restricted Diet. Foods which give a positive reaction in direct or indirect skin tests (as indicated by an immediate wheal with pseudopods, itching, and a surrounding zone of erythema) should be retested for verification; if the reaction is

again positive, they should be removed from the diet on the assumption that they are at least partially the cause of the patient's symptoms. He should be supplied with a written list not only of the foods banned, but of those permitted. A typed or printed form may be adjusted to each person's needs by crossing from the list all culpable foods that are to be avoided[46] (see Appendix, Table A-20). In the adult suffering from chronic bronchial asthma or chronic allergic enteritis or colitis, it is also advisable to have the patient avoid all flatulence-producing foods even though they are not incriminated as specific excitants.

Patients sensitive to milk, egg, wheat, or nuts must be cautioned against the use of many of the preparations and food mixes supplied by manufacturers. Such processed substances may contain the specific food excitants in quantities sufficient to produce allergic symptoms, as in the case of egg and milk in pancake mixes for home use. Since the labels on packages of such products list all the ingredients, the patient should be urged to develop the habit of reading all such labels as a protective measure. Fish-sensitive patients must be warned against acquiring the habit of licking labels. While adhesives used on postage stamps and many envelopes are not of fish origin, fish collagen is used as the adhesive upon some types of labels, stamps, and stickers.

In the diet prepared for the patient, rigid restrictions against more than one or two food items are rarely permanent. Early changes are often desirable in an effort to enlarge and simplify the diet. Once the patient becomes symptom-free, the banned foods are tried singly, at three-day intervals, in a trial-and-error procedure, as outlined subsequently. The problem of maintaining proper nutrition is simplified by providing the patient with data upon the mineral and vitamin content of important foods. Where added vitamin preparations are indicated, the synthetic varieties should be employed if possible.

The Delayed Reaction Type of Food Allergy. In those cases where the interval is prolonged, 4 to 72 hours elapsing between contact with the food and appearance of symptoms, not only is the cause usually unknown to the patient, but the allergic nature of the problem often is unknown, as well. Unfortunately in just these instances, where the skin testing procedure would be most helpful, it fails. In at least some instances, the negative results upon test are due to a lack of the proper antigen, which may not be the food itself but some digestive product requiring several hours for its appearance and its allergic effect upon the patient. This was true in Cooke's[47] case where allergic symptoms appeared several hours after the ingestion of milk. Skin tests were negative to milk itself but positive to the milk proteoses. Where neither history nor skin test affords information, but where there is reason to suspect an active food allergy, paroxysmal or continuous, an attempt at diagnosis should be made by food diary maintenance, dietary elimination, and trial-and-error methods

Food Diary. Entries should be made by the patient each day of the separate items of food, beverage, and drugs ingested at each meal, between each meal, and at bedtime. At the end of the day's entry, the patient should note any occurrence or continuance of his allergic symptoms. Once weekly the physician should attempt to correlate repetitive symptoms with repetitive ingested items, the interval of from 4 hours to 3 days being a constant for each suspected item. Should it be found, for instance, that headache occurred consistently on the third day following the ingestion of egg, that food should be suspected; but if the interval proved to vary, being 24 hours at some entries and 3 days at others, the case against egg would be weakened, as, too, it would be if headache did not occur in the majority of instances after egg was ingested. Foods suspected should be banned until subsequent verification of their allergenic importance can be attempted by trial-and-error procedure.

Simple Elimination Diets. The simplest attempt at elimination consists of removal from the diet of those foods most notorious as excitants: milk, egg (but not at the same time as milk), seafood, nuts, seeds, chocolate, orange, tomato. Care must be taken to explain to the patient the need for thorough avoidance, and he should be provided with a list of foods or food compounds in which the banned items

may be present in disguised form, as shown in Appendix, Table A-21, in the milk-poor, egg-poor, seafood-poor, wheat-poor, and nut-poor diets. Few patients object to abstinence from these food items for a 4-week period— usually sufficient for a proper evaluation. Occasionally, the chronic nature of the symptoms requires a longer period for evaluation. If promising results have been obtained from the restricted diet, the patient becoming symptom-free, the diet should be continued and, at intervals of 31 days, the several banned items should be tried separately; those showing negative results, usually the majority, should be returned to the diet.

Trial-and-Error Procedure. If the patient is so fortunate as to become symptom-free as a result either of this relatively simple dietary procedure, or of restrictions based on positive findings in the clinical history or skin test, an attempt should be made to verify the fact that the excluded foods were offenders. Each banned item, obtained from the original source and prepared as identically as possible, should be separately and cautiously introduced into the diet by feeding a small portion on an empty stomach, preferably 1 hour before the midday meal. It is helpful in eliminating the personal equation if the food can be given in a disguised form, so that the patient is unaware of its identity; however, this is often impossible. If no symptoms are induced, the food is tried again after an interval of three days, in double quantity. If no symptoms occur from the first and second attempt, it may be concluded that the food under study may be eaten without discomfort, at least in moderate amounts and infrequently, although it must be remembered that a cumulative effect is always possible. If symptoms appear, the suspected food is eliminated, to be tried again once the patient is symptom-free. The same or even a lesser amount of the food is to be eaten, depending upon the severity of the condition previously produced. The eliciting of symptoms typical of the patient's allergic complaint upon both first and second trials is presumptive evidence of a positive food cause if the patient was aware of the item under study; it may be considered positive proof if the food was fed in a disguised form. If either the first or second test alone be positive, further study is necessary.

The Rigidly Restricted Diet. When a relatively simple procedure is not successful, more austere methods may be necessary. The rigidly restricted diet is justified only in patients with severe, presumably allergic problems, such as recurrent headaches, urticaria, edema or colitis, and should not be employed in children, or in the severely ill. The choice of foods is limited to the specific items, but the quantities ingested are not curtailed. With symptoms occurring frequently, at daily or weekly intervals, the patient's preferences may be consulted in the selection, after the first day, of the three vegetables, the meat, and the three fruits to be studied. Beef or chicken may thus be substituted for lamb, and other vegetables and fruits for those listed for the first 5 days of the diet. If improvement in symptoms has occurred at the end of the week, additional food items may be attempted singly and at intervals of 3 days, by trial-and-error procedures, until the daily menu meets the nutritional requirements of the normal diet. If at the end of 2 weeks no improvement has occurred, the diet should be replaced with a similar one with entirely different food constituents. If this should prove unsuccessful, the presence of a food allergy is doubtful.

Where the symptoms ordinarily occur at intervals of 7 to 14 days or longer, symptom-free periods of 2 to 4 weeks are usually required to determine whether offending foods have been removed from the diet. In such instances, the elimination procedures of Rowe are most useful, having the advantage of offering specific dietary measures, pertinent menus[31] and recipes[48] as well. To the urban dweller, dependent upon restaurants for his meals, the use of these and all other types of restrictive diets poses a formidable problem.

Other Diagnostic Measures. No change in tissue function or tissue construction, temporary or permanent, is pathognomonic of food allergy. Food allergy is protean in its clinical manifestations and may mimic many other physical ailments due to entirely different causes. Even in gastrointestinal allergy of food origin where ingestion of a specifically exciting food produces sharp pathologic changes, demonstrable by roentgen ray such as edema of the mucous membrane, gastric retention and hypermobility with segmentation of the small intestine,[49-51] the effects are not diagnostic of allergy as pointed out by Cooke.[52]

There are no laboratory procedures of specific diagnostic importance. Even the demonstration of an eosinophilia may only suggest the presence of an allergic condition.

The Nonspecific Diet in Chronic Bronchial Asthma. The chronic adult sufferer from bronchial asthma, usually of infective origin, is frequently distressed by anorexia, nausea, abdominal distention, gaseous eructations and constipation. These disturbances he erroneously attributes to the presence of a food allergy, since the distress appears soon after a meal, and intensifies his asthmatic breathing by upward displacement of the diaphragm, with resulting diminution of the vital capacity. Such intestinal manifestations, together with constipation, are due to lowered gastrointestinal tone and are probably caused by anoxemia of the mucosa and muscularis,[52,53] as they are in congestive heart failure. Since the chronic asthmatic patient frequently suffers from an associated or secondary myocardial dysfunction, the avoidance of all flatus-producing foods is of the utmost importance. Legumes of all types, especially dried; the cabbage family; turnip; sweet potato; melon; chocolate; cheese; shellfood; nuts; and highly spiced, fried or greasy foods, including salad oils, are especially disturbing, as are carbonated beverages, artificially flavored juices, beer and ale (see Appendix, Table A-22).

The nonspecific diet is often applicable to adult cases with allergic intestinal conditions. In this diet, the restricted items are those which cause abdominal distention. The list of foods is quite similar to that prepared by Borborka[54] and mentioned by Bromer and Stroud[55] in their discussion of the dietary management of congestive heart failure. If there be any proven food excitant, it is of course also removed from the diet. Changes may be necessary in deference to any associated systemic disease such as nephritis, colitis, gastroenteritis, obesity, and rarely diabetes;

these conditions require restrictive diets of their own which usually should take precedence over the nonspecific diet here submitted, unless the two can be blended.

The asthmatic patient should eat lightly, in moderation, with between-meal supplements of fruit juices, tea, or milk, preferably fat-free. No food should be taken after 6 P.M., and he should abstain from any but the lightest foods during periods of mental stress, or acute asthmatic attacks. He should eat slowly, deliberately, and, since his ability to assimilate his food is greater in the mornings, he should make his breakfast and his lunch the chief meals of the day. A thirty-minute rest period after each meal is helpful.

Alcohol in moderate amounts is apparently helpful to the chronic allergic patient since, when taken before meals, it stimulates the appetite, eases tension, and, by the liberation of histamine, stimulates gastric secretion.[56] It is helpful in relieving the asthmatic attack and, before the advent of epinephrine and anti-asthmatic drugs, was habitually employed, especially taken hot, to control asthma[57]—a procedure which readily leads to its excessive use. Its ability to increase the permeability of the gastrointestinal mucosa may intensify the symptoms of food allergy, as is frequently observed when it is taken before a meal, and its influence in dilating the peripheral vascular system[58] may be the cause of temporarily increased nasal obstruction, coryza, and sneezing in the case of allergic coryza due to foods or to inhalants.

The Diet Indicated in Allergic Conditions. No rigid dietary measures can be established for the treatment of allergic disease, since its causes are multiple and its various manifestations may involve any of the major systems of the body. If the allergic disease is of nonfood origin no specific diet is necessary, unless one is required for an associated systemic disorder. If the allergic disease is the result of food sensitization, the diet should be one from which the foods identified as important causative factors have been banned. The nutritional requirements are the same as those of the normal nonallergic person. Far from being routine, the diet prescription for an allergic patient must be specific, individually modified and adjusted as the provocative food causes discovered may indicate.

THERAPY IN FOOD ALLERGY

Specific Measures. The complete and prolonged elimination from the diet of the identified incriminating food or foods constitutes the specific therapy in cases of food allergy. Immunization procedures with the food itself or its extract, orally or parenterally administered, are rarely successful and they are often dangerous, especially in the highly allergic individual. There should be proper substitution of other foods and the addition of necessary vitamins to maintain nutrition and to avoid monotony in the daily diet. Where food allergy is suspected and the cause has not been determined by history or skin tests, extensive trials with restricted diets, intentional feeding diets (trial-and-error procedure) and other established diets as previously outlined should be tried.

General Therapeutic Measures. The medications of value in the control of symptoms due to food allergy are the same as those used for similar symptoms in other allergic manifestations, regardless of cause. It is beyond the scope of this chapter to discuss in detail these medications and their use. Since, however, dietary measures must almost always be accompanied by some form of therapy, the most important agents will be mentioned.

Therapeutic Agents Useful in Acute Allergic Food Accidents. Although comparatively rare, unexpected allergic emergencies due to foods may sometimes involve even the most wary and experienced of patients, who are continually on their guard against chance contact with their specific food excitants. Swift, devastating, and extremely grave symptoms may result from a trace of egg in a food; mustard in salad, sauce or condiment; nut crumbs in pastry, ice cream or candy; or from accidental inhalation of the odor of a food, such as fish, banana, nut or celery. Before he realizes its nature, the fish-sensitive patient may receive parenterally a sclerosing agent of fish origin, or the egg-sensitive patient an egg-containing virus vaccine against influenza, Rocky Mountain spotted fever, typhus, or yellow fever; or the pork- or beef-sensitive patient may receive a highly disturbing injection of insulin or adreno-corticotropin (ACTH) or of liver extracts prepared from organs of the animal to whose proteins he is sensitive. Allergic reactions have been reported following the drinking of milk from cows who were given slow absorption penicillin because of mastitis. McLean[59] suggests therefore that the food and drug law be amended so that dairy cows producing milk are never given slow absorption penicillin and that milk should not be sold to the public from sick cows receiving penicillin or other antibiotics for at least 6 days from the last dose. Allergic reactions due to penicillin are appearing in increasing numbers and similar reactions following the administration of poliomyelitis vaccine which contains a small quantity of penicillin have occurred in extremely sensitive people.[60] While this is not directly a food problem, Rinkel[61] claims that it is closely related to certain foods, namely those containing yeast. He states that there is a synergism between various yeast-containing foods and a penicillin sensitization, which in some instances at least is the cause of long continued penicillin urticaria (due to cross sensitization among the molds). Therefore, penicillin-sensitive individuals should eliminate all foods containing yeast, including all fermented drinks, root beer, all cheeses, bread, vinegar and any of the cereal grain foods enriched with these products.

Ill-advised intravenous or clinical testing of the exquisitely sensitive allergic patient with his specific food excitant may swiftly cause overwhelming, even fatal effects; these may involve the respiratory, cutaneous and intestinal systems, as manifested in coryza, bronchial asthma, cyanosis, massive urticaria, edema of the lips, tongue, larynx and skin, and various gastrointestinal symptoms. In such accidents, time is of the essence. Epinephrine 1 to 1000, 0.2 to 0.5 ml, subcutaneously or intravenously, should be given and oxygen administered if available. Emergency hospitalization and tracheotomy may be required if there is edema of the larynx and asphyxia threatens.[62] Ephedrine and antihistaminic drugs are ineffectual in such situations, and the steroid hormones are often too slow in their action requiring a few hours to a day or two before their effect is produced. However, intravenous therapy with 100 mg of Solu-cortef should act rapidly enough to meet the emergency in addition to the immediate use of adrenalin. Antihistamines, epinephrine, ephedrine and oral steroids should sustain control once the critical stage has passed.[63] Morphine in 16-mg ($\frac{1}{4}$-grain) hypodermic doses may be used to control pain due to intestinal or uterine spasm, provided the possibility of an acute surgical abdomen can be excluded. Morphine is contraindicated if the patient gives evidences of respiratory distress.

Therapeutic Agents Useful in the Common Forms of Food Allergy. The antihistaminic preparations in doses recommended by their makers are especially helpful in relieving pruritus and edema of food origin, whether the distress be in the respiratory, alimentary, or cutaneous systems. Food-provoked allergic rhinitis,[64] allergic bronchitis, and even bronchial asthma (except the severe type) respond swiftly to the oral administration of antihistaminic preparations. Nausea, abdominal distention, diarrhea, and acute distress of the intestine and colon due to food allergy may often be satisfactorily controlled by these agents, as well as the pruritus and congestion of allergic dermatitis, urticaria, and angioedema. Many food-sensitive patients, fearful of attending dinner parties or banquets where their exciting agents may be served in hidden or masked forms, are reassured by the presence in purse or pocket of an antihistaminic drug.

In some instances the administration of antihistamines has been followed by numerous side reactions. All preparations are capable of producing some degree of somnolence in some persons. Additional side reactions vary with the individual and with the dose and include drowsiness, vomiting, dryness of the mouth, constipation, confusion, urinary frequency, excitability and loss of judgment. Various cutaneous manifestations have also been reported. Isolated cases of respiratory distress and more serious blood dyscrasias have been described.[65] The topical use of the antihistaminic drugs and of local anesthetics for the erythema and pruritus of allergic skin disorders should be avoided, since it has been shown that sensitization to them may be induced by their repeated application in a cream or ointment base to the skin, especially if it be inflamed or fissured.

Epinephrine, 1 to 1000, 0.3 to 1.0 ml, by subcutaneous injection, is useful in controlling the immediate and severe symptoms which follow the ingestion of a specific food excitant, whether they be those of coryza, bronchial asthma, urticaria, angioedema, or gastroenteritis. Where the symptoms are stubborn or protracted, epinephrine 1 to 500, 0.5 to 1 ml by subcutaneous injection in a slowly absorbed vehicle such as oil or gelatin,[66] is helpful; the latter vehicle is preferable where a nut or seed sensitiveness is suspected. Epinephrine 1 to 100, by nebulization, may offer relief in acute cases.

Ephedrine sulfate, 8 mg ($\frac{1}{8}$ gr), in children, or 25 mg ($\frac{3}{8}$ gr) in the adult, administered orally each 2 to 6 hours, is useful in respiratory distress; it is of little value in controlling allergic symptoms of the gastrointestinal, cutaneous, or other systems. The addition of phenobarbital in amounts equal to the ephedrine will often lessen the nervous tension produced by the latter drug.

Aminophyllin is useful in asthmatic attacks of food origin. It may be given orally each 4 to 6 hours, 0.05 gm ($\frac{3}{4}$ gr) in the child, 0.1 gm ($1\frac{1}{2}$ gr) in the adult. Aminophyllin is also available in suppository form. In acute cases it may be given intravenously each 8 to 24 hours, 0.1 gm ($1\frac{1}{2}$ gr) in the child, 0.25 gm ($3\frac{3}{4}$ gr) in the adult.

Hydrocortisone sodium succinate (Solucortef), 100 mg, and methylprednisolone sodium succinate (Solu-medrol), 40 mg, each 6 hours are given until symptoms subside, then gradually reduced according to clinical response in massive urticaria and angioedema. The steroids, given orally, may be equally effective though not as promptly. The initial daily dose of the steroid is gradually lessened, being discontinued within 7 to 10 days. In chronic debilitating cases of urticaria or angioedema due to unidentified causes, maintenance doses of the steroids may be required for much longer periods. Newer steroids have been developed during the past several years

with the aim of increasing their potency, lessening the dosage and minimizing their side effects. The currently available synthetic analogues of cortisone and hydrocortisone have as yet failed to demonstrate any physiologic effects not manifested by the parent fraction but the intensity of their biologic actions and the ratio of glucocorticoid to mineralocorticoid effects are altered. Corticosteroid therapy is not a substitute for specific treatment of allergic conditions and should be administered as a supplement to immunologic management and other well-established symptomatic measures. The steroids should be reserved for acute allergic states of a life-threatening nature, such as intractable asthma, severe serum sickness, acute angioedema in the vicinity of the glottis and drug reactions. Contraindications to the use of ACTH, corticotropins and the corticosteroids have been widely publicized. They include hypertension, diabetes, pulmonary tuberculosis (active or inactive), peptic ulcer and psychic states. Treatment with the steroids must be individualized and the well-known precautions and complications incident to their use should receive close attention.[76]

Belladonna, atropine, and products with an atropine-like effect, often combined with a barbiturate, are useful in controlling the abdominal distress resulting from the spastic intestinal muscle of allergic as well as of non-allergic origin. Paregoric is helpful in controlling the diarrhea due to food allergy; while the use of secobarbital sodium (Seconal sodium), pentobarbital sodium (Nembutal), or sodium bromide may permit a night's rest in the presence of an aggravating pruritus. Topical applications of some phenol-containing preparation may allay the itching.

Tranquilizing drugs are being used alone or in combination with other drug therapy for the relief of urticaria, anxiety, tension and insomnia in patients suffering from allergic manifestations due to foods or other causes. While these drugs are helpful in allaying some of the stress problems of the allergic patient they must be administered with caution as side reactions have been reported following their use.

The use of aspirin to relieve pain should never be suggested to the allergic person until it is quite clear that it is well tolerated. Severe, even lethal effects may be produced in the allergic by as little as 0.3 gm (5 gr). Aspirin is often present inconspicuously in the multitude of antipain and "anticold" medications and nostrums.

BIBLIOGRAPHY

1. Rosenau and Anderson: Hyg. Lab. Bull., No. 29, 1906, U.S. Govt. Printing Office.
2. Walzer: J. Immunol., *14*, 143, 1927.
3. Walzer and Walzer: Am. J. Med. Sci., *173*, 279, 1927.
4. Zinsser: *Resistance to Infectious Diseases*, New York, The Macmillan Co., 1931.
5. Ratner, Jackson and Gruehl: J. Immunol., *14*, 249, 1927.
5a. Ishizaka and Ishizaka: J. Immunol., *99*, 1187, 1967.
5b. Ishizaka, Ishizaka, Gunvar *et al.*: J. Immunol., *102*, 884, 1969.
6. Baldwin: J. Immunol., *13*, 345, 1927.
7. Coca, Walzer and Thommen: *Asthma and Hay Fever*, London, Bailliere, Tindall & Cox, 1931.
8. Anderson and Schloss: Am. J. Dis. Child., *26*, 451, 1923.
9. Gillette: J.A.M.A., *50*, 40, 1908.
10. Weaver: Arch. Int. Med., *3*, 485, 513, 1909.
11. Billard: Compt. rend. Soc. de Biol., *73*, 462, 1912.
12. Bernard, Debre and Porak: J. physiol., et path. gen., *14*, 971, 1912.
13. Ratner and Gruehl: J. Clin. Invest., *13*, 517, 1934.
14. Fink and Quinn: J. Immunol., *70*, 61, 1953.
15. Glaser and Johnstone: J.A.M.A., *153*, 620, 1953.
16. Cooke: *Allergy in Theory and Practice*, Philadelphia, W. B. Saunders Co., 1947.
17. Cooke and VanderVeer: J. Immunol., *1*, 201, 1916.
18. Spain and Cooke: J. Immunol., *9*, 521, 1924.
19. O'Keefe: Boston Med. Surg. J., *185*, 194, 1921.
20. Donnally: J. Immunol., *9*, 15, 1930.
21. Cooke: Am. J. Med., *3*, 523, 1947.
22. Spain: Proc. Connecticut M. Soc., *141*, 105, 1933.
23. Chobot: *Pediatric Allergy*, New York, McGraw-Hill Book Co., Inc., p. 3, 1951.
24. Rinkel: *Food Allergy*, Springfield, Charles C Thomas, 1951.
25. Rowe and Rowe: California Med., *69*, 261, 1948.
26. Stoesser: Minnesota Med., *23*, 412, 1943.
27. Ratner and Untracht: Am. J. Dis. Child., *63*, 309, 1952.
28. Clein: Ann. Allergy, *9*, 195, 1951.
28a. Heiner, Wilson, and Lahey: J.A.M.A., *189*, 568, 1964.
29. Glaser and Johnstone: Ann. Allergy, *10*, 443, 1952.
30. Ratner: In *Current Therapy*, Ed. by Conn, p. 506, Philadelphia, W. B. Saunders Co., 1953.
31. Rowe: *Elimination Diets and the Patient's Allergies*, 2nd ed., Philadelphia, Lea & Febiger, 1944.
32. Cannon: J. Immunol., *44*, 107, 1942.
33. Kolmer: In *Dietotherapy*, edited by Wohl, pp. 519–520, Philadelphia, W. B. Saunders Co., 1945.
34. Moen and Reimann: Arch. Int. Med., *51*, 789, 1933.
35. Richardson: J. Clin. Invest., *19*, 239, 1940.
36. Bates and Weiss: Am. J. Dis. Child., *62*, 346, 1941.
37. Wohl, Waife, Green and Clough: Proc. Soc. Exper. Biol. Med., *70*, 305, 1949.
38. Fries and Borne: Ann. Int. Med., *38*, 928, 1953.
39. Feingold: J. Pediat., *34*, 545, 1949.
40. Berg: J. Allergy, *2*, 54, 1930.
41. Fries, Borne and Barnes: J. Pediat., *32*, 532, 1948.
42. Selye: *The Physiology and Pathology of Exposure to Stress*, p. 22, Montreal, Acta, Inc., 1950.
43. Kirkendall, Hodges and January: J. Lab. Clin. Med., *37*, 771, 1951.
44. LaRoche, Richetfils and Saint-Girosis: *Alimentary Anaphylaxis*, Berkeley, Calif., University of California Press, 1930. Translated by Rowe and Rowe.
45. Prausnitz and Küstner: Centralbl. F. Bakt., *86*, 160, 1921.
46. Spain: *Food Allergy in Current Therapy*, Ed. by Conn, p. 500, Philadelphia, W. B. Saunders Co., 1953.
47. Cooke: Ann. Int. Med., *16*, 71, 1942.
48. Rowe: In *Dietotherapy*. Ed. by Wohl, p. 699, Philadelphia, W. B. Saunders Co., 1945.
49. Fries and Zizmor: Am. J. Dis. Child., *54*, 1239, 1937.
50. Fries and Mogil: J. Allergy, *14*, 310, 1943.
51. Fries: J. Allergy, *23*, 39, 1952.
52. Cooke: *Allergy in Theory and Practice*, p. 392, Philadelphia, W. B. Saunders Co., 1947.
53. Crisler, Van Liere and Booher: Am. J. Physiol., *102*, 629, 1932.
54. Borborka: *Treatment by Diet*, Ed. 4th Philadelphia, J. B. Lippincott Co., 1939.
55. Bromer and Stroud: In *Dietotherapy*, Ed: by Wohl, p. 673, Philadelphia, W. B. Saunders Co., 1945.
56. Beazell and Ivy: Quart. J. Studies in Alcohol, *1*, 45, 1940.
57. Salter: *Asthma*, New York, Wood & Co., 1882, p. 108.
58. Musser: In *Dietotherapy*, p. 512, Ed. by Wohl, Philadelphia, W. B. Saunders Co., 1945.
59. McLean: Arch. Pediat., *73*, 276, 1956.
60. Lippman: G. P., *15*, 94, 1957.

61. Rinkel: Trans. Amer. Acad. Opth. and Othol., 60, 475, 1956.
62. Fuchs: N.Y. State J. Med., 56, 2529, 1956.
63. Michelson and Lowell: N. Eng. J. Med., 258, 994, 1958.
64. Spain, Strauss and Fuchs: J. Allergy, 10, 209, 1939.
65. Harris and Shure: Practical Allergy, Philadelphia, F. A. Davis Co., p. 335, 1957.
66. Zeligman: J.A.M.A., 149, 263, 1952.

Chapter

34

Nutrition and Diseases of the Skin

W. A. KREHL

INTRODUCTION

What is so desired as a clear, soft, unblemished skin of fine, smooth texture—not too dry or too moist? "The skin you love to touch" is the goal for which millions are spent each year for myriad kinds of cosmetic, soaps, salves, vibrators, mud packs, etc. ad nauseum.

From primitive times, man has related the gloss and sheen of the hair coat and skin of his pets and herds with good dietary practices and good general health. In experimental nutrition studies, a change in the hair coat and skin of animals has often been the first and most outstanding feature of deficiency disease. Unfortunately, these skin and hair changes are so nonspecific that they rarely permit a specific diagnosis of an isolated nutritional deficiency. However, because these skin changes have appeared with poor diet, dermatologists have naturally been much influenced by the use of special diets, vitamins and minerals in nearly every conceivable dosage level and combination in an attempt to manage and treat skin diseases. Since accurate diagnosis is difficult under such conditions and since many skin diseases are of unknown etiology, much of this form of therapy has been doomed to failure and, indeed, has tended to place the role of nutrition in the therapy of skin disease in disrepute.

While dermatoses related to dietary deficiency states can appear on any part of the body, they do for the most part tend to be located over areas of irritation or excessive stimulation. Lesions are most apt to appear on the backs of the hands, on the front and backs of the wrists, on the elbows, over the face, around the neck, under the breasts, over the knees and feet, and in the perianal region. These lesions are often bilaterally symmetrical and tend to be separated from healthier appearing skin by a sharp line of demarcation. They are generally accompanied by burning, itching, and pain.[1]

The skin area in the average adult is about 1.75 square meters of a tough, yet resilient, double layered structure of skin which is the principal line of defense against the entrance of foreign substances and protects against almost every conceivable physical and chemical stress. When damaged, it has remarkable ability to repair itself, thus reflecting its dynamic metabolic activity. Through its sweat glands and blood vessels, the skin provides the principal means by which the body heat is regulated and through its nerve endings permits sensation of contact with the external environment perceiving heat, cold, pain and other stimuli. The skin also reflects the emotions, such as embarrassment, fear, anger, anxiety and, unfortunately, a person's age as well. We are even individualized by characteristic skin markings—our fingerprints.

A brief review of the structure and physiology of the skin may be helpful in understanding the changes that take place in skin diseases.[2,3] The skin is composed of three principal layers: (*a*) epidermis; (*b*) corium (dermis or true skin); and (*c*) the subcutaneous tissue.

The epidermis is a thin layer averaging about 0.2 mm in thickness, in which the greatest metabolic activity of the skin is

941

located. From the outside inward, the epidermis is composed of cell layers, i.e. (a) stratum corneum, (b) stratum granulosum, (c) prickle cell layer, and (d) the basal cell layer. Melanocytes, responsible for the production of skin pigment, are found in the basal cell layer. The epidermis overlies the corium or dermis in a wave-like pattern. The principal metabolic activity of the epidermis is the production of the protein keratin, which is the chief component of the stratum corneum layer. Keratin, by its toughness, elasticity and resistance to chemical change, provides great protection. It is structurally integrated into the flat, shrunken, non-nucleated dead cells of the stratum corneum. The process of keratinization is, therefore, concerned with the production of keratin and the gradual elaboration and replacement of the stratum corneum from the basal cell layer of the epidermis. This response is continuous and may vary with the stimuli on the epidermis.

There are two kinds of skin appendages derived from the epidermis: (a) glandular, i.e. apocrine and eccrine sweat glands, and sebaceous glands; and (b) keratinized structures, i.e. the hair follicles and hair and the nails.

The corium or secondary protective layer supports the vascular bed and peripheral nerves of the skin and the epidermal appendages. The corium is also a large potential storehouse for water, blood and electrolytes. This is well exemplified in the individual with edema.

The subcutaneous tissue provides further support and is an excellent heat insulator, a good shock absorber, and a storehouse of calories in the form of fat.

There is little doubt that the normal defense mechanisms of the skin are disrupted and break down in states of malnutrition.[4] Many of the cutaneous signs of malnutrition are characterized by inadequate or inappropriate response to mechanical, thermal or action trauma or a lack of the normal defense mechanisms against infection. Clinical examples of dermatoses which exemplify these skin changes are tropical ulcers and the skin changes of ariboflavinosis and pellagra. The localization and the morphology of these dermatoses are strongly influenced by the breakdown of skin defenses in association with inadequate intake and absorption or utilization of nutrients. Specific nutrient deficiencies may prevent the synthesis of substances which are necessary to the growth and function of the skin and its appendages.

It must also be recognized that there may be very significant cutaneous losses of nutrients; in particular, the increased losses of nitrogen, calcium, magnesium and other minerals with profuse sweating and chronic exfoliative diseases need to be considered. The importance of malnutrition occurring following extensive burns, and bullous dermatoses due to serum loss has great importance.[5-8]

PROTEIN DEFICIENCY

The proteins of plasma, especially albumin, exert an essential osmotic influence on preventing the loss of water from the vascular system. Any clinical circumstance in which the plasma level of albumin falls much below 2.5 grams per 100 cc leads to the development of edema. An adequate level of dietary protein of good biological value should be achieved in any therapeutic regimen in an edematous person with hypoalbuminemia. However, in severe cirrhosis of the liver where the ability to metabolize amino acids is seriously impaired, protein must be used with great caution to prevent the development of hepatic coma.

It has also been shown that long exposure to experimental diets low in protein results in extensive skin changes. These changes are characterized by dryness, scaliness, inelasticity, and a gray, pallid appearance, suggestive of old age. Also noticed is a blotchy, dirty, brownish pigmentation, which may appear anywhere on the body, but is generally most often seen on the face.[9]

Widespread throughout the technically underdeveloped areas of the world, and especially in children between the ages of 1 to 4, is a protein deficiency manifested in the extreme by the disease known as kwashiorkor. This disease is characterized by faulty growth, marked liver enlargement with fatty infiltration, gastrointestinal disturbances, including diarrhea, and extensive skin changes with hypopigmentation and dryness of the hair and skin.[10] Therapy for this disease is an adequate amount of protein, particularly of animal origin, although mixtures of selected vegetable protein prove quite satisfactory. The important question here is how to get into the basic diet of millions of people enough protein of proper nutritional value. This is undoubtedly the single most challenging problem to our nutritionists, economists, agriculturists, and public health workers.

LIPIDS

Several types of skin lesions, eczematous in character, have been associated with the long-term consumption of diets low in fat.[11] It has also been noted that individuals who have excessive fat losses associated with idiopathic steatorrhea frequently have erythematous eczematous lesions.[12] Difficulties arise, however, in attempting to correlate these skin lesions with any specific biochemical abnormality. For example, while there is no significant difference between the level of total blood lipids of eczematous and noneczematous infants, it has been shown that the amount of unsaturated fatty acids is considerably lower in eczematous infants, particularly the levels of arachidonic and linoleic acid.[13] This observation has encouraged the use of fats and oils rich in these two substances in the treatment of eczema in infants—unfortunately, not with uniformly good results.

Studies on the disease phrynoderma or hyperkeratosis follicularis have shown that the increased incidence of this disease is correlated with a lowered intake of essential fatty acids. While vitamin A has often been proposed in the treatment of this disease, it has been effective in relatively few cases. However, recent studies in India, where this disease is common, have shown that the administration of raw linseed oil or linoleic acid produced marked clinical improvement in two to four weeks and cured many patients in four to twenty-four weeks.[14] Even better results were obtained when pyridoxine was combined with the essential fatty acid therapy of phrynoderma.

It has been demonstrated[15] that patients with phrynoderma have significantly higher levels of trienoic acid and the ratio of trienoic to tetraenoic acids (a parameter of essential fatty acid nutritional status) in plasma was also significantly higher than for control subjects. This affords a further suggestion that phrynoderma is a manifestation of essential fatty acid deficiency and vitamins of the B-complex group (B_6 particularly) may play a significant role in the etiology and treatment of the condition.

In view of the fact that vitamin A in huge doses has been used in the treatment of certain dermatological lesions, a word of caution must be raised. Doses of 50,000 or more units per day may produce signs and symptoms of vitamin A intoxication which, in fact, resemble the lesions of vitamin A deficiency as far as the skin is concerned. In addition, bone changes take place, which reduce their density and make them brittle.

Obesity and Skin Disease. The obese patient seems to be excessively plagued with skin disorders. With obesity, one has excessive fat folds with resultant intertrigo, caused primarily by friction between the skin surfaces and by the maceration of the skin from accumulated moisture in these folds. These changes often lead to infection, particularly with staphylococcal organisms or to fungal diseases, such as dermatophytosis and moniliasis. In addition, many obese patients activate a latent diabetic tendency with all of the accompanying dermatoses associated with diabetes. Obese people, because of their thick subcutaneous layers of fat, tend to become overheated easily and sweat more profusely. This produces undesirable effects on normal skin, exaggerating areas of inflammation and skin rashes. Prickly heat or miliaria rubra is a commonly recognized evidence of sweat retention. Obviously, the therapy for this problem is correction of obesity by decreased caloric intake and increased exercise (see Chapter 22).

VITAMINS AND SKIN DISEASE

The search for vitamins has always captured the imagination of the research scientist and because deficiencies of these substances werc so often associated with skin and hair changes in experimental animals, it was an easy transition from animals to man by dermatologists and physicians eager to treat difficult dermatological problems. Hence, vitamins in every form, combination and dosage level have been used in the treatment of skin diseases with a great variety of results. These are characterized mostly by their inconsistency. The question most often raised is whether more vitamins are needed than are ordinarily present in a well-balanced diet. Frankly, there is no easy answer to this question, but it should be remembered that in skin disease as with disease in general, there is tissue pathology and presumably accompanying abnormal metabolism. Certainly adequate vitamin intake must be insured, which is most easily done by appropriate vitamin supplementation. Danger lies, however, in over-zealous specific claims for "skin cures" effected by vitamins since many dermatological problems improve without therapy and for no known reason. Certainly, claims for vitamin therapy must be made only after the closest control of experimental or clinical studies and the most conservative judgment must be exercised.

Vitamin A. Since vitamin A is intimately concerned in the maintenance of normal cell structure, one of the most characteristic changes seen in vitamin A deficiency is disintegration of epithelial surfaces followed by their replacement with a keratinized stratified epithelium.

In man, lack of vitamin A[16] may result in dryness, scaliness, furunculosis, and abscesses of the scalp and in bleaching, drying out or loss of the hair. The follicular lesions, which are most helpful in establishing diagnosis, vary in size, the maximum diameter being 5 mm. They are hard, deeply pigmented, and surrounded by a zone of pigmentation. The center of the lesion, the papule, is a scaly, pointed plug of keratinized epithelium, which, if pressed out, leaves a crater. Though comedones are common on the face, the keratinized lesions do not occur there; hence, the two are never associated, though both respond promptly to treatment with vitamin A. Histologic examination shows hyperplasia and hyperkeratinization of the related epithelium around the hair follicles, together with metaplastic changes of the sweat ducts and degeneration of the glands, accounting for the dryness of the skin. As might be anticipated, skin lesions associated with a deficient intake of vitamin A respond to therapy with this vitamin.

The use of vitamin A in the treatment of other diseases associated with excessive keratinization, particularly those involving the hair follicle, has not always yielded consistently beneficial results. This therapy has shown to be of some therapeutic value, however, in the treatment of pityriasis rubra pilaris and Darier's disease. While such treatment may provide symptomatic improvement, it is rarely curative. Again, as pointed out above, one must warn against the long-term dosage of massive amounts of vitamin A.[17] This is a potentially toxic material.

Of interest also, is the fact that an excessive intake of pro-vitamin A, carotene, produces a yellowish discoloration of the skin and carotenemia. This, at first glance, may be confused with jaundice. It represents an inability of the body to convert carotene rapidly enough to vitamin A in the face of a large carotene intake.

Vitamin B Complex Deficiencies. Experimental animal studies in which deficiencies of nearly all of the B complex vitamins have been established are all associated with some skin or hair changes ranging from mild to severe. The correlation between these changes noted in animals and various dermatological lesions seen in man remains unclear. Riboflavin, niacin, pyridoxine, and possibly pantothenic acid are the members of the B complex group of vitamins that have clinical dermatological significance for man.

Riboflavin. The symptoms of riboflavin deficiency may be divided into three groups—oral, cutaneous and ocular.[18] The oral changes are angular stomatitis and cheilosis and are not alone characteristic of riboflavin deficiency; other possible causes of these lesions must be ruled out. Tongue changes are noted in riboflavin deficiency, particularly characterized by purplish or magenta glossitis.[19] The dermatitis of riboflavin deficiency is primarily a seborrheic dermatitis with many fine greasy scales on an erythematous base.

Of considerable interest are the results of studies on nutrition in the Far East by Pollack and his co-workers.[20] These studies, carried out on Chinese Nationalist Army troops on Taiwan, clearly indicate a very high incidence of riboflavin deficiency and an interesting syndrome called the oral-genital syndrome has been described. A very high incidence of scrotal dermatitis was observed in those individuals who also had angular stomatitis, cheilosis, magenta tongue, and nasolabial seborrhea. When the biochemical findings in blood and urine were correlated with the clinical findings in the oral-genital syndrome, it was evident that a riboflavin deficiency was involved. Niacin deficiency was also noted in significant numbers in this study. Enrichment of the rice in the diet with riboflavin and niacin rapidly eliminated the signs attributable to the deficiency of these vitamins. It is now becoming more evident from nutrition surveys conducted in many areas of the world that riboflavin deficiency is one of the most common seen.

All cracks in the corners of the mouth are not due to vitamin deficiencies. In fact, most are not. The administration of riboflavin even for prolonged periods does not cure perleche. Perleche might be confused with lichen planus, discoid lupus erythematosus, and leukoplakia as well as other causes, such as physical and chemical trauma and irritation.

Niacin Deficiency—Pellagra. The earliest symptoms of pellagra may involve either the skin or the gastrointestinal tract. Premonitory evidence of skin involvement may appear as a temporary redness like that of sunburn; it clears up without a trace only to return later in severer degree. Earliest lesions are usually macular, of a light or dark red color, but these coalesce and form a dark red or purplish eruption followed by desquamation. The areas involved are those of friction and exposure. The face, neck, hands, forearms and feet are the usual sites. This early eruption may be accompanied by considerable swelling of the involved parts. In severe cases, bullae may be present, but usually these dry up, leaving crusts, though

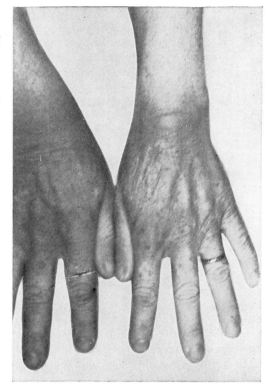

Fig. 34-1. Glove-like pigmentation of the hands in pellagra.

they may of course become infected. Ulceration has been known to occur. A highly characteristic feature of the erythema and subsequent pigmentation is the occurrence of sharp margination of the wrist or forearm producing the so-called "pellagrous glove" (Fig. 34–1). The skin manifestations present three stages: (1) congestion; (2) thickening and pigmentation; (3) atrophic thinning. Subjective symptoms are usually slight; and they consist chiefly of a burning sensation rather than an itching.

The mucous membranes are also involved. The tongue becomes swollen and denuded and is often brilliant red in color. The buccal mucous membrane may, in severe cases, have a similar appearance; the redness may at times extend to the lips, too. Sometimes the oral commissures become fissured.

Thousands of pellagrous patients have now been treated with niacin or niacinamide. Doses up to 1,000 mg daily may be safely administered, although the average dose is 100 mg t.i.d. In a day or two, the redness of the oral, pharyngeal, and vaginal mucous membranes is reduced; nausea, vomiting, and excessive salivation decrease; and bowel movements become normal. Unless the continuity of the skin is broken, the acute red lesions fade rapidly. The acute mental symptoms, varying from confusion to delirium and mania, usually disappear quickly. The addition of vitamin B_1 is necessary to improve symptoms due to involvement of the peripheral nervous system. Riboflavin may be required if there is clinical evidence of an associated riboflavin deficiency.

Diets in which corn predominates are prone to lead to niacin deficiency and pellagra especially if these diets are inadequate in proteins that contain tryptophan.[21] The niacin requirement is significantly affected by the amount of tryptophan in the diet since this amino acid is metabolically converted by the body to niacin. The approximate dietary replacement ratio is 50 or 60 mg of tryptophan to 1 mg of niacin.

Another interesting aspect of nicotinic acid therapy is the dermatological effect of producing a marked cutaneous vasodilatation with extensive flushing of the skin. This characteristic is not shared by nicotinamide.

Vitamin B_6. The effects of pyridoxine deficiency in a number of dermatoses have been studied and it is reported that certain kinds of eczema, particularly eczema of the seborrheic type, may improve, after having failed to respond to local treatment, when pyridoxine is given intravenously or subcutaneously in rather large doses of 24 to 50 mg.[22] Pyridoxine deficiency has been produced in human subjects by the use of pyridoxine antagonists and in association with this deficiency there is seen a seborrhea-like lesion about the eyes, nasolabial fold and mouth, with extension to the eyebrows and skin behind the ears. Many of these cases of seborrheic dermatitis responded well to the local application of pyridoxine in an ointment base, while but little effect was noted when the vitamin was given orally or parenterally.[23]

Vitamin C. In vitamin C deficiency there is impairment of the structure of the ground substance of the connective tissue and in scurvy the skin may show secondary changes, such as petechial hemorrhage and inelasticity. Ascorbic acid is also concerned with the metabolism of the amino acids tyrosine and phenylalanine, which are precursor substances for the formation of the melanin pigments of the skin.

Therapy with vitamin C has been proposed for a variety of skin diseases, such as allergic contact dermatitis, atopic dermatitis, psoriasis, and acne vulgaris. Unless there is associated vitamin C deficiency, no benefit is derived from the use of this vitamin in the specific treatment of the above conditions.

Pantothenic Acid, Inositol, p-Aminobenzoic Acid and Biotin. Experiments reported by Woolley[24] have shown that pantothenic acid has an influence on the growth of hair. It has also been shown that a deficiency of pantothenic acid is a factor in the graying of hair and that pantothenic acid improved the skin and decreased graying of the fur of experimental animals.[25,26] Unna, Richards and Sampson[27] have found that black rats fed a synthetic diet deficient in pantothenic acid become gray in from four to six weeks. Pantothenic acid at a level of 100 mg a day will prevent or cure this condition. On the other hand, Williams[28] found pantothenic acid to be without effect on the graying of hair. There is no evidence that pantothenic acid acts in human beings as it seems to act in various animals.

Little is known about inositol; its relation to human nutrition is still a subject for investigation. Considerable interest has been aroused by the investigations of Woolley[29] who has shown that inositol will cure alopecia in mice.

Thirty-three patients with lupus erythematosus were given 1 to 4 gm of para-aminobenzoic acid (PABA) at two- to three-hour intervals by Zarafonetis.[30] Two of 10 with chronic discoid lupus showed no improvement; 1 patient had a poor response and 7 good to excellent responses. Improvement occurred in all of 7 patients with scleroderma, the sclerodermatous areas gradually softening and becoming thinner and more pliable. PABA produced improvement in 5 patients with dermatitis herpetiformis. Toxic hepatitis, drug fever and nausea and vomiting may occasionally result from PABA, and much more careful work must be done before any serious recommendations can be made for its use in dermatological conditions.

Biotin-deficient rats develop marked loss of hair with erythema of the underlying skin. Marked periorbital hair loss is also noted which may represent in part a complication from inositol deficiency. No counterpart deficiency has been demonstrated in man.

Vitamin K, Vitamin E and Vitamin D. A deficiency of vitamin K resulting in impaired synthesis of prothrombin may result in a cutaneous purpura reflecting impairment of the coagulation mechanism.

No clear-cut cutaneous manifestations are associated with vitamin E deficiency. Indeed, only recently has this vitamin been recognized as being essential for man. As the intake of essential fatty acids increases, the need for a greater dietary supply of vitamin E becomes evident. Many oils that are recommended in substantial amounts in the management of certain skin diseases may increase the need for vitamin E in the diet. Fortunately, most vegetable oils are in fact good sources of vitamin E.

Vitamin D, the so-called "sunshine vitamin" is produced in the skin where solar rays from the far-ultraviolet region of the spectrum (wavelength, 290 to 390 millimicrons) convert the provitamin 7-dehydrocholesterol into natural vitamin D_1. A fascinating hypothesis has been put forward suggesting that variation in solar ultraviolet at different latitudes may have caused racial differentiation in man through the mechanism of skin pigment regulation of vitamin D biosynthesis in man. "The known correlation between the color of human skin and latitude is explainable in terms of two opposing positive adaptations to solar ultraviolet radiation, weak in northern latitudes in winter yet powerful the year around near the equator." . . . "Selection against the twin dangers of rickets on the one hand and toxic doses of vitamin D on the other hand would thus explain the world-wide correlations observed between skin pigmentation and nearness to the equator."[31]

Side Effects of Vitamin Therapy. Certain undesirable cutaneous side effects may be associated with the use of vitamins. These are for the most part allergic in character. Thiamin may cause urticaria, angioneurotic edema, pruritus and contact dermatitis. Niacin produces marked erythema, peripheral vasodilation and pruritus. This is quite a common reaction noted in patients who are given niacin to attempt to lower the blood cholesterol. Cutaneous reaction to niacin, interestingly, is not seen with niacinamide, which, incidentally, does not lower blood cholesterol levels.

Vitamin B_{12}, which contains cobalt, may cause reactions in cobalt-sensitive patients, especially when given by the parenteral route.

As might be expected, vitamins like other chemical substances might be anticipated to cause allergic reactions with dermatological manifestations in a certain number of individuals. Fortunately, the incidence is quite insignificant.

DIET AND OTHER DERMATOLOGICAL PROBLEMS

Allergy. Food allergy may be the cause of many skin lesions, including atopic dermatitis, urticaria, infantile dermatitis and eczema.[32] The dietary approach to this problem area has been reviewed in Chapter 33.

Dermatological Manifestations of Hyperlipoproteinemias. Considerable clinical interest has been reported in the classification of primary hyperlipoproteinemia into five basic types by Fredrickson.[33] Serum cholesterol levels are elevated in Types II, III and V, and may be normal or elevated in Type IV. Xanthomas and xanthelasma are frequently associated with severe hypercholesterolemia, particularly in Type III. The treatment of hyperlipidemias has been discussed in detail in Chapter 31.

Psoriasis. Psoriasis is a chronic inflammatory skin disease characterized by the development of reddish, erythematous patches covered with raised, silvery-white, dried scales. Cracking and fissuring of the skin in the extensive psoriatic area are quite common. The disease affects primarily the extensor surfaces of the body and the scalp, although it may be very widely disseminated.

While such patients have failed to show any

clear-cut metabolic disturbance as the underlying cause of this dermatitis, some interesting studies have been conducted. For many years it has been demonstrated that a diet free from fat or very low in protein is moderately therapeutically effective in the treatment of psoriasis.[34] Schamberg[35,36] has been the outstanding proponent of the low-protein diet and he has indicated that psoriatic individuals give definite signs of abnormal nitrogen retention. Patients with psoriasis, placed on diets containing no more than 4 or 5 gm of nitrogen per day, with an adequate caloric intake, were able to maintain their weight and experienced a gradual disappearance of the lesions of this disease. Unfortunately, when this very restricted dietary regimen is discontinued, the disease returns.

Recent findings have shown that the psoriatic scales containing keratin-like protein have an unusually high content of sulfur amino acids. In this connection, it is worth noting that the standard therapy of psoriasis with both coal tar and ultraviolet light is known to disrupt the metabolism of the sulfhydryl group and may provide a clue to understanding and therapy of this disease. It has also been reported that there is an interesting relationship between decreased urinary secretion of sulfur and of ascorbic acid in patients with psoriasis.[37] Experiments with diets containing a maximum of 250 mg of sulfur per day in patients for periods of several months have yielded inconsistent results.

Still another approach to the evaluation of amino acids in the management of psoriasis has been the use of diets low in tryptophan. The skin lesions in four cases of long-standing psoriasis cleared strikingly when the patients were placed on a low-tryptophan diet.[38] It should be remembered, however, that in a disease as complicated as psoriasis spontaneous remissions are not uncommon. In the particular study reported "none of the patients had previously experienced significant improvement even with extensive treatment."

Attempts to obtain a clear understanding of the nature of the water-soluble organic components of psoriatic scales have been reported.[39] The following abnormalities were found to be present: (a) increased soluble proteins; (b) raised sulfhydryl proteins; (c) low free amino nitrogen; (d) elevated pentoses; (e) high total phosphates; (f) increased uracil and (g) increased mucopolysaccharides. These abnormalities indicate a possible relationship between protein and mucopolysaccharide abnormal metabolism.

Acne Vulgaris. Acne vulgaris is a chronic inflammatory disease of the sebaceous glands and the pylosebaceous structures of the skin, and is almost always associated with seborrhea. This is predominantly a dermatological disease of youth, particularly teenage youth and associated with it are all of the emotional and psychological factors so prevalent in this age group. It is a rather common clinical experience that gross dietary indiscretion, particularly in the form of taking too much cake, candy, ice cream and chocolates, aggravates an existing acne and strongly suggests that the skin condition may be associated with a disturbance of carbohydrate metabolism.[40] Not all agree on this and, in fact, improvement has been reported in patients taking a high-carbohydrate diet.[41]

It is also thought that acne is made worse by diets high in fat. Unfortunately, low-fat diets have not been particularly effective in the management of this problem. It may well be that the principal effect of high-fat diets is to permit excessive weight gain in children with acne, who are often withdrawn, quiet and relatively inactive because of the emotional trauma that is associated with the stigma of this disease. It has been pointed out that the diet of the Eskimo is mostly fat and protein, but Eskimos have relatively little or no acne. One cannot doubt that psychoneurogenous factors play a significant role in producing exacerbation of this disease. In addition, fatigue and exhaustion are often predisposing factors.

In view of the fact that we have no specific knowledge as to the cause or treatment of acne, it seems most reasonable to place persons with this disease on a well-balanced diet, which does not contribute an excessive amount of calories, so that weight gain is not excessive. Such a diet should contribute all the food nutrients in the recommended daily allowances. Perhaps most important of all, the child or individual with this disease, as with all difficult dermatological diseases, must have the necessary psychological lift from the physician and from his friends and family to permit him to learn to live with his disease and to function as much like a normal individual as possible.

SUMMARY

There is little doubt that dietary deficiency, whether primary or conditioned, may be associated with dermatological lesions which can respond to specific therapy with vitamins or unusual diets.

Dermatoses are certainly associated with obesity, and since this is such a common problem in this country, therapy directed at weight reduction will probably provide the best management in related dermatological problems.

The general dermatological changes associated with under-nutrition, rather rare in this country, are extremely common in technically underdeveloped countries, and here improvement of the protein intake of the diet seems to be the most rational way of correcting this problem.

Certainly, allergies to foods may produce dermatoses and such allergies should be ruled out if suspected either on the basis of family history or by history of the patient's food intake.

It is extremely important that every patient presenting a dermatological problem should have a careful nutritional history, physical examination and, if necessary, biochemical studies carried out to rule out any evidence of nutritional abnormality.

It must be remembered that the underlying defects related to dermatoses of unknown etiology may be the result of improper nutrition and metabolic error endured over very long periods of time. Hence, their correction by diet or improved metabolism may require long and intensive therapy.

BIBLIOGRAPHY

1. Spies: Postgraduate Medicine, *17*, No. 3, 1955.
2. Pillsbury, Shelley, and Kligman: *Dermatology*, Philadelphia, W. B. Saunders Co., 1956.
3. Urbach with LeWinn: *Skin Diseases, Nutrition and Metabolism*, New York, Grune and Stratton, 1946.
4. Rothman and Lorincz: Annual Review of Medicine, *14*, 215, 1963.
5. Roe: N.Y.S. J. of Med., *62*, 3455, 1962.
6. Freedberg and Baden: J. Invest. Dermat., *38*, 277, 1962.
7. Tickner and Basit: Brit. J. Dermat., *72*, 138, 1960.
8. Rook and Walton: *Comparative Physiology and Pathology of the Skin*. Philadelphia, F. A. Davis Co., 1965.
9. Keys: J.A.M.A., *138*, 500, 1948.
10. Waterlow (Ed.): *Protein Malnutrition*, Proceedings of a Conference in Jamaica, 1953. Univ. Press, Cambridge, England, 1955.
11. Hansen and Burr: J.A.M.A., *132*, 855, 1946.
12. Konstam and Gordon: Proc. Roy. Soc. Med., *29*, 629, 1936.
13. Hansen: Proc. Soc. Exp. Biol. and Med., *31*, 160, 1933.
14. Rajagopal, Chowdhury and Chakraborty: Ind. Med. Gaz., *89*, 283, 1954.
15. Bhat and Belvady: Amer. Jour. of Clin. Nutr., *20*, 386, 1967.
16. Eddy and Dalldorf: *The Avitaminoses*, Baltimore, Williams & Wilkins Co., 1941.
17. Sultzberger and Lazar: J.A.M.A., *146*, 788, 1951.
18. Sebrell, Jr. and Butler: U.S. Public Health Reports, *53*, 2282 and *54*, 2121, 1939.
19. Youmans: J.A.M.A., *144*, 307, 1950.
20. Pollack: Metabolism, *5*, 231, 1956.
21. Krehl, Sarma and Elvehjem: J. Biol. Chem., *162*, 403, 1946.
22. Wright: Michigan State Med. J., *41*, 774, 1942.
23. Schreiner, Slinger, Hawkins and Vilter: J. Lab. and Clin. Med., *40*, 121, 1952.
24. Woolley: Proc. Soc. Exp. Biol. and Med., *43*, 660, 1940.
25. Dimik and Lepp: J. Nutrition, *20*, 413, 1940.
26. Morgan and Simms: J. Nutrition, *20*, 627, 1940.
27. Unna, Richards and Sampson: J. Nutrition, *21*, 553, 1941.
28. Williams: Science, *92*, 561, 1940.
29. Woolley: Science, *92*, 384, 1940.
30. Zarafonetis: Ann. Intern. Med., *30*, 1188, 1949.
31. Loomis: Science, *157*, 501, 1967.
32. McGovern: Borden's Review of Nutrition Research, *17*, 27, 1956.
33. Fredrickson, Levy and Lees: New Engl. J. Med., *276*, 34, 94, 148, 273, 1967.
34. Buckley: J.A.M.A., *59*, 535, 1912.
35. Schamberg: J.A.M.A., *98*, 1633, 1932.
36. Schamberg, Kolmer, Ringer and Raiziss: J. Cutaneous Dis., *31*, 698, 1913.
37. Reiss: Chinese Med. J., *53*, 141, 1938.
38. Spiera and Lefkovitis: The Lancet, *2*, 137, 1967.
39. Flesch, Hodgson and Esoda: Arch. Derm., *85*, 476, 1962.
40. Lemon and Hermann: Brit. J. Dermat., *52*, 123, 1940.
41. Crawford and Swartz: Arch. Derm. and Syph., *33*, 1035, 1936.

Chapter

35

Diet and Nutrition in the Care of the Surgical Patient

INTRODUCTION

The well-nourished and reasonably healthy patient, who is subjected to a single and relatively uncomplicated major surgical procedure, or who suffers moderately severe trauma, does well in the immediate postoperative period with a relatively simple program of parenteral infusion. This is designed to maintain circulatory volume and to provide water, salt, potassium and glucose to prevent dehydration or electrolyte imbalance. The glucose plays an important role in sparing body protein breakdown otherwise required for gluconeogenesis in starvation.[1,2] A high caloric, high protein parenteral regime can and will reduce nitrogen and weight loss that results from semi-starvation and the metabolic response to trauma. However, body reserves of protein and fat are sufficient to sustain most patients for a week or more during inadequate caloric and nitrogen intakes without serious consequences. Oral intake should be resumed as soon as it can be tolerated to permit repletion of relatively minor losses which occur on the latter regimen. The risk of either high caloric intravenous feeding or the use of tube feedings of either "elemental" or homogenized diets probably outweighs their advantages in the large majority of surgical patients.

A significant minority of surgical patients require that their nutritional program be planned as carefully as their operative procedure. These patients are of two general types: those who preoperatively are severely debilitated and malnourished as the result of chronic or subacute disease, and those who for prolonged periods of time are unwilling or unable to eat adequately, as the result of severe trauma, sepsis, or complications of surgery. Examples of patients with major preoperative debility include those with severe inflammatory disease of large or small bowel, carcinoma of the stomach or colon, chronic pancreatitis, chronic infection, particularly of lung or bone, and some forms of liver, kidney or heart disease. All of these patients have substantial weight loss with severe reduction of their skeletal muscle mass and total body protein. Most patients have an increase in relative proportion of extracellular fluid and total sodium, despite quite common hyponatremia. Two examples of the changes in body composition produced by chronic illness are shown in Figure 35–1.[3] In both cases there has been loss of body weight and relative expansion of extracellular fluid. In the patient with congestive heart failure, the body cell mass remains at normal levels while body fat has been substantially reduced and the extracellular fluid increased. In the patient with regional enteritis substantial loss of body weight is reflected by the fact that the skeleton is more than twice its normal proportion of total body weight; body cell mass is substantially reduced even on a percentage basis of the depleted body and the extracellular fluid compartment is markedly expanded. Patients with these derangements of body composition due to malnutrition and

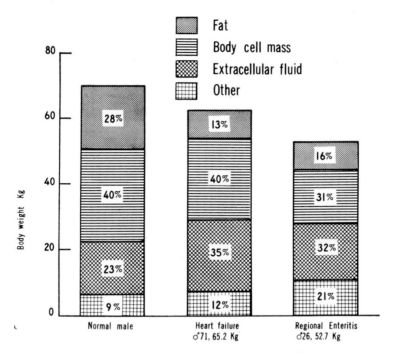

Fig. 35-1. Alteration in body composition in subacute and chronic illness. Body fat is reduced and extracellular fluid (ECF) increased with moderate weight loss as seen in heart failure. Major loss of weight in chronic illness results in both a proportional reduction of body cell mass with expansion of the ECF, and an absolute reduction of even greater magnitude, as shown by the high proportion of body weight represented by the skeleton and other extracellular non-fluid tissues. Data from F. D. Moore et al.[3]

disease represent severe operative risks and require major attention to nutritional management in the preoperative as well as the postoperative period.

More acute problems include patients with acute or subacute pancreatitis, unresolved peritonitis, high output fistulas from the gastrointestinal tract to skin, abdominal trauma, major wound sepsis, retroperitoneal hematomas, and most particularly, patients with major burns or multiple injury including femoral and pelvic fractures. Most of these patients were healthy and well nourished before the onset of their acute problem; however, because of major catabolic response to trauma and sepsis and simultaneous partial starvation, the demands on fat and especially protein are so great that expendable protein may be exhausted from within two to four weeks. Death will occur from muscle weakness resulting in pulmonary infection and respiratory failure, unless food is provided in sufficient quantity and proper qualities to spare essential body cell mass. A loss of one third of total body protein within 30 days appears to be lethal in man as well as in experimental animals.[4]

NITROGEN AND CALORIE NEEDS

In 1930 Cuthbertson[5] published data to validate and in part to explain the well-recognized clinical observation that there is an extraordinary wasting of skeletal muscle and a decrease in strength following severe skeletal trauma; such changes occur often despite a seemingly adequate oral intake of both calories and protein. Cuthbertson reported that immobilization of normal male volunteers who were on a regular diet caused only a small negative nitrogen balance (1 to 2 grams a day) which occurred within one to two days. Subsequent surgery increased the rate of nitrogen loss in these patients greater than that produced by immobilization alone despite maintenance of the same diet.

Cuthbertson's observations were confirmed and extended by J. E. Howard and his associates[6,7,8] who compared the nitrogen balance of patients in convalescence following long bone fractures to that of patients undergoing surgery on the skeleton. All the long bone fracture patients showed nitrogen losses of considerable magnitude following injury, i.e., the equivalent of an average loss of 6.6 kilograms of lean body mass in a 70-kilogram man. The peak nitrogen loss in fracture cases occurred on the sixth day after injury; the patients undergoing operations on the skeleton sustained a much smaller total nitrogen loss with an earlier peak and a much more rapid repletion. It was concluded that a high protein-high caloric diet did not exert any appreciable protein sparing effect at the peak of negative nitrogen balance following trauma in healthy and previously active patients. They did, however, observe one severely debilitated patient who, following *multiple* fractures, showed no essential change in nitrogen metabolism, and who was kept in nitrogen equilibrium one week after injury with a daily intake of 6 grams of nitrogen and 900 calories per 1.73 M^2. Studies were conducted on volunteers at bed rest who were subjected to a stepwise decrease in diet to the point of complete starvation and then stepwise repletion. Bed rest alone produced slightly more than 2 grams negative nitrogen balance per day on a basal intake of 1,600 kcalories, and 10 grams of protein nitrogen per 1.73 M^2. Abrupt starvation resulted in 12 grams nitrogen loss on the first day for each of two patients, the loss of 33 and 45 mEq of potassium, and the loss of matching amounts of phosphorus. The nitrogen, potassium and phosphorus ratios in stepwise starvation and repletion were similar to the ratio of these elements found in normal skeletal muscle. During repletion, Howard observed retention of potassium before nitrogen, and concluded that deviations from this pattern of loss of potassium, nitrogen and phosphorus as seen after injury represented a result of the injury *per se* and was different from the normal patterns of starvation.

During World War II Elman[9] and Brunschwig et al.[10] studied the effectiveness of parenteral solutions of casein hydrolysates in altering postoperative nitrogen loss in surgical patients. While there was an increased excretion of total nitrogen with the use of these preparations, there was also a reduction in the amount of patient-derived nitrogen. Neither group was able to achieve nitrogen equilibrium in any patient after major surgery when preoperative nutrition had been normal. Reigel and associates[11] and CoTui et al.[12] found that nitrogen equilibrium could be achieved in many patients postoperatively if elevated levels of protein intake and substantial additional calories were administered. The latter group was able to achieve positive nitrogen balance in patients within a very short period following surgery for duodenal ulcer by administering pureed beef into the gastrointestinal tract. However, most of the patients were relatively debilitated preoperatively which undoubtedly enhanced their ability to retain nitrogen.

Separation of the effects of starvation from the effects of trauma of surgery was further elaborated by the studies of Werner et al.[13] They showed that when patients undergoing either ventral or inguinal herniorrhaphy or elective cholecystectomy were given preoperative parenteral nutrition (consisting of 18 to 24 kcalories per kilogram per day of a 10% solution of glucose with 12.5 to 14.4 grams of nitrogen as amino acids), their slight negative nitrogen balance was increased by less than 1 gram per day following operation. When patients were subjected to partial gastrectomy for duodenal ulcer and a similar preoperative intravenous nutritional regime was used, nitrogen losses during the immediate postoperative period were larger than following herniorrhaphy or cholecystectomy. However, the losses were considerably less than those noted in another group of patients maintained postoperatively on routine parenteral fluids consisting of 5% dextrose with some sodium and potassium chlorides. They concluded that starvation played the major role in postoperative nitrogen loss under the conditions of their studies.

Hume[14] has stated that the stimuli which induce endocrine and metabolic changes following injury include pain, hemorrhage and hypovolemia, infection—particularly major sepsis, alterations in blood pH—particularly severe acidosis of a respiratory origin, anaesthetic drugs, central nervous system injury, and emotional trauma. He also pointed out that immobilization, hypoglycemia, starvation—particularly acute starvation, and withdrawal symptoms from alcohol or narcotic drugs may be involved. Hormones that are generally increased in trauma include ACTH, cortisone, renin and aldosterone (which are both activated by changes in circulating volume) and antidiuretic hormone (also stimulated by hypovolemia). Growth hormone is stimulated by hypoglycemia, as is glucagon. Hormones not changed or decreased by trauma include TSH and thyroxin, insulin, follicle-stimulating hormone, ketosteroids of either gonadal or adrenal origin, or luteinizing hormone.

Alterations in carbohydrate metabolism induced by either trauma or surgery include hyperglycemia and a mildly diabetic glucose tolerance curve and increases in pyruvic and lactic acids with some acidosis which may be noted following injury, particularly if the trauma is severe. Elevations in plasma free fat and fatty acids also occur and provide the substrate for most of the energy requirements of the body. This process occurs in spite of the fact that plasma insulin levels may be considerably higher in the post-traumatized or post-surgical patient than in simple starvation.

It has been repeatedly demonstrated that high caloric parenteral feeding can significantly reduce nitrogen loss at the peak of catabolic response and reduce or even reverse catabolism of protein and fat in the more chronic states of illness including surgical convalescence. Various studies indicate the importance and effectiveness of the provision of 35 to 50 kcalories and 0.1 to 0.2 gram nitrogen as amino acids per kilogram per day in reducing or reversing nitrogen loss in the postoperative patient.[15-19]

INTRAVENOUS WATER, ELECTROLYTES AND GLUCOSE

The requirements for parenteral therapy can be considered in three categories:

1. Base-line requirements: What does the patient require in water, electrolytes, calories, and micronutrients to minimize or to prevent dehydration and starvation which would otherwise result as a consequence of the cessation or reduction of oral intake? The calculation of base-line requirements disregards any preexisting dehydration or any abnormal losses, but base-line volumes may require modification in patients with extracellular fluid excess or dilutional hyponatremia.

2. Abnormal losses: What does the patient require in order to replace ongoing abnormal fluid and electrolyte losses resulting from the disease or its treatment, or both?

3. Deficits or excesses: What deficits (or excesses) does the patient have in water, electrolytes, blood volume, plasma proteins, and micronutrients? What should be done to correct these abnormalities, and at what rate should reconstitution be effected?

The orders written for parenteral fluid and electrolyte therapy should take into consideration these three major categories. The parenteral fluids required are the sum of base-line requirements and abnormal losses plus a part of or all the deficits existing at the time treatment is begun or minus a part or all of the excesses present when initiating treatment.

Base-Line Requirements: Water. Normal water requirements have been discussed in Chapter 7. The usual surgical patient cannot be expected to have the normal degree of renal efficiency; in addition he may be subjected to an increased solute load as the result of trauma and increased catabolism of body cell mass. Therefore, a urine volume of 1,200 to 1,500 ml/day is desirable in the average adult following operation. However, this goal for urine volume may be either excessive or inadequate with certain types of serious impairment of renal function; it may not be achievable in the early postoperative period when post-traumatic inhibition of renal free water clearance is to be expected with previously normal renal function. A patient with a normal body temperature, living in a comfortable environment of both temperature and humidity, will lose between 800 and 1,000 ml of water/day as insensible loss. The rate of loss is somewhat higher in men than in women and is proportionate to body surface area and to respiratory minute volume. There is a small insensible loss of sodium, potassium and chloride due to a combination of minimal sweating and to electrolyte lost in desquamation of the epidermis. Balance studies have suggested an insensible loss of approximately 20 mEq of sodium/day, an equal amount of chloride, and between 5 and 10 mEq of potassium.

The daily caloric requirement of the afebrile patient at bed rest will vary from 1,500 to 2,300 kcal, 400 to 500 of which are usually provided by the administration of glucose. The base-line production of endogenous water in this situation will be from 150 to 200 ml, or about 10 per cent of the total daily requirement. However, fever, trauma, infection, and immobilization greatly increase endogenous water production, and the seriously ill patient suffering from extensive trauma or massive infection may provide as much as 1,000 ml of sodium-free, potassium-rich endogenous water a day. This must be taken into account in considering fluid balance.

Normal base-line parenteral water requirements vary from 1,250 to 3,000 ml/day depending on body cell mass size, age, and sex. Table 35–1 illustrates two methods of estimating the base-line parenteral fluid requirements of surgical patients. Both these methods depend upon an estimation of the ideal body weight for height, sex, and age in those patients who are obese, since excess fat has little metabolic activity or effect other than increasing somewhat the total body surface area.

Both methods should be considered rule-of-thumb guides for base-line fluid requirements to be modified as necessary in accordance with the needs of the individual patient.

Weights of patients on restricted parenteral fluid therapy of glucose, water and electrolytes should decrease with a loss of approximately 0.3 to 0.5 per cent of body weight per day until adequate nutrition is instituted. Exceptions occur with blood transfusions, with deliberate changes in hydration, and during the first 24 to 48 hours following trauma or operation with local sequestration of fluid and increased parenteral therapy to compensate for it. The patient who otherwise gains weight while on this type of parenteral therapy is almost certainly being overhydrated. The patient who loses weight rapidly, except during the normal post-traumatic diuresis, usually has abnormal fluid losses which are being underestimated and underreplaced.

Table 35-1. Base-Line Water Requirements

Computed per day for relatively normal semi-starving patients without massive trauma, dehydration, or chronic illness.

Method 1: based on "ideal" body weight for height, sex, and age for obese patients and on actual body weight for others:

1. Children over 20 kg—1,500 ml + 30 ml/kg above 20 kg
2. Previously vigorous young adults with large muscle mass—40 ml/kg/day
3. Adults between 18 and 55 years—   35 ml/kg/day
4. Older patients with no major cardiac or renal disease—30 ml/kg/day

Method 2: for all patients except infants weighing less than 5 kg, based on "ideal" body weight for height, sex, and age for obese patients and on actual body weight for others:[*]

	ml/kg/day
First 10 kg of body weight	100
Second 10 kg of body weight	50
All weight above 20 kg	20 if < 50 years old
	15 if > 50 years old

* Modified from recommendations of Kiesewetter.[20]

Daily (or more frequent) body weight measurements are the single most important method of controlling water balance.

Factors Which Increase Base-Line Requirements. These are essentially ones which increase the insensible loss.

FEVER. Fever increases the base-line water requirements largely through hyperventilation with increased water evaporation. A patient with a fever of 103° F will require about 500 ml of additional base-line water per day. Endogenous water production is also increased.

SWEATING. A rule of thumb with respect to sweat loss is to increase the average adult base-line water requirements by 500 ml/day for each 5° above 85° F of ambient temperature. This is dependent on the humidity. Sweat is about one-third isotonic sodium chloride in the summertime and nearly two-thirds isotonic in winter, so that additional salt must be provided in base-line therapy to compensate. When the environmental temperature approaches body temperature, the seriously ill patient should be cooled, preferably by air conditioning, because insensible loss of water becomes very large when the ambient temperature exceeds body temperature.

INCREASED METABOLISM. Hyperthyroidism increases the base-line water turnover substantially, as it does caloric requirements. Hyperthyroid patients in the semi-starving state tend to consume massive amounts of lean body tissue and body fat producing unusual amounts of endogenous water; simultaneously they lose water by both respiratory evaporation and skin sublimation as well as by sweating.

Factors Which Reduce Base-Line Water Requirements. These include reduced metabolic activity, as seen in hypothyroidism, in the elderly, and in situations in which there is an excessive amount of body water with overexpanded extracellular fluid space as in cardiac edema, in hypoproteinemia with starvation, in prolonged infection, in carcinoma of the gastrointestinal tract, and in the special circumstance of acute renal failure.

Base-Line Requirements: Electrolytes. In the absence of abnormal losses or of dehydration and salt deficits, the base-line sodium requirements of the average previously healthy adult are easily met by a maximum of 500 ml of 0.9% sodium chloride with 5% dextrose. This provides 76 mEq each of sodium and chloride ion. In addition, 40 mEq of potassium chloride/day for all adults except those suffering from acute dehydration or renal insufficiency will provide sufficient base-line potassium to prevent many problems of potassium depletion. Potassium chloride should not be administered in concentrations in excess of 40 mEq/L of fluid, and therefore the base-line requirement should be dissolved in at least 1,000 ml of otherwise isotonic infusion fluid. Another approach to the administration of base-line electrolytes is to provide 3 mEq of sodium and 2 mEq of potassium/100 ml of infusion fluid in the form of chloride salts. This method is particularly useful in pediatric surgical therapy but may result in an excessive electrolyte load for base-line fluids in the adult.

In the presence of an overexpanded extracellular fluid space with excess total body sodium, the sodium chloride content of base-line fluids should be reduced or eliminated. In the presence of acute or chronic renal insufficiency or severe acidosis with elevation of the plasma potassium level, potassium should be reduced or withheld.

The remaining water requirements beyond that used to dissolve the electrolytes suggested are, of course, made up by the use of 5 or 10% glucose in distilled water.

Base-Line Requirements: Carbohydrate. The administration of 100 to 125 gm of glucose/day parenterally in the average-sized adult patient will result in the avoidance of nearly one-half of the nitrogen loss which results from the catabolism of lean body mass during starvation. In addition it will prevent the development of starvation acidosis in most patients. Unfortunately the administration of 200 or even 400 gm of glucose/day will not completely prevent the lysis of body cell mass and may create major problems.

Base-line glucose should be divided into at least two infusions a day for the average adult, as should the parenteral water requirements.

Much more substantial efforts at providing calories, protein, vitamins, and mineral are required in debilitated patients, in those with sepsis, with gastrointestinal-cutaneous fistulae, with major trauma, including burns, and in general in patients who cannot or will not eat an adequate food intake for prolonged periods of time. High caloric intravenous feeding or "parenteral alimentation" is discussed in the next chapter.

Abnormal Losses. This is the second major category for consideration in determining fluid and electrolyte requirements. It includes both external abnormal losses of water, electrolytes, and plasma protein, and internal fluid shifts with functional loss of fluids by sequestration within the body.

External abnormal loss may be in the form of excessive loss of water and electrolytes by normal routes of excretion or secretion, or losses may occur from intraluminal tubes, drains, fistulae, or wounds. The most common of the sources of external abnormal losses in surgical patients is the gastrointestinal tract; next in frequency are losses from surgical wounds, increased evaporation from the skin and respiratory tract, and burns. Sequestration of extracellular fluids into areas of traumatized or infected tissue produces a decrease in the usual distribution of extracellular fluid without external loss or change in body weight.

Losses From the Gastrointestinal Tract. The normal daily volume of secretions into the gastrointestinal tract is not precisely known but has been estimated to be 8,000 to 10,000 ml, of which saliva constitutes 1 to 2 liters; gastric juice, including both acid and mucoid secretions, about 2,500 ml; bile, 500 to 750 ml; and pancreatic juice, more than 1,000 ml. In addition, secretion of the upper small bowel contributes between 2,000 and 3,000 ml. All but 100 to 200 ml is normally reabsorbed by the small bowel and the colon.

Abnormal losses from the gastrointestinal tract include water and electrolytes, and varying amounts of protein. The electrolyte content of fluid from the gastrointestinal tract varies significantly with the level from which the bulk of the fluid is derived. Table 35-2 shows the average and the range of variation of sodium, potassium, chloride, and bicarbonate in fluid from different levels of the

Table 35-2. Electrolyte Concentration of Gastrointestinal Secretions

Source of fluid	Na, mEq/L	K, mEq/L	Cl, mEq/L	Effective HCO₃ mEq/L
Saliva, average of 3 pt (based on 1 ml/minute) *	60	20	16	50
Gastric, average†	59	9.3	89	0–1
Range	30–90	4.3–12	52–155	
Upper small bowel, average	105	5.1	99	≃10
Range	72–128	3.5–6.8	69–127	
Ileum, average	117	5.0	106	15–20
Range	91–140	3.0–7.5	82–125	
Bile, average	145	5.2	100	≃50
Range	134–156	3.9–6.3	83–110	
Pancreatic fistula, average of 3 pt	141.6	4.6	76.6	≃70

* Modified from H. W. Davenport, "Physiology of the Digestive Tract," The Year Book Medical Publishers, Inc., Chicago, 1961. Remaining data from author's publications.
† Range represents values for the middle two-thirds of a series of patients, except for gastric secretion, where a group of patients with high gastric acidity and a high Cl⁻ concentration in gastric juice has been included at the upper limit.

intestine in patients with a variety of causes for drainage. It is important to note that of all the secretions of the gastrointestinal tract only bile and pancreatic juice are approximately isotonic in their observed electrolyte content. The average calculated osmolarity of saliva is about 160 mO; of fasting gastric juice, in patients without duodenal ulcer, about 180 mO; of upper small bowel content, 220 mO; and of fluid from the distal ileum, about 240 mO. Other substances, including mucoproteins, other polysaccharides, urea, and calcium and phosphate, increase the total osmolality beyond these approximations.

The average values shown may be used for semi-quantitative replacement of gastrointestinal tract losses. When volumes exceed 2,000 ml in 24 hours or when substantial losses (1 liter or more per day) continue for more than a few days, it is wise to send an aliquot of the 24 hour drainage to the laboratory for analysis for electrolytes and protein and to determine the pH of a freshly obtained specimen. With this information more precise replacement can be made.

A significant loss of protein may occur from distended and atonic small bowel. Losses of from 20 to 30 gm of protein/liter of small bowel drainage have been observed. Larger losses of plasma protein, as well as substantial losses of whole blood, are seen in patients with severe diarrhea accompanying ulcerative colitis. A high percentage of this protein is serum albumin. Accordingly, when large volumes of bowel content are lost, replacement of lost plasma protein becomes necessary if a serious decrease in plasma protein concentration is to be avoided. If plasma, or preferably an albumin fraction is used and the patient is otherwise adequately hydrated, the water and electrolyte content of the infusate must be considered.

Internal Fluid Shifts. If the intracellular and extracellular fluid spaces are considered as the two major body fluid compartments, an abnormal "third" fluid space is created when interstitial fluid, plasma, and sometimes red blood cells are sequestered in abnormal amounts in an area of tissue injury. This sequestered fluid is in continuity with the remaining extracellular fluid from which it

was derived, yet is unavailable for restoring diminished interstitial fluid and plasma volumes. It is apparent as edema in patients with burns; it also occurs in crush injuries, in peritonitis, in pulmonary infection, in soft tissue and wound infection, and in areas distal to obstructed venous flow. Sequestered fluid is accumulated to some degree postoperatively in all surgical wounds and is substantial in retroperitoneal dissection or with visceral or muscle trauma.

A special type of internal fluid shift is seen with the development of transcellular pooling such as occurs within the gastrointestinal tract with intestinal obstruction or adynamic ileus; the volume of fluid involved may be quite large. These collections of transcellular fluid may become abnormal external losses if they are vomited or drained by intestinal intubation, or they may resolve by reabsorption as the patient recovers gastrointestinal function.

If the volume of sequestered fluid is significantly large, it must be replaced exactly as if an external loss had occurred. The major difference between development of a third space of sequestered fluid and an abnormal external fluid loss is that sequestered fluid remains within the body, so that there is no loss of weight. A gain in weight results from the necessary replacement of diminished plasma and interstitial fluid volumes of the rest of the body. Also, unlike an external loss, the sequestered fluid will eventually return to the circulation as normal function returns to the affected area—presenting a potential problem in water and electrolyte overloading.

Deficits or Excesses. The administration of water, electrolytes, calories, and vitamins as base-line therapy for replacement of abnormal external losses and for provision for internal fluid shifts is intended to help the patient to maintain normal functional volumes of body fluids, normal concentrations of electrolytes, and a normal pH of plasma and interstitial fluid. However, patients may have deficits or excesses of some or all of the component body fluids at the time when they are first seen and treatment is begun. In other patients significant abnormalities of volume, concentration, and pH may develop while the patient is under treatment. The replacement of deficits of water and electrolytes necessary to restore function when losses have occurred and the recognition and treatment of excessive fluid volumes or concentrations of electrolytes when present constitute the third major category for clinical consideration in fluid and electrolyte therapy.

Acute Dehydration. Acute change in the volume of total body water can occur either as the result of dehydration or through retention of an excessive amount of water, usually parenterally administered. There is, of course, a comparable change in body weights which, if known, greatly assists in diagnosis. Rapid weight loss due to dehydration is almost entirely extracellular fluid. A loss of 2 per cent of body weight will produce thirst and some oliguria. A loss of 4 per cent of body weight (20 per cent of extracellular fluid) causes oliguria, tachycardia, and often postural hypotension, and an acute extracellular fluid loss of 6 per cent of body weight is a life-threatening event, reducing interstitial fluid and plasma volumes by about 30 per cent and compromising both blood pressure and renal function.

TREATMENT. Replacement of acute loss of extracellular fluid or its functional loss by sequestration or transcellular pooling is best accomplished by infusion of water containing the electrolytes of extracellular fluid. Balanced salt solutions such as Ringer's lactate or a solution of 2 parts of 0.9% sodium chloride and 1 part M/6 sodium lactate are most effective. The rate of replacement can and usually should be rapid when the loss has occurred rapidly. If the loss causing the dehydration has been from vomiting, with an excess loss of hydrogen ion as hydrochloric acid, the plasma carbon dioxide content and pH will be elevated. Under these conditions the ideal fluid for rapid replacement is isotonic (0.9%) sodium chloride. If a severe metabolic acidosis is present, with a low pH and carbon dioxide content of plasma, initial infusion of 88 mEq of sodium bicarbonate or 500 ml of M/6 sodium lactate solution should precede the use of a balanced salt solution. Close monitoring of serum potassium level is indicated with addition of KCl as indicated to prevent significant

hypokalemia as potassium enters the cells with rising pH. Rapid infusion of glucose-containing solutions should be avoided to prevent a solute diuresis due to glucose overloading. Glucose solutions should be introduced somewhat later, except in treatment of diabetic ketoacidosis where glucose will be required as administered insulin becomes effective.

Chronic Dehydration. A patient who has become chronically dehydrated over a period of several days to a week or more, as a result of inadequate intake of water and food, may well lose 10 per cent or more of body weight. The loss of body water in such instances is more evenly distributed between intracellular and extracellular fluids. The effects of combined fluid depletion are less severe than those with acute extracellular fluid dehydration; hypotension and hemoconcentration are less marked, and the degree of oliguria is less.

TREATMENT. Rehydration in such a patient requires replacement of the extracellular fluid deficit in sufficient volume to raise urine volume to 25 to 50 ml/hour and to reduce the hematocrit to normal levels. A period of days rather than hours is desirable for repletion of the intracellular water and potassium deficits. Emergency surgical measures, if required, can be performed after repletion of the extracellular fluid component. Complete rehydration should not result in return to predehydration weight because of the loss of protein and fat during the period of underhydration and semi-starvation.

Dehydration by Primary Water Loss: Desiccation. This occurs as the result of excessive loss of water vapor or of very hypotonic solutions with the retention of extracellular fluid electrolytes and an increase in all the solutes of the plasma with a rise in plasma osmolality. The common clinical settings are those of excessive evaporation of water from the skin and respiratory tract, as seen with fever and hyperventilation due to metabolic acidosis. Tracheostomy and the administration of insufficiently humidified oxygen by catheter are additional respiratory causes. A high volume of dilute urine, as seen with diabetes insipidus, use of osmotic diuretics, and excessive sweating, all with inadequate water replacement, produce excessive water loss. The open treatment of burns with massive loss of water vapor from injured skin surfaces is particularly likely to produce desiccation dehydration. Oliguria, azotemia, fever, disorientation, coma, convulsions, and death will follow. Hypotension is usually a late complication.

Laboratory findings in this setting demonstrate an increase in the concentration of all the solutes of plasma, with an increase in osmolality. Serum sodium concentration is the key, and values of 160 mEq/L or more may be found, denoting osmolality of more than 325 mO. The hematocrit will rise in proportion to loss of total body water when the process takes days to develop as is usually the case; therefore it will not be as high as with acute extracellular fluid loss. Urine is highly concentrated and small in volume.

TREATMENT. Treatment consists of the administration of water as 5% glucose solution intravenously, or water by mouth in sufficient volumes to restore electrolyte concentrations and urine volume to normal. The rate of administration will depend somewhat on the rate at which water was initially lost; the more rapid the loss, the more rapid can be rehydration. Usually 1 or 2 days are required to bring the serum sodium level down to normal. Some salt may be required in the later stages of rehydration if significant amounts have been lost as the process has developed. An estimation of the volume of water required can be made from the loss of total body water necessary to raise the hematocrit and serum sodium to the levels observed. In patients who excrete large volumes of dilute urine while becoming dehydrated and hypertonic, a response to injected Pitressin tannate is both diagnostic of diabetes insipidus and therapeutic in promoting restoration of water balance.

Chronic Overexpansion of Extracellular Fluid. With chronic illnesses such as cancer, liver disease, chronic infection, starvation, or cardiac decompensation, the patient often will present with an overexpansion of the extracellular fluid space with an excess of total body sodium despite hyponatremia. Such a patient will have a decrease in the normal intracellular water because of a diminished relative volume of body cell mass. Figure 35–1 illustrates abnormalities of distribution of body water and cell mass seen in chronic illness. With the characteristic fall in body cell mass, as per cent of weight, there is a relative expansion of the extracellular fluid space. Such patients are usually hyponatremic, with serum sodium concentrations in the low 130 mEq range. Usually total body potassium is markedly depleted although the plasma concentrations of potassium may be normal or even a little high. In addition there is usually a considerable hypoproteinemia and a reduction in the normal osmolality of the plasma with the osmolality in the range of 260 to 270 mO.

Water and sodium retention are exaggerated postoperatively in such patients, and more marked hyponatremia and hyperkalemia often occurs. They have a very poor tolerance for the administration of large volumes of extracellular fluid expander such as Ringer's lactate solution or saline solution. The expanded extracellular fluid space with hyponatremia is the most common pattern of water and electrolyte abnormality seen in surgical patients and is one of the most difficult to treat once it becomes established.

TREATMENT. Treatment of this dilutional hyponatremia must *not* be by the administration of salt solutions on some formula based on unit deficit multiplied by a theoretical volume for extracellular fluid; rather it must be based on a combination of a restriction of water intake to less than that required by the normally hydrated individual and the restoration of the red cell mass and plasma volume to normal by the transfusion of blood or the infusion of plasma, or both. Since a large intracellular potassium deficit is usually present in such patients, the electrolyte need is usually for potassium rather than for sodium.

Hypertonicity Due to Solute Loading. This is usually the result of inadequate intake of water in patients who are receiving *tube feedings of mixtures which are high in protein and salt* in relation to water content. The syndrome is likely to develop in patients who have had head and neck surgical treatment, those on gastrostomy feedings, unconscious patients being tube-fed, and patients with brain stem injury. Hypertonicity due to solute loading can result from the exclusive use of an isotonic balanced salt solution such as Ringer's lactate solution given with the mistaken idea that such a solution will meet base-line requirements for patients on parenteral fluids. Unless renal function permits excretion of urine of very high specific gravity with elimination of excessive electrolyte, urea and other solutes in a volume of water smaller than that administered, both hypernatremia and azotemia will result.

Laboratory findings demonstrate an increased concentration of all plasma solutes, both electrolytes and crystalloids, which is out of proportion to changes in hematocrit. An elevated plasma sodium level in the presence of a moderate to large urine output is the key to diagnosis differentiating these patients from those with desiccation dehydration. The serum sodium may reach levels of 170 mEq/L or more in severe cases.

TREATMENT. This consists of the administration of large volumes of water orally or via the tube, or parenterally as 5% glucose in water, while at the same time eliminating, or at least reducing, the osmolar load. Caution must be exercised in order to reduce the osmolality relatively slowly. The entire body, including the cerebrospinal fluid and brain, becomes hypertonic during the solute loading period; cerebral edema, convulsions or coma may result if the extracellular fluid osmolality is reduced too rapidly. Large volumes of urine will persist for several days during solute release, and the hematocrit will not change greatly unless dehydration has also been present in significant degree.

Overhydration, Hypotonicity, and Water Intoxication. The opposite of solute overloading occurs with the excessive administration of water in the presence of antidiuresis. This condition exists in a chronic state in patients with wasting illnesses but may be seen acutely usually because of excessive and ill-advised parenteral administration of glucose and water.

Patients with cancer, heart disease, liver disease, renal insufficiency, or chronic infection are likely to have an expanded extracellular fluid before surgical treatment. They are particularly prone, as previously noted, to retain water and electrolytes and further to expand and dilute extracellular fluid.

Water intoxication is an acute form of hypotonic dilution. Drowsiness, weakness, and a fall in urine volume are early symptoms, followed by convulsions and coma. A rapid weight gain will always occur. Peripheral and pulmonary edema may appear but are not always present. Water intoxication may result from excessive administration of parenteral glucose and water, from absorption of water from the colon as the result of enemas or colon irrigations given for dis tension, or from water absorption from wounds and burns treated with hypotonic wet dressings. Water intoxication is a particular hazard of the dilute silver nitrate treatment of burns. It is particularly likely to occur in patients with inappropriate antidiuretic hormone release. (See Chapter 7.)

Laboratory findings include a low concen tration of serum sodium, usually less than 120 mEq and often less than 110 mEq/L. The urine may contain a substantial concen tration of sodium, 30 mEq/L or more despite the extremely low plasma value, due to an inappropriate sodium release in the presence of a very large extracellular fluid volume. Adrenal insufficiency and primary renal tubular disease must be excluded. The rapidity of fall of the plasma sodium concen tration is apparently of greater significance than the absolute values. Cerebral edema from a shift of water into the cerebrospinal fluid due to the difference in osmolality is the probable cause of convulsions and coma.

TREATMENT. Either total water restriction for a time or the very slow administration of a small volume of water as hypertonic glucose (20%)—not more than 500 ml over 24 hours—is required. If the patient has good cardiovascular function and central venous pressure is within normal limits, small volumes (300 ml or less) of hypertonic sodium chloride solution (5%) should be given slowly with monitoring of central venous pressure. This will begin restoration of extracellular fluid osmotic pressure and promote renal excretion of water. No attempt should be made to administer salt with a "formula" based on extracellular fluid deficit for severe overloading can result. Time and patience will result in a rising urine volume and an increase in serum sodium concentration with recovery in most cases. In an emergency hemodialysis with ultrafiltration to remove water may be desirable.

TOTAL PARENTERAL NUTRITION

This method of providing amino acids, carbohydrate calories, minerals and vitamins is of great value in the surgical patient who is incapable of utilizing his gastrointestinal tract as the avenue of adequate nutrition. The methods and materials used are discussed in detail in the chapter which follows.

NUTRITION WITH BULK-FREE CHEMICALLY DEFINED DIETS

The use of chemically formulated bulk-free diets for human nutrition is relatively new although extensive animal studies have demonstrated that such diets will support normal longevity, reproduction, growth and lactation in experimental animals.[21] In 1965 sixteen human male volunteers received between 2,100 and 3,700 calories per day of such an "elemental" diet as their sole nutritional source for a period of up to nineteen weeks.[22] Blood and balance studies during the entire test period failed to reveal abnormality of any parameter tested except for lowered plasma cholesterol levels with glucose diets which returned to normal when sucrose was added as half the carbohydrate source. Fecal elimination of all the individuals was strikingly reduced with the subjects experiencing smaller than normal bowel movements at regular intervals of five to six days.

Such diets have several advantages over presently available high caloric-high protein food supplements or liquid tube feedings of usual foods. The bulk-free and virtually fat-free composition requires minimal digestion thereby bypassing the digestive need for most pancreatic and biliary secretion. Because of the absence of indigestible material, stool volume is reduced. Diarrhea has not been much of a problem when diets are administered slowly and continuously in concentra-

tions not exceeding 25% weight volume in the adult or 10 per cent weight volume in the newborn and in infants.

Stephens and Randall[23] in 1969 reported the first known use of chemically defined liquid elemental diets for nutritional management of surgical patients in catabolic states. Since that time they have fed more than 250 patients, either substantially or completely, with chemically defined diets. Evidence continues to accumulate that such diets serve a very substantial role as an intermediate between high caloric intravenous feeding and the feeding of modified or normal diets made from normal foodstuffs. "Elemental" diets, like the high caloric parenteral mixtures which they closely resemble (except for added trace elements and the use of sucrose or oligosaccharides in some diets), permit the physician to control the caloric intake as well as water volume and electrolytes. They appear to be safer than high caloric parenteral nutrition by obviating the risk of infection caused by intravenous catheters, but have the limitation of requiring a functional section of small bowel for absorption of the sugars, minerals, and amino acids.

The nitrogen content of "elemental" diets consists either of mixtures of purified L-amino acids derived from acid hydrolysis of casein, adjusted to restore tryptophan content, or of chemically identified individual crystalline amino acids reconstituted into mixtures which provide defined amounts of essential amino acids together with nonessential amino acids. Such diets contain carbohydrate in the form of glucose, sucrose, or a mixture of glucose and partially hydrolyzed starch as the main source of calories. Electrolytes are added at a level calculated to meet base-line requirements. Fat- and water-soluble vitamins exclusive of vitamin K, and trace minerals except cobalt, are present in minimal daily requirement levels for normal man. Most diets contain either no fat or less than 1 per cent fat, a distinct advantage in patients with limited bowel function. In some instances, particularly with standard Vivonex, Jejunal, WT Low Residue Food and Flexical (Table 35–3 and Appendix, Table A–23) efforts have been made to add flavoring material to disguise or

Table 35-3. Chemically Defined Diets*
Composition per 1000 Kcalories†

	Vivonex	Vivonex HN	Jejunal	W-T Low	Flexical
Nitrogen (gm)	3.27	6.7	3.37	3.0	3.5
CH₂O source‡	Glu, Oligo	Oligo	Glu, Oligo	Oligo (Dextrin)	Corn syrup solids, Sucr, Starch
Fat, %	0.54	0.33	0.1	0.3	15
Electrolytes (mEq/L) at Normal Dilution (±25% (W/Vol)†					
Na	37.4	33.5	37. (106)§	57	15
K	29.9	17.9	22.9	33.8	38.4
Mg	16.0	9.6	7.9	0.06	0.09
Ca	22.2	13.3	34.3	28.0	50.0
Cl	50.8	52.4	62. (143)§	86	34
P	25.8	25.8	65.	54	52

* Vivonex and Vivonex HN: Eaton Laboratories, Norwich, New York.
Jejunal: Johnson and Johnson, New Brunswick, New Jersey.
W-T Low Residue: Warren Teed Pharmaceuticals, Columbus, Ohio.
Flexical: Mead Johnson Laboratories, Evansville, Indiana.
† All diets are approximately 1 kcal/ml at normal dilution.
‡ Glu = glucose; Oligo = glucose oligosaccharides; Sucr = Sucrose.
§ Jejunal broths have very high sodium and chloride concentration.

improve the rather strong organic taste and smell inherent in amino acid mixtures. Oral tolerance is fair to good at lower amino acid concentrations. It is very much less at therapeutic levels of protein equivalent of 35 to 40 grams (5.6–6.5 grams of nitrogen) per thousand calories, which is the amount necessary for adequate nutrition in most debilitated surgical patients. High nitrogen "elemental" diets now available must be tube fed to assure adequate intake.

The composition of currently available diets is shown in Table 35–3. They may be administered in a wide variety of concentrations, from 7.5% weight/volume which is best tolerated by newborn infants, to 25% weight/volume which is the concentration generally used for maintenance in adults. The latter solutions provide approximately 1 kcal per ml, while a 7.5% solution provides approximately 0.4 kcal. per ml.

Indications for Use of "Elemental" Diets. These diets have been found useful in the following types of patients where there is sufficient function of the gastrointestinal tract to permit use: 1. Persons depleted of protein reserves owing to disease of the gastrointestinal tract including ulcerative colitis and acute granulomatous disease of small and large bowel; chronic infection; carcinoma of the gastrointestinal tract particularly stomach or colon in preoperative preparation; intestinal atresia in infants and malabsorption syndromes in infants or adults. 2. Patients with partial function of the gastrointestinal tract: esophageal, gastric and duodenal cutaneous fistulas with feeding distal to the fistula; jejunal or ileal fistulas with feeding either proximal or distal depending on the level of the fistula, colonic fistula; acute pancreatitis after the ileus is cleared, and the short gut syndrome. 3. Patients with accelerated metabolic states who will not or cannot eat adequately; these include those with fractures of the jaw, long bone fractures requiring a supplement when dietary studies show caloric intake is inadequate, severe burns with inadequate caloric intake, and patients with multiple trauma.   4. Incidental uses: as a preoperative bowel preparation and for preparation for x-rays of the colon to avoid semi-starvation or excessive catharsis; as a virtually non-allergenic source of food; and as a dietary supplement. Under these circumstances the flavored varieties of diets are best tolerated by the patient, but it must be remembered that the patient receives not more than 25 grams of protein per 1000 calories.

We have found the use of "elemental" diets particularly advantageous in patients with inflammatory disease of the bowel, either Crohn's disease or ulcerative colitis. The diets are particularly useful in the acute phase where either excessive diarrhea or obstructive symptoms are predominant, and in the rehabilitation of patients who have had substantial body cell mass loss as the result of chronic malnutrition and infection.

"Elemental" diets have proved of considerable value in the management of nutritional problems in newborn and infants.[24] Infants have a much smaller fuel reserve than do adults and any delay in nutritional therapy will rapidly deplete those stores resulting in impaired wound healing and reduced resistance to infection.   Protein depletion is even more critical in infants because at birth their lean body mass is proportionately one third less than it will be as an adult.   There are probably no excess stores of protein as there are of fat and carbohydrate; therefore any nitrogen loss represents a loss or destruction of active living body cell mass.   We have shown[24] that the use of elemental diets in infants and children requires careful management and monitoring.   Infants will rapidly develop severe symptoms of osmotic dehydration if they receive a 25% weight/volume diet. These complications can be avoided if the diet is started slowly at a roughly isotonic concentration of 7 or 7.5% weight/volume and slowly increased over four or five days to the tolerance level which is usually about 10% and not more than 12%.   In children older than 10 months concentrations up to 25% weight/volume are well tolerated if the diet is started slowly as a continuous 15% weight/volume feeding in small volume and then gradually advanced in speed and concentration over several days to a week or more to allow for gastrointestinal adaptation.   It has been found that infants and young children will readily take the high nitrogen elemental diets from a nursing bottle, and that for prolonged feeding, as has been our experience with malabsorption syndromes of undefined etiology, children need not be fed with a feeding tube or gastrostomy beyond the initial adaptation phase.

Visceral cutaneous fistulas are infrequent but serious and often catastrophic complications of abdominal surgery or trauma and as the result of inflammatory disease of the bowel and as the result of cancer involving the gastrointestinal tract.   High output fistulas, 200 ml. per day or more, are likely to persist for prolonged periods of time and present major problems in management involving water and electrolyte loss, abdominal sepsis, and maintenance of adequate nutrition. Gastrointestinal-cutaneous fistulas are of three types: upper tract fistulas which include gastric duodenal and anastomotic fistulas, small bowel fistulas of the jejunum or ileum, and colonic fistulas.   Upper tract and small bowel fistulas are more difficult to manage because in general the higher the fistula the larger the output, and except for gastric fistulas, the more active and proteolytic the enzyme content of the drainage.   Reports of large series of patients from the literature indicate mortality rates of from 39 to 65 per cent in patients with high output gastrointestinal tract fistulas.   Causes of death are starvation, sepsis and carcinoma, with malnutrition playing a major role in at least 50 per cent of these patients who died.   The author and his colleagues have found the use of chemically defined diets very rewarding in the management of patients with gastrointestinal-cutaneous fistulas.   Following an initial period of intravenous nutrition, including careful attention to monitoring and electrolyte balance, elemental diets were used as the major or only source of nutrition for from 5 days to 77 days, in a series of 33 patients with a mean of 30 days and a median of 25 days. Sixteen of these patients closed their fistulas spontaneously; 6 of 12 with upper tract, 8 of 15 with small bowel, and 2 of 6 with colonic fistulas.   Six fistulas were successfully closed surgically.   Twenty-six of 33 patients had significant decrease in fistula drainage while on an elemental diet. There were 6 deaths in this series (18%); four of these died of disseminated carcinoma, one of reinfarction of the small bowel, and one of massive gastrointestinal tract hemorrhage.

Methods of Administration. *Oral.* Various flavored preparations made up as directed all yield approximately 1 calorie per ml. The liquid diets should be ingested in small amounts (100 to 150 ml) because of the high osmolality. Ingestion of 2000 or more ml. in a 16 hour day thus provides 2000 calories including approximately 40 grams of protein. Puddings and broths are also available, but strict attention should be paid to the electrolyte content of some of these since in some the sodium content is inordinately high and considerable sodium loading will result.

Intragastric Tube Feeding. This can be accomplished either with a #8 French transnasal intragastric feeding tube in an adult, or a #5 French in small children or infants. A variable-speed pump is useful in controlling the volume and rate of flow, in preference to a gravity drip which may fluctuate considerably. Diet should be drawn from a small 500 to 1000 ml. reservoir, kept at ice temperature. This is particularly important if 7 to 10 per cent dilutions are used since these are extraordinarily good culture media. Bulk diet should be kept refrigerated once reconstituted, and discarded after 24 hours. Initial concentration in the adult should be 12.5 to 15% weight/volume and should be administered initially in rates of 40 to 60 ml. per hour. If tolerated without nausea, vomiting or large gastric residue, the concentration can be increased to 25% weight/volume in 24 hours, and then the volume progressively increased by steps of approximately 500 ml. or more each day until the desired caloric and protein intake is achieved. If either nausea or diarrhea or abdominal distention occur the diet should be stopped entirely for 12 to 24 hours, then re-started slowly.

In elderly patients or unconscious patients elevation of the head of the bed to an angle of 30 degrees may forestall aspiration. It is wise to discontinue feeding at night in elderly or very weak patients who may aspirate if supine.

In all patients being fed with "elemental" diets, urine glucose levels should be checked frequently. In seriously ill patients, blood glucose levels and plasma electrolyte concentrations and pH should be checked at least twice a day during the initial period of gradual increase in diet. Diabetic patients can be fed with elemental diets if blood glucose levels are followed carefully and insulin adjusted accordingly. Dehydration from osmotic diuresis is the greatest problem.

Electrolyte, vitamin and water supplements can be given as required, either via the feeding tube, or intravenously.

DIETARY INTAKE AND OUTPUT RECORDS

Of the greatest importance in care of seriously ill surgical patients is an accurate record of intake and output. This record should include not only fluid intake but also total caloric and protein intakes. When patients are on an oral intake a daily estimate of the calories and protein taken as food (actually eaten, not just served), together with a record of any supplemental calories and protein given, should be recorded in the chart by the dietician. These data serve as an important guide to the surgeon in treating the patient.

BIBLIOGRAPHY

1. Gamble: *Chemical Anatomy, Physiology and Pathology of Extracellular Fluid.* Boston, Harvard University Press, 1947.
2. Cahill: New Eng. J. Med., *282*:668, 1970.
3. Moore, Olesen, McMurrey, et al.: *The Body Cell Mass and Its Supporting Environment. Body Composition in Health and Disease.* Philadelphia, W. B. Saunders Co., 1963.
4. Morgan, Filler, and Moore: Surgical nutrition. Med. Clin. N.A. *54*:1367, 1970.
5. Cuthbertson: Biochem J., *24*:1244, 1930.
6. Howard, Parson, Stein, et al.: Bull. Johns Hopkins Hosp. *75*:156, 1944.
7. Howard, Bigham, Jr., Eisenberg, et al.: Bull. Johns Hopkins Hosp. *75*:209, 1944.
8. Howard, Bigham, Eisenberg, et al.: Bull. Johns Hopkins Hosp., *78*:282, 1946.
9. Elman: *Parenteral Alimentation in Surgery With Special Reference to Proteins and Amino Acids.* New York, Hoeber, 1947.

10. Brunschwig, Clark, and Corbin: Ann. Surg., *115*:1091, 1942.
11. Reigel, Koop, Drew, et al.: J. Clin. Invest., *26*:18, 1947.
12. CoTui, Mulholland, Carabba, et al.: Ann. Surg., *130*:688, 1949.
13. Werner, Habif, Randall, Lockwood: Surg. Forum, *1*:458, 1951.
14. Hume: Chap. 1, *In Principles of Surgery*, Schwartz, S. I. (ed.). New York, The Blakiston Division, McGraw-Hill Book Company, 1969.
15. Holden, Kreger, Levey, and Abbott: Ann. Surg., *146*:503, 1957.
16. Abbott and Albertsen: Ann. New York Acad. Sci., *39*:941, 1963.
17. Johnston, Marino, and Stevens: Brit. J. Surg., *53*:885, 1966.
18. Larsen and Brockner: Acta Chir. Scand., *343*:191, 1966.
19. Wadstrom and Wiklund: Acta Chir. Scand., *325*:50, 1964.
20. Kiesewetter: *In Manual of Preoperative and Postoperative Care*. American College of Surgeons, Philadelphia, Pa., W. B. Saunders Co., 1967.
21. Greenstein, Otey, Birnbaum, and Winitz: Arch. Biochem. Biophys., *72*:396, 1957.
22. Winitz, Seedman, and Graff: Am. J. Clin. Nutr., *23*:525, 1970.
23. Stephens and Randall: Ann. Surg., *170*:642, 1969.
24. Stephens, Bury, DeLuca, and Randall: Am. J. Surgery, *123*:374, 1972.

Chapter

36

Total Parenteral Nutrition

Maurice E. Shils

INTRODUCTION

Knowledge of human requirements, availability of various essential nutrients, and means for their parenteral delivery over protracted periods are at a stage where nutritional status can be improved and maintained solely through intravenous feeding.[1-5] However, achievement of this goal for a given patient presents problems in logistics, in the details of formulating and preparing the fluids, in guaranteeing sterility, and in providing safe administration. Programs have been developed in various laboratories which can assist physicians and other staff to provide more easily this potentially life-saving—but not infrequently hazardous—procedure. This chapter is directed primarily to a consideration of the nutritional and practical aspects of this form of intravenous feeding.

The basic problem associated with conventional intravenous feeding (*i.e.*, 5 or 10 per cent glucose solutions with electrolytes) is the inability to provide sufficient calories to permit utilization of administered amino acids unless very large volumes of water are infused. Persistent negative caloric and nitrogen balances result in gradual loss of tissue and, if protracted, to debilitation with its multiple problems. Conventional parenteral feeding is, therefore, incapable of either maintaining the well-nourished for prolonged periods or of improving the already malnourished individual.

Aspects of the history of the development and rational use of fluids have been reviewed by various authors.[6-8] During and shortly after World War II there was much activity

directed toward achieving adequate nutrition by parenteral means; by the end of that decade the important relationships among caloric intake, nitrogen intake and nitrogen utilization were well recognized by clinicians knowledgeable in the field.[9,10] Provision of very hypertonic glucose solutions through catheters inserted in central veins became fairly common in managing severe renal failure in the period prior to the advent of simplified hemodialysis.[11] The combination of indwelling catheters, hypertonic glucose, protein hydrolysates and other nutrients was successfully utilized in the decade of 1955–65 by individual clinicians on a limited basis with or without the use of intravenous fat (I.V. Lipomul). This fat preparation suffered from the drawback that it could produce serious side effects with prolonged daily use;[1,7] it eventually was withdrawn from the market.

The term "hyperalimentation" appeared in the clinical literature in 1965 relating to supplementary intravenous feeding of fat.[12] It has been used extensively as a general term for total parenteral nutrition since the University of Pennsylvania group published their excellent studies on dogs and patients which re-awakened widespread interest and activity in this field.[2,13] It is my opinion that the term "hyperalimentation" may be mistakenly interpreted as meaning that *all* patients being maintained in adequate nutritional status solely by intravenous means require solutions providing calories, amino acids and other nutrients in amounts much larger than those indicated for normal body weight maintenance. To the contrary, patients dependent on parenteral nutrition who may be overweight will actually benefit by some caloric deficit in situations where wound healing is normal and other nutrient intakes are adequate. Many other patients in an acceptable weight range will do quite well at maintenance caloric levels. Those individuals with prior significant weight loss or with serious hypermetabolic problems will require additional calories and certain other nutrients. The aim of parenteral nutrition, like that of diet therapy by oral or tube-fed routes, is the provision of the calories and nutrients required by the specific patient. The phrases "total parenteral nutrition" and "total parenteral alimentation" appear more accurate and inclusive than does the term "hyperalimentation." The latter, if utilized, should refer to the administration of calories appreciably in excess of those usually required.

INDICATIONS FOR TOTAL PARENTERAL NUTRITION

The primary purpose of total parenteral nutrition is to maintain an adequate nutritional state or to improve it in a previously undernourished individual. Its use is indicated only when oral or tube feeding (nasoesophageal, gastrostomy or jejunostomy) is contraindicated or inadequate, and when conventional parenteral support is no longer sufficient for the needs of the patient. With these indications and with the guidelines indicated below, this form of nutrition may be life-saving in a variety of clinical situations, including obstructing lesions of the gastrointestinal tract where surgical intervention must be delayed, massive bowel resections prior to instituting tube or oral feeding, gastrointestinal fistulas, hypermetabolic states associated with extensive burns, major trauma, severe infections where oral or tube feeding is not feasible, acute stages of inflammatory bowel disease, severe uncontrolled malabsorptive states with undernutrition, congenital anomalies in the neonate prior to surgery, prolonged coma where hope for recovery is entertained and the danger of aspiration negates tube feeding, and in patients with

acute renal failure where dialysis is contraindicated during a critical period.

When the basis for impaired nutrition has been diagnosed (i.e., bowel obstruction, multiple intestinal fistulas, etc.), the availability of total parenteral therapy should not be an excuse for procrastination in initiating more definitive therapy when this can be done without a significant increase in risk to the patient. Deficits of hemoglobin, albumin, water, electrolytes, vitamins and minerals can usually be replaced in a matter of days and so permit surgery to proceed in the majority of cases.

The development of a postoperative complication precluding oral or tube feeding cannot be predicted. When such complications do occur, there is a tendency to hope for the best and to delay initiation of adequate parenteral feeding until very serious weight loss or actual debilitation occurs. *Nutritional rehabilitation of the wasted patient is a slow affair.* Furthermore, the debilitated patient is prone to infection, skin breakdown, and fluid and electrolyte problems—all of which complicate recovery.

The making of a decision to undertake total parenteral nutrition requires the weighing of a number of factors (outlined below) and due consideration for the patient's diagnosis and prognosis. At the present time intravenous fat is not generally available in the United States; therefore, large amounts of glucose must serve as the major source of calories with obligatory use of an indwelling central venous catheter. Hence, a long-term commitment to a potentially hazardous, expensive and time-consuming procedure is involved. When the clinical situation is such that prolonged maintenance or improvement in nutritional status will assist in achieving recovery of the patient or will permit significant palliation of underlying disease, the program has obvious merit and should be pursued vigorously. It has no place in prolonging life in the hopelessly ill patient or in routine postoperative care.

Each patient will require a decision based on his specific needs. Unfortunately, there are no accepted guidelines for deciding on the *time* of initiating the program. Assuming that the criteria mentioned in the preceding paragraphs have been met, I initiate the program in either of the two following situations: (*a*) The patient's edema-free body weight has fallen to approximately 10 per cent below his ideal body weight and there is no immediate prospect for improvement in the underlying condition or (*b*) conventional intravenous feeding has been utilized for approximately 3 to 4 weeks as the primary source of nutrition and there is no immediate prospect for improvement in the underlying situation. Total parenteral nutrition is then undertaken in the latter situation even though edema-free body weight is at or above ideal weight. The 3- to 4-week span is an arbitrary one based on observations of clinical behavior of previously well-nourished individuals. During this interval sustained conventional parenteral feeding will reduce soft tissue loss and permit prolonged use of fat stores. The waiting period should be shortened if the patient's clinical status so indicates, *e.g.*, when there is poor wound healing, development of marked hypermetabolic state, exhaustion of suitable peripheral veins or other special circumstances where it is apparent early that prolonged intravenous therapy will be required. "Prevent debilitation while minimizing risk" would seem to be the appropriate aphorism in deciding when to institute total parenteral nutrition.

During the period of conventional intravenous infusion, thought must be given to conservation of the vessels which may be required at a later date for central venous catheters.

ROUTES OF ADMINISTRATION

When total intravenous feeding is deemed necessary, an indwelling central venous catheter is essential for infusion of the necessary hypertonic solutions. This catheter, with its tip in the superior vena cava or atrium, permits the prolonged administration of the nutrient solutions directly into a region of high blood flow where rapid dilution occurs; this minimizes the occurrence of phlebitis and thrombosis.

The use of an indwelling central venous catheter imposes significant risks to the patient. These may be reduced by aseptic techniques in its insertion and maintenance, in its proper placement (checked by x-ray study *prior* to use) and in delivery of sterile solutions. Insertion of the catheter should be treated as an important surgical procedure. Techniques for catheterization of the superior vena cava or right atrium by way of the subclavian or external jugular veins have been published.[2,3,14,15]

The greatest hazard associated with indwelling catheters is bacterial infection, and fungal septicemia has an unexpectedly high occurrence.[16,20] The incidence of infections has been related to the length of time the catheter remains in place. This aspect must be weighed against the critical fact that the number of veins suitable for insertion of the catheter is limited; thus, it is essential to maintain a given catheter as long as possible, consistent with the overall welfare of the patient. Our experience and that of others[2,3,14] indicate that, with aseptic technique and proper maintenance, indwelling catheters may remain safely in place for weeks to months without infection. The situation is less sanguine in patients with chronic infection, debility or diseases affecting immune mechanisms. When infection is apparent or suspected, blood from the catheter and from peripheral veins should be cultured for fungi as well as bacteria.

When indwelling catheters can no longer be used because of exhaustion of suitable veins, internal or external arteriovenous (AV) shunts should be considered for long-term infusion of hypertonic solutions.[4,15,21] In the external technique, an AV shunt of the type used in hemodialysis is inserted and, after adequate flow is assured, a sidearm is placed between the arterial and venous arms to receive the infusion. The hypertonic solution is diluted with flowing blood in the shunt before it reaches the cannulated vein. High-flow shunts are desirable since they minimize clotting: long-term heparinization may be necessary to permit prolonged use of relatively low-flow shunts. Details of a delivery system utilizing external AV shunts have been published.[4,15,21] As with indwelling catheters, infection and clotting have been the factors eventually causing removal. Utilization of an internal AV fistula[22] for parenteral feeding has been proposed[4,15] and reports of limited experience have been published.[15] Its usefulness in permitting administration of hypertonic solutions for prolonged periods without serious complications requires further exploration.

DELIVERY SYSTEMS

The nutrient solutions may be delivered from bottles or plastic bags by gravity flow or by a propulsion pump utilizing infusion tubing leading into indwelling catheters or AV shunts.

Hydrostatic pressure allows infusion of large volumes of hypertonic solution through the catheter. To assure an even flow rate, to overcome the increased resistance of filters of small porosity (especially with continued use) and to minimize the likelihood of clotting at the catheter tip, the utilization of a constant-flow propulsion pump is desirable. However, pumping of fluids—even from systems with collapsible bags—presents the danger of air embolism; hence, it must be used only when there is constant supervision, or, preferably, when the pump has proven safeguards, such as a controlling photoelectric monitor attached to the drip chamber[4] or a weight-sensing device.

Although there is no uniformity of agreement on their value, in-line cellulose-ester membrane filters have been used in an effort to provide greater assurance of sterile delivery of parenteral fluids[2,4,16] and to prevent introduction of particulate matter. Details have been presented elsewhere.[16,23]

The use of pliable plastic bags[4,23] eliminates the danger of breakage, simplifies transportation and storage and greatly reduces storage space requirements prior to and after filling, as compared to formed glass or plastic bottles. One-liter and 2-liter bags are available.[23] If albumin, lipids or blood is avoided in these bags, the usual water solutions of nutrients do not extract measurable amounts of plasticizers or stabilizers used in their manufacture.[23–25]

Empty standard IV bottles may be obtained, sterilized and used for preparing and storing formulas. "Partial-fill" bottles of 1 liter with protein hydrolysate are available; 50 per cent glucose and other solutions can be added. Two-liter sterile evacuated bottles, originally designed for storing plasma, are useful; while large and heavy, they are less expensive than plastic bags, allow easier initiation of transfer of fluid and fill much more rapidly because of the negative pressure.

NUTRITIONAL CONSIDERATIONS

General Requirements. Approximately 30 kcalories (kcal) per kg of body weight per day should be sufficient to maintain weight for the patient who is in an acceptable weight range with restricted activity and has little or no fever or other significant hypermetabolic condition.[8,35] Calories should be increased appropriately to permit weight gain in individuals who are significantly underweight or to meet other needs. All of the essential and sufficient nonessential amino acids should be provided in amounts needed for adequate protein synthesis. Mineral and vitamin intakes should meet individual requirements without excessive wastage or toxicity. These nutritional requirements are discussed in detail below. Water should be administered in volumes consistent with the renal and cardiovascular requirements of the patient and adequate to cover abnormal fluid losses.

Energy Sources and Requirements. Glucose is the most commonly used carbohydrate for caloric replacement and in the United States is the major source of energy. It is readily available and relatively inexpensive, can be given in high concentrations and in large total amounts which are well tolerated by most patients after a period of adaptation. It should be noted that glucose in parenteral fluids is glucose monohydrate; 1 gram provides 3.4 kcal. Infrequent but potentially serious complications may develop with hypertonic solutions. These include coma attributable to hyperosmolar nonketotic hyperglycemia,[26] acidosis,[27,28] convulsions secondary to acute osmotic changes and osmotic diuresis with sodium loss and dehydration. Fructose offers no obvious advantage and is more expensive; when administered rapidly, it has induced increased blood lactate levels and corresponding acidosis.[29] Fructose or xylitol infusions can decrease serum phosphate and raise lactate, urate and bilirubin.[30] Serious other side effects have been reported with xylitol in clinical trials;[31,32] however, it has been suggested that these effects were caused by contamination from the bottle closure. Intravenous maltose is metabolized[33] but has not been evaluated for its utility or safety in parenteral nutrition. Other disaccharides and the polysaccharides are not hydrolyzed significantly and, hence, are not available for metabolism.

The availability of a parenteral fat emulsion providing approximately 1000 or more kcal per liter and capable of being given safely for prolonged periods will assist greatly in meeting caloric needs by eliminating the need for large fluid volumes and high glucose concentrations; it may also eliminate the need for deep vein catheters. While certain preparations are widely used in Europe, FDA-approved intravenous fat is no longer available in the United States for general use. New emulsions are presently undergoing clinical trial and hopefully will be available shortly. Although the European experience is encouraging,[5] further experience is required to learn whether they will overcome the problems of previous emulsions.[1,7]

Alcohol is sometimes used as a source of calories. It cannot be given in large concentrations, and it has been my experience that older debilitated patients often do not tolerate even dilute solutions well. Increasing evidence for a direct pharmacologic effect on liver[34] makes its use questionable.

Where significant losses of lean tissue have occurred and replenishment is indicated, caloric intake (primarily as glucose) may be proportionately increased from the usual 30 kcal/kg to 50 kcal per kg or more. Caloric requirements above resting levels may be imposed by trauma and inflammation. Kinney et al.[35] note that major skeletal injury (this excludes uncomplicated elective surgery) commonly results in increases of 10 to 30 per cent above normal for 1 to 3 weeks, followed by a reduction to values of 10 to 20 per cent below normal, as a reflection of the tissue depletion which has occurred. Infection in a major serous cavity usually produces increases of 15 to 50 per cent above normal, with some elevation persisting as long as the inflammation remains. Extensive burn may cause an increase of metabolism of 40 to 100 per cent for weeks at a time; the older figures of 5000 to 6000 kcal per day are not accepted. As these and other authors[36] point out, the catabolism of infection and trauma is not related to lack of energy sources in the body. Soft tissue breakdown continues despite fat reserves and glucose infusion. The need for control of infection and optimum treatment of trauma is obvious in reducing catabolic activity.

Amino Acids. Achievement of nitrogen equilibrium or positive nitrogen balance requires sufficient essential amino acids and nonessential amino acids (or a source of nitrogen for synthesis of the latter) together with adequate calories to avoid utilization of the amino acids for caloric purposes.[7] The use of blood, plasma, or plasma protein fractions solely to provide amino acids is a wasteful and expensive procedure;[1] administration of blood or plasma also invites the risk of hepatitis. Presently, the cheapest sources of amino acids are protein hydrolysates, which are solutions of free amino acids and short-chain peptides. Two main types are available, casein hydrolyzed by porcine pancreas and beef blood fibrin hydrolyzed by acid. Both types have added amino acids to give a more balanced amino acid pattern. A large proportion (approximately $\frac{1}{3}$) of the nitrogen in the hydrolysates is present as peptides, a proportion of which is believed to be metabolically unavailable and excreted in the urine. The free amino acids are available for protein synthesis: their absolute and relative amounts are important in metabolism and tissue synthesis.[37] Purified L-amino acids preparations are currently entering into clinical use. Whether their general usefulness and cost will result in them replacing the hydrolysates remains to be seen. Solutions of essential amino acids with glucose appear to have special value in patients with severe renal failure being maintained by intravenous nutrition where dialysis is undesirable at that time.[38]

Hydrolysate nitrogen daily intakes capable of inducing weight in infants has been reported at approximately 4.5 gm of hydrolysate per kg of body weight (equivalent to 0.6 to 0.7 gm of nitrogen);[2,3] these were supplemented periodically, in many patients, with blood and plasma. Dudrick et al.[2] give a base solution to adults supplying 685 ml of 5 per cent fibrin hydrolysate per 1000 ml and 1000 kcal. When this formula is utilized, the nitrogen and caloric intakes are proportional. There are experimental data and our own experience to suggest that amino acid requirements for wound healing and weight maintenance are met with a total of approximately 20 ml of 5 per cent hydrolysate per kg of body weight (equivalent to 0.140 gm of hydrolysate nitrogen or 1 gm of hydrolysate per kg of body weight) when (a) caloric and other needs are being met, (b) there is no significant extra loss of protein from the body and (c) infection, other hypermetabolic states and malignancy are controlled.

Very prolonged intravenous feeding has been noted, in our experience, to be associated with fatty liver. Whether this is related to some deficiency or imbalance in the amino acid supply or to some other nutritional deficit or imbalance is not known.

It is of interest to consider the additional nitrogen requirements imposed by accretion of lean body mass in previously depleted or debilitated patients. There is good experimental evidence that previously protein-depleted animals[39] and man[36,40] utilize amino acids more efficiently than do normal animals. When metabolic conditions are favorable for anabolism in patients, an average daily accretion rate for nitrogen (positive nitrogen balance) appears to be approximately 4 gm, representing 20 to 26 gm of protein or 90 to 120 gm of lean body mass.[2,41] This is 0.057 gm of nitrogen per kg of body weight for a 70-kg man. This, incidentally, would require further retention of approximately 10 mEq of potassium and 2 mEq of magnesium. Assuming that about two-thirds of the amino acids of the hydrolysate are available and are utilized, an additional 10 ml of hydrolysate per kg should permit good net protein synthesis. Thus, when persistent lean tissue renewal is required, a total of 30 ml of 5 per cent hydrolysate per kg should be adequate, up to a maximum of 2 liters per day, administered with hypertonic glucose and other nutrients. Physical therapy of the bedridden patient and mobilization where possible will assist in muscle renewal and prevent other undesirable consequences of bed rest. When the infused nitrogen is inadequate and a significant chronic acidosis is present, ammonia excretion in the urine will increase at the expense of body protein.[42]

It is to be noted that protein hydrolysate and amino acid solutions have nutrients other than amino acids and glucose. Representative analyses from our laboratory are given in Table 36–1. It should be noted that casein hydrolysate has appreciably more sodium, calcium and phosphate than fibrin hydrolysate. Fre-amine has essentially no potassium, calcium, phosphate or magnesium.

Vitamins. The vitamin dosages used by various investigators in parenteral feeding of infants appear adequate for growth.[2,3,28] However, it should be emphasized that, in most of the pediatric studies, the patients were infused for less than 6 weeks. The daily use of a multiple vitamin infusion (MVI, U.S.V. Pharmaceutical) by these investigators presents certain problems. It contains vitamins A and D in moderately large amounts, vitamin E in small amounts, and has many but not all water-soluble vitamins present in high concentrations. Vitamins K, B_{12} and folic acid were added. Increasing the

Table 36-1. Average Composition of Intravenous Amino Acid Solutions

		Fibrin Hydrolysate (Aminosol) (per L)	Casein Hydrolysate (Amigen) (per L)	Fre-amine (8.5%) (per 0.5 L)
Na	mEq	2.5	33.0	5.0
Cl	mEq	10.2	17.0	7.5
K	mEq	17.0	19.0	0.0
Ca	mg	20.0	115‡	0.0
P free*	mg	10.0	220	0.15
P total†	mg	10.0	460	0.30
Mg	mEq	2.2	2.2	0.27
Nitrogen	g	7.4	6.8	6.3

* As free inorganic orthophosphate
† As determined after dry ashing and heating in N/1 HCl
‡ Range of 100–125 mg/L

Table 36-2. Composition of Basic Formula Nutrient Solution[23]*

Bag/Bottle	Sodium Chloride (0.9%) (ml)	Protein Hydro-lysate (5%) Dextrose (ml)†	Glucose (50%) (ml)	Magnesium Sulfate (50%) (ml)	Calcium Gluconate (10%) (ml)	Potassium Chloride (mEq)	Potassium Phosphate (ml)§	Trace Element Solution (ml)	Vitamins
A	350	1000	650	4	20 (10)‡	40	0	1‖	+¶
B	150	500	350	0	0	20	5 (0.0)‡	0	0

* From Shils[23] JAMA; reprinted with permission.

† Total composition with fibrin hydrolysate (*e.g.* Aminosol): calories, 2150; sodium, 80 mEq; potassium, 99 mEq; chloride, 150 mEq; calcium, 215 mg; magnesium, 20 mEq; phosphorus (as inorganic phosphate), 356 mg. Total composition with casein hydrolysate (*e.g.* Amigen): calories, 2150; sodium, 134 mEq; potassium, 100 mEq; chloride, 160 mEq; calcium, 295 mg; magnesium, 20 mEq; phosphorus (as free inorganic phosphate), 350 mg.

‡ When casein hydrolysate (*e.g.* Amigen) is used, a reduction is made in calcium gluconate and potassium phosphate as indicated in parentheses.

§ Potassium phosphate, sterile solution contains 3 mEq of potassium and 68 mg of phosphorus as inorganic phosphate per ml.

‖ Trace element solution: zinc chloride, 0.62 gm; cupric sulfate .5H$_2$O, 0.60 gm; manganous sulfate .H$_2$0, 0.20 gm and sodium iodide, 0.01 gm are dissolved in 150 ml sterile saline, transferred to sterile vials through a 0.22 μ Millipore filter and sterilized by autoclaving: 1 ml supplies 2.0 mg of zinc, 0.4 mg of copper, 0.2 mg of manganese and 0.056 mg of iodide ions. Iron is given intramuscularly (as the dextran, Imferon) or intravenously (as the dextrin, Astrafer) as indicated.

¶ Vitamins: Berocca C, 2 ml twice/wk; Folbesyn, 1 vial/wk; MVI, 10 ml twice/wk; Aquamephyton, 5 mg/wk (see Table 36-3).

vitamin E with this preparation means giving more vitamins A and D. There may be a basis for concern about giving extra vitamin D when intravenous calcium and phosphate are also being administered. This preparation does not contain folic acid, B_{12}, biotin or vitamin K. Information is needed as to whether biotin is necessary when intestinal flora may be markedly altered or absent.

Our program utilizes four different preparations (footnote, Table 36–2) to obtain what is presumed to be adequate amounts of all known vitamins, with the possible exception of vitamin E. Multiple sources are necessary, since no single suitable parenteral vitamin preparation is available. The average daily intake with this vitamin combination is compared with the Recommended Dietary Allowances (RDA)[43] in Table 36–3. Attempting to meet requirements for all vitamins by using the preparations mentioned is not entirely satisfactory, since the amounts of some vitamins are high while the amount of vitamin E is low. The fact that some of the water-soluble vitamins are present in amounts much larger than the RDA does not mean that blood levels will be proportionally higher, since the excess will be excreted, if kidney

Table 36-3. Average Daily Adult Vitamin Intake with Basic Formula and Recommended Daily Dietary Allowances (RDA)[43]

Vitamin	Basic Formula	RDA*
Thiamine mg	18.6	1.3
Riboflavin mg	7.1	1.7
Niacinamide mg	33.6	17
Pyridoxine mg	10.7	2
Pantothenate mg	14.3	5–10†
Folic acid mg	0.4	0.4
Vitamin B_{12} μg	2.1	5
Biotin μg	57.0	150–300†
Ascorbic acid mg	215.0	60
Vitamin A IU	2860.0	5000‡
Vitamin D IU	286.0	—
Vitamin E IU	1.4	30†
Vitamin K mg	0.7	—

* For adult males—age 35–55.

† RDA not established; amounts considered to be adequate in usual dietary intake.

‡ Activity includes carotene

Table 36-4. Minerals of Interest in TPN

MACRO (> 200 mg or 5 mM/day)	MICRO (Trace) (< 5 mg/day)
1. Sodium	1. Iron
2. Chloride	2. Zinc
3. Bicarbonate	3. Copper
4. Potassium	4. Iodide
5. Calcium	5. Fluoride
6. Magnesium	6. Chromium*
7. Phosphate	7. Cobalt†
8. Sulfate	8. Manganese*
	9. Molybdenum*
	10. Selenium*
	11. Vanadium*
	12. Nickel*
	13. Tin*

* Human requirement not established.

† Cobalt other than that in vitamin B_{12}.

function is normal. Analyses of blood levels of vitamins in patients on prolonged parenteral feedings have not been published. Unpublished data on a patient with prolonged AV shunt feeding[4] indicate that, of eleven fat- and water-soluble vitamins measured, all were within a normal range after 13 months, with the exception of vitamin E. Although the parenteral requirements for vitamin E for man are unknown and the consequences of its depletion are still unclear, further supplementation appears desirable.

Minerals. These ions may be divided into two broad groups on the basis of their quantitative requirements (Table 36–4).

Macronutrients. Probably the most critical aspect of total parenteral nutrition on a day-by-day basis concerns the requirements for the electrolytes, sodium, potassium and chloride, and for water. No matter how well constructed is the overall formulation, it must be reviewed daily, and sometimes more frequently, when administered to patients with serious problems in fluid and electrolyte balance. Requirements for these ions will depend on the cardiovascular, renal, gastrointestinal and endocrine status of the patient. They have been discussed in detail in Chapters 7 and 35. Ranges used in various formulations have been presented elsewhere.[44]

Calcium and Phosphorus. Neonates on breast feeding ingest in the range of 34 to 44 mg of calcium and 21 to 24 mg of phosphorus per kg per day with absorptions of 55 and 89 per cent, respectively.[44] Most intravenous formulations contain significantly higher levels for pediatric use. There have been two points of view about addition of these two ions to solutions for adults. One position has been to add them routinely, calcium in the range of 200 to 400 mg per 2,500 kcal per day and phosphorus as potassium ortho-phosphate at 300 to 350 mg.[44] The other attitude has been to omit them, while follow-ing serum levels, and then to supply one or both "as indicated." The latter position is no longer tenable with respect to phosphorus. The desirable amount and frequency of calcium administration cannot be answered with certainty. The goal is maintenance of adequate bone mineralization without induc-ing soft tissue calcification. Factors to be taken into account in deciding on calcium administration include parathyroid status, age, state of bone mineralization, heparin usage, magnesium repletion, and degree of mobilization. The decision reached will also determine which protein hydrolysate will be used, since calcium is added to certain products (Table 36–1). Unless there is a contraindication, such as hypercalcemia, cal-cium gluconate is routinely added to our basic formula to meet calcium needs and to avoid hypocalcemia, which may occur as the result of rapid phosphate infusion.

Hypophosphatemia has been noted to de-velop in patients on prolonged feeding unless phosphate is included, either with casein hydrolysate or as an additive in the nutrient solution. The clinical significance of hypo-phosphatemia and phosphate depletion has begun to be appreciated. The importance of phosphate in very many stages of inter-mediary metabolism, in bone formation, and as a constituent of nucleic acids, phospho-proteins and phospholipids makes it desirable to maintain normal levels without waiting for hypophosphatemia to develop. The observations of Lotz *et al.* on the effects of phosphate depletion are suggestive, although the symptoms were variable and nonspecific.[45] Further support for the value of phosphate is

indicated by increasing reports in hypophos-phatemic patients of reduced red cell gly-colysis, decreased concentrations of 2-3 di-phosphoglycerate and ATP, increased hemo-globin-oxygen affinity[46,47] and reversible hemolytic anemia.[48] Avoidance of soft tissue calcification with calcium and phosphate infusions must be an important consideration in giving these ions parenterally for long periods. Some reassurance of the safety of the formulation given below in this regard is obtained by the observation of an absence of nephrocalcinosis in a patient after 16 months of infusion.

The importance of magnesium in human nutrition is well established[49] (Chapter 6B). There is no known direct efficient hormonal control of the serum level of this ion; control will depend on a balance resulting from the amounts administered and released from tissue breakdown, renal excretion, and gastrointestinal losses. The requirements for this ion by the I.V. route are not known with certainty. It is suggested[44] that 0.3 mEq per kg per day is adequate for infants and young children, although a wide range has been given in practice. Similarly adult formula-tions vary widely, from 4 to 25 mEq per 2,500 kcal.

There is an apparent solubilizing effect of magnesium on urinary calcium.[50] If this is a real factor, it may be desirable to provide sufficient magnesium in the paren-teral dose to allow a good urine level which I arbitrarily suggest at 5 or more mEq per day. Renal insufficiency in a patient will require careful monitoring of serum mag-nesium, potassium, phosphorus and calcium. Periodic determinations of serum and urine levels of these ions will afford a basis for evalu-ating the need for possible revision of dosages.

Sulfur. This element is present in tissues as methionine, cysteine, taurine, certain mucopolysaccharides and glycolipids and as sulfate esters of various metabolites. The sul-fur content in the two amino acids is appar-ently sufficient for formation of the other S-containing compounds when the amino supply is adequate. Sulfur enters into taurine along the metabolic pathway of cysteine and into sulfated compounds from inorganic sul-fate derived from cysteine. The sulfate is incorporated into 3'phosphoadenosine-5'phosphosulfate which serves as a general agent for esterification of sulfate.

Microminerals (trace elements). Most physicians have made an effort to supply these nutrients (Table 36–4) in a qualitative way by periodically infusing plasma or blood and by giving parenteral iron.

Iron. Pre-existing iron deficiency anemia should be corrected with intravenous or intramuscular iron. Maintenance iron in infants or children may be given once weekly or biweekly; a suggested dose is approximately 1 mg of iron per day (Table 36–5). Adult iron requirements are given in Chapter 6C. Serial determinations of hemoglobin, red cell indices, serum iron and iron-binding capacity will permit further evaluation of iron requirements, which can be met by parenteral iron every month or two unless iron losses are severe and chronic. Suggested dosage is indicated in Table 36–5.

Other trace elements have been discussed in Chapters 8A and 8B. Objective data on the requirements for these trace elements in parenteral nutrition are essentially non-existent. A trace element mixture (footnote Table 36–2) has been given daily for a year to one patient[4] who remained in good clinical state. The use of purified solution of these elements appears more desirable than periodic administration of blood or plasma with the attendant danger of hepatitis. A review of requirements and tentative suggested intravenous dosages have been given elsewhere[44] and summary data are reproduced here (Table 36–5). The very tentative nature of many of the dosage figures is indicated by a question mark. There are few data indicating the quantities of various of these microminerals which are present in intravenous solutions as contaminants.

Polyunsaturated Fatty Acid (essential fatty acids). Their nutritional and metabolic roles are described in Chapter 4. A parenteral form of these fatty acids is not available in the United States, because of the lack of an approved intravenous fat emulsion with its polyunsaturated fat. With prolonged administration of fat-free formulations, depletion of body stores of these fatty acids may be expected to occur, especially in infants. Re-

Table 36–5. Suggested Approximate Daily Intravenous Requirements for Minerals*

	Infants & Young Children per kg/day	Adults per day
Sodium mEq	3–5	60 and up*
Potassium mEq	3–5	60 and up*
Magnesium mEq	0.3–0.5	8–20
Calcium mg	20–40	200–400+
Phosphorus mg	20–40	300–400
Sulfur	++	++
Iron mg	1†/day	1—males and nm females‡ 2—m females‡
Zinc mg	0.02–0.04(?)	2–4(?)
Copper mg	0.01–0.02(!)	0.5–1.0
Fluoride mg	0.001/ml	1–2(?)
Iodide mcg	3–5(?)	1–2/kg
Manganese mg	0.01–0.02(??)	1–2(??)

* For patients without significant cardiovascular-renal dysfunction or intestinal or renal losses. The upper range is suggested for those with rapid growth rate. The upper ranges for sodium and potassium are very variable and will depend on individual status.
+ Suitability of daily calcium administration in adult will depend on many factors including those affecting bone resorption and soft tissue calcification.
++ Supplied as cysteine and methionine.
† May be given weekly or biweekly after correcting deficiency.
‡ May be given monthly or bimonthly after correcting deficiency; nm = non-menstruating females; m = menstruating females.
(?) Inadequate data—range very uncertain.
(??) Human requirement probable but not definite —range very uncertain.

ports to this effect are beginning to appear. Dermatitis, as well as abnormal tissue fatty acid levels, has been reported in infants.[51,52] After 16 months of parenteral feeding, the types and quantities of fatty acids present in serum, erythrocytes and adipose tissue were similar to the pattern described as occurring in essential fatty acid deficiency in experimental animals.[53] Where available, relatively small amounts of a suitable fat emulsion should be sufficient for this purpose.

It should be emphasized that the empirical aspects of total parenteral nutrition have advanced ahead of our basic knowledge of human long-term intravenous nutritional requirements.

Formulation and Preparation of Solutions. Formulation of the contents of parenteral solutions must be based on a combination of sound nutritional principles and the particular needs of the individual patient. Two approaches in general formulation are

possible. One is the development of a basic unit solution providing a standard amount of kcalories and nutrients per unit volume; the number of units supplied will depend upon individual needs. Adherence to this unit approach involves supplying calories and the constituent nutrients without regard to specific fluid requirement or to the lack of relationship between total calories and cer-

Table 36-6. Preparation of Hyperalimentation Solutions for Adults*

	Bulk method (pharmacy)	Single unit method (ward or pharmacy)
Unit composition of base solution		
Composition	165 g of anhydrous glucose (U.S.P.) + 860 ml 5% glucose in 5% fibrin hydrolysate	350 ml of 50% glucose + 750 ml of 5% glucose in 5% fibrin hydrolysate.
Preparation	Sterilization through 0.22 μ membrane filter under laminar flow, filtered air hood	Aseptic mixing technique under laminar flow, filtered air hood
Volume (ml)	1000	1100
Calories (kcal)	1000	1000
Glucose (g)	208	212
Hydrolysates (g)	43	37
Nitrogen (g)	6.0	5.25
Sodium (mEq)	8	7
Potassium (mEq)	14	13

Additions to each unit of base solution†

Routine
  Sodium (⅔ chloride, ⅓ bicarbonate)   40–50 mEq
  Potassium (chloride)   30–40 mEq
  Magnesium (sulfate)   4–10 mEq
Optional
  Calcium (gluconate)   4– 5 mEq
  Phosphate (potassium acid salt)   4– 5 mEq

Additions to only one unit daily (average adult)†

Routine
  Multiple vitamin infusion   10 ml
Optional
  Vitamin K   5–10 mg
  Vitamin B₁₂   10–30 μg
  Folic acid   0.5–1.5 mg
  Iron (dextriferron)   2.0–3.0 mg

* From Dudrick and Ruberg[55]; reprinted with permission.
† Micronutrients such as zinc, copper, manganese, cobalt, and iodine are present as contaminants in hydrolysate solutions, but may be given in plasma transfusion once or twice weekly if desired.

tain nutrient requirements. The other approach is the individual formulation where the overall daily fluid, caloric and amino acid requirements are estimated and combined with other nutrients. This requires daily review of patient needs prior to preparation and leads to a different prescription for each patient. The basic unit method is the one most widely used as a consequence of the publications of Dudrick et al.[2,13,54,55] Either method will work well if there is the necessary careful daily evaluation of the patient and flexibility in modifying the formulation as the clinical situation demands.

The solutions can be prepared in large-scale procedures in a manufacturing pharmacy, utilizing bulk chemicals and large volume filtering, sterilizing and bottling devices.[54] An alternative method is a smaller-scale preparation utilizing commercial sterile intravenous solutions which are then mixed by open, or preferably, by closed procedures.[2,4,23,56] Strict and persevering adherence to sterile precautions with routine microbiologic monitoring is essential regardless of method.

Examples of formulations based on a basic unit composition are given for adults (Table 36-6) and young children (Table 36-7). An example of a formulation based on an individual prescription but which has fairly broad usefulness is given in Table 36-2.

In this latter formulation the solution is divided between two containers to permit flexibility in fluid volume and to separate calcium and magnesium from phosphate and bicarbonate ions in order to prevent precipitation when these ions are utilized. Details of simple and sterile closed system preparation using plastic bags or bottles are given elsewhere.[23] Such small-scale procedures would appear to have general usefulness in most hospitals and are even applicable for home use after suitable training of the visiting nurse or family members. The relatively large fluid volume in the adult formulas is predicated upon the experience that many

Table 36-7. **Preparation of Pediatric Hyperalimentation Solutions***

Unit composition of base solution			
400 ml	5% Glucose in 5% fibrin hydrolysate	160 kcal	{ 20 g of hydrolysates
250 ml	50% Glucose	500 kcal	{ 20 g of glucose
650 ml		660 kcal	

Additions to each unit of base solution				
Sodium	20 mEq	Sodium chloride (2 mEq/ml)	10	ml
Potassium	25 mEq }	Potassium acid phosphate (2 mEq/ml)	12.5	ml
Phosphorus	25 mEq }			
Calcium	20 mEq	Calcium gluconate, 10% (0.45 mEq/ml)	44	ml
Magnesium	10 mEq	Magnesium sulfate, 50% (4 mEq/ml)	2.5	ml
Multiple vitamin infusion			4	ml
Vitamin K }				
Vitamin B12 }		Added to solution daily or weekly or given		
Folic acid }		intramuscularly	1	ml
Iron }				
Trace elements		Added to solution daily or given as 10 ml/kg plasma twice weekly	1	ml
			75	ml

Base solution	650 ml	
Additives	75 ml	
Final solution†	725 ml	

* From Dudrick and Ruberg;[55] reprinted by permission.
† Given at rate of 145 ml per kg per day, equivalent to 130 kcal per kg per day.

patients requiring parenteral nutrition have appreciable fluid losses from the gastrointestinal tract. Even without such losses, this volume is usually well tolerated. If less fluid is desired without sacrificing caloric content, a 13 per cent volume reduction is achieved by substituting 90 ml of 5 per cent sodium chloride for 500 ml of 0.9 per cent salt solution in the formula. Further volume reduction can be achieved by reducing the quantities of hydrolysate or of glucose or by using more concentrated hydrolysates or amino acids when commercially available. When increased volume is required without additional calories, this is achieved by diluting the formula with saline or sterile water as needed or, more simply, by running in sterile normal saline in "piggy back" fashion.

Additional calories may be given by replacing 0.9 per cent saline with 10 per cent dextrose in saline, by increasing the 50 per cent glucose solution or by giving supplementary bottles of 20 per cent glucose. Smaller caloric intake is achieved by decreasing the volume of 50 per cent glucose.

Electrolytes may be increased or decreased by simple addition or omission from specified bottles. Significant amounts of sodium chloride may be added in relatively small volume by using 5 per cent sodium chloride solution; this may be added accurately by use of a sterile buret-type administration set with calibrated chamber. Crystalline amino acid solutions (with dextrose) are supplied as the chlorides and, therefore, impose a load of chloride ions; sufficient sodium should, therefore, be supplied in the form of bicarbonate, acetate or lactate rather than as the chloride to prevent acidosis.

ADMINISTRATION

There are a number of precautions relating to administration. Many of these (and others where indicated) should be incorporated in prepared medical orders by the physician for guidance and instruction of the house- and nursing staffs. Prior to initiating total parenteral nutrition, the patient's nutritional requirement must be evaluated; in addition, the tolerance for fluid, nitrogen, glucose and minerals, especially potassium and sodium,

must be reviewed in the light of the cardiovascular, renal, gastrointestinal and endocrine status of the individual. Re-evaluation should be made daily on the basis of serial clinical and biochemical evaluations until the patient is known to be stable, then laboratory tests may be made less frequently. Following insertion of the central venous catheter, roentgenologic evidence of its correct position must be obtained, prior to initiating the hypertonic solutions.

Testing the patient's ability to adjust to a large glucose load is essential. It is recommended that for the first 2 to 4 days the glucose content of the formula be halved. Fractional urines should be tested for glucose every 6 hours. Water balance data and daily weight should be obtained. Since most patients develop a good tolerance to glucose, it is our policy to give insulin only for 3+ or 4+ glycosuria or ketonuria, or where glycosuria leads to an osmotic diuresis causing dehydration or where blood sugars are persistently elevated despite minimal glycosuria. Except in diabetics with insulin requirements, relatively small doses of insulin are given initially (4 units for 3+ and 8 units for 4+ without ketones) and modified as experience dictates. Monitoring blood sugar twice daily in the early days will help avoid potentially dangerous hyperosmolar nonketotic coma. When the patient manifests good tolerance or the insulin requirement is fairly well established with a given glucose load, the full amount of glucose may be given with fractional urines being monitored until assurance is obtained that the patient is very well stabilized and utilizing the glucose well, with or without exogenous insulin. In some patients tolerance will develop late. Physicians and nurses caring for the patient receiving insulin must be cautioned against (a) excessive insulin dosage and frequency and (b) replacing hypertonic glucose solutions with isotonic glucose or saline while exogenous insulin is still active.

It will be noted that there is an excess of chloride ion relative to sodium in most formulas. This is no problem for the adult patient with normal renal function or for one with gastric secretory losses. However, in certain individuals this imbalance may cause acidosis and may require addition of sodium bicarbonate or equivalent. Where Cl⁻ salts of crystalline amino acids replace hydrolysate, sodium as bicarbonate, acetate or lactate should replace some of the NaCl.

Filters tend to clog with use and impede or stop infusion rate by gravity flow or propulsion pump. They should be changed not less than every third or fourth day.

A critical aspect of care involves the insurance of sterile precautions when inserting tubing and filters, in making connections and in caring for the CVP catheter and skin at its entry. Tubing from container to filter should be changed daily and preferably with each new container. When a filter is changed, the tubing connecting it to the CVP catheter should be changed simultaneously; its reinsertion to the catheter should be made with prior alcohol or other antiseptic treatment of the joints and use of sterile gloves. A CVP catheter introduced by subclavian approach poses the possibility of an air embolus if accidentally detached. All joints must be firmly connected with sterile tape and insurance taken against direct tension on the catheter.

Catheters must be sutured in place to minimize to-and-fro movements at the skin opening. Opinion differs on the value of antiseptic treatment and use of antibiotics at this entry site. I apply betadine, followed by antibacterial and antifungal ointments every 2 days with fresh sterile dressings utilizing paper tape.

A TEAM FOR TOTAL PARENTERAL NUTRITION

It is apparent from the preceding discussion that this potentially life-saving and morbidity-reducing procedure is a complex one posing multiple problems in patient care, nutrition, safety and equipment. It is constantly changing as new information and supplies become available. Experience indicates that the optimum care of the patient requiring this form of nutritional therapy is most adequately assured by a team approach. The minimum team should include a physician knowledgeable in clinical nutrition and physiology and technique, one or more nurses skilled in the various procedural aspects to supervise administration to the patient and to assist and educate floor nurses, and one or more pharmacists or nurses or other personnel trained in solution preparation. It is desirable for the team physician(s) either to insert the catheters or to have responsibility for insuring that only surgeons trained in catheter insertion are permitted to do so. It is advisable that the hospital medical board formally designate the team and issue a clear statement of its mission and responsibility.

BIBLIOGRAPHY

1. Shils: Postgrad. Med., *36*, A99, 1964; J.A.M.A., *220*, 1721, 1972.
2. Dudrick, Wilmore, Vars, *et al.*: Ann. Surg. *169*, 974, 1969.
3. Filler, Eraklis, Rubin, *et al.*: New Engl. J. Med., *287*, 589, 1969.
4. Shils, Wright, Turnbull and Brescia: New Engl. J. Med., *283*, 341, 1970.
5. Meng and Law (eds.): *Parenteral Nutrition.* Springfield, Charles C Thomas, 1970.
6. Elman: *Parenteral Nutrition in Surgery.* New York, Paul B. Hoeber, 1947, pp. 1–13.
7. Geyer: Physiol. Rev., *40*, 150, 1960.
8. Mengoli: Am. J. Surg., *121*, 311, 1971.
9. Ellison, McCleery, Zollinger and Case: Surgery, *26*, 374, 1949.
10. Rice, Orr, Treloar and Strickler: Arch. Surg., *61*, 977, 1950.
11. Merrill: *The Treatment of Renal Failure.* New York, Grune and Stratton, 1955, pp. 88–89.
12. Watkin and Steinfeld: Am. J. Clin. Nutrition, *16*, 182, 1965.
13. Dudrick, Wilmore, Vars and Rhoads: Surgery, *64*, 134, 1968.
14. Wilmore and Dudrick: Arch. Surg., *98*, 256, 1969.
15. Atkins, Vizzo, Cole, *et al.*: Trans. Am. Soc. Artif. Int. Organs, *16*, 260, 1970.
16. Wilmore and Dudrick: Arch. Surg., *99*, 462, 1969.
17. Corso, Agostinelli and Brandriss: J.A.M.A., *210*, 2075, 1969.
18. Bolasny, Shepard and Scott: Surg. Gyn. Obst., *130*, 342, 1970.
19. Ashcraft and Leape: J.A.M.A., *212*, 454, 1970.
20. Curry and Quie: New Engl. J. Med., *285*, 1221, 1971.
21. Scribner, Cole, Christopher, *et al.*: J.A.M.A., *212*, 457, 1970.
22. Brescia, Cimino, Appel *et al.*: New Engl. J. Med., *275*, 1089, 1966.
23. Shils: J.A.M.A., *220*, 1721, 1972.
24. Jaeger and Rubin: Science, *170*, 460, 1970.
25. Rubin: *In* Proc. A.M.A. Symp. Total Parenteral Nutrition, Nashville, Tenn., 1/18/72. A.M.A. Council on Foods and Nutrition, Chicago, Ill., 1972.

26. Wyrick, Rea and McClelland: J.A.M.A., *211*, 1697, 1970.
27. Winters, Scaglione, Nahas, *et al.*: J. Clin. Invest., *43*, 647, 1964.
28. Kaplan, Mares, Quintana, *et al.*: Arch. Surg., *99*, 567, 1969.
29. Bergström, Hultman and Roch-Norlund: Acta Med. Scand., *184*, 359, 1968.
30. Schumer: *In* Nahas and Fox (eds.): *Body Fluid Replacement in the Surgical Patient.* New York, Grune and Stratton, 1970, pp. 326–333.
31. Thomas and Edwards: New Engl. J. Med., *283*, 437, 1970 (Letter).
32. Schumer: Metabolism, *20*, 345, 1971.
33. Young and Weser: J. Clin. Invest., *50*, 986, 1971.
34. Rubin and Lieber: Science, *172*, 1097, 1971.
35. Kinney, Long and Duke: *In* Nahas and Fox (eds.): *Body Fluid Replacement in the Surgical Patient.* New York, Grune and Stratton, 1970, pp. 296–300.
36. Cahill, Felig and Marliss: *In* Nahas and Fox (eds.): *Body Fluid Replacement in the Surgical Patient.* New York, Grune and Stratton, 1970, pp. 286–293.
37. Harper: *In* Munro and Allison (eds.): *Mammalian Protein Metabolism.* New York, Academic Press, 1964, Vol. 2, Chap. 13, pp. 87–134.
38. Dudrick, Steiger and Long: Surgery, *68*, 180, 1970.
39. Allison: Am. J. Med., *5*, 419, 1948.
40. Werner: Ann. Surg., *126*, 175, 1947.
41. Moore: *Metabolic Care of the Surgical Patient.* Philadelphia, W. B. Saunders, 1959, p. 46.
42. Owen, Felig, Morgan, *et al.*: J. Clin. Invest., *48*, 574, 1969.
43. Nat. Res. Council, Food & Nutrition Board: Recommended Dietary Allowances 7th ed., 1968, Pub. #1694, Nat. Acad. Sci., Washington, D.C.
44. Shils: *In* Proc. A.M.A. Symp. Total Parenteral Nutrition, Nashville, Tenn., 1/17/72. A.M.A. Council on Foods and Nutrition, Chicago, Ill., 1972.
45. Lotz, Zisman and Bartter: New Engl. J. Med., *278*, 409, 1968.
46. Lichtman, Miller, Cohen and Waterhouse: Ann. Int. Med., *74*, 562, 1971.
47. Travis, Sugarman, Ruberg, *et al.*: New Engl. J. Med., *285*, 763, 1971.
48. Jacob and Amsden: New Engl. J. Med., *285*, 1446, 1971.
49. Shils: Medicine, *48*, 61, 1969.
50. Miller, Vermeulen and Moore: J. Urol., *79*, 607, 1958.
51. Holman: Chap. 8 *In Progress in the Chemistry of Fats and Other Lipids.* Holman (ed.) Vol. 9 Pt. 2. New York, Pergamon Press, 1968, pp. 275–348.
52. Paulsrud, Pensler and Whitten, *et al.*: Am. J. Clin. Nutrition, *25*, 897, 1972.
53. Shils: Gastroenterology, *60*, 734, 1971 (abstract).
54. Flack, Gans, Serlick and Dudrick: Am. J. Hosp. Pharmacy, *28*, 326, 1971.
55. Dudrick and Ruberg: Gastroenterology, *61*, 901, 1971.
56. Burke: *In* Proc. A.M.A. Symp. Total Parenteral Nutrition, Nashville, Tenn., 1/18/72. A.M.A. Council on Foods and Nutrition, Chicago, Ill., 1972.

Chapter

37

Nutrition and Neoplasia

MAURICE E. SHILS

NUTRITION AS AN ETIOLOGIC FACTOR IN TUMOR DEVELOPMENT

Modification by Calories and Nutrients of Spontaneous Tumor Development in Experimental Animals. Various manipulations of dietary components have been utilized to test the effects of their intake. In some experiments, the diets have been adequate in all components, but the major caloric contribution in the control diet, usually carbohydrate, has been partially withheld from the experimental group leading to inadequate caloric intake, designated as "caloric restriction."[1] Another approach to calorie deficit has involved restricting all components of the control diet: this has been termed "underfeeding."[1] In most studies of these types the experimental animals were allowed to ingest only 50 to 70 per cent as much as their fully fed controls. The development of spontaneous tumors in mice and rats was inhibited by such restriction; however, the magnitude of inhibition was influenced by tumor type, the degree of restriction and the presence of carcinogenic agents.[1]

Several more recent long-term studies in rats confirm the older studies, but provide some exceptions and new data. When a commercial diet was compared to four purified diets varying in protein (casein), carbohydrate (sucrose) or in total calories in male rats, total tumor risk was found to be directly and exponentially related to caloric intake. Within each dietary group, rats of heavier weight had greater tumor risk than lighter rats. Occurrence and malignancy of certain

tumors correlated with the level of protein intake; malignant lymphomas were predominant in rats with high protein intake, whereas fibromas and fibrosarcomas predominated in those with low protein intake. Lowest incidence, greatest delay in time of occurrence, absence of malignant epithelial tumors and greatest life expectancy were observed when intakes of protein, carbohydrate and total calories were low.[2] In another study 10, 22 or 51 per cent casein in isocaloric diets was fed to male rats on an *ad libitum* or caloric-restricted basis. With *ad libitum* intake, the highest incidence of chromophobe adenomas of the anterior pituitary gland was found to be associated with the dietary group having the highest intake of food. Under restricted conditions tumor incidence was directly related to the protein level in the diet. Restriction in both caloric and protein intakes depressed the incidence to the greatest extent. Among all six dietary groups, body weight of the rat early in life correlated directly with the tumor prevalence in later life.[3]

Vitamin and Mineral Deficiencies and Tumor Development. There are important exceptions to the preceding evidence for decreased tumor incidence with restrictions of calories and major dietary components. Deficiencies of certain micronutrients have been associated with an *increased* incidence of spontaneous tumors in rats. Thus, vitamin A deficiency has been related to the development of odontomas[4] and salivary gland tumors;[5] a cereal-type diet low in iodide to increased frequency of thyroid tumors and pituitary enlargement;[6]

magnesium deficiency to thymoma, resembling lymphoma,[7,8] or to chronic myelogenous leukemia.[9] The development of cirrhosis and hepatoma which was noted to occur in rats on choline-deficient diets[10a] is now believed also to be related to the concomitant exposure to aflatoxin which was unknown at the time of the original experiments.[10b]

Nutrient Intake Modifies Carcinogens. The possible relation of food additives, food contaminants and naturally occurring toxic constituents, *per se*, to neoplastic development will not be discussed here. However, evidence is at hand which associates nutritional factors with modification of the action of carcinogenic substances.

Endoplasmic reticulum (or its fragments, the microsomes) of various organs, especially the liver, contains enzyme systems which can convert many drugs and foreign chemicals into more polar compounds.[11] Also, treatment of an animal with certain drugs causes the animal to acquire an increased capacity to metabolize a wide range of drugs administered later.[12] Genetic and developmental factors play a role, but the extent of the drug-metabolizing enzymes inducibility appears to be influenced principally by hormones and by environmental factors: the latter include dietary and nutritional factors. There is evidence that the activities of these enzymes are depressed by protein deficiency,[13,14] starvation,[15] fat-free diets[16] and certain vitamin deficiencies.[17]

One of the most intensively studied carcinogens whose action is strongly influenced by nutritional factors is the azo dye, p-dimethylaminoazobenzene (DMAB). In the 1930's, Japanese investigators observed that rats subsisting on rice developed liver cancer when given the dye. Addition of yeast or liver prevented the tumors. It was found by others that riboflavin and casein, together, markedly reduced tumor incidence when added to the rice diet. An ameliorating influence of nutritional factors has also been observed even after the initiating effect of the dye has been operating for some time;[18] however, once adenomatous hyperplasia of the bile ducts, cholangioma or hepatoma was present, improvement in diet was without effect. Demethylation of DMAB by drug-

metabolizing enzymes results in loss of carcinogenicity.[19] It is possible that deficiencies, such as those of protein and riboflavin, may depress the activities of these enzymes, with resultant persistence of carcinogenicity.

Aflatoxins, a family of mycotoxins produced by certain strains of *Aspergillus flavus*, may contaminate peanuts, cereals and other foods.[20] Diets low in protein have had variable effects on aflatoxin toxicity and carcinogenicity.[21,22] Although malnutrition and aflatoxins coexist in many areas of the world where liver cancer is prevalent, animal experiments thus far have not precisely duplicated the disease syndrome and morphologic picture observed in man.[23] Acute toxicity of aflatoxin B is appreciably *less* in rats on a diet marginally low in lipotropes as compared to those on a control diet; however, following a carcinogenic dose, abnormal hepatocytes and hepatic carcinoma appeared much earlier in the experimental than in control rats.[23] Demethylating and hydroxylating enzymes were reduced in the livers of rats on the low lipotrope diet and the former were not induced by aflatoxin B.

A somewhat similar situation appears to occur with protein deficiency and dimethylnitrosoamine.[24] Protein deficiency protects rats against the acute lethal effects of the chemical but increases the late carcinogenic actions, leading to kidney cancer. It is postulated that the metabolizing enzyme in liver is suppressed by a low protein diet, thus decreasing the rate of metabolism of the toxic product and decreasing acute mortality, but, at the same time, resulting in prolonged exposure of the kidney with increased methylation of DNA and increased carcinogenesis.

Examples of the opposite effect have been noted where increased amounts of nutrients augment carcinogens. Addition of tryptophan or other indoles to 2-acetylaminofluorene markedly increased the incidence of bladder tumors in rats.[25] Extra thiamin, given to rats on a grain diet with bracken fern, increased the incidence of bladder tumor, without affecting the high incidence of intestinal tumors occurring in animals subsisting on the basic diet with the carcinogen.[26] A single injection of streptozotocin, a naturally occurring nitrosourea, when given with two injections of large doses of nicotinamide, resulted in the appearance of insulin-secreting pancreatic islet cell tumors in 92 per cent of male rats 226 to 547 days later; streptozotocin by itself caused a 4 per cent tumor incidence; nicotinamide by itself had no effect.[27]

Dietary Deficiencies and Tumor Growth. It has been concluded that caloric intake can retard the establishment and growth of transplanted tumors only when the host weight diminishes.[1] Similarly, protein deprivation and other deficiencies are inhibitory only when caloric intake is decreased with resultant poor growth or weight loss.[1] An exception to this may occur with zinc deficiency in rats, where Walker 256 transplanted tumor growth was significantly reduced despite only small growth differences with weight-matched controls.[28] Variation in the proportion of dietary fat appears to have no consistent effect on transplant take and growth. When protein intakes of 0, 18 and 30 per cent were fed to rats for 2 weeks and Walker carcinosarcoma 256 injected intraportally, it was noted that the greater the protein intake, the greater the number of animals demonstrating hepatic metastases and the larger the tumors present. The level of hepatic protein influenced the growth of metastases rather than the "take" of tumor cells. The incidence and size of metastases were no greater in fatty livers caused by a high-fat choline-free diet than in normal livers on choline-containing or low-fat diets.[29]

Amino Acids. Omission of many but not all of the essential amino acids from the diets of rats with Walker 256 transplants[30] and of sarcoma-180 bearing mice[31] inhibited growth of the tumors but also resulted in loss of host body weight. There have been a small number of limited and unsatisfactory clinical trials with diets low in phenylalanine and tyrosine.[32] While not considered to be an essential amino acid, nutritional requirements have been found to exist for L-asparagine by certain neoplastic cells in tissue culture, because of a deficiency of L-asparagine synthetase. A number of studies[33] have resulted in the finding that the enzyme L-asparaginase (which deaminates L-asparagine to aspartic acid) has antitumor action in

neoplasms of the mouse, rat and dog. A wide variety of human neoplasms have been treated with L-asparginase derived from *E. coli*; however, at this time, acute lymphocytic leukemia appears to be the most sensitive, with a high percentage of remissions which are not sustained.[33,34]

Amino acid analogs have been tested as inhibitors of tumor growth, but, with the possible minimal usefulness of the glutamine antagonists azaserine and diazo-oxo-norleucine (DON), these have not been clinically useful.

Vitamins. Deficiencies of folic acid,[35] of pyridoxine[36] or of riboflavin[37] have each been found to result in significant inhibition of the growth of certain tumors beyond the effect of the vitamin deficiency *per se.* Studies of the vitamin composition of various experimental tumors indicate that there is no specific qualitative difference as compared to normal tissues. While a number of tumors tend to be low in certain vitamins, values as low or even lower are noted in some normal tissues. Various vitamin antimetabolites have been tested against human neoplasms. To date, the only clinically useful analog is methotrexate, which plays an important role in the treatment of acute leukemias and metastatic choriocarcinoma. Pyridoxine-low diets, combined in some cases with 4-deoxypyridoxine, had no definite antitumor effect in patients with advanced neoplastic diseases.[38] Possible new approaches utilizing nutritional factors in cancer chemotherapy have been discussed recently.[32,39]

The inhibition of tumor genesis by dietary means involves a potentially very complex and poorly understood problem. Dietary restriction, or specific deficiency, leads to many changes in the animal body. With endocrine-sensitive tumors, such as spontaneous mammary tumors, the principal effect may be related to reduced estrogen production. A general phenomenon may be involved, such as that suggested by Bullough, who postulated that inhibition is secondary to a decrease in the mean mitotic activity of the tissue.[40] Where a deficiency leads to tumor development, the converse may occur, with increased mitotic activity of certain cells with neoplastic potential.

Human Epidemiologic Data Relating Neoplasia to Dietary Practices. From the earliest medical records to the present, physicians and laymen have postulated an association (either protective or predisposing) between diet and the development of cancer.[41] This has proved a fertile area for a wide range of speculation extending from food faddists to epidemiologists. An objective approach views diet composition and practices in food preparation as among the possible environmental factors which may influence tumor development. Gastrointestinal neoplasms have been of special interest, since the incidence of malignancy in both the upper and lower areas of the alimentary tract is often high and the survival rate is low. Possible relations to diet are briefly discussed by anatomical division of the alimentary tract.

Oropharyngeal and Esophageal Carcinoma. An association has been noted between the occurrence of Plummer-Vinson syndrome and cancer of the hypopharynx in Swedish women.[42] The syndrome is believed to be secondary to iron deficiency, but vitamin deficiencies are also involved.

Esophageal carcinoma has an extremely high incidence (especially among males) in certain areas, including France,[43,44] India,[43,45] parts of the Soviet Union,[43] Finland,[43,44] China and Hong Kong,[43] West Indies[43] and parts of Africa.[43,46] It is practically unknown in West Africa but is very common in East and South Africa; the high frequency in certain areas seems to be a development of the past 30 or 40 years.[46] An epidemiologic study of patients with carcinoma of the esophagus in New York City, as compared with equal numbers of controls with tumors in other organs, indicated that the males with esophageal cancer tended to be heavier smokers and drinkers and consumed less milk, eggs and green and leafy vegetables than their controls.[47]

Gastric Cancer. There are large demographic differences in the prevalence of this malignancy. Japan, Chile, Austria, Finland, and Iceland, among others, have rates (predominately in males) four or more times those of U.S. Caucasians.[43,44] In the U.S.[44,48] and in Europe,[49] higher rates are noted for gastric as well as esophageal cancer among low income groups. Certain ethnic groups in the U.S. appear to have increased risk.[44,48] Studies of dietary practices in patients with gastric cancer have yielded few[48] or no significant differences[50,51] from control groups. An association with alcohol intake has been suggested[52] and denied.[48,50] The increased use of laxatives[48] or mineral oil[53] in affected individuals has been noted. It has been suggested, but remains unproven, that the high incidence of this tumor in Iceland is related to the large intake of smoked food, perhaps in association with a low intake of vitamin C.[54a] It has been pointed out that Japanese prefer talc-dusted rice, and that the talc may contain asbestos.[54b] The latter is implicated in the development of gastrointestinal cancer, especially gastric cancer.[54c] It is postulated that the asbestos-contaminated talc on rice is the carcinogen or co-carcinogen responsible for the high incidence of stomach cancer in Japan.[54b]

Colon Cancer. Death rates for carcinoma of the large bowel have a strong negative correlation with those of gastric cancer, the one being common where the other is rare. In the U.S. and England, colon cancer is second only to lung cancer in numbers of deaths, accounting for approximately 14 and 12 per cent respectively of all deaths from malignancy. It has been suggested that cancer of the colon in New Yorkers is associated with their high fat intake.[55] In Japan, where colonic cancer is uncommon, fat intake is about 12 per cent of calories and mostly of an unsaturated type, compared to the 40 to 44 per cent figure in the U.S. Japanese immigrants, and especially their children born in the U.S., have a much higher incidence of this disease than Japanese in Japan. The same trend has been noted for Puerto Ricans living in Puerto Rico and on the mainland. Japanese with colon cancer have a higher socioeconomic status than those with rectal cancer and tend to eat diets with more calories in the form of fats and fresh fruit.[56] Czechs have approximately twice the U.S. rate for gastric carcinoma and about one-half the U.S. rate for intestinal cancer.[57] Their dietary intake is appreciably lower in animal-derived protein and fat and in vitamins;

the caloric intake is the same and obtained to a greater degree from vegetable sources than is the American diet. Contrary to the observations with carcinoma of the esophagus and stomach, the incidence of colon cancer in the U.S. does not vary appreciably with color or socioeconomic status.[43,44]

Various authors have pointed out that populations in areas with a high incidence of colonic tumors tend to consume diets relatively high in refined foods and low in unabsorbed cellulose ("fiber"), whereas those where the incidence is low subsist largely on vegetarian diets with relatively little animal products. The refined diets result in relatively small stool volumes and prolonged intestinal transit times (primarily in the colon), whereas large stools and more rapid transit is associated with high cellulose diets.[58-62] There are also differences in the bacterial flora associated with the two types of diets.[62] Consumers of "Western" type diets were found to have higher concentrations of fecal steroids, which also tended to be more degraded, than those on vegetarian diets. It was suggested that certain metabolites of bile salts may be carcinogenic.[62] There appears to be some disagreement on the relative amounts of certain fecal bile salts in groups on vegetarian diets.[63] Assuming that carcinogens are produced by bacterial action, delayed colon transit time would permit increased formation and epithelial exposure.

Liver. Primary hepatic carcinoma is a major problem in certain population groups, especially males, in Africa, South China, Hawaii, Romania and elsewhere.[43,46,64,65] In sub-Saharal Africa this is the most common of all forms of cancer, representing 10 to 30 per cent of all male tumors in most series.[46] In Bantu males in Laurenco Marques, Mozambique, it accounts for two-thirds of tumors in men (sex ratio about 3.4 to 1), with a rate approximately 500 times that observed in the United States in the 24 to 34 year age group.[64] In the U.S. the overall rate is about 2.4 per 100,000;[64] Negro males have a higher rate than Caucasian males; the rates in females of both races are about the same.[65] The variation in liver cancer is confined primarily to tumors of the hepatocytes, adenocarcinoma remaining constant, except in areas in Asia where infection with *Clonorchis sinensis* is common.[64] It has been suggested that the high frequency in Africa and Asia is the result of a high proportion of cirrhotic livers developing neoplastic changes and that a similar trend is occurring elsewhere.[64] Although fatty liver is a common finding in protein-calorie malnutrition in children in areas where primary liver cancer is common, there is no good evidence suggesting a causal relation between the two occurrences.[64] A role for aflatoxin is possible but remains unproven at this time.[23,66]

Cancer and Fat Intake. An 8-year comparison of mortality in elderly men, in an institution in California, subsisting on either conventional diets or on one high in polyunsaturated fat and low in saturated fat and cholesterol was conducted. An intriguing finding was a decreased incidence of fatal atherosclerotic events in the group on the high polyunsaturated-low saturated fat diet, associated with an increase in fatal carcinomas of various types.[67] The significance of this observation is still uncertain and has been called into question by retrospective analyses done elsewhere.[67a] It recalls a preliminary study where the incidences of tumors and mortality were increased in female (but not male) C3H mice and in male rats when dietary fat was increased and especially when highly unsaturated fats were incorporated in the diets at 5 and 10 per cent by weight.[68]

Relation of Body Weight to Cancer Incidence in Man. Tannenbaum[1] has summarized statistics derived from life insurance records. In the study by Dublin of records between 1887 and 1921 of men purchasing insurance at and past age 45 years, whose weight was known at issue of policy, there was a positive correlation between incidence of cancer of all types and increasing weight. In the few studies in which an attempt was made to correlate cancer according to site, there was suggestive evidence that cancer of the intestinal tract, liver, gallbladder and genitourinary tract was positively associated with weight to a greater degree than that in other sites.[1] A statistically significant association has been noted between obesity and carcinoma of the large bowel in men, but not in women.[55]

There is good evidence that cancer of the uterus occurs more frequently in overweight women[69,70] and that obesity is also associated with hypertension, diabetes and irregular menstrual bleeding; these may reflect a fundamental constitutional abnormality related to pituitary function. There are no data on the obvious question of the possible beneficial effect of persistent weight reduction on incidence of tumor development.

NUTRITIONAL EFFECTS INDUCED BY CANCER

General Systemic Effects. A striking and presently unexplained effect of active neoplastic disease in a significant number of patients is the marked anorexia and wasting not attributable to obvious intestinal obstruction, sepsis, endocrine disorder or other causative anatomical lesions. Such observations have led to the belief that the disease process is capable of inducing profound alterations in the metabolism of the host.

A century ago Pettenkofer and Voit noted high energy production in a leukemic patient. Since 1914 a number of clinical studies have reported elevation of basal metabolic rate in patients with various malignancies; however, this was not a universal finding, since in some patients the basal metabolic rate was in the normal range. On the other hand, there are few reports of significantly lowered rates in the presence of active disease. Thus, increased energy requirement in the face of anorexia and reduced food intake appears to be a factor in the weight loss observed so frequently.

In attempting to ascertain what other nutritional-metabolic effects occur in patients with active cancer, it is noteworthy that the number of such patients who have been investigated during controlled metabolic studies is relatively small. The problem is complicated also by differences in the types of malignancies involved and variability in the neoplastic activity. However, with these serious limitations, certain interesting facts emerge which have been confirmed and extended in studies with experimental animals. Some patients with active disease who are losing weight have been found to be in

nitrogen equilibrium or even in positive nitrogen balance, suggesting that the growing tumor is retaining nitrogen while the host tissues are losing it. Metabolic studies with a relatively few patients have indicated that nitrogen incorporated into the tumors may be derived not only from the diet but also from normal tissues.[71] Furthermore, the situation changes as the activity of the disease changes, and, with effective therapy, nitrogen retention by normal tissue again occurs. There is suggestive evidence that, during tumor regression, some of the nitrogen derived from the neoplasm is incorporated into the host tissues.

A number of studies with isotopically labeled amino acids in experimental animals have demonstrated the marked capacity of tumor tissue for protein synthesis; the labeled amino acids tend to stay in the tumor, in contrast to their turnover in certain normal tissues.[72,73] It has also been demonstrated that various rapidly growing transplanted rodent tumors develop at the expense of host tissues; some obtain enough nitrogen for growth from the host tissues when the diet contains very little nitrogenous substance.[73,74] These and other observations have given rise to the concept of the tumor as a "nitrogen trap," i.e., incorporation of amino acids into tumor is essentially a one-way passage from metabolic pool to the tumor.[75] More recent evidence indicates that experimental tumors are not entirely autonomous, and, depending on their type and growth phase, are influenced both nutritionally and metabolically by the host; furthermore, an interchange of nitrogen between tumor and host may occur. With certain tumors, improved nutrition in terms of protein and calories favors the host in terms of weight and nitrogen content, even though the experimental tumor also grows larger.[76] Eventually, however, circumstances develop when even forced feeding is unable to prevent loss of normal host tissues.[77] Goodlad has summarized these and other relationships between protein metabolism and the growth of experimental tumors.[78]

With reference to the anorexia developing in tumor-bearing animals, it has been found that Walker tumor transplanted in rats previously made hyperphagic by lesions in the ventromedial hypothalamus resulted in depression of food intake, indicating that this tumor effect is not mediated by this center.[79]

Would an effort toward increasing caloric and protein intake benefit those patients with active disease who are in negative balance? Surprising as it may seem, there are insufficient data to allow an unequivocal answer to this important question. Pareira *et al.*[80] have stressed the possibility of temporarily reversing to a significant degree the cancer cachexia of terminal patients by tube feeding. Terepka and Waterhouse[81] have also observed large gains in body weight during forced feeding of patients with active widespread malignancies; however, they found that the increase was due predominantly to an accumulation of large quantities of intracellular fluid and that weight loss was rapid upon discontinuation of forced feeding. Some of the patients appeared to have acceleration of the malignancy during and after the feeding program.

Others have also suggested that increased calories may be undesirable on the basis of possible increased disease activity.[82,83] High protein and calorie intakes during an active phase of neoplastic disease, when protein turnover is already high, may increase energy and protein metabolism without inducing net nitrogen retention.[84] In order to test this hypothesis, patients with neoplastic disease and those with other chronic illnesses were compared for their reactions to prolonged daily infusions of an I.V. fat preparation while consuming a constant diet identical to that taken during a control period. In general, the patients without neoplasia responded better to the supplementation than did those with cancer, in terms of weight gain, caloric balance and nutrient retention. The response of the latter group was inversely proportional to the activity of the disease process; a rapidly growing tumor was associated with increased caloric expenditure during hyperalimentation, whereas a patient with a slow-growing tumor retained nutrients and calories and had a greater albumin synthesis during fat infusion.[85]

Based on these relatively few studies, it would appear that forced feeding or hyperalimentation by parenteral means is not necessarily beneficial to the patient with widespread active disease and may actually be deleterious. With less active disease, the response is more likely to be favorable. Additional information in this area is highly desirable.

Table 37-1. Some Effects of Neoplastic Diseases on Nutritional Status

1. Cachexia secondary to anorexia.
2. Malnutrition associated with impaired food intake secondary to obstruction.
3. Malabsorption associated with:
    a. Deficiency of pancreatic enzymes or bile salts.
    b. Infiltration of small bowel by neoplasms, such as lymphoma or carcinoma.
    c. Fistulous bypass of small bowel.
    d. Gastric hypersecretion inhibiting pancreatic enzymes (in Zollinger-Ellison syndrome).
    e. Blind loop secondary to partial upper small bowel obstruction.
4. Protein-losing enteropathy (*e.g.*, in gastric carcinoma, lymphoma or with lymphatic obstruction).
5. Electrolyte and fluid balance disturbances associated with:
    a. Persistent vomiting in obstruction.
    b. Vomiting secondary to increased intracranial pressure from tumors.
    c. Small bowel fluid losses from fistula.
    d. Diarrhea associated with hormone-secreting tumors (*e.g.*, carcinoid, medullary thyroid carcinoma) and villous adenoma of the colon.
    e. Inappropriate antidiuretic hormone secretion associated with certain tumors.
    f. Hyperadrenalism secondary to excessive corticotropin or corticosteroid production by tumors.

Malabsorption, Fluid, Electrolyte and Vitamin Disturbances. In addition to the systemic effects of cancer there are a number of more localized effects of various neoplasms leading to nutritional problems. Some of these are listed in Table 37-1.

By far the most common causes of malnutrition in this general category are interferences with food intake as a result of partial or complete obstruction of some portion of the gastrointestinal tract. Relief of obstruction by radiation or surgical means is necessary, with intravenous alimentation or nasogastric-gastrostomy, or jejunostomy, tube feeding as indicated, until normal oral feedings can be re-instituted.

Involvement of the pancreas, pancreatic duct or common bile duct may lead to impaired digestion and absorption of fats and fat-soluble vitamins: in addition, proteins and electrolytes may be much less efficiently absorbed with serious pancreatic insufficiency. The use of oral or parenteral vitamin K and other fat-soluble vitamins is often helpful in restoring the patient to the best possible nutritional state for surgical procedure. Insufficient bile salts also depress fat absorption.

Malabsorption of various nutrients may occur to a significant degree when a leukemia, lymphoma or other solid tumor infiltrates the small bowel wall, obstructs lymphatic outflow, or modifies the mucosa.[86-89] In addition, protein-losing enteropathies have been described in cases of lymphoma and of carcinoma of the stomach.[90,91]

Villous abnormalities have been noted in individuals with carcinoma of the small intestine;[92-95] some of whom have been discovered to have concomitant gluten-enteropathy or sprue syndrome.[94,95] There is evidence suggesting an association between this disorder and the development of carcinoma.[96,97] Abnormal changes in the small bowel villi, with impaired absorption, have been described in patients with malignancies arising outside of and not involving the small intestine.[98-100] Other investigators have not confirmed findings of abnormal mucosa.[101-103]

Bypass of small bowel as a result of gastrocolic or jejunocolic fistulas may also occur in the course of abdominal cancer, with significant malabsorption and electrolyte and fluid disturbances.

An area of expanding interest concerns the secretion by tumors of a variety of potent pharmacologic substances, including trophic hormones, steroids, small molecular weight hormone polypeptides, kinins and prostaglandins.[104,105] A wide variety of nutritional-metabolic problems may develop in patients with such secreting neoplasia, some of which may produce more than one active agent. Diarrhea may occur with gastrin-secreting pancreatic islet adenomas (Zollinger-Ellison syndrome),[106,107] malignant carcinoid tumors of the intestine[108,109] and bronchus,[109] medullary carcinoma of the thyroid,[110] villous adenoma[111,112] and ganglioneuroma.[109] Losses of potassium with the Zollinger-Ellison syndrome and fluid and electrolyte depletion with villous adenoma may be severe. Steatorrhea occurs in the Zollinger-Ellison syndrome: this has been attributed partly to inactivation of pancreatic lipase by excessive acid production in the stomach and partly to villous damage.[113] While the diarrhea of carcinoid is usually of the watery type, cases of steatorrhea have been reported.[114] Hyponatremia, fluid retention and increased urinary sodium losses attributable to inappropriate antidiuretic hormone secretion have been described, most commonly in association with, but not restricted to, bronchogenic and oat cell carcinoma.[115] Medullary carcinoma of the thyroid gland secretes excessive amounts of calcitonin[116] as well as prostaglandins[110] and histamine[117] and may be associated with pheochromocytoma.[118] The calcitonin may result in hypocalcemia but patients are usually normocalcemic, presumably secondary to parathyroid hormone stimulation. Hypercalcemia secondary to secretion of parathormone-like substance occurs with a variety of tumors.[119] Electrolyte disturbances and increased nitrogen losses may occur in the hyperadrenal state, induced either by the secretion of adrenal cortical carcinoma or, less frequently, by corticotropin secreted by certain solid tumors, especially those in the lung.[120]

The major causes of electrolyte disturbance in cancer patients are vomiting and diarrhea, secondary to partial or complete obstruction, and gastric and small bowel fluid losses through a fistula. Electrolyte losses, including sodium, chloride, potassium and magnesium, may be serious.

Hypoalbuminemia and anemia are also frequently noted in advanced cancer cases: they are unresponsive to ordinary nutritional therapy.

Fluid and electrolyte imbalances are seen in patients with widespread hepatic metastases, ascites and liver failure, with cardiac metastases and failure, with metastatic ovarian carcinoma and ascites, with renal failure secondary to obstruction of the urinary tract by tumor, and with obstruction of lymphatic or venous drainage in major areas.

Abnormalities in folate metabolism may occur in acute and chronic leukemias. Increased retention of this vitamin by such patients has been noted,[121,122] in association with a tendency for increased vitamin content of leukocytes, especially in acute leukemias and chronic myeloid leukemia.[123] Patients with leukemias, disseminated lymphomas[124,125] and various metastatic carcinomas[102,126] tend to have low serum folate levels. Malabsorption of folate appears to be restricted to individuals with lymphomatous involvement of the small intestine.[103] Serum vitamin B_{12} levels are elevated in leukemias[127,128] and in a significant percentage of patients with solid tumors, especially in the presence of metastatic liver disease.[103]

Contradictory reports of jejunal mucosal changes in patients with malignancies outside of the gastrointestinal tract (vide supra) are reflected in similarly varying reports of the presence[98–100] or absence[103] of steatorrhea in such subjects. We have observed normal fat and xylose absorption prior to surgery in a number of patients with esophageal carcinoma not involving other portions of the intestinal tract.[129,130] Caution is to be exercised in interpreting urinary xylose data in patients with neoplasms, since blood levels may indicate adequate absorption.[103] Malabsorption of vitamin B_{12} is not uncommon, although its etiology is uncertain.[103]

Abnormalities of vitamin B_6 and tryptophan metabolism in significant numbers of patients with Hodgkin's disease and in some with carcinoma of the breast and of the bladder have been reported; this literature has been reviewed recently.[131] Plasma levels of pyridoxal phosphate were depressed in 8 of 14 untreated patients with Hodgkin's disease, and 14 of 21 excreted increased quantities of at least one of the metabolic intermediates of tryptophan. The incidence of these abnormalities was correlated with the severity of the disease. The tests were normal in patients in remission after chemotherapy. All eight patients with low pyridoxal phosphate were anergic. Pyridoxine administration raised the plasma pyridoxal phosphate but did not uniformly restore tryptophan metabolism to normal; this suggests that factors other than vitamin B_6 deficiency (perhaps increased secretion of corticosteroid) contribute to abnormal tryptophan metabolism.[131]

Reversal for any significant period of the undesirable systemic, metabolic and nutritional changes described depends primarily upon removal or destruction of the malignancy entirely or in large part. However, the physician frequently faces the problem of having to correct significant malnutrition and fluid and electrolyte imbalances in patients requiring surgical procedure or in those who need to be maintained in the best possible state for as long as possible in order to permit a therapeutic trial of radiation or chemotherapy. For such patients careful attention and a positive approach to correction of all abnormalities are indicated. As with all chronic wasting diseases, one cannot and should not expect to restore significant amounts of tissue in a short period of time, nor should urgent surgical intervention wait upon this goal. Correction of acute or chronic vitamin and mineral deficiencies, blood loss, and electrolyte and fluid imbalances can often be accomplished within a matter of days and this achievement improves the surgical risk. When operation is performed for removal of malignancy or for palliation in a debilitated patient and when there is a prolonged period of little or no oral intake of food, an attempt to restore caloric, nitrogen and other balances toward the positive side by adequate parenteral administration or tube feeding may be an aid to survival or a decreased period of convalescence.

NUTRITIONAL PROBLEMS ARISING FROM THE TREATMENT OF CANCER

Significant nutritional problems may arise as the result of the specific treatment given to control the neoplastic disease. This section discusses briefly some of the more common problems in this area (Table 37–2).

Radiation. A moving account by a physician relating her subjective reactions to the effects of destruction of the sense of taste following radiotherapy for cancer of the pharynx serves to emphasize the need on the part of the attending physician to understand the profound psychological, physiological, and nutritional aftereffects which may occur with varied treatments.[132] In the case of

---

Table 37-2. Consequences of Cancer Treatment Predisposing to Nutrition Problems

1. Radiation Treatment.
    a. Radiation of oropharyngeal area.
        (1) Destruction of sense of taste and impaired intake.
    b. Radiation of abdomen and pelvis.
        (1) Bowel damage, acute and chronic, with diarrhea, malabsorption, stenosis and obstruction.

2. Surgical Treatment.
    a. Radical resection of oropharyngeal area.
        (1) Dependency on tube feeding.
    b. Esophagectomy and esophageal reconstruction.
        (1) Gastric stasis secondary to vagotomy.
        (2) Malabsorption.
        (3) Fistula development or stenosis with long-term dependency on tube feeding.
    c. Gastrectomy.
        (1) Dumping syndrome.
        (2) Malabsorption.
        (3) Hypoglycemia.
    d. Intestinal resection.
        (1) Jejunum.
            (a) Decreased efficiency of absorption of many nutrients.
        (2) Ileum.
            (a) Vitamin B_{12} deficiency.
            (b) Bile salt losses.
        (3) Massive bowel resection.
            (a) Malabsorption.
            (b) Malnutrition.
        (4) Ileostomy and colostomy.
            (a) Complications of salt and water balance.
    e. Blind loop syndrome.
    f. Pancreatectomy.
        (1) Malabsorption.
        (2) Diabetes mellitus.
    g. Ureterosigmoidostomy.
        (1) Hyperchloremic acidosis.
        (2) Potassium depletion.

3. Chemotherapy Treatment.
    a. Corticosteroids and other hormones.
        (1) Fluid and electrolyte problems.
    b. Antimetabolites and other agents.
        (1) Gastrointestinal damage.
        (2) Anemias.

"mouth blindness" resulting from loss of taste sensation, and in other situations reducing food acceptance and leading to anorexia, improper food preparation and serving create a serious situation since "the patients are not hungry anyway, and it is easier to starve." When all food becomes tasteless, appearance and aroma become much more important, as do supplementary liquid feedings.

Radiation damage to small and large bowel occurs in a small but significant number of patients receiving external or internal radiation therapy. The epithelium of the small bowel is second only to bone marrow in its sensitivity to radiation. Altered intestinal function may occur during therapy and usually disappears. In those in whom significant "late" radiation changes are developing, symptoms recur usually within the year, but sometimes not for 10 or more years. Flattening and ulceration of the mucosa, telangiectasis, fibrosis, endarteritis of small vessels and stenosis of the bowel develop and these changes are often progressive. Obstruction and fistula formation may occur and require bowel resection, which complicates preexisting diarrhea and malabsorption. While the damaged tissue may make operation difficult, the obstructive symptoms may be caused by a local stenosis; consequently, exploratory laparotomy is recommended before malnutrition increases the risk. In our experience, patients with severe radiation damage and previous resection are more difficult to manage than patients with massive small bowel resection alone. Intermittent obstruction, diarrhea, malabsorption and chronic intestinal and bladder blood loss create a multitude of problems in nutrition and electrolyte balance. However, with close follow-up and attention to nutritional requirements, these patients often do very well.

Surgery. The effects of ablative surgery may be varied and many. Most of these procedures and their sequelae are, of course, not peculiar to surgery for cancer. However, certain resections are much more common or limited almost entirely to patients with cancer (*e.g.*, extensive resection of the head and neck, total esophagectomy in the adult, total gastrectomy, or ureterosigmoidostomy).

Surgery of the Head and Neck. Radical surgery of the head and neck region, including partial or total glossectomy and/or mandibulectomy, often interferes with mastication and swallowing. With some training or with laryngectomy, which prevents aspiration of fluids and food, oral food intake is possible. In others, prolonged tube feeding may be required. Liquid diets are prepared by blending the types of food ordinarily consumed by the family, having made certain that the pattern is nutritious. Where the personal situation does not permit this, simple and inexpensive tube formulas may be used (see Appendix). Many elderly individuals do not tolerate the large amounts of milk or milk powder often recommended for liquid formulas, nor do they tolerate large amounts of fluids. The composition of the formula should be modified as concomitant cardiovascular, renal, or endocrine disease indicates. Attention should be paid to psychologic aspects of food with tube feedings; *e.g.*, the aroma of a separate cup of coffee may be important.

Surgery of the Digestive Tract. Esophagectomy often induces significant malabsorption of fat.[129,130] The cause of this peculiar dysfunction appears to be the bilateral vagotomy inherent in the procedure; however, the precise intestinal mechanism causing the steatorrhea is unknown. The previously recognized sequelae of vagotomy—gastric stasis (necessitating a drainage procedure) and diarrhea—also occur in esophagectomized patients. Carbohydrate absorption is normal. The use of medium-chain triglycerides (MCT) as a major portion of fat intake diminishes the steatorrhea.[129]

Gastrectomy. The physiologic and nutritional consequences of subtotal and total gastrectomy have been reviewed in Chapter 28, Section A. It suffices to state here that clinical problems increase proportionately to the extent of the resection. In addition to the well-known occurrences of dumping syndrome, hypoglycemia, steatorrhea, afferent loop syndrome and loss of intrinsic factor, emphasis is needed on the long-term consequences of loss of the stomach with the insidious development of various vitamin and mineral deficiencies.[133–136] Serious and persistent attention by the physician to prevention of these nutritional problems is essential for long-term health, when the underlying disease leading to the need for operation is benign or malignancy has been eradicated.

Intestinal Resection. Clinical studies in normal subjects and in those with ablation of varying portions of small intestine indicate that all nutrients studied, with the exception of vitamin B_{12}, are most efficiently and (in the usual dietary amounts) rather completely absorbed in the proximal small bowel.[137,138] However, with jejunal resection, the ileum, with its reserve absorptive capacity, can absorb these nutrients in good degree.

Massive small bowel resection, with a residual of three feet or less, presents very serious and long-term problems in maintaining adequate nutrition, including water and electrolytes. If there is additional loss of the ileocecal valve and portions of the colon, the problems are intensified. However, the application of present knowledge with respect to care of these patients will permit a successful outcome. These principles include the following:

1. The postoperative period is often a stormy one complicated by infection, ileus, and weight loss. During this period, it is essential that all factors tending to weight loss and malnutrition be combatted vigorously. This includes preparation at operation for long-term parenteral nutrition with sterile insertion of an indwelling catheter or A–V shunt and the formation of a feeding gastrostomy.[139–141]

2. Absorptive capacity of many of these patients improves with time,[142–143] so that patience and a carefully developed nutritional program, designed to meet the changing needs, often achieve a successful outcome. Our supply of intravenous nutrients is now sufficient to permit good nutrition by this route alone for periods of months, provided the vascular route can be kept open. As gastrointestinal function returns, special gastrostomy feedings can be initiated, utilizing round-the-clock feedings, if indicated, with hydrolyzed protein or amino acids and other nutrients capable of rapid absorption. This route is increasingly utilized as conditions improve, to the point where I.V. feedings are discontinued and eventually oral intake commences, supplemented by gastrostomy feedings when necessary. Protracted and meticulous care is essential for survival.

3. A marked reduction in the intake of long-chain fats reduces diarrhea and decreases fecal calcium, magnesium and other electrolyte losses.[144] The use of medium-chain triglycerides (MCT) in increasing amounts (as tolerated by the patient and consistent with an acceptable level of diarrhea) is often of value in increasing calories.[145] This product, in significant amounts, will cause some ketosis and acidosis which may require additional sodium bicarbonate.[146]

4. The acidosis associated with malabsorption and diarrhea will tend to increase calcium and potassium losses in urine and should be watched for and treated on a continuing basis.

5. *Persistent* gastric hypersecretion may occur in occasional patients, and this possibility should be investigated. When it does occur, without spontaneous improvement, vagotomy (preferably selective) and pyloroplasty may be helpful in decreasing fistula or fecal losses.[147] In our experience, this is a rare occurrence.

6. When the distal ileum has been resected, physiologic doses of vitamin B_{12} cannot be absorbed and periodic injections of this vitamin are necessary.

7. The terminal ileum is also the site of absorption of conjugated bile salts. Hence, the usual enterohepatic circulation of these emulsifying agents is disrupted and their concentration in the intestine is decreased, since the liver is incapable of making up the massive loss. Administration of conjugated bile salts to such patients may make the diarrhea worse.[148] Attempting to chelate the bile salts with cholestyramine (to minimize possible deleterious effects on the large bowel) is apparently without effect in those with major ileal resection (>100 cm), and the treatment may result in complications.[149]

8. Resection of the terminal ileum may be associated with the development of hyperoxaluria and oxalate stone in the kidney. Cholestyramine reduces urinary oxalate excretion.[149a]

9. The surgeon should retain the ileocecal valve whenever possible, since it appears to

slow the exit of small bowel contents and, hence, improve absorption and perhaps act to hinder retrograde movement of colonic bacteria. The use of an antiperistaltic segment of bowel as a replacement for the valve has been recommended with more or less enthusiasm.[150,151] The inherent danger posed by the possibility of sacrificing further absorptive surface in a patient with massive bowel resection, together with the danger of obstruction, must be carefully considered before such a procedure is done.

Ileostomy is usually followed by large sodium and water losses but, within 7 to 10 days, these usually decrease to the range which will characterize the otherwise healthy individual on a stable diet. Generally, these stabilized individuals lose 300 to 600 ml of water daily, with 40 to 100 mEq of sodium and 2.5 to 10 mEq of potassium, emphasizing the physiologic role of the colon in absorbing water and sodium and in exchanging potassium for sodium. Gastroenteritis, partial intestinal obstruction and prolonged excessive sweating impose additional losses. Studies in man and in dogs during sodium depletion have demonstrated a reduction in sodium concentration of ileostomy material as depletion progressed, accompanied by increased potassium concentration.[152,153]

Pancreatectomy with consequent loss of digestive enzymes leads to loss into the stool not only of fats and of protein, but also of significant amounts of various vitamins and minerals. Since pancreatectomy necessitates partial gastrectomy, this is a complicating factor.

Pancreatic enzyme insufficiency may be effectively replaced by potent pancreatic extracts given with meals or at 2-hour intervals: occasionally, sodium bicarbonate supplements are helpful.[154] The diabetes mellitus following the resection is usually of the "brittle" type, requiring relatively small amounts of insulin and rather difficult to control with precision. Hence, tolerance of some glycosuria is safer than the hypoglycemic episodes which may occur with achievement of glucose-free urine.

Ureterosigmoidostomy, performed on certain patients in whom the bladder must be removed with implantation of the ureters into the sigmoid colon, often leads to significant disturbances in acid-base balance with development of a hyperchloremic acidosis.[155] Potassium depletion may occur in association with the acidosis. These abnormalities occur significantly less in patients with ileal bladder construction.

Chemotherapy. *Hormones.* Hormones and other chemotherapeutic agents may also lead to disturbances in nutrition. The effects of adrenocortical steroids are well known and include losses of protein, calcium, and potassium; these may be significant, depending on the type of steroid, dosage, and duration of treatment.

Most of the present chemotherapeutic agents, aside from hormones, inhibit one or more key steps in the intermediary metabolism of cells—normal as well as neoplastic.[156] Since the epithelial cells of the small intestine have a relatively rapid turnover, it is to be expected that many of these drugs will adversely affect intestinal functions to a degree depending on drug, dosage, duration of treatment, altered rates of excretion and metabolism, and individual susceptibility.

Antimetabolites. A major effect of folic acid antagonists is exerted on the gastrointestinal mucosa and the bone marrow. The morphologic changes induced in the intestines of experimental animals are similar to those seen in sprue.[157,158] These morphologic changes are accompanied by alterations in metabolism and decreased absorptive ability for xylose and presumably other nutrients.[159,160] In man, a single intravenous injection of methotrexate (2 to 5 mg per kg body weight) is followed by the inhibition of mitotic activity in the jejunal mucosa, as well as by marked fine structural changes in the cells observable with the electron microscope.[161] These pathologic changes may be prevented or reversed by Leucovorin.

The fluorinated pyrimidines have a marked action on gastrointestinal mucosa.[162,163] In patients receiving an adequate course of 5-fluorouracil the bone marrow may become megaloblastic, with associated changes in various epithelial and cancer cells: these morphologic changes are similar to those found in pernicious and other megaloblastic anemias resulting from nutritional deficiencies.[164] Actinomycin D also induces marked gastrointestinal changes.[165] Malabsorption of fat and other nutrients has been observed in rats following its administration.[166]

Intestinal mucosal changes with associated changes in intestinal function have been noted in experimental animals and/or in man with other agents, including glutamine antagonists, hydroxyurea, daunomycin, Vinca alkaloids, and polyfunctional alkylating agents.[156]

BIBLIOGRAPHY

1. Tannenbaum: Nutrition and Cancer, In *Physiopathology of Cancer*, 2nd ed. F. Homberger, ed. New York, Hoeber-Harper, Chap. 13, pp. 517–562, 1959.
2. Ross and Bras: J. Nutrition, *87*, 245, 1965.
3. Ross, Bras and Ragbeer: J. Nutrition, *100*, 177, 1970.
4. Orten, Burn and Smith: Proc. Soc. Exp. Biol. Med., *36*, 82, 1937.
5. Rowe, Grammer, Watson and Nickerson: Cancer, *26*, 436, 1970.
6. Axelrad and Leblond: Cancer, *8*, 339, 1955.
7. Jasmin: Rev. Canad. Biol., *22*, 383, 1963.
8. Bois, Sandborn and Messier: Cancer Res., *29*, 763, 1969.
9. Battifora, McCreary, *et al.*: Arch. Path., *86*, 610, 1968.
10a. Copeland and Salmon: Am. J. Path., *22*, 1059, 1946.
10b. Butler and Newberne: Cancer Res., *29*, 236, 1969.
11. Gillette: Adv. Pharmacol., *4*, 219, 1966.
12. Conney: Pharmacol. Rev., *19*, 317, 1967.
13. Kato, Oshima and Tomizawa: Jap. J. Pharmacol., *18*, 356, 1968.
14. Marshall and McLean: Biochem. Pharmacol., *18*, 153, 1969.
15. Dixon, Shultice and Fouts: Proc. Soc. Exp. Biol. Med., *103*, 333, 1960.
16. Wattenberg, Leong and Strand: Cancer Res., *22*, 1120, 1962.
17. Kanda and Tanaka: Kumanoto Med. J., *21*, 149, 1968.
18. Sugiura: J. Nutrition, *44*, 345, 1951.
19. Conney, Miller and Miller: Cancer Res., *16*, 450, 1956.
20. Wogan: Progr. Exp. Tumor Res., *11*, 134, 1969.
21. Newberne, Harrington and Wogan: Lab. Invest., *15*, 662, 1966.
22. Madhaven and Gopalan: Arch. Path., *80*, 123, 1965.
23. Rogers and Newberne: Nature, *229*, 62, 1971.
24. McLean and Magee: Br. J. Exp. Path., *51*, 587, 1970.
25. Dunning, Curtis and Mann: Cancer Res., *10*, 454, 1950.
26. Pamukcu, Yalciner, Price and Bryan: Cancer Res., *30*, 2671, 1970.
27. Rakieten, Gordon, Beaty, Cooney, Davis and Schein: Proc. Soc. Exp. Biol. Med., *137*, 280, 1971.
28. DeWys, Pories, Richter and Strain: Proc. Soc. Exp. Biol. Med., *135*, 17, 1970.
29. Fisher and Fisher: Cancer, *14*, 547, 1961.
30. Sugimura, Birnbaum, Winitz and Greenstein: Arch. Biochem. Biophys., *81*, 439, 1959.
31. Skipper and Thompson: In *Amino Acids and Peptides with Antimetabolic Activity*, Ciba Fdn. Symp., Wolstenholme and O'Connor eds. London, J. & A. Churchill, Ltd., pp. 38–58, 1958.
32. Bertino and Nixon: Cancer Res., *29*, 2417, 1969.
33. Cooney and Handschumacher: Ann. Rev. Pharmacol., *10*, 421, 1970.
34. Capizzi, Bertino and Handschumacher: Ann. Rev. Med., *21*, 433, 1970.
35. Rosen, Sotobayashi and Nichol: Proc. Am. Assoc. Cancer Res., *5*, 54, 1964.
36. Rosen, Mihich and Nichol: Vitamins and Hormones, *22*, 609, 1964.
37. Morris and Robertson: J. Nat. Cancer Inst., *3*, 479, 1943.
38. Gailani, Holland, Nussbaum and Olson: Cancer, *21*, 975, 1968.
39. Nichol: Cancer Res., *29*, 2422, 1969.
40. Bullough: Brit. J. Cancer, *4*, 329, 1950.
41. Hoffman: *Cancer and Diet*, Baltimore, The Williams & Wilkins Co., 1937, 767 pp.
42. Ahlbom: Acta Radiol., *18*, 163, 1937.
43. Doll, R.: In *Tumors of the Alimentary Tract in Africans*, Nat. Cancer Inst. Monogr. No. 25, Washington, D.C., U.S. Govt. Print. Off., 1967, pp. 173–190.
44. Bailar: In *Carcinoma of the Alimentary Tract*. W. J. Burdette, ed. Salt Lake City, Univ. Utah Press, 1965, pp. 3–14.
45. Desai, Borges, Vohra and Paymaster: Cancer, *23*, 979, 1969.
46. Cooke and Burkitt: Brit. Med. Bull., *27*, 14, 1971.
47. Wynder and Bross: Cancer, *14*, 389, 1961.
48. Graham, Lilienfeld and Tidings: Cancer, *20*, 224, 1967.
49. Langman: Gut, *8*, 315, 1967.
50. Acheson and Doll: Gut, *5*, 126, 1964.
51. Higginson: J. Nat. Cancer Inst., *37*, 527, 1966.
52. Wynder, Kmet, Dungal and Segi: Cancer, *16*, 1461, 1963.
53. Boyd and Doll: Brit. J. Cancer, *8*, 231, 1954.
54a. Dungal and Sigurdjonsson: Brit. J. Cancer, *21*, 270, 1967.
54b. Merliss: Science, *173*, 1141, 1971.
54c. Selikoff, Churg and Hammond: J.A.M.A., *188*, 22, 1964.
55. Wynder and Shigematsu: Cancer, *20*, 1520, 1967.
56. Wynder, Kajitani, Ishikawa, Dodo and Takano: Cancer, *23*, 1210, 1969.
57. Gregor, Toman and Prusova: Gut, *10*, 1031, 1969.

58. Oettle: In *Symposium on Tumors of the Alimentary Tract in Africans*. Nat. Cancer Inst. Monogr. No. 25. Washington, D.C. U.S. Govt. Print. Off., 1967, pp. 97–109.
59. Burkitt: Lancet, 2, 1229, 1969.
60. Walker, Walker and Richardson: Br. Med. J., 3, 48, 1970.
61. Bremner and Ackerman: Cancer, 26, 991, 1970.
62. Hill, Crowther, *et al.*: Lancet, 1, 95, 1971.
63. Walker: Lancet, 1, 593, 1971.
64. Higginson: Gastroenterology, 57, 587, 1969.
65. UICC: *Cancer Incidence in Five Continents*. Vol. II Doll, Muir and Waterhouse. eds., New York, Springer, 1970.
66. Purchase: S. Afr. Med. J., 41, 406, 1967.
67. Pearce and Dayton: Lancet, 1, 464, 1971.
67a.Ederer, Leren, Turpeinen and Frantz: Lancet, 2, 203, 1971.
68. Harmon: Proc. 7th Internat. Congr. Gerontology, Vol. 5, Vienna, June 1966, p. 259.
69. Moss: Am. J. Roentgenol., 58, 203, 1947.
70. Garnet: Am. J. Obst. Gynecol., 76, 11, 1958.
71. Fenninger, Waterhouse and Keutmann: Cancer, 6, 930, 1953.
72. Le Page *et al.*: Cancer Res., 12, 153, 1952.
73. Henderson and Le Page: Cancer Res., 19, 887, 1959.
74. White: J. Nat. Cancer Inst., 5, 265, 1945.
75. Mider: Cancer Res., 11, 821, 1951.
76. Allison, Wannemacher, Prosky and Crossley: J. Nutrition, 60, 297, 1956.
77. Stewart, quoted by Fenninger and Mider: Adv. Cancer Res., 2, 229, 1954.
78. Goodlad: In *Mammalian Protein Metabolism*, Munro and Allison, ed. New York, Academic Press, 19, Vol. 2, pp. 415–444, 1964.
79. Baille, Millar and Pratt: Am. J. Physiol., 209, 296, 1965.
80. Pareira *et al.*: Cancer, 8, 803, 1955.
81. Terepka and Waterhouse: Am. J. Med., 20, 225, 1956.
82. Levenson and Watkin: Fed. Proc., 18, 1155, 1959.
83. Watkin: Am. J. Clin. Nutrition, 9, 446, 1961.
84. Tschudy *et al.*: J. Clin. Invest., 38, 892, 1959.
85. Watkin and Steinfeld: Am. J. Clin. Nutrition, 16, 182, 1965.
86. Fairley and Mackie: Brit. Med. J., 1, 375, 1937.
87. Sleisenger, Almy and Barr: Am. J. Med., 15, 666, 1953.
88. Pitney, Joske and MacKinnon: J. Clin. Path., 13, 440, 1960.
89. Kent: Arch. Path., 78, 97, 1964.
90. Jarnum and Schwartz: Gastroenterology, 38, 769, 1960.
91. Werdegar, Adler and Washington: Ann. Intern. Med., 59, 207, 1963.
92. Joske: Gastroenterology, 38, 810, 1960.
93. Blackwell: Gut, 2, 377, 1961 (Abstract).
94. Moertel and Hargraves: J.A.M.A., 176, 612, 1961.
95. Fric, Bednar, Niederle and Lepsik: Gastroenterology, 44, 330, 1963.
96. Harris, Cooke, Thompson and Waterhouse: Am. J. Med., 42, 899, 1967.
97. Brzechwa-Ajdukiewicz *et al.*: Gut, 7, 572, 1966.
98. Creamer: Brit. Med. J., 2, 1435, 1964; Loehry and Creamer, ibid, 1, 827, 1966.
99. Dymock *et al.*: Brit. J. Cancer, 21, 505, 1967.
100. Deller, Murrell and Blowes: Austral. Ann. Med., 16, 236, 1967.
101. Girdwood: Brit. Med. J., 2, 1592, 1964 (Letter).
102. Fischer *et al.*: Cancer, 18, 1278, 1965.
103. Klipstein and Smarth: Am. J. Digest. Dis., 14, 887, 1969.
104. Hall and Nathanson: CA, 18, 322, 1968.
105. Sircus: Gut, 10, 506, 1969.
106. Zollinger and Ellison: Ann. Surg., 142, 709, 1955.
107. McGuigan and Trudeau: New Eng. J. Med., 278, 1308, 1968.
108. Sjoerdsma, Weissbach and Udenfriend: Am. J. Med., 20, 520, 1956.
109. Sandler, Karim and Williams: Lancet, 2, 1053, 1968.
110. Williams, Karim and Sandler: Lancet, 1, 22, 1968.
111. McKittrick and Wheelock: *Carcinoma of the Colon*. Springfield, Charles C Thomas, 1954, pp. 94.
112. Da Cruz, Gardner and Peskin: Am. J. Surg., 115, 203, 1968.
113. Shimoda, Saunders and Rubin: Gastroenterology, 55, 705, 1968.
114. Kowlessar, Law and Sleisenger: Am. J. Med., 27, 673, 1959.
115. Kleeman: Ann. Rev. Med., 21, 259, 1970.
116. Tashjian and Melvin: New Eng. J. Med., 279, 279, 1968.
117. Baylin, Beaven, Engelman and Sjoerdsma: New Eng. J. Med., 283, 1239, 1970.
118. Schimke, Hartmann, Prout and Rimoin: New Eng. J. Med., 279, 1, 1968.
119. Munson, Tashjian and Levine: Cancer Res., 25, 1062, 1965.
120. Liddle, Givens, Nicholson and Island: Cancer Res., 25, 1057, 1965.
121. Swendseid, Swanson, Meyers and Bethell: Blood, 7, 307, 1952.
122. Spray and Witts: Clin. Sci., 12, 385, 1953.
123. Swendseid, Bethell and Bird: Cancer Res., 11, 864, 1951.
124. Rao, Lagerlöf, Einhorn and Reizenstein: Lancet, 1, 1192, 1963.
125. Rose: J. Clin. Path., 19, 29, 1966.
126. Magnus: Cancer Res., 27, 490, 1967.
127. Beard, Pitney and Sanneman: Blood, 9, 789, 1954.
128. Hall and Finkler: Blood, 27, 611, 1966.
129. Shils and Gilat: Gastroenterology, 50, 347, 1966.
130. Shils: Surg. Gyn. Obstet., 132, 709, 1971.
131. Chalner, DeVita, Livingstone and Oliverio: New Eng. J. Med., 282, 838, 1970.

132. MacCarthy-Leventhal: Lancet, *2*, 1138, 1959.
133. Hines, Hoffbrand and Mollin: Am. J. Med., *43*, 555, 1967.
134. Deller *et al.*: Gut, *5*, 218, 1964.
135. Geokas and McKenna: Canad. Med. Assoc. J., *96*, 411, 1967.
136. Eddy: Am. J. Med., *50*, 442, 1971.
137. Booth: Postgrad. Med. J., *37*, 725, 1961.
138. Stewart *et al.*: Quart. J. Med., *36*, 425, 1967.
139. Wilmore and Dudrick: Arch. Surg., *98*, 256, 1969.
140. Shils *et al.*: New Eng. J. Med., *283*, 341, 1970.
141. Atkins *et al.*: Trans. Am. Soc. Artif. Int. Org., *16*, 260, 1970.
142. Weinstein *et al.*: Arch. Surg., *69*, 560, 1969.
143. Dowling: Brit. Med. Bull., *23*, 275, 1967.
144. Booth, MacIntyre and Mollin: Quart. J. Med., *33*, 401, 1964.
145. Bochenek, Rogers and Balint: Ann. Intern. Med., *72*, 205, 1970.
146. Bergen, Hashim and van Itallie: Diabetes, *15*, 723, 1966.
147. Frederick, Sizer and Osborn: New Eng. J. Med., *272*, 509, 1965.
148. Hardison and Rosenberg: New Eng. J. Med., *277*, 337, 1967.
149. Hoffman and Poley: New Eng. J. Med., *281*, 397, 1969.
149a.Smith, Fromm and Hofmann: New Eng. J. Med., *286*, 1371, 1972.
150. Wilmore and Johnson: Arch. Surg., *97*, 784, 1968.
151. Winchester and Dorsey: Surg. Gyn. and Obstet., *132*, 131, 1971.
152. Smiddy *et al.*: Lancet, *1*, 14, 1960.
153. Gallagher, Harrison and Skyring: Gut, *3*, 219, 1962.
154. Littman and Hanscom: New Eng. J. Med., *281*, 201, 1969.
155. Ferris and Odel: J.A.M.A., *142*, 634, 1950.
156. Dowling, Krakoff and Karnofsky: In *Chemotherapy of Cancer*. W. H. Cole, ed. Philadelphia, Lea & Febiger, 1970, pp. 1–74.
157. Thiersch and Philips: Proc. Soc. Exp. Biol. Med., *71*, 484, 1949.
158. Ryback: Gastroenterology, *42*, 306, 1962.
159. Vitale *et al.*: J. Lab. Clin. Med., *43*, 583, 1954.
160. Small *et al.*: Am. J. Dig. Dis., *4*, 700, 1959.
161. Trier: Gastroenterology, *43*, 407, 1962.
162. Heidelberger *et al.*: Cancer Res., *18*, 305, 1958.
163. Muggia *et al.*: Am. J. Path., *42*, 407, 1963.
164. Brennan, Vaitkevicius and Rebuck: Blood, *16*, 1535, 1960.
165. Philips *et al.*: Ann. N.Y. Acad. Sci., *89*, 348, 1960.
166. Yeh and Shils: Fed. Proc., *25*, 322, 1966.

Chapter

38

Nutrition in Ophthalmology

J. J. STERN

CONJUNCTIVA, CORNEA AND SCLERA

Vitamin A Deficiency. *Signs and Symptoms.* The ocular changes due to vitamin A deficiency range from simple xerosis conjunctivae to the fully developed picture of keratomalacia. The latter type is seldom seen any more in economically sound countries. Xerosis is more frequent, particularly in undernourished infants, where improper diet after weaning is a common cause of its appearance.

In xerosis conjunctivae, the bulbar conjunctiva presents a peculiar dry aspect, described as "lack of luster." Light reflection from the conjunctiva is interfered with. This becomes easily detectable when the lids are kept open for ten to twenty seconds. In the very early stages, the conjunctival changes are patchy, becoming confluent when the condition progresses. The deeper conjunctival and episcleral vessels take on a bluish tinge or become invisible because of the diminished transparency of the epithelium. Loss of elasticity causes a wrinkling of the conjunctiva which can be provoked by pushing the bulbar conjunctiva towards the limbus with a finger pressed over the lower lid. Later, the folds appear spontaneously, forming concentric circles and showing dry, lusterless tops and moist furrows when the eyes are moved sideways.

Another common sign is the appearance of Bitôt's spots: white, elevated, sharply outlined patches not wetted by tears and covered with material resembling dried foam. They are usually triangular in shape, the base facing the limbus, and most frequently occupy the temporal side of the conjunctiva, within the lid aperture. The foam-like substance can be scraped away but reforms. It consists of epithelial debris, fatty globules, and frequently masses of xerosis bacilli. The latter are saprophytes and have neither diagnostic nor etiologic significance. It should be pointed out, however, that lesions resembling Bitôt spots have been reported from several tropical countries in persons with normal vitamin A blood levels and no other signs of vitamin A deficiency; the role of Bitôt spots as a pathognomonic sign of vitamin A deficiency is becoming increasingly doubtful.[1]

In the Orient a certain type of conjunctival pigmentation has been described in avitaminosis A.[2-8] It first occupies the lower part of the bulbar conjunctiva, the lower fornix, and the semilunar folds; these areas become yellowish, then gray, finally bluish mauve. Later on, the same changes may appear in the upper lid and fornix. The pigment is melanin, and it usually remains for some time after all other evidence of the condition has responded to therapy.

A smoky discoloration of the bulbar conjunctiva, attributed to vitamin A deficiency, has been described in colored races. It is due to an outward migration of chromatophores from the limbal pigment ring.[1a] The same phenomenon has been produced experimentally in rabbits fed a diet deficient in vitamin A. Only animals with pigment showed it; there was no development of new chromatophores.[2]

In severe cases of xerosis all signs are

accentuated. The bulbar conjunctiva becomes thick, opaque, thrown into large folds
and furrows. At the same time the cornea
becomes involved. The first signs here are
loss of luster, dryness on exposure to air, and
reduced sensitivity. The latter suggests
nerve involvement and will be discussed later.
When the condition progresses unchecked,
patchy areas resembling Bitôt's spots appear
on the cornea, sometimes as a continuation
of the conjunctival spots; sometimes as
crescents along the limbus, and occasionally
as isolated areas in the center. If the process
advances further, true keratomalacia sets in.
The cornea becomes dull, central or peripheral infiltrates form, and the periphery
becomes vascularized. The epithelium over
the infiltrates is shed, ulcers form and become
infected, and the cornea finally perforates.
The vascularization of the cornea is morphologically different from that seen in riboflavin
deficiency and may be secondary to necrosis
of the corneal epithelium.

Kruse[3] described the occurrence of conjunctival spots in chronic vitamin A deficiency in a large number of seemingly
healthy subjects. The lesions are "grossly
perceptible elevated spots of distinctive color
and characteristic location." They disappeared or at least receded after many
months' treatment and with very large
doses of vitamin A (100,000 units daily). It
is noteworthy that only few subjects showed
high adaptometer readings and most of them
had normal blood vitamin A levels. Whether
the lesions described by Kruse are senile or
presenile alterations, or are due to chronic
mild vitamin A deficiency remains to be
proven.

Diagnosis. Xerosis or thickening of the
conjunctiva is one of the early signs of
avitaminosis A. This was confirmed in a
nutritional survey in Newfoundland,[4] where
thickening of the conjunctiva was observed to
be very common in children of grade school
age, and always associated with low serum
vitamin A levels. Four years later, the same
observers found a statistically significant
improvement in the same age group. Within
those four years, the government had introduced the fortification of oleomargarine with
vitamin A and the enrichment of bread.

There is some evidence of lack of correlation between dietary intake of vitamin A or
vitamin A blood level and conjunctival
lesions.[5,6] Likewise, large doses of vitamin A,
given over a period of two years, failed to
influence various degrees of opaqueness of
the conjunctiva and pinguecula-like spots in
a group of subjects.[7,7a] The most recent and
probably most comprehensive experimental
work done on human volunteers[8] resulted in
the same negative findings: no conjunctival or
corneal changes occurred after as long as 25
months of vitamin A depletion, in spite of an
early drop in the carotenoid level of the blood
and a drop of the vitamin A level after about
eight months. This discrepancy between
clinical and experimental findings will have
to be explained before a final evaluation of
the situation can be made.

Pathogenesis. The mechanism of the epithelial damage in vitamin A deficiency is
by no means clear. Anatomically, the
changes can be described as atrophy of the
epithelium, reparative proliferation of the
basal cells, and growth and differentiation of
these new products into a stratified keratiniz-
ing epithelium.[9] In avitaminosis A, the
mitotic rate of a healing corneal wound is
reduced by 30 per cent.[10] The mechanism
has been claimed to be essentially neuro-
trophic. Of particular interest are degenerative changes in the myelin sheath of the
trigeminal nerve,[11] reduced corneal sensitivity
in xerosis and the finding of thickened corneal
nerves at an early stage of the disease,[12]
together with degeneration of the Gasserian
and ciliary ganglia.[13] Thus, peripheral
nerve involvement may play an important
role in the pathogenesis of xerophthalmia.
It is known also that O_2 flows in the cornea
from front to rear and CO_2 from rear to
front; the sclerosis of the superficial corneal
epithelium caused by vitamin A deficiency
brings on anoxia of the corneal stroma
which becomes cloudy.

Prevalence. Xerosis conjunctivae is not
infrequently seen in patients suffering from
liver disease—particularly in infants who
have not yet accumulated stores of vitamin A
in the liver—because the diseased organ is
unable to store or mobilize vitamin A.

While keratomalacia is practically unknown

in economically sound communities, where even simple xerosis is uncommon, it causes havoc in large areas of the Orient and other regions where severe malnutrition is prevalent. Keratomalacia was frequent in Malaya before World War II, because condensed milk was so cheap that many mothers substituted it for breast-feeding. During the Japanese occupation, when condensed milk was unobtainable, breast-feeding was resorted to, and keratomalacia almost disappeared. Now, with condensed milk available again, the incidence of keratomalacia is once more on the increase.[14]

Treatment. PREVENTIVE TREATMENT. An allowance of 5,000 i.u. (based upon two-thirds as carotene) daily for normal adults has been adopted in the Recommended Daily Allowances.[15] The Medical Research Council of Great Britain[8] recommends 2,500 i.u. daily as a mimimum maintenance dose.

CURATIVE TREATMENT. Deficiency signs make their appearance only when the body stores of vitamin A have reached a very low level. In order to replenish the depleted stores at a fast rate, it is advisable to administer the vitamin in amounts far greater than the maintenance requirement. It is therefore the general practice to give 25,000, 50,000 or even 100,000 i.u. daily, until results are obtained. Treatment has to be adapted to special conditions like liver disease or intestinal disorders. Where utilization of dietary carotene is impaired, it is advisable to substitute preformed vitamin A for carotene.

LOCAL THERAPY. Vitamin A and carotene have been used locally in a number of eye conditions, such as corneal injuries, superficial neuroparalytic and interstitial keratitis, and Mooren's ulcer. Local therapy with vitamin A does not seem rational, and should be replaced either by systemic administration of vitamin A, if a deficiency is suspected, or by appropriate local treatment.

Ariboflavinosis. *Signs and Symptoms.* Corneal vascularization is probably the earliest and most constant sign of riboflavin deficiency. Its development is preceded by injection of the bulbar and palpebral conjunctiva and the fornix, circumcorneal injection, and engorgement of the limbic plexus. Later, there may be superficial and interstitial in-

filtration of the cornea, sometimes patchy, sometimes diffuse. Finally, congestion of the sclera, and even of the iris, may occur. The subjective symptoms include itching and burning, roughness of the eyes, photophobia, and impairment of visual acuity. In the more commonly observed early stages, the discrepancy between the patient's complaints and the paucity of clinical signs is characteristic.

The diagnosis is facilitated by the presence of other clinical signs of ariboflavinosis: cheilosis, glossitis and dyssebacia.

Pathology. Corneal vascularity is a compensatory process bringing blood into closer contact with the deeper layers of the corneal epithelium when the cornea is suffering from riboflavin deprivation. The corneal epithelium shows a surprisingly high metabolic rate, while that of the stroma is relatively low.[16–19] Riboflavin, as the phosphoric acid ester, in combination with adenylic acid, forms a flavin-adenine-dinucleotide which is the prosthetic group of Warburg's yellow respiratory enzyme. It acts as dehydrogenase in anaerobic glycolysis. This mechanism is essential for the respiratory process of the cornea and other avascular tissues.

The oxygen consumption of the cornea of riboflavin-deficient rats is lowered. When vascularization of the cornea is present, the oxygen uptake of the corneal stroma is elevated; in the absence of vascularization it is rather low. The increased oxygen uptake of the stroma must therefore be the result of the vascularization, and perhaps of the cellular infiltration.

Differential Diagnosis. Circumcorneal injection is undoubtedly an early sign of ariboflavinosis, but it also occurs in many other ocular disturbances. Thus, riboflavin cannot be expected to exert a therapeutic influence on every case of circumcorneal injection. Familiarity with the variations of the normal limbus as visualized by the slit lamp is essential for the detection of corneal vascularity: a condition in which newly formed blood vessels leave the limbic plexus and centripetally enter the subepithelial space of the true cornea. This state, and nothing less, is acceptable as corneal vascularity.

The limbus is not a line, but a band about

1 mm wide. This area is plentifully provided with blood vessels which comprise the limbic plexus. This plexus is not always visible in the living eye, as the vessels are frequently empty and cannot be seen. The plexus responds readily to mechanical or chemical irritation that causes conjunctival hyperemia and opens the vessels of the limbus. This hyperemia is entirely nonspecific. The sprouting out of new vessels from the limbic plexus is preceded by engorgement and increased activity of the plexus itself. This condition will or will not respond to riboflavin administration, according to its etiology. For practical clinical purposes it must be insisted upon that vessels appear in the cornea before one can speak of corneal vascularity.

The corneal vascularity of well-developed riboflavin deficiency always occurs in the entire circumference of the cornea. This fact is important for correct diagnosis. Both eyes usually show equal vascularity, but there are exceptions to this rule. Disease or trauma may condition vascularization of the cornea of one eye when the degree of riboflavin deficiency is insufficient to produce signs in the other eye.

Invasion of the cornea by blood vessels occurs in several pathologic conditions. In rosacea keratitis it is usually most marked in the upper quadrants of the cornea and preceded by subepithelial infiltrates which progress towards the center of the cornea and the deeper layers of the stroma. Eventually, the epithelium over these areas becomes eroded, and the ensuing ulcers attract blood vessels which form a vascularization of the fascicular type. This clinical picture is different from that of the ariboflavinotic type of corneal vascularity. There is disagreement in regard to the beneficial effect of riboflavin in rosacea keratitis claimed by some writers.[20-23] The possibility of a conditioned deficiency must be taken into consideration. It may be that coincidental riboflavin deficiency can aggravate rosacea keratitis, in which case benefit may be derived from riboflavin administration.

Another condition associated with corneal vascularization is phlyctenular or eczematous keratoconjunctivitis. Here the situation is quite different; this disease is actually nothing but a manifestation of true ariboflavinosis against an allergic background. Patients suffering from it make a dramatic recovery with riboflavin by mouth, without any local treatment, while the usual treatment with yellow oxide of mercury, atropine, and cod-liver oil is in many cases a very tedious affair. The condition occurs mainly in under-nourished children who show stigmata of "scrofulous" diathesis. Patients with eczematous keratoconjunctivitis show low ribo flavin values in the urine.[24] This, together with the therapeutic effect of riboflavin, certainly suggests that eczematous keratitis is a manifestation of ariboflavinosis, released by nonspecific stimuli of an allergic nature in predisposed individuals. The prompt therapeutic effect of cortisone in eczematous keratoconjunctivitis observed by Thygeson and Fritz[25] does not invalidate this contention. Cortisone is a very effective agent in combating allergic manifestations of any kind by blocking the inflammatory reaction, but it has no specific effect.

Another disease characterized by corneal vascularization is trachoma. Typical trachomatous pannus is limited to the upper part of the cornea and cannot be confused with ariboflavinotic vascularity. There are cases, however, in which a marked discrepancy exists between the appearance of the active pannus and that of the smooth and well-cicatrized palpebral conjunctiva. The patients complain of watering, itching, and burning, and sometimes even exhibit marked photophobia. The palpebral conjunctiva is inactive and not amenable to treatment. Nonspecific treatment with atropine alleviates the symptoms but cannot prevent relapses. On careful examination with the slit lamp, the cornea is frequently found to be vascularized not only in its upper half or third, as in classical trachomatous pannus, but in its entire circumference, as in ariboflavinosis. Treatment with riboflavin promptly relieves the condition.[26] The therapeutic success in such "intractable" cases of trachomatous pannus means that they are provoked by ariboflavinosis, causing typical vascularization of the cornea. The vessels of the trachomatous pannus never leave the cornea entirely but remain visible through the slit lamp as minute, empty channels. If riboflavin deficiency occurs at this stage of trachoma, the well-known response of the cornea sets in: the limbic plexus becomes flushed, and newly-formed capillaries encroach upon the cornea. In the upper half of the cornea, where the old channels of the trachomatous pannus are still present, there is no new formation of vessels, but the vessels of the pannus become engorged and present the picture of active trachomatous pannus. Adequate provision of riboflavin will then, of course, exert its beneficial effect on the old pannus as well as on the newly formed vessels.

Corneal vascularity of the same type as that found in ariboflavinosis occurs in rats on diets deficient in protein or in any of the essential amino acids. It is probably due to some metabolic upset in the corneal cells caused by the absence of these substances. A similar type of vascularization occurs in zinc deficiency,[27] sodium deficiency,[28] and thallium poisoning.[29] Although this vascularity is of the same type as that in ariboflavinosis, it seems to occur only under experimental conditions unlikely to be encountered in clinical practice, hence, it need rarely, if ever, be considered in the differential diagnosis.

It seems that a low intake of riboflavin must continue for a prolonged period of time before anatomical signs of the deficiency, and particularly corneal vascularization, make their appearance. This is surprising in view of the fact that riboflavin is water-soluble and might be expected to be washed out of the organism in a short time in a deficiency state. It can perhaps be explained by assuming that riboflavin is bound in the organism to the protein of enzymes and cells. In rats on a riboflavin-deficient diet, the first signs of corneal vascularization appear only when the riboflavin concentration of the cornea falls to less than 50 per cent of normal. In rats on a comparatively riboflavin-free diet, this stage is reached in 3 weeks; but in animals on a diet containing only slightly less than the optimum, it takes a considerably longer period of time.[19]

A deficiency disease may be caused not primarily by an inadequate diet, but rather by interference with absorption or utilization of essential nutrients, or by increased requirements, destruction, or excretion. Jolliffe has termed these states "conditioned" malnutrition,[30] and Kruse has given this concept an important place in the science of nutrition.[31] Cases of corneal vascularity after surgical trauma to the cornea (corneal transplantation) are an example.[32] Here, the trauma is to be regarded as the conditioning factor. The healing process after trauma causes increased activity of the corneal epithelium and stroma, with a correspondingly high oxygen requirement. Thus, a degree of riboflavin deficiency which remains subclinical under normal conditions may lead to corneal vascularization when other pathologic conditions increase the corneal metabolism. In experimental animals, prolonged deprivation of riboflavin definitely handicaps the healing process of experimental corneal lesions.[33] This, then, is the answer to the question as to why not every case of dietary riboflavin deficiency displays signs of corneal vascularity.

Treatment. The recommended dietary allowance for adult humans is 1.5 to 1.7 mg of riboflavin per day (more during pregnancy and lactation). Supply of the normal demand should be sufficient to establish a well-balanced function. Empirically, however, it has been found that it is advisable to give therapeutically at least 5 to 10 times the amount required physiologically for a limited time.

Vascularity of the cornea can be cured clinically with riboflavin alone; it is, however, safe to assume that the other B factors are also lacking to a certain degree, and it would seem advisable to treat these cases not with riboflavin alone but with the whole vitamin B complex. It is quite possible that in partial avitaminosis the cumulative damage to the important epithelial structures of the eye may lower their vitality, favor the incidence and prolong the activity of infection, and precipitate degenerative changes on a wider scale than is yet realized.[34]

Acute Manifestations. In the preceding section, the ocular signs of ariboflavinosis were described as they occur in cases taking a more or less chronic course. This is not always the case. The condition can assume the aspect of a violent, acute disease.[35,36] Such cases present very marked photophobia and intense hyperemia, mainly of the bulbar conjunctiva. No mucous or purulent discharge is present, but lacrimation is profuse. The conjunctival smear is sterile or shows harmless saprophytes. With the slit lamp, the limbic plexus is seen to be maximally engorged. The loops, transformed into tiny convolutions of capillaries, send out fine vessels 3, 4, or more millimeters into the subepithelial corneal layers. The newly formed capillaries sometimes stand out plastically from the corneal epithelium. The epithelium covering the vascularized part of the cornea is edematous and shows cyst-like vesicles filled with clear fluid. These may break down and produce small ulcers that stain with fluorescein.

Gross dietary deficiency can be found in the history and, in some cases, the condition is provoked by acute infections such as tonsillitis. Mild signs of other deficiencies of the vitamin B complex are often observed, such as pellagroid pigmentation of the skin and overactive tendon reflexes. These cases represent acute exacerbations of long-standing chronic deficiency states, provoked by a sudden deterioration of the general state of health. Acute infectious diseases, gastrointestinal disorders, or similar occurrences will almost always be found in the history.

The condition looks so alarming that hesitation may be felt about limiting therapy to riboflavin. The prompt response of the eyes to this medication is, however, most gratifying, and local treatment is generally superfluous.

Amino Acid Deficiency. *Etiology.* Rats on a tryptophan-deficient diet which receive sufficient amounts of vitamin B complex develop vascularity of the cornea.[37,38] Most of the other essential amino acids produce the same effect when absent from the diet of experimental animals: leucine,[39,40] histidine,[39,41] lysine,[42] methionine,[43,44] isoleucine,[39] threonine, valine, arginine and phenylalanine.[39,45]

Pathology. The ocular reaction to any of these deficiencies is a congestion of the scleral conjunctiva and engorgement of the limbic plexus, followed by slight thickening and diffuse corneal clouding; capillary "sprouts" shoot from the marginal limbic vessels and these new capillaries invade the clear cornea.

This corneal vascularity resembles closely that observed in riboflavin deficiency; however, deep vascularization and keratinization of the epithelium frequently distinguish it from ariboflavinotic vascularity. This keratinization has been termed "nutritional corneal dystrophy."[40,41] It is reversible if treated in time with the missing amino acid. It is important to note that it does not respond to riboflavin administration. Amino acid deficiency must, therefore, exert some direct effect upon the cornea, rather than acting by inducing a deficiency of riboflavin.

Prevalence. In rats, general protein deficiency, not only deficiency of a single amino acid, may result in the appearance of corneal vessels. In man, however, this has never been observed. A clear-cut deficiency of a single amino acid is unlikely to occur clinically in man, and it is doubtful whether it ought to be taken into consideration in the differential diagnosis of corneal vascularity. This problem is, however, far from being settled. Givner[46] has observed two cases of exfoliative dermatitis with corneal changes similar to those seen in experimental valine deficiency. Administration of amino acids parenterally and aminoids and protein by mouth was followed by clearing of the cornea and, finally, by complete recovery.

Local Application. Amino acids have been applied externally to one experimentally injured cornea of guinea pigs, while the other cornea with a similar injury was treated with isotonic saline as control. Regeneration of the cornea in the eye treated with amino acids was much more rapid.[47]

Angular Blepharoconjunctivitis. *Pyridoxine* (vit. B$_6$) has been shown to be a factor in angular blepharoconjunctivitis. Patients with this condition have a low pyridoxine level in the urine, and the causative organism, Hemophilus duplex (Morax-Axenfeld bacillus), survives longer in the conjunctiva of pyridoxine-deficient rabbits than in normal controls.[47a] While the condition is doubtless of bacterial origin, pyridoxine deficiency seems to play a role in its establishment, and it can be cured by pyridoxine without any local therapy.[47b,47c]

Keratoconus. The etiology of keratoconus is not established. It has been shown that lack of vitamin E in the diet of rats occasionally causes keratoconus as well as other ocular disturbances; they could be cured by administering the missing vitamin. Progressive cases of keratoconus in man have been treated with some benefit with vitamins E, D, and calcium.[48-51] The results, however, have not been confirmed.

Interstitial Keratitis. Vitamin E was reported to be beneficial in syphilitic interstitial keratitis.[52] The addition of riboflavin appeared to have some effect on the corneal vascularity, rapidly improving interstitial syphilitic keratitis.[53] Antisyphilitic treatment was, of course, also given.

Spring Catarrh. Riboflavin and nicotinamide are reported to alleviate the subjective complaints of patients with spring catarrh, without, however, appreciably influencing the anatomical changes.[54,55] Spring catarrh undoubtedly is an allergic condition.

Vitamin Treatment of a Variety of Corneal Diseases. *Riboflavin.* Certain corneal diseases, such as superficial punctate keratitis, corneal ulcer, and catarrhal infiltrates, have occasionally been reported to be favorably influenced by riboflavin.[56-58]

Thiamin. Favorable results have been claimed for thiamin therapy of herpetic infections of the eye, like herpetic keratitis, disciform keratitis, punctate keratitis and ophthalmic herpes.[59-62]

Vitamin C. Corneal inflammations like superficial keratitis, chronic infiltrates, and ulcers have been reported to improve strikingly on oral vitamin C therapy.[63] It has also been claimed that the addition of vitamin C to the routine treatment of hypopyon ulcers made the hypopyon disappear more rapidly.[64]

That vitamin C may be of importance for the cornea is suggested by the observation that the vitamin C content of the cornea increases in rats suffering from keratomalacia due to vitamin A deficiency.[65] Vitamin C is also necessary for the formation of collagen in the cornea.[66] In scorbutic animals, thermal injuries to the cornea are followed by corneal vascularization at a significantly higher rate than in controls. It can be assumed that the accumulation of metabolites leads to edema and opening of the corneal lamellae, which permits the blood vessels to approach the injured parts of the cornea.[67]

LENS AND AQUEOUS HUMOR

Vitamin C in Ocular Biology. *Presence of Vitamin C in Lens and Aqueous Humor.* The crystalline lens occupies a unique place in physiology. Devoid of nerves and vascular supply, it is freely suspended in the aqueous humor on which it depends for its nutrition. It represents an isolated metabolic system, the respiratory processes of which are mediated by a system of relatively simple chemical compounds; these are able to transport hydrogen and oxygen and thus maintain oxidation and reduction activities. In 1932, Müller[68] reported that ascorbic acid in the lens is responsible for reversible oxidation-reduction processes. Quantitative analysis brought out the fact that the amount of ascorbic acid in the lens and the aqueous was 10 or 20 times higher than in any other part of the body, except the adrenals, the sex glands, and the hypophysis.

The Function of Vitamin C in the Eye. The function of vitamin C in the crystalline lens and its surrounding fluid seems to be the mediation—together with glutathione and cystine—of the oxygen uptake of the lens.

Source of Vitamin C in the Eye. There are two possible sources of vitamin C in the eye. (1) It may be brought to the eye by the circulation and accumulated by the lens and the aqueous. (2) It may be formed in the lens and retained there and in the anterior chamber.

The lens of the ox is capable of synthesizing ascorbic acid.[69] A reaction which has been shown to occur *in vitro* may also occur in the living eye. Intravenous injection of glucose is likewise followed by a rise of the ascorbic acid content in the aqueous.[70]

Further proof that at least part of the ascorbic acid in the aqueous is produced by the lens is the fact that the high vitamin C content of the aqueous in man is maintained only when the lens is present and intact. In cataract and aphakia the percentage of ascorbic acid in the aqueous falls almost to its level in the blood.[71] When the lens is intact, ascorbic acid in the aqueous is present in an oxidized form; in eyes with cataract it is found in a reversibly reduced form.[72] Ascorbic acid is brought into the anterior chamber where, in the presence of a healthy lens, it becomes converted by dehydrogenation into the oxidized form, thus playing a part in the oxidation-reduction system of the lens.

The blood-aqueous barrier is usually permeable to reversibly oxidized ascorbic acid in the direction blood→aqueous, while it is impermeable in the opposite direction. The high content of ascorbic acid of the aqueous is therefore caused, at least partly, by the following mechanism: (1) supply of oxidized ascorbic acid from the blood, (2) reduction of ascorbic acid by the lens, (3) retention of the reduced ascorbic acid by the blood-aqueous barrier.

Vitamin C in Ocular Pathology. Vitamin C plays an important role in the respiratory processes of the lens. In pathologic conditions these processes are altered, and the vitamin C metabolism reflects this disturbance. As the lens ages, its respiration becomes less intense, and the lens nucleus contains less vitamin C than the biologically more active cortex. If the respiratory processes of the lens are suppressed by cataract or absence of the lens, ascorbic acid is found in the aqueous in the reversibly reduced form alone; it is, in contradistinction to oxidized ascorbic acid, easily reabsorbed into the blood, and its concentration in the eye is thus equal to that in the blood.

Cataract. In senile cataract, the vitamin C content of the lens and the aqueous drops to almost zero. Whether the absence of vitamin C in the cataractous lens is a cause or a consequence of the lens alteration is not known. From all the evidence at hand it seems likely that the absence of vitamin C in the aqueous and lens in cataract is secondary to, and not the cause of, the lens changes.

The question of the curative effect of vitamin C on lens opacities has likewise not been settled. Improvement of early lens opacities has been claimed by some, and complete absence of any therapeutic effect by others.

It is remarkable that diseases like uveitis, glaucoma, and retinitis pigmentosa, which are known occasionally to cause cataract, are accompanied by low vitamin C values in the aqueous and the lens prior to visible lens changes.[73–76] Naphthalene poisoning of rabbits causes first a decrease of ascorbic acid in the aqueous and only later cataracts,[77,78] but while large doses of vitamin C prevent the fall of ascorbic acid concentration in the anterior chamber, they do not prevent the appearance of cataract.[77] X-ray irradiation of the eye, a procedure which ultimately causes cataract, provokes a fall in the vitamin C content of the aqueous.[77,79]

Postoperative Hemorrhage. Vitamin C has been shown to be necessary for the healing of wounds. It has been tried, therefore, as a preventive of postoperative hemorrhage following cataract extraction with iridectomy. There is no convincing evidence that the occurrence of hyphema following cataract extraction is influenced by administration of vitamin C.

Various Conditions. The occurrence of hemorrhage into different parts of the eye in scurvy is well known. Hemorrhages have been described in the conjunctiva, iris, and retina, and in rare cases exophthalmos has resulted from hemorrhage into the orbit.

A variety of conditions have been ascribed to avitaminosis C or have been treated with vitamin C: ocular tuberculosis, retinal hemorrhages, and anaphylactic ocular disease. Much further work needs to be done in order to arrive at conclusive evidence of its value in ophthalmic therapy.

Cataract. *Riboflavin.* Contrary to previous claims correlating the presence of riboflavin in the lens with its transparency, riboflavin is found in the lens only in insignificant amounts. In the 1930's, however, many workers reported that uncomplicated experimental vitamin G (or B_2) deficiency caused cataract in rats, mice, and chicks. On the other hand, when better riboflavin-free diets were devised, fewer experimental animals developed cataract.[80] Young animals seem to be more liable to develop nutritional cataract than older ones. While cataract may occur in certain animals on a certain diet, it is probable that the essential disturbance is due to a combination of several deficiencies, or to a factor as yet unidentified.[81] It is certainly not riboflavin, which has been shown to be practically nonexistent in the lens and to have no therapeutic or preventive effect.

Amino Acids. The essential amino acids, deficiencies of which are known to cause corneal vascularization, seem also to be necessary in the metabolism of the lens. A certain percentage of animals on diets deficient in one of the essential amino acids (tryptophan) develop cataracts; the process can be reversed by feeding the missing nutrient, provided the changes are not too far advanced.[82] Lenticular changes to some extent are also seen in general protein deficiency.

It is of interest that during the war years in Russia it was observed[83] that the age incidence of cataract was much lower than prior to the war. All patients showed signs of deficiencies of vitamin A and B complex, and while vitamin treatment was inconclusive, it was thought that those presenile cataracts were due, in part, to avitaminosis. It has also long been known that in India, where malnutrition is frequent, cataract is more prevalent and occurs at an earlier age than in other countries.

Diabetic Cataract. It is not uncommon to find cataractous lens changes in diabetes. True diabetic cataract has a characteristic appearance and is rare. More frequently, a type of cataract is observed which is morphologically identical with the senile type, but occurs at an earlier age and progresses more rapidly.

Two mechanisms are generally accepted as responsible for the production of cataract: one is the decrease in the permeability of the lens capsule in the presence of glucose and ketone bodies; the other is the disturbance of the tissue-fluid equilibrium causing, by osmotic influences, hydration of the lens.

TREATMENT. Treatment of early true diabetic cataract can be quite effective if it is started before denaturation of the proteins in the lens has set in and only edema is present. Adequate control of the diabetes can then result in complete disappearance of the lens opacities.

Presenile cataract in older diabetics does not respond to medical treatment. Surgery must be resorted to sooner or later, and, while complications must be feared more than in nondiabetics, the disease itself is no contraindication.

Galactosemia. Galactosemia is a congenital and hereditary error of carbohydrate metabolism. The usual symptoms, occurring within a few days after birth, consist of vomiting, lethargy, fever and failure to gain weight. The clinical signs include jaundice, ascites, hepatomegaly and splenomegaly. Bruck and Rapoport[84] published a report of an interesting case of galactosemia causing cataracts, and the occurrence of this ocular complication has been reported with increasing frequency. Galactosemia is due to the absence of a specific enzyme, uridyl transferase, necessary for the utilization of galactose. This leads to an accumulation of an intermediary metabolic product, galactose-1-phosphate,[85] which probably has a toxic effect on such tissues as liver, spleen, brain and crystalline lens. Treatment consists in withdrawing milk and instituting galactose- and lactose-free diets which usually lead to rapid recovery and prevention of cataracts (see Chapter 39).

RETINA, OPTIC NERVE AND VISUAL DISTURBANCE

Night Blindness. *Signs and Symptoms.* One of the first symptoms of vitamin A deficiency is night blindness. Unfortunately, two diametrically opposed terms—etymologically—are used for this condition, hemeralopia and nyctalopia; however, the term night blindness is expressive, unequivocal and should be used.

Vitamin A deficiency is only one of the several causes of night blindness. It occurs in all conditions that prevent the rods, cones, or both from participating to their full capacity in the visual process, conditions in which retinal disease has resulted in destruction or dysfunction of the nervous elements. The adaptation curve will become abnormal according to the kind of elements most affected—rods or cones—and the degree of impairment. The rods are the elements responsible for light discrimination in reduced illumination, and, while the function of the cones is also affected in vitamin A deficiency, it has been established that for practical purposes the best single criterion is the final rod threshold. Deterioration of dark adaptation is also accompanied by changes in the color sensitivity of the retina. The fields for blue and red may become diminished or even inverted, and a shrinking of the field for yellow may be observed. Concentric constriction of the visual fields may occur, a sign probably indicating involvement of the cones as well as of the rods.

The role of vitamin A in the visual process has been the subject of intense study since Wald[87–89] demonstrated that it is an essential constituent of visual purple and this is discussed in some detail in Chapter 5, Section A.

The reason for a vitamin A deficiency may be twofold: either inadequate intake or absorption of the provitamin or the vitamin from vegetable or animal sources, or else a disturbance of the process of synthesis of vitamin A in the human organism due to gastrointestinal or liver disease. The role of liver disease in the etiology of night blindless is demonstrated by the fact that dark adaptation is frequently disturbed in such conditions.[90] There may be a significant relationship between other nutritional deficiencies and impaired dark adaptation. Riboflavin,[91,92] thiamin,[93] and nicotinic acid amide[94] have been reported to be effective in alleviating night blindness and other vitamin A deficiency signs when vitamin A alone failed to bring on recovery. The vitamin B complex may thus play a role in the utilization of vitamin A. Another possible relationship is suggested by reports of a beneficial effect of ascorbic acid on night blindness.[95,96] Certain amino acids, chiefly l-glutamic acid and l-cysteine, have also been shown to improve the curve and the threshold of dark adaptation.[97]

Age seems to play a physiologic part in dark adaptation, and a progressive deterioration of this capacity has been charted, amounting to about 0.12 log units for an increase of 10 years.[98]

Considerable difficulty was experienced in the attempt to establish experimentally the period of reduced vitamin A intake required to cause disturbances of the light sense. Several factors have to be taken into consideration. The most important one seems to be the storage of vitamin A in the liver. As long as this was disregarded in experiments, the results were unreliable. Many persons respond to an experimental vitamin A deficiency with a prompt rise of the rod threshold, while in others it takes weeks or months before deviations of the normal adaptation curve can be observed. The latter response seems to be the more frequent one.

The development of disturbances of dark adaptation in vitamin A deficiency is governed by the previous dietary history of the individual and the amount of vitamin A stored in the liver. This storage is probably not entirely related to the amount recently ingested, but is more intimately connected with as yet undefined metabolic capacities which differ among different persons.

Any condition which increases the metabolic need for vitamin A (some of the known ones are: fever, infection, elevated basal metabolic rate, rapid growth, pregnancy)[99] may cause impairment of dark adaptation in spite of a seemingly adequate daily intake of vitamin A. Interference with absorption in the gastrointestinal tract may have the same effect.

Pathology. Avitaminosis A of long duration has been claimed to provoke fundus changes analogous to those characterizing retinitis punctata albescens and Wilson's disease; the fundus changes disappeared on therapy with vitamin A.[100] This observation is unconfirmed.

The question has been approached experimentally by Myra L. Johnson,[101] who produced vitamin A deficiency in rats and examined the retina histologically. Severe deficiency for only a short time failed to produce any structural changes except edema; deficiency over a longer period, however, resulted in degeneration, beginning in the visual cells and progressing through the retina to the inner nuclear layer. The outer segments of rods with slight degenerative changes showed a remarkable degree of repair after only twenty-four hours on vitamin A therapy, and complete recovery after 21 to 28 days. When the outer segments of the rods were completely degenerated, they were shown to be capable of regeneration after 10 to 18 weeks. If the degeneration had progressed to the outer nuclear layer or further, no repair could be observed. In night blindness due to vitamin A deficiency a total or almost total loss of the b-potential is found in the electro-retinogram. Treatment with massive doses of vitamin A leads to complete restoration of the rod system functions, indicated by a normalization of the electrical response of the retina.[102]

Prevalence. Night blindness caused by vitamin A deficiency is common in many countries. It is endemic in regions where vitamin A-deficient diets are habitually consumed. It is common in persons who, due to faulty dietary habits or for economic reasons, subsist on inadequate amounts of vitamin A-containing foods.

Severe vitamin A deficiency is, however, rare in Western countries. In Britain, it has been shown[103] that, of those school children who received two-thirds of a pint of milk a day in school, 67 per cent had normal dark adaptation, while only 37 per cent of others receiving only one-third of a pint of milk or less daily showed normal dark adaptation curves. Measurements of dark adaptation may be used to assess nutritional levels in respect to vitamin A either by the determination of the effect of vitamin A on dark adaptation, or by the comparison of the values of dark adaptation in various groups. The latter method, while not providing such conclusive evidence as the former, may sometimes provide presumptive evidence of the relative nutritional status in respect to vitamin A, and for technical reasons it may be the only feasible procedure.[104]

Differential Diagnosis. There can be no doubt that wide physiologic variations in the light sense occur; there are individuals with a normal level of vitamin A in the plasma who have a physiologically low sense of light which cannot be improved with vitamin A. Moreover, psychic factors, age, fatigue, depression, or ocular lesions all play a part. Derangements in the light sense cannot,

therefore, be used as an exclusive test for vitamin A deficiency; chemical estimations of vitamin A in the blood are necessary. Only when the vitamin A concentration falls below a certain limit is there a measurable deficiency in the sense of light. Subjective night vision disturbances, however, begin only with a much lower vitamin level.

With normal blood values, the light sense is usually good. Of subjects with normal average values of light sense, a rather small percentage improves on vitamin A therapy. These individuals have probably an exceptionally good light sense and happen to suffer from a slight degree of avitaminosis A; there is nothing to suggest that hypervitaminosis increases the light sensitivity.

Treatment. It seems that recovery from disturbances of dark adaptation is relatively slow. Short-term therapy with high doses of vitamin A has only a slight effect and is followed, at best, by a transitory, incomplete recovery. Complete recovery is a matter of weeks and months. This slow recovery rate indicates some deep-seated lesion, the development of which may be peculiarly favored by the sudden and acute onset in experimental depletion of vitamin A, the long continuance of a deficiency diet, and also, perhaps, by the sharp restriction of vitamin A alone. Prolonged ingestion of large doses of vitamin A can result in an intoxication with severe general symptoms as loss of hair, skin rashes, skin desquamation, arthritic pains, and hepatomegaly. The eye signs may include papilledema with retinal hemorrhages, muscle pareses, diplopia and exophthalmos. The signs and symptoms clear rapidly upon withdrawal of the medication.

The Role of Riboflavin in Vision. The pigment epithelium of the retina of fish and mammals contains a substance that shows a green fluorescence and changes into lumi-flavin under the influence of light. This property is typical of riboflavin and it is reasonable to assume that this vitamin exists in the retina. It has been suggested that riboflavin has a special function during twilight, transforming light of short wavelength into light of a wave frequency for which the eye has a maximum sensitivity.[105] This postulate can be upheld by certain clinical observations. Cases have been described of impaired night vision and reduced vitamin A level in the blood which failed to respond to vitamin A, but reacted with both improved night vision and raised vitamin A plasma levels when riboflavin was administered.[106–109] These observations suggest that riboflavin plays a part in the utilization of vitamin A.

Diabetic Retinopathy. There is some evidence that nutritional imbalance plays a part in the pathogenesis of diabetic retinopathy. The oxygen consumption of the isolated retina of alloxan-diabetic rabbits is significantly lowered,[110] and the same fact has been observed in experimental thiamin deficiency;[111] improper diet and B-complex avitaminosis have been accused of being partly responsible for the typical retinal involvement, with hemorrhages and exudates.

Diabetic patients have been found to have levels of carotene and vitamin A outside the range established for healthy persons. Thiamin may be reduced in the blood and the gastric juice of diabetics, and it has been stated that this vitamin enhances the effect of small insulin doses, decreases the blood sugar of normal dogs, and depresses the blood sugar curve in dogs after glucose intake.[112]

Some of these statements need confirmation. Diabetic retinopathy has come under particularly close scrutiny lately, and there are certainly other factors involved more important than the nutritional ones enumerated above. But there can be no doubt that experimental diabetes is increased in severity by deficiencies of the vitamin B complex, and that diabetics with concomitant vitamin deficiency symptoms respond to vitamin therapy with amelioration of the severity of their diabetes and its retinal manifestations (see Chapter 29).

Nutritional Amblyopia. During and after World War II, numerous cases of serious neurologic and metabolic disturbances were seen among prisoners of war and internee camp inmates. They nearly always showed ocular changes. The greatest number of serious cases were observed in the unfortunate victims of the Japanese prison camps, but less severe cases were also described in others. In retrospect, these cases are clinically comparable to those observed earlier in the malnourished population of tropical countries.

Early Japanese writings on beriberi indicate that retrobulbar neuritis, scotomata, and oculomotor palsies have been encountered with varying frequency in Oriental beriberi. Involvement of the optic nerve with pallor of the nerve head and relative central scotomata have also been described in pellagra. Vitamin B complex has a beneficial effect on such cases.

Retrobulbar neuritis is a not uncommon effect of malnutrition in tropical countries, and vitamin B complex has often been reported as being beneficial in its treatment. Progressive loss of vision with temporal pallor of the optic disc, as seen in India, frequently responds to vitamin A therapy.[113]

Visual disturbances in prisoners of war were characterized by a retrobulbar neuritis; when it existed for any length of time, permanent damage to the optic nerve resulted. The highly sensitive papillomacular bundle, in particular, suffered to a marked degree.

The majority of observers accept a serious deficiency of the vitamin B complex as the etiologic factor in this condition. Protein deficiency, a hypothetical toxin from moldy rice, and general malnutrition probably contribute to its development.

The mottling of the macular retina in nutritional amblyopia is similar in appearance to the fundus changes of solar retinopathy occurring in people who observe a solar eclipse without adequate protection; the retinal damage of nutritional amblyopia may be attributable to the action of the tropical sun upon a tissue that has become sensitized to light by a dietary deficiency, as in pellagra or beriberi.

Toxic Amblyopia. The nutritional amblyopia in the tropics and among prisoners of war seems to be closely related to the retrobulbar neuritis—toxic amblyopia due to alcohol and nicotine. Toxic amblyopia is considered to be the result of a toxic action of nicotine and alcohol on poorly-nourished nerve cells. It is possible to cure toxic amblyopia by placing the patient on an adequate diet or by giving him thiamin, even without depriving him of the habitual intake of alcohol or the use of tobacco. This points to thiamin deficiency as being a factor in the pathogenesis of toxic retrobulbar neuritis. Evidence also has been presented that the retina or the optic nerve is unduly sensitive to tobacco in even mild vitamin B_{12} deficiency. Amblyopia may precede other manifestations of the deficiency, and parenteral administration of cyanocobalamin improves visual acuity and reverses the field changes.[114] Vitamin B_{12} has been used successfully in other optic nerve diseases.[115]

While the ultimate goal in the treatment of these patients is, of course, to discontinue completely the abuse of alcohol and tobacco, serious nervous complications can be prevented by the prompt institution of adequate dietary and vitamin therapy.[116]

Vitamin B complex and thiamin have also been used at times with good results in the treatment of retrobulbar neuritis of unknown origin; however, the role of thiamin in these conditions is not very well understood.

Another instance of a conditioned affection of the optic nerve is the retrobulbar neuritis occasionally encountered in pregnancy. The increased vitamin requirement in pregnancy and hyperemesis gravidarum, impairing vitamin intake, are probably the conditioning factors. Thiamin has been used with benefit in retrobulbar neuritis of pregnancy. The same may be true for the rare cases of retrobulbar neuritis following unduly prolonged breast-feeding without adequate replenishing of the vitamin stores of the mother.

Pathology. There is scanty information available concerning the anatomical changes in the optic nerve of thiamin-deficient animals. Co-carboxylase is important in the oxidation of pyruvic acid in the nerve tissue. There is no proof, however, that the damage is really due to any toxic action of pyruvic acid. The optic nerve of thiamin-deficient pigeons with beriberi shows edema and interruptions of the myelin sheath.[117] Degeneration of the myelin sheath manifests itself by the formation of lipoid granules, particularly in the papillomacular bundle.[118]

The first evidence that vitamin A is necessary for normal functioning of the nerve tissue was offered by the finding of severe degenerative changes in the optic, sciatic, and femoral nerves of young pigs fed a vitamin A-deficient diet from the time of weaning.[119] Pigs, calves, or rats whose mothers are fed a diet deficient in vitamin A are born with anophthalmos or microphthalmos.[120] These conditions are attributed to a malformation of the optic nerve, either primary or due to a stenosis of the optic canal.[121–123] Young dogs fed a diet deficient in vitamin A develop degeneration of the spinal cord, the eighth nerve and also the optic nerve.[124] Optic nerve degenerations were also observed in rats on a diet deficient in vitamin A,[125] and much more severe changes occurred when the avitaminotic animals were exposed to various poisons and bacterial toxins.[126]

Prevalence. It is to be borne in mind that the experimental results were obtained in animals exposed to an extremely vitamin A-deficient diet. Vitamin A-deficient animals whose litters were born with malformations of the eyes had vitamin A serum levels of one-tenth or less of the normal. Such extremely low levels are not likely to occur in man.

Myopia. Experimental and clinical evidence has been presented that the animal protein content of the diet can influence the state of refraction in the growing animal[126a] and child.[126b] A group of nearsighted children received, in a carefully conducted controlled study, extra animal protein; the rate of increase in myopia was much less than in a control group whose diet was not changed. While other factors must be at work as well, the course of myopia in children and adolescents may be beneficially modified by dietary means.

Wernicke's Syndrome. In Wernicke's syndrome an ophthalmoplegia is observed, associated with clouding of consciousness, ataxia, and other manifestations of central nervous system involvement. The basic pathology of this syndrome consists of small foci of degeneration, varicose blood vessels, and petechial hemorrhages in the cerebral cortex and the region of the nuclei of the third, fourth, and sixth cranial nerves. The etiology of the syndrome is complex, but thiamin deficiency seems to be the cause of the ophthalmoplegia, and thiamin administration may cure it promptly.[127–131]

BIBLIOGRAPHY

1. McLaren: *Malnutrition and the Eye*, New York, Academic Press, 1963.
1a. Collins: Tr. Ophth. Soc. U. K., *50*, 201, 1930.
2. Mann, *et al.*: Am. J. Ophth., *29*, 801, 1946.
3. Kruse: Milbank Mem. Fund Quart., xix, *3*, 207, 1941.
3a. Paton and McLaren: Am. J. Ophth., *50*, 568, 1960.
4. Aykroyd, *et al.*: Can. Med. Assn. J., *60*, 1, 1949.
5. Darby and Milam: Am. J. Pub. Health, *35*, 1014, 1945.
6. Calvo, *et al.*: J. Am. Diet. Assn., *22*, 297, 1946.
7. Robertson and Morgan: J. Nutrition, *31*, 471, 1946.
7a. Ferguson: Trans. Ophth. Soc. U. K., *66*, 108, 1946.
8. Medical Research Council: Spec. Rep. Series No. 264, His Majesty's Stationery Office, London, 1949.
9. Wolbach and Bessey: Phys. Rev., *22*, 233, 1942.
10. Friedenwald, *et al.*: J. Nutrition, *29*, 299, 1945.
11. Mellanby: Brit. Med. J., *1*, 677, 1930; Brain, *54*, 247, 1931; Edinburgh Med. J., *40*, 197, 1933; J. Path. Bact., *38*, 391, 1934.
12. Pillat: China Med. J., *43*, 907, 1929.
13. Cirincione: Richerche sulla Xerosi Congiunctivale, Pavia, 1891.
14. Williamson: Med. J. Malaya, *3*, 68, 1948.
15. National Research Council: Recommended Daily Dietary Allowances, Revised 1968.
16. Kohra: Acta Soc. Ophth. Japan, *40*, 1595, 1936.
17. Orzalesi: Bull. d'Ocul., *17*, 509, 1939.
18. Gundersen: Arch. Ophth., *21*, 76, 1939.
19. Bessey and Lowry: J. Biol. Chem., *155*, 635, 1944.
20. Johnson and Eckardt: Arch. Ophth., *23*, 899, 1940; *24*, 1001, 1940.
21. Johnson: Am. J. Ophth., *24*, 1233, 1941.
22. Connors, *et al.*: Arch. Ophth., *29*, 956, 1943.
23. Sohr: Klin. Monatsbl. Augenh., *11*, 389, 1944.
24. Stern and Landau: Am. J. Ophth., *31*, 1619, 1948.
25. Thygeson and Fritz: Am. J. Ophth., *34*, 357, 1951.
26. Landau and Stern: Am. J. Ophth., *31*, 952, 1948.
27. Follis, *et al.*: J. Nutrition, *22*, 223, 1941.
28. Orent-Keiles and McCollum: J. Biol. Chem., *133*, 75, 1940.
29. Buschke: Arch. f. Derm. und Syphilis, *116*, 477, 1913.
30. Jolliffe: J.A.M.A., *122*, 299, 1943.
31. Kruse: Milbank Mem. Fund Quart., *27*, 5, 1949.
32. Stern: Am. J. Ophth., *33*, 1127, 1950.
33. Lowry and Bessey: J. Nutrition, *30*, 285, 1945.
34. Duke-Elder: *Text Book of Ophthalmology*, Vol. II, St. Louis, C. V. Mosby Co., p. 1424, 1946.
35. Mann: Am. J. Ophth., *28*, 243, 1945.
36. Stern: Ophthalmologica, *114*, 103, 1947.

37. Chang, *et al.*: Chin. J. Phys., *16*, 241, 1941.
38. Totter and Day: J. Nutrition, *24*, 159, 1942.
39. Sydenstricker, *et al.*: Proc. Soc. Exp. Biol. & Med., *64*, 59, 1947.
40. Maun, *et al.*: Arch Path., *40*, 173, 1945.
41. ———: Arch. Path., *41*, 25, 1946.
42. Hock, *et al.*: Fed. Proc., *4*, 155, 1945.
43. Sydenstricker, *et al.*: Science, *103*, 194, 1946.
44. Berg, *et al.*: J. Nutrition, *33*, 271, 1947.
45. Sydenstricker, *et al.*: J. Nutrition, *34*, 481, 1947.
46. Givner: New York State J. Med., *48*, 2700, 1948.
47. Schaeffer: Proc. Soc. Exp. Biol. & Med., *61*, 165, 1946.
47a. Irinoda, K., *et al.*: Arch. Ophth., *60*, 303, 1958.
47b. Hinokuma, S., *et al.*: Ganka Rinsho Iho, *44*, 58, 1950, quoted in 47a.
47c. Asahinga, Y., *et al.*: Acta Soc. Ophth. Japon., *47*, 938, 1943, quoted in 47a.
48. Demole and Knapp: Ophthalmologica, *101*, 65, 1941.
49. Mandach: Schweiz. Med. Wochenschr., *21*, 673, 1941.
50. Carreras: La Prensa Med. Argent., *34*, 37, 1764, 1947.
51. Knapp: J.A.M.A., *110*, 1933, 1938; Am. J. Ophth., *22*, 289, 1939.
52. Stone: Arch. Ophth., *30*, 467, 1943.
53. Kruse, *et al.*: U. S. Publ. Health Rep., *55*, 157, 1940.
54. Castellanos: Arch. Ophth., *31*, 214, 1944.
55. Stern: Am. J. Ophth., *32*, 1553, 1949.
56. McKay: Med. Ann. Columbia, *10*, 290, 1949.
57. Cosgrove, *et al.*: Am. J. Ophth., *25*, 5, 544, 1942.
58. Conners, *et al.*: Arch. Ophth., *29*, 956, 1943.
59. Nitzulescu and Triandaf: Brit. J. Ophth., *21*, 654, 1937.
60. Grandi: Bull. d'Ocul., *18*, 208, 1939.
61. Cantuliera: Arch. de la Soc. Oft. Hisp.-Am., *5*, 776, 1945.
62. Gross: Brit. Med. J., *115*, 834, 1947.
63. Lyle and McLean: Brit. J. Ophthal., *30*, 129, 1941.
64. Summers: Brit. J. Ophth., *30*, 129, 1946.
65. Maestro: Rass. Ital. Ottal., *10*, 487, 1941.
66. Wolbach: Am. J. Path., 9 Suppl., p. 689, 1937.
67. Campbell and Ferguson: Brit. J. Ophth., *34*, 329, 1950.
68. Müller: Ber. 49ste Zus. Ophth. Ges. Heidelberg, *49*, 168, 1932.
69. Fischer: Klin. Wochenschr., *13*, 596, 1934.
70. Müller: Bull. Soc. Belge d'Opht., *69*, 65, 1934; Arch. f. Augenheilk., *109*, 304, 434, 1935.
71. Müller and Buschke: Arch. f. Augenheilk., *108*, 368, 1934.
72. ———: Arch. f. Augenheilk., *108*, 592, 1934.
73. Müller, *et al.*: Klin. Wochenschr., *13*, 20, 1934.
74. Bietti and Carteni: Boll. S. Ital. Biol. Speriment, *9*, 983, 1934.
75. Nakamura and Nakamura: Graefe's Arch., *134*, 197, 1935.
76. Yamagami: Kekkagu (Abstr. Sect.), *13*, 42, 1935.

77. Müller and Buschke: Arch. f. Augenheilk., *108*, 597, 1934.
78. Carteni and Basile: Boll. Soc. Ital. Biol. Speriment., *12*, 686, 1937.
79. Cavalacci: Arch. di Ottal., *52*, 149, 1935.
80. Harris: Bioch. J., *29*, 776, 1935.
81. Duke-Elder: *Text Book of Ophthalmology*, Vol. III, St. Louis, C. V. Mosby Co., p. 3146, 1939.
82. Schaeffer and Geiger: Proc. Soc. Exp. Biol. & Med., *66*, 309, 1947.
83. Torokhova: Vestnik Opt., *25*, 33, 1949.
84. Bruck and Rapoport: J. Dis. Child., *70*, 267, 1945.
85. Holzel, A., *et al.*: Am. J. Med., *22*, 703, 1957.
86. Adler: *Clinical Physiology of the Eye*, 4th Ed. St. Louis, C. V. Mosby Co., 1965.
87. Wald: Nature, *132*, 316, 1933; *134*, 65, 1934; Am. J. Phys., *109*, 107, 1934.
88. ———: Nature, *139*, 1017, 1937.
89. ———: Gener. Physiol., *22*, 775, 1939.
90. Wohl and Feldman: Am. J. Digest. Dis., *8*, 464, 1941.
91. Kimble and Gordon: J. Biol. Chem., *128*, Proc. 52, 1939.
92. Sloan: Am. J. Ophth., *30*, 705, 1946.
93. De Felice: Probl. Aliment, II, 5, 1941.
94. Hosoya, *et al.*: Tokoku J. Exp. Med., *53*, 103, 1950.
95. Gorczycki: Schweiz. Med. Wochenschr., *12*, 250, 1937.
96. Stewart: J. Phys., *96*, 28, 1939.
97. Cambiaggi: Boll. Ocul., *32*, 271, 1953.
98. Robertson and Yudkin: J. Phys., *103*, 1, 1944.
99. Wohl and Feldman: Endocrinology, *24*, 389, 1939.
100. Pillat: Zeitschr. f. Augenheilk., *80*, 189, 1933.
101. Johnson: Arch. Ophth., *29*, 793, 1943.
102. Dhanda: Arch. Ophth., *54*, 841, 1955.
103. Harris and Abassy: Lancet, *2*, 1299, 1355, 1939.
104. Robertson and Yudkin: Brit. J. Ophth., *28*, 556, 1944.
105. Euler and Adler: Zentralbl. Phys. Chem., *228*, 1, 1934.
106. Kimble and Gordon: J. Biol. Chem., *28*, Proc. 2, 1939.
107. Pock-Steen: Geneesk. Tijdschr. voor Nederl. Indie, *79*, 1986, 1939.
108. Boulanger and Swyngedauw: Bull. Ac. Méd. Paris, *126*, 394, 1942.
109. Pollak: Brit. J. Ophth., *29*, 288, 1945.
110. Illing and Gray: J. Endocrinol., 7, 242, 1951.
111. Alajmo: G. Ital. Oftalmol., *4*, 195, 1951.
112. Tislowitz: Klin. Wochenschr., *1*, 226, 1937.
113. Kempner: Ophth. Ibero-Amer., *13*, 41, 1951.
114. Heaton, J. M., *et al.*: Lancet, *2*, 286, 1958.
115. Rehak, S., *et al.*: Ophthalmologica, *135*, 951, 1958.
116. Carrol, F. D.: Arch. Ophth., *76*, 406, 1966.
117. Barletta: Rass. Ital. Ott., *1*, 210, 1932.
118. Marchesini and Papagno: Ann. Ott., *63*, 81, 1935.
119. Hughes, *et al.*: J. Nutrition, *2*, 183, 1929.
120. Novaes: Hora Medica, *11*, 84, 1939.
121. Moore, *et al.*: J. Nutrition, *9*, 533, 1935.
122. Mellanby: Edinburgh Med. J., *40*, 197, 1933.
123. Moore: J. Nutrition, *17*, 443, 1939.
124. Mellanby: Brain, *54*, 247, 1931.
125. Lee and Sure: Arch. Pathol., *24*, 430, 1937.
126. Imachi and Takamasa: Act. Soc. Ophth. Japan, *42*, 1024, 1938.
126*a*.Gardiner, P. A., *et al.*: Clin. Sci., *16*, 435, 1957.
126*b*.Gardiner, P. A.: Lancet, *1*, 1152, 1958.
127. Wortis, *et al.*: Arch. Neurol. & Psychiat., *47*, 215, 1942.
128. Jolliffe: *Vitamin B₁₂*, Chicago, Univ. of Chicago Press, p. 43, 1942.
129. Jolliffe, *et al.*: J. Neurol. & Ment. Dis., *93*, 218, 1941.
130. Barrie: Lancet, *253*, 278, 1947.
131. Wardener and Lennox Lancet, *252*, 11, 1947.

Chapter

39

Inborn Errors of Metabolism *

Paul Wing-Kon Wong

AND

David Yi-Yung Hsia†

In the Croonian Lectures delivered at the Royal Society of Physicians in 1908, Garrod[1] suggested that four metabolic disorders—albinism, alkaptonuria, cystinuria, and pentosuria—had certain features in common. First, in all four conditions, the onset of the particular abnormality could be dated from the first days or weeks of life, especially when a special effort was made to do so. A second characteristic was their familial occurrence in a considerable number of cases. A third feature was that the conditions were relatively benign and compatible with a normal life-expectancy. A fourth feature, noted by other clinicians in Garrod's day, was the frequency with which these disorders occurred among the offspring of consanguineous marriages.

Up to the present, some 270 "inborn errors of metabolism"[2] have been described in man. Of these, some conditions can be treated either by eliminating certain substances from the diet or adding certain nutrients to the diet as shown in Table 39–1. The diseases which can be influenced by diet will be discussed in terms of disturbances in the metabolism of amino acids, carbohydrates, lipids, renal transport, and muscle.

DISTURBANCES IN AMINO ACID METABOLISM[3]

Phenylketonuria (PKU). This is a hereditary metabolic disease characterized

by mental deficiency and the presence of phenylpyruvic acid in the urine.[4] The condition is transmitted by an autosomal recessive gene. The heterozygous carriers have a delayed clearance of plasma phenylalanine during oral tolerance tests. The condition is caused by a deficiency of phenylalanine hydroxylase in the liver, resulting in an excessive accumulation of phenylalanine in the plasma (Fig. 39–1). Phenylketonuria is

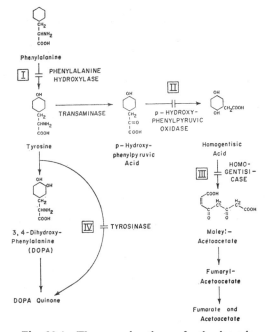

Fig. 39-1. The normal pathways for the degradation of phenylalanine and tyrosine in man. The known metabolic defects are: I. phenylketonuria, II. tyrosinemia, III. alkaptonuria, IV. albinism.

* These studies were aided by grants from the U.S. Public Health Service and the Illinois Mental Health Fund.

† Deceased, January 27th, 1972.

Table 39-1. Inborn Errors of Metabolism which can be Treated by Diet

Elimination from Diet	Addition to Diet
Disturbances in amino acid metabolism	
1. Phenylketonuria	14. Cystathioninuria
2. Tyrosinemia	15. Pyridoxine dependency
3. Maple syrup urine disease	16. Pyridoxine deficiency
4. Hypervalinemia	17. Hydroxykynureninuria
5. Propionicacidemia	
6. Methylmalonicacidemia	
7. Carbamylphosphate synthetase deficiency	
8. Ornithine transcarbamylase deficiency	
9. Citrullinemia	
10. Argininosuccinicaciduria	
11. Arginase deficiency	
12. Lysine intolerance	
13. Homocystinuria	
Disturbances of carbohydrate metabolism	
1. Hereditary fructose intolerance	5. von Gierke's disease
2. Galactosemia	6. Deficiency of glycogen synthetase
3. Disturbances of intestinal enzymes	
4. Glucose-galactose malabsorption	
Disturbances in lipid metabolism	
1. Disturbances of lipoprotein metabolism	
2. Cystic fibrosis of the pancreas	
Disturbances in renal transport mechanisms	
1. Nephrogenic diabetes insipidus	
2. Vitamin D resistant rickets	
3. Cystinuria	
4. Hartnup disease	
Disturbances in muscle metabolism	
1. Familial periodic paralysis	

usually detected during the newborn period by blood screening tests using either the Guthrie bacterial inhibition test or the McCaman-Robbins fluorimetric technique for determining excessive phenylalanine levels.

Elevations of serum phenylalanine can be effectively controlled by reducing the content of this amino acid in the diet (Fig. 39–2). Complete elimination is not indicated, since phenylalanine is an essential amino acid and sufficient amounts must be supplied to insure normal physical growth. Natural protein contains about 5 per cent of this compound, so an artificial replacement for dietary protein is necessary. The most commonly used preparation is Lofenalac (Mead Johnson) made from hydrolyzed casein supplying dietary nitrogen as amino acids. It contains only between 0.06 to 0.1 per cent phenylalanine and is supplemented with tyrosine which is an essential amino acid for these patients. Lofenalac is fortified with vitamins, iron and other minerals and, in normal dilution, supplies 20 calories per ounce. While the taste is rather unpalatable, we have had no trouble in persuading any child under 3 years of age to take it, although problems in this area have been reported. The most common problem is diarrhea which appears promptly after the first few feedings.

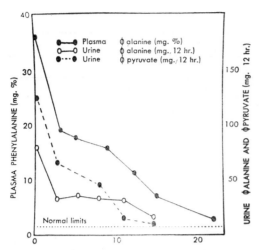

Fig. 39-2. Reduction of plasma phenylalanine levels after administration of low-phenylalanine diet in patient with phenylketonuria. The reduction in urine phenylpyruvate and urine phenylalanine excretion also parallels that of the plasma phenylalanine. (Hsia, Postgrad. Med., 22, 209, 1957.)

This rarely causes difficulty and disappears after a few days. In addition to the basic formula, these children are allowed limited quantities of normal foodstuffs, mainly those low in protein. Most fruits, vegetables and cereals can be introduced at the usual age.

The first step in management is education of the parents. Unless they understand the principles underlying treatment of PKU, medical efforts are doomed. While it is impossible to give a course on biochemistry and nutrition to parents without any such background, immediately following diagnosis, it is most important to start their indoctrination in a simple fashion as soon as possible. Institution of the diet is best performed on an outpatient basis. There is no advantage in admitting a PKU infant except further disruption of the parents' feelings. Any mother can make up Lofenalac and most feel immediately better once they discover this and observe that the infant takes it without protest. The formula may be offered ad lib, the aim being to produce a satisfied infant with good weight gain and a serum phenylalanine level between 2 and 5 mg per cent. However, the phenylalanine content of the 20 to 24 ounces the average 7-pound infant consumes is unlikely to be adequate for the demands of this active growth phase. Serum phenylalanine levels must be checked at weekly intervals during the first 3 months, and should the level be persistently below 2 mg per cent, or the weight gain unsatisfactory, addition of small amount of evaporated or cow's milk may be indicated to increase the phenylalanine intake. Solid foods may be introduced at the usual age, or for the normal indications as in an unaffected child. From the age of 3 months, blood levels should be checked bimonthly until 6 months, and monthly thereafter. During this period, the disease and its treatment will become familiar to the family and the parents more confident in coping with it. A useful concept where solids are concerned is the equivalent, *i.e.*, an amount of a certain food containing 15 mg of phenylalanine, *e.g.* 16 tablespoons of applesauce contain 15 mg of phenylalanine or 1 equivalent, 1 medium baked potato contains 120 mg of phenylalanine or 8 equivalents. Using a dietary prescription based on the amount of phenylalanine a specific child requires and a list of suitable foods, a mother can develop some variety for her child. In addition, the Lofenalac powder can be used to make puddings and cookies that are perhaps more palatable to him as he gets older, and a special low-protein flour from which a loaf of bread containing 45 mg of phenylalanine (3 equivalents) may be made is available. In treating a child or infant who has already been on a regular diet, milk is replaced by Lofenalac and the dietary prescription based on 25 mg of phenylalanine per kg may be used as a base line for allowances of solid food. Serial blood tests and weight records will indicate whether or not this amount is adequate.

In spite of a theoretically correct dietary prescription, high serum phenylalanine levels are not at all uncommon, and may be due to any one of the following causes:

A. *Excessive Intake.* Many children whose control has been excellent during the first year, start running much higher phenylalanine levels as soon as they become mobile and are able to help themselves to forbidden food. They become expert at this, even going so far as to eat from the garbage can. They are not motivated primarily by hunger, but by the frustrations of a limited diet, especially when there are other normal children in the family. Less frequently, excessive intake is due to other relatives, siblings, and neighbors feeding the child. An educated environment and extreme care on the part of the parents are the only way of managing this problem.

B. *Febrile Illnesses.* Febrile illnesses place additional stress on these individuals and increased tissue catabolism causes the phenylalanine to rise. The dietary intake should be increased during these episodes and careful follow-up is necessary to re-establish good control.

C. *Phenylalanine Deficiency.* The deficiency presents initially with persistently low (below 2 mg per cent) phenylalanine levels associated with anorexia and lethargy. This is succeeded by a rise to between 10 and 15 mg per cent in association with weight loss. This in turn leads to persistent levels below 1 mg per cent and severe illness with acidosis, hypoglycemia, extensive skin rash, microcytic anemia, and overwhelming infection may follow. This situation again can be prevented and treated by increasing the dietary phenylalanine, even placing the child on a normal diet when adequate monitoring is possible. Since a large deficit may be present, several days, or even weeks, may be necessary before

significant elevations are again recorded even with a normal intake of phenylalanine.

As yet, there is no agreement about the length of time the diet should be continued. Suggestions have varied from dietary control for the first 2 years of life only, for the first 5 years, and for the first 15 years. So far there is no evidence that regression occurs following cessation of good control regardless of the age. However, one cannot say that further improvement might not have occurred had restrictions been continued. Since the brain achieves 90 per cent of its adult size by approximately 5 years and 95 per cent by 10 years, either of these dates merits consideration. We have discontinued the diet in several of our patients over the age of 5 years, in whom a stable I.Q. existed before this time, and in whom control was not considered satisfactory. As far as family, school and formal psychologic reporting are concerned, no marked change has been noted in these children during follow-up periods of up to 4 years.

In infants diagnosed before 2 months of age, the low phenylalanine diet appears to result in normal or near normal intelligence.[5] In those diagnosed between 2 months and 3 years of age, a progressively lower expectation of intellectual development can be anticipated

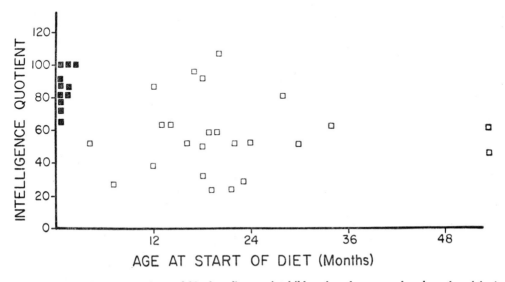

Fig. 39-3. Intelligence quotients of 32 phenylketonuric children based on age when low phenylalanine diet was started. The patients in GROUP I (started on diet prior to 2 months) are represented by closed squares, those in GROUP II (started on diet after 2 months) by open squares.[5]

(Fig. 39–3). A PKU child who, at 2 years of age, does not walk alone, can be expected to start walking soon after institution of good control, but normal intellectual development is most unlikely to occur. In general, any child 3 years of age or under is entitled to a trial on dietary therapy, since the hyperactivity and irritability so characteristic of untreated PKU's is distinctly improved by the diet and better behavior may allow a retarded child to respond to stimuli which otherwise did not penetrate to him before. For children past the age of 3 years in whom behavior problems are severe, again treatment with Lofenalac may be indicated in an effort to maintain the child in a home environment and avoid institutionalization if the parents so wish.

Hyperphenylalanemic Variants. With the nationwide blood-screening of newborn infants for the detection of PKU, some 400 infants with persistent hyperphenylalanemia may be expected each year. Approximately two-thirds of these have the "classical" form of PKU but the remaining one-third do not fit the definitions of the classical phenylketonuria. Although there may be several different variants, there are no definitive clinical features or laboratory tests which can be used to differentiate one subgroup from another. For the purpose of dietary management, these may be considered as a single group.

Patients with hyperphenylalanemic variants are physically and mentally normal.[6] The increased plasma phenylalanine is a manifestation of a partial deficiency of *phenylalanine hydroxylase*. Apparently the residual enzyme activity is sufficient to lower the plasma phenylalanine concentration to a degree so that none of the clinical manifestations and only some of the biochemical abnormalities are present. As a "working rule," patients with persistent plasma phenylalanine levels over 25 mg per cent should be treated as "classical" PKU with dietary therapy. Patients with plasma phenylalanine below 15 mg per cent do not require treatment with low-phenylalanine diet; since long-term follow-up of these untreated children has revealed no signs of physical or mental damage. The patients who have persistent plasma phenylalanine levels between 15 mg per cent and 25 mg per cent may be treated in the same manner as the "classical" PKU. Subsequent decision to continue or abandon the dietary therapy should be reassessed with the following considerations: family history, clinical course, phenylalanine tolerance tests and the ease of management with the diet. However, none of these is a very precise parameter.

Hyperphenylalanemia Associated with Tyrosinemia. While the phenylalanemic variants tend to show normal or decreased plasma tyrosine levels, infants with a physiological delay in the maturation of p-hydroxyphenylpyruvic oxidase system (Fig. 39–1) have increased plasma levels of both phenylalanine and tyrosine. Depending on the protein content in the milk, hyperphenylalanemia associated with tyrosinemia may be observed in 50 per cent of low birth weight infants and 5 per cent of infants with normal birth weight. The syndrome is transient and seldom lasts more than a few weeks.[7] Daily administration of 100 mg of ascorbic acid will generally bring both the tyrosine and phenylalanine levels down to normal.

Maternal Phenylketonuria. All of the offspring of untreated phenylketonuric mothers have a degree of intrauterine growth retardation. All except one of the reported nonphenylketonuric offspring of PKU mothers show mental retardation. Some are found to have various congenital malformations. At least three PKU mothers have been treated with low-phenylalanine diet during pregnancy. They have tolerated the diet well, and their offspring have shown normal physical and mental development.[8]

Tyrosinemia. Different conditions associated with tyrosinemia have been described:

(1). Hereditary tyrosinemia is an autosomal recessive metabolic disorder of tyrosine metabolism, characterized by multiple renal tubular defects and nodular cirrhosis of the liver.[9] Infants with this disorder generally appear to be well until the second or third month of life when they develop liver failure manifested by anorexia, vomiting, diarrhea and abdominal distension. These are followed by hepatomegaly, splenomegaly, ascites and hemorrhagic tendencies. Most of the infants die at an early age. Those who survive continue to show chronic liver disease and may have recurrent episodes of hypoglycemia. Most of the patients develop renal tubular defects characterized by glycosuria, generalized aminoaciduria and phosphaturia with rickets.

Liver enzyme studies show that these patients have a marked decrease of p-hydroxyphenylpyruvic oxidase activity (Fig. 39–1), accounting for the increased tyrosine in the blood and the excessive tyrosyluria. In addition, Gaull *et al.* have presented evidence showing a decrease of both the methionine-activating enzyme and cystathionine synthase (Fig. 39–7) in the livers of their patients. These observations may account for the irregular finding of increased plasma methionine in some of the patients. At the present, the primary defect in this condition is not certain.

Hereditary tyrosinemia may be detected in the newborn period by blood-screening. Because of the high incidence of transient tyrosinemia in low birth weight infants and full-term infants on high protein milk, the diagnosis of hereditary tyrosinemia must be made with caution.[10] It may be confirmed by family history and the persistence of tyrosinemia and tyrosyluria despite ascorbic acid therapy.

Treatment of these patients by restriction of dietary tyrosine and phenylalanine to a degree compatible with normal growth and development is of definite value.[11] Such treatment will prevent the development of liver disease in young infants and may correct the renal tubular dysfunction in older children. Reduction of methionine intake may also have theoretical merit. An artificial formula suitable for young infants may be prepared similar to that described for patients with maple syrup urine disease.

(2). Neonatal tyrosinemia is a physiological and transient deficiency of p-hydroxyphenylpyruvic oxidase. These infants show an elevation of tyrosine in blood and excessive tyrosyluria. However, unlike hereditary tyrosinemia, the biochemical abnormalities in neonatal tyrosinemia disappear within a few days or weeks. The correction of the biochemical abnormalities may be facilitated by adminis-

tering 100 mg of ascorbic acid daily. Dietary restriction of tyrosine and phenylalanine is not required. At the present, there is no convincing evidence that transient neonatal tyrosinemia produces damage in these infants.

(3). Tyrosine transaminase deficiency has been observed in the "soluble" but not in the mitochondrial fractions from the liver of one patient with tyrosinemia. The patient with "tyrosinosis" described by Medes may have a similar biochemical defect.

Maple Syrup Urine Disease (MSUD). In 1954 Menkes *et al.* described a new syndrome characterized by cerebral symptoms and an odor of the urine similar to that of maple syrup. All the affected infants show clinical symptoms in the first few days of life. There is difficulty in feeding, an absence of the Moro reflex, and the development of irregular, jerky respirations. These are followed by signs of spasticity, opisthotonus and coma. There is usually a rapid deterioration and the infants die within a few weeks or months. The condition is transmitted by an autosomal recessive gene. MSUD is caused by a block in the oxidative decarboxylation of the keto-acids of the branched-chain amino acids—valine, leucine and isoleucine—as shown in Figure 39–4. This results in the accumulation of the branched-chain amino acids and the corresponding α-keto-acids — α-ketoisovaleric acid, α-ketoisocaproic acid, α-keto-β-methyl-valeric acid, as well as alloisoleucine.

Maple syrup urine disease can be detected through newborn screening using either a bacterial inhibition assay or paper chromatography for plasma amino acids. The diagnosis can be readily confirmed by showing an excess of the branched-chain amino acids using ion-exchange chromatography or showing an excess of the corresponding α-keto-acids using gas-liquid chromatography. Once the diagnosis is made or suspected, dietary treatment must be immediately started to prevent death or permanent neurological damage.

Treatment should be initiated with an artificial formula free of valine, leucine and isoleucine.[12] This should produce a reasonably prompt reduction of these branched-

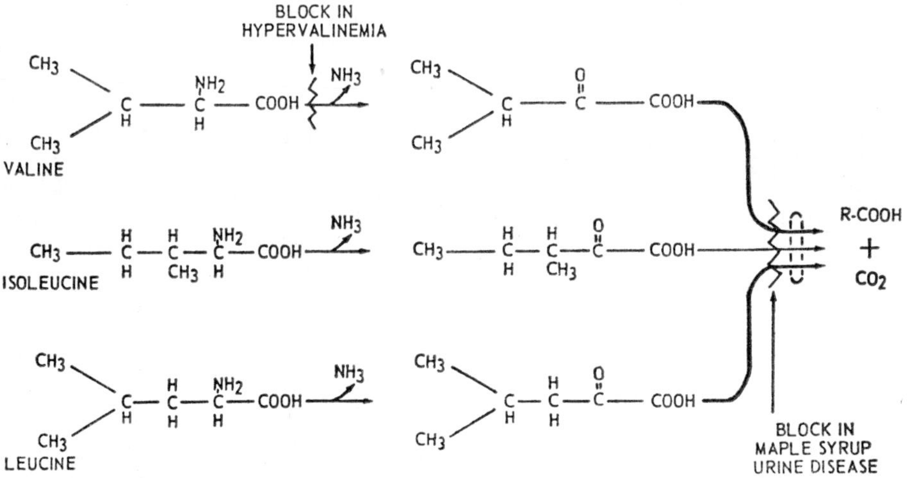

BLOCK IN
HYPERVALINEMIA

VALINE

ISOLEUCINE

LEUCINE

R-COOH
+
CO_2

BLOCK IN
MAPLE SYRUP
URINE DISEASE

Fig. 39-4. Metabolic lesion in hypervalinemia and maple syrup urine disease. (Tada *et al.*: Am. J. Dis. Child., *113*, 64, 1967.)

chain amino acids in the blood and improvement in the clinical symptoms. Initially, plasma amino acids should be closely monitored by repeated quantitative tests every 2 or 3 days. As the branched chain amino acids in the plasma return to normal levels, each of them should be successively added to and its quantity adjusted in the formula to maintain normal levels in the blood. Relatively small changes in the intake of the branched-chain amino acids may produce rather large fluctuations of their concentrations in the plasma. In this respect, maple syrup urine disease is more difficult to control by dietary means than phenylketonuria, as each of the

Table 39-2. Lofenalac Base
(per 100 gm of Z-618)

Protein	None
Carbohydrate	72 gm
Fat	22 gm
Calories	489 kcal
Calcium	750 mg
Potassium	574 mg
Phosphorus	330 mg
Magnesium	68 mg
Zinc	3.6 mg
Copper	0.55 mg
Iodine	58 mg
Manganese	1.8 mg
Choline	80 mg

Table 39-3. Vitamin Premix (Z-619)
(per quart of formula)

Vitamin A, (U.S.P. Units)	2000
Vitamin D, (U.S.P. Units)	400
Vitamin E, (Int. Units)	6.5*
Vitamin C, (mg)	52
Vitamin B$_1$, (mg)	0.6
Vitamin B$_2$, (mg)	1.0
Vitamin B$_6$, (mg)	0.5
Vitamin B$_{12}$, (mcg)	2.5
Niacin, (mg)	8
Folic acid, (mcg)	50
Pantothenic acid, (mg)	30
Vitamin K, (mcg)	100
Inositol, (mg)	100
Iron (mg)	13

* Amount in Premix. Additional vitamin E is supplied by other ingredients in the product (corn oil).

branched-chain amino acids has to be individually adjusted and the patients are more sensitive to smaller changes in dietary intake.

A complete formula[13] consisting of 20 calories per ounce can be made by mixing 800 gm of Z-618 (Table 39-2), 1.9 gm of Z-619 (Table 39-3), 4 gm of sodium chloride, 151 gm of amino acid mixture (Table 39-4) and 7 liters of water. In practice, a smaller equivalent amount of thoroughly mixed

Table 39-4. Amino Acid Mixture (gm)*

L-alanine	5.3
L-arginine	9.2
L-aspartic acid	17.6
L-cystine	4.3
L-glutamic acid	35.1
L-glycine	4.1
L-histidine	3.5
L-lysine HCl	14.2
L-methionine	3.4
L-phenylalanine	9.8
L-proline	12.2
L-serine	10.7
L-threonine	9.2
L-tyrosine	9.2
L-tryptophan	3.4

* (From Holt and Snyderman;[14] courtesy of J.A.M.A.)

powder is added to water for the daily requirement of the infant. Variable amounts of valine, leucine and isoleucine are added to the formula according to the requirement of essential amino acids in infancy established by Holt and Snyderman[14] (Table 39–5). Further adjustment of the intake of the individual branched chain amino acid is necessary according to serial determinations of plasma amino acids. These infants will thrive better when small quantities of cow's milk are given daily. Criteria used to assess the adequacy of therapy include weight gain, hemoglobin, serum protein—particularly albumin—neurological and developmental evaluation.

As the infant becomes older, the approach suggested by Westall[15] may be used. Gelatin is used as a significant source of protein since it contains relatively low quantities of the branched chain amino acids. A mixture of amino acids to compensate for the deficiency of gelatin in a number of other essential amino acids is also required. In addition, sucrose, glucose, low protein fruits, vegetables and products made from gluten-free flour are used to provide more variety in the diet.

Education of the parents on the nature of the disease, the early signs and symptoms and prompt medical attention during intercurrent illnesses are essential for the successful management of these patients.

Intermittent Branched-chain Ketonuria.
A variant of maple syrup urine disease has been described by Dancis.[16] Patients with intermittent branched-chain ketonuria appear normal under usual circumstances. The symptoms and the characteristic odor of the urine are intermittent. The onset may be delayed for months or years until the patients are challenged with large protein loads, surgical stress or infections. There may be a complete lack of neurological damage between the symptomatic episodes, but these attacks may be lethal. Prompt treatment of these patients during the symptomatic periods is essential.

Thiamin-responsive Maple Syrup Urine Disease. Recently, Scriver et al.[17] described a patient with MSUD who had delayed milestones, an abnormal EEG but a benign clinical course. Thiamin hydrochloride (10 mg per day) corrected the abnormal plasma concentrations of the branched-chain amino acids within 48 hours. Thiamin therapy should be tried in all patients with MSUD when their clinical conditions warrant a short period of normal protein intake.

Hypervalinemia. In 1963, Wada et al.[18] described a patient with a metabolic defect in valine metabolism (Figure 39–4). This patient had vomiting shortly after birth, muscular hypotonia, failure to thrive and mental retardation. The excess of valine in the serum and urine unaccompanied by abnormal increase of leucine or isoleucine represents a deficiency of valine transaminase.

Table 39-5. Essential Amino Acid Requirement of Infants (mg/kg/day)

Histidine	16–34
Isoleucine	102–119
Leucine	76–229
Methionine (in presence of cystine)	33–45
Phenylalanine (in presence of tyrosine)	47–90
Threonine	45–87
Tryptophan	15–22
Valine	85–105
Lysine	88–103

(From Holt and Snyderman;[14] courtesy of J.A.M.A.)

A low-valine formula prepared in a manner similar to that for the treatment of maple syrup urine disease may be used.

Propionicacidemia with Hyperglycinemia. Patients with this disorder present with periodic episodes of vomiting, lethargy, dehydration, acidosis and ketosis.[19] They may succumb during these attacks or may survive with developmental retardation. The condition is transmitted as an autosomal recessive trait. It has been demonstrated that the metabolic abnormalities are the consequences of a deficiency of propionyl-CoA carboxylase (Figure 39–5). Life-threatening episodes of ketoacidosis with marked accumulation of propionic acid in the blood and the urine are the hallmark of this disease. Such episodes may be aggravated or precipitated by high protein intake or the administration

of isoleucine, threonine and methionine. Hyperglycinemia and hyperglycinuria are not constant findings. When the disease is suspected, the diagnosis can be confirmed by the presence of large quantities of propionic acid in the blood and the urine and the absence of abnormal quantities of methylmalonic acid using gas-liquid chromatography. Alternatively enzyme studies of white blood cells may serve the same purpose.

Some patients with propionicacidemia have been reported to respond to biotin, the cofactor of propionyl-CoA carboxylase. Biotin, 5 mg twice daily, may correct the biochemical abnormalities.[20] However, whether such treatment will prevent neurological damage is unknown. Other patients do not respond to biotin and have to be treated with dietary means. An artificial formula with low con-

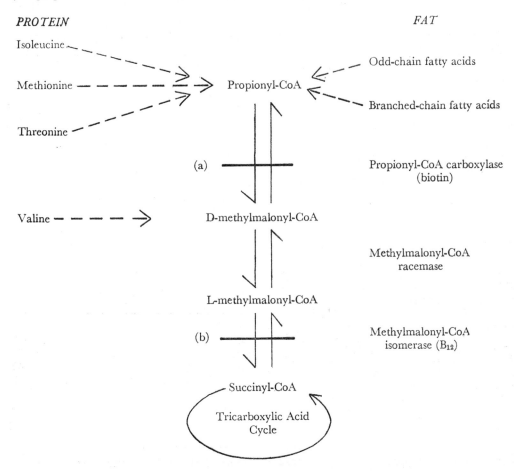

Fig. 39-5. Metabolic defects in (a) propionicacidemia and (b) methylmalonicacidemia.

tents of the "offending" amino acids (similar to that for maple syrup urine disease) may be used. It must be pointed out that restriction of these amino acids alone cannot prevent the accumulation of propionic acid and the appearance of clinical symptoms. Restriction of the total quantities of all amino acids or total protein intake is required. Initially, the equivalent of 0.5 gm of protein per kg per day may be given. Since such severe restriction for prolonged period of time will undoubtedly produce protein malnutrition, total protein intake should be gradually increased according to serial determinations of plasma propionic acid and clinical evaluation. The long-term effect of such treatment remains to be evaluated.

Methylmalonicacidemia with Hyperglycinemia. Clinically, the patients with methylmalonicacidemia[21] cannot be differentiated from those with propionicacidemia. The diagnosis has to be established either with gas-liquid chromatography of the blood and urine or with enzyme studies in white blood cells. In these patients, there is a deficiency of methylmalonyl-CoA isomerase, resulting in accumulation of methylmalonic acid (Figure 39–5). Some of these patients respond to vitamin B_{12} therapy (the co-factor of the deficient enzyme). Daily injection of 1,000 μg of B_{12}, representing some 200 times the requirement in normal individual, results in improvement of the clinical and biochemical abnormalities. Another variant of the disease does not respond to vitamin B_{12} therapy.[22] Treatment of these patients requires the restriction of the offending amino acids—valine, isoleucine, threonine and methionine—as well as the total protein intake similar to that for patients with propionicacidemia. The adequacy of treatment is assessed by periodic determinations of methylmalonic acid, plasma amino acids, hemoglobin, serum albumin, weight gain, and clinical and developmental evaluations.

Urea Cycle Disorders. An inborn error of metabolism has been described in each of the five enzymatic steps of the urea cycle: (1) carbamyl phosphate synthetase deficiency, (2) ornithine transcarbamylase deficiency, (3) citrullinemia (argininosuccinate synthetase deficiency), (4) argininosuccinicaciduria (argininosuccinate lyase deficiency), and (5) lysine intolerance (arginase deficiency). In all these conditions, it seems likely that the common factor of hyperammonemia may be responsible for damage to the developing nervous system. Figure 39–6 shows the Krebs-Henseleit cycle of urea synthesis and associated pathways.

Carbamyl Phosphate Synthetase Deficiency. In 1964, Freeman et al.[23] described an infant with periods of vomiting, lethargy, flaccidity, dehydration and acidosis. There was marked increase of ammonia concentration in the blood and cerebrospinal fluid. Plasma glycine was also elevated. Liver biopsy showed a reduction in hepatic carbamyl phosphate synthetase (Figure 39–6). Low protein diet (1 gm protein per kg of body weight per day) resulted in disappearance of the symptoms and normal development.

Ornithine Transcarbamylase Deficiency. In 1962, Russell et al.[24] described a patient suffering from episodes of vomiting, agitation, lethargy, stupor and coma. These attacks could be precipitated by the administration of a diet high in protein and they were accompanied by marked increase of blood ammonia. There was also hypotonia, failure to thrive and slow mental development.

Liver biopsy showed a decrease of ornithine transcarbamylase (Figure 39–6). A low protein diet (1.5 gm per kg of body weight) was effective in reducing ammonia concentration in the blood and CSF with clinical improvement. However, it was not known if such treatment from the newborn period might prevent the cerebral atrophy observed in these patients.

Citrullinemia. In 1963, McMurray et al.[25] discovered this disease in a mentally retarded child. It was characterized by persistent vomiting, developmental regression, semicoma and convulsions. There was chemical evidence compatible with hepatic dysfunction. Citrulline concentration in the urine, blood, and cerebrospinal fluid was markedly increased. Blood ammonia after meals or after protein loading might be elevated above the normal range. Enzyme studies in liver biopsy and skin fibroblasts demonstrated a deficiency of argininosuccinic acid synthetase. A low protein diet (0.5 to 1 gm per

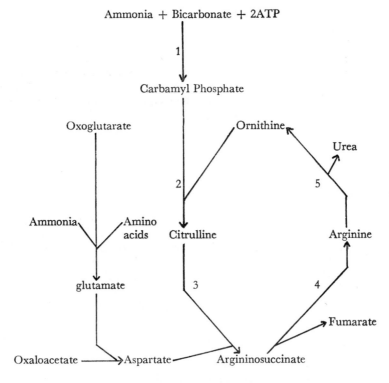

Ammonia + Bicarbonate + 2ATP

Carbamyl Phosphate

Enzymes: 1. Carbamyl phosphate synthetase
          2. Ornithine transcarbamylase
          3. Argininosuccinate synthetase
          4. Argininosuccinate lyase
          5. Arginase

Fig. 39-6. Urea cycle and associated pathways.

pound of body weight) was used for treatment with clinical improvement.[26]

Argininosuccinicaciduria. Patients with this disorder are characterized by mental retardation and the presence of argininosuccinic acid in the urine and blood.[27] Argininosuccinic acid is a intermediate metabolite of the urea cycle, but is not detected in normal urine or blood. Other symptoms and signs include vomiting, ataxia, convulsions, brittle hair (trichorrhexis nodosa) and evidence of liver dysfunction. There is a deficiency of argininosuccinase (or argininosuccinic lyase) in the liver and other tissues. It is generally considered that the abnormalities in this disease are most probably due to ammonia accumulation and that a low protein diet may be of value as an approach to treatment.

Arginase Deficiency. In 1969, Terheggen *et al.*[28] described two siblings with spastic diplegia, epileptic seizures, and severe mental retardation who showed elevated ammonia levels in the blood and the disulfides of cysteine and homocysteine in the urine. Plasma arginine was markedly increased. The activity of arginase in the red cells was very low (Fig. 39–6). Treatment with a low protein diet of 1.5 gm per kg per day resulted in a lowering of blood ammonia.

Lysine Intolerance. In 1964, Colombo and his associates[29] described a 3-month-old infant suffering from episodes of vomiting, seizures and coma. Her blood ammonia concentration was markedly increased during coma and was correlated with the amount of protein intake. On a low protein diet, the patient remained well. There was evidence that lysine degradation was defective, resulting in its accumulation in the blood. Since lysine is a potent inhibitor of arginase, it has been postulated that ammonia detoxication and urea formation are impaired. A low protein diet (1.6 to 1.8 gm per kg per day) or a low lysine diet may be used for treatment.

Homocystinuria. This condition was first described by Carson and her co-workers.[30] Patients with homocystinuria show a consistent picture of mental retardation, ectopia lentis, fine fair hair, malar flush, thromboembolic episodes, scoliosis, long extremities and arachnodactyly. Mudd and his co-workers have demonstrated a deficiency of cystathionine synthase in the liver, resulting in the accumulation of methionine and the appearance of homocystine and the disulfide of cysteine and homocysteine in the blood and urine (Figure 39-7). Formation of cystathionine and cysteine from methionine is lacking. To these patients, cystine is an essential amino acid. The disease is transmitted by an autosomal recessive gene, and the parents of the patients have a reduced hepatic cystathionine synthase activity.

In 1967, Barber and Spaeth[31] demonstrated that administration of large doses of pyridoxine to some patients resulted in the elimination of homocystine, reduction of methionine and restoration of cystine concentrations in the blood towards normal. During pyridoxine therapy, these patients showed improved methionine tolerance after oral methionine loading tests. Liver biopsies performed during pyridoxine therapy showed 3 to 4 per cent cystathionine synthase activity as compared with 1 to 2 per cent enzyme activity without treatment.[32] Pyridoxine may be used in a dosage of 150 to 500 mg per day without dietary restriction. However, whether pyridoxine can prevent all the clinical abnormalities remains to be determined.

Newborn infants with homocystinuria and older patients who do not respond to pyridoxine therapy, should be treated with a diet low in methionine and supplemented with cystine. An artificial formula, similar to that used for the treatment of patients with maple syrup urine disease, may be made by varying the methionine content according to the requirement of the young patients.[33] In older patients soybean products may be used as the main source of protein. Starch, fruit and vegetable of low protein content may be given. However, all food of animal origin must be excluded. In addition, 30 to 300 mg of L-cysteine per kg per day in divided doses must be given.[34] The limited observations available suggest that dietary therapy may prevent the clinical abnormalities.

Since the thromboembolic episodes may occur at any age and in any vital organ, treatment of these patients should be carried on indefinitely from the newborn period.

Cystathioninuria. In 1959, Harris and his co-workers[35] described an elderly imbecile who excreted about 500 mg of cystathionine per day. Subsequently, primary cystathioninuria has been described in a number of normal and healthy people.[36] This leads us to believe that the condition is a benign one. Cystathioninuria is due to a deficiency of

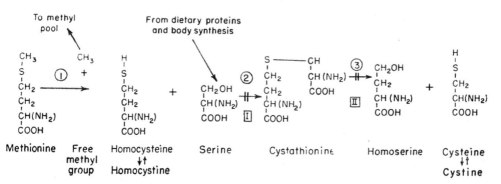

Fig. 39-7. Pathways for the degradation of methionine. The known sites of metabolic defects are I, Homocystinuria, II, Cystathioninuria.

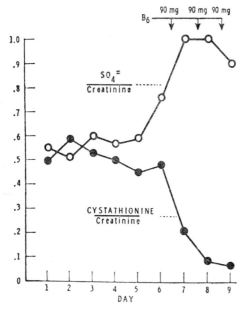

Fig. 39-8. Effect of pyridoxine administration on the urinary excretion of cystathionine in cystathioninuria. (Frimpter, Haymovitz, and Horwith, New Engl. J. Med., *268*, 333, 1963.)

cystathionase in the liver (Figure 39–7). In most patients, the metabolic defect can be corrected by the administration of 100 mg of vitamin B_6 daily (Figure 39–8). However, such treatment is probably not indicated.

Pyridoxine Dependency Syndrome. In 1954, Hunt and his co-workers[37] described a female infant who started to have intractable convulsions within 3 hours after birth. These seizures could be controlled only by the use of large doses of pyridoxine. Since then about 40 cases of this syndrome have been described. In the majority of cases, the seizures begin within the first days of life and consist of severe generalized convulsions, accompanied by hyperirritability and hyperacusis. Ultimately a decrease in growth rate occurs. The electroencephalograms tend to show low-voltage waves and rudimentary biphasic spikes. Microscopic examination of the brain at post mortem in these infants reveals some nonspecific neuronal degeneration, indistinguishable from changes due to hypoxia. The condition is probably transmitted as an autosomal recessive trait. Scriver[38] has presented evidence that pyri-

doxine dependency syndrome represents a true and persistent need for supplementary vitamin B_6 for the control of seizures. It would appear that these patients have some form of pyridoxine dependency not unlike those described for some patients with homocystinuria and cystathioninuria. Presumably, there is a mutation at the locus which codes for an apoenzyme, and the deleterious effect of such a mutation is overcome by increasing the availability of the coenzyme. The apoenzyme responsible for this particular syndrome has not yet been identified although there is some suggestion that glutamate decarboxylase may be responsible. Oral or parenteral administration of 10 to 50 mg of pyridoxine daily can prevent the irritability and convulsions in these patients.

Vitamin B_6 Deficiency Syndrome. During 1952, a peculiar phenomenon occurred among infants characterized by epileptiform convulsions unassociated with any signs of illness and devoid of either physical findings or laboratory data indicative of or suggesting an etiological factor. These infants were normal at birth and were in good health until 8 to 16 weeks of age when suddenly generalized convulsions occurred, usually several times a day. Careful investigations showed that these infants were receiving inadequate amounts of pyridoxine in their milk formula.

Scriver and Hutchinson[39] have made a distinction between patients with pyridoxine "deficiency" and pyridoxine "dependency." In patients with the "deficiency" syndrome, there is a diffuse interference with pyridoxal phosphate availability at reactive apoenzyme sites. The pathways for the metabolism of tryptophan are given in Figure 39–9. These investigators showed that a patient with this syndrome after a tryptophan load excreted a marked excess of xanthurenic acid and little 5-hydroxyindoleacetic acid in the urine. As the vitamin B_6 intake was increased, there was a decline in xanthurenic acid excretion and an increase in 5-hydroxyindoleacetic acid formation. The decarboxylase enzymes were more affected by vitamin B_6 depletion than were the transaminases. The estimated daily requirement for vitamin B_6 in this infant was 2.25 mg, as compared with 0.2 mg in normal infants. In contrast, the "depen-

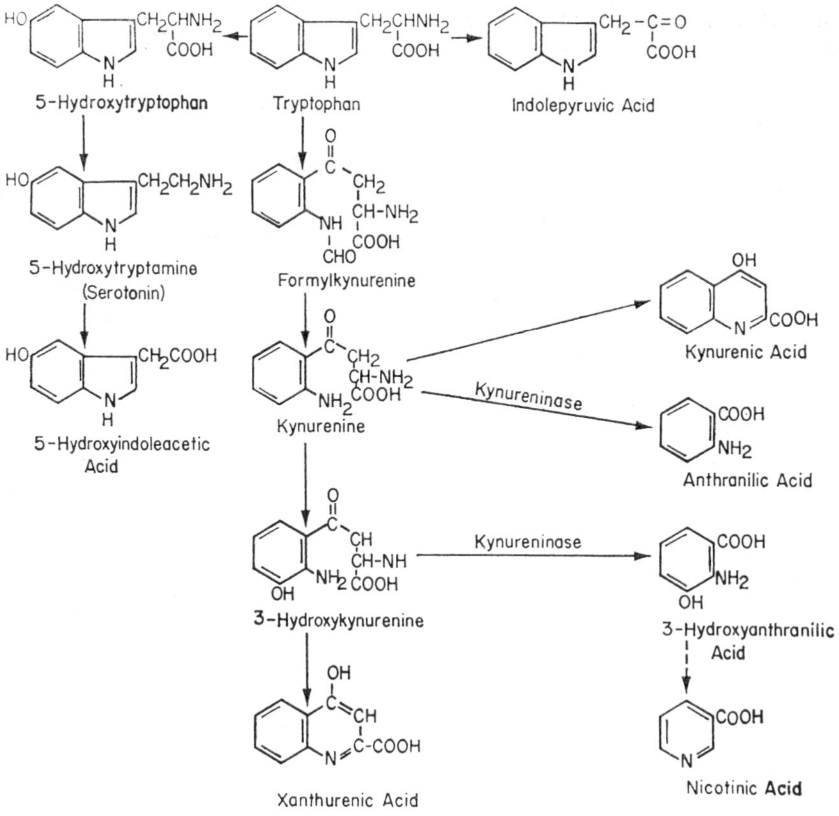

Fig. 39-9. The metabolism of tryptophan.

dency" syndrome involves a true and persistent need for supplementary vitamin B_6 for the control of seizures. Since no systemic biochemical disturbances of pyridoxal phosphate-dependent reactions have been detected, there appears to be a primary abnormality of vitamin B_6 coenzyme synthesis or distribution in the brain, or alternatively, an abnormality of coenzyme binding by a pyridoxal phosphate-dependent system in the brain which exists from birth.

Early treatment of pyridoxine "deficiency" syndrome with 2 to 10 mg of pyridoxine hydrochloride daily will prevent convulsions and the deterioration associated with seizures.

Hydroxykynureninuria. In 1964, Komrower and co-workers[40] described a new syndrome characterized by clinical signs of nicotinic acid deficiency and an excess of kynurenine, 3-hydroxykynurenine, and xanthurenic acid in the urine. The patient with this

defect showed reddening of the buttocks with some desquamation, mild stomatitis, gingivitis, and loose stools at a young age. Although the patient's symptoms improved somewhat with various dietary regimens, she remained short in stature, her I.Q. was 78 at 8 years and she had migraine headaches, which improved with nicotinic acid. She was the only child. Her mother showed an exaggerated response to a tryptophan load and excreted 3 or 4 times more xanthurenic acid than normal controls. Although no direct enzyme assays have been carried out, the patient probably suffered from kynureninase deficiency, which would account for her accumulating large quantities of kynurenine, 3-hydroxykynurenine, and xanthurenic acid, and lack of excessive excretion of anthranilic acid and 3-hydroxyanthranilic acid (Figure 39–9). Komrower and co-workers[40] have found that the administration of 10 mg of niacin daily is helpful in preventing symptoms.

DISTURBANCES OF CARBOHYDRATE METABOLISM

Hereditary Fructose Intolerance. Fructosuria has long been regarded as a benign, asymptomatic condition characterized by impaired fructose metabolism. In 1959, however, Froesch and his co-workers[41] reported a new error of fructose metabolism differing from essential fructosuria in the occurrence of severe intolerance to fructose. Episodes of pallor, sweating, cyanosis, nausea, vomiting, tremor, confusion, coma and convulsion occurred after ingestion of fruit or cane sugar in several members of a Swiss family. Fructose tolerance tests showed a profound hypoglycemia (as low as 8 mg per 100 ml) lasting 5 to 6 hours, accompanied by a sharp rise in blood fructose levels. The fall in blood glucose was accompanied by a steep drop in serum phosphorus levels. This severe hypoglycemia was followed by a slight and transient icterus, albuminuria and aminoaciduria.

The normal rapid conversion of fructose in the liver does not occur in patients with fructose intolerance. Hers has described decreased aldolase activity in liver tissue from these patients. This enzyme is normally more active with fructose-1-6-diphosphate as substrate than with fructose-1-phosphate, but is equally active on both in the presence of substrate saturation. In fructose intolerance, however, aldolase activity with fructose-1-6-diphosphate is reduced to 25 per cent of normal and to 4 per cent of normal with fructose-1-phosphate. This produces an accumulation of the latter compound (step 2, Fig. 39–10), which has been shown to inhibit fructose phosphorylation in normal liver homogenate. Hereditary fructose intolerance is transmitted by an autosomal recessive gene.

Treatment of these patients consists of complete exclusion of fruit and cane sugar from the diet to prevent hypoglycemia. Early diagnosis and treatment are most important in view of the possible cerebral damage which may follow the hypoglycemia.

Galactosemia. During recent years, con-

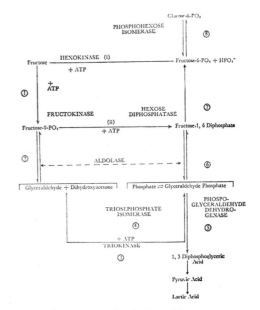

Fig. 39-10. Metabolism of fructose.

siderable knowledge has been gained concerning the degradation of galactose in man. Generally, galactose is ingested as lactose, which is the main carbohydrate component in milk. In the microvilli of the small intestine, the disaccharide is split into its two monosaccharide components—galactose and glucose—and these are absorbed. The studies of Leloir and Kalckar have shown that the pathways of galactose metabolism in mammalian systems involve steps shown in Figure 39–11. A rare type of galactosemia is due to a deficiency of galactokinase. The classical galactosemia and its variants are due to a deficiency of galactose-1-phosphate uridyl transferase.

Galactokinase Deficiency.[42] The first known patient affected with this disorder was reported, in 1933 at the age of 9, as having a rare condition of "galactose intolerance" or "galactose diabetes." Nuclear cataract comprises the only striking feature of the disease. This has been noted as very discrete opacities along the posterior lens sutures early in life. There is no milk intolerance, liver disease, renal dysfunction and mental retardation. It is transmitted as an autosomal recessive trait. The diagnosis of this disease may be confirmed by assaying galactokinase and galactose-1-phosphate uridyl transferase

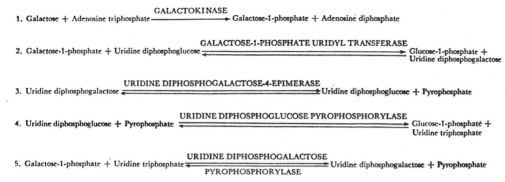

GALACTOKINASE
1. Galactose + Adenosine triphosphate ⟶ Galactose-1-phosphate + Adenosine diphosphate

GALACTOSE-1-PHOSPHATE URIDYL TRANSFERASE
2. Galactose-1-phosphate + Uridine diphosphoglucose ⇌ Glucose-1-phosphate + Uridine diphosphogalactose

URIDINE DIPHOSPHOGALACTOSE-4-EPIMERASE
3. Uridine diphosphogalactose ⇌ Uridine diphosphoglucose + Pyrophosphate

URIDINE DIPHOSPHOGLUCOSE PYROPHOSPHORYLASE
4. Uridine diphosphoglucose + Pyrophosphate ⇌ Glucose-1-phosphate + Uridine triphosphate

URIDINE DIPHOSPHOGALACTOSE
5. Galactose-1-phosphate + Uridine triphosphate ⇌ Uridine diphosphogalactose + Pyrophosphate
PYROPHOSPHORYLASE

Fig. 39-11. Metabolism of galactose.

in the red blood cells. The former is deficient and the latter is normal in these patients. Exclusion of lactose and galactose from the diet will prevent the development of cataracts.

Classical Galactosemia. This is a hereditary condition resulting from a disturbance of galactose metabolism.[43] Infants with this condition usually appear to be normal at birth, but after milk feeding begin to vomit, become lethargic, fail to gain weight and show enlargement of the liver. Proteinuria and aminoaciduria may be found. Prolonged jaundice during the neonatal period is a common finding, and ascites and edema may develop. In severe cases, death occurs owing to malnutrition and wasting in the first few months of life. Those who survive are usually malnourished and dwarfed, with cataracts and mental retardation occurring in some instances. Very early institution of therapy may stop or completely reverse early cataract formation. Not all galactosemic patients present in this way: a few escape the severe infantile illness, leading healthy lives in spite of their metabolic block, and are usually diagnosed during a family survey of a symptomatic case.

In 1956, Schwarz *et al.* showed that an accumulation of galactose-1-phosphate occurs in the red cells of these patients. Since then, this metabolite has been identified in the brain, kidney, liver, lens and heart of galactosemic patients on post-mortem examination. In the same year, Kalckar *et al.* demonstrated that galactose-1-phosphate uridyl transferase is deficient. Subsequently, it

has been shown that this condition is transmitted as an autosomal recessive trait.

Treatment of patients with classical galactosemia consists of rigid exclusion of lactose and galactose from the diet. The design of the diet free from lactose in the very young infant is not easy. Holzel *et al.*[44] recommended a formula based on Moll and Stransky's diet for intestinal disorders:

RECIPE. (Moll's pudding)
6 oz. lactose-free cereal (*e.g.* baby rice)
14 oz. water
2 eggs, separated
3 oz. glucose
Pinch of salt, sodium bicarbonate
Vegetable margarine
Mix cereal with water. Beat yolks and sugar together. Beat egg whites with salt and sodium bicarbonate until stiff. Mix all these ingredients together and place in top part of double boiler that has been greased with margarine. Boil for 20 to 30 minutes.
To make the feed, dilute 1 part of pudding with 4 parts of boiled water or weak tea, mix and strain before giving to the baby.
The concentration of the pudding may be increased with age of the infant, as may the amount of margarine. The latter may rise to 1 ounce before mixed feeding is introduced and should be added to the pudding before cooking. One ounce of the pudding contains approximately 30 calories.

This provides a high calorie formula for the affected infant, but initially may produce diarrhea. It is wise to start with feedings more dilute than that given above and to increase the concentration gradually. Since the pudding is low in calcium, supplementary calcium chloride or gluconate should be given as well as the usual vitamins. The lactose content of all tablets and medicinal preparations should be checked before prescription, since lactose is often used as a packing agent in their manufacture.

Other workers in America have used proprietary preparations such as Nutramigen and Mull-soy. It is felt that the small amounts of lactose present in these products are not dangerous to the infant. Holzel, however, considers that even such minute quantities may be detrimental to the nervous system and should be avoided. Further, he feels that any food containing substances such as stachyose, found in soybeans and peas, should also be avoided, since it has not been proved unequivocally that these are not hydrolyzed in the intestine to galactose.

As an alternate diet for the galactosemic infant, Meat Base Formula has produced a satisfactory clinical response. It consists of beef heart extract, sucrose, tapioca and additional minerals and vitamins. One ounce of normal dilution contains 22 calories.

As the child becomes older, it is easier to design a balanced diet, and mixed feeding should be introduced as soon as possible. All unprocessed fish and animal products except "brains" and mussels are galactose-free. Fresh fruits and vegetables, except peas, are allowed. Creamed cheese often contains lactose, but cheddar cheeses do not. Caution should be used in the selection of canned preparations since lactose is added to many during production. It is wise to advise the mother to study the manufacturer's label on each product and to avoid those containing lactose. Bread and rolls generally contain milk, but those made from cracked wheat and "Vienna bread" are exceptions.

In infants, as soon as a lactose-free formula is introduced, vomiting and diarrhea promptly subside, and if hepatic damage is not severe, liver histology, size and function return to normal. The result of dietary restriction on the cataracts is less obvious. In our series of 20 patients with cataracts, 13 eventually required surgical excision. Little is known about the effect of a lactose-free diet on the mental defect. The age at which the diet is started does not appear to affect the eventual intelligence quotient level attained, but those patients in whom firm dietary control is practiced have higher intelligence quotient levels than those with poor or no control.

There is no doubt that lactose restriction is invaluable in treatment of the initial stage of the disease when the child is often very ill. It should be continued at least for 3 years while the central nervous system is developing and, since there is evidence that in older children small amounts of lactose may cause symptoms, probably for life. This problem is frequently resolved by the patients themselves, many of whom dislike and avoid foods containing lactose.

Galactosemia Variants. In 1968, Segal and his co-workers[45] discovered a Negro variant with the usual clinical signs of liver disease and failure to thrive during infancy. These patients subsequently developed cataracts. Although their red blood cells are deficient in galactose-1-phosphate uridyl transferase, they can oxidize considerable amounts of intravenously administered ^{14}C galactose to ^{14}C O_2 in expired air. A liver biopsy of a patient with this variant shows some 5 per cent of enzyme activity.

In 1971, Chacko and his co-workers[46] described an Indiana variant in an 18-month-old female who excreted galactose in the urine whenever she drank milk, but was otherwise free of the characteristic symptoms of galactosemia. The red cell galactose-1-phosphate uridyl transferase activities were highly variable, ranging from 0 to 11.0 units (μm UDP consumed/hr/gm Hb). An older sister had died 6 weeks after birth following a stormy clinical course characterized by jaundice, diarrhea, vomiting, hepatomegaly, cataracts and albumin in the urine. Transferase from this patient was demonstrated to be labile. Both the Indiana variant and Negro variant should be treated with galactose-free diet.

The Duarte variant was discovered by Beutler and his co-workers.[47] Transferase activity in the red cells of these patients are below that usually seen in heterzygotes but above that usually seen in homozygotes of classical galactosemia. Individuals with the Duarte variant are free of clinical signs and symptoms and do not require dietary therapy.

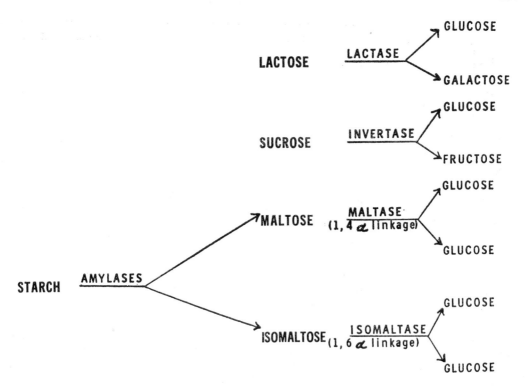

Fig. 39-12. Intestinal disaccharidases.

Intestinal Disturbances of Carbohydrate Metabolism. Recently, several specific human intestinal disaccharidases have been isolated and identified (Fig. 39–12). A deficiency of these sugar-splitting enzymes or the malabsorption of their products has been shown to cause chronic diarrhea and failure to thrive. Four syndromes have been described; the treatable conditions are discussed.

(1) *Hereditary Lactose Malabsorption (hereditary alactasia).* In 1959, Holzel, *et al.*[48] reported on two siblings who had a selective intolerance to lactose. Additional examples of this defect have been observed and it appears that these infants differ from those with more generalized intolerance to other disaccharides.

These patients present with flatulence, colic, and diarrhea in infancy. Although they appear relatively well and have had an adequate quantity of breast milk, they do not gain weight well. Frequently, this condition improves markedly when cereals are introduced with an associated reduction in the lactose intake. In normal individuals, oral lactose loading results in a characteristic increase of glucose and galactose in the blood. In these patients, after lactose loading, the normal increase of glucose and galactose in blood is absent. However, a normal increase of glucose and galactose is observed when these sugars are administered simultaneously. There is a marked reduction of lactase activity in the morphologically normal intestinal mucosa. These observations indicate that the breakdown of lactose is impaired but the absorption of its products is normal. This condition is probably transmitted as an autosomal recessive trait. Infants with this defect should avoid lactose in their diet.

(2) *Hereditary Disaccharide Intolerance.* In 1960, Weijers and his co-workers[49] reported on 3 children who showed a clinical picture which was very similar to hereditary lactose malabsorption. However, upon further investigation, they were found to have a flat sucrose tolerance curve but a normal glu-

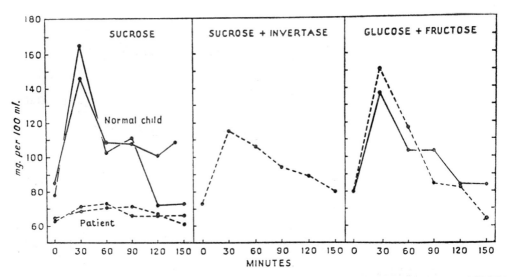

Fig. 39-13. Sucrose tolerance test in a patient with invertase deficiency as compared with a normal child. (Weijers *et al.*,[49] courtesy of Lancet.)

cose and fructose tolerance curve (Fig. 39–13), suggesting that they had a deficiency of intestinal sucrase. Furthermore, the symptoms improved upon supplementation of the diet with sucrase.

Subsequent studies showed that a patient with sucrase deficiency, had a flat maltose tolerance curve which could be corrected by supplemental maltase. Finally, Prader and his associates have described patients with sucrose intolerance who also had diarrhea after the ingestion of starch or dextrin-maltose mixture. These patients were found to have normal amylase activity; but there was virtual absence of sucrase and isomaltase and an 80 per cent decrease of maltase in the morphologically normal intestinal mucosa. Bacterial action on the unabsorbed disaccharides resulted in the formation of organic acid and liquid, frothy acid stools. The condition is transmitted as an autosomal recessive trait. Treatment consists of avoiding the offending carbohydrates. Dramatic improvement after the removal of sucrose and starch from the diet is the rule.

(3) *Glucose-Galactose Malabsorption.* In 1962 Lindquist and Meeuwisse[50] reported a syndrome in which the patients had an impaired absorption of glucose and galactose but not of fructose. The symptoms are essentially the same as in congenital lactase deficiency. Infants with this syndrome develop chronic diarrhea from the first few days of life. In spite of taking normal amounts of milk, they lose weight, become severely dehydrated and sometimes require intravenous fluid therapy. As long as the infants receive lactose, dextrin-maltose and sucrose, the symptoms will persist, but they disappear when fructose is used as the only carbohydrate source. Glucosuria is usually present even when blood sugar is normal. The intestinal mucosa from these patients are normal and contain normal disaccharidases activity. After oral glucose or galactose tolerance tests, blood sugar shows a flat curve. Later on in life, the symptoms are generally milder, consisting of colic and flatulence after ingestion of moderate amount of carbohydrates other than fructose. Infants with this disease should be fed a formula containing fructose as the only carbohydrate. Later on, a diet low in starch and milk may be introduced.

Disorders of Glycogen Metabolism.[51] Of the seven well-defined hereditary disorders of glycogen metabolism, two are amenable to dietary therapy.

(1) *Glycogen Storage Disease of the Liver and Kidneys (Type I, von Gierke's Disease).* In 1928, van Creveld and von Gierke independently reported on a condition characterized by excessive enlargement of the liver and

other organs during infancy owing to the accumulation of glycogen. Initially, the infants appear to be completely well, but may develop anorexia, weight loss, and vomiting, and in the later stages hypoglycemia, convulsions and coma.

These patients have a low resistance to infection, and some retardation of growth and development is a frequent finding. In many instances, death ensues in the first 2 years of life, but some patients may reach adult life and do moderately well.

Since it is essential to differentiate this form of glycogen storage disease from other types, Holt has recommended five criteria that should be met to establish the diagnosis: (1) marked enlargement of the liver; (2) rapid development of hypoglycemia and ketosis when food is withheld; (3) subnormal or absent response of the blood glucose to an injection of epinephrine; (4) glycogen content of the liver representing 12 to 16 per cent

of the wet weight and no marked increase in fat; (5) an abnormal stability of the liver glycogen *in vitro* and after death.

In 1952, Cori and Cori showed that this condition is due to a deficiency of glucose-6-phosphatase (Fig. 39–14). Consequently, the patients are unable to convert liver glycogen to blood sugar after epinephrine or glucagon injection but produce large amounts of lactic acid. Similarly, after intravenous galactose infusion, blood glucose shows a flat curve. Since the synthesis and breakdown of liver glycogen are normal, there is no abnormality in the structure of glycogen. von Gierke's disease is transmitted by an autosomal recessive gene.

The management of this condition should concentrate on maintaining glucose homeostasis and avoiding the secondary consequences of hypoglycemia. In severe cases, frequent feedings every 3 to 4 hours are sometimes required. The diet should be relatively

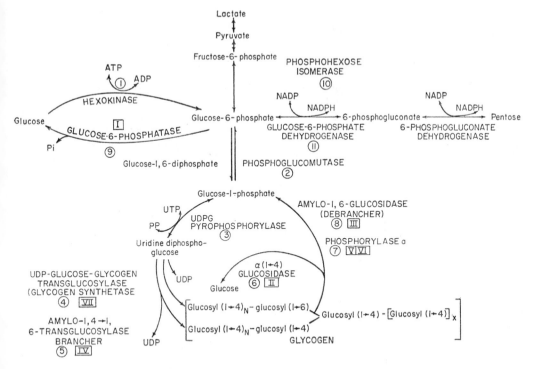

Fig. 39-14. The synthesis and breakdown of glycogen. The known metabolic defects are: I. Glycogen storage disease of the liver and kidneys (von Gierke's disease); II. Glycogen storage disease of the heart (Pompe's disease); III. Debrancher deficiency (limit dextrinosis); IV. Diffuse glycogenosis with hepatic cirrhosis; V. Myophosphorylase deficiency glycogenosis; VI. Hepatophosphorylase deficiency glycogenosis; and VII. Deficiency of glycogen synthetase. (From Hsia.[2])

normal in protein, low in fat, and not excessive in total calories. Obviously, the source of carbohydrate should be glucose or its polymers because both galactose and fructose (*e.g.* from lactose and sucrose, respectively) are converted to glycogen and to lactic acid in the liver. In patients with high blood lactate levels and acidosis, oral sodium bicarbonate should be administered. Glucagon or epinephrine are of no value. The prognosis in glycogen storage disease Type I is variable. The patients may succumb to acidosis, hypoglycemia and intercurrent infections. After infancy, the children seem to do much better, and after adolescence, such patients are seldom bothered by the disease.

(2) *Deficiency of Glycogen Synthetase (Type VII)*. In 1963, Lewis *et al.* described a pair of identical twins who consistently developed profound hypoglycemia after an overnight fast. In these patients, the abnormality was first noted at 8 months of age, when the mother observed that before early morning feeding, one of the twins was sometimes pale and showed transient strabismus. These were corrected rapidly after a feeding. When the child was 9 months of age, one of these episodes developed into a generalized convulsion. Subsequently, the infant was found to have a fasting blood glucose of 7 mg per 100 ml. It was found that the hypoglycemia could be readily prevented in the twins by giving them an additional meal at night.

Liver biopsy revealed that the patient had a reduced glycogen content of 0.45 per cent and enzyme studies revealed undetectable glycogen synthetase activity. More recently Cornblath and his colleagues have demonstrated a deficiency of glycogen synthetase activity in red blood cells.

Dietary control with high protein feedings is effective in the mildly affected patients. When hypoglycemia is persistent and severe, glucocorticoid therapy is indicated.

DISTURBANCES IN LIPID METABOLISM

Disturbances of Lipoprotein Metabolism. These are discussed in detail in Chapter 31.

Cystic Fibrosis of the Pancreas. Cystic fibrosis of the pancreas is a hereditary defect in which the clinical picture of celiac syndrome, resulting from pancreatic exocrine insufficiency, is combined with severe pulmonary disease and disturbances in the secretion of the sweat and salivary glands.[52]

The gastrointestinal symptoms consist of foul-smelling, bulky stools and failure to gain weight despite adequate food intake. The concentration of sodium and chloride in the sweat of these infants is 2 to 4 times that of normal controls. In hot weather, they may suffer from heat prostration due to excessive loss of water and sodium chloride in the sweat.

In addition to the treatment of the pulmonary disease, management of these patients should consist of the following: (1) A high-protein diet with moderate restriction of excessively fatty food is advisable; medium-chain triglycerides may be given in place of ordinary fat. (2) Pancreatic enzymes substitution should be given to improve digestion and absorption of fats and proteins; in our hands, Viokase, Cotazym and pancreatin have proved to be of great value. (3) A high water-soluble multivitamin intake is also recommended. (4) During hot weather, febrile periods, and periods of strenuous physical exertion, when sweating is profuse, the addition of salt to the dietary intake is advisable. (5) N-Acetyl cysteine has recently been shown to reduce the viscosity of tracheobronchial secretions.

DISTURBANCES IN RENAL TRANSPORT MECHANISMS

Nephrogenic Diabetes Insipidus. In nephrogenic diabetes insipidus there is a congenital failure of the renal tubules to reabsorb water, a condition which does not respond to antidiuretic hormone. The disease becomes apparent in early infancy, characterized by failure of the infant to thrive and develop normally. Polyuria may not be so noticeable as in an older child, although the mother may remember, in retrospect, that the baby's diapers always seem to be wet. Thirst, too, is not an easily recognizable symptom in young infant, although water, if offered between feedings, may be taken avidly. There is a continual excretion of large volume of dilute urine, as well as excessive thirst; and if sufficient water is not consumed, the patient will rapidly become dehydrated and feverish. During hot weather, the infant may die from dehydration. Mental and physical retardation has been noted frequently among patients with this disorder. It is transmitted as an X-linked trait.

Although there is no specific treatment for this disease, a diet designed to decrease obligatory water loss by reducing the solute load has proved helpful in infants and children. Initially, dietary protein is restricted to between 1 and 2 gm per kg per day, most of which is supplied in the formula. Similac PM 60/40 powder (Ross Laboratories) provides a high calorie, low protein milk; the content of 100 ml of normal dilution is 7.3 per cent lactose, 3.4 per cent fat, and 1.5 per cent protein, and 0.21 per cent minerals. An alternate formula, designed by Hillman,[53] consists of 7 ounces of whole milk, 2 ounces of 40 per cent cream, and 23 ounces of water. This contains 274 calories with 87 milliosmols of solute in comparison with an isocaloric standard evaporated milk formula, which contains 296 milliosmols of solute. The milk may be supplemented with unlimited amounts of most common cooked or fresh fruits and vegetables. A limited quantity of foods such as white bread (salt-free), puffed wheat, noodles, cauliflower, and orange juice may be given, depending on the daily protein allowance. Meat, eggs, milk and most milk products (except salt-free butter), fish and soups are forbidden. Salt is also restricted, a few grains only being allowed for cooking. Water should be offered ad lib.

It is usually necessary to maintain strict dietary control for about 1 year. Although the low protein content of the diet may result in poor weight gain, this is a small price to pay for the relief of symptoms and avoidance of repeated dehydration. As the child becomes older and more able to satisfy fluid requirement himself, a more liberal diet may be introduced, and eventually the patient will be able to regulate his intake satisfactorily without too much supervision.

In the treatment of severe dehydration, 5 per cent dextrose in water should be avoided since it may increase the existing hyperosmolality. A satisfactory clinical response is produced by 2.5 to 3 per cent dextrose.

Vitamin D-Resistant Rickets (*Familial Hypophosphatemia*). This disorder is characterized by the development of rickets in spite of vitamin D in doses usually considered adequate for prevention. The clinical and radiologic pictures are similar to those of vitamin D-deficiency rickets; the main difference is that tetany never occurs. Biochemically these patients show (1) a low serum phosphorus (usually 2 mg per 100 ml or less in the child), (2) normal serum calcium, and (3) a raised blood level of alkaline phosphatase. Decreased renal tubular reabsorption of inorganic phosphate has been demonstrated, and impaired intestinal absorption of calcium probably occurs also. In the majority of instances, this condition is transmitted as an X-linked dominant.

In children with obvious bone disease, treatment is most urgent to ensure proper growth and minimal deformities. Massive doses of vitamin D (usually as calciferol) are necessary, starting with 25,000 to 50,000 I.U. daily.[54] This is increased by 25,000 I.U. daily at intervals of about 4 weeks, depending on the degree of healing seen on x-ray film and on the rate of fall of the serum alkaline phosphatase level. The eventual dose of vitamin D required may be as high as 150,-000 to 250,000 I.U. daily.

The main problem in treatment is that the therapeutic dose necessary to heal the bone lesions may be close to toxic, and the risk of hypervitaminosis D is great. Usually the dosage is gradually adjusted to maintain the serum inorganic phosphorus above 2.5 mg per 100 ml, the serum calcium no higher than 11.5 mg per 100 ml, and the urinary excretion of calcium below 400 mg per 24 hours. For this, careful biochemical control is necessary. On this regimen adequate growth is obtained but these children are often rather short in adult life.

In adults with symptoms of osteomalacia, the dosage of vitamin D required is the same as in infants, and the same possibility of toxicity exists. Although symptoms may be relieved by treatment, deformities will not be affected.

Cystinuria. The term is used to describe three genetically distinct types of transport disorders of dibasic amino acids, involving the renal tubules and intestinal mucosa. Investigations in patients with cystinuria and renal stones have shown that the abnormality in the urine is not limited to cystine alone but that three other dibasic amino acid are also involved. On the average, a patient with cystinuria will, in the course of the day, excrete 0.73 gm of cystine, 1.8 gm of lysine, 0.83 gm of arginine, and 0.37 gm of ornithine; these amounts persist throughout his life relatively uninfluenced by dietary intake. Cystine stone formation occurs in such patients because it is the least soluble of the amino acids. When the urine volume decreases, particularly at night, this amino acid is likely to come out of solution, and renal calculi may form. Since lysine, arginine, and ornithine are freely soluble, they do not become incorporated in stones.

Although Rosenberg has demonstrated three types of cystinurics biochemically, all the homozygous persons excrete large quantities of cystine and other dibasic amino acids and cannot be differentiated from one another clinically.

Therapy should be directed toward decreasing the formation of cystine stones in the kidneys. This can be done by making the urine alkaline with sodium bicarbonate or lactate. Dent and Senior[55] are of the opinion that alkali therapy is not necessary if adequate diuresis is maintained. They showed that a typical patient excretes cystine at the rate of about 500 μg per minute. When the urine flow is at the rate of 2.0 ml per minute in the day hours, the urine is undersaturated with cystine. However, at night, when the urine flow is reduced to 0.7 ml per minute, the cystine concentration rises to about 700 μg per ml, the urine becomes supersaturated, and cystine crystals form. To avoid this, Dent and Senior recommend drinking two glasses of water at bedtime and two more at 2:00 A.M.

Hartnup Disease. In 1956, Baron and his associates[56] described a disease characterized by "hereditary pellagra-like skin rash with temporary cerebellar ataxis, constant renal aminoaciduria, and other bizarre biochemical features." They named it Hartnup disease, after the surname of the family. The clinical features are quite variable, depending on the patient and the season of the year. Most of the affected individuals have skin lesions, best described as a scaly red rash affecting the exposed areas of the body and identical in appearance with that of classical pellagra. They also develop a severe but fully reversible cerebellar ataxia, which tends to occur when the skin rash is most severe. During these attacks, they walk with an unsteady gait and wide base; nystagmus and double vision are sometimes present. In addition, psychologic disturbances, ranging from emotional instability to delirium with hallucinations, can occur, but there is little evidence to suggest that there is intellectual deterioration with these attacks. The condition is transmitted as an autosomal recessive trait.

In these patients, there is a generalized renal aminoaciduria. Similar defects in the absorption of amino acids are also observed in the small intestine. The most prominent effect of this excessive loss of amino acids is a decreased supply of tryptophan for endogenous formation of nicotinamide (Fig. 39–9), resulting in pellagra-like symptoms. Oral administration of nicotinamide (40 to 200 mg of nicotinamide or nicotinic acid daily) will improve the dermatitis.[57] Avoidance of excessive exposure to sunlight is also helpful.

DISTURBANCES IN MUSCLE METABOLISM

Familial Periodic Paralysis. Familial periodic paralysis is characterized by intermittent attacks of flaccid paralysis of muscles of the extremities and loss of deep tendon reflexes. Three types of this syndrome have been described.

(1) *Familial Hypokalemic Periodic Paralysis.*[58] Patients with this condition suffer from acute attacks of paralysis. These are frequently preceded by a prodromal period when the patients feel tired or irritable, or have a sense of apprehension for several hours before the

attack. In typical cases, paralysis begins peripherally in the legs and progresses centrally until the patient becomes completely helpless and unable to move. The deep reflexes of the involved parts are greatly diminished or absent during these episodes. In some instances, paralysis of the respiratory muscles leads to suffocation and death. Most commonly, the attacks occur during the early morning hours or in the forenoon, then disappear late in the day. An attack can sometimes be induced following strenuous exercise, the ingestion of a high carbohydrate meal, or by the injection of epinephrine.

After a few hours the muscles begin to recover gradually, starting with the central muscles, which are the last to become affected, and followed by the peripheral ones. Some residual stiffness or soreness may persist for a few days after an attack.

The condition is transmitted as an autosomal dominant with complete penetrance. Most of the attacks begin between the ages of 7 and 21 years, with a few occurring in early infancy.

It has been shown that during the development of an attack the potassium moves into the muscle and that during recovery the potassium is released slowly back into the blood stream. Moreover, certain agents that can induce an attack, such as glucose, insulin, deoxycorticosterone acetate and 9-α-fluorohydrocortisone, exert their influence by lowering the serum potassium level. Between attacks the exchangeable body potassium levels are either low normal or low.

Oral administration of 2 to 10 gm of KCl is effective in stopping an acute attack. The episodes can also be prevented by taking frequent low carbohydrate meals and administering KCl at regular intervals.

(2) *Familial Hyperkalemic Periodic Paralysis (Adynamia Episodica Hereditaria)*. In 1956, Gamstorp reported on a series of patients with periodic paralysis who showed normal or increased potassium levels in the serum.[59] In these patients, the attacks of weakness usually start at an earlier age and tend to occur more often by day than by night. They are less widespread, less severe, and shorter than the hypokalemic variety. These attacks can be precipitated by the administration of KCl, induced by hunger and relieved by taking a meal. The condition is transmitted as an autosomal dominant with complete penetrance.

During a clinical attack, there is a rise of serum potassium level without any diminution in the urinary excretion. Striking weakness will sometimes occur with a potassium level of 4.5 mEq per liter or less, and severe paralysis may develop at levels of 7 mEq per liter or less. This is followed by a fall in the serum potassium level during recovery, when potassium returns intracellularly to the muscles. Usually, no treatment is indicated. Intravenous administration of 5 to 20 ml of 10 per cent calcium gluconate appears to shorten the attacks.

(3) *Familial Normokalemic Periodic Paralysis*. In 1961, Poskanzer and Kerr[60] reported on a third form of periodic paralysis characterized by normal potassium levels. The illness starts in the first decade of life and is characterized by episodes of paralysis at intervals of 1 to 3 months, lasting 2 days to 3 weeks. There is often a severe paralysis of all four limbs and weakness in the muscles of mastication, but no involvement of the facial and respiratory muscles. These episodes are provoked by rest after physical exertion; in addition, alcohol intake, cold and dampness, and mental stress will predispose a susceptible person to such an attack. The condition is transmitted as an autosomal dominant.

The plasma potassium is normal during attacks. Administration of KCl brings on, or increases the muscular paralysis. Oral or intravenous NaCl (5 to 10 gm) will stop an attack. The use of 9-α-fluorohydrocortisone and acetazolamide in combination has proved to be effective in preventing symptoms.

BIBLIOGRAPHY

1. Garrod: *Inborn Errors of Metabolism*, London, Henry Frowde, 1909.
2. Hsia: *Inborn Errors of Metabolism*, 2nd ed., Chicago, Year Book Medical Publisher Inc., 1966.
3. Symposium on treatment of amino acid disorders. Chicago, Sept. 3–4, 1966. Hsia, D. Y. Y., editor. Amer. J. Dis. Child., *113*, 1–178, 1967.
4. Fölling: Z. Physiol. Chem., *227*, 69, 1934.
5. Hsia: Pediatrics, *38*, 173, 1966.
6. Berman and Ford: J. Pediatrics, *77*, 764, 1970.

7. Hsia *et al.*: New Eng. J. Med., *267*, 1067, 1962.
8. Arthur and Hulme: Pediatrics, *46*, 235, 1970.
9. Gjessing (ed.): *Symposium on Tyrosinosis.* Oslow: Universitetsforlagets Trykningssentral, 1966.
10. Wong *et al.*: Develop. Med. Child. Neurol., *9*, 551, 1967.
11. Gentz *et al.*: Amer. J. Dis. Child., *113*, 31, 1967.
12. Snyderman: Amer. J. Dis. Child., *113*, 68, 1967.
13. Wong *et al.*: J. Clin. Genet., *3*, 1, 1972.
14. Holt and Snyderman: J.A.M.A., *175*, 100, 1961.
15. Westall: Amer. J. Dis. Child., *113*, 58, 1967.
16. Dancis: *Amino Acid Metabolism and Genetic Variation.* (Nyhan, W. L., Ed.) New York, McGraw-Hill Book Co., 1967.
17. Scriver *et al.*: Lancet, *1*, 310, 1971.
18. Wada *et al.*: Tohoku J. Exp. Med., *81*, 46, 1963.
19. Hsia *et al.*: Lancet, *1*, 757, 1969.
20. Barness *et al.*: Lancet, *2*, 244, 1970.
21. Oberholzer *et al.*: Arch. Dis. Child., *42*, 492, 1967.
22. Hsia *et al.*: Pediatrics, *46*, 497, 1970.
23. Freeman *et al.*: J. Pediat., *65*, 1039, 1964.
24. Russell *et al.*: Lancet, *2*, 699, 1962.
25. McMurray *et al.*: Pediatrics, *32*, 347, 1963.
26. Marrow: Amer. J. Dis. Child., *113*, 157, 1967.
27. Westall: Amer. J. Dis. Child., *113*, 160, 1967.
28. Terheggen *et al.*: Lancet, *2*, 748, 1969.
29. Colombo *et al.*: Lancet, *1*, 1014, 1964.
30. Carson *et al.*: J. Pediatrics, *66*, 565, 1965.
31. Barber and Spaeth: Lancet, *1*, 337, 1967.
32. Mudd *et al.*: J. Clin. Invest., *49*, 1762, 1970.
33. Komrower *et al.*: Arch. Dis. Child., *41*, 666, 1966.
34. Perry: *Inherited Disorders of Sulphur Metabolism* (Carson, N. A. J. and Raine, D. N., editors). Edinburgh, Churchill Livingstone, 1971, page 245.
35. Harris *et al.*: Ann. Human Genet., *23*, 442, 1959.
36. Perry *et al.*: New Eng. J. Med., *278*, 590, 1968.
37. Hunt *et al.*: Pediatrics, *13*, 140, 1954.
38. Scriver: Pediatrics, *26*, 62, 1960.
39. Scriver and Hutchison: Pediatrics, *31*, 240, 1963.
40. Komrower *et al.*: Arch. Dis. Child., *39*, 250, 1964.
41. Froesch *et al.*: Helvet. Paediat. Acta, *14*, 99, 1959.
42. Gitzelmann: Pediat. Res., *1*, 14, 1967.
43. Hsia (editor): *Galactosemia.* Springfield, Charles C Thomas, 1969.
44. Holzel *et al.*: Mod. Prob. Paed., *3*, 359, 1957.
45. Segal and Cuatrecacas: Amer. J. Med., *44*, 340, 1968.
46. Chacko *et al.*: J. Pediat., *78*, 454, 1971.
47. Beutler *et al.*: J. Lab. Clin. Med., *68*, 646, 1966.
48. Holzel *et al.*: Lancet, *1*, 1126, 1959.
49. Weijers *et al.*: Lancet, *2*, 296, 1960.
50. Lindquist and Meeuwise: Acta Paed., *51*, 674, 1962.
51. Field: In *The Metabolic Basis of Inherited Disease* (Stanbury, Wyngaarden & Fredrickson, eds.). New York, McGraw-Hill Book Co., 3rd ed., 1972.
52. Lawson (editor): *Proceedings of the 5th International Cystic Fibrosis Conference* (London: Cystic Fibrosis Research Trust, 1969), pages 1–420.
53. Hillman *et al.*: Pediatrics, *21*, 430, 1958.
54. Dent and Harris: J. Bone and Joint Surg., *38*-B, 204, 1956.
55. Dent and Senior: Brit. J. Urol., *27*, 317, 1955.
56. Baron *et al.*: Lancet, *2*, 421, 1956.
57. Wong *et al.*: Arch. Dis. Child., *42*, 642, 1967.
58. Talbott: Medicine, *20*, 85, 1941.
59. Gamstorp: Acta Paed., *108*, (Suppl.) 1, 1956.
60. Poskanzer and Kerr: Amer. J. Med., *31*, 328, 1961.

Chapter

40

Nutrition and Alcoholism

ROBERT E. OLSON

Chronic alcoholism may be regarded as a psychosomatic disease with both psychologic and physiologic determinants. There are, of course, many controversies about the significant factors of both physiologic and psychologic origin.[1] Nonetheless, this definition of alcoholism serves as a hypothesis for the current study of its etiology and pathogenesis. Present knowledge of its causes may be discussed within the framework of the traditional agent-host-environment triangle of the epidemiologist.

AGENT

The agent of chronic alcoholism is ethyl alcohol. It is, of course, an essential but not sufficient cause. Ethanol which contains 7 calories per gm is a food as well as a drug. The agent is normally present in mammals in trace quantities[2] and hence addiction to alcohol is dose-dependent. The effect of alcohol on the human host is well understood in biologic terms although the biochemical mechanisms responsible for these effects are obscure. Alcohol is a depressant drug and not a stimulant, exerting its toxic action primarily on the central nervous system, although many other organs such as liver and heart are affected. It is estimated that approximately 60,000,000 Americans drink alcohol but only about 5,000,000 can be considered alcoholics.

HOST

The variation in host response to the ingestion of ethanol varies enormously. Some human subjects are very sensitive to the acute action of ethanol and become giddy and unsteady with the intake of less than 1 ounce. Others, by contrast, may ingest several ounces in one dose with much less subjective as well as objective effects. There also appear to be genetic factors that predispose to alcoholism. Cruz-Coke *et al.*[3,4] have presented evidence to suggest that proneness to alcoholism is a sex-linked recessive characteristic. A relatively high percentage of alcoholism in males as opposed to females would support this view particularly if it is accepted that alcoholism is an example of genetic polymorphism. Furthermore, the wide variation of response to ethanol is determined in part by sex and ethnic group.

Knight[5] has classified alcoholics from the psychologic point of view into three general categories: (1) essential; (2) reactive; (3) symptomatic. Essential alcoholics are those in whom the onset of disease is early and without apparent overt reason; reactive alcoholics are those in whom an unusually trying social or emotional upheaval precedes the onset of heavy drinking; and finally, the symptomatic alcoholics are those who take alcohol as a simple narcotic or analgesic to overcome the somatic pain associated with such maladies as tic douloureux or terminal cancer.

ENVIRONMENT

Environment contributes to the pathogenesis of alcoholism in several ways. First, the agent is derived from the environment. Secondly, social and cultural factors favoring drinking versus non-drinking play a role in increasing exposure of the population at risk to alcohol. Finally, malnutrition, infection or drug ingestion may alter susceptibility to alcoholism. A variety of other factors derived from the environment play an important role in this ecologic triad.

ETIOLOGY

It is thus seen that chronic alcoholism is a disease of multiple etiology in which the agent is only one of the causes. Other causes intrinsic to the nutrition, metabolism and genetic endowment of the host and those related to the social environment of the host may be more critical in the pathogenesis of the disease than the agent, notwithstanding the essentiality of ethanol.

NUTRITION AND THE METABOLISM OF ALCOHOL

When ethanol is ingested by the mammal, it distributes in total body water. Ratios of alcohol concentration among blood, body tissues and body secretions may thus be predicted from their water content. In a 70-kg man, 1 highball containing 1.5 ounces of 90 proof whiskey will produce a maximum concentration of 30 mg per cent in the blood. Larger amounts produce proportionately higher levels. Most persons are drunk at blood levels greater than 150 mg per cent (which is the blood level signifying medical-legal evidence of intoxication) and in danger of respiratory arrest at 400 to 500 mg per cent. The linear fall in blood alcohol levels with time is due to the fact that the enzymes responsible for the initial oxidation step (conversion of alcohol to acetaldehyde) represent the limiting step in the removal of alcohol (Fig. 40–1). The principal enzyme oxidizing alcohol is alcohol dehydrogenase, a cytoplasmic NAD-linked dehydrogenase, which appears to be saturated at 2 mM alcohol or about 10 mg per cent. More recently, it has been shown that two other enzyme systems in liver are capable of oxidizing alcohol. One is the catalase system depending upon hydrogen peroxide which converts alcohol to acetaldehyde[6] and the other is a microsomal

ethanol-oxidizing (MEO) system.[7] The relative extent to which these two systems oxidize alcohol to acetaldehyde is not yet certain. Lieber[7] claims that as much as one third of the total alcohol oxidation can be accounted for by the microsomal system which appears to be a typical mixed function oxidase requiring cytochrome P_{450} and NADPH. The microsomal system furthermore appears to be adaptive to alcohol feeding and its activity has been found to be doubled in vitro after feeding alcohol to rats. It is believed that ethanol tolerance in alcoholics may be increased above normal and conceivably this inductive system may account for this adaptation to high alcohol intakes although this assumption is controversial.[8]

The subsequent reactions of acetaldehyde generated by these systems are outlined in Figure 40–1. The pathway involves two enzyme systems in the mammal. The pyruvate dehydrogenase, which converts pyruvate to acetyl coA, will also metabolize acetaldehyde to hydroxyethylthiamin pyrophosphate. The acetaldehyde group is then transferred to lipoic acid to form acetyl lipoate whose acyl group is finally transferred to coA. This system is probably a minor system accounting for the oxidation of about 10 per cent of acetaldehyde but it has been demonstrated[2] in rat liver systems.

The second pathway involves aldehyde dehydrogenase and produces acetic acid. In order to be further metabolized, the acetic acid must be converted to acetyl coA by means of ATP and the specific thiokinase. Free acetic and acetoacetic acids appear in the hepatic venous blood after administration of alcohol.[9,10] It has been shown in rats by Schulman, Zurek and Westerfeld[10] that the specific activities of such acetyl derivatives as fatty acids and cholesterol are 2 to 3 times higher when alcohol 1–[14]C is the source of carbon than when acetate-1-^{14}C is, suggesting that the acetyl coA formed from alcohol does not mix completely with that from acetate. This result is consistent with the conversion of acetaldehyde directly to hydroxyethylthiamin pyrophosphate via the pyruvic oxidase system. Flavine enzymes such as xanthine oxidase also oxidize alde-

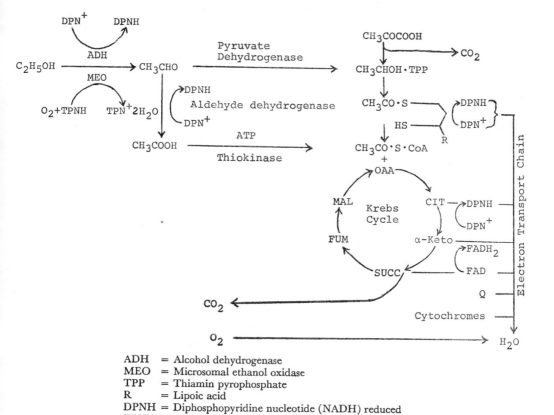

ADH   = Alcohol dehydrogenase
MEO   = Microsomal ethanol oxidase
TPP   = Thiamin pyrophosphate
R   = Lipoic acid
DPNH = Diphosphopyridine nucleotide (NADH) reduced
TPNH = Triphosphopyridine nucleotide (NADPH) reduced

Fig. 40-1. Metabolism of ethanol.

hydes but appear to play a minor role in the metabolism of alcohol.

It is now established that ethanol is a trace normal constituent of mammalian tissues as the result of the reversibility of the two reactions between hydroxyethylthiamin pyrophosphate and ethanol. It has been shown by McManus, Contag and Olson[2] that pyruvate-2-^{14}C is converted to ethanol-1-^{14}C in liver slices *in vitro*. This reaction is increased greatly by anaerobiosis. Although it has been generally believed that, because of the tight binding of acetaldehyde to the pyruvic oxidase, the fermentation of glucose to ethanol is nil in the mammal, it is now established that the rate of this fermentation is low but not zero. It results in the formation and catabolism of between 1 and 10 gm of alcohol per day in the human being. Endogenous ethanol has been identified in the breath of abstainers by gas phase chromatog-raphy[11,12] in concentrations which suggest that the steady state concentration in the blood is between 0.01 and 0.23 mg per cent.

From the involvement of vitamin-containing coenzymes in the oxidation of the alcohol, it follows that vitamin deficiency could impair the rate of alcohol oxidation and thus increase the retention of alcohol in the blood of malnourished chronic alcoholic subjects. Actually, there is little evidence for this assumption either in animals or in man. Since the rate of alcohol oxidation is limited by the amount of alcohol dehydrogenase present and tends to be slow normally, the effect of vitamin deficiency upon the alcohol oxidation rate has not been spectacular. Berg, Stotz, and Westerfeld[13] showed that the rate of alcohol metabolism was not decreased in thiamin-deficient dogs, even though blood pyruvate was found to be elevated. Vitale *et al.*[14] also reported that thiamin deficiency in rats had no effect upon alcohol-1-^{14}C oxidation rates as measured by the rate of decline in blood alcohol and the rate of appearance of [14]CO$_2$. They did observe, however, that the simultaneous administration of pyruvate or acetate reduced the rate of appearance of [14]CO$_2$, and the rate of alcohol disappearance in normal but not thiamin-deficient animals. These data further support the reversibility of the reaction between hydroxyethylthiamin pyrophosphate and alcohol, suggesting that, when the pyruvic oxidase system is loaded with pyruvate as a preferred substrate, the rate of uptake of acetaldehyde is reduced, with secondary inhibition of alcohol dehydrogenase.

The substitution of alcohol isocalorically for carbohydrate in the diet of animals on thiamin-deficient diets may delay the onset of clinical disease. This was observed by Lowry, Sebrell, Daft, and Ashburn[15] in rats, and by Westerfeld and Doisy[16] in pigeons. This effect may be due to the sparing of the thiamin requirement by ethanol via the aldehyde-dehydrogenase shunt. Butler and Sarett[17] found in human subjects that such replacement of carbohydrate by alcohol increased the urinary excretion of thiamin and N-methyl nicotinamide. They interpreted this result to indicate that less vitamin has been utilized in a metabolic process and more was available for excretion.

It would appear, however, that the nutritional effects upon alcohol metabolism are relatively small because of the highly limiting effect of alcohol dehydrogenase on the over-all oxidation process. Secondly, it would appear that two opposite effects of alcohol upon nutritional status may be discerned. The first is a metabolic sparing action which may delay the onset of symptoms. The second is a diuretic effect promoting vitamin loss which may actually deplete stores. It is difficult to decide whether either of these effects, in the long run, will make a chronic alcoholic more or less susceptible to deficiency disease when subsisting on suboptimal diets.

NUTRITION AND THE ETIOLOGY OF CHRONIC ALCOHOLISM

Although argument exists on the role of somatic factors in the etiology of chronic alcoholism, it seems reasonable to assume that such factors exist. Social scientists have not identified a unique social or interpersonal conflict which is specific for chronic alcoholism.[18] Attempts to define the somatic trait or biochemical profile essential for the development of chronic alcoholism, have not, as yet, been convincing. There have been many suggestions that specific endocrine, biochemical, or nutritional factors, either hereditary or acquired, may play a role in predisposing a given subject to this disease.

The most outspoken exponent for a "genetotrophic view" of chronic alcoholism has been R. J. Williams[19] who has proposed that alcoholics have an unduly high requirement for B-complex vitamins. He recommends, furthermore, that therapeutic doses of B-complex vitamins be given to chronic alcoholics as a means of preventing compulsive drinking. The evidence in support of this hypothesis is very weak although it has called attention to genetic variation in humans and the possibility of a somatic trait for the disease. Williams has produced evidence in experimental animals to provide partial support for this hypothesis.[20] He found that rats placed on diets deficient in one or more B vitamins selected alcohol instead of ordinary drinking water within a short period of time. Rats on diets abundantly supplied with all nutrients did not consume alcohol. Similar results have been obtained by Mardones, Segovia, and Onfray[21] and by Brady and Westerfeld.[22]

Trulson, Fleming and Stare[23] found no evidence in man to support the view that vitamin therapy reduced addiction to alcohol. There seems little evidence[24] to support the view that vitamin deficiency is a cause for alcoholism or that alcoholics have an unusually high requirement for vitamins. They appear to develop deficiency disease at the usual rates expected from their dietary histories.

Other suggestions have been made regarding the possible role of metabolic error in the predilection of patients to chronic alcoholism. Olson, Gursey, and Vester[25] reported that the conversion of tryptophan to 5-hydroxyindoleacetic acid was reduced in a group of 34 chronic alcoholics who had been repleted nutritionally and were abstinent at the time of the study. The rate of formation of nicotinic acid from tryptophan was in the normal range. Although the idea that serotonin formation was depressed in chronic alcoholics had behavioral implications, it was recognized that this could be an acquired incidental trait.

J. J. Smith[26] has proposed that alcoholics as a group have adrenocortical hypofunction and that a lack of adrenal corticoids provides a physiologic and psychologic basis for a craving for alcohol. This hypothesis has not been generally confirmed and, in fact, it has been observed that many chronic alcoholics may have marked increased plasma 17-hydroxycorticoids and a typical stress reaction after a prolonged drinking bout.[27]

Alcoholics as a group are peptic ulcer-prone and manifest a higher than normal average serum pepsinogen.[28] This appears not to provide a basis for taking alcohol although it is a definitely associated trait. Much further study is needed to clarify the somatic traits for chronic alcoholism.

EFFECTS OF ALCOHOL ON METABOLISM AND NUTRITION

Acute Effects of Ethanol upon Metabolism and Nutritional Status. Because alcohol is a readily oxidized, hydrogen-rich substrate, the administration of ethanol to animals increases the DPNH/DPN in the cytoplasm of liver which has a number of significant effects. First is the reduction of pyruvate to lactate. Lactate levels have been shown to rise considerably higher after ethanol administration than after glucose.[29] Alcohol is a better source of hepatic DPNH than glucose because there is no phosphorylation barrier to the entrance of alcohol hydrogen into the pyridine nucleotide pool. A second consequence of a heightened DPNH/DPN (and TPNH/TPN) ratio in the liver cell is the generation of reduced synthetic products of acetate such as fatty acids and cholesterol. In liver slices incubated with cold ethanol acetate-1-^{14}C, incorporation into fatty acids was increased and oxidation to $^{14}CO_2$ was decreased, consistent with a diversion of carbon from the oxidative to the synthetic pathway. In addition, increased reduction

of dihydroxyacetone phosphate to α-glycerophosphate occurs, which promotes triglyceride synthesis.[30] These changes in lipid metabolism may contribute to the pathogenesis of the fatty liver associated with alcohol intake. Ethanol appears to have an inconsistent effect upon the mobilization of fatty acids from adipose tissue, in some instances increasing, in some instances decreasing, the level of plasma nonesterified fatty acids. It has been shown that hepatotoxins, such as chloroform and carbon tetrachloride, markedly reduce the ability of the liver to secrete lipoproteins. Since ethanol is "hepatotoxic" to subjects with an immediate past history of hepatitis or a drinking bout,[31] it is possible that such effects may also influence lipoprotein release with resulting accumulation of liver fat. This type of fatty liver is not antagonized by choline[32] and does not occur in the absence of the adrenals.[33] The subject of alcoholic fatty liver will be discussed further under chronic effects of ethanol intake.

The rise in blood lactate which occurs when ethanol is given, particularly to fasted persons, causes secondary effects upon renal function. It has been shown by Lieber et al.[34] that the excretion of urate was markedly reduced when the lactate level reaches ca 20 mg per cent. This may account for the classic association of gout and gouty attacks with intake of alcoholic beverages. Galactose tolerance is also markedly diminished by ethanol and this has been shown by Isselbacher and Krane[35] to be due to the inhibitory effect of the increased liver cell DPNH/DPN ratio upon the uridine diphosphate galactose 4-epimerase reaction.

Other acute effects of ethanol have been demonstrated on the metabolism of biogenic amines. A reduction in the formation of serotonin from 5-OH-tryptophan[36] and a similar reduction in monoamine oxidase activity[37] has been demonstrated in mice. These authors also observed that single doses of ethanol stimulated urinary tryptamine excretion and suggested that ethanol might release stores of bound amines as well as inhibit monoamine oxidase activity. A reduced excretion of 5-HIAA in humans given 100 gm of ethanol has been observed by Rosenfeld.[38] He also observed the inhibition of serotonin metabolism in mice given ethanol.

Effects of Chronic Alcohol Intake on Metabolism and Nutritional Status. Although nutritional deficiency disease has traditionally been associated with chronic alcoholism, evidence obtained in this country since the end of World War II suggests that frank deficiency disease in alcoholics is now relatively uncommon in the United States. Whereas 30 pellagrins per 1000 alcoholics were seen in the Cook County Hospital in 1939, in 1942 the figure dropped to 5.8 and in 1944 to zero. At the Boston City Hospital, the prevalence of pellagra was 7.0 per 1000 alcoholics in 1939, whereas in 1944 it dropped to 2.6. The prevalence of cirrhosis per 1000 alcoholics did not change in either hospital over that 5-year period.[39] This marked decline in the rate of pellagra has been attributed to the fortification of bread with vitamins. In a study of 451 alcoholics newly admitted to the Correction House of the City of Chicago in 1948, only 2.2 per cent had clinical evidence of avitaminosis. Of 426 patients admitted to the Alcoholic Research Ward of the University of Pittsburgh at St. Margaret Memorial Hospital from 1954–58, only 2.1 per cent were observed to have frank vitamin deficiency disease. Caloric malnutrition was not relevant to this problem since 30 per cent of the Chicago group were underweight, whereas 25 per cent of the Pittsburgh group were underweight.

In the current American environment, which is probably typical of most of the developed countries, the prevalence of mild malnutrition in chronic alcoholics, detected by biochemical examination of nutrient stores, probably does not exceed 20 per cent, with frank deficiency disease being less than 3 per cent. This improvement in the nutritional status of alcoholics over the past 20 years is no doubt partially due to the fortification of foods with B-complex vitamins, but is also due to the generally better economic status of the population and the availability of foods. It is to be remembered that chronic alcoholics generally are not continuous drinkers. They are intermittent drinkers and, although they eat poorly or not at all when drinking, they may eat adequately during periods of sobriety. Such intermittent feeding and fasting may still provide nutrient stores sufficient to prevent malnutrition during the drinking period. Nonetheless, it is still important for the physician to recognize both subclinical and frank malnutrition and to treat them vigorously when they occur in the chronic alcoholic. Case studies are available to indicate that the deficiency diseases to which alcoholics are most prone are those of protein, water-soluble vitamins, particularly those of the B-complex, thiamin, niacin, riboflavin, pyridoxine, and folic acid, and the minerals magnesium, potassium, and zinc. These will be discussed in the following section.

Protein Deficiency. Chronic alcoholics with a long history of subsistence on diets poor in protein and accompanying large intakes of ethanol develop manifestations of protein deficiency. These include the appearance of fatty liver, hypoalbuminemia, hypocholesterolemia, edema, and normocytic anemia. These manifestations are not so severe as those seen in kwashiorkor, the disease of protein deficiency in infants, because the requirements for essential amino acids and total nitrogen are considerably lower in adults than in children. Nonetheless, the syndromes are related and are discernible, in a small percentage of chronic alcoholics, apart from liver disease. The association of alcoholism with liver disease, from benign fatty liver on through the spectrum of serious disorders to cirrhosis, complicates the interpretation of many of the ordinary signs of protein deficiency in alcoholics. For example, the appearance of fatty liver and the depression of plasma proteins may be a result of deteriorating liver function in a cirrhotic liver, rather than an effect of high ethanol and low protein intake *per se*. The pathogenesis of cirrhosis of liver in alcoholics is still not settled, because many factors, including previous virus hepatitis, may contribute to the final end state of Laennec's cirrhosis. Animal studies suggest that long-standing fatty infiltration of the liver from any cause may lead to elaboration of fibrous tissue, necrosis and regeneration of liver cells and the full histologic picture of cirrhosis. Disability from alcoholism may thus range from elevated titers of serum glutamic oxaloacetic transaminase in otherwise normal persons to hepatic coma as a result of terminal liver failure in jaundiced, edematous, terminal cirrhotics.

The precise biochemical etiology and pathogenesis of fatty liver in the alcoholic are still a matter of dispute. A number of factors exist which may provide an increase in liver fat in alcoholics. The increased hepatic DPNH levels, which result from ingestion of alcohol, increase fatty acid synthesis and may alter the amount of liver fat produced. Starvation may lead to mobilization of nonesterified fatty acids from the depots, which creates an additional load of lipid to be disposed of by the liver. The effect of lipotropic factors in controlling the liver fat content of animals is well known.[40] Harper[41] has summarized his studies of amino acid imbalance in rats and has shown that, when dietary protein is relatively low, the addition of one or more amino acids may either increase or decrease liver fat content. These effects of amino acids upon liver fat are not lipotropic effects in the sense of providing additional choline or choline precursors. The situation in man, however, is far from clear.

Gabuzda[42] has summarized the factors that may play a role in the etiology of fatty liver of alcoholism. He points out that the fatty liver of the alcoholic may result in part from "toxic" properties of ethanol, from accompanying starvation, from the consumption of diets low in protein, or high in calories, in which most calories are derived from nonprotein nonprotective sources, or from pituitary-adrenal discharge because of prolonged stress. All these factors no doubt contribute in given cases. It has become clear, however, that the lipotropic factors which are active in animal experiments in correcting the fatty liver of choline deficiency are not important in humans. The evidence that choline and methionine as sources of "labile methyl groups" are essential nutrients for man is not convincing. When choline is administered to alcoholics on low-protein or protein-free diets, it does not result in the significant mobilization of liver fat. In Figure 40–2, a study of an alcoholic given alcohol and choline on a low-protein diet for 30 days is presented. During the time on this regimen his liver fat,

as determined by biopsy, increased until he was given a diet containing adequate amounts of protein and alcohol was withdrawn. It is not clear, furthermore, that protein deficiency alone is determining for the onset of cirrhosis. There was no difference in the protein intake in a group of chronic alcoholics with cirrhosis studied in our clinic. This suggests that other factors than protein intake play a role although it does not rule out protein deficiency as important.

In contrast to the developed western countries in which alcohol intake bears a significant relationship to diffuse hepatic fibrosis and cirrhosis, the condition is common among adults in tropical countries who, because of poverty or religious scruples, do not drink alcohol. In these countries, cirrhosis is also common in children.[43] Evidence is strong that hepatic fatty infiltration, like that in alcoholics, is dependent upon the habitual consumption of a deficient diet. It affects only the native races who are malnourished and then only the poorer classes of these, particularly after weaning in children, where it takes the form of kwashiorkor. The Gillman brothers[44,45] reported that such cases are not relieved by lipotropic doses of methionine but are ameliorated by liver extract or powdered hog stomach.

Vitamin Deficiency Diseases. The clinical induction of vitamin deficiency disease occurs most rapidly when the calorie/vitamin ratio is high. This form of asymmetric malnutrition is encouraged in alcoholics who may ingest up to 2400 kcal daily from ethanol with little or no intake of vitamins. Since the fat-soluble vitamins are stored somewhat better than the water-soluble ones, the alcoholic is likely to develop biochemical evidence of unsaturation of the water-soluble vitamins, and then clinical manifestations of these deficiency diseases. For some reason, scurvy is found rarely in alcoholics, and when found, it generally reflects an altered food intake for other reasons. Nonetheless, alcoholics tend to be somewhat unsaturated in their ascorbic acid stores as might be expected.[46] The more prevalent deficiency diseases in alcoholics are those of the B-complex, particularly thiamin, riboflavin, niacin, pyridoxine, and folic acid.

Thiamin Deficiency. Thiamin deficiency is the most common vitamin deficiency seen in chronic alcoholics in our country at the present time. Clinical manifestations of thiamin deficiency in alcoholism are variable, depending upon the severity of the deprivation of the vitamin. In all degrees of deficiency, they involve muscle and/or nerve tissue. The most serious form of thiamin deficiency in alcoholics is Wernicke's syndrome. This serious disorder corresponds to complete restriction of thiamin in laboratory

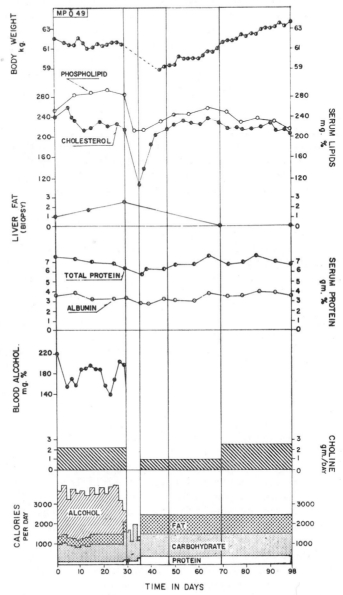

Fig. 40-2. Fatty liver—effect of feeding alcohol plus choline upon fatty liver in man. This clinical course illustrates that, on a regimen containing 25 gm protein and 2 gm choline per day and approximately 2000 calories from alcohol, this 49-year-old subject continued to deposit liver fat, as measured by biopsy. Upon withdrawal of alcohol and increase in dietary protein the liver fat disappeared. There was no appreciable effect of this regimen upon total serum protein or serum albumin concentrations. A period of parenteral therapy followed withdrawal from alcohol.

animals. This syndrome is characterized by opthalmoplegia, 6th nerve palsy, nystagmus, ptosis, ataxia, confusion, and coma, which frequently terminates in death. It may be associated with other manifestations of thiamin deficiency, such as peripheral neuropathy or cardiac failure, but it is a distinct syndrome with a prognosis so grave that it must be quickly recognized and vigorously treated with thiamin and supportive measures, if the patient is to survive. Oftentimes the confusional state persists after treatment of the acute thiamin deficiency. This persistent amnesic confabulatory state is known as Korsakoff's psychosis.[47]

The next most severe form of thiamin deprivation, similar to Oriental beriberi, is seen in alcoholics who have minimal amounts of thiamin in their diet. Alcoholic beriberi is manifested by symmetrical foot drop and wrist drop associated with great tenderness of muscles and a mild disturbance of general sensations over characteristic areas of the outer aspects of the legs, the thighs, and the abdomen. Achilles tendon reflexes first increase and then decrease, followed by severe weakness and paralysis of the muscles of the legs, particularly the peroneal and quadriceps femoris, resulting in difficulty in rising from the squatting postion.[48,49]

This degree of deficiency also affects cardiac muscle metabolism and, particularly under conditions of salt retention or other forms of venous loading, it may result in congestive heart failure, of the high output type. Cardiac catheterization of such patients has revealed no uptake of either pyruvate or lactate by the myocardium, despite elevated values in the blood and a cardiac respiratory quotient of 0.7 consistent with exclusive use of fatty acids as a source of energy. In experimental animals with thiamin deficiency, the oxygen consumption of the heart is limited due to the lack of thiamin pyrophosphate as a coenzyme for α-keto-acid oxidation, and arrest of the Krebs tricarboxycyclic acid cycle occurs at the α-ketoglutarate stage.[50]

The mildest and most common form of thiamin deficiency is the polyneuropathy affecting only the lower extremities of the chronic alcoholic. This disorder is manifested by depressed tendon reflexes, muscle cramps, and weakness, paresthesias, and pains and discomforts in the feet. Foot drop is occasionally seen. This mild form is also the least specific in the sense that other disorders, such as diabetic neuropathy, porphyria, and arsenic poisoning, may mimic these findings. All forms of thiamin deficiency respond to thiamin treatment unless the pathology is irreversible and this is not infrequently found with polyneuropathy.

The biochemical criteria of thiamin deficiency are seen in alcoholics in proportion to the severity of thiamin deprivation. In Wernicke's disease, for example, the blood pyruvate is universally elevated and red blood cell transketolase depressed,[51] whereas in chronic mild polyneuropathy the chemical changes may be minimal. The urinary excretion of thiamin is a good guide to the extent of depletion. Only values less than 30 μg/gm of creatinine indicate serious depletion of vitamin.

Pellagra. Alcoholic pellagra, like endemic pellagra, is the result of a lack of nicotinic acid and/or its precursor tryptophan. Since the incubation period of pellagra is longer than beriberi, and since the likelihood of avoiding both animal protein and fortified bread is very low, pellagra is less prevalent than beriberi in alcoholics these days.

Clinically, alcoholic pellagra does not differ in any appreciable way from endemic pellagra seen prior to 1930 in the southern United States. It is characterized by a bilateral photosensitive dermatitis, stomatitis, gastritis, diarrhea, encephalopathy, and peripheral neuropathy. Lesions may appear on extensor surfaces of both hands and feet despite the lack of overt evidence of exposure to sunlight. Interestingly, in alcoholics the "Casal's necklace" is often absent. The tongue in pellagra is bright red with flattened papillae. The mucous membranes of the mouth and the epithelium of the whole gastrointestinal tract may be involved with characteristic diarrhea in 50 per cent. Alcoholics, of course, manifest changes in the tongue which may reflect general disturbance in gastrointestinal function with lesser degrees of deficiency. The encephalopathy of pellagra may simulate any mental disease although depression and suicidal tendency usually predominate. Disorientation, hallucinosis, and delirium, sometimes difficult to distinguish from *delirium tremens*, may be observed. A fulminating form of pellagrous encephalopathy characterized by progressive stupor, grasping and sucking reflexes, and cogwheel rigidity of the extremities has been described.[52] The peripheral neuropathy features a chronic sensory disturbance with prominent burning paresthesias of the feet. On adequate diets, the excretion of N-methyl-nicotinamide in adult humans varies from 5 to 20 mg per day. In alcoholic pellagrins it falls to values less than 1 mg per day, and this change in excretion of a metabolic end product of pyridine nucleotide metabolism serves as a useful chemical index of nicotinic acid depletion.

Riboflavin Deficiency. Ariboflavinosis due to reduced riboflavin intake may complicate alcoholic pellagra. It is rarely seen as a distinct entity. Many of its manifestations are part of the pellagra syndrome: dermatitis, particularly in the nasolabial and scrotal areas, angular stomatitis and cheilosis. A urinary excretion of less than 50µg per day is required to make a diagnosis of riboflavin deficiency.

Pyridoxine Deficiency. Pyridoxine deficiency has been reported in chronic alcoholism as a cause for withdrawal convulsions ("rum fits") in alcoholics who tend, in the recovery phase, to be unduly sensitive to convulsive stimuli.[53] Pyridoxine deficiency in humans is characterized by a vague syndrome of nervousness, irritability, insomnia, mild ataxia and skin lesions, which imitate those of riboflavin deficiency.[54] In human subjects, given deoxypyridoxine as an antagonist, seborrheic lesions around the eyes, nasolabial folds and intertriginous areas, together with cheilosis, glossitis, and stomatitis, were noted. In pyridoxine-deficient alcoholics the pyridoxic acid drops from an average of about 0.6 mg to less than 0.1 mg per day. Xanthurenic acid excretion is elevated above 25 mg per day. The administration of 100 mg of pyridoxine daily to alcoholics in the acute phase of recovery from a drinking bout has been reported to abolish the incidence of withdrawal convulsions.[55]

Folic Acid Deficiency. It has been discovered that one of the major causes for macrocytic anemia in alcoholic patients is folic acid deficiency.[56] The finding of spontaneous reticulocytosis upon admission of the chronic alcoholic to the hospital has suggested, furthermore, that cessation of alcohol ingestion itself improves hemopoiesis. Recent observations indicate the minimal daily oral requirement for folic acid to be in the range of 50 µg per day, and serum folate values less than 3 mµg/ml may be considered presumptive evidence of deficiency.[57] Sullivan and Herbert[58] have studied the effect of folate supplements with and without added alcohol in folic acid-deficient alcoholics. When normal diets containing about 100 µg of folic acid per day were administered to these anemic alcoholics, a reticulocyte shower occurred in the absence of alcohol, but not in its presence. When larger amounts of folate were given, a reticulocyte response occurred despite continued alcohol ingestion. The marrow did not revert completely from megaloblastic to normoblastic unless alcohol was stopped. These data suggest that, with folate supplies low, alcohol inhibits the utilization of folic acid for marrow DNA synthesis via *de novo* methyl biosynthesis. A case illustrating these phenomena is shown in Figure 40–3. It clearly illustrates in serial manner the effect of 75 µg folic acid per day in stimulating reticulocytosis and of alcohol in suppressing it, with a reciprocal effect on serum iron during reticulocytosis.

Mineral Deficiencies. After prolonged drinking bouts, chronic alcoholics suffer from a number of mineral deficiencies, including sodium, chloride, potassium, magnesium, and zinc. General dehydration accompanies such mineral deficiencies and mild to severe acidosis may also be present, further evidence of a deficit in total body base. In severe cases, the ions of the extracellular phase, sodium and chloride, are usually restored by prompt intravenous therapy, but the deficits of the intracellular compartment may be overlooked. The evidence for these will be discussed in more detail.

Magnesium Deficiency. Flink *et al.*[59] first noted that low serum magnesium levels were associated with *delirium tremens* in alcoholics. The most severe alcoholics averaged 1.29 ±0.27 mEq/L compared to a control group

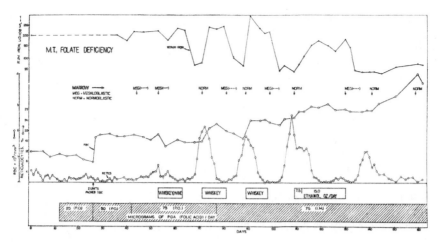

Fig. 40-3. Folic acid deficiency. Response of a chronic alcoholic with folic acid deficiency anemia to administration of folic acid with and without ethyl alcohol. Note the reciprocal relationship with serum iron and reticulocytosis. The condition of the marrow during each response is indicated in the middle of the chart. (From Sullivan and Herbert.[58])

of 1.91 ± 0.20 mEq/L. They suggested that the hypomagnesemia might be etiologically related to the *delirium tremens*, particularly since the tremor responded in most cases to parenteral MgSO₄ therapy.

Heaton *et al.*[60] reported that the incidence of hypomagnesemia in a group of 50 chronic alcoholics was 25 per cent. Johannes Nielsen[61] also found that patients with *delirium tremens* had lower serum magnesium values than other alcoholics, although there was a considerable overlap in the values. They showed, however, that treatment of hypomagnesemia was not essential for the treatment of *delirium tremens*. McCollister *et al.*[62] showed that ethanol promoted magnesium excretion in man, a conclusion confirmed by Heaton.[60] This renal effect, coupled with diets inadequate in magnesium, causes significant magnesium depletion in chronic alcoholics.

Potassium Deficiency. Dietary potassium deficiency exists in most chronic alcoholics when drinking heavily. This, coupled with the obligatory daily loss of K⁺ in the urine, provides ample basis for potassium deficiency in such drinkers. Martin *et al.*[63] observed that 10 of 30 acutely ill chronic alcoholics had reduced serum potassium levels. Practically one-third showed hypernatremia and hyperchloremia. Amatuzio *et al.*[64] have made

similar observations in alcoholics with portal cirrhosis. Depressed electrolyte intake, poor gastrointestinal absorption, and accelerated urinary loss of electrolytes contribute to the loss of these intracellular cations.

Zinc Deficiency. Zinc is associated with a variety of dehydrogenase enzymes including alcohol dehydrogenase. Vallee *et al.*[65,66] have reported decreased plasma zinc content to 60 per cent of normal, coupled with increased urinary zinc excretion, in chronic alcoholics with cirrhosis. The normal zinc excretion was found to be 457 ± 120 μg/day, whereas in chronic alcoholics with cirrhosis the values ranged from 884 to 1396. Sullivan[67] found that the administration of 1000 ml of 5 per cent alcohol to alcoholics and nonalcoholic subjects did not increase the excretion of zinc appreciably. He observed, however, that, whereas his normal subjects excreted 402 ± 150 μg of zinc daily, most of the chronic alcoholics demonstrated increased rates of urinary zinc excretion (295 to 3960 μg/day). Increased zincuria occurred in the group that had no physical evidence of hepatic disease, other than hepatomegaly, and normal liver function tests. The highest zinc excretion rates, however, where found in patients with overt cirrhosis with ascites and variable degrees of jaundice. Excess zincuria, occurring in 5 of the 6 alcoholic patients with mimimal evidence of hepatic disease suggested that increased urinary zinc excretion may occur early in the development of liver cirrhosis, or as a consequence of long-standing alcohol intake. Zinc deficiency in man has been reported in hypogonadic dwarfs in the Near East by Prasad *et al.*[68] Plasma and total body zinc were reduced appreciably in these patients. Although a clear causal relationship between the hypogonadism and the zinc depletion has not yet been established, it is interesting to speculate whether or not the hypogonadism occasionally seen in alcoholics and usually attributed to lack of estrogen inactivation may be related to zinc deficiency.

Cardiac Myopathy. For many years, it has been believed that chronic alcoholism can lead to cardiac failure associated with a cardiomyopathy different from that seen in beriberi and not responsive to thiamin therapy. A recent report[69] further documents this belief. In this series, 39 of 119 patients with chronic alcoholism under 50 years of age referred to a cardiac clinic were found to have evidence of primary myocardial disease after exclusion of arteriosclerotic, hypertensive, and other less common types of non-valvular heart disease. Alcohol was presumed to be related to the etiology. The patients presented a picture of undernutrition, cardiac hypertrophy, right ventricular failure, nonspecific electrocardiographic abnormalities, and gallop rhythm. Eight patients who underwent biopsy showed interstitial myocardial fibrosis usually with myocardial hypertrophy. The disease did not respond to nutritional supplementation but improved after cessation of alcohol intake. Generalized myopathy has also been seen in alcoholism[70] characterized by muscle tenderness, cramping, increased creatine phosphokinase in the blood, diminished ability after ischemic exercise to develop appropriate lactic acid levels. In one case, a woman with tender painful legs after intense drinking bout developed myoglobinuria and elevation of LDH and CPK in her blood. Light and electron microscopy showed evidence of chronic myopathy. It was reasoned that the principal change may be increased membrane permeability.

The evidence is clear that chronic alcohol intake in some patients induces serious forms of cardiac and skeletal myopathy, which respond only to withdrawal of alcohol. In advanced cases, withdrawal of alcohol may not reverse the process. The pathogenesis is obscure.

A very special problem of cardiac myopathy associated with alcohol intake is the toxic myocardiopathy reported by Sullivan *et al.*[71,72] in Omaha; Kesteloot *et al.*[73] in Louvain, Belgium; and Morin *et al.*[74] in Quebec. The syndrome occurred only in those who drank large quantities of beer, and it was characterized by rapid onset of cardiac failure and high mortality. In 28 cases from Omaha, age 25 to 75 years of age, there was no family history of cardiac disease and 11 of the 28 died. The Quebec mortality was 41 per cent of 48 patients. The congestive failure was unresponsive to thiamin, digitalis or diuretics. Gallop rhythm was invariably present as was tachycardia, hypotension, venous distension, edema, pericardial effusion, polycythemia and thromboembolism. Neuropathy was infrequent and arrhythmias were rare. It was discovered in epidemiologic study that the offending agent was a cobalt-containing antidetergent which had been added to improve the foaming properties in beer in all the breweries in areas where the epidemic occurred. Cobalt was suspected because of the high incidence of polycythemia and histologic changes of epithelial hyperplasia and scanty colloid in the thyroid glands in 13 of the Quebec fatalities. The intake from 24 pints of beer was calculated to be 8 mg of cobalt sulfate per day which is a very low dose, since up to 300 mg of cobalt salts have been given therapeutically without cardiotoxic effects in other patients treated for hyperthyroidism.

It is now known that cobalt and nickel ions inhibit excitation-contraction coupling in cardiac muscle competitively with calcium.[75] Since only a few of the subjects exposed to the high cobalt beer developed this form of cardiac failure, it is likely that host factors increasing the competitiveness of cobalt ions with Ca^{++} were operative in those who developed cardiac failure.

NUTRITIONAL THERAPY OF CHRONIC ALCOHOLICS

It is evident from the foregoing that chronic alcoholics by virtue of their use of alcohol as a food as well as a drug are constantly in danger of protein, B-complex vitamin, and mineral malnutrition. Despite the fact that the clinical manifestations of vitamin deficiency disease have nearly disappeared since World War II, the physician treating the chronic alcoholic must be cognizant of the fact that his patient undergoes depletion of these nutrients every day that he drinks without eating. The extent of desaturation in given cases will depend upon the length of the drinking spree, the amount of food taken during the spree (which is uniformly lower than that taken when sober and sometimes nil) and the quality of the diet the patient takes when he is not drinking. Approximately 300 chronic alcoholic males admitted to the Alcoholic Research Ward of the St. Margaret Memorial Hospital at University of Pittsburgh had an average daily intake of 2800 calories, 105 gm protein, 1.6 mg thiamin, 2.1 mg of riboflavin and 17 mg of nicotinic acid when not drinking. During drinking bouts, these same men averaged 850 calories, 35 gm protein, 0.5 mg thiamin, 0.7 mg riboflavin, and 6 mg of nicotinic acid per day.[76]

Although intravenous and oral fluids, tranquilizing drugs, high protein, polymineral and polyvitamin therapy is traditional for the chronic alcoholic hospitalized in the acute withdrawal state, it is important to encourage these patients to seek dietary advice in a clinical setting during the periods of sobriety. Consultation with a nutritionist at regular intervals in an outpatient clinic has proved useful in our hands. In this manner a preventive approach to the inevitable depletion of nutrients during the drinking bout can be planned.

BIBLIOGRAPHY

1. Kruse, editor: *Alcoholism as a Medical Problem*, New York, Paul B. Hoeber Inc., 1956.
2. McManus, Contag and Olson: J. Biol. Chem., *241*, 349, 1966.
3. Cruz-Coke: Lancet, *1*, 1131, 1965.
4. Cruz-Coke and Varela: Lancet, *2*, 1282, 1966.
5. Knight: J. Nerv. and Ment. Dis., *86*, 538, 1937.
6. Warren, Johnson and Ziegler: Biochem. Biophys. Res. Commun., *28*, 78, 1965.
7. Lieber and DeCarli: J. Biol. Chem., *245*, 2505, 1970.
8. Tephly, Tinelli and Watkins: Science, *166*, 627, 1969.
9. Forsander and Raiha: J. Biol. Chem., *235*, 34, 1960.
10. Schulman, Zurek and Westerfeld: In *Alcoholism —Basic Aspects and Treatment*. Edited by H. E. Himwich, pp. 29–37, AAAS—pub. 47, 1957.
11. Lester: Quart. J. Alc. Studies, *22*, 554, 1961.
12. Eriksen and Kulkarni: Science, *141*, 639, 1963.
13. Berg, Stotz and Westerfeld: J. Biol. Chem., *152*, 51, 1944.
14. Vitale, Hegsted, McGrath, Grable and Zamcheck: J. Biol. Chem., *210*, 753, 1953.
15. Lowry, Sebrell, Daft and Ashburn: J. Nutr., *24*, 73, 1942.
16. Westerfeld and Doisy, Jr.: J. Nutr., *30*, 127, 1945.
17. Butler and Sarett: J. Nutr., *35*, 539, 1948.
18. Fleming and Tillotson: New England J. Med., *221*, 741, 1939.
19. Williams: *Nutrition and Alcoholism*, Norman, University of Oklahoma Press, 1951.
20. Williams: Am. J. Clin. Nutr., *1*, 32, 1952.
21. Mardones, Segovia and Onfray: Arch. Bioch., *9*, 401, 1946.
22. Brady and Westerfeld: Quart. J. Alc. Studies, *7*, 499, 1947.
23. Trulson, Fleming and Stare: J.A.M.A:, *155*, 114, 1954.
24. Goodhart: Am. J. Clin. Nutr., *5*, 612, 1957.
25. Olson, Gursey and Vester: New Eng. J. Med., *263*, 1169, 1960.
26. Smith: New York State J. Med., *50*, 1704, 1950.
27. Olson: Unpublished work.
28. Mirsky: Am. J. Digestive Dis., *3*, 285, 1958.
29. Lieber and Davidson: Am. J. Med., *33*, 319, 1962.
30. Nikkila and Ojala: Proc. Soc. Exptl. Biol. and Med., *113*, 814, 1963.
31. Bang, Iversen, Jagt and Madsen: J.A.M.A., *168*, 156, 1958.
32. DiLuzio: Am. J. Physiol., *194*, 453, 1958.
33. Mallov and Bloch: Am. J. Physiol., *184*, 29, 1956.
34. Lieber, Jones, Losowsky and Davidson: J. Clin. Invest., *41*, 1863, 1962.
35. Isselbacher and Krane: J. Biol. Chem., *236*, 2394, 1961.
36. Maynard and Schenker: Int. J. Neuropharmacol., *2*, 303, 1964.
37. ————: Nature, *196*, 575, 1962.
38. Rosenfeld: Proc. Soc. Exptl. Biol. and Med., *103*, 144, 1960.
39. Figueroa, Sargent, Imperiale, Morey, Paynter, Vorhaus and Kark: Am. J. Clin. Nutr., *1*, 179, 1953.
40. Best and Lucas: In *Clinical Nutrition*. Edited by Norman Jolliffe, 2nd ed., New York, Paul B. Hoeber, 1962.

41. Harper: Am. J. Clin. Nutr., *6*, 242, 1958.
42. Gabuzda: Am. J. Clin. Nutr., *6*, 280, 1958.
43. Himsworth: *Lectures on the Liver and its Diseases*, Cambridge, Harvard University Press, 1947.
44. Gillman and Gillman: Arch. Path., *40*, 239, 1945.
45. ———: J.A.M.A., *129*, 12, 1945.
46. Lester, Buccino and Bizzocco: J. Nutr., *70*, 278, 1960.
47. Victor and Adams: Am. J. Clin. Nutr., *9*, 379, 1961.
48. Denny-Brown: Med., *26*, 41, 1947.
49. ———: Fed. Proc., *17*, Suppl. 2, p. 35, 1958.
50. Olson: Fed. Proc., *17*, Suppl. 2, p. 26, 1958.
51. Dreyfus: New England J. Med., *267*, 596, 1962.
52. Jolliffe and Bowman: J.A.M.A., *114*, 307, 1940.
53. Lerner, DeCarli and Davidson: Proc. Soc. Exptl. Biol. & Med., *98*, 841, 1958.
54. Vilter, Mueller, Glazer, Jarrold, Abraham, Thompson and Hawkins: J. Lab. Clin. Med., *42*, 335, 1953.
55. Lunde: J. Nerv. and Mental Dis., *131*, 77, 1960.
56. Herbert, Zalusky and Davidson: Ann. Int. Med., *58*, 977, 1963.
57. Herbert: Arch. Int. Med., *110*, 649, 1962.
58. Sullivan and Herbert: J. Clin. Invest., *43*, 2048, 1964.
59. Flink, Stutzman, Anderson, Konig and Fraser: J. Lab. & Clin. Med., *43*, 169, 1954.
60. Heaton, Pyrah, Beresford, Bryson and Martin: Lancet, 2, 802, 1962.
61. Nielsen: Danish Med. Bull., *70*, 225, 1963.
62. McCollister, Prasad, Doe and Flink: J. Lab. & Clin. Med., *52*, 928, 1958.
63. Martin, McCuskey, Jr. and Tupikova: Am. J. Clin. Nutr., 7, 191, 1959.
64. Amatuzio, Stuzman, Shrifter and Nesbitt: J. Lab. & Clin. Med., *39*, 26, 1952.
65. Vallee, Wacker, Bartholomay and Robin: New England J. Med., *255*, 403, 1956.
66. Vallee, Wacker, Bartholomay and Hoch: New England J. Med., *257*, 1055, 1957.
67. Sullivan: Quart. J. Alc. Studies, *23*, 216, 1962.
68. Prasad, Schulert, Mialc, Farid and Sandstead: Am. J. Clin. Nutr., *12*, 437, 1963.
69. Tobin, Driscoll, Lim, Sutton, Szanto, and Gunnar: Circulation, *35*, 754, 1967.
70. Perkoff, Hardy and Velez-Garcia: New Engl. J. Med., *274*, 1277, 1966.
71. Sullivan, Egan, George, and McDermott: J. Lab. Clin. Med., *68*, 1022, 1966.
72. McDermott, Delaney, Egan, and Sullivan: J. Am. Med. Assn., *198*, 253, 1966.
73. Kesteloot, Terryn, Bosmans, and Joossens: Acta Cardiol., *21*, 341, 1966.
74. Morin, Foley, Martineau, and Roussel: Canad. Med. Assn. J., *97*, 881, 1967.
75. Fleckenstein: In *Calcium and the Heart*. Harris and Opie, Eds., Academic Press, New York, p. 135, 1971.
76. Neville, Eagles, Samson and Olson: Am. J. Clin. Nutr., *21*, 1329, 1968.

Appendix

ABBY STOLPER BLOCH, MARTHA H. MILES, AND MAURICE E. SHILS

The major portion of this Appendix provides information about diets and supplements to implement recommendations in the text for dietary management of specific disease entities. Because detailed and extensive tables of food composition are easily available, inclusion of this type of data has been limited. A printed diet may require modification in accordance with the clinical status and reactions of the individual patient. Comments on clinical experience with specific diets will be welcome.

Table A-1. Recommended Daily Dietary Allowances (Revised 1968). Food

Recommended Daily

	Age[2] Years From — Up to	Weight kg	Weight lb	Height cm	Height in	K calories	Protein gm	Fat Soluble Vitamins Vitamin A Activity I.U.	Vitamin D I.U.	Vitamin E Activity I.U.
Infants	0 — 1/6	4	9	55	22	kg × 120	kg × 2.2[3]	1500	400	5
	1/6 — 1/2	7	15	63	25	kg × 110	kg × 2.0[3]	1500	400	5
	1/2 — 1	9	20	72	28	kg × 100	kg × 1.8[3]	1500	400	5
Children	1 — 2	12	26	81	32	1100	25	2000	400	10
	2 — 3	14	31	91	36	1250	25	2000	400	10
	3 — 4	16	35	100	39	1400	30	2500	400	10
	4 — 6	19	42	110	43	1600	30	2500	400	10
	6 — 8	23	51	121	48	2000	35	3500	400	15
	8 — 10	28	62	131	52	2200	40	3500	400	15
Males	10 — 12	35	77	140	55	2500	45	4500	400	20
	12 — 14	43	95	151	59	2700	50	5000	400	20
	14 — 18	59	130	170	67	3000	60	5000	400	25
	18 — 22	67	147	175	69	2800	60	5000	400	30
	22 — 35	70	154	175	69	2800	65	5000	—	30
	35 — 55	70	154	173	68	2600	65	5000	—	30
	55 — 75+	70	154	171	67	2400	65	5000	—	30
Females	10 — 12	35	77	142	56	2250	50	4500	400	20
	12 — 14	44	97	154	61	2300	50	5000	400	20
	14 — 16	52	114	157	62	2400	55	5000	400	25
	16 — 18	54	119	160	63	2300	55	5000	400	25
	18 — 22	58	128	163	64	2000	55	5000	400	25
	22 — 35	58	128	163	64	2000	55	5000	—	25
	35 — 55	58	128	160	63	1850	55	5000	—	25
	55 — 75+	58	128	157	62	1700	55	5000	—	25
Pregnancy						+200	65	6000	400	30
Lactation						+1000	75	8000	400	30

and Nutrition Board National Academy of Sciences-National Research Council

Dietary Allowances[1] (Revised 1968)

Water Soluble Vitamins							Minerals				
Ascorbic Acid mg	Folacin[4] mg	Niacin mg equiv[5]	Ribo-flavin mg	Thiamine mg	Vitamin B_6 mg	Vitamin B_{12} μg	Calcium gm	Phos-phorus gm	Iodine μg	Iron mg	Mag-nesium mg
35	0.05	5	0.4	0.2	0.2	1	0.4	0.2	25	6	40
35	0.05	7	0.5	0.4	0.3	1.5	0.5	0.4	40	10	60
35	0.1	8	0.6	0.5	0.4	2	0.6	0.5	45	15	70
40	0.1	8	0.6	0.6	0.5	2	0.7	0.7	55	15	100
40	0.2	8	0.7	0.6	0.6	2.5	0.8	0.8	60	15	150
40	0.2	9	0.8	0.7	0.7	3	0.8	0.8	70	10	200
40	0.2	11	0.9	0.8	0.9	4	0.8	0.8	80	10	200
40	0.2	13	1.1	1.0	1.0	4	0.9	0.9	100	10	250
40	0.3	15	1.2	1.1	1.2	5	1.0	1.0	110	10	250
40	0.4	17	1.3	1.3	1.4	5	1.2	1.2	125	10	300
45	0.4	18	1.4	1.4	1.6	5	1.4	1.4	135	18	350
55	0.4	20	1.5	1.5	1.8	5	1.4	1.4	150	18	400
60	0.4	18	1.6	1.4	2.0	5	0.8	0.8	140	10	400
60	0.4	18	1.7	1.4	2.0	5	0.8	0.8	140	10	350
60	0.4	17	1.7	1.3	2.0	5	0.8	0.8	125	10	350
60	0.4	14	1.7	1.2	2.0	6	0.8	0.8	110	10	350
40	0.4	15	1.3	1.1	1.4	5	1.2	1.2	110	18	300
45	0.4	15	1.4	1.2	1.6	5	1.3	1.3	115	18	350
50	0.4	16	1.4	1.2	1.8	5	1.3	1.3	120	18	350
50	0.4	15	1.5	1.2	2.0	5	1.3	1.3	115	18	350
55	0.4	13	1.5	1.0	2.0	5	0.8	0.8	100	18	350
55	0.4	13	1.5	1.0	2.0	5	0.8	0.8	100	18	300
55	0.4	12	1.5	0.9	2.0	5	0.8	0.8	90	18	300
55	0.4	10	1.5	0.9	2.0	6	0.8	0.8	80	10	300
60	0.8	15	1.8	+0.1	2.5	8	+0.4	+0.4	125	18	450
60	0.5	20	2.0	+0.5	2.5	6	+0.5	+0.5	150	18	450

[1] The allowance levels are intended to cover individual variations among most normal persons as they live in the United States under usual environmental stresses. The recommended allowances can be attained with a variety of common foods, providing other nutrients for which human requirements have been less well defined.

[2] Entries on lines for age range 22–35 years represent the reference man and woman at age 22. All other entries represent allowances for the mid-point of the specified age range.

[3] Assumes protein equivalent to human milk. For proteins not 100 percent utilized factors should be increased proportionately.

[4] The folacin allowances refer to dietary sources as determined by *Lactobacillus casei* assay. Pure forms of folacin may be effective in doses less than 1/4 of the RDA.

[5] Niacin equivalents include dietary sources of the vitamin itself plus 1 mg equivalent for each 60 mg of dietary tryptophan.

Table A-2. Nutrient Intakes Recommended for Adults of Different Body Size and Degree of Activity (Canada)*

Weight lb[1]	Activity	Calories	Protein gm[2]	Calcium gm	Iron mg	Vitamin A I.U.[3]	Vitamin D I.U.	Ascorbic Acid mg	Thiamine mg	Riboflavin mg	Niacin mg
MALES:											
144	Maintenance	2150	44	0.5	6	3700	—	30	0.6	1.1	6
	A	2650	44	0.5	6	3700	—	30	0.8	1.3	8
	B	3400	44	0.5	6	3700	—	30	1.0	1.7	10
	C	4000	44	0.5	6	3700	—	30	1.2	2.0	12
	D	4600	44	0.5	6	3700	—	30	1.4	2.3	14
158	Maintenance	2300	48	0.5	6	3700	—	30	0.7	1.2	7
	A	2850	48	0.5	6	3700	—	30	0.9	1.4	9
	B	3650	48	0.5	6	3700	—	30	1.1	1.8	11
	C	4250	48	0.5	6	3700	—	30	1.3	2.1	13
	D	4900	48	0.5	6	3700	—	30	1.5	2.5	15
176	Maintenance	2500	54	0.5	6	3700	—	30	0.8	1.3	8
	A	3100	54	0.5	6	3700	—	30	0.9	1.5	9
	B	3950	54	0.5	6	3700	—	30	1.2	2.0	12
	C	4600	54	0.5	6	3700	—	30	1.4	2.3	14
	D	5350	54	0.5	6	3700	—	30	1.6	2.7	16

* Canadian Bulletin on Nutrition, Vol. 6, No. 1, March 1964 (Protein, revised 1968). Dietary Standard for Canada, pp. 72–74.

FEMALES:

111	Maintenance	1750	35	0.5	10	3700	—	30	0.5	0.9	5
	A	2200	35	0.5	10	3700	—	30	0.7	1.1	7
	B	2800	35	0.5	10	3700	—	30	0.8	1.4	8
	C	3300	35	0.5	10	3700	—	30	1.0	1.7	10
	D	3800	35	0.5	10	3700	—	30	1.2	1.9	12
124	Maintenance	1900	39	0.5	10	3700	—	30	0.6	1.0	6
	A	2400	39	0.5	10	3700	—	30	0.7	1.2	7
	B	3000	39	0.5	10	3700	—	30	0.9	1.5	9
	C	3550	39	0.5	10	3700	—	30	1.1	1.8	11
	D	4100	39	0.5	10	3700	—	30	1.2	2.0	12
136	Maintenance	2050	43	0.5	10	3700	—	30	0.6	1.0	6
	A	2550	43	0.5	10	3700	—	30	0.8	1.3	8
	B	3250	43	0.5	10	3700	—	30	1.0	1.6	10
	C	3800	43	0.5	10	3700	—	30	1.1	1.9	11
	D	4400	43	0.5	10	3700	—	30	1.3	2.2	13
Pregnancy—during 3rd trimester add		up to 500	9	0.7	3	500	400	10	0.15	0.25	1.5
Lactation—add		500 to 1000	23	0.7	3	1500	400	20	0.3	0.5	3

[1] Weights include indoor clothing without shoes. Weights illustrated are the 25th, 50th and 75th percentiles of the 25- to 29-year age group in the Canadian population.

[2,3] See footnotes [1] and [2] in last section of this table.

Table A-2. (Continued)　Recommended Daily Nutrient Intakes for Boys and Girls (Canada)

Sex	Age yrs	Weight lb	Activity Category	Calories	Protein gm[1]	Calcium gm	Iron mg	Vitamin A I.U.[2]	Vitamin D I.U.	Ascorbic Acid mg	Thiamine mg	Riboflavin mg	Niacin mg
Both	0–1	7–20	Usual	360–900	7–13	0.5	5	1000	400	20	0.3	0.5	3
Both	1–2	20–26	Usual	900–1200	12–16	0.7	5	1000	400	20	0.4	0.6	4
Both	2–3	31	Usual	1400	17	0.7	5	1000	400	20	0.4	0.7	4
Both	4–6	40	Usual	1700	20	0.7	5	1000	400	20	0.5	0.9	5
Both	7–9	57	Usual	2100	24	1.0	5	1500	400	30	0.7	1.1	7
Both	10–12	77	Usual	2500	30	1.2	12	2000	400	30	0.8	1.3	8
Boy	13–15	108	Usual	3100	40	1.2	12	2700	400	30	0.9	1.6	9
Girl	13–15	108	Usual	2600	39	1.2	12	2700	400	30	0.8	1.3	8
Boy	16–17	136	B[3]	3700	45	1.2	12	3200	400	30	1.1	1.9	11
Girl	16–17	120	A[4]	2400	41	1.2	12	3200	400	30	0.7	1.2	7
Boy	18–19	144	B[3]	3800	47	0.9	6	3200	400	30	1.1	1.9	11
Girl	18–19	124	A[4]	2450	41	0.9	10	3200	400	30	0.7	1.2	7

[1] Protein recommendation is based on normal mixed Canadian diet. Vegetarian diets may require a higher protein content.

[2] Vitamin A is based on the mixed Canadian diet supplying both vitamin A and carotene. As the preformed vitamin A the suggested intake would be about ⅔ of that indicated.

[3] Expenditure assessed as being 113 per cent of that of a man of same weight and engaged in same degree of activity.

[4] Expenditure assessed as being 104 per cent of that of a woman of the same weight and engaged in the same degree of activity.

Table A-3. Desirable Weights for Men and Women Aged 25 and Over*
(in pounds according to height and frame, in indoor clothing)

Height†		Small Frame	Medium Frame	Large Frame
		MEN		
Feet	Inches			
5	2	112–120	118–129	126–141
5	3	115–123	121–133	129–144
5	4	118–126	124–136	132–148
5	5	121–129	127–139	135–152
5	6	124–133	130–143	138–156
5	7	128–137	134–147	142–161
5	8	132–141	138–152	147–166
5	9	136–145	142–156	151–170
5	10	140–150	146–160	155–174
5	11	144–154	150–165	159–179
6	0	148–158	154–170	164–184
6	1	152–162	158–175	168–189
6	2	156–167	162–180	173–194
6	3	160–171	167–185	178–199
6	4	164–175	172–190	182–204
		WOMEN		
4	10	92– 98	96–107	104–119
4	11	94–101	98–110	106–122
5	0	96–104	101–113	109–125
5	1	99–107	104–116	112–128
5	2	102–110	107–119	115–131
5	3	105–113	110–122	118–134
5	4	108–116	113–126	121–138
5	5	111–119	116–130	125–142
5	6	114–123	120–135	129–146
5	7	118–127	124–139	133–150
5	8	122–131	128–143	137–154
5	9	126–135	132–147	141–158
5	10	130–140	136–151	145–163
5	11	134–144	140–155	149–168
6	0	138–148	144–159	153–173

* Prepared by Metropolitan Life Insurance Co.; data derived primarily from Build and Blood Pressure Study, 1959, Society of Actuaries.
† Height in shoes.

Table A-4. Nutrients in Alcoholic Beverages*
per 100 ml

	kcal	Na‡	K
		mEq	mEq
Beer, Lager	45	0.30	1.02
Wine			
Red	80	0.34	2.02
Rosé	78	0.69	1.71
Dry White	75	0.47	2.00
Sweet White	91	0.43	1.79
Vermouth			
Sweet	167 }	0.47	1.58–3.07
Dry	105 }		
Dessert Wines			
Dry Sherry	130	0.30	1.82
Sweet Sherry	153	0.34	2.07
Port	161	0.39	2.41
Muscatel	163	0.60	1.97
Champagne	83	0.30	1.89
Distilled Spirits†	239	—	0.10

* Averages of data taken from Leake and Silverman: Alcoholic Beverages in Clinical Medicine, Year Book Medical Publishing, Inc., Chicago, 1966.
† Based on 86 proof alcohol concentration for whiskey, gin, vodka, and 80 proof brandy and most rums.
‡ Na content varies greatly in wine. European wines are lower than U.S. wines due to water Na content. Brandy contains 2.0 mg (0.08 mEq). For a more complete list see Newborg: Arch. Intern. Med., *123*:693, 1969.

Table A-5. Cholesterol Content of Commonly Used Foods*

(mg per 100 grams edible portion)

Food and Description	mg	Food and Description	mg
Beef, lean, cooked total edible	91	Herring, flesh only	85
		Ice cream, 10% fat	40
Brains, raw	>2,000	Ice milk	20
Butter	250	Lamb, cooked, total edible	98
Buttermilk, from skim milk	2	Lard	95
Cake, chocolate	48	Liver	
Cheese		Beef, calf, hog, lamb, cooked	438
American, pasteur. processed	90	Chicken, cooked	746
Cheddar, natural	99	Margarine	
Cottage, creamed 4% fat	19	All vegetable fat	0
Cottage, uncreamed	7	$\frac{2}{3}$ animal fat—$\frac{1}{3}$ vegetable fat	50
Cream	111	Mayonnaise, commercial	70
Parmesan, grated	113	Milk	
Swiss, pasteur. processed	93	Dry non-fat	22
Chicken		Low fat, 1% fat	6
Breast, cooked, total edible	80	Whole fluid	14
Drumstick, cooked, total edible	91	Pork, cooked, total edible	89
Chicken fat	65	Salmon, raw, canned	35
Clams	50	Sausage, all meat, cooked	62
Crab meat	101	Shrimp, raw, flesh only	150
Cream		Sweetbreads, cooked	466
Light	66	Tuna, drained solids	65
Sour	66	Turkey, cooked	
Eggs		Light meat, no skin	77
Whole	504	Dark meat, no skin	101
White	0	Veal, cooked, total edible	101
Yolk	1,480	Yogurt	
Frankfurter, all meat, cooked	62	Plain or vanilla	8
Flounder, flesh only	50	Fruit, all kinds	7
Haddock, flesh only	60		
Halibut, flesh only	50		

* Data from Feeley et al: Cholesterol content of foods. *J. Amer. Diet. Assoc.*, *61*:134–149, 1972.

Table A-6. Fatty Acid Composition of Selected Fats and Oils

| | Saturated Fatty Acids | | | | | | | | | Unsaturated Fatty Acids | | | | P/S | References† |
| | Butyric | Caproic | Caprylic | Capric | Lauric | Myristic | Palmitic | Stearic | C20 & Higher | Palmitoleic | Oleic | Linoleic | Linolenic | Ratio* | |
	C4	C6	C8	C10	C12	C14	C16	C18		C16	C18	C18	C18		
Butter Fat	3.5	1.4	1.7	2.6	4.5	14.6	30.2	10.5	1.6	5.7	18.7	2.1		1:34	2
Lard							31.0	7.0			46.0	10.0	1.0	1:34	4
Meat Fat						2.6	23.4	13.9	38.4	1.5	41.9	3.3		1:24	
Hydrog. Veg. Solid Shortening							14.0	6.0			65.0	7.0	Trace	1:2.8	4
Coconut Oil		(2) 0.8	(2) 5.4	(2) 8.4	42.4	15.5	10.7	2.7		0.5	6.8	1.6		1:54	
Soybean Oil						(2) 0.4	9.7	4.0	(2) 2.4	(2) 1.0	24.2	51.7	7.9	1:0.3	
Corn Oil					0.1	(2) 0.2	11.4	2.0	(2) 0.2	(2) 0.5	27.5	57.1	1.5	1:0.2	
Cottonseed Oil						(2) 1.4	11.4	2.0	(2) 1.3	0.6	16.0	59.6	0.1	1:0.3	
Peanut Oil					0.1		11.1	3.0		0.1	52.1	27.8	0.5	1:0.5	
Safflower Oil							7.1	2.2			12.4	77.3	0.1	1:0.1	
Olive Oil							13.3	2.9		1.1	74.6	7.0	1.0	1:2.0	
Sesame Oil							8.0	4.0			38.0	42.0		1:0.3	4
Corn Oil Margarine							9.1	5.4			27.2	32.2		1:0.45	5
MCT Oil		1	75	23	1			Trace						0/100	3

* P/S Ratio: The ratio of polyunsaturated to total saturated fatty acids. Monounsaturated fatty acids are not included in this ratio.

† All values are from Ref. 1 unless otherwise designated by number

REFERENCES:

1. Altman, Dittmer: Metabolism. Fed. Amer. Soc. Exp. Biol. Bethesda, Md., pp. 47–52, 1968.
2. Brink, Balsley, Speckman: *The Amer. J. Clin. Nutrition*, 22:168–180, 1969.
3. *Medium Chain Triglycerides:* Senior, J. R. (Ed.), p. 193, 1968, Univ. of Penna. Press.
4. *New Jersey Diet Manual, Rev. 1967:* N.J. State Dept. Health, Trenton, N.J.
5. Miljanich and Ostwald: *J. Amer. Diet Assoc.*, 56:29–30, 1970.

Table A-7. Diets for Weight Reduction and Diabetes Control Based on Exchange Lists* †

	Kcal per day			
	800	*1200*	*1800*	*2400*
TOTAL DAILY INTAKE				
Carbohydrate gm	90	120	185	250
Protein 〃	55	65	80	100
Fat 〃	25	55	80	110
Total Exchanges for one day				
Milk	2 skim	2 whole	2 whole	4 whole
Meat, lean	5	5	7	7
(Liver one weekly)				
Bread	2	4	7	9
Vegetables				
A		— as desired —		
B	1	1	2	2
Fruit	3	3	4	5
Fat	0	1	5	7
SAMPLE MEAL PATTERN	Servings based on Exchanges—Table A-8			
Breakfast				
Fruit	1	1	1	1
Egg	1	1	1	1
Bread	1	1	3	3
Coffee, Tea		— as desired —		
Fat	0	1	2	2
Milk	0	0	0	1 whole
Lunch				
Meat, lean	2	2	3	3
Vegetables				
A (salad)		— as desired —		
B	0	0	$\frac{1}{2}$ cup	$\frac{1}{2}$ cup
Bread	1	2	2	2
Fruit	1	1	1	1
Milk	1 skim	1 whole	1 whole	1 whole
Fat	0	0	2	2
Coffee, Tea		— as desired —		
Dinner				
Meat, lean	2	3	3	3
Vegetable				
A		— as desired —		
B	$\frac{1}{2}$ cup	$\frac{1}{2}$ cup	$\frac{1}{2}$ cup	$\frac{1}{2}$ cup
Fruit	1	1	1	1
Bread	0	1	2	3
Fat	0	0	1	2
Milk	1 skim	1 whole	1 whole	1 whole
Coffee, Tea		— as desired —		
8 PM				
Fruit			1	1
Milk				1 whole
Bread				1
Fat				1

* For high polyunsaturated fat diet see Table A-9.   Exchange lists in Table A-8.
† Modified from Diet Manual, Memorial Sloan-Kettering Cancer Center, New York, N.Y. Revised 1967.

Table A-8. Food Exchange Lists*

LIST I.—MILK

Carbohydrate 12 gm, protein 8 gm, fat 10 gm per serving.   170 kcal.

Food	Approximate Measure 1 Exchange	Weight gm
Milk†	1 cup (8 oz)	240
Milk, evaporated	½ cup	120
Milk, powder, whole	¼ cup (3 tbsp level)	35
Buttermilk†	1 cup	240
Milk, skim†	1 cup	240

† Add 2 fat exchanges if fat free.

LIST II.—VEGETABLES

A. *Vegetables.* Negligible carbohydrate, protein, and fat in amounts ordinarily used.

If more than one cup in cooked form is used at one meal, it should be calculated as one serving of a Group B vegetable.

Asparagus	Mushrooms	Water cress
Broccoli	Okra	Greens:
Brussels sprouts	Parsley	Beet greens
Cabbage	Pepper, green	Chard
Cauliflower	Radish	Collards
Celery	Romaine	Dandelion
Chicory	Rhubarb	Kale
Cucumber	Sauerkraut	Mustard
Escarole	String beans, young	Poke
Eggplant	Summer squash	Spinach
Lettuce	Tomatoes	Turnip greens

B. *Vegetables.* Carbohydrate 7 gm, protein 2 gm, fat negligible per serving. 35 kcal.

1 exchange = ½ measuring cup = 100 gm

Beets	Peas, green	Squash, winter
Carrots	Pumpkin	Turnip
Onions	Rutabagas	

* The American Dietetic Association, Chicago, Ill., and American Diabetes Association, Inc., New York, N.Y. Meal Planning with Exchange Lists, Revised 1956.

Table A-8. Food Exchange Lists (*Continued*)

List III.—Fruits

Fresh, cooked, canned or frozen *unsweetened*.
Carbohydrate 10 gm per exchange, protein and fat negligible.   40 kcal.

Fruit	Approximate Measure 1 Exchange	Weight gm
Apple, 1 small	2″ diameter	80
Applesauce	½ cup	100
Apricots, fresh	2 medium	100
Apricots, dry	4 halves	20
Banana	½ small	50
Berries (blackberries, raspberries and strawberries)*	1 cup	150
Blueberries	⅔ cup	100
Cantaloupe*	½ (6″ diameter)	200
Cherries	10 large or 15 small	75
Dates	2	15
Figs, dried	1 small	15
Figs, fresh	2 large	50
Grapefruit*	½ small	125
Grapefruit juice*	½ cup	100
Grapes	12	75
Grape juice	¼ cup	60
Honeydew melon	¼ (7″ diameter)	150
Mango	½ small	70
Nectarines	1 medium	100
Orange*	1 small	100
Orange juice*	½ cup	100
Papaya	⅓ medium	100
Peach	1 medium	100
Pear	1 small	100
Pineapple	½ cup, cubed	80
Pineapple juice	⅓ cup	80
Plums	2 medium	100
Prunes, dried	2 medium	25
Raisins	2 tbsp. level	15
Rhubarb	(See List II A)	
Tangerine*	1 large	100
Watermelon	1 cup diced	
	1 slice 3″ × 1½″	175

* These fruits are rich sources of vitamin C; use at least one serving each day.

Table A-8. Food Exchange Lists (*Continued*)

LIST IV.—BREAD EXCHANGES

Carbohydrate 15 gm, protein 2 gm, fat negligible.   70 kcal.

Food	Approximate Measure 1 Exchange	Weight gm
Bread, baker's	1 slice	25
Biscuit, roll	2″ diameter	35
Muffin	2″ diameter	35
Cornbread	1½″ cube	35
Cereals, cooked	½ cup, cooked	100
Cereals, dry (flakes, puffed and shredded varieties)	¾ cup, scant	100
Rice, macaroni, noodles, spaghetti	½ cup, cooked	100
Flour	2½ tbsp.	20
Crackers:		
Graham	2 (2½″ × 2¾″)	20
Oyster	20 (½ cup)	20
Saltines	5 (2″ square)	20
Soda	3 (2½″ × 2½″)	20
Round, thin varieties	6–8 (½″ diameter)	20
Vegetables:		
Beans, peas, dried (cooked) Includes: limas, navy, kidney beans, black-eyed, cowpeas and split peas, etc.	½ cup, scant	100
Corn	⅓ cup or ½ ear	80
Parsnips	½ cup	125
Potatoes:		
White, baked	2″ diameter	100
White, boiled, mashed	½ cup	100
Sweet or yam	¼ cup	50
Ice cream, vanilla*	⅛ quart	70
Sponge cake, no icing	1½″ cube	25

* Omit 2 fat exchanges

LIST V.—MEAT EXCHANGES

Carbohydrate negligible, protein 7 gm, fat 5 gm per serving. 75 kcal. *Note:* All items expressed in cooked weight. One or more fat exchanges from the diet may be used to cook or season these foods.

Food	Approximate Measure 1 Exchange	Weight gm
Meat:		
Beef, fowl, lamb, veal (medium fat), liver, pork, ham (lean)	1 oz.	30
Cold cuts:		
Salami, minced ham, bologna, cervelat, liver sausage, luncheon loaf	1 slice, 4½″ diam. × ⅛″	45
Frankfurter (8-9 per lb.).	1	50

Table A-8. Food Exchange Lists (*Continued*)

List V.—Meat Exchanges (*Continued*)

Food	Approximate Measure 1 Exchange	Weight gm
Fish:		
Cod, haddock, halibut, herring, etc. . . .	1 oz.	30
Salmon, tuna, crabmeat, lobster	1 oz.	30
Shrimp, clams, oysters (medium)	5	45
Sardines	3 medium	30
Cheese:		
Cheddar type	1 oz.	30
Cottage	3 tbsp. level	45
Peanut butter*	2 tbsp. scant	30
Egg	1	50

* Limit to one serving per day unless adjustment is made to balance carbohydrate content.

List VI.—Fat Exchanges

Carbohydrate and protein negligible, fat 5 gm per serving.   45 kcal.

Food	Approximate Measure 1 Exchange	Weight gm
Avocado	4″ diam.	30
Butter or margarine	1 tsp. level	5
Bacon, crisp	1 slice	10
Cream, light, sweet or sour—20%	2 tbsp. level	30
Cream, heavy—40%	1 tbsp. level	15
Cream, cheese	1 tbsp. level	15
French dressing	1 tbsp. level	15
Mayonnaise	1 tsp. level	5
Nuts	2 tsp.	6
Oil or cooking fat	1 tsp. level	5
Olives	5 small	50

Foods that do not need to be measured are:

Coffee	Rennet tablets
Tea	Pickles, sour
Clear broth	Pickles, unsweetened dill
Bouillon (without fat)	Cranberries
Gelatin, unsweetened	Rhubarb

Table A-9. Diets for Weight Reduction and for Diabetes Control (High Polyunsaturated Fat Diets) *

Total Daily Intake		kcal per day		
		1200	1800	2500
Carbohydrate	gm	135	195	275
Protein	gm	60	80	118
Fat	gm	45	70	100
P/S ratio		2:1	2:1	2.5:1
Total Exchanges for One Day				
Skim milk		2	3	3
Vegetable A		——— as desired ———		
Vegetable B		1	1	2
Fruit		3	3	5
Bread		4	7	10
Meat†		5	6	10
Unsaturated Fat		4	8	10
Sample Meal Pattern		Servings based on exchanges—Table A-8		
Breakfast				
Fruit		1	1	1
Bread		1	2	3
Meat†		0	1	1
Fat, unsaturated		1	2	3
Milk, skim		1	1	1 + 1 mid-meal snack
Tea/Coffee		——— as desired ———		
Lunch				
Meat†		2	2	3
Vegetable A		——— as desired ———		
Vegetable B		0	0	1
Bread		2	2	3
Fat, unsaturated		2	3	3
Fruit		1	1	2
Milk, skim		1	1	1
Tea/Coffee		——— as desired ———		
Dinner				
Meat†		3	3	4
Vegetable A		——— as desired ———		
Vegetable B		1	1	1
Bread		1	2	2
Fat, unsaturated		1	3	3
Fruit		1	1	2
Tea/Coffee		——— as desired ———		
Evening				
Meat†		0	0	2
Bread		0	1	2
Milk, skim		0	1	0
Fat, unsaturated		0	0	1
Tea/Coffee		——— as desired ———		

* Data courtesy of: Beth Israel Medical Center, New York, N.Y.
† 11 of 14 main meals/week should contain 6 oz of poultry (without skin), fish, lean veal, uncreamed cottage cheese or skim milk yogurt. Remaining meals may include 3 oz servings of lean beef, lamb or pork. No more than 3 egg yolks should be taken per week (eating and cooking).

Table A-10. Sodium-Restricted Diets*

Degree of Restriction:		Strict†	Moderate	Mild
Na in mg	=	500	1,000	2,400 —4,500
Na in mEq	=	21.7	43.4	104.3— 195.6
NaCl in gm	=	1.2	2.5	6.1— 11.5
Approximate Composition	*Unit*			
Carbohydrate	gm	291	327	339
Protein	gm	84	147	111
Fat	gm	65	84	96.5
Calories		1,925	2,500	2,589.2
Calcium	mg	811	1,182	1,193
Phosphorus	mg	1,337	2,094	1,932
Iron	mg	12.7	19.5	15.8
Sodium	mg (mEq)	455 (20)	891 (44)	2,444 (106)
Potassium	mg (mEq)	3,840 (98)	4,765 (122)	4,267 (109)
Vitamin A	I.U.	6,178	7,222	7,358
Thiamine	mg	1.2	1.6	1.4
Riboflavin	mg	1.9	2.9	2.6
Niacin-equivalents	mg	21.7	35.6	23.2
Ascorbic Acid	mg	206	208	158

ADEQUACY: This diet meets the 1968 Recommended Dietary Allowances of the National Research Council except for calories which are low for an active individual. The calculations are based on the sample meal plan.

The use of water-softeners may add significant amounts of sodium to the water supply.

* Modified from Diet Manual, Memorial Sloan-Kettering Cancer Center, New York, N.Y. Revised 1967; courtesy Dietary Department.
† This strict diet can be modified to 250 mg sodium by eliminating regular milk and using only low sodium milk and eliminating all commercial sherbets and ice cream.

Table A-10. Sodium-Restricted Diets (*Continued*)

GENERAL RULES:

1. Avoid the use of all salt, baking soda and/or baking powder in cooking and for table use.
2. Avoid medicines, laxatives, and salt substitutes unless prescribed by physician.
3. Read labels carefully for sodium or salt content of packaged foods.

Type of Food	*Amount**		*Foods Included*	*Foods Excluded*
Milk	Strict	*2 cups	Evaporated, non-fat dry milk; skim milk; unsalted buttermilk and whole milk. *Additional milk must be low sodium, fluid or powdered.	Cultured buttermilk; condensed milk; and all milk drinks prepared with malt, chocolate syrup and ice cream; yogurt; more than two cups of regular milk daily.
	Moderate Mild }	3 cups		
	Mild			(*Mild*—No restriction except limit to 3 cups)
Other beverages	Strict	2–3 cups	Cocoa prepared with milk allowance; coffee, instant and regular; Postum; Sanka; tea; fresh and frozen fruitades; carbonated beverages limit to one 8 oz. bottle daily of Coca-Cola or Orange Crush.	Ginger ale; commercial choc. syrup, fountain beverages; instant cocoa and all powdered beverage mixes; all those not listed as allowed; alcoholic beverages allowed with physician's permission.
	Moderate Mild }	as desired		
	Mild	″ ″		(*Mild*—Only Dutch process cocoa and alcoholic beverages without physician's permission.)
Soup		1 cup (8 oz. per cup)	Unsalted broth; unsalted vegetable soup made with allowed vegetables; unsalted cream soup made from butter and milk allowance; unsalted tomato bouillon.	All canned, dehydrated, and frozen soups containing salt; bouillon cubes; consomme and other commercial meat extract soups.

* Varying amounts of foods included relate to degrees of restriction.

Table A-10. Sodium-Restricted Diets (Continued)

Type of Food	Amount		Foods Included	Foods Excluded
Meat, poultry and fish	Strict—	4 oz.	Fresh, unsalted frozen or unsalted canned meats, fish and poultry such as: beef; chicken; duck; lamb; liver (beef, calves or chicken liver allowed once every two weeks); pork; fresh tongue; turkey; veal; *use fresh fish only* such as: bass; bluefish; cod; flounder; halibut; oysters; perch; salmon; snapper; sole; trout; tuna; sweetbreads and salt-free peanut butter. (Mild—Reg. tuna, salmon, shellfish)	All salted, koshered, smoked, corned, and canned (with salt) meats; fish; and poultry; bacon; brains; kidneys; luncheon meats; chipped or corned beef; ham; frankfurters; anchovies; caviar; sardines; herring; regular canned tuna; salmon and shellfish; clams; crabs; lobsters; scallops; shrimps and regular peanut butter
	Moderate—	10 oz.		
	Mild—	6 ozs.		
	Mild			
Cheese		1 svg. (1 oz.)	Unsalted cottage cheese, unsalted cream cheese and unsalted American cheese. (Mild—Amer. cheese, cheddar, Swiss, cottage, cream)	All other cheese not listed as allowed.
Eggs	Strict—	Limit to 1 a day	Boiled; poached; scrambled or fried in unsalted butter.	None except in excess of amount allowed.
	Moderate Mild	2 a day		
Potato or substitute		2 svgs. (½ cup per svg.)	Potatoes, white or sweet; macaroni; noodles; rice and spaghetti.	Potato chips and prepared potato products.
Bread	Strict—	4 svgs.	Unsalted bread and unsalted crackers such as melba toast and plain Passover or thin tea matzoth.	Regular bread; rolls; biscuits; muffins and cereal products prepared with salt or soda; commercial mixes; graham crackers; saltines; soda crackers; salted matzoth and self-rising flour
	Moderate—	6 svgs.		
	Mild	4 svgs.	(Mild—regular bread; graham crax; biscuits; muffins)	
Cereals	Strict— Moderate	1 svg. (½ cup per svg.)	Unsalted slow cooking unenriched cereals; barley; cornmeal; cornstarch; grits; tapioca; dry cereals; puffed rice; puffed and shredded wheat.	Quick cooking and enriched cereals; dry cereals except those listed as allowed. (Mild—None)
	Mild			

Table A-10. Sodium-Restricted Diets (*Continued*)

Type of Food	Amount	Foods Included	Foods Excluded
Vegetables	Strict— Moderate } 3 svgs. (½ cup per svg.) Mild 4 svgs.	All fresh, frozen and unsalted canned vegetables except those listed under Food Excluded; dried lima beans, lentils, split peas and soybeans. (Mild—All fresh, unsalted, canned and unsalted, frozen vegetables.	Canned vegetables and vegetable juices to which salt has been added; artichokes; beets; beet greens; carrots; celery; collards; swiss chard; dandelion greens; kale; mustard greens; sauerkraut; spinach; white turnips; frozen vegetables processed with salt such as lima beans, peas and mixed vegetables.
Fruit and fruit juice	Strict— Moderate } 3 svgs. (½ cup per svg.) Mild	Any fruit or fruit juice; fresh, frozen or canned except those listed under Food Excluded. Include one citrus fruit or juice daily.	Cantaloupe; crystallized or glazed fruit; dried figs or raisins; tomato juice; all fruits to which sodium coloring, sodium flavoring or sodium benzoate has been added. (Mild—None)
Butter or fat	Strict— 6 svgs. (1 tsp. per svg.) Moderate 6 svgs. Mild 5 svgs.	Unsalted butter; unsalted margarine; unsalted salad and cooking fats such as corn, cottonseed, Crisco, olive oil, Spry; unsalted French and mayonnaise dressings; unsalted gravy; sweet & sour cream, limit 2 tbsps. per day. (Mod.—3 pats may be salted, 6 tsp. sw/or sour cream) (Mild—3 oz. butter; margarine; mayonnaise; French dressing; oil; plus 3 oz cream)	Salted butter and salted margarine; all commercial salad and mayonnaise dressings; bacon and pork fat; salted meat gravy. (Mild—bacon, bacon fat, excess of amount allowed)

Table A-10.   Sodium-Restricted Diets *(Continued)*

Type of Food	Amount	Foods Included	Foods Excluded
Dessert	Strict— } 1 svg. Moderate } (1 svg. = ½ c.)	Fruit ice, gelatin made with fresh fruit juices; unsalted desserts made from milk and egg allowance such as custard, tapioca, cornstarch, and rice pudding; unsalted fruit crisps and unsalted fruit pies; junket except chocolate; unsalted sugar cookies. * Commercial ice cream and sherbet must be used as milk allowance. (Mild—cake; cookies and pies)	All commercial cakes; cookies; pies; puddings; Jell-O; chocolate junket; rennet tablets; all dessert made with baking powder, salt or soda; commercial ice cream and sherbet when not taken as milk allowance, gingersnaps, sandwich type cookies, any dessert prepared with nuts.
	Mild 3 svgs.		
Sweets	As desired	Sugar, white and brown; honey; jams; jellies made without the addition of sodium benzoate; hard candy; maple syrup and gum drops.	Commercial candies and syrups; chocolate syrups; molasses; saccharin and sucaryl.
Spices	As desired	All except those listed in Foods Excluded.	Accent; dried or fresh celery leaves; celery salt; celery seed; garlic salt; horseradish prepared with salt; onion salt; salt substitutes unless recommended by your physician; all seasonings with salt added.
Miscellaneous	As desired	Dietetic catsup, low sodium dietetic meat extracts and tenderizers; cream of tartar; yeast; unsalted popcorn; unsalted nuts; sodium free baking powders if allowed by physician.	Regular catsup; chili sauce; meat extracts; meat tenderizers; meat sauces; prepared mustard; olives; pickles; relishes; soy sauce; worcestershire sauce; salted pretzels and popcorn; Fritos and all *snacks* containing salt; salted nuts.

Example of DIETARY PATTERN for Strict Na Restriction (21.7 mEq)

Breakfast	*Serving Portion*	*Sample Menu*
Fruit	½ cup	Orange juice
Cereal	½ cup	Unsalted Wheatena
Egg	1	Soft cooked egg
Bread	2 slices	Low sodium toast
Fat	1 tsp.	Unsalted butter
Milk	½ cup	Milk
Beverage	1 cup	Coffee
Sugar	1 tbsp.	Sugar
Lunch		
Meat or substitute	2 oz.	Unsalted broiled chicken
Potato	1	Baked potato
Vegetable	½ cup	Unsalted asparagus
Salad	½ cup	Sliced tomato
Dressing	1 tbsp.	Unsalted French dressing
Dessert	½ cup	Lime ice
Bread	1 slice	Low sodium bread
Fat	1 tsp.	Unsalted butter
Milk	½ cup	Milk
Beverage	1 cup	Coffee or tea
Sugar	2 tsp.	Sugar
Dinner		
Soup	1 cup	Unsalted broth
Meat	2 oz.	Unsalted roast beef
Potato	1	Unsalted boiled potato
Vegetable	½ cup	Unsalted Brussels sprouts
Fruit	½ cup	Canned apricots
Bread	1 slice	Low sodium bread
Fat	1 tsp.	Unsalted butter
Beverage	1 cup	Coffee or tea
Sugar	2 tsp.	Sugar
8:00 P.M.		
Milk	1 cup	Milk
Fruit	½ cup	Applesauce

Table A-11. Sources of Information on Low-Sodium Food Products

1. American Heart Association:
   a. Your 500 Milligram Sodium Diet—Strict Sodium Restriction, New York, 1968.
   b. Your 1,000 Milligram Sodium Diet—Moderate Sodium Restriction, New York, 1969.
   c. Your Mild Sodium Restricted Diet, New York, 1969.

2. Payne, Alma Smith, and Callahan, Dorothy: *Low-Sodium-Fat Controlled Cookbook*, 3rd Edition, Boston, Little, Brown and Company, 34 Beacon Street, Boston, Mass., 1966. Price $5.95.

3. *The Cookbook for Low Sodium Diets*. The Massachusetts Heart Association, 85 Devonshire Street, Boston, Mass., 1965. Price $0.25.

4. *The Salt-Free Diet Cookbook*. Conason, Emil, G., and Metz, Ella, Grosset and Dunlap, New York, 1969. Price $1.45.

Local Public Health Departments or Extension Services should be contacted for bulletins and brochures.

Individual food companies may be contacted for specific dietary information on their products.

Table A-12. Diet Information for Control of Renal Failure

Diet management of renal disease varies from patient to patient. References, lists of foods with specific nutrient values and basic dietary concepts are available for such dietary management.[1,2,3] The U.S.D.A. publication on "Composition of Foods: Raw, Processed, Prepared"[4] gives a complete listing of foods commonly used with their protein, nitrogen and mineral values. A selected short list is given in Table A-13.

Three types of renal diets based on national menus have been published. These are:

(a) Giordano-Giovanetti diet.[5] This is a two-part regimen for use when blood urea nitrogen is elevated above 100 mg% on a normal protein diet. Initially, the diet includes 1800–3200 calories, low sodium, no protein of animal origin, 3–4 grams protein of vegetable origin. When the blood urea nitrogen falls, 12–40 grams animal and vegetable protein are given by using two eggs or the equivalent as milk, chicken or veal.

(b) A modified Giordano-Giovanetti diet developed in England by Shaw et al.[6] supplies 2000 calories and 18 grams of protein of various origins supplying the daily requirements of essential amino acids except methionine.

(c) A modified Giordano-Giovanetti diet has been developed in Poland by Polec et al.[7] Potato, butter, sugar, vegetables and fruits are permitted. All exogenous amino acids except methionine are provided in addition to adequate calorie supply.

Less rigid dietary control based on equivalent lists is now the most acceptable approach for those patients currently being managed on dialysis programs.[3]

Hospital manuals may also provide a good source of diet patterns for special regimens. Large food companies offer technical data about their dietary preparations.

Special products of interest for this purpose include:

(a) Wheat products: Wheat starch flour, Chicago Dietetic Supply House, Inc.; Paygel-P (a high purity wheat starch) and Dietetic Paygel Baking Mix (formerly Resource Baking Mix). Aproten (3 varieties of pasta), General Mills, Chemical Division, Minn., Minn.; self-rising wheat starch flour, 100 gm = 529 mg (23 mEq) sodium, 13 mg (0.33 mEq) potassium, MacDowell Brothers, Ogdensburg, N.Y. and Brockville, Ontario, Canada.

(b) Substitutes for light or whipped cream: Rich's Coffee Rich or Cafe-Lite, 0.8% protein, 0.25% sodium, trace potassium, $\frac{1}{4}$ cup = 88 kcal > 0.4 gm protein; Coffee Mate (Carnation), 3 gm = 16 kcal > 0.1 gm protein, 26.2 mg potassium, 3.6 mg sodium; Praise (Carnation) reconstituted, 1 fluid oz = 29 kcal > 0.13 grm protein, 3.6 mg potassium, 6.0 mg sodium; Praise (Carnation) whipped, $\frac{1}{4}$ cup = 50 kcal > 0.21 gm protein, 7.2 mg potassium, 12 mg sodium; Rich's Whipped Topping = 0.00% protein, 0.25% sodium, trace potassium.

(c) High carbohydrate-low protein and electrolyte drinks: Hy-Cal, Beecham-Massengill Pharmaceuticals, Bristol, Tenn. 4 oz = 295 kcal > 0.03% protein, 0.74 mg (0.02 mEq) potassium, 16.3 mg (0.71 mEq) sodium; Cal Power, General Mills, Minn., Minn., 8 oz. carton = > 0.3 gm protein, 30 mg (1.3 mEq) sodium, 12 mg (0.31 mEq) potassium; Controlyte, low protein, low electrolyte, high calorie dietary supplement, The Doyle Pharmaceutical Co., Minn., Minn.; dietetic portion-controlled salad dressings, condiments and jellies, William J. Elwood, Inc., New York, N.Y.

REFERENCES

1. de St. Jeor, S. T., Carlston, B. J., Christensen, S., Maddock, Jr., R. K., and Tyler, F. H.: Low Protein Diets for the Treatment of Chronic Renal Failure. University of Utah Press, Salt Lake City, Utah, 1970.
2. Margie, J. D., Anderson, C. F., Nelson, R. A., and Hunt, J. C.: The Mayo Clinic Renal Diet Cookbook, Western Publishing Co., New York, N.Y. (in press).
3. Lewis, E. J., and Magill, J. W. (eds): Conference on the Nutritional Aspects of Uremia. *Amer. J. Clin. Nutrition, 21*:547–641, 1968.
4. Watt, B. D., and Merrill, A. L.: Composition of Foods: Raw, Processed, Prepared. Agriculture Handbook No. 8, U.S. Dept. Agriculture, Washington, D.C., 1963.
5. Giovanetti, S. and Maggiore, O.: A low nitrogen diet with proteins of high biological value for severe chronic uremia. *The Lancet, 1*:1000, 1965.
6. Shaw, A. B., Bazzard, F. J., Booth, E. M., Nilwarangkur, S., and Berlyne, G. M.: The Treatment of Chronic Renal Failure by a Modified Giovanetti Diet. *Quart. J. Med., 34*:237, 1965.
7. Polec, R.: Potato Diet in the Treatment of Chronic Renal Failure. *Polish Med. J., 6*:43–53, 1967.

Table A-13. Protein, Sodium, and Potassium Contents of Common Foods*

	Amount	Protein (grams)	Potassium (mEq)	Sodium (mEq)
Dairy Products				
Eggs, large or extra large	1	6.5	1.70	2.70
Cottage cheese, salt free	1 ounce	4.1	1.10	0.50
Cream, light	1 ounce	0.9	0.90	0.50
Cream, sour	1 ounce	0.9	0.90	0.50
Milk, butter (fluid culture)	1 ounce	1.0	1.00	1.60
Milk, regular	1 ounce	1.0	1.10	0.70
Milk, skimmed	1 ounce	1.1	1.10	0.70
Milk, low sodium	1 ounce	1.0	1.80	0.04
Butter or Fat				
Butter, sweet	1 pat	0.03	0.01	0.02
Corn or olive oil		—	—	—
Crisco	1 tsp			
French dressing, low-calorie	1 tsp	0.04	0.20	3.40
Margarine, salt free	1 pat	—	0.03	0.02
Mayonnaise	1 tsp	0.17	0.08	2.70
Cereal				
Bran flakes, 40%	½ cup	1.0	—	4.00
Corn flakes	½ cup	0.8	0.30	4.40
Cream of rice, salt free	1 serving	0.9	0.60	0.05
Cream of wheat, salt free	1 serving	1.8	0.30	0.01
Farina, salt free	1 serving	1.7	0.30	0.01
Oatmeal	1 serving	2.1	1.30	0.01
Puffed rice	½ cup	0.6	0.30	0.10
Puffed & shredded wheat	½ cup	1.5	0.90	0.10
Rice flakes	½ cup	0.6	0.50	4.30
Rice krispies	½ cup	0.6	0.30	0.10
Tapioca, salt free	1 serving	0.1	0.10	0.03
Bread, Cookies, Crackers				
Bread, regular	1 slice	1.7	0.50	4.40
Bread, salt free	1 slice	1.7	0.50	0.30
Bread, whole wheat	1 slice	2.1	1.40	4.60
Crackers, graham	2 squares	0.8	1.00	2.90
Crackers, salt free	3 squares	3.1	0.30	0.04
Crackers, saltines	1 square	0.4	0.10	1.90
English muffin	½	2.0	0.50	5.00
Roll, hard	½	1.5	0.60	6.80
Roll, soft	1	2.0	0.60	5.50
Roll, soft, salt free	1	1.7	0.50	0.30
Vanilla wafers	4	0.5	0.20	1.10

* Data from Watt, B. D., and Merrill, A. L. Composition of Foods—Raw, Processed, Prepared. U.S. Department of Agriculture Handbook No. 8, revised 1963.

Table A-13. (*Continued*)

	Amount	Protein (grams)	Potassium (mEq)	Sodium (mEq)
Meat, Fish				
Boiled beef, cooked	1 ounce	7.8	2.80	0.80
Chopped beef, lean	1 ounce	5.8	2.70	0.90
Filet Mignon	1 ounce	5.8	2.70	0.90
Chicken, dark, cooked	1 ounce	8.4	2.50	1.10
Chicken, white, cooked	1 ounce	9.7	2.30	0.60
Lamb, loin, raw	1 ounce	6.0	2.30	1.00
Turkey, dark, cooked	1 ounce	9.0	3.10	1.30
Turkey, white, cooked	1 ounce	9.8	3.10	1.00
Veal, lean, cooked	1 ounce	5.9	2.40	1.10
Bass, raw	1 ounce	5.6	†	†
Bluefish, raw	1 ounce	6.1	†	1.00
Cod, raw	1 ounce	5.2	2.90	0.90
Halibut, raw	1 ounce	5.9	†	†
Snapper, raw	1 ounce	5.9	2.40	0.80
Sole, raw	1 ounce	5.0	2.60	1.00
Tuna, regular	1 ounce	7.4	2.30	10.40
Tuna, salt free	1 ounce	8.4	2.10	0.50
Sweets				
Candy, hard, sour balls (Schrafft's)	—	—	—	—
Honey	½ tsp	—	0.10	0.01
Ice cream, regular	1 serving	2.3	2.40	1.40
Ice milk	1 serving	2.4	2.50	1.50
Jams	½ tsp	—	0.10	0.10
Sherbet (fruit ice)	1 serving	0.5	0.30	0.20
Sugar, brown		—	2.60	0.30
Sugar, white		—	—	—
Juices	3½ *ounces*			
Apple		0.1	2.59	0.04
Apricot		0.3	3.90	0.25
Cranberry		0.1	0.46	0.13
Grape		0.2	2.90	0.08
Grapefruit		0.5	4.10	0.04
Lemon		0.5	3.60	0.04
Orange, canned		0.8	5.10	0.04
Orange, fresh		0.6	5.82	0.04
Pear nectar		0.3	1.00	0.04
Pineapple		0.4	3.82	0.04
Prune		0.4	6.00	0.09
Raisin, cooked, liquid	(1 ounce)	0.4	2.70	0.16
Tomato		0.9	5.82	8.70
Tomato, salt free		0.8	5.82	0.13

† Data are inadequate or variable

Table A-13.　(*Continued*)

	Amount	Protein (grams)	Potassium (mEq)	Sodium (mEq)
Vegetables				
Asparagus	¾ cup or 1 serving	2.4	4.25	10.26
Asparagus, salt free	"	2.6	4.25	0.13
Beans, green	"	1.4	2.43	10.26
Beans, green, salt free	"	1.5	2.43	0.09
Beans, wax	"	1.4	2.43	10.26
Beets	"	1.0	4.28	10.26
Beets, salt free	"	0.9	4.28	2.00
Broccoli	"	3.1	5.64	0.52
Cabbage	"	0.5	2.05	0.30
Carrots	"	0.8	3.06	10.26
Carrots, fresh	"	1.1	8.74	2.04
Carrots, salt free	"	0.8	3.06	1.70
Celery, fresh	"	0.9	8.70	5.48
Cucumber, fresh	"	0.6	4.10	0.26
Peas, green	"	4.6	2.40	10.30
Peas, green, salt free	"	4.4	2.40	0.13
Tomato, fresh	"	1.1	6.25	0.13
Potato, boiled	"	2.1	10.50	0.13
Noodles, cooked	"	2.6	0.69	0.04
Rice, cooked	"	1.5	0.80	0.08
Fruits				
Apple	1 med/small	0.2	2.80	0.04
Applesauce	⅓ cup	0.2	1.70	0.09
Apricots, canned	3 halves	0.6	5.90	0.04
Banana	1 small 6"	1.1	9.50	0.04
Blueberries, frozen	1 ounce	0.2	0.50	0.01
Cherries, frozen	1 ounce	0.3	1.00	0.01
Grapefruit	½ med.	0.5	3.40	0.04
Orange, fresh	1 small	1.3	5.00	0.04
Peach, canned	2 halves	0.4	3.30	0.09
Pear, canned	2 halves	0.2	2.10	0.04
Pineapple, canned	1 large sl.	0.3	2.40	0.04
Strawberries, fresh	10 large	0.7	4.20	0.04
Strawberries, frozen	½ cup	0.5	2.90	0.04

Table A-14. Protein-Restricted and Potassium-Restricted Diets*

(30 gm. Protein, 20 mEq Potassium)

PURPOSE: This diet is designed for use in the feeding of patients with advanced renal disease where control of elevated blood urea and plasma phosphorus and potassium by dietary means is indicated.

Approximate Composition	Unit	Amount
Carbohydrate	gm	244
Protein	gm	30
Fat	gm	36
*Calories		1,350
Calcium	mg	178
Phosphorus	mg	385
Iron	mg	7.8
Sodium	mg. or mEq.	1,074 or 46.6
Potassium	mg. or mEq.	676.9 or 17.3
Vitamin A	I.U.	12,818.7
Thiamine	mg	.5
Riboflavin	mg	.6
Niacin-equivalents	mg	6.2
Ascorbic Acid	mg	75

ADEQUACY: This diet does not meet the 1968 Recommended Dietary Allowance of the National Research Council except for vitamin A and ascorbic acid. A vitamin supplement should be ordered by the physician. The calculations are based on the sample menu.

NOTE: To increase protein to 50–60 gm while maintaining restricted potassium add:

3½ oz. cheese: American, parmesan, Swiss or

2 oz. light meat chicken or

2 eggs or suitable combinations thereof.

* If additional calories are desired the following liquid formula or tapioca pudding may be advisable:

Liquid Formula: 125 gms. dextrose; 50 gms. egg; 40 gms. corn oil; 50 gms. lemon juice or other flavors; 20 gms. corn starch and 750 cc water may be ordered. This amount of formula will supply 1,000 calories, 6.7 gms. of protein, 3 mEq of potassium and 2 mEq. of sodium.

Pudding: 120 gms. tapioca; 100 gms. of dextrose; 120 gms. of sweet butter; 100 gms. of egg; 0.5 of methionine; 360 ml. of water and flavoring. This will supply: 1,855 calories, 14.3 gms. of protein, 4 mEq. of potassium and 6 mEq of sodium.

These preparations may be used by the physician to replace the diet in whole or in part as the clinical situation warrants. Sodium or other nutrients must be ordered as indicated.

* Modified from Diet Manual, Memorial Sloan-Kettering Cancer Center, New York, N.Y. Revised 1967, courtesy Dietary Department.

Table A-14.   (*Continued*)

Type of Food	*Amount*	*Food Included*	*Food Excluded*
Milk	None	None	Whole milk; skim milk; buttermilk; malted milk
Other beverages	2 cups	Ginger ale; Pepsi Cola; root beer; Seven Up; Koolade (unrestricted amounts)	Coca Cola; cocoa; * coffee; Postum; Sanka; tea * One cup of coffee may be included if ordered by physician.
Soup	None	None	All soups
Meat, poultry, fish	1½	Beef; chicken; lamb; pork; turkey; beef; calves and chicken liver; beef heart; beef kidney; cooked bacon (6 slices); sweetbreads; canned salmon; canned tunafish; codfish; clams; canned crabmeat; lobster; haddock; perch; oysters; shad; shrimp; red snapper; whitefish; whiting	Meat extracts; halibut; canned sardines; scallops; veal. All others not listed as allowed
	And		
Cheese	¼ cup	Cottage cheese	All others not listed as allowed
	Or		
	1½ oz.	Cheddar cheese; cream cheese; Camembert cheese; Swiss cheese	All others not listed as allowed
	Or		
Eggs	1 (in place of cheese)	Any type prepared without milk.	None
Potato substitute	1 serving ½ cup	Enriched white rice; macaroni; noodles; spaghetti	All potatoes—white; sweet; canned potatoes; potato chips; brown rice
Bread	3 slices	Enriched white bread; saltines (5 only)	Rye bread; whole wheat bread; all those not listed as allowed

Table A-14. (*Continued*)

Type of Food	Amount	Food Included	Food Excluded
Cereal	1 serving $\frac{1}{2}$ cup	Cream of wheat; farina; hominy grits all served without milk	All others not listed as allowed
Vegetables	2 servings $\frac{1}{2}$ cup	Cooked or raw cabbage; fresh, frozen or canned green beans; canned carrots; cucumbers (6 slices); lettuce (2 leaves); canned peas; fresh or canned wax beans	All others not listed as allowed
Fruit	2 servings ($\frac{1}{2}$ cup)	Canned—applesauce; blueberries; Royal Anne cherries; peaches; pears; pineapple; grapefruit sections; fresh—blackberries; raspberries; strawberries; pineapple; grapes; apple; cherries; frozen—raspberries; strawberries; cranberry sauce	All dried fruits; all others not listed as allowed
Fruit juice	2 servings $\frac{1}{2}$ cup	Cranberry juice; frozen lemonade; frozen limeade	All others not listed as allowed
Butter or fat	6 tsp.	Butter; margarine; mayonnaise; corn oil (unrestricted amounts)	Cream gravies; all others not listed as allowed
Desserts	1 serving $\frac{1}{2}$ cup	Gelatin made with Koolade and sugar; dietetic gelatin (D'Zerta); lime ice	Commercial Jell-O; all others not listed as allowed
Sweets	In moderation	Gum drops; hard candy; marshmallows; white sugar; white syrup	Brown sugar; maple syrup; chocolate; molasses; jams; jellies; all others not listed as allowed
Spices	As desired	White pepper; vanilla; vinegar; peppermint extract; salt; nutmeg; cinnamon; mace	All others not listed as allowed
Miscellaneous			Nuts; olives; pickles; catsup; coconut; peanut butter; baker's yeast

Example of DIETARY PATTERN for Protein and Potassium Restricted Diet

30 gm. Protein, 20 mEq Potassium

Breakfast	Serving Portion	Sample Menu
Fruit	$\frac{1}{2}$ cup	Cranberry juice
Cereal	$\frac{1}{2}$ cup cooked	Farina
Bread	1 slice	Enriched white toast
Fat	2 tsps.	Butter or margarine
Sugar	1 tbsp.	Sugar

Lunch		
Meat substitute	1 medium	Soft cooked egg
Potato substitute	$\frac{1}{2}$ cup cooked	Unsalted white rice
Vegetable	$\frac{1}{2}$ cup	Green beans
Bread	1 slice	Enriched white bread
Fat	2 tsps.	Butter or margarine
Beverage	1 cup	Pepsi Cola
Dessert	$\frac{1}{2}$ cup	Canned blueberries

Dinner		
Meat	$1\frac{1}{2}$ oz.	Roast beef
Vegetable	$\frac{1}{2}$ cup	Canned carrots
Fruit	$\frac{1}{2}$ cup	Applesauce
Bread	1 slice	Enriched white bread
Fat	2 tsps.	Butter or margarine
Dessert	$\frac{1}{2}$ cup	Lime ice

8 P.M.		
Fruit Juice	$\frac{1}{2}$ cup	Frozen lemonade

Table A-15. Diet I for Peptic Ulcer Therapy*

PURPOSE: To minimize gastric acid secretion and activity in a patient with acute bleeding peptic ulcer or one who is severely ill with ulcer symptoms. This milk or milk and cream diet is given for a limited number of days to be specified by the physician.

Approximate Composition	Unit	Gastric I (skim milk) 1,400 ml	Gastric I (milk) 1,400 ml	Gastric I (milk & cream) 700 ml & 700 ml
Carbohydrate	gm	71	69	64
Protein	gm	50	49	45
Fat	gm	1.4	49	169
Calories		500	911	1,958
Calcium	mg	1,694	1,652	1,540
Phosphorus	mg	1,330	1,302	1,211
Iron	mg	trace	trace	trace
Sodium	mg(mEq)	708(31)	702(31)	6,408(28)
Potassium	mg(mEq)	2,074(53)	2,020(52)	1,856(48)
Magnesium	mg(mEq)	196(16)	182(15)	168(14)
Vitamin A	I.U.	trace	1,960	6,860
Thiamine	mg	.5	.4	.4
Riboflavin	mg	2.6	2.4	2.3
Niacin equivalents	mg	1.4	1.4	1.4
Ascorbic acid	mg	14	14	14

ADEQUACY: These diets do not meet the 1968 Recommended Dietary Allowances of the National Research Council for any of the nutrients except calcium and riboflavin and for vitamin A when whole milk or cream is used.

Diet I (with milk, skim or whole): This routine consists solely of milk. When this routine is ordered 90 ml of milk are served on the hour from 7 A.M. to 10 P.M., inclusive, totaling 1400 ml daily.

Diet I (with milk & cream): This routine consists solely of milk and light cream (half & half). When this routine is ordered 45 ml of milk and 45 ml light cream are served on the hour from 7 A.M. to 10 P.M., inclusive, totaling 1400 ml daily.

* Modified from Diet Manual, Memorial Sloan-Kettering Cancer Center, New York, N.Y. Revised 1969, courtesy Dietary Department.

Table A-16. Diet II for Peptic Ulcer Therapy*

PURPOSE: To advance the symptomatic peptic ulcer patient to a more nutritious diet for a *limited* period. When hyperlipidemia or pyloric obstruction with gastric retention is of concern, skim milk is recommended.

This routine consists of 120 ml milk or 60 ml milk and 60 ml light cream given hourly from 7 A.M. to 10 P.M. inclusive, plus 1, 3 or 6 supplements as ordered by the physician. Sugar and salt are permitted in moderation.

When 1 or 3 supplements are ordered they are served at meal time and are selected from the following list:

> Eggs—poached or soft cooked
> Cream of Wheat, Farina, strained oatmeal
> Milk toast
> Junket, custard and gelatin desserts without fruit
> Strained cream soup, prepared without meat stock

When 6 supplements are ordered they are served at meal hours as well as at 10 A.M., 3 and 8 P.M. Additional foods are selected from the following list:

> Cottage cheese
> White toast and butter
> Vanilla ice cream, blanc mange, rice, tapioca, bread and cream puddings, except chocolate
> Vanilla wafers
> Plain soda crackers and
> Steamed rice with butter

---

* From Diet Manual, Memorial Sloan-Kettering Cancer Center, New York, N.Y. Revised 1969, courtesy Dietary Department.

Table A-17. Bland Six-Feeding Diet with Increased Polyunsaturated Fats*

PURPOSE: A diet with decreased saturated and increased polyunsaturated fats which is low in spices and other gastric secretagogues; it is designed for use in gastrointestinal disturbances such as peptic esophagitis, peptic ulcer or gastritis.

Approximate Composition	Unit	Amount
Carbohydrate	gm	280
Protein	gm	112
Fat	gm	69
Calories		2,134
Calcium	mg	1,443
Phosphorus	mg	1,890
Iron	mg	12.9
Sodium	mg or mEq	2,235 or 97
Potassium	mg or mEq	3,833 or 98
Vitamin A	I.U.	11,540
Thiamine	mg	1.4
Riboflavin	mg	2.9
Niacin-equivalents	mg	22.5
Ascorbic acid	mg	143

ADEQUACY: This diet meets all 1968 Recommended Dietary Allowances of the National Research Council for adults. The calculations are based on sample meal plan.

* Modified from Diet Manual, Memorial Sloan-Kettering Cancer Center, New York, N.Y. Revised 1969, courtesy Dietary Department.

GENERAL INSTRUCTIONS:

1. Eat slowly.
2. Meals at same hour each day.
3. If possible, relax a few minutes before and after each meal.
4. Eat frequent small meals, never skip meals.
5. In-between nourishments must be included.

Bland Six Feeding

Type of Food	Amount	Food Included	Food Excluded
Bread	4 svgs.	White bread; white rolls without seeds, plain or toasted; soda crackers; saltines; melba toast; rusk, zwieback; skim milk toast	Whole wheat and rye bread; biscuits; cornbread; English muffins; rolls or muffins to which seeds, raisins, coconut or nuts have been added; whole grain crackers
Cereal	1 svg.	Refined such as rice, Cream of Wheat, Farina, hominy grits, cornmeal; cornflakes; Rice Krispies; puffed rice; Corn Kixs; strained oatmeal	Whole grain cereals; bran; all those not listed as allowed
Vegetables	2 svgs. include 1 green or yellow	Soft cooked asparagus tips; beets; carrots; green or wax beans; peas; pumpkin (not spiced); spinach; winter squash; tomato or vegetable juice without added spices; pureed lima beans, tomatoes, corn	Raw vegetables; all cooked vegetables except those listed as allowed
Fruit and fruit juice	3 svgs.	Cooked or canned without skin or seeds; apples; apricots; peaches; pears; cooked or canned Royal Anne or Bing cherries; fruit puree; ripe banana; avocado; all juices. Include one citrus daily: ex. orange, grapefruit or tangerine juice taken at end of meal.	Cooked or canned fruits with skin or seeds; canned grapefruit, orange and pineapple; raw and frozen fruits except banana and avocado; melons; berries; dried fruits unless pureed; all those not listed as allowed
Butter or fat	4 svgs.	Polyunsaturated margarine; vegetable oils; homemade mayonnaise without mustard or spices.	Spiced salad dressings; commercial mayonnaise; cream; butter
Dessert	1 svg.	Plain rice, tapioca, white bread-puddings and custard made with skim milk; blanc mange; plain and flavored gelatin; junket, vanilla, banana, lemon; ice milk sherbets; and ices (eaten slowly); plain or iced cakes; sugar cookies; vanilla wafers; sponge cake; angel food cake; pound cake	Pies; pastries; cakes; cookies and desserts containing fruits as listed above, raisins, coconut, seeds, nuts or chocolate; all those not listed as allowed
Sweets	Used in moderation	Sugar; sugar syrup; honey; molasses; jelly; gumdrops; marshmallows and fruit flavored hard candy occasionally after meals; strained cranberry jelly	Chocolate; preserves; jams; rich sauces; excessive amounts of sweets

Bland Six Feedings *(Continued)*

Type of Food	*Amount*	*Food Included*	*Food Excluded*
Spices		Cinnamon; lemon; parsley; salt; vanilla; other spices taken only with physician's permission	Spices and condiments such as pepper; catsup; chili sauce; vinegar; mustard; garlic; horseradish; Worcestershire sauce; all others not listed as allowed
Miscellaneous		Cream sauces without added spices, made with skim milk and polyunsaturated margarine; smooth peanut butter in moderation	Olives; pickles; Fritos; popcorn; pretzels; potato chips; nuts; fried foods; gravies; ice; all those not listed as allowed. Very hot or very cold foods or fluids should be avoided.
Milk	1 qt.	Fat-free buttermilk; skim milk; skim milk beverages; non-dairy coffee whiteners	Whole milk; chocolate flavored beverages; cocoa
Other beverages	As desired	Postum; weak tea and Sanka if allowed by physician	Coffee, tea and Sanka if not permitted by physician; cocoa; carbonated beverages; chocolate; beer; wine; all alcoholic drinks
Soup	1 svg. $\frac{1}{2}$ cup	Strained creamed soup only, prepared with allowed vegetables and skim milk	Broth; all canned, dried and frozen soups
Meat, fish, poultry	1 svg. 3 oz	Tender beef; lamb; with visible fat removed, liver; sweetbreads; cooked medium to well done, chicken or turkey without skin; fish and shellfish, fresh, frozen or canned without bones or skin; crisp bacon	Smoked, pickled or cured meat or seafood; fried meats, poultry, fish or seafood; pork; luncheon meats; frankfurters and sausages; clams; all those not listed as allowed.
Cheese	As desired	Skim milk or fat-free cottage, ricotta, farmer and pot cheese; low-fat cream cheese; mild cheese; cheddar cheese may be used in cooking	Sharp or spicy cheeses
Eggs	One	Poached, medium or hard cooked; soft scrambled in double boiler; baked omelet	Fried eggs
Potato or substitute	2 svgs.	Potatoes, baked (served without skin), boiled, mashed, with skim milk riced; mashed sweet potatoes or yams; white rice; macaroni, noodles, spaghetti with vegetable margarine, plain or tomato puree	Skin of potato; fried potatoes; whole grain rice; potato chips; lentils

Example of DIETARY PATTERN for Bland Six Feeding Diet

Breakfast	*Serving Portions*	*Sample Menu*
Fruit	½ cup	Orange juice
Cereal	½ cup	Farina, enriched
Egg	1	Soft cooked egg
Bread	1 slice	White toast, enriched
Polyunsaturated margarine	1 tsp	Polyunsaturated margarine
Skim milk	½ cup	Skim milk
Beverage	1 cup	Postum
Sugar	1 tbsp	Sugar
10 A.M.		
Bread	1 slice	White toast, enriched
Polyunsaturated margarine	1 tsp	Polyunsaturated margarine
Skim milk or fat-free buttermilk	½ cup	Skim milk or fat-free buttermilk
Lunch		
Lean meat	3 oz	Broiled chicken
Potato	1	Baked potato (no skin)
Vegetable	½ cup	Asparagus tips
Fruit	½ cup	Canned cherries
Bread	1 slice	White bread, enriched
Polyunsaturated margarine	1 tsp	Polyunsaturated margarine
Skim milk or fat-free buttermilk	½ cup	Skim milk or fat-free buttermilk
3 P.M.		
Fruit	½ cup	Applesauce
Skim milk or fat-free buttermilk	1 cup	Skim milk or fat-free buttermilk
Dinner		
Soup	½ cup	Strained cream of mushroom soup, made with skim milk
Lean meat	3 oz	Roast beef
Potato	1 serving	Boiled potato
Vegetable	½ cup	Carrots
Bread	1 slice	White gread, enriched
Polyunsaturated margarine	1 tsp	Polyunsaturated margarine
Skim milk or fat-free buttermilk	½ cup	Skim milk or fat-free buttermilk
8 P.M.		
Dessert	1 serving	White cake
Skim milk or fat-free buttermilk	1 cup	Skim milk or fat-free buttermilk

Table A-18. Gluten-Low Diet*

PURPOSE: This diet is designed for the treatment of patients with gluten enteropathy (i.e. sprue, celiac disease), a malabsorption syndrome caused by sensitivity to gluten or its products. Gluten is a protein-fraction present in all cereals other than rice and corn, therefore, gluten-containing cereals must be eliminated.

Approximate Composition	Unit	Amount	
Carbohydrate	gm	245	
Protein	gm	109	
Fat	gm	86	
Calories		2,148	
Calcium	mg	1,217	
Phosphorus	mg	1,688	
Iron	mg	13.2	
Sodium	mg (mEq)	2,536	(110.2)
Potassium	mg (mEq)	4,389	(112.5)
Vitamin A	I.U.	11,006	
Thiamine	mg	1.4	
Riboflavin	mg	2.2	
Niacin-equivalents	mg	23.7	
Ascorbic acid	mg	216.5	

ADEQUACY: This diet meets the 1968 Recommended Dietary Allowances for adults of the National Research Council. The calculations are based on the sample menu.

CAUTION: Gluten may be present in foods either as a basic ingredient or as a result of preparation or processing. *READING LABELS CAREFULLY IS VERY IMPORTANT.* However, the label alone cannot be fully relied upon as gluten may be present as an incidental ingredient. AVOID any food or seasoning that lists as ingredients: hydrolyzed vegetable protein, malt and malt flavorings, starch (unless specified as corn, tapioca or potato starch). Flavorings, vegetable gum, hydrolyzed plant protein, emulsifiers and stabilizers may be derived from or contain wheat, rye, oats, or barley. Foods of unknown composition should be omitted, the manufacturer should be contacted for complete ingredient information, or inquiry may be made to Mrs. Elaine I. Hartsook, Metabolic Research Dietitian, Clinical Research Center—RC-14, University Hospital, University of Washington, Seattle, Washington, 98105. Mrs. Hartsook has compiled a detailed list and evaluation of commercial preparations for gluten content.

* From Diet Manual, Memorial Sloan-Kettering Cancer Center, New York, N.Y. Revised 1969, courtesy Dietary Department.

Table A-18.   Gluten-Low Diet   *(Continued)*

Read labels on all packaged and prepared foods.

Type of Food	*Food Included*	*Food Excluded*
Milk	Milk; skim milk; buttermilk; yogurt; flavored, if desired	Malted milk; beverage made with chocolate; cocoa and cocoa syrup if wheat flour has been added; ovaltine
Other beverages	Coffee (made from ground coffee); tea; carbonated beverages; alcoholic beverages, except beer and ale	Postum, beer, ale; read labels on instant coffee to see that no wheat flour has been added
Soup	All clear and vegetable soups; cream or milk soups thickened with corn-starch or potato flour only	All canned soups except clear broth; all cream soups unless thickened with cornstarch or potato flour
Meat, poultry	All meat; poultry or fish; creamed or served with thickened gravy if made with cornstarch or potato flour	Meat patties; or meat; fish or chicken loaf made with bread or bread crumbs; croquettes; breaded meats, fish or chicken; chili con carne and other canned meat dishes. Cold cuts unless guaranteed pure meat; bread stuffings. All gravies or cream sauces thickened with wheat flour
Cheese	All cheeses	None
Egg	All types	None
Potato or substitute	Potato or rice, prepared any way; creamed only if cream sauce is made with cornstarch or potato flour	Macaroni; noodles; spaghetti; dumplings and any others not listed as allowed
Bread	Bread made from rice;* corn; soy beans; arrowroot and gluten-free wheat starch only	All bread; rolls; crackers; cake and cookies made from wheat or rye; Rye-Krisp; muffins; biscuits, waffles; pancake flour and other prepared mixes; rusks; zweiback; pretzels; any product containing oatmeal; barley or buckwheat. Breaded foods; bread crumbs; arrowroot crackers and cookies unless made with wheat-free starch.

* Rice bread recipe is given at the conclusion of this section

Table A-18. Gluten-Low Diet *(Continued)*

Type of Food	Food Included	Food Excluded
Cereal	Cornmeal; hominy; cream of rice; puffed rice; rice and tapioca	All wheat; oat and rye cereals, wheat germ; barley; oatmeal; buckwheat; kasha; cornflakes; Rice Krispies
Vegetables	All cooked, canned, frozen or raw including one dark green leafy or yellow. Creamed only if cream sauce is made with cornstarch or potato flour	Any prepared with cream sauce except when thickened with cornstarch or potato flour; any prepared with bread crumbs
Fruit and fruit juice	All, including one citrus fruit or juice daily	None
Butter or fat	Butter; cream; margarine; oils; cooking fats; pure mayonnaise and homemade salad dressing which does not contain flour	Commercial salad dressings except pure mayonnaise. Read labels
Dessert	Jell-O; fruit Jell-O; ice or sherbet; ice cream that is gluten free (Sealtest; Breyer's; Schrafft's); custard; junket; rice pudding; cornstarch pudding (homemade) or blanc mange, if thickened with cornstarch	Cakes; cookies; pastry containing gluten. Other commercial ice cream; ice cream cones; prepared mixes; puddings. All homemade puddings thickened with wheat flour
Sweets	Sugar; white or brown; molasses; jellies; jams; honey; corn syrup	Commercial candies containing cereal products; cocoa and chocolate (read label)
Spices	Salt; spices; accent; (monosodium glutamate)	Soy sauce; Worcestershire sauce
Miscellaneous		Mushrooms, nuts, peanut butter, malt

Example of DIETARY PATTERN for Gluten-Low Diet

Breakfast	*Sample Menu*
Fruit	Orange juice
Cereal	Puffed rice
Egg	Soft cooked egg
Bread	Rice bread
Fat	Butter or margarine
Milk	Milk
Beverage	Coffee
Sugar	Sugar

Lunch	
Meat or substitute	Broiled chicken
Potato or substitute	Baked potato
Vegetable	Asparagus
Salad	Sliced tomato
Dessert	Custard
Bread	Rice bread
Fat	Butter or margarine
Milk	Milk
Beverage	Coffee
Sugar	Sugar

Dinner	
Soup	Bouillon
Meat or substitute	Roast beef
Potato or substitute	Boiled potato
Vegetable	Brussels sprouts
Salad	Carrot sticks
Fruit	Canned apricots
Fat	Butter or margarine
Beverage	Coffee
Sugar	Sugar

8 P.M.	
Fruit	Applesauce
Bread	Rice bread
Cheese	American cheese
Vegetable	Leaf lettuce

Rice Bread—Low Gluten*

Ingredients	Measure	Grams
Rice flour	2 cups	300
Salt	1 tsp	7
Baking powder (Royal)	6 tsp	28
Corn oil	8 tbsp	100
Sugar	8 tbsp	100
Egg yolks	4	70
Milk	1 cup	258
Egg whites	4	112

Per —	CH_2O	33.0 gm	K	2.8 mEq
100	Protein	6.2 gm	Na	36.6 mEq
gms.	Fat	12.6 gm	P	117.8 mg
	Ca	80.0 mg	Cl	36.6 mEq
	Mg	2.0 mg	N	1.0 gm

Directions: Beat egg yolks until thick and creamy; slowly beat in sugar and corn oil. Mix dry ingredients: salt, rice flour and baking powder. Add alternately, milk and dry ingredients. Beat all together; fold in stiffly beaten egg whites. Pour into greased pan. Bake in pre-heated oven, 400°, approximately 20–25 minutes. Wet weight of batter, 975 gms; after baking approximately 800 gms.

* Courtesy: Metabolic Research Kitchen, Memorial Sloan-Kettering Cancer Center, New York, N.Y.

Table A-19. Fat Restricted Diets, 20 and 40 gm* †

PURPOSE: These diets are designed for patients with serious diseases of the biliary tract or pancreas or with malabsorption syndromes other than that caused by gluten sensitivity where a reduced fat intake may decrease diarrhea and nutrient losses. Medium-chain-length triglycerides (MCT) may be added to this diet in various recipes**. Pancreatic extract should be given where indicated.

Approximate Composition	Unit	20 Gm.	40 Gm.
Carbohydrate	gm	391	369
Protein	gm	91	98
Fat	gm	21	42
Saturated fatty acid	gm	6	14
Unsaturated fatty acid	gm	7	19
Calories		2,057	2,198
Calcium	mg	979	925
Phosphorus	mg	1,370	1,490
Iron	mg	14	16
Sodium	mg (mEq.)	2,744 (115)	2,740 (115)
Potassium	mg (mEq.)	3,272 (84)	3,422 (88)
Vitamin A	I.U.	12,000	13,000
Thiamine	mg	1.5	1.5
Riboflavin	mg	2.2	2.4
Niacin equivalents	mg	19	23
Ascorbic acid	mg	122	123

ADEQUACY: These diets meet the 1968 Recommended Dietary Allowances for adults of the National Research Council. The calculations are based on the sample menu with an average weekly figure used for protein foods.

  † The 20 gm Restricted Fat Diet contains approximately 6 gm saturated fatty acids or 27.9% of the total fat; 7 gm polyunsaturated fatty acids or 34% of the total fat. The 40 gm. Restricted Diet contains 14 gm saturated fatty acids or 33% of the total fat, 19 gm. polyunsaturated fatty acids or 44.8% of the total fat.

  The 40 gm will be decreased to 20 gm by omitting the egg and 1 teaspoon fat, reducing the meat allowance from 6 oz to 3 oz and adding 4 oz fat free cottage cheese.

  ** MCT oil may be added to this diet to increase calories as potentially absorbable fat. For information and recipes on MCT see: Medium-Chain-Triglycerides, Senior, J. R. (ed.), Univ. of Penna. Press, 1968.

* From Diet Manual, Memorial Sloan-Kettering Cancer Center, New York, N.Y. Revised 1969, courtesy Dietary Department.

Table A-19   (*Continued*)

20 and 40 Gm. Fat Diets

Type of Food	Amount	Food Included	Food Excluded
Milk	1 Pt.	Skim milk; fat-free buttermilk	Whole milk; cultured buttermilk; chocolate milk; yogurt
Other beverages	As desired	Coffee; tea; Sanka; Postum; carbonated beverages	All alcoholic beverages; Ovaltine; chocolate; flavored drinks; cocoa
Soup	As desired	Fat free bouillon or broth; tomato bouillon; vegetable soup; skim milk soup	Any soup containing cream, fat or whole milk
Meat, poultry	6 oz. cooked weights for 40 gm. diet; 2 oz. for 20 gm. diet	All broiled, boiled, baked or cooked without fat in a Teflon pan. All visible fat must be removed	Pork; ham; bacon; duck; goose; salami; pastrami; bologna; frankfurter; sausages; luncheon meats; frozen or canned meat dishes
OR			
Fish		Meat and fish may be wrapped in foil before broiling or baking in order to retain juices	
		Lean cuts of beef; Canadian bacon; lamb; liver; veal; white meat of chicken and turkey, remove skin before cooking; organ meats	
		All fish, including canned pink salmon and sardines in tomato sauce, except those listed as not allowed	Fish canned in oil (sardines, tunafish); frozen fish sticks; fresh or frozen salmon
Cheese	40 gm diet: as desired; 20 gm diet: additional 4 oz to replace meat portion	Fat free cottage cheese, pot cheese; other skim milk cheese	All others
Eggs	40 gm diet: 1 daily; omit on 20 gm diet	Medium or hard cooked; poached; scrambled in double boiler; cooked without fat in a Teflon pan; egg whites as desired	More than 1 daily; eggs fried in fat
Potato or substitute	2–3 svgs.	Baked; boiled; mashed without whole milk or fat; rice; spaghetti; macaroni; hominy	Escalloped or creamed potatoes; fried potatoes; potato chips; oven browned potatoes; egg noodles

Table A-19. *(Continued)*

20 and 40 Gm. Fat Diets—*Continued*

Type of Food	Amount	Food Included	Food Excluded
Bread	5 svgs.	White; whole wheat; rye; French; hard rolls; soft rolls; matzoth; rye crisp; saltines; Uneeda biscuits, melba toast	All other breads and rolls quickbreads; biscuits; popovers; muffins; egg matzoth; butter-crackers
Cereals	1 svg.	All cooked and dry cereals	None
Vegetables	3 or more svgs. including 1 green or yellow	All fresh; frozen or canned vegetables prepared without cream sauce; fats or oils	Creamed vegetables or vegetables prepared with fat or oil
Fruit and fruit juice	4 or more svgs. including citrus or tomato	All fresh; frozen; canned and stewed except avocado and coconut, all fruit juices	Avocado and coconut
Butter or Fats	40 gm diet, 1 tsp. if tolerated; 20 gm diet omit	One of the following may be substituted for 1 tsp. of butter or margarine: light cream 2 tbsp. heavy cream 1 tbsp. French dressing 1 tbsp. mayonnaise 1 tsp. oil 1 tsp.	More than 1 teaspoon of butter or margarine, no gravies
Dessert	In moderation	Plain angel food cake, vanilla wafers, lady-fingers, arrowroot-cookies, graham crackers, meringues, jello, junket, cornstarch, rice and tapioca pudding made with skim milk and egg-whites. Water ices, fruit whips made with gelatin or egg whites	All other cakes, pies, doughnuts, cookies, puddings, pastry, ice cream, puddings made with whole milk and egg yolks, or eggs
Sweets	In moderation	Sugar, honey, jelly, jam, marmalade, molasses, maple syrup and sugar, sour balls, gum drops, jelly beans, marshmallows, hard candy and fondant	Chocolate, chocolate candy, chocolate syrup, candy made with cream, cocoa fats and nuts
Spices		Salt, paprika, herbs, mustard, nutmeg	Pepper
Miscellaneous		Catsup, chili sauce, vinegar, pickles, garlic, unbuttered popcorn, white sauce made with skim milk, vanilla	Olives, nuts, peanut butter, apple butter, cream sauces, gravies, buttered popcorn, waffles, pancakes, fritters

Example of DIETARY PATTERN for 40 Gm. Fat Diet

Breakfast	*Serving Portion*	*Sample Menu*
Fruit	½ cup	Orange Juice
Cereal	½ cup	Wheatena
Egg	1	Soft Boiled
Bread	2 slices	White Bread
Jelly	1 tbsp.	Jelly
Milk, Skimmed	1 cup	Skim Milk
Beverage	As desired	Coffee
Sugar	1 tbsp.	Sugar

Lunch		
Meat	3 ounces	Sliced White Chicken
Potato Substitute	1 cup	Rice
Vegetables	1 serving	Carrots
Salad	1 serving	Sliced Tomato
Bread	2 slices	White Bread
Fat	1 teaspoon	Mayonnaise
Skimmed Milk	½ cup	Skim Milk
Beverage	1 cup	Tea
Sugar	1 tbsp	Sugar
Dessert	1 serving	Canned Peaches

Dinner		
Soup	½ cup	Bouillon
Meat	3 ounces	Broiled Steak
Potato	1 serving	Baked Potato
Vegetables	1 serving	Steamed Green Beans
Salad	1 serving	Celery Hearts
Bread	1 serving	Hard Roll
Jelly	1 tablespoon	Honey or Jelly
Skimmed Milk	½ cup	Skim milk
Beverage	1 cup	Coffee
Sugar	1 tablespoon	Sugar
Dessert	1 serving	Raspberry Jell-O

9 P.M.		
Fruit	1	Raw Apple

Table A-20. Diet List to be Given Allergic Patient

This diet is not to be continued indefinitely without supervision. (Report for a possible revision at the end of 4 weeks.)

Avoid those foods which have been crossed out. Use all other foods.

Dairy Products

Milk, cream, ice cream, sherbets, milk soups and other milk-containing foods (see Milk-poor Diet below).

Butter, cheese, except cream cheese and cottage cheese.

Egg, unless hard boiled for ten minutes, and egg-containing foods, as griddle cakes, waffles, egg sauce, etc. (see Egg-poor Diet below).

Meat and Fish

Chicken, duck, goose, turkey.
Bacon, crisp; smoked ham.
Fresh pork and pork sausage, lard.
Lamb (roast, chops, kidneys).
Beef (roast, steak, calves liver, chipped beef); all beef products.
Veal (roast, chops, kidneys).
Shellfish, except oyster.
Fish (see Seafood-free Diet below).

Cereals or Breadstuffs

Wheat and wheat products, as macaroni, noodles, spaghetti, Cream of Wheat, Wheatena, Shredded Wheat, Bran Flakes, cookies, cakes, etc. (see Wheat-poor Diet below).

Rye (pure rye bread, Rye Krisp).
Corn (cornmeal muffins, cornflakes, Farina, hominy).
Rice (also Rice Flakes, Cream of Rice cereal).
Oats, oatmeal
Barley
Soybean flour
Arrowroot
Tapioca

Vegetables

Artichokes	Eggplant	Pumpkin
Asparagus	Endive	Radish, horse
Beans, all types	Green pea	radish
Beets	Green pepper	Spinach
Broccoli	Lentils	Squash
Brussels sprouts	Lettuce	String beans
Cabbage, sauer-	Mushroom	Sweet corn
kraut	Mustard	Sweet potato
Carrots	Okra	Tomato
Cauliflower	Onion (baked or	Turnip
Celery	boiled)	Watercress
Chicory	Parsley	White potato
Cucumber	Parsnip	(baked)

Fruits

Apples	Grapefruit	Plums
Apricots	Grapes	Prunes
Avocado	Honeydew melon	Raisins
Banana	Lemon	Rhubarb
Berries	Lime	Strawberry
Cherries	Orange	Tangerine
Cranberries	Peaches	Watermelon
Cantaloupe	Pears	
Date	Pineapple	
Fig		

Table A-20. Diet List to be Given Allergic Patient (*Continued*)

Beverages

All alcoholic drinks, including beer, ale, wine.
Chocolate, cocoa.
Coffee, tea, cola drinks.

Miscellaneous

Nuts, peanut butter (see Nut-poor Diet below).
Condiments, highly spiced foods.
Foods fried in vegetable oils such as cottonseed, peanut and corn oils.
Excessively sweet foods.
Intensely cold foods or drinks.
Olives, pure olive oil.
Gelatin.
Permitted foods should not be used constantly, but, whenever possible, in rotation.

Milk-poor Diet

Avoid:

Milk, buttermilk, cream, as such and in prepared foods, as ice cream, sodas, milk
   sherbet, Bavarian cream mousses, custards, gravies, cream sauces, soups,
   chowders.
Prepared flour mixes for home cooking.
Malted milk, hot chocolate or cocoa prepared with milk.
Cheese.
Evaporated, powdered, condensed milk (bakery products, as pies, breads and cakes
   containing small amounts of cooked milk can often be tolerated).
Butter and oleomargarine can usually be permitted in modest amounts.
Study the label on packaged foods for evidence of milk or milk products content.

Egg-poor Diet

Avoid:

Eggs: Fresh, frozen, powdered, cooked in any form.
Egg-containing foods, such as:
   Soups, broths made with egg.
   Prepared flour mixes for home cooking.
   Waffles, doughnuts, pretzels.
   Pancakes, griddle cakes, pastries, French toast.
   Macaroons, meringues, frostings.
   Cakes, cookies, unless known to be egg-free.
   Breads with glazed crust.
   Foods breaded with egg mixture.
   Sausages, croquettes, meat cakes, containing egg as binder.
   Poultry, especially chicken, if fricasseed or in broth.
   Salad dressings, unless known to be egg-free; Hollandaise, mayonnaise, and egg
      sauces.
   Ice cream and sherbets, unless known to be egg-free.
   Custards, cream candies, fondants, Bavarian cream.
   Marshmallows.
   Baking powder containing egg white.
   Prepared drinks containing egg or egg powder for insomnia or underweight.
   Study the labels on packaged foods for evidence of egg in any form.
   Avoid vaccine made in egg, as for influenza, spotted fever, yellow fever.

Table A-20. Diet List to be Given Allergic Patient *(Continued)*

Seafood-free Diet

Avoid:

Fish, shellfish, fresh, canned, smoked, pickled; fish liver oils, and concentrates in vitamin preparations.

Fish and shellfish stews, bisques, broths, soups, salad, hors d'oeuvres, caviar.

Avoid licking labels, which may contain a fish glue adhesive.

Avoid injections of fish origin in the treatment of varicose veins.

Wheat-poor Diet

Avoid:

White, whole wheat, cracked wheat flour in breads, waffles, griddle cakes, doughnuts, muffins, pastries, pies, cakes, crackers, spaghetti, macaroni, dumplings, pretzels, zwieback, noodles.

Corn bread, unless known to be wheat-free.

Soy bread, unless known to be wheat-free.

Rye bread, unless known to be wheat-free.

Gluten bread.

Breakfast cereals, dry or cooked, containing wheat, whole wheat, cream soups, Farina or bran.

Custards, gravies, sauces containing wheat.

Breaded foods prepared with wheat.

Coffee substitutes containing wheat; beer; ale.

Prepared meats, as sausages, frankfurters, meat loaf, croquettes made with wheat.

Prepared mixes for biscuits, muffins, pastries, pie crusts, cookies.

Study the label on prepared foods for evidences of wheat or wheat product content.

Nut-poor Diet

Avoid:

Nuts, of all types, also peanuts (although a member of the bean family), cottonseed meal in health and laxative breads, soybean bread.

Nut crumbs on cookies, cake icings, ice cream.

Candies containing nuts.

Salad oils, lard substitutes, margarines made of cocoanut, soybean, cottonseed or peanut oils (many are so made). (Olive oil permitted.)

Individuals highly sensitive to nuts are often allergic to seeds, such as cottonseed, flaxseed, mustard (by external application in poultices, as well as when ingested as foods), beans, peas. Legumes, such as peas, beans, lentils, are often allergenic factors in the patient sensitive to nuts, but some patients tolerate legumes, such as peanuts, despite high degrees of nut sensitivity.

Table A-21. Rowe Allergy Diets

General Rules:

1. The series consists of four diets, each one containing certain types of food.
2. The patient should follow each diet for at least ten days in order to make certain whether any sensitivity to the food exists.
3. Eventually, it is possible to determine from the series which foods to eliminate or desensitize.

Diet I	*Diet II*	*Diet III*
Rice or Rice Krispies	Corn	Tapioca
Tapioca	Rye	White and sweet potato
Rice bread	Corn pone	Lima bean potato bread
Rice biscuit	Corn rye muffin	Soya bean lima bean
Lettuce	Rye bread	bread
Spinach	Rye-Krisp	Beets
Carrot	Tomato	Carrots
Beet	Squash	Lima beans
Artichoke	Asparagus	String beans
Olives	Peas	Tomato
Lamb	String beans	Olives
Lemon	Chicken	Beef
Grapefruit	Bacon	Bacon
Pears	Pineapple	Lemon
Cane sugar	Peaches	Grapefruit
Wesson Oil	Apricots	Peaches
Olive oil	Prunes	Apricots
Gelatin	Gelatin	Cane Sugar
Salt	Cane sugar	Olive oil
Syrup made of maple	Karo corn syrup	Wesson Oil
sugar or cane sugar	Mazola Oil	Gelatin
flavored with maple-	Wesson Oil	Salt
leine or maple sugar	Salt	Maple syrup or syrup
Pear butter		made with cane sugar
		and flavored with
		maple

Diet IV

Milk

Milk should be taken up to two or three quarts a day. Tapioca cooked with milk and sugar also may be taken.

Table A-22. Nonspecific Diet in Chronic Bronchial Asthma

Avoid

Milk, cream, ice cream
Cheese, except cream cheese and cottage cheese
Shellfish

Vegetables	*Vegetables (cont.)*	*Fruits*
Beans, all types, except string beans	Green pepper	Apples, raw
	Lentils	Avocado pear
Broccoli	Mustard	Cantaloupe
Brussels sprouts	Onion	Honeydew melon
Cabbage	Parsley	Raisins
Cauliflower	Radish, horse radish	Strawberry
Celery	Sweet potato	Watermelon
Cucumber	White potato	
Green pea	Turnip	

Miscellaneous

Nuts, peanut butter
Coffee
Tea
Chocolate, cocoa
Beer, ale
Carbonated drinks as cola drinks, ginger ale, etc.
Condiments, highly spiced foods and artificially flavored juices
Oleomargarines, salad oils as French dressing or mayonnaise prepared from
    vegetable oils
Foods fried in vegetable oils such as cottonseed, soy, peanut and corn oils
Excessively sweet or salty foods
Intensely cold foods or drinks

INTRODUCTION TO SECTION ON LIQUID FORMULAS
Tables A-23—A-28

When a physician or his surrogate places a patient on a liquid formula as the sole or major source of nutrients for periods longer than a few weeks, he or she assumes a serious responsibility. It is mandatory that the prescription be nutritionally adequate, that it meet special clinical requirements and that it is properly prepared and consumed. Reasonably close follow-up is required with the flexibility to modify the formula as clinical, nutritional and psychosocial needs of the patient dictate. It is suggested that the patient's tolerance for a specific complete formula be tested under close supervision with relatively slow administration initially with some dilution with water; progression to the total undiluted formula should follow as rapidly as tolerance permits.

The data in Table A-23 are worthy of examination when one or more of these preparations is used as a total or major constituent of diet. Nutrient sources and milk, lactose and fiber contents should be noted. The fluid and salt content must always be evaluated in relation to individual need. A number of formulas contain very large amounts of certain minerals which may be excessive under certain conditions. Space does not permit statements of osmolality and vitamin content; these should be reviewed prior to prescription. Cost to the patient should also be considered in relation to nutritional content and clinical and nutritional requirements.

Attention to psychosocial needs of the patient restricted to formula feeding is very important. These include prior explanation of the medical value of the formula, in-hospital use of insulated containers, in-hospital food service related temporally to that of other patients, mechanical assistance in holding funnels, education in avoidance of air entrapment in the feeding tube and separate serving of desired beverages such as coffee, tea, cocoa and alcoholic beverages.

Table A-23. Nutrient Content of Complete Formulas for Oral and Tube-Feeding (Commercially Available)

(Per 1,000 Kcalories)

	Prot gm	Fat gm	CH₂O gm	Ca mg	P mg	Na mEq	K mEq	Mg mEq	Fe mg	Base*	Dilution†
Compleat-B, Doyle (liquid)	40	40.0	120	625	1375	60	37	18	11	MF	1000 ml
Flexical, Mead-Johnson	22	33.9	155	500	450	15	38	15	5	P	227 gm to 1000 ml
Gerber MBF, Gerber (liquid)	50	57.0	72	1747	1165	14	19	6	27	MF	698 ml
Instant Breakfast diluted with water (powder)	65	1.8	175	853	1029	46	75	15	19	MB	270 gm to 2100 ml
Instant Breakfast diluted with milk, skimmed (powder)	79	1.9	165	2919	2249	54	87	249	17	MB	166 gm to 1148 ml
Jejunal, Johnson & Johnson (powder)	3.4‡	0.9	213	685	685	37	23	8	53	CD	274 gm to 1140 ml
Meritene, Doyle (liquid)	60	33.0	115	1400	1250	40	43	24	17	MB	1000 ml
Meritene, Doyle (powder)	90	0.5	160	2740	2192	60	98	22	41	MB	274 gm to 950 ml
Nutri-1000, Syntex (liquid)	34	55.0	106	1200	900	22	36	15	6	MB	1000 ml

Product											
Portagen, Lactose-Free, Mead-Johnson (powder)	35	48.0	115	104	833	27	40	17	19	P	215 gm to 1000 ml
Precision LR, Doyle (powder)	22	0.7	226	409	410	27	20	15	9	P	268 gm to 900 ml
Precision High Nitrogen, Doyle	42	0.5	207	267	267	41	22	10	6	P	276 gm to 1000 ml
Sustacal, Mead-Johnson (liquid)	60	23.0	138	1500	1330	48	44	12	17	MB	1000 ml
Sustacal, Mead-Johnson (powder)	64	1.5	182	2361	2250	41	72	41	30	MB	270 gm to 1810 ml
Sustagen, Mead-Johnson (powder)	60	8.6	171	1829	1314	30	53	17	10	MB	256 gm to 640 ml
Vivonex 100, Eaton (powder)	3.3‡	0.7	226	443	444	56	30	7	6	CD	266 gm to 1000 ml
Vivonex 100 HN, Eaton (powder)	6.6‡	0.4	210	266	266	34	18	10	3	CD	266 gm to 1000 ml
W-T Low Residue Food, Warren-Teed (powder)	20	0.8	227	556	556	56	30	19	10	CD	266 gm to 1000 ml

* MB — milk-based
CD — chemically defined
MF — mixed foods
P — partially chemically defined
† Powdered formulas diluted according to manufacturer's directions
‡ Amino Acid Nitrogen

36

Table A-24. Oral Semi-Purified Formula*

Purpose: This is an example of a non-commercial palatable oral formula composed almost entirely of purified foods; it has a very low residue and contains only small amounts of lactose. It is useful as a dietary supplement for those patients who have difficulty with solid foods, who require a very low residue intake or who have moderate to severe malabsorption. This formula requires supplementation with magnesium salts and modification of sodium chloride according to the patient's individual needs. It is suggested that the magnesium be taken separately in capsule or tablet form in order to maintain palatability. For those with significant malabsorption, MCT oil may be included; for those capable of utilizing long-chain fats, corn oil may be used. Supplementary iron and vitamins should be given.

Preparation: Cook dextrose, cornstarch and egg in about 2 cups of the $5\frac{1}{2}$ cups of measured water. Place into blender and add all other ingredients. Blend for two minutes at high speed, strain and pour into container. Store in refrigerator.

Ingredients for 1,800 ml:

70	gm	Calcium Caseinate
10	gm	Gevral Protein (Lederle)
60	gm	Oil (Corn or MCT as indicated)
9	gm	Sanka Powder (optional— for flavor)
180	gm	Dextrose
90	gm	Cornstarch
100	gm	Egg
50	ml	KCl solution 9%
1,390	ml	Water
2	gm	NaCl

Nutritive Analysis per 1,800 ml:

Kcal		$\begin{cases} 2{,}026\ (\text{corn oil}) \\ 1{,}966\ (\text{MCT}) \end{cases}$
Protein	gm	83
Fat (egg)	gm	12
MCT or C.O.	gm	60
CH_2O	gm	262
Ca	mg	1,475
Mg	mEq	6
K	mEq	82
Na	mEq	50
P	mg	802
Nitrogen	gm	13
Osmolality		880 mOsm

* Formula DeR #8—Shils, M.; Miles, M.; DeSimone, R., and Bloch, A., Memorial Sloan-Kettering Cancer Center, New York, N.Y.

Table A-25. Simple Oral or Tube Formula of Non-Perishable Foods*

Purpose: This formula is nutritionally complete, is composed of ingredients which require no prior refrigeration and is easily prepared. It may be used for oral or tube feeding and is especially useful for patients on formula feeding who must travel. It contains skim milk and may not be satisfactory for those with lactose or milk intolerance. It is very low in residue and tends to be constipating. The materials are easily available and relatively inexpensive. Fruit juices, coffee or other beverages may be taken separately. The water volume will depend on the fluid requirements of the patient. Changes in kcalories are accomplished by modifying the amounts of Karo syrup and corn oil. Sweetness may be modified by varying the amounts of Karo syrup or omitting Gevral Protein.

Preparation: Mix well in a blender at low speed or shake in a jar. Refrigerate. For better chocolate flavor use one or two packages of chocolate with one package of vanilla.

Ingredients for 2,400 ml:	*Nutritive Analysis:*		
321 gm (Nine packages) of Instant Breakfast	Kcal		2,073
90 gm (¼ cup) Karo syrup, dark	Protein	gm	80
6 gm (1 tbsp) Gevral Protein (Lederle Labs)	Fat	gm	72
	CH₂O	gm	276
70 gm (3 oz) corn oil	Ca	mg	1,157
2,160 ml (9 cups) water	P	mg	1,277
	Na	mEq	59
	K	mEq	94
	Mg	mEq	19
	Fe	mg	2.5

* Modified by Shils, M. E. and Bloch, A. S. from a formula suggested by Mr. John Dewitt Norton and designated here as N-#2.

Table A-26. Commercially Available Oral Supplements

Supplementary formulas which are listed below are composed of two or more nutrients and may be of value as dietary adjuncts to the regular diet. *These are not nutritionally complete and are to be used only as supplements.* The formulas listed under the section on Complete Formulas may also be used as supplementary diets. Space does not permit a detailed analysis of these formulas. The physician and dietitian are advised to familiarize themselves with the specific contents before recommending them for clinical use.

Name	*General Composition*
Casec	Dried calcium caseinate.
Controlyte	Partial enzymatic hydrolysate of cornstarch, vegetable oil, emulsifier and BHA. Restricted protein and electrolyte content.
Gevral Protein	Calcium caseinate, lactose, artificial flavoring, malt extract, sucrose, vitamins and minerals added.
Lambase	Lamb heart and corn oil. Milk-free.
Lonalac	Casein, coconut oil. Lactose, vitamins and minerals added, low sodium.
Mullsoy	Soy flour, soy oil, sugar. No milk (liquid has added vitamins).
Nutramigen	Casein hydrolysate, dextri-maltose, corn oil, milk-free, added calcium, phosphorus, iron.
Probana	Milk, casein hydrolysate, banana powder, dextrose, lactic acid. Vitamin E added.
Provimalt	Non-fat dry milk solids, calcium caseinate, vegetable protein.
ProSobee	Soy flour, soy and coconut oils. Vitamins added.
Somagen	Milk protein, yeast and liver.

Table A-27. Low Sodium Supplementary Formula*

(71 gm protein; 169 gm fat; 221 gm carbohydrate; 5.7 mEq sodium; 95 mEq potassium; 2690 kcal.)

Ingredients	*Gm*	*Ounces*	*Approximate Measure*
Low sodium milk	750	25	3 cups
Heavy cream	200	$6\frac{2}{3}$	$\frac{3}{4}$ cup
"Lonalac"	150	10	$1\frac{1}{4}$ cups
"Controlyte"	100	$3\frac{1}{2}$	1 cup
Sugar	50	$1\frac{2}{3}$	$\frac{1}{4}$ cup
Vanilla	10	$\frac{1}{3}$	2 tsp
TOTAL VOLUME	1000		

* Courtesy of Charles S. Davidson, M.D., Harvard Medical School

Table A-28. General Tube-Feeding Formula*

Purpose: For patients who need to be fed by naso-esophageal, gastrostomy or jejunostomy tubes. It is relatively low in milk to meet the needs of those with known or suspected milk or lactose intolerances. Milk or any other ingredient may be increased as tolerated and indicated. It is equally satisfactory for jejunostomy feedings; when given into the jejunum it should be given by slow drip initially, preferably by a pump to insure controlled rate of feeding and to prevent symptoms of "dumping." This general formula is easily modified to meet specific clinical needs; examples are given in the Addendum to this table.

Preparation and Administration: Blend ingredients until finely homogenized and pour through a medium-sized strainer. Store formula in refrigerator. Before administering, mix thoroughly and warm to body temperature. Feeding should be given slowly through a funnel or by slow drip.

Wt.	Ingredients:	Household Measures	Nutritive Analysis: 2,000 kcal†		
240 gm	Cooked Enriched Farina	1 cup	Protein	80	gm
135 gm	Egg, Boiled	3	Fat	86	gm
40 gm	Skim Milk Powder	4 tbsp	CH_2O	229	gm
210 gm	Ground Beef, Defatted, Cooked	7 oz			
90 gm	Canned Carrots	½ cup	Ca	866	mg
60 gm	Canned Wax Beans, may be fresh	½ cup	P	1,218	mg
60 gm	Corn Oil	2 oz	Na	95	mEq
360 gm	Orange Juice	1½ cups	K	75	mEq
180 gm	Dark Karo Syrup	½ cup	Mg	243/20	mg/mEq
3 gm	Salt	½ tsp	Fe	12	mg
1 Tablet	Multivitamins (Poly-Vi-Sol + Fe)†		Vit A	11,382	I.U.
750 ml to make 2000 ml	Water or Juice from Canned Vegetables	3 cups	B_1	0.9	mg
			B_2	2.4	mg
			Niacin	14	mg
			Vit C	193	mg
			Osmolality	440	mOsm

* From Diet Manual, Memorial Sloan-Kettering Cancer Center, New York, N.Y. Revised 1969, courtesy Dietary Department.

† One tablet of Multivitamins + Iron provides the following *additional* vitamins and iron: Vit A 3,500 USP Units; Vit D 400 USP Units; Vit E 4 IU; Vit C 75 mg; B_1 1.1 mg; B_2 1.2 mg; Niacin 15 mg; B_6 1.2 mg; B_{12} 5 mcg; Folic Acid 0.1 mg; Panto. acid 7 mg; Iron 12 mg.

Table A-28 Addendum. Modifications of General Tube-Feeding Formula for Special Clinical Conditions

MCT Oil: Eliminate 60 gm corn oil. Substitute 67 gm MCT oil (to maintain 2,000 kcal). Various proportions of both oils may be added as indicated by patient's condition.

Low Fat: Eliminate 60 gm corn oil. Add 135 gm sugar (to maintain 2,000 kcal). Meat must be very lean. Fat = 26 gm.

Low Na: Eliminate 3.0 gm salt (44 mEq Na). If a severely restricted Na intake is indicated substitute SF carrots, SF wax beans for regular. Na will be less than 10 mEq.

Low protein, potassium and sodium: The restrictions of this diet are substantial and require close clinical supervision. Modifications should be made as soon as the patient's condition permits. An example of such a diet follows:

Wt.	Ingredients:	Household Measures	Nutritive Analysis:	2,287 kcal*	
240 gm	Cooked Enriched Farina	1 cup	Protein	17	gm
45 gm	Egg, boiled	1	Fat	95	gm
20 gm	Skim Milk Powder	2 tbsp	CH$_2$O	339	gm
45 gm	Carrots, salt free	$\frac{1}{4}$ cup			
60 gm	Wax Beans, salt free	$\frac{1}{2}$ cup	Ca	363	mg
90 gm	Corn Oil	3 oz.	P	329	mg
300 gm	Glucose	2 cups	Na	176/8	mg/mEq
	Water up to 2,000 ml		K	535/14	mg/mEq
	volume or as indicated		Fe	2.8	mg
			Vit A	7,347	I.U.	plus
			B$_1$	0.24	mg	those
			B$_2$	0.97	mg	in
			Niacin	1.54	mg	multivitamin
			Vit C	17.9	mg	mineral supplement

* Does not meet 1968 RDA except for Vitamin A. When multivitamin and mineral prescriptions are given, vitamin and mineral allowances may be achieved.

Index

Page numbers in *italics* refer to illustrations; page numbers followed by t refer to tables.

Nitrogen balance, 39, 48, 65, 72–73
  in aged, protein requirement for, 55
  anabolic steroids and, 44–*45*, 690
  in cancer, 986, 987
  corticoids and, 44–*45*
  growth hormone and, 77
  in massive resection of small intestine, 787
  protein intake and, 53
  riboflavin requirement and, 195
  RNase levels and, *44, 45, 46*
  in semi-starvation, 74
  in starvation, 952
  of surgical patient, 951–952
Noma, 764, *765*
Nonspecific diet for bronchial asthma, 1100t
Nontropical sprue, *562*
Nor-di-hydroguaiaretic acid, 118
Norepinephrine, 66, 250
  in fat metabolism, 468–469
Norethandrolone, 883
Norite eluate factor, 222
NPU. See *Net protein utilization.*
Nuclear fission yields, 446t
Nuclear fuel, 448
Nuclear reactors, 448, 452
Nucleoproteins, 106, 114
Nucleotide, 59–60
Nutramigen, 1028
Nutrition, total parenteral. See *Total parenteral nutrition.*
Nutritional gerontology, 684–685
Nutrition for National Defense, Interdepartmental Committee on, 574
Nutrition Program of the Center for Disease Control, 574
Nutrition status, anthropometric evaluation, 577–580
  blood data interpretation, 587t
  clinical evaluation of, 572–592
  examiner bias in, 580
  genetic factor, 678
  historical evaluation in, 575–577
  human variability, 526
  laboratory assessment, 584–589
  physical examination for, 580–581t
  population sampling, 574
  population survey data, 572–574, 573t
Nyctalopia. See *Night blindness.*

Obesity, 2, 131. See also *Body weight.*
  in adolescence, 677
  adopted children research, 632–633
  in adults, 628–629
    treatment, 636–642
  in children, 628
    treatment, 642–643
  coronary heart disease and, 900
  criterion for, 627–628t
  definition, 475, 625
  in diabetes mellitus, 844–847
  diagnosis, 625–626
  eating habits and, 634
  emotional factor, 633, 634, 636
  endocrine disturbances and, 637
  environmental factor, 633–634
  estimation of, 625–626

Obesity—(*Continued*)
  ethnic factor, 631
  etiology, 630t
  exercise and, 634
  experimental, 633
  familial occurrence, 631
  genetic factor, 630–633
  heart disease and, 889
  history in, 636
  hypertension and, 637, 866–867
  hypothalamic, 477–478
  in infants, 666
  insurance data, 629t–630
  metabolic, 634, 636, 637
  in osteoarthritis, 921
  pathogenesis, 634, 636
  peptic ulcer and, 778
  phases, 637
  prevalence, 628–630
  regulatory, 634
  reproduction and, 637–638
  respiration in, 636–637
  risks of, 9, 635t, 636, 637–638
  satiety cues in, 491
  sex ratios, 632
  skin disease and, 943
  somatotype and, 633
  tissue, 13–15t, 16t
  total body water in, 329
  traumatic factor, 633
  twins research, 632
Ochromonas danica assay, 531, 532, 533
Ochromonas malhamensis assay, 525, 539, 540–541
Ochronosis, 67
Octopus, 426
Ocular hemorrhage, 1004
Odoratism, 420, 421
Oils and fats, fatty acid composition of, 1060t
Oleic acid, 898
Oligophrenia phenylpyruvica, 67
Ophthalmia, 192
Ophthalmology. See *Eye; specific structures and diagnoses.*
Ophthalmoplegia, 595
  thiamin deficiency and, 1009
Opsin, 149, 150
Optic atrophy, 237
Optic nerve, cyanocobalamin and, 1009
  thiamin deficiency and, 1009
  vitamin A and, 1005–1007, 1008, 1009
Oral-genital syndrome, 945
Orange peel, 414
Organic arsenicals, 439
Organophosphorus compounds, 436
Organ rejuvenation, 59
Ornithine, 62, 63
Ornithine cycle, 62
Oropharyngeal carcinoma, 984
Orotic acid, 130
Osmolality, 337–338
Osmole, 337
Osmometers, freezing point depression, 338
Osmotic equilibrium, in malnutrition, 82
Osmotic pressure, 337–338
  in tissue nutrition, 338–340

Succinoxidase, 80, 686
Succinyl CoA, 204
Sucrase, 99
Sucrose, 408, 640, 698
 coronary heart disease and, 898
 dental caries and, 739
Sucrose-isomaltose intolerance, 802
Sucrose tolerance test, 1029–*1030*
Sugar(s), in iron absorption, 300
 nitrogen-sparing action, 57
 simple, 112–114
"Sugar baby," 607, 613
Sugar-Na$^+$ carrier, 102
Sulfaguanidine, 257
Sulfasuxidine, 257
Sulfate-creatinine ratio, 586
Sulfhydryl groups, in aminoaciduria, 71
Sulfolipids, 122
Sulfur intake, in total parenteral nutrition, 974–975
Sunlight, dental caries and, 745–746
Supermineralization, 663
Surgery, 991–993
 protein catabolism after, 74–75
Surgical patient, 950–965
 abnormal fluid and electrolyte losses, 956–957
 body water, component deficits or excesses, 957–961
  shifts in, 957
 bulk-free chemically defined diets for, 961–964
 calorie requirement, 951–953, 954
 carbohydrate metabolism in, 953
 carbohydrate requirement, 955–956
 electrolyte requirement, 955–961
 glucose for, 950, 954, 955
 intake and output records, 964
 nitrogen balance, 951–952
 nitrogen requirement, 951–953
 parenteral feeding. See *Parenteral nutrition.*
 protein losses, 957
 total parenteral nutrition, 961. See also *Total parenteral nutrition.*
 tube feeding, 959
 urine volume, 953
 water requirement, 953–961, 954t
 weight loss, 954–955
Survival, protein stores and, 104
 rations, 56
Swayback, 379
Sweat. See *Perspiration.*
Swede turnips, 416
Sweeteners, artificial, 640
Sweet pea, 420
Sweet tooth, 675
Swiss chard, 417
Synkavite, 171
Syphilis, 551

Tachycardia, 189
Taricha torosa, 427
Taste, 479
Taurine, 66
Teart, 380, 395
Temperature, calorie allowances and, 407
 environmental. See *Environmental temperature.*
Teratogenesis, 440

Terramycin, 257
Testosterone, 78, 463
Tetany, 272, 292
 hypocalcemic, 160
Tetrahydrofolic acid, 224, 225
Tetrahymena pyriformis assay, 533, 534, 535, 536, 537, 538
Texturizing agents, 438
Thalassemia, 314
 major, 321
Thiamin, 111, 186–190, *187*, 594
 biological functions, 187–188
 chemistry, 186–187
 in corneal disease, 1003
 excretion, 588t
 lethal dose, 189–190
 metabolism, 190
 synthesis, 187
 toxicity, 189–190
 urine metabolites, 532
Thiaminase, 415–416
Thiamin assay, 188–189, 530–533
 erythrocyte transketolase, 530, 531
 excretion tests, 532, 533
  load, 532
 microbial, 188, 531, 532
 protozoan, 531, 532
 rat, 189
 thiochrome, 188, 189, 530
Thiamin deficiency, 189, 499
 in alcoholism, 1044–1045
 diagnosis, 595–596
 ethanol oxidation and, 1039–1040
 ophthalmoplegia and, 1009
 optic nerve and, 1009
Thiamin intake, heat and, 724
 laboratory assessment, 588t
 requirement, 189
 sources, 189, 212t–213t
 work and, 718–719, 720
Thiamin monophosphate, 188
Thiamin propyl disulfide, 532
Thiamin pyrophosphate, 187, 188, 204
Thiamin-responsive maple syrup urine disease, 1019
Thiazole, 187
Thiochrome, *187*
Thiokinase, 120, 127
Thirst, 341, 410
Thirst center, 341
Threonine, 40
Thrombocytopenia, 313
Thyrocalcitonin, 161
Thyroglobulin, 363
Thyroid, 271
 in carbohydrate absorption, 104
 in malnutrition, 584
 protein and, 75–76
 radiation exposure, 449–450
Thyroid function tests, 367–368
 radioiodine uptake, 367
 thyroid hormone blood concentration, 367–368
 thyroid scanning, 367
 thyrotropic hormone blood concentration, 368
Thyroid hormone, blood concentration, 367–368